YO-AUZ-381

IMPORTANT

HERE IS YOUR REGISTRATION CODE TO ACCESS MCGRAW-HILL
PREMIUM CONTENT AND MCGRAW-HILL ONLINE RESOURCES

For key premium online resources you need THIS CODE to
gain access. Once the code is entered, you will be able to
use the web resources for the length of your course.

Access is provided only if you have purchased a new book.

If the registration code is missing from this book, the registration screen on our
website, and within your WebCT or Blackboard course will tell you how to obtain
your new code. Your registration code can be used only once to establish access.
It is not transferable.

To gain access to these online resources

1. **USE** your web browser to go to: **www.mhhe.com/insel10e**

2. **CLICK** on "First Time User"

3. **ENTER** the Registration Code printed on the tear-off bookmark on the right

4. After you have entered your registration code, click on "Register"

5. **FOLLOW** the instructions to setup your personal UserID and Password

6. **WRITE** your UserID and Password down for future reference. Keep it in a safe place.

If your course is using WebCT or Blackboard, you'll be able to use this code to
access the McGraw-Hill content within your instructor's online course.

To gain access to the McGraw-Hill content in your instructor's WebCT or
Blackboard course simply log into the course with the user ID and Password provided by your instructor. Enter the registration code exactly as it appears to the
right when prompted by the system. You will only need to use this code the first
time you click on McGraw-Hill content.

These instructions are specifically for student access. Instructors are not required
to register via the above instructions.

All Mc. Q's

REGISTRATION CODE

SBJG-LFSU-NYWV-UER4-8X3T

Thank you, and welcome to your
McGraw-Hill Online Resources.

0-07-297234-3 t/a
Insel
Core Concepts in Health, 10e

The McGraw-Hill Companies

McGraw Hill Higher Education

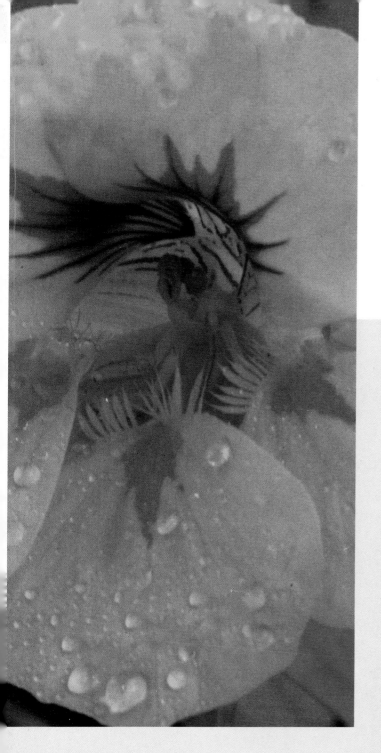

TENTH EDITION

Core Concepts in Health

Paul M. Insel
Walton T. Roth
Stanford University

Kirstan Price
Developmental Editor

Boston   Burr Ridge, IL   Dubuque, IA   Madison, WI   New York
San Francisco   St. Louis   Bangkok   Bogotá   Caracas   Kuala Lumpur
Lisbon   London   Madrid   Mexico City   Milan   Montreal   New Delhi
Santiago   Seoul   Singapore   Sydney   Taipei   Toronto

Published by McGraw-Hill, an imprint of The McGraw-Hill Companies, Inc., 1221 Avenue of the Americas, New York, NY 10020. Copyright © 2006. All rights reserved. No part of this publication may be reproduced or distributed in any form or by any means, or stored in a database or retrieval system, without the prior written consent of The McGraw-Hill Companies, Inc., including, but not limited to, in any network or other electronic storage or transmission, or broadcast for distance learning.

This book is printed on acid-free paper.

1 2 3 4 5 6 7 8 9 0 VNH/VNH 0 9 8 7 6 5

ISBN 0-07-297230-0

Editor in chief: *Emily Barrosse*
Publisher: *William R. Glass*
Executive editor: *Nicholas R. Barrett*
Director of development: *Kathleen Engelberg*
Executive marketing manager: *Pamela S. Cooper*
Senior developmental editor: *Kirstan A. Price*
Editorial assistant: *Sarah Hill*
Managing editor: *Melissa Williams*
Senior production editor: *Brett Coker*
Manuscript editor: *Darlene Bledsoe*
Art director: *Jeanne M. Schreiber*
Senior design manager and cover designer: *Violeta Díaz*
Text designer: *Mark Ong*
Art manager: *Robin Mouat*
Illustrator(s): *John and Judy Waller, Susan Seed, Kevin Sommerville*
Manager, photo research: *Brian J. Pecko*
Lead production supervisor: *Randy Hurst*
Senior supplements coordinator: *Louis Swaim*
Development editor for technology: *Julia D. Ersery*
Senior media producer: *Lance Gerhart*
Senior media project manager: *Ron Nelms*
Composition: *GTS, Los Angeles*
Printing: *45# Pub Matte Plus, by Von Hoffmann Graphics*

Cover: © *Zach Holmes Photography*

Library of Congress Cataloging-in-Publication Data

Core concepts in health / [edited by] Paul M. Insel, Walton T. Roth; Kirstan Price, developmental editor.—10th ed.
    p. cm.
Includes bibliographical references and index
ISBN 0-07-297230-0 (alk. paper)
1. Health—Handbooks, manuals, etc. I. Insel, Paul M. II. Roth, Walton T. III. Price, Kirstan.

RA776.C83 2005b
613—dc22

The Internet addresses listed in the text were accurate at the time of publication. The inclusion of a website does not indicate an endorsement by the authors or McGraw-Hill, and McGraw-Hill does not guarantee the accuracy of the information presented at these sites.

www.mhhe.com

Brief Contents

PART ONE

Establishing a Basis for Wellness

Chapter 1   Taking Charge of Your Health   1
Chapter 2   Stress: The Constant Challenge   31
Chapter 3   Psychological Health   63

PART TWO

Understanding Sexuality

Chapter 4   Intimate Relationships and Communication   95
Chapter 5   Sex and Your Body   123
Chapter 6   Contraception   151
Chapter 7   Abortion   183
Chapter 8   Pregnancy and Childbirth   203

PART THREE

Making Responsible Decisions: Substance Use and Abuse

Chapter 9   The Use and Abuse of Psychoactive Drugs   235
Chapter 10   The Responsible Use of Alcohol   269
Chapter 11   Toward a Tobacco-Free Society   297

PART FOUR

Getting Fit

Chapter 12   Nutrition Basics   327
Chapter 13   Exercise for Health and Fitness   377
Chapter 14   Weight Management   411

PART FIVE

Protecting Yourself from Disease

Chapter 15   Cardiovascular Health   445
Chapter 16   Cancer   479
Chapter 17   Immunity and Infection   515
Chapter 18   Sexually Transmitted Diseases   547

PART SIX

Accepting Physical Limits

Chapter 19   Aging: A Vital Process   581
Chapter 20   Dying and Death   603

PART SEVEN

Living Well in the World

Chapter 21   Conventional and Complementary Medicine: Skills for the Health Care Consumer   629
Chapter 22   Personal Safety: Protecting Yourself from Unintentional Injuries and Violence   661
Chapter 23   Environmental Health   693

Appendix A   Nutritional Content of Popular Items from Fast-Food Restaurants   A-1
Appendix B   A Self-Care Guide for Common Medical Problems   A-5
Credits   C-1
Index   I-1

iii

Contents

PART ONE

Establishing a Basis for Wellness

1 Taking Charge of Your Health 1

WELLNESS: THE NEW HEALTH GOAL 2
The Dimensions of Wellness 2
New Opportunities, New Responsibilities 3
National Wellness Goals: The Healthy People
Initiative 5
Health Issues for Diverse Populations 6

CHOOSING WELLNESS 11
Factors That Influence Wellness 11
A Wellness Profile 12

HOW DO YOU REACH WELLNESS? 14
Getting Serious About Your Health 14
Building Motivation for Change 15
Enhancing Your Readiness to Change 20
Developing Skills for Change: Creating
a Personalized Plan 21
Putting Your Plan into Action 24
Staying with It 24

BEING HEALTHY FOR LIFE 25
Making Changes in Your World 25
What Does the Future Hold? 26
Tips for Today 27
Summary 27
Take Action 27
For More Information 28
Selected Bibliography 29

2 Stress: The Constant Challenge 31

WHAT IS STRESS? 32
Physical Responses to Stressors 32
Emotional and Behavioral Responses
to Stressors 35
The Stress Experience as a Whole 38

STRESS AND DISEASE 38
The General Adaptation Syndrome 39
Allostatic Load 40

Psychoneuroimmunology 40
Links Between Stress and
Specific Conditions 40

COMMON SOURCES OF STRESS 42
Major Life Changes 42
Daily Hassles 42
College Stressors 43
Job-Related Stressors 44
Social Stressors 45
Environmental Stressors 46
Internal Stressors 47

TECHNIQUES FOR MANAGING STRESS 47
Social Support 47
Communication 47
Exercise 47
Nutrition 48
Sleep 49
Time Management 49
Strive for Greater Spirituality 51
Confide in Yourself Through Writing 51
Cognitive Techniques 51
Relaxation Techniques 53
Counterproductive Coping Strategies 56

CREATING A PERSONAL PLAN
FOR MANAGING STRESS 57
Identifying Stressors 57
Designing Your Plan 58
Getting Help 58
Tips for Today 58
Summary 58
Take Action 59
For More Information 59
*Behavior Change Strategy: Dealing with
Test Anxiety 60*
Selected Bibliography 61

3 Psychological Health 63

WHAT PSYCHOLOGICAL HEALTH IS NOT 64

DEFINING PSYCHOLOGICAL HEALTH 64
Realism 65
Acceptance 65

Autonomy   65
A Capacity for Intimacy   66
Creativity   66

MEETING LIFE'S CHALLENGES   66

Growing Up Psychologically   66
Achieving Healthy Self-Esteem   68
Being Less Defensive   70
Being Optimistic   71
Maintaining Honest
   Communication   72
Dealing with Loneliness   73
Dealing with Anger   73

PSYCHOLOGICAL DISORDERS   74

Anxiety Disorders   74
Mood Disorders   78
Schizophrenia   82

**MODELS OF HUMAN NATURE AND
THERAPEUTIC CHANGE   84**

The Biological Model   84
The Behavioral Model   85
The Cognitive Model   86
The Psychodynamic Model   87
Evaluating the Models   87

GETTING HELP   88

Self-Help   88
Peer Counseling and Support
   Groups   88
Professional Help   88

Tips for Today   90
Summary   90
*Behavior Change Strategy:
   Dealing with Social Anxiety*   91
Take Action   92
For More Information   92
Selected Bibliography   93

PART TWO

Understanding Sexuality

4   Intimate Relationships and Communication   95

DEVELOPING INTIMATE RELATIONSHIPS   96

Self-Concept and Self-Esteem   96
Friendship   97
Love, Sex, and Intimacy   97
Challenges in Relationships   99
Successful Relationships   101

Unhealthy Relationships   102
Ending a Relationship   102

COMMUNICATION   102

Nonverbal Communication   102
Communication Skills   103
Gender and Communication   103
Conflict and Conflict Resolution   103

PAIRING AND SINGLEHOOD   106

Choosing a Partner   107
Dating   107
Living Together   107
Same-Sex Partnerships   110
Singlehood   112

MARRIAGE   112

Benefits of Marriage   113
Issues in Marriage   113
The Role of Commitment   114
Separation and Divorce   114

FAMILY LIFE   114

Becoming a Parent   114
Parenting   115
Single Parents   117
Stepfamilies   117
Successful Families   117

Tips for Today   119
Summary   119
Take Action   120
For More Information   120
Selected Bibliography   121

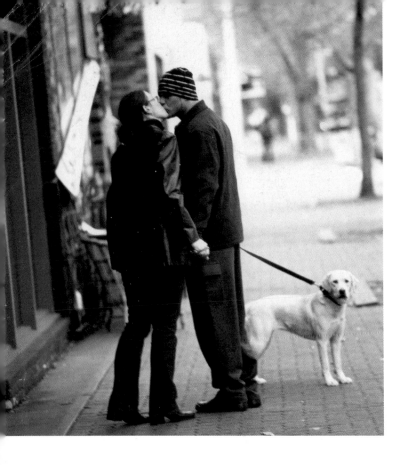

Tips for Today   147
Summary   147
Take Action   148
For More Information   148
Selected Bibliography   149

6   Contraception   151

PRINCIPLES OF CONTRACEPTION   152

REVERSIBLE CONTRACEPTION   154

Oral Contraceptives: The Pill   154
Contraceptive Skin Patch   156
Vaginal Contraceptive Ring   157
Contraceptive Implants   158
Injectable Contraceptives   158
Emergency Contraception   159
The Intrauterine Device (IUD)   160
Male Condoms   161
Female Condoms   162
The Diaphragm with Spermicide   164
Lea's Shield   166
The Cervical Cap   166
The Contraceptive Sponge   166
Vaginal Spermicides   167
Abstinence, Fertility Awareness,
   and Withdrawal   168
Combining Methods   169

PERMANENT CONTRACEPTION: STERILIZATION   170

Male Sterilization: Vasectomy   171
Female Sterilization   172

ISSUES IN CONTRACEPTION   174

When Is It OK to Begin Having
   Sexual Relations?   174
Contraception and Gender Differences   175
Sexuality and Contraception Education
   and Teenagers   176

WHICH CONTRACEPTIVE METHOD IS RIGHT FOR YOU?   177

Tips for Today   179
Summary   179
Take Action   180
For More Information   180
Selected Bibliography   181

7   Abortion   183

THE ABORTION ISSUE   184

The History of Abortion in
   the United States   184

5   Sex and Your Body   123

SEXUAL ANATOMY   124

Female Sex Organs   124
Male Sex Organs   125

HORMONES AND THE REPRODUCTIVE LIFE CYCLE   127

Differentiation of the Embryo   127
Female Sexual Maturation   128
Male Sexual Maturation   132
Aging and Human Sexuality   132

SEXUAL FUNCTIONING   132

Sexual Stimulation   133
The Sexual Response Cycle   133
Sexual Problems   135

SEXUAL BEHAVIOR   137

The Development of Sexual Behavior   137
Sexual Orientation   141
Varieties of Human Sexual Behavior   142
Atypical and Problematic
   Sexual Behaviors   144
Commercial Sex   144
Responsible Sexual Behavior   146

Current Legal Status   184
Moral Considerations   186
Public Opinion   186
Personal Considerations   189
Current Trends   190

METHODS OF ABORTION   192

Suction Curettage   194
Manual Vacuum Aspiration   194
Abortion After the First Trimester   195
Medical Abortion   195

COMPLICATIONS OF ABORTION   196

Possible Physical Effects   196
Possible Psychological Effects   196

**DECISION MAKING AND UNINTENDED
PREGNANCY   197**

Tips for Today   199
Summary   199
Take Action   199
For More Information   200
Selected Bibliography   200

8   Pregnancy and Childbirth   203

PREPARATION FOR PARENTHOOD   204

Deciding to Become a Parent   204
Preconception Care   205

UNDERSTANDING FERTILITY   206

Conception   206
Infertility   208

PREGNANCY   212

Pregnancy Tests   212
Changes in the Woman's Body   212
Emotional Responses
   to Pregnancy   214
Fetal Development   214
The Importance of Prenatal Care   220
Complications of Pregnancy
   and Pregnancy Loss   224

CHILDBIRTH   226

Choices in Childbirth   226
Labor and Delivery   226
The Postpartum Period   229

Tips for Today   231
Summary   231
Take Action   232
For More Information   232
Selected Bibliography   233

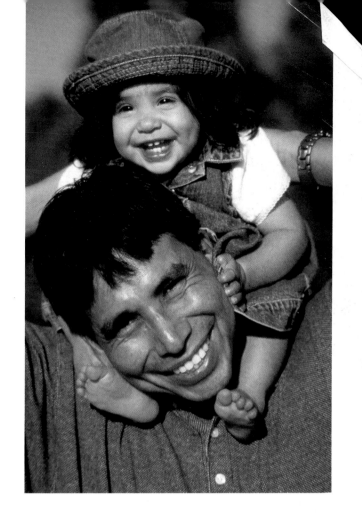

PART THREE

Making Responsible Decisions: Substance Use and Abuse

**9   The Use and Abuse of
Psychoactive Drugs   235**

ADDICTIVE BEHAVIOR   236

What Is Addiction?   236
Characteristics of Addictive Behavior   237
The Development of Addiction   237
Characteristics of People with
   Addictions   237
Examples of Addictive Behaviors   238

DRUG USE, ABUSE, AND DEPENDENCE   239

The Drug Tradition   239
Drug Abuse and Dependence   240
Who Uses Drugs?   241
Why Do People Use Drugs?   242
Risk Factors for Dependence   243
Other Risks of Drug Use   244

HOW DRUGS AFFECT THE BODY   246

Changes in Brain Chemistry   246
Drug Factors   246
User Factors   247
Social Factors   248

REPRESENTATIVE PSYCHOACTIVE DRUGS   248

Opioids   248
Central Nervous System
    Depressants   250
Central Nervous System Stimulants   250
Marijuana and Other Cannabis
    Products   254
Hallucinogens   255
Inhalants   257

DRUG USE: THE DECADES AHEAD   258

Drugs, Society, and Families   258
Legalizing Drugs   258
Drug Testing   260
Treatment for Drug Dependence   260
Preventing Drug Abuse   262
The Role of Drugs in
    Your Life   263
Tips for Today   264
Summary   264
*Behavior Change Strategy:
    Changing Your Drug Habits*   265
Take Action   265
For More Information   266
Selected Bibliography   267

10   The Responsible Use of Alcohol   269

THE NATURE OF ALCOHOL   270

The Chemistry of Alcohol   270
Absorption   270
Metabolism and Excretion   271
Alcohol Intake and Blood Alcohol
    Concentration   271

ALCOHOL AND HEALTH   273

The Immediate Effects of Alcohol   273
Drinking and Driving   275
The Effects of Chronic Use   277
The Effects of Alcohol Use During
    Pregnancy   278
Possible Health Benefits of Alcohol   279

ALCOHOL ABUSE AND DEPENDENCE   280

Alcohol Abuse   280
Binge Drinking   280
Alcoholism   282
Gender and Ethnic Differences   286
Helping Someone with an
    Alcohol Problem   288

DRINKING BEHAVIOR AND RESPONSIBILITY   288

Examine Your Attitudes About
    Alcohol Use   288
Examine Your Drinking Behavior   288
Drink Moderately and Responsibly   290
Promote Responsible Drinking in Others   290
Tips for Today   292
Summary   292
*Behavior Change Strategy: Developing Responsible
    Drinking Habits*   293
Take Action   294
For More Information   294
Selected Bibliography   295

11   Toward a Tobacco-Free Society   297

WHY PEOPLE USE TOBACCO   298

Nicotine Addiction   298
Social and Psychological Factors   301
Genetic Factors   301
Why Start in the First Place?   301
Who Uses Tobacco?   303

HEALTH HAZARDS   304

Tobacco Smoke: A Toxic Mix   304
The Immediate Effects of Smoking   307
The Long-Term Effects of Smoking   307
Other Forms of Tobacco Use   311

THE EFFECTS OF SMOKING ON THE NONSMOKER   313

Environmental Tobacco Smoke   314
Smoking and Pregnancy   315
The Cost of Tobacco Use to Society   315

WHAT CAN BE DONE?   317

Action at the Local Level   317
Action at the State and Federal Levels   317
International Action   317
Action in the Private Sector   318
Individual Action   318
Controlling the Tobacco Companies   319

HOW A TOBACCO USER CAN QUIT   319

The Benefits of Quitting   319
Options for Quitting   320
Tips for Today   322
*Behavior Change Strategy:
    Kicking the Tobacco Habit   322*
Summary   323
Take Action   324
For More Information   324
Selected Bibliography   325

PART FOUR

Getting Fit

12   Nutrition Basics   327

NUTRITIONAL REQUIREMENTS: COMPONENTS OF A HEALTHY DIET   328

Proteins—The Basis of Body Structure   329
Fats—Essential in Small Amounts   330
Carbohydrates—An Ideal Source of Energy   334
Fiber—A Closer Look   337
Vitamins—Organic Micronutrients   338
Minerals—Inorganic Micronutrients   340
Water—Vital but Often Ignored   340
Other Substances in Food   340

NUTRITIONAL GUIDELINES: PLANNING YOUR DIET   343

Dietary Reference Intakes (DRIs)   343
Dietary Guidelines for Americans   344
USDA's MyPyramid   350
The Vegetarian Alternative   354
Dietary Challenges for Special Population
    Groups   356

A PERSONAL PLAN: MAKING INFORMED CHOICES ABOUT FOOD   357

Reading Food Labels   357
Reading Dietary Supplement Labels   357

Protecting Yourself Against Foodborne
    Illness   360
Environmental Contaminants and
    Organic Foods   363
Additives in Food   364
Food Irradiation   365
Genetically Modified Foods   365
Food Allergies and Food Intolerances   366
Staying Committed to a Healthy Diet   366
Tips for Today   368
Summary   368
*Behavior Change Strategy: Improving Your Diet
    by Choosing Healthy Beverages   369*
Take Action   369
For More Information   370
Selected Bibliography   371

13   Exercise for Health and Fitness   377

WHAT IS PHYSICAL FITNESS?   378

Cardiorespiratory Endurance   378
Muscular Strength   379
Muscular Endurance   380
Flexibility   380
Body Composition   380

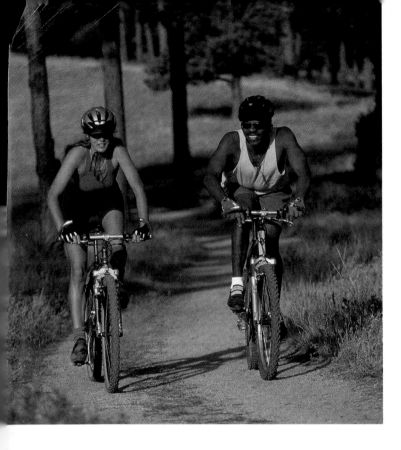

Managing Your Fitness Program   400
Tips for Today   405
Summary   405
*Behavior Change Strategy: Planning
   a Personal Exercise Program*   406
Take Action   407
For More Information   408
Selected Bibliography   409

14   Weight Management   411

BASIC CONCEPTS OF WEIGHT MANAGEMENT   412

Body Composition   412
Energy Balance   413
Evaluating Body Weight and Body Composition   414
Excess Body Fat and Wellness   416
What Is the Right Weight for You?   419

FACTORS CONTRIBUTING TO EXCESS BODY FAT   419

Genetic Factors   419
Physiological Factors   420
Lifestyle Factors   421
Psychosocial Factors   423

ADOPTING A HEALTHY LIFESTYLE FOR SUCCESSFUL WEIGHT MANAGEMENT   423

Diet and Eating Habits   423
Physical Activity and Exercise   427
Thinking and Emotions   427
Coping Strategies   428

APPROACHES TO OVERCOMING A WEIGHT PROBLEM   428

Doing It Yourself   428
Diet Books   430
Dietary Supplements and Diet Aids   430
Weight-Loss Programs   433
Prescription Drugs   433
Surgery   434
Psychological Help   435

BODY IMAGE   435

Severe Body Image Problems   435
Acceptance and Change   436

EATING DISORDERS   437

Factors in Developing an Eating Disorder   437
Anorexia Nervosa   438
Bulimia Nervosa   438
Binge-Eating Disorder   439
Borderline Disordered Eating   439
Treating Eating Disorders   439
Today's Challenge   439

THE BENEFITS OF EXERCISE   380

Improved Cardiorespiratory Functioning   380
More Efficient Metabolism   380
Improved Body Composition   381
Disease Prevention and Management   382
Improved Psychological and Emotional
   Wellness   383
Improved Immune Function   383
Prevention of Injuries and
   Low-Back Pain   383
Improved Wellness over the Life Span   384

DESIGNING YOUR EXERCISE PROGRAM   384

Physical Activity and Exercise for Health
   and Fitness   386
First Steps   388
Cardiorespiratory Endurance
   Exercises   391
Developing Muscular Strength
   and Endurance   393
Flexibility Exercises   395
Training in Specific Skills   397
Putting It All Together   397

GETTING STARTED AND STAYING ON TRACK   398

Selecting Instructors, Equipment,
   and Facilities   398
Eating and Drinking for Exercise   400

Tips for Today 440
Summary 440
*Behavior Change Strategy: A Weight-Management
    Program* 441
Take Action 442
For More Information 442
Selected Bibliography 443

PART FIVE

Protecting Yourself from Disease

15 Cardiovascular Health 445

THE CARDIOVASCULAR SYSTEM 446

RISKS FACTORS FOR CARDIOVASCULAR
DISEASE 447

Major Risk Factors That Can Be Changed 448
Contributing Risk Factors That Can
    Be Changed 453
Major Risk Factors That Can't
    Be Changed 455
Possible Risk Factors Currently Being
    Studied 456

MAJOR FORMS OF CARDIOVASCULAR
DISEASE 460

Atherosclerosis 460
Heart Disease and Heart Attack 461
Stroke 464
Peripheral Arterial Disease 466
Congestive Heart Failure 467
Other Forms of Heart Disease 467

PROTECTING YOURSELF AGAINST
CARDIOVASCULAR DISEASE 469

Eat Heart-Healthy 469
Exercise Regularly 472
Avoid Tobacco 472
Know and Manage Your Blood
    Pressure 472
Know and Manage Your Cholesterol
    Levels 472
Develop Effective Ways to Handle Stress
    and Anger 473
Manage Other Risk Factors and Medical
    Conditions 474
Tips for Today 474
Summary 474
Take Action 474
*Behavior Change Strategy: Reducing the Saturated
    and Trans Fat in Your Diet* 475
For More Information 475
Selected Bibliography 477

16 Cancer 479

WHAT IS CANCER? 480

Benign Versus Malignant Tumors 480
How Cancer Spreads: Metastasis 481
Types of Cancer 481
The Incidence of Cancer 482

COMMON CANCERS 484

Lung Cancer 484
Colon and Rectal Cancer 485
Breast Cancer 485
Prostate Cancer 487
Cancers of the Female Reproductive Tract 488
Skin Cancer 490
Oral Cancer 493
Testicular Cancer 493
Other Cancers 493

THE CAUSES OF CANCER 495

The Role of DNA 495
Dietary Factors 498
Inactivity and Obesity 500
Microbes 501
Carcinogens in the Environment 501

DETECTING, DIAGNOSING, AND
TREATING CANCER 503

Detecting Cancer 503
Diagnosing Cancer 505
Treating Cancer 505
Living with Cancer 507

PREVENTING CANCER 507

Avoiding Tobacco 507
Controlling Diet and Weight 509
Regular Exercise 509
Protecting Skin from the Sun 509

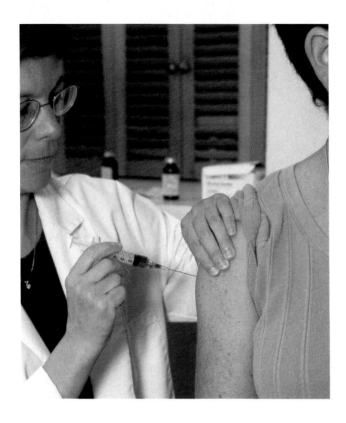

Fungi   537
Protozoa   538
Parasitic Worms   539
Prions   539
Emerging Infectious Diseases   539
Other Immune Disorders: Cancer and
    Autoimmune Diseases   541

**GIVING YOURSELF A FIGHTING CHANCE:
HOW TO SUPPORT YOUR IMMUNE
SYSTEM   542**

Tips for Today   543
Summary   543
Take Action   544
For More Information   544
Selected Bibliography   545

18   Sexually Transmitted Diseases   547

THE MAJOR STDS   548

HIV Infection and AIDS   548
Chlamydia   562
Gonorrhea   565
Pelvic Inflammatory Disease   565
Human Papillomavirus Infection
    (Genital Warts)   566
Genital Herpes   569
Hepatitis B   570
Syphilis   571

OTHER STDS   572

WHAT YOU CAN DO   573

Education   573
Diagnosis and Treatment   574
Prevention   575

Tips for Today   577
Summary   577
Take Action   578
For More Information   578
Selected Bibliography   579

Avoiding Environmental and Occupational
    Carcinogens   509
Recommended Screening Tests   509

Tips for Today   510
Summary   510
Take Action   510
*Behavior Change Strategy: Incorporating More Fruits
    and Vegetables into Your Diet   511*
For More Information   511
Selected Bibliography   512

17   Immunity and Infection   515

THE CHAIN OF INFECTION   516

Links in the Chain   516
Breaking the Chain   517

THE BODY'S DEFENSE SYSTEM   517

Physical and Chemical Barriers   517
The Immune System   518
Immunization   521
Allergy: The Body's Defense System
    Gone Haywire   523

**THE TROUBLEMAKERS: PATHOGENS
AND DISEASE   525**

Bacteria   526
Viruses   531

PART SIX

Accepting Physical Limits

19   Aging: A Vital Process   581

GENERATING VITALITY AS YOU AGE   582

What Happens as You Age?   582
Life-Enhancing Measures:
    Age-Proofing   582

CONFRONTING THE CHANGES OF AGING 586

Planning for Social Changes 586
Adapting to Physical Changes 587
Handling Psychological and Mental Changes 590

AGING AND LIFE EXPECTANCY 592

Factors Influencing Life Expectancy 592
Theories on Aging 592

LIFE IN AN AGING AMERICA 593

America's Aging Minority 594
Family and Community Resources
for Older Adults 595
Government Aid and Policies 597
Changing the Public's Idea of Aging 598

Tips for Today 599
Summary 599
Take Action 600
For More Information 600
Selected Bibliography 601

20 Dying and Death 603

WHY IS THERE DEATH? 604

UNDERSTANDING DEATH AND DYING 604

Defining Death 604
Learning About Death 605
Denying Versus Welcoming Death 605

PLANNING FOR DEATH 606

Making a Will 606
Considering Options for End-of-Life Care 608
Deciding to Prolong Life or Hasten Death 608
Completing an Advance Directive 611
Becoming an Organ Donor 612
Planning a Funeral or Memorial Service 614

COPING WITH DYING 616

Awareness of Dying 616
The Tasks of Coping 617
The Trajectory of Dying 617
Supporting a Dying Person 619

COPING WITH LOSS 619

Experiencing Grief 619
Supporting a Grieving Person 621
Helping Children Cope with Loss 623

COMING TO TERMS WITH DEATH 623

Tips for Today 624
Summary 624
Take Action 625

For More Information 625
Selected Bibliography 626

PART SEVEN

Living Well in the World

21 Conventional and Complementary
Medicine: Skills for the Health Care
Consumer 629

**SELF-CARE: MANAGING MEDICAL
PROBLEMS** 630

Self-Assessment 630
Decision Making: Knowing When
to See a Physician 630
Self-Treatment: Many Options 631

**PROFESSIONAL MEDICAL AND HEALTH CARE:
CHOICES AND CHANGE** 633

CONVENTIONAL MEDICINE 634

Premises and Assumptions of Conventional
Medicine 634
The Providers of Conventional Medicine 635
Choosing a Primary Care Physician 637
Getting the Most Out of Your Medical Care 638

COMPLEMENTARY AND ALTERNATIVE MEDICINE   643

Alternative Medical Systems   643
Mind-Body Interventions   646
Biological-Based Therapies   648
Manipulative and Body-Based Methods   648
Energy Therapies   649
Evaluating Complementary and Alternative Therapies   651
Why Do Consumers Use Complementary Medicine?   652

PAYING FOR HEALTH CARE   653

The Current System   653
Health Insurance   654
Choosing a Policy   656

Tips for Today   656
Summary   656
Behavior Change Strategy: Complying with Physicians' Instructions   657
Take Action   658
For More Information   658
Selected Bibliography   659

22   Personal Safety: Protecting Yourself from Unintentional Injuries and Violence   661

UNINTENTIONAL INJURIES   662

What Causes an Injury?   662
Motor Vehicle Injuries   664
Home Injuries   668
Leisure Injuries   671
Work Injuries   672

VIOLENCE AND INTENTIONAL INJURIES   673

Factors Contributing to Violence   673
Assault   676
Homicide   676
Gang-Related Violence   676
Hate Crimes   677
School Violence   677
Workplace Violence   678
Terrorism   678
Family and Intimate Violence   678
Sexual Violence   683
What You Can Do About Violence   686

PROVIDING EMERGENCY CARE   687

Tips for Today   688
Summary   688
Behavior Change Strategy: Adopting Safer Habits   689
Take Action   689
For More Information   690
Selected Bibliography   691

23   Environmental Health   693

CLASSIC ENVIRONMENTAL HEALTH CONCERNS   694

Clean Water   695
Waste Disposal   696
Food Inspection   698
Insect and Rodent Control   698

POPULATION GROWTH   699

How Many People Can the World Hold?   699
Factors That Contribute to Population Growth   700

POLLUTION   701

Air Pollution   701
Chemical Pollution   708
Radiation   711
Noise Pollution   713

HEALING THE ENVIRONMENT   714

Tips for Today   715
Summary   715
Take Action   716
For More Information   716
Selected Bibliography   717

APPENDICES

A

Nutritional Content of Popular Items
from Fast-Food Restaurants A-1

B

A Self-Care Guide for Common
Medical Problems A-5

Credits C-1

Index I-1

BOXES

In the News

Medical Innovations in the Twenty-First
  Century 13
Coping After Terrorism or Mass Violence 46
Antidepressant Use in Young People 86
Same-Sex Marriage and Civil Unions 111
Cybersex 145
Future Methods of Contraception 175
Timeline of Selected Key Abortion Decisions and
  Legislation 185
Reproductive Technology 211
Medical Marijuana 256
College Binge Drinking 283
After the Master Settlement Agreement 316
America's Poor Eating Habits 367
Drugs and Supplements for Improved
  Athletic Performance 396
The Growing American Waistline 413
Sudden Death in Young Athletes 468
Putting Cancer Risks in Perspective 502
The Next Influenza Pandemic—When,
  Not If? 534
Half of Americans Will Have an STD by
  Age 25 567
Stem Cells 583
Profound Trauma and Loss 622
Prescription Drug Use and Regulation:
  Lessons from Vioxx 640
Emergency Preparedness 680
Climate Change: Politics and Science 705

Mind/Body/Spirit

Ten Warning Signs of Wellness 4
Stress and Your Brain 42
Healthy Connections 48
Paths to Spiritual Wellness 69
Are Intimate Relationships Good for Your Health? 113
Sexual Decision Making 139
Stress and Pregnancy 219
Spirituality and Drug Abuse 244
Tobacco Use and Religion: Global Views 300
Eating Habits and Total Wellness 330
Exercise and the Mind 384
Exercise, Body Image, and Self-Esteem 428
Anger, Hostility, and Heart Disease 455
Religion and Wellness 473
Coping with Cancer 508
Immunity and Stress 542
Stress and Genital Herpes 570
Help Yourself by Helping Others 587
In Search of a Good Death 618
Expressive Writing and Chronic Conditions 631
The Power of Belief: The Placebo Effect 647
Nature and the Human Spirit 695

Take Charge

Motivation Boosters 26
Overcoming Insomnia 50
Meditation and the Relaxation Response 54
Breathing for Relaxation 55
Realistic Self-Talk 71

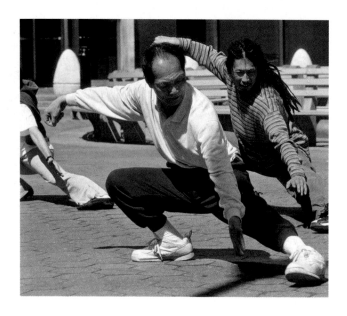

Being a Good Friend   98
Strategies for Enhancing Support in Relationships   101
Guidelines for Effective Communication   104
Online Relationships   109
Strategies of Strong Families   118
Communicating About Sexuality   146
Talking with a Partner About Contraception   174
Healthy Eating During Pregnancy   221
If Someone You Know Has a Drug Problem . . .   263
Dealing with an Alcohol Emergency   274
Building Motivation to Quit Smoking   302
Helping a Friend or Partner Stop Using Tobacco   318
Setting Intake Goals for Protein, Fat,
   and Carbohydrate   334
Choosing More Whole-Grain Foods   336
Eating for Healthy Bones   342
Reducing the Saturated and Trans Fat in Your Diet   348
Judging Serving Sizes   353
Eating Strategies for College Students   358
Safe Food Handling   363
Becoming More Active   387
Determining Your Target Heart Rate Range   392
Safe Weight Training   395
Maintaining Your Exercise Program   405
Strategies for Successful Weight Management   429
If Someone You Know Has an Eating
   Disorder   440
What to Do in Case of a Heart Attack, Cardiac Arrest,
   or Stroke   463
Breast Self-Examination   487
Testicle Self-Examination   494
Protecting Yourself Against Tickborne and
   Mosquitoborne Infections   529
How to Keep Yourself Well   543
Preventing HIV Infection and Other STDs   563
Don't Wait—Early Treatment of STDs
   Really Matters   575

Talking About Condoms and Safer Sex   576
Communication and Care for the Older Adults
   in Your Life   596
Tasks for Survivors   616
Coping with Grief   623
Recognizing the Potential for Abusiveness
   in a Partner   681
Preventing Date Rape   684
Staying Safe on Campus   687
Making Your Letters Count   715

Critical Consumer

Evaluating Sources of Health Information   18
Alternative Remedies for Depression   83
Choosing and Evaluating Mental Health
   Professionals   89
Dietary Supplements and PMS   131
Obtaining a Contraceptive from a Health Clinic
   or Physician   156
Buying and Using Over-the-Counter
   Contraceptives   163
Making a Birth Plan   227
Choosing a Drug-Treatment Program   262
Alcohol Advertising   291
Smoking Cessation Products   321
Using Food Labels   359
Using Dietary Supplement Labels   361
Choosing Exercise Footwear   401
Evaluating Fat and Sugar Substitutes   426
Is Any Diet Best for Weight Loss?   431
Choosing and Using Sunscreens and
   Sun-Protective Clothing   492
Avoiding Cancer Quackery   506
Preventing and Treating the Common Cold   532
Tattoos and Body Piercing   537
Getting an HIV Test   557
Choosing a Place to Live   597
A Consumer Guide to Funerals   615
Evaluating Health News   636
Avoiding Health Fraud and Quackery   644
Choosing a Health Care Plan   656
Choosing a Bicycle Helmet   669
How to Be a Green Consumer   698

Dimensions of Diversity

Factors Contributing to Health Disparities
   Among Ethnic Minorities   10
Diverse Populations, Discrimination, and Stress   45
Ethnicity, Culture, and Psychological Disorders   75
Interfaith and Intrafaith Partnerships   108
Are There Ethnic Differences in Sexual Decision
   Making and Behavior?   142
Contraceptive Use Among American Women   173
Abortions Around the World   193

Ethnicity and Genetic Diseases   207
Drug Use and Ethnicity: Risk and
    Protective Factors   259
Metabolizing Alcohol: Our Bodies
    Work Differently   272
Smoking Among U.S. Ethnic Populations   305
Ethnic Foods   346
Exercise for People with Disabilities and
    Other Special Health Concerns   385
Overweight and Obesity Among U.S. Ethnic
    Populations   422
Ethnicity and CVD   458
Ethnicity, Poverty, and Cancer   496
Poverty, Ethnicity, and Asthma   525
HIV Infection Around the World   550
HIV/AIDS Among African Americans and Latinos   555
Multicultural Wisdom About Aging   599
Día de los Muertos: The Day of the Dead   607
Who Are the Uninsured?   654
Violence and Health: A Global View   679
Poverty and Environmental Health   709

 Gender Matters

Women's Health/Men's Health   8
Women, Men, and Stress   39
Depression, Anxiety, and Gender   80
Gender and Communication   105
Sexual Differentiation, Hormones, and the Brain   128
Men's Involvement in Contraception   176
Pregnancy Tasks for Fathers   215
Gender Differences in Drug Use and Abuse   243
Gender and Alcohol Use and Abuse   287
Gender and Tobacco Use   311
How Different Are the Nutritional Needs
    of Women and Men?   356
Gender Differences in Muscular Strength   393
Gender, Ethnicity, and Body Image   436
Women and CVD   457
Gender and Cancer   483
Women and Autoimmune Diseases   541
Women Are Hit Hard by STDs   564
Suicide Among Older Men   592
Why Do Women Live Longer?   593
Grief and Gender   620
Health Care Visits and Gender   638
Injuries Among Young Men   663
Gender and Environmental Health   711

 Assess Yourself

Wellness: Evaluate Your Lifestyle   16
What Stage of Change Are You In?   21
How High Is Your Stress Level?   33
Are You Suffering from a Mood Disorder?   78
Love Maps Questionnaire   100

Your Sexual Attitudes   140
Which Contraceptive Method Is Right for You
    and Your Partner?   178
Creating a Family Health Tree   209
Do You Have a Problem with Drugs?   245
Do You Have a Problem with Alcohol?   289
Nicotine Dependence: Are You Hooked?   299
Your Diet Versus MyPyramid Recommendations   355
The 1.5-Mile Run-Walk Test   402
What Triggers Your Eating?   424
Are You at Risk for CVD?   470
What's Your UV Risk?   491
Do Your Attitudes and Behaviors Put You
    at Risk for STDs?   573
Personal Health Profile   640
Are You an Aggressive Driver?   665
Environmental Health Checklist   714

 In Focus

Headaches: A Common Symptom
    of Stress   43
Shyness   77
Myths About Suicide   81
Relationship Styles and Conflict Resolution   106
Myths About Contraception   153
The Opposing Views: Pro-Choice   187

The Opposing Views: Pro-Life   188
The Adoption Option   191
Personal Decisions About Abortion   198
Club Drugs   251
Children of Alcoholics   284
Diabetes   418
Genetic Testing for Breast Cancer   498
Are All Diseases Infectious?   535
College Students and STDs   568
Alzheimer's Disease   591
Hospice: Comfort and Care for the Dying   609
What Can Be Done About the Shortage
   of Organ Donors?   613
Herbal Remedies: Are They Safe?   650
Cellular Phones and Distracted Driving   666
Carpal Tunnel Syndrome   674
Natural Ecosystems and Biodiversity   700

TOPICS OF SPECIAL CONCERN TO WOMEN

Aging among women, 132, 584, 587
Alcoholism, patterns among women, 286–287

Alcohol metabolism in women, 271
Alcohol use, special risks for women, 275, 278–279
Amenorrhea, 419, 438
Anxiety disorders, 76, 80
Arthritis, 385, 529, 542, 588–589
Asthma, 314–315, 524–525
Autoimmune disorders, 541
Bacterial vaginosis, 572–573
Body composition, 381–382, 398, 412, 415
Body image, negative, 435–436
Breast cancer, 209, 485–487, 498, 504
Breast self-examinations, 486–487, 504
Cancer, rates and risk factors, 482, 483, 488–490
Cardiovascular disease, risk among women, 456–457, 459, 461
Caregiving for older adults, 595–596, 619
Carpal tunnel syndrome, 674
Causes of death among women, 5, 8, 593
Cervical cancer, 155, 311, 488–489, 504, 566, 569
Communication styles among women, 103, 105
Contraception, female methods, 154–161, 162–168, 172, 174
Contraceptive use and roles and responsibilities, 173, 175–176
Cybersex, 144–145
Depression, risk among women, 76, 79–80
Dietary recommendations for
   women, 334, 337, 344, 353, 356, 372–374
Drug use, rates of and special risks for
   women, 243, 247, 252, 253, 255
Eating disorders 437–439
Ectopic pregnancy, 196, 224–225
Environmental health risks, 709, 710, 711
Family violence, 678–680
Female athlete triad, 419
Female genital mutilation, 138
Financial planning for retirement, 587
Folic acid, 206, 220, 338, 339, 344, 357, 471, 485, 500
Gender roles, 39, 96, 137–138, 663
Grief, pattern among women, 620
Health care visits, 638
Health concerns and status, general, 7–8, 638
Heart attack risk among women, 456–457, 461
HIV infection rates and transmission, 550, 552, 554
Hormone replacement therapy, 132, 457, 485, 589, 590
Hormones, female, 127–132
Infertility, female, 210
Life expectancy of women, 593
Marital status, 112
Menopause, 132, 457, 589
Menstrual cycle, 128–132, 212, 344, 419, 589
Migraine, 43
Muscular strength, development of, 393
Obesity in women, 422, 423, 501
Osteoporosis, 340, 357, 383, 385, 589–590
Ovarian cancer, 489–490
Pap tests and pelvic exams, 155, 156, 488, 489
Parenting, single, by women, 117
Pelvic inflammatory disease, 135, 158, 160, 210, 563, 566
Physical activity levels, 378
Post-traumatic stress disorder, 41–42, 77–78, 80
Poverty rates among older women, 594
Pregnancy and childbirth, 203–226
Premenstrual syndrome and premenstrual dysphoric
   disorder, 130–132
Psychological disorders among women, 76, 79–80
Rape, 683–685

Sexual anatomy, female, 124–125
Sexual health problems and dysfunctions, female, 135, 137
Sexual functioning, female, 133–135
Sexual harassment, 686
Sexually transmitted diseases and
    pregnancy, 222–223, 550, 559–560, 563–564, 565, 568, 571
Sexually transmitted diseases, symptoms and special risks
    among women, 563–569, 572
Stalking and cyberstalking, 680–682
Sterilization, female, 172–174
Stressors and responses to stress among women, 38, 39, 593
Tobacco use, rates and special risks among
    women, 311, 315, 448
Uterine cancer, 489, 504
Violence against women, 675, 678–685, 686
Yeast infections, 538

TOPICS OF SPECIAL CONCERN TO MEN

Aging among men, 132, 584
Alcohol abuse and dependence, patterns among men, 286–287
Alcohol metabolism in men, 271
Bladder cancer, 494
Body composition, 381–382, 398, 412, 415
Body image, negative, 435–436
Cancer, rates and risk factors, 482, 483
Cardiovascular disease risk among men, 456, 461
Causes of death among men, 5, 8, 593
Cigars and pipes, 312–313
Circumcision, 126–127, 489, 552
Cluster headaches, 43
Communication styles among men, 103, 105
Contraception, male methods, 161–162, 169, 171–172
Contraceptive roles and responsibilities, 175–176
Cybersex, 144–145
Dietary recommendations for men, 334, 337, 353, 356, 372–374
Drug use, rates of, 243
Environmental health, 711
Family violence, 678–680
Firearm-related injuries, 671, 676, 686–687
Gambling, 238
Gender roles, 39, 96, 137–138, 663
Grief, pattern among men, 620
Health care visits, 638
Health concerns and status, general, 7–8
Heart attack risk among men, 456, 459, 461
HIV infection rates and transmission, 550, 552, 554
Homicide, rates among men, 663, 675, 676
Hormones, male, 127–128, 593, 663
Infertility, male, 210
Injuries, rates of, 663
Life expectancy of men, 593
Marital status, 112
Motorcycle and moped injuries, 667–668
Motor vehicle injuries, 664–668
Muscular strength, development of, 393
Obesity in men, 422, 423, 501
Oral cancer, 312–313, 493, 499, 509
Parenting, single, by men, 117
Physical activity levels, 378
Poverty rates among older men, 594
Pregnancy, men's roles, 214, 215, 224
Prostate cancer, 487–488, 496, 499, 504–505

Psychological disorders among men, 76, 79–80
Rape, 683–684
Schizophrenia, 76, 82–84, 536
Sexual anatomy, male, 125–127
Sexual health problems and dysfunctions, male, 135–136
Sexual functioning, male, 133–135
Sexual harassment, 686
Sexually transmitted diseases, symptoms and special risks
    among men, 563, 564, 565, 567
Spit tobacco, 298–299, 305, 311–312, 313, 316, 493
Stalking and cyberstalking, 680–682
Sterilization, male, 171–172
Stomach cancer, 493–494, 496, 501
Stressors and responses to stress among men, 38, 39
Suicide, 8, 79–80, 592, 676
Testicular cancer, 135, 493
Testicular self-examination, 494
Tobacco use, rates and special risks among men, 304, 311–313
Violent behavior among men, 675, 676, 678–685
Violent deaths of men, 675

Note: The health issues and conditions listed here include those that disproportionately influence or affect women or men. For more information, see the Index under gender, women, men, and any of the special topics listed here.

DIVERSITY TOPICS RELATED TO ETHNICITY

Aging, attitudes toward, 592, 599
Alcohol abuse patterns, 286–287
Alcohol metabolism, 272
Alcohol use patterns, 286–287
Asthma, 525, 709
Body image, 436

Cancer, rates and risk, 487–488, 489, 490, 493, 495, 496
Cardiovascular disease patterns and
    risks, 449, 456, 458, 461, 467
Contraceptive use, patterns of, 173
Cystic fibrosis, 207
Death, attitudes toward, 607
Diabetes, 417–418, 422, 453, 458
Dietary patterns and considerations, 338, 346, 349, 471
Discrimination and health, 10, 45, 458, 496, 709
Drug use, risk and protective factors, 259
Environmental health, 709
Ethnic foods, 346
Fetal alcohol syndrome, 222, 278–279
Genetic disorders, 206, 207, 209
Glaucoma, 588
Hate crimes, 677
Health disparities, general, 5–7, 8–10
Health insurance status, 10, 654
Health status and concerns, general, 8–10
Heart disease, 458
Hemochromatosis, 207
HIV/AIDS rates, 553–554, 555
Homicide rates, 676
Hypertension, 349, 449, 456, 458, 471
Infant mortality, 225
Lactose intolerance, 207, 347, 366
Lead poisoning, 709

Lupus, 541
Marketing, targeted, 303, 305
Metabolic syndrome, 458
Osteoporosis, 342, 589–590
Overweight/obesity, rates and trends, 422
Poverty rates among older adults, 594
Prostate cancer, 487–488, 496, 504
Psychological disorders, symptoms and rates, 75
Rheumatic heart disease, 467–468
Sexual decision making and behavior, 142
Sexually transmitted diseases, rates of, 562
Sickle cell disease, 155, 207
Single-parent families, 117
Smoking rates, 304, 305, 307
Stress and discrimination, 38, 45
Suicide rates, 79, 592
Tay-Sachs disease, 207
Thallasemia, 207
Tobacco use, 304, 305, 307
Violence, rates of, 674, 676
Vitamin deficiencies, 338

Note: The health issues and conditions listed here include those that disproportionately influence or affect specific U.S. ethnic groups or for which patterns may appear along ethnic lines. For more information, see the Index under ethnicity, culture, names of specific population groups, and any of the topics listed here.

Preface

Core Concepts in Health has maintained its leadership in the field of health education for more than 25 years. Since we pioneered the concept of self-responsibility for personal health in 1976, hundreds of thousands of students have used our book to become active, informed participants in their own health care. Each edition of Core Concepts has brought improvements and refinements, but the principles underlying the book have remained the same. Our commitment to these principles has never been stronger than it is today.

OUR GOALS

Our goals in writing this book can be stated simply:

- To present scientifically based, accurate, up-to-date information in an accessible format
- To involve students in taking responsibility for their health and well-being
- To instill a sense of competence and personal power in students

The first of these goals means making expert knowledge about health and health care available to the individual. Core Concepts brings scientifically based, accurate, up-to-date information to students about topics and issues that concern them—exercise, stress, nutrition, weight management, contraception, intimate relationships, HIV infection, drugs, alcohol, and a multitude of others. Current, complete, and straightforward coverage is balanced with user-friendly features designed to make the text appealing. Written in an engaging, easy-to-read style and presented in a colorful, open format, Core Concepts invites the student to read, learn, and remember. Boxes, tables, artwork, photographs, and many other features highlight areas of special interest throughout the book.

Our second goal is to involve students in taking responsibility for their health. Core Concepts uses innovative pedagogy and unique interactive features to get students thinking about how the material they're reading relates to their lives. We invite them to examine their emotions about the issues under discussion, to consider their personal values and beliefs, and to analyze their health-related behaviors. Beyond this, for students who want to change behaviors that detract from a healthy lifestyle, we offer guidelines and tools, ranging from samples of health journals and personal contracts to detailed assessments and behavior change strategies.

Perhaps our third goal in writing Core Concepts in Health is the most important: to instill a sense of competence and personal power in the students who read the book. Everyone has the ability to monitor, understand, and affect his or her health. Although medical and health professionals possess impressive skills and have access to a huge body of knowledge that benefits everyone in our society, people can help to minimize the amount of professional care they actually require in their lifetime by taking care of themselves—taking charge of their health—from an early age. Our hope is that Core Concepts will continue to help young people make this exciting discovery—that they have the power to shape their futures.

ORGANIZATION AND CONTENT OF THE TENTH EDITION

The organization of the book as a whole remains essentially the same as in the ninth edition, with some improvements. The book is divided into seven parts: Part One, Establishing a Basis for Wellness, includes chapters on taking charge of your health (Chapter 1), stress (Chapter 2), and psychological health (Chapter 3). Part Two, Understanding Sexuality, opens with an exploration of communication and intimate relationships, including friendship, intimate partnerships, marriage, and family (Chapter 4), and then moves on to discuss physical sexuality (Chapter 5), contraception (Chapter 6), abortion (Chapter 7), and pregnancy and childbirth (Chapter 8). As in previous editions of Core Concepts, we devote a separate chapter to abortion to reflect both the importance of this issue and our belief that abortion is not a form of contraception and should not be included in the chapter on that topic.

Part Three, Making Responsible Decisions: Substance Use and Abuse, opens with a discussion of addictive behavior and the different classes of psychoactive drugs (Chapter 9), followed by chapters on alcohol (Chapter 10) and tobacco (Chapter 11). Part Four, Getting Fit, includes a detailed discussion of nutrition (Chapter 12), exercise (Chapter 13), and weight management (Chapter 14).

Part Five, Protecting Yourself from Disease, deals with the most serious health threats facing Americans today—cardiovascular disease (Chapter 15), cancer (Chapter 16), infectious diseases (Chapter 17), and sexually transmitted diseases (Chapter 18). Part Six, Accepting Physical Limits, explores aging (Chapter 19) and dying and death (Chapter 20).

Part Seven, Living Well in the World, includes the topics covered in the final two parts of the ninth edition. In response to reviewer feedback, the coverage of health care has been integrated and streamlined into a single chapter that looks at both conventional and complementary medicine (Chapter 21). It is followed by chapters on injury prevention (Chapter 22) and environmental health (Chapter 23).

Taken together, the chapters of the book provide students with a complete guide to promoting and protecting their health, now and through their entire lives, as individuals, as participants in a health care community and system, and as citizens of a planet that also needs to be protected if it is to continue providing human beings with the means to live healthy lives.

For the tenth edition, all chapters were carefully reviewed, revised, and updated. The latest information from scientific and health-related research is incorporated in the text, and newly emerging topics and issues are discussed. The following list gives a sample of some of the current concerns addressed in the tenth edition:

- 2005 Dietary Guidelines for Americans and the USDA MyPyramid food guidance system
- Physical activity guidelines from the USDA, Surgeon General, ACSM, and other organizations
- Prescription drug safety issues
- Ecstasy, GHB, and other club drugs
- Health problems associated with overweight and obesity, and popular approaches to weight loss
- HIV/AIDS testing and treatment
- Emergency contraception, the patch, the ring, extended cycle oral contraceptives, and other new contraceptive methods
- Tobacco promotion, additives, and quitting strategies
- Glycemic index and response
- Trans fat labeling requirements
- Pre-diabetes and diabetes
- Links between lifestyle and risk of illness and death
- Food safety issues, including mad cow disease and chemical contamination of fish
- Eating disorders and disordered eating
- CVD risk factors, including psychological and social factors and metabolic syndrome
- Avian influenza, SARS, West Nile virus, and other emerging infections
- Parenting styles, conflict resolution, and interfaith partnerships

- Online relationships and cybersex
- Dietary supplement safety and labeling
- Effects of profound trauma and loss
- Emergency preparedness

The tenth edition continues to emphasize the development of total wellness, with expanded coverage of spiritual wellness and the close connections between mind and body. Key topics include paths to spiritual wellness; global religious views on tobacco use; the effects of stress on the brain, the immune system, and the course of pregnancy; the use of journal writing and spiritual practices to cope with stress; the benefits of volunteering; and the advantages of close connections with others. Chapter 4 includes information on the benefits of intimate relationships and strategies for building and maintaining healthy interpersonal relationships. Suggested journal writing activities on the Web site that accompanies the book help students to further explore their feelings and values.

Many other areas of special concern to students have also been expanded and updated in the tenth edition. Chapters 2, 3, and 20 include expanded information on how to cope after terrorism, mass violence, or natural disasters and how to recognize and deal with post-traumatic stress disorder. Chapter 2 also includes a new section on stressors common to nontraditional students. The coverage of drugs in Chapter 9 includes updated material on club drugs, oxycodone, medical marijuana, and ephedrine. The latest guidelines for healthy nutrient intakes and recommended patterns of physical activity are described in Chapters 12–14, along with expanded coverage of popular diets. Chapters 14 and 15 examine the health risks associated with diabetes, pre-diabetes, and insulin resistance, along with strategies for prevention and treatment. Chapter 17 includes a new discussion of safety issues related to body art (tattoos and body piercing), and Chapter 18 provides an expanded look at the high rate of STDs among young adults. Prescription drug safety issues are highlighted in Chapter 21, including direct-to-consumer advertising and postapproval surveillance. Chapter 22 looks at terrorism and the magnitude and impact of interpersonal and collective violence worldwide.

Core Concepts takes care to address the health issues and concerns of an increasingly diverse student population. Although most health concerns are universal—we all need to eat well, exercise, and manage stress, for example—certain differences among people have important implications for health. These differences can be genetic or cultural, based on factors such as ethnicity, socioeconomic status, and age. Where such differences are important for health, they are discussed in the text or in highlight boxes called Dimensions of Diversity (described in greater detail below). For the tenth edition, coverage of ethnic diversity has been expanded. Diversity topics in the tenth edition include factors underlying health disparities, links between ethnicity and certain genetic diseases, the effects of culture on the expression of psychological disorders, high rates of HIV/AIDS among certain groups, and the relationships among ethnicity, poverty, educational attainment, and such risk factors as smoking, overweight, and exposure to pollutants.

Topics related to gender are also given special attention in the tenth edition of *Core Concepts*. Key gender differences as well as issues of particular importance to women or men are discussed in the text and in new highlight boxes called Gender Matters (described below). New and expanded gender-related topics include differences in such areas as responses to stress, risk of depression and suicide, communication styles, health effects from tobacco and alcohol use, heart attack symptoms, cancer rates and risk factors, life expectancy, dietary needs, body image, grief, and risk of unintentional injuries and violence.

The health field is dynamic, with new discoveries, advances, trends, and theories reported every week. Ongoing research—on the role of diet in cancer prevention, for example, or on new treatments for HIV infection—continually changes our understanding of the human body and how it works in health and disease. For this reason, no health book can claim to have the final word on every topic. Yet within these limits, *Core Concepts* does present the latest available information and scientific thinking on innumerable topics.

To aid students in keeping up with rapidly advancing knowledge about health issues, *Core Concepts* also includes coverage of the Internet, a key source of up-to-date information. Each chapter includes an annotated list of World Wide Web sites that students can use as a launching point for further exploration of important topics. Chapter 1 includes important information about evaluating health-related Web sites.

 Each chapter in the tenth edition is also closely tied to the Web site developed as a companion to the text. Elements marked with the World Wide Web icon have corresponding links and activities on the *Core Concepts in Health* Online Learning Center (www.mhhe.com/insel10e). The Web site and other online supplements are described below in greater detail.

FEATURES OF THE TENTH EDITION

This edition of *Core Concepts in Health* builds on the features that attracted and held our readers' interest in the previous editions. One of the most popular features has always been the **boxes**, which allow us to explore a wide range of current topics in greater detail than is possible in the text itself. The boxes are divided into eight categories, each in a different color and marked with a distinctive icon and label. Refer to the table of contents for a complete list of all the boxes in each category.

 In the News boxes focus on current health issues that have recently been highlighted in the media. Most of the In the News boxes are new to the tenth edition; new topics include same-sex marriage, medical innovations, reproductive technology, individual and environmental influences on eating habits, medical marijuana, the next influenza pandemic, problems with antidepressant use in children, and the science and politics of climate change. Each In the News box is accompanied by the World Wide Web icon, indicating that the *Core Concepts* Online Learning Center has links to Internet resources students can use to learn more about the topic of the box.

 Mind/Body/Spirit boxes focus on spiritual wellness and the close connections between people's feelings and states of mind and their physical health. Included in Mind/Body/Spirit boxes are topics such as paths to spiritual wellness, religious views of tobacco use, benefits of being a volunteer, sexual decision making and personal values, the placebo effect, how exercise fosters emotional wellness, and how stress can affect pregnancy and the immune system. Mind/Body/Spirit boxes emphasize that all the dimensions of wellness must be developed for an individual to achieve optimal health and well-being.

 Take Charge boxes distill from each chapter the practical advice students need in order to apply information to their own lives. By referring to these boxes, students can easily find ways to foster friendships, for example; to become more physically active; to enhance support in their relationships; to reduce the amount of saturated and trans fats in their diets; to perform deep-breathing exercises for stress reduction; and to help a friend who has a problem with tobacco, drugs, or an eating disorder.

Critical Consumer boxes emphasize the key theme of critical thinking by helping students develop and apply critical thinking skills, thereby allowing them to make sound choices related to health and well-being. Critical Consumer boxes provide specific guidelines for evaluating health news and advertising, using food labels to make dietary choices, choosing a bicycle helmet, avoiding quackery, selecting exercise footwear, evaluating dietary supplements, choosing smoking-cessation products, making environmentally friendly shopping choices, and so on.

Dimensions of Diversity boxes are part of our commitment to reflect and respond to the diversity of the student population. These boxes give students the opportunity to identify any specific health risks that affect them because of who they are as individuals or as members of a group. Most Dimensions of Diversity boxes focus on issues related to U.S. ethnic groups, but some look at other dimensions, including socioeconomic status, age, and ability. Topics covered in these boxes include factors contributing to health disparities among ethnic minorities, diverse populations and stress, ethnic and cultural influences on psychological disorders, risk and protective factors for drug use related to ethnicity, rates of smoking and alcohol use among ethnic populations, ethnic foods, suicide among older men, exercise for people with special health concerns, and links between poverty and asthma.

In addition, some Dimensions of Diversity boxes highlight health issues and practices in other parts of the world, allowing students to see what Americans share with people in other societies and how they differ. Students have the opportunity to learn about laws and attitudes toward abortion in other countries, tobacco control around the world, the global pattern of HIV infection, and other topics of interest.

 Gender Matters boxes, new to the tenth edition, highlight key gender differences related to wellness as well as areas of particular concern to men or women. An overview of key gender-related wellness concerns is provided in Chapter 1. Topics covered in later chapters include gender differences in rates of anxiety, depression, drug use, and cancer; in the symptoms and course of heart attack and STDs; and in responses to stress and grief. Other boxes look at the higher rates of autoimmune disorders in women and the higher rates of injuries in men.

 Assess Yourself boxes give students the opportunity to examine their behavior and identify ways that they can change their habits and improve their health. By referring to these boxes, students can, for example, examine their eating habits, evaluate their fitness level, discover if they are at increased risk for cancer or cardiovascular disease, evaluate their driving habits, determine what triggers their eating, and examine their drinking and drug-taking behavior. These self-assessments are also included on the *Core Concepts in Health* Online Learning Center.

 In Focus boxes highlight current wellness topics of particular interest. Topics include diabetes, Alzheimer's disease, headaches, genetic testing for cancer, carpal tunnel syndrome, and shyness. In addition to the boxes, many carefully refined features are included in the tenth edition of *Core Concepts.*

Each chapter opens with **Test Your Knowledge**—a series of 4 to 6 multiple choice and true-false questions, with answers. These self-quizzes facilitate learning by getting students involved in a variety of wellness-related issues. The questions emphasize important points, highlight common misconceptions, and spark debate.

Vital Statistics tables and figures highlight important facts and figures in a memorable format that often reveals surprising contrasts and connections. From tables and figures marked with the Vital Statistics label, students can learn about drinking and drug use among college students, alternative medicine use in the United States, world population growth, prevalence of psychological disorders, trends in public opinion about abortion, and a wealth of other information. For students who grasp a subject best when it is displayed graphically, numerically, or in a table, the Vital Statistics feature provides alternative ways of approaching and understanding the text. In addition, for each Vital Statistics table and figure, the *Core Concepts* Online Learning Center has links to sites where students can find the latest statistics and information.

Core Concepts features a wealth of attractive and helpful **illustrations.** The anatomical art, which has been prepared by medical illustrators, is both visually appealing and highly informative. These illustrations help students understand such important information as how blood flows through the heart, how the process of conception occurs, and how to use a condom. Other topics illustrated in the tenth edition include diabetes, the effects of cocaine use on brain chemistry, the allergic response, the process of tumor development, osteoarthritis, the Healthy Eating Pyramid, and trends in global temperature. These lively and abundant illustrations will particularly benefit those students who learn best from visual images.

Chapter-ending **Tips for Today** sections provide brief distillations of the major message of each chapter, followed by suggestions for a few simple things that students can try right away. Tips for Today are designed to encourage students and to build their confidence by giving them easy steps they can take immediately to improve their wellness.

Take Action, appearing at the end of every chapter, suggests hands-on exercises and projects that students can undertake to extend and deepen their grasp of the material. Suggested projects include interviews, investigations of campus or community resources, and experimentation with some of the behavior change techniques suggested in the text. Special care has been taken to ensure that the projects are both feasible and worthwhile.

The **Behavior Change Strategies** that conclude many chapters offer specific behavior management/modification plans relating to the chapter's topic. Based on the principles of behavior management that are carefully explained in Chapter 1, these strategies will help students change unhealthy or counterproductive behaviors. Included are strategies for dealing with test anxiety, quitting smoking, developing responsible drinking habits, planning a personal exercise program, phasing in a healthier diet, and many other practical plans for change.

Two quick-reference appendixes provide students with resources they can keep and use for years to come:

- **Appendix A,** "Nutritional Content of Popular Items from Fast-Food Restaurants," provides information on commonly ordered menu items.
- **Appendix B,** "Self-Care Guide for Common Medical Problems," provides information to help students assess and manage common symptoms, including fever, sore throat, indigestion, headache, and cuts and scrapes.

"Steps for Choking Emergencies" from the Red Cross appears inside the back cover of the text, providing information that can save lives.

Several features from previous editions of *Core Concepts in Health* have been moved to the Online Learning Center. There, you'll find Communicate! exercises, which suggest strategies and activities for improving communication skills to enhance wellness; Journal Entry activities, which help students deepen their understanding of their wellness-related behaviors and become more skilled critical thinkers; and information about finding and evaluating Internet resources, formerly located in Appendix C.

LEARNING AIDS

Although all the features of *Core Concepts in Health* are designed to facilitate learning, several specific learning aids have been incorporated in the text. Learning objectives labeled **Looking Ahead** appear on the opening page of each chapter, identifying major concepts and helping guide students in their reading and review of the text. Important terms appear in boldface type in the text and are defined in a **running glossary,** helping students handle a large and complex new vocabulary.

Chapter summaries offer a concise review and a way to make sure students have grasped the most important concepts in the chapter. **For More Information** sections contain annotated lists of books, newsletters, hotlines, organizations, and Web sites that students can use to extend and broaden their knowledge or pursue subjects of interest to them. Also found at the end of every chapter are **Selected Bibliographies.** A complete **Index** at the end of the book includes references to glossary terms in boldface type.

TEACHING TOOLS

Available with the tenth edition of *Core Concepts in Health* is a comprehensive package of supplementary materials designed to enhance teaching and learning.

Interactive Instructor's CD-ROM

The **Interactive Instructor's CD-ROM** (ISBN 0-07-297232-7) presents key teaching resources in an easy-to-use format. It is organized by chapter and works in both Windows and Macintosh environments. It includes the following teaching tools:

- The **Course Integrator Guide** includes learning objectives, extended chapter outlines, suggested activities, and lists of additional resources. It also describes all the print and electronic supplements available with the text and shows how to integrate them into lectures and assignments for each chapter. For the tenth edition, the guide was prepared by Cathy Kennedy, Colorado State University.

- The **test bank** includes more than 3000 true-false, multiple choice, and short essay questions; it also includes two 100-question multiple choice tests that cover the content of the entire text. The answer key lists the page number in the text where each answer is found. Contributors to the tenth edition test bank are Phil Kelly, Salem State University; Karen Vail-Smith, East Carolina University; and Kathy McGinnis, San Diego City College. Special thanks also go to our test bank reviewer panel: Phil Kelly; Betty Shepherd, Virginia Western Community College; Charla Blumell, East Carolina University; and Susan Moore, Western Illinois University.

The test bank is available on the Instructor's CD-ROM as Word files and with the EZ Test **computerized testing software.** EZ Test provides a powerful, easy-to-use test maker to create printed quizzes and exams. EZ Test runs on both Windows and Macintosh systems. For secure online testing, exams created in EZ Test can be exported to WebCT, Blackboard, PageOut, and (beginning fall 2005) EZ Test Online. The EZ Test CD is packaged with a Quick Start Guide; once the program is installed, users have access to the complete User's Manual, including multiple Flash tutorials. Additional help is available at www.mhhe.com/eztest.

- The **PowerPoint slides,** expanded for the tenth edition, provide a lecture tool that you can alter or expand to meet the needs of your course. The slides include key lecture points and images from the text and other sources. For the tenth edition, the PowerPoint presentations were created by Andrew Shim, Indiana University of Pennsylvania. As an aid for instructors who wish to create their own presentations, a complete **image bank,** including all the illustrations from the text, is also included on the Instructor's CD-ROM.

- **Transparency masters and handouts**—more than 150 in all—are provided as additional lecture resources. The transparency masters feature tables showing key statistics and data, illustrations from the text and other sources, and key points from the text. Illustrations of many body systems are also provided. The student handouts provide additional information and can be used to extend student knowledge on topics such as pre-diabetes, glycemic index, yoga for relaxation, and dealing with alcohol emergencies.

• A complete set of **Wellness Worksheets** (ISBN 0-07-297649-7), a student learning aid described below, is also included on the Instructor's CD-ROM.

Printed versions of key supplements—the Course Integrator Guide, test bank, transparency masters, handouts, and Wellness Worksheets—are also available (ISBN 0-07-310563-5). The printed supplements are loose-leaf and three-hole-punched, ready to be placed in a binder.

Video and Other Visual Resources

A variety of visual resources is available for use with *Core Concepts in Health*.

• **Resource Presentation Manager CD-ROM** (ISBN 0-07-310531-7), new for the tenth edition, is a pre-sentation tool with chapter-specific video clips and images designed to engage students and promote critical thinking and dialogue on relevant topics in personal health. The searchable library contains contemporary student interviews, news clips, and historical health videos on body image, depression, stress, genetics, spirituality, and many other topics. Each video clip is accompanied by an Instructor Guide that describes the objective of the clip and gives critical thinking questions to ask before the clip is shown and discussion questions to use for follow-up.

• A set of 80 color **Transparency Acetates** (ISBN 0-07-310562-7) is available as a lecture resource. The acetates are not duplicates of the transparency masters on the Instructor's CD-ROM; many are from sources other than the text.

Videos from Films for Humanities are also available.

Digital Solutions

The *Core Concepts in Health* Online Learning Center (www.mhhe.com/insel10e) provides many additional resources for both instructors and students. Instructor tools include downloadable versions of the Course Integrator Guide and all the PowerPoint slides, links to professional resources, and a guide to using the Internet. For students, there are learning objectives, self-quizzes and glossary flashcards for review, interactive Internet activities, and extensive links. The Online Learning Center also includes many tools for wellness behavior change, such as interactive versions of the Wellness Worksheets and a workbook for behavior change. Through the Online Learning Center, students can also access **PowerWeb** (www.dushkin.com/online)

resources, including articles on key health topics, self-scoring quizzes, interactive exercises, study tips, and a daily news feed.

The **Online Wellness Workbook** (ISBN 0-07-310530-9), developed in collaboration with Quia™, offers an electronic version of assessments and quizzes compiled from the text and its main supplements. This new online supplement provides students with interactive assessments, self-scoring quizzes, and instant feedback. Benefits for instructors include a gradebook that automatically scores, tracks, and records students' results; it also offers instructors the opportunity to review individual and class performance and customize activities and features for their course. Access to the Quia™ Online Wellness Workbook can be packaged with the text for a small additional fee.

Classroom Performance System (CPS) brings interactivity into the classroom or lecture hall. CPS is a wireless response system that gives instructors and students immediate feedback from the entire class. Each student uses a wireless response pad similar to a television remote to respond instantly to polling or quiz questions. Contact your local sales representative for more information about using CPS with *Core Concepts in Health*.

PageOut (www.pageout.net) is a free, easy-to-use program that enables instructors to quickly develop Web sites for their courses. PageOut can be used to create a course home page, an instructor home page, an interactive syllabus that can be linked to elements in the Online Learning Center, Web links, online discussion areas, an online gradebook, and much more. Instructors can combine Online Learning Center resources with popular **course-management systems**. The McGraw-Hill Instructor Advantage program offers access to a complete online teaching Web site called the Knowledge Gateway, toll-free phone support, and unlimited e-mail support directly from WebCT and Blackboard. Instructors who use 500 or more copies of a text can enroll in the Instructor Advantage Plus program, which provides on-campus, hands-on training from a certified platform specialist.

For more information about McGraw-Hill's digital resources, including how to obtain passwords for PageOut and PowerWeb, contact your local representative or visit McGraw-Hill on the Internet (www.mhhe.com/solutions).

Student Resources Available with *Core Concepts in Health*

Students who purchase a new copy of *Core Concepts* receive free access to **premium resources on the Online Learning Center.** These premium resources include interactive self-assessments, articles on health and human performance, and a daily news feed. Students who purchase a used copy of the text can purchase access to the premium resources by visiting the Online Learning Center (www.mhhe.com/insel10e).

Many other resources are available to help students learn and apply key concepts; contact your local representative to find out more about packaging any of the following with *Core Concepts in Health*.

- More than 100 **Wellness Worksheets** (ISBN 0-07-297649-7) are available to help students become more involved in their wellness and better prepared to implement successful behavior change. The worksheets include assessment tools, Internet activities, and knowledge-based reviews of key concepts. They are available shrink-wrapped with the text in an easy-to-use pad and in the premium resources section of the Online Learning Center.

- **NutritionCalc Plus** (ISBN 0-07-292126-9) is a dietary analysis program with an easy-to-use interface that allows users to track their nutrient and food group intakes, energy expenditures, and weight control goals. It generates a variety of reports and graphs for analysis, including comparisons with the latest Dietary Reference Intakes (DRIs). The ESHA database includes thousands of ethnic foods, supplements, fast foods, and convenience foods, and users can add their own foods to the food list. NutritionCalc Plus is available on CD-ROM (Windows only) or as an online version.

- **The Daily Fitness and Nutrition Journal** (ISBN 0-07-284432-9) is a handy booklet that guides students in planning and tracking a fitness program. It also helps students assess their current diet and make appropriate changes.

- The **Health and Fitness Pedometer** (ISBN 0-07-320933-3) can be packaged with copies of the text. It allows students to count their daily steps and track their level of physical activity.

- The interactive **HealthQuest CD-ROM** (ISBN 0-07-295117-6) helps students explore and change their wellness behavior. It includes tutorials, assessments, and behavior change guidelines in such key areas as stress, fitness, nutrition, cardiovascular disease, cancer, tobacco, and alcohol.

Additional supplements and many packaging options are available; check with your McGraw-Hill sales representative.

A NOTE OF THANKS

The efforts of innumerable people have gone into producing this tenth edition of *Core Concepts in Health*. The book has benefited immensely from their thoughtful commentaries, expert knowledge and opinions, and many helpful suggestions. We are deeply grateful for their participation in the project.

Academic Contributors

Virginia Brooke, Ph.D., University of Texas Medical Branch at Galveston
Aging: A Vital Process

Theodore C. Dumas, Ph.D., Institute of Neuroscience, University of Oregon
Stress: The Constant Challenge

Thomas D. Fahey, Ed.D., California State University, Chico
Exercise for Health and Fitness

Samuel Goth, Ph.D., Center for Children's Environmental Health, University of California, Davis
Immunity and Infection

Michael R. Hoadley, Ph.D., Assistant Vice-President for Academic Affairs, Center for Academic Technology Support, Eastern Illinois University
Personal Safety: Protecting Yourself from Unintentional Injuries and Violence

Paul M. Insel, Ph.D., Stanford University
Taking Charge of Your Health

Nancy Kemp, M.D.
The Responsible Use of Alcohol; Sexually Transmitted Diseases

Charles Ksir, Ph.D., University of Wyoming
The Use and Abuse of Psychoactive Drugs

Howard Lee, M.D., M.P.H., Health Officer, Colusa County Department of Health and Human Services
Cancer

Tova Marx, Ph.D.
Intimate Relationships and Communication

Nancy E. Mason, M.D., Department of Gynecology and Obstetrics, Stanford University School of Medicine
Abortion; Pregnancy and Childbirth

David Quadagno, Ph.D., Florida State University
Sex and Your Body

Jacob W. Roth, M.D., Dana Farber Cancer Institute, Harvard University
Dying and Death

Walton T. Roth, M.D., Stanford University
Psychological Health

James H. Rothenberger, M.P.H., University of Minnesota
Environmental Health

Judith Sharlin, Ph.D., R.D., Department of Nutrition, Simmons College
Weight Management

David S. Sobel, M.D., M.P.H., Director of Patient Education and Health Promotion, Kaiser Permanente Northern California
Conventional and Complementary Medicine: Skills for the Health Care Consumer

Mae V. Tinklenbeg, R.N., N.P., M.S.
Contraception

Jennifer A. Tremmel, M.D., S.M., Department of
Cardiovascular Medicine, Stanford University
Medical Center
Cardiovascular Health

R. Elaine Turner, Ph.D., R.D., University of Florida
Nutrition Basics

Patrick Zickler, Senior Science Writer, Masimax Resources, Inc.
Toward a Tobacco-free Society

Academic Advisers and Reviewers of the Tenth Edition

Charlene Brown, Western Michigan University

Mary V. Brown, Utah Valley State College

Susan T. Burge, Cuyahoga Community College

Laura Burger, Grossmont College

Karen Camarata, Eastern Kentucky University

Jacquie Cottingham, Confederation College

Paula J. Dahl, Bakersfield College

Kathi Deresinski, Triton College

P. K. Doyle-Baker, University of Calgary

Maqsood M. Faquir, Palm Beach Community College

Kathi Fuller, Western Michigan University

Cathy Hammond, Morehead State University

Mary E. Iten, University of Nebraska at Kearney

Belinda L. Jones, North Carolina Central University

Roland J. Lamarine, California State University, Chico

Teresa A. Lyles, University of Florida

Susan A. Lyman, University of Louisiana at Lafayette

Lori S. Mallory, Johnson County Community College

Tom Pestolesi, Irvine Valley College

Roseann L. Poole, Tallahassee Community College

Donna Jeanne Pugh, Florida Metropolitan University

Bruce M. Ragon, Albany State University

Priscilla Rice, Bucks County Community College

Leah E. Robinson, Bucks County Community College

Stafford C. Rorke, Oakland University

Andrew Shim, Indiana University of Pennsylvania

Carol A. Smith, Elon University

Phillip B. Sparling, Georgia Institute of Technology

Debra Tavasso, East Carolina University

Finally, we would like to thank the members of the *Core Concepts* book team at McGraw-Hill Higher Education. First, we are indebted to Kirstan Price for her dedication and her extraordinary creative energies, which have helped to make this book such a success. Thanks also go to Nick Barrett, executive editor; Julia Ersery, developmental editor for technology; Pam Cooper, senior marketing manager; Sarah Hill, editorial assistant; Lance Gerhart, media producer; Ron Nelms, media project manager; Brett Coker, production editor; Randy Hurst, production supervisor; Violeta Díaz, design manager; Robin Mouat, art manager; Brian Pecko, photo researcher; and Marty Granahan, permissions editor. To all we express our deep appreciation.

Paul M. Insel
Walton T. Roth

A Guided Tour of *Core Concepts in Health*

Are you looking for ways to improve your health behaviors and quality of life? Do you need help finding reliable wellness resources online? Would you like to boost your grade? *Core Concepts in Health* can help you do all this and much more!

ASSESS YOURSELF BOXES

Assess Yourself boxes give you the opportunity to evaluate your current level of wellness and pinpoint lifestyle behaviors that you can change. Assess Yourself boxes are marked with a World Wide Web icon to indicate that you can find them in an interactive format on the *Core Concepts in Health* Online Learning Center (www.mhhe.com/insel10e). Look for this icon throughout the text to identify elements that have corresponding activities and links on the Online Learning Center. For courses using the Quia™ Online Wellness Workbook, the self-assessments from the text are also available in the Workbook.

BEHAVIOR CHANGE STRATEGIES

Behavior Change Strategies provide specific behavior change plans for particular areas of wellness. Included are strategies for dealing with test anxiety, developing responsible drinking habits, quitting tobacco use, improving diet, planning a personal exercise program, and many other practical plans for change.

CRITICAL CONSUMER BOXES

Critical Consumer boxes are designed to help you develop and apply critical thinking skills so you can make sound choices related to wellness. Included are guidelines for evaluating health news and advertising, popular diets, and food and supplement labels; for choosing smoking cessation products, exercise footwear, and bicycle helmets; for making environmentally friendly shopping choices; and much more.

Using Food Labels

Food labels are designed to help consumers make food choices based on the nutrients that are most important to good health. In addition to listing nutrient content by weight, the label puts the information in the context of a daily diet of 2000 calories that includes no more than 65 grams of fat (approximately 30% of total calories). For example, if a serving of a particular product has 13 grams of fat, the label will show that the serving represents 20% of the daily fat allowance. If your daily diet contains fewer or more than 2000 calories, you need to adjust these calculations accordingly.

Food labels contain uniform serving sizes. This means that if you look at different brands of salad dressing, for example, you can compare calories and fat content based on the serving amount. (Food label serving sizes may be larger or smaller than MyPyramid serving size equivalents, however.) Regulations also require that foods meet strict definitions if their packaging includes the terms *light*, *low-fat*, or *high-fiber* (see the sample label). Claims such as "good source of dietary fiber" or "low in saturated fat" on packages are signals that those products can wisely be included in your diet. Overall, the food label is an important tool to help you choose a diet that conforms to MyPyramid and the Dietary Guidelines.

Selected Nutrient Content Claims and What They Mean

Healthy A food that is low in fat, has no more than 360–480 mg of sodium and 60 mg of cholesterol, *and* provides 10% or more of the Daily Value for vitamin A, vitamin C, protein, calcium, iron, or dietary fiber per serving.

Light or lite One-third fewer calories or 50% less fat than a similar product.

Reduced or fewer At least 25% less of a nutrient than a similar product; can be applied to fat ("reduced fat"), saturated fat, cholesterol, sodium, and calories.

Extra or added 10% or more of the Daily Value per serving when compared to what a similar product has.

Good source 10–19% of the Daily Value for a particular nutrient per serving.

High, rich in, or excellent source of 20% or more of the Daily Value for a particular nutrient per serving.

Low calorie 40 calories or less per serving.

High fiber 5 g or more of fiber per serving.

Good source of fiber 2.5–4.9 g of fiber per serving.

Fat-free Less than 0.5 g of fat per serving.

Low-fat 3 g of fat or less per serving.

Saturated fat-free Less than 0.5 g of saturated fat and 0.5 g of trans fatty acids per serving.

Low saturated fat 1 g or less of saturated fat and no more than 15% of total calories.

Cholesterol-free Less than 2 mg of cholesterol and 2 g or less of saturated fat per serving.

Low cholesterol 20 mg or less of cholesterol and 2 g or less of saturated fat per serving.

Low sodium 140 mg or less of sodium per serving.

Very low sodium 35 mg or less of sodium per serving.

Lean Cooked seafood, meat, or poultry with less than 10 g of fat, 4.5 g or less of saturated fat, and less than 95 mg of cholesterol per serving.

Extra lean Cooked seafood, meat, or poultry with less than 5 g of fat, 2 g of saturated fat, and 95 mg of cholesterol per serving.

NOTE: As of April 2005, the FDA had not yet defined nutrient claims relating to carbohydrate, so foods labeled low- or reduced-carbohydrate do not conform to any approved standard.

1. Serving size: Determine how many servings there are in the food package and compare it to how much you actually eat. You may need to adjust the rest of the nutrient values based on your typical serving size.

2. Calories and calories from fat: Note whether a serving is high in calories and fat. The sample food shown here is low in fat, with only 30 of its 235 calories from fat.

3. Daily Values: Based on a 2000-calorie diet, Daily Value percentages tell you whether the nutrients in a serving of food contribute a lot or a little to your total daily diet.
5% or less is low
20% or more is high

4. Limit these nutrients: Look for foods low in fat, saturated fat, trans fat, cholesterol, and sodium. (Trans fat content must be included on the label by January 2006 for any food with more than 0.5 g trans fat per serving.)

5. Get enough of these nutrients: Look for foods high in dietary fiber, vitamin A, vitamin C, calcium, and iron.

Nutrition Facts
Serving Size 1 cup (265g)
Servings per Container 2

Amount per Serving	
Calories 235	Calories from Fat 30

	% Daily Value*
Total Fat 3g	5%
Saturated Fat 1g	5%
Trans Fat 0.5g	
Cholesterol 30mg	10%
Sodium 775mg	32%
Total Carbohydrate 34g	11%
Dietary Fiber 9g	36%
Sugars 5g	
Protein 18g	

Vitamin A 25%	•	Vitamin C 0%	
Calcium 12%	•	Iron 20%	

*Percent Daily Values are based on a 2,000 calorie diet. Your daily values may be higher or lower depending on your calorie needs.

	Calories	2,000	2,500
Total Fat	Less than	65g	80g
Sat Fat	Less than	20g	75g
Cholesterol	Less than	300mg	300mg
Sodium	Less than	2,400mg	2,400mg
Total Carbohydrate		300g	375g
Dietary Fiber		25g	30g

Calories per gram
Fat 9 • Carbohydrate 4 • Protein 4

Note: This section shows recommended daily intake for two levels of calorie consumption and values for dietary calculations; it's the same on all labels.

TURKEY CHILI

Maintaining Your Exercise Program

- *Set realistic goals.* Unrealistically high goals will only discourage you.
- *Sign a contract and keep a fitness journal.* A journal can help keep your program on track, identify sources of problems, and give you a continuing sense of accomplishment.
- *Start slowly, and increase your intensity and duration gradually.* Overzealous exercising can result in discouraging discomforts and injuries. Your program is meant to last a lifetime. The important first step is to break your established pattern of inactivity.
- *Make your program fun.* Participate in a variety of different activities that you enjoy. Vary the routes you take walking, running, or biking.
- *Exercise with a friend.* The social side of exercise is an important factor for many regular exercisers.
- *Focus on the positive.* Concentrate on the improvements you obtain from your program, how good you feel during and after exercise.
- *Revisit and revise.* If your program turns out to be unrealistic, revise it. Expect to make many adjustments in your program along the way.

- *Expect fluctuation.* On some days your progress will be excellent, whereas on others you'll barely be able to drag yourself through your scheduled activities.
- *Expect lapses.* Don't let lapses discourage you or make you feel guilty. Instead, feel a renewed commitment to your exercise program.
- *Plan ahead for difficult situations.* Think about what circumstances might make it tough to keep up with your fitness routine, and develop strategies for sticking with your program. For example, devise a plan for your program during vacation, travel, bad weather, and so on.
- *Reward yourself.* Give yourself frequent rewards for sticking with your program.
- *Renew your attitude.* If you notice you're slacking off, try to list the negative thoughts and behaviors that are causing noncompliance. Devise a strategy to decrease the frequency of negative thoughts and behaviors. Make changes in your program plan and reward system to help renew your enthusiasm and commitment.
- *Review your goals.* Visualize what it will be like to reach them, and keep these pictures in your mind as an incentive to stick to your program.

Physical activity and exercise offer benefits in nearly every area of wellness, helping you generate energy, manage stress, control your weight, improve your mood, and, of course, become physically stronger and healthier. Building a program of regular exercise into your life is well worth the effort, even if it seems complicated or difficult at first. Even a low-to-moderate level of activity provides valuable health benefits. The important thing is to get moving. When in doubt, exercise!

Right now you can

- Get up and stretch.
- Go outside and take a brisk walk.
- Look at your calendar for the rest of the week and write in some physical activity—such as walking, running, biking, skating, swimming, hiking, or playing Frisbee—on as many days as you can; schedule the activity for a specific time, and stick to it.
- If you don't yet use the gym or fitness facility on your campus, go there now and begin planning how to use it.
- Call a friend and invite him or her to start a regular exercise program with you.

SUMMARY

- The five components of physical fitness most important to health are cardiorespiratory endurance, muscular strength, muscular endurance, flexibility, and body composition.
- Exercise improves the functioning of the heart and the ability of the cardiorespiratory system to carry oxygen to the body's tissues. It also increases the efficiency of the body's metabolism and improves body composition.
- Exercise lowers the risk of cardiovascular disease by improving blood fat levels, reducing high blood pressure, and interfering with the disease process that causes coronary artery blockage.
- Exercise reduces the risk of cancer, osteoporosis, and diabetes. It improves immune function and psychological health and helps prevent injuries and low-back pain.
- Everyone should accumulate at least 30–60 minutes per day of moderate endurance-type physical activity. Additional health and fitness benefits can be achieved through longer or more vigorous activity.
- Cardiorespiratory endurance exercises stress a large portion of the body's muscle mass. Endurance exercise should be performed 3–5 days per week for a total of 20–60 minutes per day. Intensity can be evaluated by measuring the heart rate.

TAKE CHARGE BOXES

Take Charge boxes present the practical advice you need to apply information from the text to your own life and to take charge of your health. Take Charge topics include breathing techniques for relaxation; guidelines for dealing with an alcohol emergency; and strategies for judging portion sizes, increasing physical activity, and improving communication.

Help Yourself by Helping Others

Choosing to help others—whether as a volunteer for a community organization or through spontaneous acts of kindness—can enhance emotional, social, spiritual, and physical wellness. Surveys and studies indicate that the sense of purpose and service and the feelings of generosity and kindness that go with helping others may be as important a consideration to wellness as good nutrition and regular exercise. Older adults who volunteer have higher levels of emotional and social wellness and lower rates of death.

In a national survey of volunteers from all fields, helpers reported the following benefits:

- Helper's high—physical and emotional sensations such as sudden warmth, a surge of energy, and a feeling of euphoria that occur immediately after helping
- Feelings of increased self-worth, calm, and relaxation
- A perception of greater physical health
- Fewer colds and headaches, improved eating and sleeping habits, and some relief from the pain of chronic diseases such as asthma and arthritis

Just how might helping benefit the health of the helper? By helping others, we may relieve our own distress and guilt over their problems. We focus on things other than our own problems, and we get a special kind of attention from the people we help. Helping others can be effective at banishing a bad mood or a case of the blues. Helping may block physical pain because we can pay attention to only a limited number of things at a given time. Helping others can also expand our perspective and enhance our appreciation for our own lives. Helping may benefit physical health by providing a temporary boost to the immune system and by combating stress and hostile feelings linked to the development of chronic diseases.

Helping others doesn't require a huge time commitment or a change of career. To get the most out of helping, keep the following guidelines in mind:

- *Make contact.* Choose an activity that involves personal contact.
- *Help as often as possible.* If your schedule allows, volunteer at least once a week. But, as with many parts of a wellness lifestyle, any amount of time helping is better than none.
- *Make helping voluntary.* Voluntary helping has positive results, whereas obligatory helping situations can actually increase stress.
- *Volunteer with others.* Working with a group enables you to form bonds with other helpers who can support your interests and efforts. Studies have found that the health benefits of volunteering are strongest for people

who otherwise have low levels of social interaction.

- *Focus on the process, not the outcome.* We can't always measure or know the results of our actions.
- *Practice random acts of kindness.* Smile, let people go ahead of you in line, pick up litter, and so on.
- *Adopt a pet.* Several studies suggest that pet owners enjoy better health, perhaps by feeling needed or by having a source of unconditional love and affection.
- *Avoid burnout.* Recognize your own limits, pace yourself, and try not to feel guilty or discouraged. Take pride in being a volunteer or caregiver.

You can experience "helper's high" and the other personal rewards of volunteering as soon as you begin helping others. In addition to the benefits for you, volunteering has the added bonus of having a positive impact on the wellness of others. It fosters a sense of community and can provide some practical help for many of the problems facing our society today.

SOURCES: Shmotkin, D.; T. Blumstein, and B. Modan. 2003. Beyond keeping active: Constraints of being a volunteer in old-old age. *Psychological Aging* 18(3): 602–607; adapted with permission from Sobel, D. S., M.D., and R. Ornstein, Ph.D. 1996. *The Healthy Mind, Healthy Body Handbook.* Los Altos, Calif.: DRx.

Financial planning for retirement is especially critical for women. American women are much less likely than men to be covered by pension plans, reflecting the fact that many women have lower-paying jobs or work part-time during their childbearing years. They tend to have less money vested in other types of retirement plans as well. Although the gap is narrowing, women currently outlive men by about 5–6 years, and they are more likely to develop chronic conditions that impair their daily activities later in life. The net result of these factors is that older women are almost twice as likely as older men to live in poverty. Women should investigate their retirement plans and take charge of their finances to be sure they will be provided for as they get older.

Adapting to Physical Changes

As described earlier in the chapter, there are many things a person can do to avoid or minimize the effects of the physical changes associated with aging. However, some changes in physical functioning are inevitable, and successful aging involves anticipating and accommodating these changes.

Decreased energy and changes in health mean that older people have to develop priorities for how to use their energy. Rather than curtailing activities to conserve energy, they need to learn how to generate energy. This usually involves saying yes to enjoyable activities and paying close attention to the need for rest and sleep.

MIND/BODY/SPIRIT BOXES

Mind/Body/Spirit boxes focus on the close connections among people's feelings, states of mind, and physical health. Topics include religious views of tobacco use, effects of stress on the brain, sexual decision making and personal values, benefits of being a volunteer, expressive writing, and characteristics of a good death.

GENDER MATTERS

New to the tenth edition, Gender Matters boxes highlight key gender differences related to wellness as well as areas of particular concern to men or women. Topics include gender differences in rates of anxiety, depression, drug use, and cancer; in the symptoms and course of heart attack and STDs; in styles of communication; and in responses to stress and grief.

Women, Men, and Stress

Special Stressors for Men and Women

Women are more likely than men to find themselves balancing multiple roles—student, employee, parent, spouse, caregiver to aging parents. Women who work outside of the home still do most of the housework, and time-related stress can be severe. All of these stressors can contribute to higher levels of stress-related health problems. Social forces can also undermine opportunities for women and cause stress. Women now make up more than half of the workforce but hold only 5% of the top leadership jobs. On average, women make less money than men with comparable jobs and are more likely to face sexual harassment. Disparity in domestic responsibilities, lack of integration into dominant organization coalitions, and even being considered excessively "nice" can all reduce the chances of being considered for leadership positions. The more women view themselves as fitting the traditional feminine gender stereotype, the less likely they are to report leadership aspirations.

Men who fit a traditional male gender role may feel the need to be active and in charge in all situations. They may have a communication style that is competitive and aggressive, causing stress in many interpersonal situations and limiting their ability to build social support networks. The responsibility to support a family may be felt very keenly among men with a traditional male gender role.

Physiological Differences and Stress

Due to hormonal differences, men are considered to be more biologically vulnerable to certain diseases. For example, because of a rise in circulating testosterone levels, from puberty onward, males have higher blood pressure than do age-matched females. Along with other risk factors, including fewer physician visits, the rise in testosterone produces greater wear and tear on the male circulatory system over time, leading to greater risk for cardiovascular disease. A part of the brain responsible for regulating fear and emotional balance, the amygdala, is very sensitive to testosterone. Thus, having more circulating testosterone may predispose men to see social situations as more threatening than

a woman would see them, creating more frequent activation of the stress response.

Women, on the other hand, have higher levels of the hormone oxytocin and are more likely to respond to stressors by seeking social support. The tend-and-befriend response among women may give them a longevity advantage compared with men by decreasing the risk of stress-related disorders.

Gender and Stress Among College Students

Gender role development is a significant source of stress during college for both men and women, but there are gender differences in key stressors and coping strategies. College women are more likely than men to report having roommate conflicts and personal appearance issues. Men have more difficulty relating to and meeting other students, making friends, and dealing with peer pressure. College women report significantly higher emotional resources and ability to give and receive social support than do men. College men more frequently utilize physical coping resources than do women.

The General Adaptation Syndrome

Biologist Hans Selye, working in the 1930s and 1940s, was one of the first scientists to develop a comprehensive theory of stress and disease. Selye coined the term **general adaptation syndrome (GAS)** to describe what he believed was a universal and predictable response pattern to all stressors. He recognized that stressors could be pleasant, such as attending a party, or unpleasant, such as getting a flat tire or a bad grade. He called stress triggered by a pleasant stressor **eustress** and stress triggered by an unpleasant stressor **distress**. The sequence of physical responses associated with GAS is the same for both eustress and distress and occurs in three stages: alarm, resistance, and exhaustion (Figure 2-3).

Alarm This stage includes the complex sequence of events brought on by the activation of the sympathetic nervous system and the endocrine system—the fight-or-flight reaction. During this stage, the body is more susceptible to disease or injury because it is geared up to deal with a crisis. A person in this phase may experience headaches, indigestion, anxiety, and disrupted sleeping and eating patterns.

Resistance With continued stress, Selye theorized, the body developed a new level of homeostasis in which it was more resistant to disease and injury than it normally would be. During the resistance stage, a person can cope with normal life and added stress.

Exhaustion As you might imagine, both the mobilization of forces during the alarm reaction and the maintenance of homeostasis during the resistance stage require a considerable amount of energy. If a stressor persists or if several stressors occur in succession, general exhaustion results. This is not the sort of exhaustion people complain

Terms

gender role A culturally expected pattern of behavior and attitudes determined by whether a person is male or female.

general adaptation syndrome (GAS) A pattern of stress responses consisting of three stages: alarm, resistance, and exhaustion.

eustress Stress resulting from a pleasant stressor.

distress Stress resulting from an unpleasant stressor.

IN THE NEWS BOXES

In the News boxes focus on current health issues that have recently been highlighted in the media, including such topics as same-sex marriage, medical marijuana, prescription drug safety, influenza pandemics, stem cells, and reasons behind poor eating habits among Americans. In the News boxes are marked with the Web icon to indicate that the Online Learning Center has links to Web sites you can use to learn more about In the News topics.

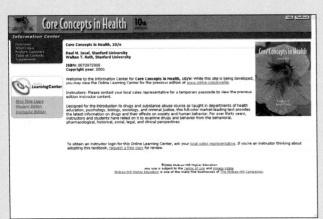

Vw CORE CONCEPTS IN HEALTH ONLINE LEARNING CENTER

Visit the *Core Concepts in Health* Online Learning Center (www.mhhe.com/insel10e) for resources to help improve your grade and your level of wellness. You'll find chapter objectives and quizzes, flashcards, and many more study aids. You'll also find behavior change tools, Internet activities, and links to reliable wellness-related sites. A password granting access to additional premium online resources is available free with each new copy of the text; these premium resources include interactive self-assessments, articles on health and human performance, and a daily news feed.

Core Concepts in Health

Looking AHEAD

After reading this chapter, you should be able to

- Describe the six dimensions of wellness and a wellness lifestyle

- Identify major goals of the national Healthy People initiative

- Explain the importance of personal decision making and behavior change in achieving a wellness lifestyle

- Describe the steps in creating a behavior management plan to change a health-related behavior

- Describe the influence of gender, ethnicity, income, disability, family history, and environment on health

- Discuss the available sources of health information and how to think critically about them

Taking Charge of Your Health

Knowledge

1. **In 1900, infectious diseases such as pneumonia and tuberculosis were responsible for more than one-third of all deaths in the United States.**
   True or false?

2. **The leading cause of death among Americans age 15–34 is unintentional injuries (accidents).**
   True or false?

3. **Which of the following lifestyle factors is the leading preventable cause of death for Americans?**
   a. alcohol abuse
   b. cigarette smoking
   c. poor dietary habits and lack of exercise

4. **Only 50% of health-related Web sites are nonpromotional and based on scientific information.**
   True or false?

5. **More than two-thirds of all college students make which of the following positive lifestyle choices?**
   a. using safety belts
   b. not drinking and driving
   c. using contraception (if sexually active)
   d. eating two or fewer high-fat foods per day
   e. not using tobacco

ANSWERS

1. TRUE. A century later, infectious diseases cause only about 2% of all deaths; heart disease, cancer, and stroke are now responsible for more than 50% of all deaths among Americans.

2. TRUE. Homicide and suicide round out the top three leading causes of death for 15–34-year-olds; in this age group, the death rate for males is more than twice that of females.

3. B. Smoking causes about 435,000 deaths each year; poor diet and inactivity are responsible for about 365,000 deaths, and alcohol, more than 80,000.

4. FALSE. The number is closer to 35%. Most health-related Web sites sell products and/or are not based on scientific information.

5. ALL FIVE. However, the majority of students do not exercise regularly, do not wear bicycle helmets, and eat few fruits and vegetables. There are many areas in which college students can change their behavior to improve their health.

Visit the *Core Concepts in Health* Online Learning Center (www.mhhe.com/insel10e) for study aids and many additional resources.

1

A first-year college student resolves to meet the challenge of making new friends. A long-sedentary senior starts riding her bike to school every day instead of taking the bus. A busy part-time student organizes a group of coworkers to help plant trees in a blighted inner-city neighborhood. What do these people have in common? Each is striving for optimal health and well-being. Not satisfied to be merely free of major illness, these individuals want more. They want to live life actively, energetically, and fully, in a state of optimal personal, interpersonal, and environmental well-being. They have taken charge of their health and are on the path to wellness.

WELLNESS: THE NEW HEALTH GOAL

Wellness is an expanded idea of health. Many people think of health as being just the absence of physical disease. But wellness transcends this concept of health—for example, when individuals with serious illnesses or disabilities rise above their physical or mental limitations to live rich, meaningful, vital lives. Some aspects of health are determined by your genes, your age, and other factors that may be beyond your control. But true wellness is largely determined by the decisions you make about how to live your life. In this book, we will use the terms *health* and *wellness* interchangeably to mean the ability to live life fully—with vitality and meaning.

The Dimensions of Wellness

No matter what your age or health status, you can optimize your health in each of the following six interrelated dimensions. Wellness in any dimension is not a static goal but a dynamic process of change and growth (Figure 1-1).

Physical Wellness Optimal physical health requires eating well, exercising, avoiding harmful habits, making responsible decisions about sex, learning about and recognizing the symptoms of disease, getting regular

medical and dental checkups, and taking steps to prevent injuries at home, on the road, and on the job. The habits you develop and the decisions you make today will largely determine not only how many years you will live, but also the quality of your life during those years.

Emotional Wellness Optimism, trust, self-esteem, self-acceptance, self-confidence, self-control, satisfying relationships, and an ability to share feelings are just some of the qualities and aspects of emotional wellness. Emotional health is a dynamic state that fluctuates with your physical, intellectual, spiritual, interpersonal and social, and environmental health. Maintaining emotional wellness requires monitoring and exploring your thoughts and feelings, identifying obstacles to emotional well-being, and finding solutions to emotional problems, with the help of a therapist if necessary.

Intellectual Wellness The hallmarks of intellectual health include an openness to new ideas, a capacity to question and think critically, and the motivation to master new skills, as well as a sense of humor, creativity, and curiosity. An active mind is essential to overall wellness, for learning about, evaluating, and storing health-related information. Your mind detects problems, finds solutions, and directs behavior. People who enjoy intellectual wellness never stop learning. They relish new experiences and challenges and actively seek them out.

Spiritual Wellness To enjoy spiritual health is to possess a set of guiding beliefs, principles, or values that give meaning and purpose to your life, especially during difficult times. Spiritual wellness involves the capacity for love, compassion, forgiveness, altruism, joy, and fulfillment. It is an antidote to cynicism, anger, fear, anxiety, self-absorption, and pessimism. Spirituality transcends the individual and can be a common bond among people. Organized religions help many people develop spiritual health. Many others find meaning and purpose in their lives on their own—through nature, art, meditation, political action, or good works.

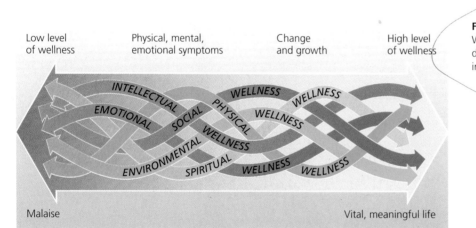

Figure 1-1 The wellness continuum. Wellness is composed of six interrelated dimensions, all of which must be developed in order to achieve overall wellness.

Low level of wellness — Physical, mental, emotional symptoms — Change and growth — High level of wellness

INTELLECTUAL WELLNESS WELLNESS
EMOTIONAL SOCIAL PHYSICAL WELLNESS
ENVIRONMENTAL WELLNESS SPIRITUAL WELLNESS WELLNESS

Malaise — Vital, meaningful life

With wellness come health and vitality throughout the life span.

Interpersonal and Social Wellness Satisfying relationships are basic to both physical and emotional health. We need to have mutually loving, supportive people in our lives. Developing interpersonal wellness means learning good communication skills, developing the capacity for intimacy, and cultivating a support network of caring friends and/or family members. Social wellness requires participating in and contributing to your community, country, and world.

Environmental or Planetary Wellness Increasingly, personal health depends on the health of the planet—from the safety of the food supply to the degree of violence in a society. Other examples of environmental threats to health are ultraviolet radiation in sunlight, air and water pollution, lead in old house paint, and secondhand tobacco smoke in indoor air. Wellness requires learning about and protecting yourself against such hazards—and doing what you can to reduce or eliminate them, either on your own or with others.

The six dimensions of wellness interact continuously, influencing and being influenced by one another. Making a change in one dimension often affects some or all of the others. For example, regular exercise (developing the physical dimension of wellness) can increase feelings of well-being and self-esteem (emotional wellness), which in turn can increase feelings of confidence in social interactions and your achievements at work or school (interpersonal and social wellness). Maintaining good health is a dynamic process, and increasing your level of wellness in one area of life often influences many others (see the box "Ten Warning Signs of Wellness" on p. 4).

New Opportunities, New Responsibilities

Wellness is a relatively recent concept. A century ago, people considered themselves lucky just to survive to adulthood. A child born in 1900, for example, could expect to live only about 47 years. Many people died as a result of common **infectious diseases** and poor environmental conditions (unrefrigerated food, poor sanitation, air and water pollution). However, since 1900, the average life span has increased by more than 60%, thanks largely to the development of vaccines and antibiotics to prevent and fight infectious diseases and to public health campaigns to improve environmental conditions (Figure 1-2, p. 4).

But a different set of diseases has emerged as our major health threat, and heart disease, cancer, and stroke are now the top three causes of death in the United States (Table 1-1 on p. 5). Treating these and other **chronic diseases** has proved enormously expensive and extremely difficult. It has become clear that the best treatment for these diseases is prevention—people having a greater awareness about their own health and about taking care of their bodies.

The good news is that people do have some control over whether they develop heart disease, cancer, and other chronic diseases. People make choices every day that either increase or decrease their risks for these diseases—lifestyle choices involving behaviors such as exercise, diet, smoking, and drinking. When researchers look at the lifestyle factors that contribute to death in the United States, it becomes clear that individuals can profoundly influence their own health risks (see Table 1-2 on p. 6 and the last column in Table 1-1). Smoking is the leading preventable cause of death among Americans, responsible for about 435,000 deaths each year; it is followed by poor diet and inactivity (about 365,000 deaths per year) and alcohol use (about

Terms

wellness Optimal health and vitality, encompassing physical, emotional, intellectual, spiritual, interpersonal and social, and environmental well-being.

infectious disease A disease that is communicable from one person to another; caused by invading microorganisms such as bacteria and viruses.

chronic disease A disease that develops and continues over a long period of time; usually caused by a variety of factors, including lifestyle factors.

Ten Warning Signs of Wellness

1. The persistent presence of a support network

2. Chronic positive expectations; the tendency to frame events in a constructive light

3. Episodic outbreaks of joyful, happy experiences

4. A sense of spiritual involvement

5. A tendency to adapt to changing conditions

6. Rapid response and recovery of stress response systems to repeated challenges

7. An increased appetite for physical activity

8. A tendency to identify and communicate feelings

9. Repeated episodes of gratitude and generosity

10. A persistent sense of humor

SOURCE: Ten warning signs of good health. 1996. *Mind/Body Health Newsletter* 5(1).

Mind/Body/Spirit

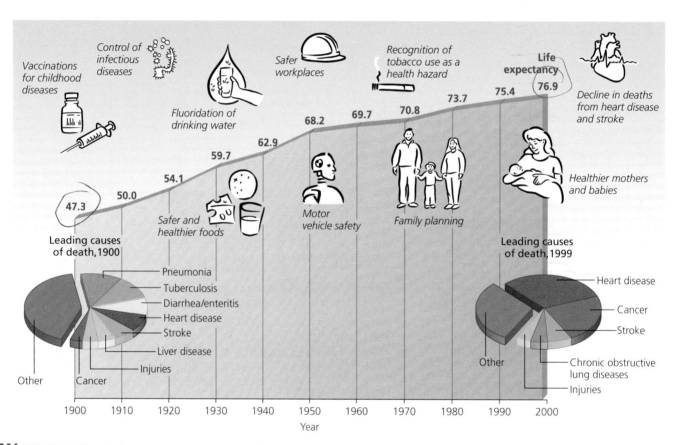

VITAL STATISTICS

Figure 1-2   Public health achievements of the twentieth century.   During the twentieth century, public health achievements greatly improved the quality of life for Americans, and life expectancy rose from 47 to 77. A dramatic shift in the leading causes of death also occurred, with deaths from infectious diseases declining from over 33% of all deaths to just 2.2%. Heart disease, cancer, and stroke are now responsible for over 50% of all deaths among Americans.

SOURCES: National Center for Health Statistics. 2004. *Health, United States, 2004, with Chartbook on Trends in the Health of Americans.* Hyattsville, Md.: National Center for Health Statistics; Centers for Disease Control and Prevention. 1999. Ten great public health achievements—United States, 1900–1999. *Morbidity and Mortality Weekly Report* 48(50): 1141.

Table 1-1 Leading Causes of Death in the United States

[handwritten: Know Top 5]

Rank	Cause of Death	Number of Deaths	Percent of Total Deaths	Female/Male Ratio[a]	Lifestyle Factors
1	Heart disease	684,462	28.0	51/49	D I S A
2	Cancer[b]	554,643	22.7	48/52	D I S A
3	Stroke	157,803	6.5	61/39	D I S A
4	Chronic lower respiratory diseases	126,128	5.2	51/49	S
5	Unintentional injuries (accidents) *[handwritten: young people]*	105,695	4.3	35/65	I S A
6	Diabetes mellitus	73,965	3.0	53/47	D I S
7	Influenza and pneumonia	64,847	2.7	56/44	S
8	Alzheimer's disease	63,343	2.6	71/29	
9	Kidney disease	42,536	1.7	52/48	D I S A
10	Septicemia (systemic blood infection)	34,243	1.4	56/44	A
11	Intentional self-harm (suicide)	30,642	1.3	20/80	A
12	Chronic liver disease and cirrhosis	27,201	1.1	36/64	A
13	Hypertension (high blood pressure)	21,841	0.9	62/38	D I S A
14	Parkinson's disease	17,898	0.7	43/57	
15	Pneumonia due to aspiration	17,457	0.7	50/50	
	All causes	2,443,930			

Key **D** Cause of death in which diet plays a part   **S** Cause of death in which smoking plays a part *[handwritten: Biggest Factor]*
I Cause of death in which an inactive lifestyle plays a part   **A** Cause of death in which excessive alcohol consumption plays a part

[a]Ratio of females to males who died of each cause. For example, about the same number of women and men died of heart disease, but only about half as many women as men died of unintentional injuries and four times as many men as women committed suicide.
[b]Among people under age 85, cancer is the leading cause of death. Decreased rates of smoking have reduced deaths from both heart disease and cancer, but among ex-smokers, heart disease risk declines more quickly and to a greater degree than cancer risk.

Note: Although not among the overall top 15 causes of death, homicide (17,096 deaths) and HIV/AIDS (13,544 deaths) are major killers; both are among the 10 leading causes of death among Americans age 15–44 years.

SOURCE: National Center for Health Statistics. 2005. Deaths: Preliminary data for 2003. *National Vital Statistics Report* 53(15); Jemal, A., et al. 2005. Cancer statistics, 2005. *CA: A Cancer Journal for Clinicians* 55(1): 10–30.

85,000 deaths per year). From these figures, it is clear that wellness cannot be prescribed; physicians and other health care professionals can provide information, advice, and encouragement—but the rest is up to each of us.

National Wellness Goals: The Healthy People Initiative

You may think of health and wellness as personal concerns, goals that you strive for on your own for your own benefit. But the U.S. government also has a vital interest in the health of all Americans. A healthy population is the nation's greatest resource, the source of its vitality, creativity, and wealth. Poor health, in contrast, drains the nation's resources and raises national health care costs. As the embodiment of our society's values, the federal government also has a humane interest in people's health.

The U.S. government's national Healthy People initiative seeks to prevent unnecessary disease and disability and to achieve a better quality of life for all Americans. Healthy People reports, published first in 1980 and revised every decade, set national health goals based on 10-year agendas.

Each report includes both broad goals and specific targets in many different areas of wellness. The latest report, *Healthy People 2010,* proposes two broad national goals:

- *Increase quality and years of healthy life.* The life expectancy of Americans has increased significantly in the past century; however, people can expect poor health to limit their activities and cause distress during the last 15% of their lives (Figure 1-3, p. 6). Health-related quality of life reflects a personal sense of physical and mental health and the ability to react to factors in the physical and social environments. It calls for a full range of functional capacity to enable people to work, play, and maintain satisfying relationships. This national goal stresses the importance of health status and quality of life, not just longevity.

- *Eliminate health disparities among Americans.* Many health problems today disproportionately affect certain American populations—for example, ethnic minorities, people of low socioeconomic status or educational attainment, and people with disabilities. *Healthy People 2010* calls for eliminating disparities in health status, health risks, and use of preventive services among all population groups within the next decade.

Table 1-2 Actual Causes of Death Among Americans, 2000

	Number of Deaths Per Year	Percent of Total Deaths Per Year	Change in Number of Deaths Per Year Since 1990
Tobacco	435,000	18.1	+
Poor diet/physical inactivity	365,000	15.2	+
Alcohol consumption	85,000	3.5	−
Microbial agents	75,000	3.1	−
Toxic agents	55,000	2.3	−
Motor vehicles	43,000	1.8	+
Firearms	29,000	1.2	−
Sexual behavior	20,000	0.8	−
Illicit drug use	17,000	0.7	−

Note: Actual causes of death are defined as lifestyle and environmental factors that contribute to the leading killers of Americans, including heart disease, cancer, and stroke. Microbial agents include bacterial and viral infections like influenza and pneumonia; toxic agents include environmental pollutants and chemical agents such as asbestos. Comparable calculations on actual causes of death were done for 1990 and 2000, and deaths from some causes increased (+) while for others, deaths declined (−). Calculation of the number of deaths due to poor diet/physical inactivity (obesity) is an area of ongoing controversy and debate.

SOURCE: Mokdad, A. H., et al. 2005. Correction: Actual causes of death in the United States, 2000. *Journal of the American Medical Association* 293(3): 293–294. Mokdad, A. H., et al. 2004. Actual causes of death in the United States, 2000. *Journal of the American Medical Association* 291(10): 1238–1245.

Giving substance to these broad goals are hundreds of specific objectives—measurable targets for the year 2010—in many different focus areas that relate to wellness, including fitness, nutrition, safety, substance abuse, health care, and chronic and infectious diseases. Specific Healthy People targets serve as the basis for national monitoring and tracking of the health status and health risks of Americans and our use of health services. They encompass individual actions as well as larger-scale changes in environment and medical services. Examples of health promotion objectives from *Healthy People 2010,* as well as estimates of our progress toward these targets, appear in Table 1-3.

Healthy People 2010 reflects the changing attitude of Americans: an emerging sense of personal responsibility as the key to good health. This new perspective is seen in our concern about smoking and drug abuse, for example;

in our emphasis on physical and emotional fitness; in our interest in good nutrition; and in our concern about the environment. The primary concerns of *Healthy People 2010* are the principal topics covered in this book. In many ways, personal wellness goals are no different from the national aspirations.

Health Issues for Diverse Populations

Americans are a diverse people. Our ancestry is European, African, Asian, Pacific Islander, Latin American, and Native American. We live in cities, suburbs, and rural areas and work at every imaginable occupation. In no other country in the world do so many diverse people live and work together every day. And in no other country are the understanding and tolerance of differences so much a part of the political and cultural ideal. We are at heart a nation of diversity, and, though we often fall short of our goal, we strive for justice and equality among all.

When it comes to health, most differences among people are insignificant; most health issues concern us all equally. We all need to eat well, exercise, manage stress, and cultivate satisfying personal relationships. We need to know how to protect ourselves from heart disease, cancer, sexually transmitted diseases, and injuries. We need to know how to use the health care system.

But some of our differences, as individuals and as members of groups, do have important implications for health. Some of us, for example, have a genetic predisposition for developing certain health problems, such as high cholesterol. Some of us have grown up eating foods that raise our risk of heart disease or obesity. Some of us live in an environment that increases the chance that we will smoke

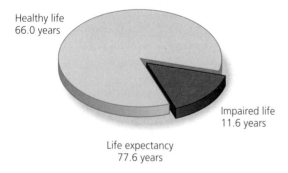

Healthy life
66.0 years

Impaired life
11.6 years

Life expectancy
77.6 years

Figure 1-3 Quantity of life versus quality of life. Years of healthy life as a proportion of life expectancy in the U.S. population. SOURCES: National Center for Health Statistics. 2005. Deaths: Preliminary data for 2003. *National Vital Statistics Reports* 53(15); National Center for Health Statistics. 2001. *Healthy People 2000 Final Review.* Hyattsville, Md.: Public Health Service.

| Table 1-3 | Selected *Healthy People 2010* Objectives |

Objective	Estimate of Current Status (%)	Goal (%)
Increase the proportion of people age 18 and older who engage regularly in moderate physical activity.	32	50
Increase the proportion of people age 2 and older who consume at least three daily servings of vegetables, with at least one-third being dark-green or orange vegetables.	3	50
Increase the prevalence of healthy weight among all people age 20 and older.	34	60
Reduce the proportion of adults 18 and older who use cigarettes.	22	12
Reduce the proportion of college students reporting binge drinking during the past 2 weeks.	39	20
Increase the proportion of pregnancies that are intended.	51	70
Increase the proportion of adults who take protective measures to reduce the risk of skin cancer (sunscreens, sun-protective clothing, and so on).	58	75
Increase the use of safety belts by motor vehicle occupants.	75	92
Increase the number of residences with a functioning smoke alarm on every floor.	87	100
Increase the proportion of people with health insurance.	83	100

SOURCE: National Center for Health Statistics. 2004. *DATA2010: The Healthy People 2010 Database: November 2004 Edition* (http://wonder.cdc.gov/data2010/obj.htm; retrieved February 16, 2005).

cigarettes or abuse alcohol. These health-related differences among individuals and groups can be biological—determined genetically—or cultural—acquired as patterns of behavior through daily interactions with our families, communities, and society. Many health conditions are a function of biology and culture combined. A person can have a genetic predisposition for a disease, for example, but won't actually develop the disease itself unless certain lifestyle factors are present, such as stress or a poor diet.

When we talk about health issues for diverse populations, we face two related dangers. The first is the danger of stereotyping, of talking about people as groups rather than as individuals. It's certainly true that every person is an individual with a unique genetic endowment and unique life experiences. But many of these influences are shared with others of similar genetic and cultural background. Statements about these group similarities can be useful; for example, they can alert people to areas that may be of special concern for them and their families.

The second danger is that of overgeneralizing, of ignoring the extensive biological and cultural diversity that exists among peoples who are grouped together. Groups labeled Latino or Hispanic, for example, include Mexican Americans, Puerto Ricans, people from South and Central America, and other Spanish-speaking peoples. Similarly, the population labeled American Indian includes hundreds of recognized tribal nations, each with its own genetic and cultural heritage. It's important to keep these considerations in mind whenever you read about culturally diverse populations.

Health-related differences among groups can be identified and described in the context of several different dimensions. Those highlighted in *Healthy People 2010* are gender, ethnicity, income and education, disability, geographic location, and sexual orientation.

Sex and Gender   Sex and gender profoundly influence wellness. The World Health Organization (WHO) defines **sex** as the biological and physiological characteristics that define men and women; these characteristics are related to chromosomes and their effects on reproductive organs and the functioning of the body. Menstruation in women and the presence of testicles in men are examples of sex-related characteristics. **Gender** is defined as roles, behaviors, activities, and attributes that a given society considers appropriate for men and women. A person's gender is rooted in biology and physiology, but it is shaped by experience and environment—how society responds to individuals based on their sex. Examples of gender-related characteristics that affect wellness include higher rates of smoking and drinking among men and lower earnings among women (compared with men doing similar work).

Terms

sex The biological and physiological characteristics that define men and women.

gender The roles, behaviors, activities, and attributes that a given society considers appropriate for men and women.

Men and women have different life expectancies, different reproductive concerns, and different incidences of many diseases. They have different patterns of health-related behaviors, and they respond differently to medications and other medical treatments. The lists below highlight just a few of the many gender differences that can affect wellness.

Women

- Women live longer than men but have higher rates of disabling health problems like arthritis, osteoporosis, and Alzheimer's disease.

- On average, women are shorter, have a lower proportion of muscle, and tend to have a "pear" body shape, with excess body fat stored in the hips.

- Women score better on tests of verbal fluency, speech production, fine motor skills, and visual and working memory.

- Women experience heart attacks, on average, about 10 years later than men, but they have a poorer 1-year postattack survival rate. Women are more likely to experience atypical heart attack symptoms such as fatigue and difficulty breathing.

- Women are more likely to have a stroke or to die from a stroke, but women are also more likely to recover language ability after a stroke affecting the left side of the brain.

- Women have lower rates of smoking but have a higher risk of lung cancer at a given level of exposure to cigarette smoke.

- Women become more intoxicated at a given level of alcohol intake.

- Women have stronger immune systems and are less susceptible to infection by certain bacteria and

viruses, but they are more likely to develop autoimmune diseases like lupus.

- Women are more likely to react to stressors with a response called tend-or-befriend that involves social support; this response may give women a longevity advantage by reducing the risk of stress-related disorders.

- Women are more likely to suffer from depression and to attempt suicide.

- Women are more likely to suffer from migraine headaches and chronic tension headaches.

- Women are more likely to be infected with a sexually transmitted disease (STD) during a heterosexual encounter, and they are more likely to suffer severe and long-term effects from STDs, including chronic infection and infertility.

Men

- Men have a shorter life expectancy than women, but they have lower rates of disabling health problems.

- On average, men are taller, have a higher proportion of muscle, and tend to have an "apple" body shape, with excess body fat stored in the abdomen.

- Men score better in tests of visual-spatial ability—for example, the ability to imagine the relationships between shapes and objects when rotated in space.

- Men experience heart attacks, on average, about 10 years earlier than women, but they have a better 1-year postattack survival rate. Men are more likely to have classic heart attack symptoms like chest pain.

- Men are less likely to die from a stroke but are also more likely to

have permanent loss of language ability following a stroke affecting the left side of the brain.

- Men have higher rates of smoking, spit tobacco use, and alcohol use and abuse.

- Men have higher rates of death from causes linked to intoxication, risk-taking behavior, and firearms: unintentional injuries (car crashes, drowning), homicide, and suicide.

- Men are more likely to be exposed to toxic or cancer-causing chemicals on the job.

- Men have weaker immune systems and are more susceptible to infection by certain bacteria and viruses, but they are less likely to develop auto-immune diseases like lupus.

- Men are more likely to react to stressors with an aggressive or hostile response, a pattern that may increase the risk of stress-related disorders.

- Men have lower rates of depression and are less likely to attempt suicide; however, men are much more likely to succeed at suicide, and many more men than women die each year from suicide.

- Men are more likely to suffer from cluster headaches.

- Men are less likely to be infected with an STD during a heterosexual encounter.

SOURCES: World Health Organization. 2004. *Gender and HIV/AIDS* (http://www.who.int/gender/hiv_aids/en; retrieved August 13, 2004); Entering a new age of gender medicine. 2003. *Consumer Reports on Health*, December; Institute of Medicine. 2001. *Exploring the Biological Contributions to Human Health: Does Sex Matter?* Washington, D.C.: National Academy Press.

The effects of sex and gender on wellness can be difficult to separate—but both are important. For example, rates of smoking among American women increased following changes in culturally defined ideas of appropriate behavior for women. This increase in smoking, combined with women's greater biological vulnerability to the cancer-causing agents in tobacco smoke, has led to a substantial increase in the number of deaths from lung cancer among

women. See the box "Women's Health/Men's Health" for more on gender differences that impact wellness; throughout the text, boxes labeled Gender Matters focus on key wellness concerns for women and men.

Ethnicity Achieving the *Healthy People 2010* goal of eliminating all health disparities will require a national effort to identify and address the underlying causes of ethnic health disparities. Compared with the U.S. population as a whole, American ethnic minorities have higher rates of death and disability from many causes. These disparities result from a complex mix of genetic variations, environmental factors, and health behaviors.

Some genetic diseases are concentrated in certain gene pools, the result of each ethnic group's relatively distinct history. Sickle-cell disease is most common among people of African ancestry. Tay-Sachs disease afflicts people of Eastern European Jewish heritage and French Canadian heritage. Cystic fibrosis is more common among Northern Europeans. In addition to biological differences, many cultural differences occur along ethnic lines. Ethnic groups may vary in their traditional diets; their patterns of family and interpersonal relationships; their attitudes toward tobacco, alcohol, and other drugs; and their health beliefs and practices. All of these factors have important implications for wellness.

The federal government collects population and health information on five broad ethnic minority groups in American society (Figure 1-4 shows the current ethnic distribution of the United States). Each group has some specific health concerns:

• *Latinos* are a diverse group, with roots in Mexico, Puerto Rico, Cuba, and South and Central America; many Latinos are of mixed Spanish and American Indian descent or of mixed Spanish, Indian, and African American descent. Latinos on average have lower rates of heart disease, cancer, and suicide than the general population, but higher rates of infant mortality and a higher overall birth rate; other areas of concern include gallbladder disease and obesity. At current rates, about one in two Latinas will develop diabetes in her lifetime.

• *African Americans* have the same leading causes of death as the general population, but they have a higher infant mortality rate and lower rates of suicide and osteoporosis. Areas of special concern for African Americans include high blood pressure, stroke, diabetes, asthma, and obesity. African American men are at significantly higher risk of prostate cancer than men in other groups, and early screening is recommended for them.

• *Asian Americans* include people who trace their ancestry to countries in the Far East, Southeast Asia, or the Indian subcontinent, including Japan, China, Vietnam, Laos, Cambodia, Korea, the Philippines, India, and Pakistan. Asian Americans have a lower death rate and a longer life expectancy than the general population. They have lower rates of coronary heart disease and obesity. However, health differences exist among these groups. For example, Southeast Asian men have higher rates of smoking and lung cancer, and Vietnamese American women have higher rates of cervical cancer.

• *American Indians and Alaska Natives* typically embrace a tribal identity, such as Sioux, Navaho, or Hopi. American Indians and Alaska Natives have lower death

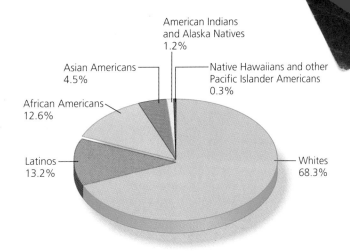

Note: Census respondents can choose more than one category, so percentages reflect both those who report one category and the approximately 2% of Americans who report two or more categories.

VITAL STATISTICS

Figure 1-4 Distribution of the U.S. population. SOURCE: U.S. Census Bureau. 2004. *Annual Estimates of Population by Race Alone or in Combination and Hispanic or Latino Origin for the United States.* Washington, D.C.: U.S. Census Bureau.

rates from heart disease, stroke, and cancer than the general population, but they have higher rates of early death from causes linked to smoking and alcohol use, including injuries and cirrhosis. Diabetes is a special concern for many groups; for example, the Pimas of Arizona have the highest known prevalence of diabetes of any population in the world.

• *Native Hawaiian and Other Pacific Islander Americans* trace their ancestry to the original peoples of Hawaii, Guam, Samoa, and other Pacific Islands. Pacific Islander Americans have a higher overall death rate than the general population and higher rates of some diseases, including diabetes and asthma. High rates of smoking and high prevalence of overweight and obesity are special concerns for this group.

It is often difficult to separate factors related to ethnicity from those associated with socioeconomic status and educational attainment. See the next section and the box "Factors Contributing to Health Disparities Among Ethnic Minorities" on page 10 for more information.

Income and Education Inequalities in income and education underlie many of the health disparities among Americans. Income and education are closely related, and groups with the highest poverty rates and least education have the worst health status. People with low incomes and less education have higher rates of infant mortality, traumatic injury and violent death, and many diseases, including heart disease, diabetes, tuberculosis, and HIV infection. They are more likely to eat poorly, be overweight, smoke, drink, and use drugs. They are exposed to more stressors

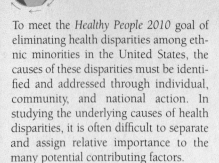

To meet the *Healthy People 2010* goal of eliminating health disparities among ethnic minorities in the United States, the causes of these disparities must be identified and addressed through individual, community, and national action. In studying the underlying causes of health disparities, it is often difficult to separate and assign relative importance to the many potential contributing factors.

Income and Education

Poverty and low educational attainment are the most important factors underlying health disparities. People with low incomes and less education have higher rates of death from all causes, especially chronic disease and injury, and they are less likely to have preventive health services such as vaccinations and Pap tests. They are more likely to live in an area with a high rate of violence, higher levels of pollutants, and many more environmental stressors. They also have higher rates of unhealthy behaviors such as tobacco and alcohol use, poor diet, and inactivity.

It is important to note that although ethnic disparities in health are significantly reduced when comparing groups with similar incomes and levels of education, they are not eliminated. For example, people living in poverty report worse health than people with higher incomes; but, within the latter group, African Americans and Latinos rate their health as worse than do whites (see figure). Infant mortality rates go down as the education level of mothers goes up; but among mothers who are college graduates, African Americans have significantly higher rates of infant mortality than whites, Latinos, and Asian Americans. These variations point to the complex nature of factors that contribute to health disparities.

Access to Appropriate Health Care

People with low incomes are less likely to have health insurance and more likely to have problems paying for health care and arranging for transportation and time away from family responsibilities in order to access care. They are also more likely to lack information about available services and appropriate lifestyle choices and preventive care. But disparities persist even at higher income levels; for example, among nonpoor Americans, many more Latinos than whites or African Americans report having no insurance, no usual source of health care, and no health care visits within the past year. Possible contributing factors include the following:

• *Local and regional differences in the availability of high-tech health care and specialists.* Minorities, regardless of income, may be more likely to live in medically underserved areas of the country.

• *Problems with communication and trust.* People whose primary language is not English are more likely to be uninsured and to have trouble communicating with health care providers; they may also have problems interpreting health information from public health education campaigns. Language barriers and lack of culturally competent care may be exacerbated by an underrepresentation of minorities in the health professions.

• *Cultural preferences relating to health care.* Groups may vary in their assessment of when it is appropriate to seek medical care and what types of invasive tests and treatments are acceptable.

• *State and federal laws and programs.* Eligibility for Medicaid (a form of government insurance) varies by state and group. For example, Puerto Ricans are U.S. citizens and Cubans are classified as refugees, so people from these groups are immediately eligible for Medicaid; emigrants from other countries may not be able to access public insurance programs until 5 years after they enter the United States.

Culture and Lifestyle

As described in the chapter, ethnic groups may vary in health-related behaviors such as diet, tobacco and alcohol use, coping strategies, and health practices—and these behaviors can have important implications for wellness, both positive and negative. For example, African Americans are more likely to report consuming five or more servings of fruits and vegetables per day than people from other ethnic groups. American Indians report high rates of smoking and smoking-related health problems. Cultural background can be an important protective factor, as seen by the fact that low income doesn't affect all groups equally. For example, poverty is strongly associated

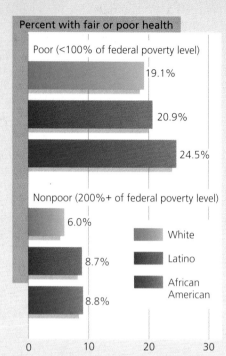

Percent with fair or poor health

Poor (<100% of federal poverty level)

- White — 19.1%
- Latino — 20.9%
- African American — 24.5%

Nonpoor (200%+ of federal poverty level)

- White — 6.0%
- Latino — 8.7%
- African American — 8.8%

Self-rated health status. Respondents were asked to rate their health as excellent, very good, good, fair, or poor. Poverty is strongly associated with negative health status, but disparities persist even among nonpoor Americans.

with increased rates of depression; but some groups, including Americans born in Mexico or Puerto Rico, have lower rates of mental disorders at a given level of income and appear to have coping strategies that provide special resilience.

Discrimination

Racism and discrimination are stressful events that can cause psychological distress and increase the risk of physical and psychological problems. Social discrimination can contribute to lower socioeconomic status and all its associated risks. Bias or discrimination in medical care can directly affect treatment and health outcomes.

SOURCES: National Center for Health Statistics. 2004. *Health, United States, 2004, with Chartbook on Trends in the Health of Americans.* Hyattsville, Md.: National Center for Health Statistics; Centers for Disease Control and Prevention. 2004. REACH 2010 surveillance for health status in minority communities. *MMWR Surveillance Summaries* 53(SS-6); Kaiser Family Foundation. 2003. *Key Facts: Race, Ethnicity, and Medical Care.* Menlo Park, Calif.: Kaiser Family Foundation; U.S. Department of Health and Human Services. 2001. *Mental Health: Culture, Race, and Ethnicity.* Rockville, Md.: U.S. Department of Health and Human Services.

and have less access to health care services. Poverty and low educational attainment are far more important predictors of poor health than any ethnic factor. However, they are often mixed with other factors in a way that makes it difficult to distinguish what causes what.

Disability People with disabilities are those who have activity limitations, need assistance, or perceive themselves as having a disability. About one in five people in the United States has some level of disability, and the rate is rising, especially among younger segments of the population. People with disabilities are more likely to be inactive and overweight. They report more days of depression and fewer days of vitality than people without activity limitations. Many people with disabilities also lack access to health care services.

Geographic Location About one in four Americans currently lives in a rural area—a place with fewer than 2500 residents. People living in rural areas are less likely to be physically active, to use safety belts, or to obtain screening tests for preventive health care. They have less access to timely emergency services and much higher rates of injury-related death than people living in urban areas. They are also more likely to lack health insurance.

Sexual Orientation The 1–5% of Americans who identify themselves as homosexual or bisexual make up a diverse community with varied health concerns. Their emotional wellness and personal safety are affected by factors relating to personal, family, and social acceptance of their sexual orientation. Gay, lesbian, and bisexual teens are more likely to engage in risky behaviors such as unsafe sex and drug use; they are also more likely to be depressed and to attempt suicide. HIV/AIDS is a major concern for gay men, and gay men and lesbians may have higher rates of substance abuse, depression, and suicide.

In this book, topics and issues in health that affect different American populations are given special consideration. Look for these discussions in the text and in boxes labeled Dimensions of Diversity. Also discussed in Dimensions of Diversity boxes are health issues and practices in other parts of the world. Explorations beyond the borders of the United States broaden our view, showing us both what we share with people in other societies and how we differ, our common concerns and our divergent solutions. All these discussions are designed to deepen our understanding of the core concepts of wellness in the context of ever-growing diversity.

CHOOSING WELLNESS

Each of us has the option and the responsibility to decide what kind of future we want—one characterized by zestful living or one marked by symptoms and declining energy.

The message of this book is that wellness is something everyone can have. Achieving it requires knowledge, self-awareness, motivation, and effort—but the benefits last a lifetime. Optimal health comes mostly from a healthy lifestyle, patterns of behavior that promote and support your health now and as you get older. In the pages that follow, you'll find current information and suggestions you can use to build a better lifestyle. You'll also find tools for assessing yourself, for improving your communication skills, and for planning and carrying out specific behavior changes. You can use this book as a guide for taking charge of your health and improving the quality of your life.

Factors That Influence Wellness

Our behavior, our family health history, the environment we live in, and whether we have access to adequate health care are all important influences on wellness. These factors, which vary for both individuals and groups, can interact in ways that produce either health or disease. For example, a sedentary lifestyle combined with a genetic predisposition for diabetes can greatly increase a person's risk of developing the disease. If this person also lacks adequate health care, he or she is much more likely to suffer dangerous complications from diabetes and have a lower quality of life. On the flip side, regular physical activity and a healthy diet can delay or prevent the development of the most common form of diabetes.

Health Habits Scientific research is continuously revealing new connections between our habits and emotions and the level of health we enjoy. For example, heart disease, the nation's number-one killer, is associated with cigarette smoking, high levels of stress, habitually hostile and suspicious attitudes toward people and the world, a diet high in saturated and trans fat and low in fiber, and a sedentary way of life. Other habits are beneficial. Regular exercise, for example, can help prevent heart disease, high blood pressure, diabetes, osteoporosis, and depression and may reduce the risk of colon cancer, stroke, and back injury. A balanced and varied diet provides the energy and nutrients we need to live a vital life and also helps prevent many chronic diseases. As we learn more about how our actions affect our bodies and minds, we can make informed choices for a healthier life.

Heredity/Family History Your **genome** consists of the complete set of genetic material in your cells; it contains about 25,000 genes, half from each of your parents. **Genes**

control the production of proteins that serve both as the structural material for your body and as the regulators of all your body's chemical reactions and metabolic processes. The human genome varies only slightly from person to person, and many of these differences do not affect health. However, some differences do have important implications for health, and knowing your family health history can help you determine which conditions may be of special concern for you. Chapter 8 includes more information about how to put together and evaluate a family health tree.

Errors in our genes are responsible for about 3500 clearly hereditary conditions, including sickle-cell disease and cystic fibrosis. Altered genes also play a part in heart disease, cancer, stroke, diabetes, and many other common conditions. However, in these more common and complex disorders, genetic alterations serve only to increase an individual's risk, and the disease itself results from the interaction of many genes with other factors. For example, researchers have identified genes that clearly increase a woman's risk for breast cancer, but these genes explain only a small proportion of cases. In the small number of inherited cases, genetic alterations that increase the risk of cancer are present at birth in the genes of all the cells in the body. In the majority of cases, however, cancer results from genetic changes that occur after birth within particular cells—usually in response to behavioral and environmental factors. Another example of the power of behavior and environment can be seen in the more than 60% increase in the incidence of diabetes that has occurred among Americans since 1990. This huge increase is not due to any sudden change in our genes; it is the result of increasing rates of obesity caused by poor dietary choices and lack of physical activity (Figure 1-5).

Environment   Your environment includes not only the air you breath and the water you drink but also substances and conditions in your home, workplace, and community. Are you frequently exposed to environmental tobacco smoke or the radiation in sunlight? Do you live in an area with poor air quality or high rates of crime and violence? Has alcohol or drug abuse been a problem in your family? These and other environmental factors all have an impact on wellness.

Access to Health Care   Adequate health care helps improve both quality and quantity of life through preventive care and the treatment of disease. For example, vaccinations prevent many dangerous infections, and screening tests help identify key risk factors and diseases in their early, treatable stages. As described earlier in the chapter, inadequate access to health care is tied to factors such as low income and lack of health insurance. Cost is one of many issues surrounding the development of advanced health-related technologies; see the box "Medical Innovations in the Twenty-First Century."

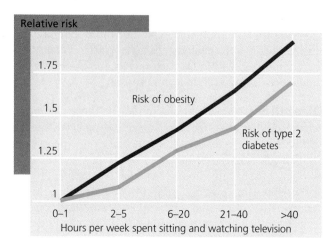

Figure 1-5   Sedentary lifestyle and risk of obesity and type 2 diabetes.   Heredity and environment can play a role in the development of obesity and diabetes, but health habits are very important. SOURCE: Hu, F. B., et al. 2003. Television watching and other sedentary behaviors in relation to risk of obesity and type 2 diabetes mellitus in women. *Journal of the American Medical Association* 289(14): 1785–1791. From Thomas D. Fahey, Paul M. Insel, Walton T. Roth, *Fit and Well,* 6th ed., Fig. 1.3a, p. 6. McGraw-Hill, 2004. Copyright © 2004 The McGraw-Hill Companies, Inc. Reprinted with permission.

Health Habits *Can* Make a Difference   In many cases, behavior can tip the balance toward good health, even when heredity or environment is a negative factor. For example, breast cancer can run in families, but it also may be associated with being overweight and inactive. A woman with a family history of breast cancer is less likely to develop and die from the disease if she controls her weight, exercises regularly, performs breast self-exams, and has regular mammograms to help detect the disease in its early, most treatable stage.

Similarly, a young man with a family history of obesity can maintain a normal weight by being careful to balance calorie intake against activities that burn calories. If your life is highly stressful, you can lessen the chances of heart disease and stroke by learning ways to manage and cope with stress. If you live in an area with severe air pollution, you can reduce the risk of lung disease by not smoking. You can also take an active role in improving your environment. Behaviors like these enable you to make a difference in how great an impact heredity and environment will have on your health.

A Wellness Profile

What does it mean to be healthy today? A basic list of important behaviors and habits includes the following:

- Having a sense of responsibility for your own health and taking an active rather than a passive stance toward your life
- Learning to manage stress in effective ways
- Maintaining high self-esteem and mentally healthy ways of interacting with other people

Imagine the following: Each person's DNA has been processed onto computer chips to identify individual disease risks. Vaccines boost the immune system's ability to attack cancerous tumors. Natural hormones stimulate the growth of new blood vessels to bypass clogged arteries feeding the heart. Gene therapies encourage cancer cells to self-destruct or protect nerves from damage following a stroke. Cows are genetically engineered to produce beneficial drugs in their milk. Genetically modified bacteria absorb toxic chemical spills. Science fiction? Not at all! These and many other health-promoting innovations are currently being studied and tested.

Stem Cells

Many chronic diseases could be cured if damaged cells could be restored. Stem cells are undifferentiated cells that can develop into any type of cell in the body. Stem cells are already being used to replace cancerous cells destroyed in the treatment of leukemia and other cancers, and scientists hope to develop many more therapies. For example, stem cells could potentially be used to replace damaged neurons in people with Parkinson's disease or spinal cord injuries and damaged insulin-producing cells in people with diabetes. See Chapter 19 for more on stem cells and their potential uses.

Gene Therapy

The manipulation of gene expression in human cells, known as gene therapy, is a potential treatment or cure for genetic diseases and cancer. For gene therapy to succeed, new genes must be delivered to defective cells without disturbing the overall functioning of the cells. In the treatment of cancer, gene therapy would "turn off" the genes responsible for causing the cells to divide rapidly and become malignant.

Bioengineering

Can we build new organs in the laboratory? Can artificial materials stand in for the body's natural molecules in tissue repair? Bioengineers are developing biodegradeable compounds that can serve as scaffolding for human tissues grown in the laboratory. Stem cells created from a cell donor could be placed on scaffolding and induced to differentiate into specific organ tissue, such as kidney or liver tissue. Once the new organ begins to develop, it could be transplanted into the original cell donor, where it could grow to full size with no danger of organ rejection.

Ethical Questions, Potential Limits, and Unforeseen Consequences

Although full of promise, the development of innovative medical technologies brings up many potentially troubling issues. For example, the use of human embryos to obtain stem cells is highly controversial. Serious, unforeseen side effects occurred in early gene therapy trials. The expense of developing these technologies and providing them to a growing population is another concern: Cost already limits access to even relatively inexpensive medications and treatments. Privacy and discrimination are other issues: If genetic testing can identify years in advance who is likely to get sick and who is not, employers and health insurance companies could save millions of dollars by not hiring or enrolling people whose genes show them to be at increased risk for disease.

Other questions relate to potential uses of tools for altering the genome. Do we have enough information to know how knocking out "bad" genes will affect our species? For example, the gene alteration that causes sickle-cell disease must be present in both copies of the gene for a person to develop the disease; people who inherit only one copy of the altered gene from their parents have an increased resistance to malaria. If the gene for sickle-cell disease were eliminated, would many more people succumb to malaria? Researchers have found similar links in the genetic mutation that causes cystic fibrosis and protection from cholera and in the genetic mutation that causes Tay-Sachs disease and protection from tuberculosis. Tinkering with the genome could have unknown negative effects.

Wellness in the Information Age

Perhaps the most important technological advance is the information revolution. A growing number of informative and interactive technologies can help you learn about healthy lifestyle behaviors and preventive medicine as well as aid you in changing your unhealthy habits. The availability of these tools gives each individual the responsibility of making the best use of new information to optimize health. Only you can enhance your ability to make choices that promote wellness in an era of innovation and technological change.

- Understanding your sexuality and having satisfying intimate relationships
- Avoiding tobacco and other drugs; using alcohol responsibly, if at all
- Eating well, exercising, and maintaining healthy weight
- Knowing the facts about cardiovascular disease, cancer, infections, sexually transmitted diseases, and injuries and using your knowledge to protect yourself against them
- Understanding the health care system and using it intelligently

- Knowing when to treat your illnesses yourself and when to seek help
- Understanding the natural processes of aging and dying and accepting the limits of human existence
- Understanding how the environment affects your health and taking appropriate action to improve it

Incorporating these behaviors into your daily life may seem like a tall order, and in a sense it is the work of a lifetime. But the habits you establish now are crucial: They tend to set lifelong patterns. Some behaviors do more than set up patterns—they produce permanent changes in your health. If you become addicted to drugs or alcohol at age 20, for example, you may be able to kick the habit, but you will always face the struggle of a recovering addict. If you contract gonorrhea, you may discover later that your reproductive organs were damaged without your realizing it, making you infertile or sterile. If you ruin your knees doing the wrong exercises or hurt your back in an automobile crash, you won't have them to count on when you're older. Some things just can't be reversed or corrected.

HOW DO YOU REACH WELLNESS?

Your life may not resemble the one described by the wellness profile at all. You probably have a number of healthy habits and some others that place your health at risk. Maybe your life is more like this:

> It's Tuesday. Simon wakes up feeling blue, not really wanting to get out of bed. He wishes he knew what he wanted to do with his life. He wishes he'd meet someone new and fall in love. No time for breakfast, so he grabs a cup of coffee to drink during his first class. He hasn't done the reading and stares blankly at the teacher during the lecture. Later he goes to the student union and has a sugary doughnut and some more coffee; he lights up his first cigarette of the day. Lunch is a fast-food cheeseburger, french fries, and a shake. He spends the afternoon at the library desperately researching a paper that's due the next day, finally quitting at 6:00 and heading to the student union for a beer. He meets up with some buddies and joins them for pizza instead of having dinner at the dorm. By 11:00 he's tired, but he's written only one page of his paper, so he takes an upper to keep going. It makes his heart race and floods his head with so many ideas he has difficulty sorting them all out. He works feverishly and finally finishes at 4:00 the next morning. Exhausted, he falls asleep in his clothes. The next thing he knows, it's Wednesday morning, time to start a new day.

This is hardly an ideal lifestyle, but it's not unusual. Simon functions OK, meets his commitments, and shows some self-discipline. On the other hand, time gets away from him, and he doesn't get much exercise, doesn't eat as well as he could, and flirts with the dangers of taking drugs. Overall, he is low on energy and has little control over his life. He could be living a lot better.

Simon isn't alone in neglecting or abusing his health; many people fall into a lifestyle that puts their health at risk. Some aren't aware of the damage they're doing to themselves; others are aware but aren't motivated or don't know how to change; still others want to change but can't seem to get started. All of these are very real problems, but they're not insurmountable. If they were, there would be no ex-smokers, recovering alcoholics, or successful graduates of weight-loss programs. People can and do make difficult changes in their lives.

Taking big steps toward wellness may at first seem like too much work, but as you make progress, it gets easier. At first you'll be rewarded with a greater sense of control over your life, a feeling of empowerment, higher self-esteem, and more joy. These benefits will encourage you to make further improvements. Over time, you'll come to know what wellness feels like—more energy; greater vitality; deeper feelings of curiosity, interest, and enjoyment; and a higher quality of life.

Getting Serious About Your Health

Before you can start changing a health-related behavior, you have to know that the behavior is problematic and that you *can* change it. To make good decisions, you need information about relevant topics and issues, including what resources are available to help you change your behavior. You also need knowledge about yourself—how you relate to the wellness profile and what strengths you can draw on to change your behavior and improve your health.

Examining Your Current Health Habits   Have you considered how your current lifestyle is affecting your health today and how it will affect your health in the future? Do you know which of your current habits enhance your health and which detract from it? Begin your journey toward wellness with self-assessment: Think about your own behavior and talk with friends and family members about what they've noticed about your lifestyle and your health.

Many people start to consider changing a behavior when they get help from others. An observation from a friend, family member, or physician can help you see yourself as others do and may get you thinking about your behavior in a new way. For example, Jason has been getting a lot of stomachaches lately. His girlfriend Anna notices other changes as well and suggests that the stress of classes plus a part-time job and serving as president of the school radio station might be causing some of Jason's problems. Jason never thought much about trying to control the stressors in his life, but with encouragement from Anna, he starts noticing what events trigger stress for him.

Landmark events can also get you thinking about behavior change. A birthday, the birth of a child, or the death of someone close to you can be powerful motivators for thinking seriously about behaviors that affect wellness. New information can also help you get started. As you read this text, you may find yourself reevaluating some of your health-related behaviors. This could be a great opportunity to make healthful changes that will stay with you for the rest of your life. To help determine whether your current health habits promote wellness, take the quiz in the box "Wellness: Evaluate Your Lifestyle" on page 16. Use the results to identify behaviors you could change to improve your health and well-being.

Choosing a Target Behavior A careful examination of your current lifestyle may reveal a number of habits that are candidates for change. To maximize your chances of success, don't try to change all your problem behaviors at once—to quit smoking, give up high-fat foods, start jogging, avoid drugs, get more sleep. Working on even one behavior change will make high demands on your energy. Concentrate on one behavior that you want to change, your **target behavior,** and work on it systematically. Start with something simple, like snacking on candy between afternoon classes or always driving to a particular class instead of walking or biking.

Obtaining Information About Your Target Behavior Once you've chosen a target behavior, you need to find out more about it. You need to know its risks and benefits for you—both now and in the future. How is your target behavior affecting your level of wellness today? For what diseases or conditions does this behavior place you at risk? What effect would changing your behavior have on your health?

You also need enough information to set an overall target for change. For some behaviors, this is simple. For example, if your target behavior is smoking, your goal will be to quit. But if your target behavior is something like a poor diet or an inactive lifestyle, you may need additional information to set an appropriate goal. Further investigation can help you determine that you should consume the equivalent of 4 cups of fruits and vegetables each day, for example, or that you should add 30–60 minutes of brisk walking to your daily routine.

To evaluate your target behavior and set an appropriate target for change, you'll need accurate information. As a starting point, use material from this text and from the resources listed in the For More Information section at the end of each chapter. See the box "Evaluating Sources of Health Information" for tips on becoming a critical consumer of health information from a wide variety of sources.

Finding Outside Help Have you identified a particularly challenging target behavior, such as alcohol addiction, excessive overeating, or depression, that interferes with your ability to function or places you at a serious health risk? Outside help is often needed for changing behaviors or conditions that may be too deeply rooted or too serious for a self-management approach. If this is the case, don't be stopped by the seriousness of the problem—there are many resources available to help you solve it. On campus, the student health center or campus counseling center may be a source of assistance. Many communities offer a variety of services through adult education, health departments, and private agencies. Consult the yellow pages, your physician, your local health department, or the United Way; the last often sponsors local referral services.

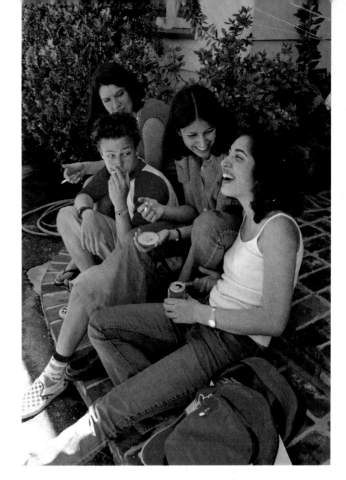

Changing powerful, long-standing habits requires motivation, commitment, and a belief that we are in control of our own behavior. To quit smoking, these young people must overcome a habit that is supported by their addiction to nicotine and by their social environment.

Building Motivation for Change

Knowledge is a necessary ingredient for behavior change, but it isn't usually enough to make people act. Millions of people smoke or have sedentary lifestyles, for example, even though they know it's bad for their health. To succeed at behavior change, you need strong motivation. Strategies for building motivation include examining the pros and cons of change, boosting self-efficacy, and overcoming key barriers to change.

Examining the Pros and Cons of Change
Health behaviors have short-term and long-term benefits and costs associated with them. For example, in the short term, an inactive lifestyle allows for more time to watch TV and hang out with friends but leaves a person less able to participate in recreational activities. Over the long term, it increases the risk of heart disease, cancer, stroke, and

Term V̄w

target behavior An isolated behavior selected as the object of a behavior change plan.

All of us want optimal health. But many of us do not know how to achieve it. Taking this quiz, adapted from one created by the U.S. Public Health Service, is a good place to start. The behaviors covered in the quiz are recommended for most Americans. (Some of them may not apply to people with certain diseases or disabilities or to pregnant women, who may require special advice from their physician.) After you take the quiz, add up your score for each section.

Tobacco Use

If you never use tobacco, enter a score of 10 for this section and go to the next section.

		Almost Always	Sometimes	Never
1.	I avoid using tobacco.	2	1	0
2.	I smoke only low-tar/nicotine cigarettes *or* I smoke a pipe or cigars *or* I use smokeless tobacco.	2	1	0

Tobacco Score: _____

Alcohol and Other Drugs

		Almost Always	Sometimes	Never
1.	I avoid alcohol *or* I drink no more than 1 (women) or 2 (men) drinks a day.	4	1	0
2.	I avoid using alcohol or other drugs as a way of handling stressful situations or problems in my life.	2	1	0
3.	I am careful not to drink alcohol when taking medications, such as for colds or allergies, or when pregnant.	2	1	0
4.	I read and follow the label directions when using prescribed and over-the-counter drugs.	2	1	0

Alcohol and Other Drugs Score: _____

Nutrition

		Almost Always	Sometimes	Never
1.	I eat a variety of foods each day, including seven or more servings of fruits and vegetables.	3	1	0
2.	I limit the amount of total fat and saturated and trans fat in my diet.	3	1	0
3.	I avoid skipping meals.	2	1	0
4.	I limit the amount of salt and sugar I eat.	2	1	0

Nutrition Score: _____

Exercise/Fitness

		Almost Always	Sometimes	Never
1.	I engage in moderate exercise for 20–60 minutes, 3–5 times a week.	4	1	0
2.	I maintain a healthy weight, avoiding overweight and underweight.	2	1	0
3.	I do exercises to develop muscular strength and endurance at least twice a week.	2	1	0
4.	I spend some of my leisure time participating in physical activities such as gardening, bowling, golf, or baseball.	2	1	0

Exercise/Fitness Score: _____

Emotional Health

		Almost Always	Sometimes	Never
1.	I enjoy being a student, and I have a job or do other work that I like.	2	1	0
2.	I find it easy to relax and express my feelings freely.	2	1	0
3.	I manage stress well.	2	1	0

premature death. For successful behavior change, you must believe that the benefits of changing outweigh the costs.

Do a careful analysis of the short-term and long-term benefits and costs of continuing your current (target) behavior and of changing to a new, healthier behavior. Focus on the effects that are most meaningful to you, including those that are tied to your personal identity and values. For example, if you see yourself as an active person who is a good role model for others, then adopting behaviors such as regular physical activity and adequate sleep would support your personal identity. If you value independence and control over your life, then quitting smoking would be consistent with your values and goals. To complete your analysis, ask friends and family

	Almost Always	Sometimes	Never
4. I have close friends, relatives, or others I can talk to about personal matters and call on for help.	2	1	0
5. I participate in group activities (such as church and community organizations) or hobbies that I enjoy.	2	1	0

Emotional Health Score: _____

Safety

	Almost Always	Sometimes	Never
1. I wear a safety belt while riding in a car.	2	1	0
2. I avoid driving while under the influence of alcohol or other drugs.	2	1	0
3. I obey traffic rules and the speed limit when driving.	2	1	0
4. I read and follow instructions on the labels of potentially harmful products or substances, such as household cleaners, poisons, and electrical appliances.	2	1	0
5. I avoid smoking in bed.	2	1	0

Safety Score: _____

Disease Prevention

	Almost Always	Sometimes	Never
1. I know the warning signs of cancer, diabetes, heart attack, and stroke.	2	1	0
2. I avoid overexposure to the sun and use a sunscreen.	2	1	0
3. I get recommended medical screening tests (such as blood pressure checks and Pap tests), immunizations, and booster shots.	2	1	0
4. I practice monthly breast/testicle self-exams.	2	1	0
5. I am not sexually active *or* I have sex with only one mutually faithful, uninfected partner *or* I always engage in safer sex (using condoms) *and* I do not share needles to inject drugs.	2	1	0

Disease Prevention Score: _____

What Your Scores Mean

Scores of 9 and 10 Excellent! Your answers show that you're aware of the importance of this area to wellness. More important, you are putting your knowledge to work for you by practicing good health habits. As long as you continue to do so, this area should not pose a serious health risk. It's likely that you are setting an example for your family and friends to follow. Since you scored high on this part of the quiz, you may want to focus on other areas where your scores indicate room for improvement.

Scores of 6–8 Your health practices in this area are good, but there is room for improvement. Look again at the items you answered with "Sometimes" or "Never." What changes can you make to improve your score? Even a small change can often help you achieve better health.

Scores of 3–5 Your health risks are showing! You may need more information about the risks you're facing and about why it's important for you to change these behaviors. Perhaps you need help in deciding how to successfully make the changes you want.

Scores of 0–2 Your answers show that you may be taking serious and unnecessary risks with your health. Perhaps you are not aware of the risks and what to do about them. You can easily get the information and help you need to improve, if you wish. The next step is up to you.

members about the effects of your behavior on them. For example, a roommate may tell you that he never ate candy in the evening until he started living with you, or a younger sister may tell you that your smoking habit influenced her decision to take up smoking.

Pay special attention to the short-term benefits of behavior change, as these can be an important motivating force. Although some people are motivated by long-term goals, such as avoiding a disease that may hit them in 30 years, most are more likely to be moved to action by shorter-term, more personal goals. Feeling better, doing better in school, improving at a sport, reducing stress, and increasing self-esteem are common short-term benefits of health behavior change. Many wellness behaviors are

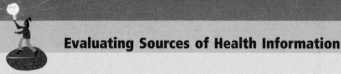

General Strategies

A key first step in sharpening your critical thinking skills is to look carefully at your sources of health information. Critical thinking involves knowing where and how to find relevant information, how to separate fact from opinion, how to recognize faulty reasoning, how to evaluate information, and how to assess the credibility of sources.

• *Go to the original source.* Media reports often simplify the results of medical research. Find out for yourself what a study really reported, and determine whether it was based on good science. What type of study was it? Was it published in a recognized medical journal? Was it an animal study, or did it involve people? Did the study include a large number of people? What did the authors of the study actually report in their findings? (You'll find additional strategies for evaluating research studies in Chapter 21.)

• *Watch for misleading language.* Reports that feature "breakthroughs" or "dramatic proof" are probably hype. Some studies will find that a behavior "contributes to" or is "associated with" an outcome; this does not imply a proven cause-and-effect relationship. Information may also be distorted by an author's point of view.

• *Distinguish between research reports and public health advice.* If a study finds a link between a particular vitamin and cancer, that should not necessarily lead you to change your behavior. But if the Surgeon General or the American Cancer Society advises you to eat less saturated fat or quit smoking, you can assume that many studies point in this direction and that this is advice you should follow.

• *Remember that anecdotes are not facts.* Sometimes we do get helpful health information from our friends and family. But just because your cousin Bertha lost 10 pounds on Dr. Amazing's new protein diet doesn't mean it's a safe, effective way for you to lose weight. Before you make a big change in your lifestyle, verify the information with your physician, this text, or other reliable sources.

• *Be skeptical, and use your common sense.* If a report seems too good to be true, it probably is. Be especially wary of information contained in advertisements. The goal of an ad is to sell you something, to create a feeling of need for a product where no real need exists. Evaluate "scientific" claims carefully, and beware of quackery (see Chapter 21).

• *Make choices that are right for you.* Your roommate swears by swimming; you prefer aerobics. Your sister takes a yoga class to help her manage stress; your brother unwinds by walking in the woods. Friends and family members can be a great source of ideas and inspiration, but each of us needs to find a wellness lifestyle that works for us.

Internet Resources

Evaluating health information from online sources poses special challenges; when reviewing a health-related Web site, ask the following questions:

• *What is the source of the information? Who is the author or sponsor of the Web page?* Web sites maintained by government agencies, professional associations, or established academic or medical institutions are likely to present trustworthy information. Many other groups and individuals post accurate information, but it is important to look at the qualifications of the people who are behind the site. (Check the home page or click on an "about us" or "who we are" link.)

• *How often is the site updated?* Look for sites that are updated frequently. Also check the "last modified" date of any specific Web page on a site.

• *What is the purpose of the page? Does the site promote particular products or procedures? Are there obvious reasons for bias?* Be wary of information from sites that sell specific products, use testimonials as evidence, appear to have a social or political agenda, or ask for money.

• *What do other sources say about a topic?* Be cautious of claims or information that appears at only one site or comes from a chat room or bulletin board.

• *Does the site conform to any set of guidelines or criteria for quality and accuracy?* Look for sites that identify themselves as conforming to some code or set of principles, such as those set forth by the Health on the Net Foundation or the American Medical Association. These codes include criteria such as use of information from respected sources and disclosure of the site's sponsors.

Additional strategies for locating and assessing health-related information from the Internet can be found on the *Core Concepts in Health* Web site (http://www.mhhe.com/insel10e).

associated with immediate improvements in quality of life. For example, surveys of Americans have found that nonsmokers feel healthy and full of energy more days each month than do smokers, and they report fewer days of sadness and troubled sleep; the same is true when physically active people are compared with sedentary people. Over time, these differences add up to a substantially greater quality of life for people who engage in healthy behaviors.

You can further strengthen your motivation by engaging your emotions and raising your consciousness about your problem behavior. This will enable you to focus on the current negatives of the behavior and to imagine the consequences if you don't make a change. Ask yourself: What do I want for myself, now and in the future?

For example, Ruby has never worried much about her smoking because the problems associated with it seem so far away. But lately she's noticed her performance on the volleyball team isn't as good as it used to be. Over the summer she visited her aunt, who has emphysema from smoking and can barely leave her bed. Ruby knows she wants to have children and a career as a teacher, and seeing her aunt makes her wonder if her smoking habit could make it difficult for her to reach these goals. She starts to wonder whether her smoking habit is worth the short- and long-term sacrifices.

Social pressures can also increase the motivation to make changes. In Ruby's case, anti-smoking ordinances keep her from smoking in her dorm and in many public places. The inconvenience of finding a place to smoke and the pressure from her roommate, who doesn't like the smoky smell of Ruby's clothes in their room, are among the short-term costs of Ruby's smoking habit that can add to her motivation to quit.

Boosting Self-Efficacy When you start thinking about changing a health behavior, a big factor in your eventual success is whether you have confidence in yourself and in your ability to change. **Self-efficacy** refers to your belief in your ability to successfully take action and perform a specific task. Self-efficacy varies with each behavior and depends on many factors, including your level of self-esteem and your past experiences with your target behavior. Strategies for boosting self-efficacy include developing an internal locus of control, using visualization and self-talk, and obtaining encouragement from supportive people. Developing specific skills for change, discussed later in this chapter, is also critical for improving self-efficacy.

LOCUS OF CONTROL Who do you believe is controlling your life? Is it your parents, friends, or school? Is it "fate"? Or is it you? **Locus of control** refers to the figurative "place" a person designates as the source of responsibility for the events in his or her life. People who believe they are in control of their own lives are said to have an internal locus of control. Those who believe that factors beyond their control—heredity, friends and family, the environment, fate, luck, or other outside forces—are more important in determining the events of their lives are said to have an external locus of control. Most people are not purely "internalizers" or "externalizers"; their locus of control changes in response to the situation.

For lifestyle management, an internal locus of control is an advantage because it reinforces motivation and commitment. An external locus of control can actually sabotage efforts to change behavior. For example, if you believe you are destined to die of breast cancer because your mother died from the disease, you may view breast self-exams and regular checkups as a waste of time. In contrast, an internal locus of control is an advantage. If you believe you can take action to reduce your hereditary risk of breast cancer, you will be motivated to follow guidelines for early detection of the disease.

People who tend to have an external locus of control can learn to view the events in their lives differently and increase their feelings of self-efficacy. If you find yourself attributing too much influence to outside forces, gather more information about your target behavior. Make a list of all the ways that behavior change will improve your health. If you recognize and accept that you are in charge of your life, you're well on your way to wellness.

VISUALIZATION AND SELF-TALK One of the best ways to boost your confidence and self-efficacy is to visualize yourself successfully engaging in a new, healthier behavior. Imagine yourself turning down cigarettes, going for a regular after-dinner walk, or choosing healthier snacks. Also visualize yourself enjoying all the short-term and long-term benefits that behavior change will bring. Create a new self-image: What will you and your life be like when you become a nonsmoker, a regular exerciser, or a healthy eater?

You can also use self-talk, the internal dialogue you carry on with yourself, to increase your confidence in your ability to change. Counter any self-defeating patterns of thought with more positive or realistic thoughts: "Behavior change is difficult, but if I work at it, I will succeed," or "I am a strong, capable person, and I can maintain my commitment to change." Refer to Chapter 3 for more on self-talk.

ROLE MODELS AND OTHER SUPPORTIVE INDIVIDUALS Social support can also make a big difference in your level of motivation and your chances of success. Perhaps you know people who have reached the goal you are striving for; they could be role models or mentors for you, providing information and support for your efforts. Talk to them about how they did it. What were the most difficult parts of changing their behavior? What strategies worked for them? Gain strength from their experiences, and tell yourself, "If they can do it, so can I."

In addition, find a buddy who wants to make the same changes you do and who can take an active role in your behavior change program. For example, an exercise buddy can provide companionship and encouragement for times when you might be tempted to skip that morning jog. Or you and a friend can watch to be sure that you both have only one alcoholic beverage at a party. If necessary, look beyond your current social network at possible new sources of help, such as a support group. Later in this chapter, you'll learn some specific strategies for involving other people in your behavior change program.

Terms **V i w**

self-efficacy The belief in one's ability to take action and perform a specific behavior.

locus of control The figurative "place" a person designates as the source of responsibility for the events in his or her life.

Identifying and Overcoming Key Barriers to Change Have you tried and failed to change your target behavior in the past? Don't let past failures discourage you; they can be a great source of information you can use to boost your chances of future success. Make a list of the problems and challenges you faced in your previous behavior change attempts; to this add the short-term costs of behavior change that you identified in your analysis of the pros and cons of change. Once you've listed these key barriers to change, develop a practical plan for overcoming each one. For example, if one of your key barriers for physical activity is that you believe you can't make time for a 40-minute workout, look for ways to incorporate shorter bouts of physical activity into your daily routine. If you always smoke when you're with certain friends, practice in advance how you will turn down the next cigarette you are offered. Developing strategies to cope with difficult situations is one of the most important factors in successful behavior change. You'll find additional advice and examples later in the chapter in the section "Developing Skills for Change."

Self-talk can also help overcome barriers. Make behavior change a priority in your life, and plan to commit the necessary time and effort. Ask yourself: How much time and energy will behavior change *really* require? Isn't the effort worth all the short- and long-term benefits?

Enhancing Your Readiness to Change

The transtheoretical, or "stages of change," model, developed by psychologists James Prochaska and Carlo DiClemente, has been shown to be an effective approach to lifestyle self-management. According to this model, you move through six well-defined stages as you work to change your target behavior. It is important to determine what stage you are in now so that you can choose appropriate strategies for progressing through the cycle of change (see the box "What Stage of Change Are You In?"). Using this approach can help you enhance your readiness and intention to change.

Precontemplation People at this stage have no intention of changing their behavior. They may be unaware of the risks associated with their behavior, or they may deny that their behavior will have any serious consequences for them. They may have tried unsuccessfully to change in the past and may now feel demoralized and think the situation is hopeless. They may also blame others for their problems.

If you are in the precontemplation stage, begin to move forward by raising your consciousness of your target behavior and its effects on you and those around you. Obtain accurate information about your behavior, and ask yourself what has prevented you from changing in the past. Enlist friends and family members to help you become more aware of your behavior and your reasons for continuing an unhealthy habit. Also find out more about the campus and community resources available to help you with behavior change.

Contemplation People at this stage are aware that they have a problem and have started to think and learn about it. They acknowledge the benefits that behavior change will have for them but are also very aware of the costs of changing. They wonder about possible courses of action but may feel stuck and unsure of how best to proceed.

At this stage, it's a good idea to begin keeping a written record of your target behavior—to help you learn more about it and to use when you begin to plan the specifics of your behavior change program. Work on your analysis of the pros and cons of change: Expand your list of the benefits, and problem-solve to overcome the key barriers on your list of the costs of changing. To be successful, you must believe that the benefits of change outweigh the costs. Engage your emotions and boost self-efficacy through visualization, self-talk, and the support of other people.

Preparation People at this stage plan to take action within a month and may already have begun to make small changes in their behavior. If you are in the preparation stage, your next step is to create a specific plan for change that includes a start date, realistic goals, rewards, and information on exactly how you will go about changing your behavior. You'll also want to prepare yourself emotionally and socially by practicing visualization and self-talk and by involving the people around you in your efforts at change. A step-by-step plan for developing a successful behavior change program is included in the next section of the chapter.

Action During the action stage, people outwardly modify their behavior and their environment. The action stage requires the greatest commitment of time and energy, and people in this stage are at risk for reverting to old, unhealthy patterns of behavior. If you are in the action stage, you'll need to use all the plans and strategies that you developed during earlier stages. In particular, be sure to plan ahead to overcome temptations and deal with problem situations.

Maintenance People at this stage have maintained their new, healthier lifestyle for at least 6 months. To guard against slips and relapses, they continue with all the positive strategies they used in earlier stages. Their confidence and self-efficacy increase. The maintenance stage typically lasts from 6 months to about 5 years.

Termination People at this stage have exited the cycle of change and are no longer tempted to lapse back into their old behavior. They have a new self-image and total self-efficacy with regard to their target behavior. This

To determine your stage, circle true or false for each of the following statements:

T F **1.** I changed my target behavior more than 6 months ago.

T F **2.** I changed my target behavior within the past 6 months.

T F **3.** I intend to take action within the next month and have already made a few small changes in my behavior.

T F **4.** I intend to take action on my target behavior within the next 6 months.

Find the stage that corresponds to your responses:

False for all four statements = Precontemplation

True for statement 4, false for statements 1–3 = Contemplation

True for statements 3 and 4, false for statements 1 and 2 = Preparation

True for statement 2, false for statement 1 = Action

True for statement 1 = Maintenance

SOURCE: Prochaska, J. O., C. A. Redding, and K. E. Evers. 2002. The transtheoretical model and stages of change. In *Health Behavior and Health Education: Theory, Research, and Practice,* 3rd ed. San Francisco: Jossey-Bass.

---

stage applies to some behaviors, such as addictions, but may not be appropriate for others.

Lapses are a natural part of the process at all stages of change. Many people lapse and must recycle through earlier stages, although most don't go back to the first stage. If you lapse, use what you learn about yourself and the process of change to help you in your next attempt at behavior change.

Next, we'll take a closer look at the specific steps and skills involved in creating and implementing a plan for change.

Developing Skills for Change: Creating a Personalized Plan

Once you are committed to making a change, it's time to put together a detailed plan of action. Your key to success is a well-thought-out plan that sets goals, anticipates problems, and includes rewards.

1. Monitor Your Behavior and Gather Data

Begin by keeping careful records of the behavior you wish to change (your target behavior) and the circumstances surrounding it. Keep these records in a health journal, a notebook in which you write the details of your behavior along with observations and comments. Note exactly what the activity was, when and where it happened, what you were doing, and what your feelings were at the time. In a journal for a weight-loss or dietary-change plan, for example, you would typically record how much food you ate, the time of day, the situation, the location, your feelings, and how hungry you were (Figure 1-6). If your goal

is to start an exercise program, use your journal to track your daily activities to determine how best to make time for your workouts. Keep your journal for a week or two to get some solid information about the behavior you want to change.

2. Analyze the Data and Identify Patterns

After you have collected data on the behavior, analyze the data to identify patterns. When are you hungriest? When are you most likely to overeat? What events seem to trigger your appetite? Perhaps you are especially hungry at midmorning or when you put off eating dinner until 9:00. Perhaps you overindulge in food and drink when you go to a particular restaurant or when you're with certain friends. Be sure to note the connections between your feelings and external cues such as time of day, location, situation, and the actions of people around you. Do you always think of having a cigarette when you read the newspaper? Do you always bite your fingernails when you're studying?

3. Set Realistic, Specific Goals
Don't set an impossibly difficult overall goal for your program—going from a sedentary lifestyle to running a marathon within 2 months, for example. Working toward more realistic, achievable goals will greatly increase your chances of success. Your goal should also be specific and measurable, something you can easily track. Instead of a vague general goal such as improving eating habits or being more physically active, set a specific target—eating eight servings of fruits and vegetables each day or walking or biking for 30 minutes at least 5 days per week.

Date	November 5				Day	M	TU	W	TH	F	SA	SU		

Time of day	M/S	Food eaten	Cals.	H	Where did you eat?	What else were you doing?	How did someone else influence you?	What made you want to eat what you did?	Emotions and feelings?	Thoughts and concerns?
7:30	M	1 C Crispix cereal 1/2 C skim milk coffee, black 1 C orange juice	110 40 — 120	3	home	reading newspaper	alone	I always eat cereal in the morning	a little keyed up & worried	thinking about quiz in class today
10:30	S	1 apple	90	1	hall outside classroom	studying	alone	felt tired & wanted to wake up	tired	worried about next class
12:30	M	1 C chili 1 roll 1 pat butter 1 orange 2 oatmeal cookies 1 soda	290 120 35 60 120 150	2	campus food court	talking	eating w/ friends; we decided to eat at the food court	wanted to be part of group	excited and happy	interested in hearing everyone's plans for the weekend
	M/S = Meal or snack			H = Hunger rating (0–3)						

Figure 1-6 Sample health journal entries.

Whatever your ultimate goal, it's a good idea to break it down into a few small steps. Your plan will seem less overwhelming and more manageable, increasing the chances that you'll stick to it. You'll also build in more opportunities to reward yourself (discussed in step 4), as well as milestones you can use to measure your progress. If you plan to lose 15 pounds, for example, you'll find it easier to take off 5 pounds at a time. If you want to start an exercise program, begin by taking 10- to 15-minute walks a few times per week. Take the easier steps first and work up to the harder steps. With each small success, you'll build your confidence and self-efficacy.

4. Devise a Strategy or Plan of Action Next, you need to develop specific strategies and techniques that will support your day-to-day efforts at behavior change.

OBTAIN INFORMATION AND SUPPLIES Identify campus and community resources that can provide practical help—for example, a stop-smoking course or a walking club. Take any necessary preparatory steps, such as signing up for a stress-management workshop or purchasing walking shoes, nicotine replacement patches, or a special calendar to track your progress.

MODIFY YOUR ENVIRONMENT As you write in your health journal, you gather quite a lot of information about your target behavior—the times it typically occurs; the situations in which it usually happens; the ways sight, smell, mood, situation, and accessibility trigger it. You can probably trace the chain of events that leads to the behavior and perhaps also identify points along the way where making a different choice would mean changing the behavior.

You can be more effective in changing behavior if you control the environmental cues that provoke it. This might mean not having cigarettes or certain foods or drinks in the house, not going to parties where you're tempted to overindulge, or not spending time with particular people, at least for a while. If you always get a candy bar at a certain vending machine, change your route so you don't pass by it. If you always end up taking a coffee break and chatting with friends when you go to the library to study, choose a different place to study, such as your room.

It's also helpful to control other behaviors or habits that seem to be linked to the target behavior. You may give in to an urge to eat when you have a beer (alcohol increases the appetite) or when you watch TV. Try substituting some other activities for habits that seem to be linked with your target behavior, such as exercising to music instead of plopping down in front of the TV. Or, if possible, put an exercise bicycle in front of the set and burn calories while you watch your favorite show.

You can change the cues in your environment so they trigger the new, target behavior instead of the old one. Tape a picture of a cyclist speeding down a hill on your TV screen. Leave your exercise shoes in plain view. Put a chart of your progress in a special place at home to make your goals highly visible and inspire you to keep going. When you're trying to change an ingrained habit, small cues can play an important part in keeping you on track.

REWARD YOURSELF Another very powerful way to affect your target behavior is to set up a reward system that will reinforce your efforts. Most people find it difficult to

Your environment contains powerful cues for both positive and negative lifestyle choices. Identifying and using the healthier options available to you throughout the day is a key part of a successful behavior change program.

change long-standing habits for rewards they can't see right away. Giving yourself instant, real rewards for good behavior along the way will help you stick with a plan to change your behavior.

Carefully plan your reward payoffs and what they will be. In most cases, rewards should be collected when you reach specific objectives or subgoals in your plan. For example, you might treat yourself to a movie after a week of avoiding extra snacks. Don't forget to reward yourself for good behavior that is consistent and persistent—such as simply sticking with your program week after week. Decide on a reward after you reach a certain goal, or mark off the sixth week or month of a valiant effort. Write it down in your health journal and remember it as you follow your plan—especially when the going gets rough.

Make a list of your activities and favorite events to use as rewards. They should be special, inexpensive, and preferably unrelated to food or alcohol. Depending on what you like to do, you might treat yourself to a concert, a ball game, a new CD, a long-distance phone call to a friend, a day off from studying to take a long hike in the woods—whatever is rewarding to you.

INVOLVE THE PEOPLE AROUND YOU Rewards and support can also come from family and friends. Tell them about your plan, and ask for their help. Encourage them to be active, interested participants. Ask them to support you when you set aside time to go running or avoid second helpings at Thanksgiving dinner. You may have to remind them not to do things that make you "break training" and not to be hurt if you have to refuse something when they forget. To help friends and family members who will be involved in your program respond appropriately, you may want to create a specific list of dos and don'ts. Getting encouragement, support, and praise from important people in your life can powerfully reinforce the new behavior you're trying to adopt.

PLAN AHEAD FOR CHALLENGING SITUATIONS Take time out now to list situations and people that have the potential to derail your program and to develop possible coping mechanisms. For example, if you think that you'll have trouble exercising during finals week, schedule short bouts of physical activity as stress-reducing study breaks. If a visit to a friend who smokes is likely to tempt you to lapse, plan to bring nicotine patches, chewing gum, and a copy of your behavior change contract to strengthen your resolve.

5. Make a Commitment by Signing a Personal Contract Once you have set your goals and developed a plan of action, make your plan into a personal contract. A serious personal contract—one that commits your word—can result in a higher chance of follow-through than will a casual, offhand promise. Your contract can help prevent procrastination by specifying the important dates and can also serve as a reminder of your personal commitment to change.

Your contract should include a statement of your goal and your commitment to reaching it. Include details of your plan: the date you'll begin, the steps you'll use to measure your progress, the concrete strategies you've developed for promoting change, and the date you expect to reach your final goal. Have someone—preferably someone who will be actively helping you with your program—sign your contract as a witness.

A Sample Behavior Change Plan Let's take the example of Michael, who wants to improve his diet. By monitoring his eating habits in his health journal for several weeks, he gets a good sense of his typical diet—what he eats and where he eats it. Through self-assessment and investigation, he discovers that he currently consumes only about one serving of fruit per week, much less than the recommended three to five servings per day. He also finds out that fruit is a major source of fiber, vitamins, minerals, and other substances important for good health. He sets the target of eating three servings of fruit per day as the overall goal for his behavior change plan. Then Michael develops a specific plan for change that involves several changes in his behavior and his environment, which he describes in a contract that commits him to reaching his goal (Figure 1-7). Once Michael has signed his contract, he's ready to take action.

. You can apply the general behavior change planning framework presented in this chapter to any target behavior. Additional examples of behavior change plans are presented in the Behavior Change Strategy sections that appear at the end of many chapters. In these, you'll find specific plans and advice for overcoming test anxiety (Chapter 2), reducing caffeine consumption (Chapter 9), quitting smoking (Chapter 11), beginning an exercise program (Chapter 13), eating more fruits and vegetables (Chapter 16), and many other positive lifestyle changes.

Putting Your Plan into Action

The starting date has arrived, and you are ready to put your plan into action. This stage requires commitment, the resolve to stick with the plan no matter what temptations you encounter. Remember all the good reasons you have for making the change—and remember that *you* are the boss.

Use all your strategies to make your plan work. Substituting behaviors is often very important—go for a walk after class instead of eating a bag of chips. Make sure your environment is change-friendly by keeping cues that trigger the problem behavior to a minimum. Also be sure to obtain as much support and encouragement from others as possible.

Use your health journal to keep track of how well you are doing in achieving your ultimate goal. Record your daily activities and any relevant details, such as how far you walked or how many calories you ate. Each week, chart your progress on a graph and see how it compares to the subgoals on your contract. You may want to track more than one behavior, such as the time you spend exercising each week and your weight.

If you don't seem to be making progress, analyze your plan to see what might be causing the problem. Possible barriers to success are listed in the section "Staying with It," along with suggestions for addressing them. Once you've identified the problem, revise your plan.

Be sure to reward yourself for your successes by treating yourself as specified in your contract. And don't forget to give yourself a pat on the back—congratulate yourself, notice how much better you look or feel, and feel good about how far you've come and how you've gained control of your behavior.

Staying with It

As you continue with your program, don't be surprised when you run up against obstacles; they're inevitable. In fact, it's a good idea to expect problems and give yourself time to step back, see how you're doing, and make some changes before going on again. If you find your program is grinding to a halt, try to identify what is blocking your progress. It may come from one of these sources.

My Personal Contract for Eating Three Servings of Fruit per Day

I agree to increase my consumption of fruit from one serving per week to three servings per day. I will begin my program on __10/5__ and plan to reach my final goal by __12/7__. I have divided my program into three parts, with three separate goals. For each step in my program, I will give myself the reward listed.

1. I will begin to have a serving of fruit with breakfast on __10/5__.
   (Reward: __baseball game_____)
2. I will begin to have a serving of fruit with lunch on __10/26__.
   (Reward: __music CD_____)
3. I will begin to substitute fruit juice for soda for one snack each day on__11/16__.
   (Reward: __concert_____)

My plan for increasing fruit consumption includes the following strategies:

1. Keeping my refrigerator stocked with easy-to-carry fruit and fruit juice.
2. Packing fruit in my book backpack every day.
3. Placing reminders to buy, carry, and eat fruit in my room, backpack, and wallet.
4. Buying lunch at a place that serves fruit or fruit juice.

I understand that it is important for me to make a strong personal effort to make the change in my behavior. I sign this contract as an indication of my personal commitment to reach my goal.

Michael Cook 9/28

Witness: *Katie Lim* 9/28

Figure 1-7   A sample behavior change contract.

Social Influences   Take a hard look at the reactions of the people you're counting on, and see if they're really supporting you. If they come up short, try connecting and networking with others who will be more supportive.

A related trap is trying to get your friends or family members to change *their* behaviors. The decision to make a major behavior change is something people come to only after intensive self-examination. You may be able to influence someone by tactfully providing facts or support, but that's all. Focus on yourself. If you succeed, you may become a role model for others.

Levels of Motivation and Commitment   You won't make real progress until an inner drive leads you to the stage of change at which you are ready to make a personal commitment to the goal. If commitment is your problem, you may need to wait until the short-term costs of your target behavior make your life more unhappy or unhealthy; then your desire to change it will be stronger. Or you may find that changing your goal will inspire you to keep going. If you really want to change but your motivation comes and goes, look at your support system and at your own level of confidence. Building these up may be the key to pushing past a barrier. For more ideas, refer to the box "Motivation Boosters" on page 26.

Choice of Techniques and Level of Effort

Your plan may not be working as well as you thought it would. Make changes where you're having the most trouble. If you've lagged on your running schedule, for example, maybe it's because you really don't like running. A group exercise class might suit you better. There are many ways to move toward your goal. Or you may not be trying hard enough. You do have to push toward your goal. If it were easy, you wouldn't need to have a plan.

Stress Barriers

If you've hit a wall in your program, look at the sources of stress in your life. If the stress is temporary, such as catching a cold or having a term paper due, you may want to wait until it passes before strengthening your efforts. If the stress is ongoing, try to find healthy ways to manage it. For example, taking a half-hour walk after lunch may help. You may even want to make stress management your highest priority for behavior change (see Chapter 2).

Games People Play

Procrastinating, rationalizing, and blaming—even when they want to change, people hold on fiercely to what they know and love (or know and hate). You may have very mixed feelings about the change you're trying to make, and your underlying motives may sabotage your conscious ones if you keep them hidden from yourself. Try to detect the games you might be playing with yourself so that you can stop them.

If you're procrastinating ("It's Friday already; I might as well wait until Monday to begin"), try breaking down your plan into still smaller steps that you can accomplish one day at a time. If you're rationalizing or making excuses ("I wanted to go swimming today, but I wouldn't have had time to wash my hair afterward"), remember that the only one you're fooling is yourself and that when you "win" by deceiving yourself it's not much of a victory. If you're wasting time blaming yourself or others ("Everyone in that class talks so much that I don't get a chance to speak"), recognize that blaming is a way of taking your focus off the real problem and denying responsibility for your actions. Try refocusing by taking a positive attitude and renewing your determination to succeed.

BEING HEALTHY FOR LIFE

Your first few behavior change projects may never go beyond the planning stage. Those that do may not all succeed. But as you taste success by beginning to see progress and changes, you'll start to experience new and surprising

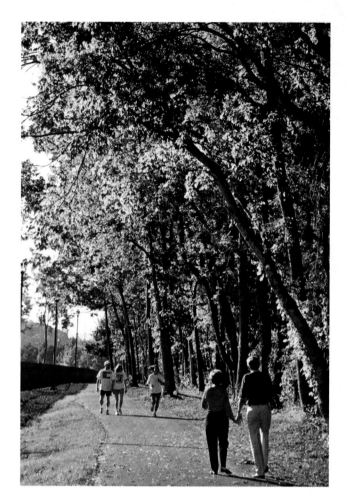

A beautiful day and a spectacular setting contribute to making exercise a satisfying and pleasurable experience. Choosing the right activity and doing it the right way are important elements in a successful health behavior change program.

positive feelings about yourself. You'll probably find that you're less likely to buckle under stress. You may accomplish things you never thought possible—winning a race, climbing a mountain, quitting smoking. Being healthy takes extra effort, but the paybacks in energy and vitality are priceless.

Once you've started, don't stop. Remember that maintaining good health is an ongoing process. Tackle one area at a time, but make a careful inventory of your health strengths and weaknesses and lay out a long-range plan. Take on the easier problems first, and then use what you have learned to attack more difficult areas. Keep informed about the latest health news and trends; research is constantly providing new information that directly affects daily choices and habits.

Making Changes in Your World

You can't completely control every aspect of your health. At least three other factors—heredity, health care, and environment—play important roles in your well-being. After you quit smoking, for example, you may still be

Changing behavior takes motivation. But how do you get motivated? The following strategies may help:

- Write down the potential benefits of the change. If you want to lose weight, your list might include increased ease of movement, energy, and self-confidence.

- Now write down the costs of not changing.

- Frequently visualize yourself achieving your goal and enjoying its benefits. If you want to manage time more effectively, picture yourself as a confident, organized person who systematically tackles important tasks and sets aside time each day for relaxation, exercise, and friends.

- Discount obstacles to change. Counter thoughts such as "I'll never have time to shop for and prepare healthy foods" with thoughts such as "Lots of other people have done it and so can I."

- Bombard yourself with propaganda. Subscribe to a self-improvement magazine. Take a class dealing with the change you want to make. Read books and watch talk shows on the subject. Post motivational phrases or pictures on your refrigerator or over your desk. Listen to motivational tapes in the car. Talk to people who have already made the change you want to make.

- Build up your confidence. Remind yourself of other goals you've achieved. At the end of each day, mentally review your good decisions and actions. See yourself as a capable person, in charge of your health.

- Create choices. You will be more likely to exercise every day if you have two or three types of exercise to choose from, and more likely to quit smoking if you've identified more than one way to distract yourself when you crave a cigarette. Get ideas from people who have been successful, and adapt some of their strategies to suit you.

- If you slip, keep trying. Research suggests that four out of five people will experience some degree of backsliding when they try to change a behavior. Only one in four succeeds the first time around. If you retain your commitment to change even when you lapse, you still are farther along the path to change than before you made the commitment. Try again. And again, if necessary.

inhaling smoke from other people's cigarettes. Your resolve to eat better foods may suffer a setback when you can't find any healthy choices in vending machines.

But you can make a difference—you can help create an environment around you that supports wellness for everyone. You can help support nonsmoking areas in public places. You can speak up in favor of more nutritious foods and better physical fitness facilities. You can include nonalcoholic drinks at your parties.

You can also work on larger environmental challenges: air and water pollution, traffic congestion, overcrowding and overpopulation, depletion of the atmosphere's ozone layer, toxic and nuclear waste, and many others. These difficult issues need the attention and energy of people who are informed and who care about good health. On every level, from personal to planetary, we can all take an active role in shaping our environment.

What Does the Future Hold?

Sweeping changes in lifestyle have resulted in healthier Americans in recent years and could have even greater effects in the years to come. In your lifetime, you can choose to take an active role in the movement toward increased awareness, greater individual responsibility and control, healthier lifestyles, and a healthier planet. Your choices and actions will have a tremendous impact on your present and future wellness. The door is open, and the time is now—you simply have to begin.

This retiree spends leisure time cross-country skiing. If you want to enjoy vigor and health in *your* middle and old age, begin now to make the choices that will give you lifelong vitality.

You are in charge of your health! Many of the decisions you make every day have an impact on the quality of your life, both now and in the future. By making positive choices, large and small, you help ensure a lifetime of wellness.

Right now you can

- Go for a 15-minute walk.

- Have an orange, a nectarine, or a plum for a snack.

- Call a friend and arrange a time to catch up with each other.

- Start thinking about whether you have a health behavior you'd like to change. If you do, consider the elements of a behavior change strategy. For example,

    - Begin a mental list of the pros and cons of the behavior.

    - Think of one or two rewards that will be meaningful to you as you reach interim goals.

    - Think of someone who will support you in your attempts to make a behavior change—either someone who might want to make the same change you're contemplating or someone you can trust to provide you with encouragement. Talk to that person about your plan, get feedback, and ask for support.

SUMMARY

- Wellness is the ability to live life fully, with vitality and meaning. Wellness is dynamic and multidimensional; it incorporates physical, emotional, intellectual, spiritual, interpersonal and social, and environmental dimensions.

- As chronic diseases have become the leading cause of death in the United States, people have recognized that they have greater control over, and greater responsibility for, their health than ever before.

- The Healthy People initiative seeks to achieve a better quality of life for all Americans. The broad goals of the *Healthy People 2010* report are to increase quality and years of healthy life and to eliminate health disparities among Americans.

- Health-related differences among people that have implications for wellness can be described in the context of gender, ethnicity, income and education, disability, geographic location, and sexual orientation.

- Although heredity, environment, and health care all play roles in wellness and disease, behavior can mitigate their effects.

- Behaviors and habits that reinforce wellness include (1) taking an active, responsible role in your health; (2) managing stress; (3) maintaining self-esteem and good interpersonal relationships; (4) understanding sexuality and having satisfying intimate relationships; (5) avoiding tobacco and other drugs and restricting alcohol intake; (6) eating well, exercising, and maintaining healthy weight; (7) knowing about diseases and injuries and protecting yourself against them; (8) understanding and wisely using the health care system; (9) knowing when to seek treatment for an illness; (10) understanding and accepting the processes of aging and dying; and (11) understanding how the environment affects your health and working to improve the environment.

- To make lifestyle changes, you need information about yourself, your health habits, and resources available to help you change.

- You can increase your motivation for behavior change by examining the benefits and costs of change, boosting self-efficacy, and identifying and overcoming key barriers to change.

- The "stages of change" model describes six stages that people move through as they try to change their behavior: precontemplation, contemplation, preparation, action, maintenance, and termination.

- A specific plan for change can be developed by (1) monitoring behavior by keeping a journal; (2) analyzing the recorded data; (3) setting specific goals; (4) devising strate-gies for modifying the environment, rewarding yourself, and involving others; and (5) making a personal contract.

- To start and maintain a behavior change program you need commitment, a well-developed plan, social support, and a system of rewards.

- Although we cannot control every aspect of our health, we can make a difference in helping create an environment that supports wellness for everyone.

Take Action

1. **Start a health journal.** Use a daily planner or PDA as your health journal throughout the course; use it to track your behavior, your emotions, and other factors related to wellness. As a first journal activity, create lists of the positive lifestyle behaviors that enhance your well-being and the behaviors that detract from wellness. Use these lists as the basis for self-evaluation as you proceed through the book. (Visit the Online Learning Center for health journal activities for each chapter.)

2. **Interview older family members.** Ask older members of your family (parents or grandparents) what they recall about patterns of health and disease when they were young. Did any of their friends or relatives die at an early age or of a disease that can now be treated? How have health concerns changed during their lifetime?

3. **Find a wellness role model.** Choose someone you consider to have embraced a wellness lifestyle. How is that person's overall health reflected in each of the dimensions of wellness? What can you borrow from her or his experiences and strategies for success in building a wellness lifestyle?

4. **Locate community resources.** Your school and community may present challenges to making healthy lifestyle choices, but they also have resources that can help you. Find out what local resources are "on your side" and can support your efforts at change; examples include free fitness facilities, stress-management workshops, and stop-smoking programs. As you become more aware of local resources and issues, you may also begin to identify ways that you could become involved to improve your community and its ability to promote wellness for all.

5. **Start building a family health history.** To help get started on your family health history, visit the site for the U.S. Surgeon General's Family History Initiative (www.hhs.gov/familyhistory). The instructions and forms from this site will help you organize your family tree and help you identify common diseases that may run in your family. Share the results with your health care provider. (For additional information on family health history, refer to Chapter 8.)

For More Information

Books

Komaroff, A. L., ed. 2005. *Harvard Medical School Family Health Guide.* New York: Free Press. *Provides consumer-oriented advice for the prevention and treatment of common health concerns.*

Prochaska, J. O., J. C. Norcross, and C. C. DiClemente. 1994. *Changing for Good: The Revolutionary Program That Explains the Six Stages of Change and Teaches You How to Free Yourself from Bad Habits.* New York: Morrow. *Outlines the authors' model of behavior change and offers suggestions and advice for each stage of change.*

Smith, P. B., M. MacFarlane, and E. Kalnitsky. 2002. *The Complete Idiot's Guide to Wellness.* Indianapolis, Ind.: Alpha Books. *A concise guide to healthy habits, including physical activity, nutrition, and stress management.*

Newsletters

Consumer Reports on Health (800-234-2188; http://www.ConsumerReportsonHealth.org)

Harvard Health Letter (800-829-9045; http://www.health.harvard.edu)

Harvard Men's Health Watch (877-649-9457)

Harvard Women's Health Watch (877-699-9457)

Mayo Clinic Health Letter (866-516-4974)

University of California at Berkeley Wellness Letter (800-829-9170; http://www.wellnessletter.com)

Organizations, Hotlines, and Web Sites

The Internet addresses (also called uniform resource locators, or URLs) listed here were accurate at the time of publication. Up-to-date links to these and many other wellness-oriented Web sites are provided on the links page of the *Core Concepts in Health* Web site (www.mhhe.com/insel10e).

Agency for Healthcare Research and Quality: Consumer Information. Provides materials on health plans and quality of care, prescription drugs, prevention and wellness, and consumer versions of evidence-based clinical practice guidelines for common conditions.
http://www.ahrq.gov/consumer

Centers for Disease Control and Prevention. Through phone, fax, and the Internet, the CDC provides a wide variety of health information.
800-311-3435
http://www.cdc.gov

Federal Trade Commission: Consumer Protection—Diet, Health, and Fitness. Includes online brochures about a variety of consumer health topics, including fitness equipment, generic drugs, and fraudulent health claims.
http://www.ftc.gov/bcp/menu-health.htm

FirstGov for Consumers: Health. Provides links to online brochures from a variety of government agencies.
http://www.consumer.gov/health.htm

Go Ask Alice. Sponsored by the Columbia University Health Service, this site provides answers to student questions about stress, sexuality, fitness, and many other wellness topics.
http://www.goaskalice.columbia.edu

Healthfinder. A gateway to online publications, Web sites, support and self-help groups, and agencies and organizations that produce reliable health information.
http://www.healthfinder.gov

Healthy People 2010. Provides information on Healthy People objectives and priority areas.
http://www.healthypeople.gov

MedlinePlus. Provides links to news and reliable information about health from government agencies and professional associations; also includes a health encyclopedia and information on prescription and over-the-counter drugs.
http://www.medlineplus.gov

MedlinePlus: Evaluating Health Information. Provides background information and links to sites with guidelines for finding and evaluating health information from the Web.
http://www.nlm.nih.gov/medlineplus/evaluatinghealthinformation.html

National Health Information Center (NHIC). Puts consumers in touch with the organizations that are best able to provide answers to health-related questions.
800-336-4797
http://www.health.gov/nhic

National Institutes of Health. Provides information about all NIH activities as well as consumer publications, hotline information, and an A to Z listing of health issues with links to the appropriate NIH institute.
http://www.nih.gov

National Women's Health Information Center. Provides information and answers to frequently asked questions.
800-994-WOMAN
http://www.4woman.gov

NOAH: New York Online Access to Health. Provides consumer health information in both English and Spanish.

http://www.noah-health.org

Office of Minority Health Resource Center. Promotes improved health among racial and ethnic minority populations.

http://www.omhrc.gov

Student Counseling Virtual Pamphlet Collection. Provides links to more than 400 pamphlets produced by different student counseling centers on a variety of wellness topics.

http://counseling.uchicago.edu/vpc

Surgeon General. Includes information on activities of the Surgeon General and the text of many key reports on such topics as tobacco use, physical activity, and mental health. You can also visit the site for the Surgeon General's Family History Initiative.

http://www.surgeongeneral.gov
http://www.hhs.gov/familyhistory

World Health Organization (WHO). Provides information about health topics and issues affecting people around the world.

http://www.who.int

The following are just a few of the many sites that provide consumer-oriented information on a variety of health issues:

FamilyDoctor.Org: http://www.familydoctor.org
InteliHealth: http://www.intelihealth.com
MayoClinic.com: http://mayoclinic.com
WebMD: http://webmd.com

The following sites provide daily health news updates:

CNN Health: http://www.cnn.com/health
MedlinePlus News: http://www.nlm.nih.gov/medlineplus/newsbydate.html
Yahoo Health News: http://dailynews.yahoo.com/h/hl

Selected Bibliography

American Cancer Society. 2005. *Cancer Facts and Figures—2005.* Atlanta: American Cancer Society.

American Heart Association. 2005. *2005 Heart and Stroke Statistical Update.* Dallas: American Heart Association.

Calle, E. E., et al. 2003. Overweight, obesity, and mortality from cancer in a prospectively studied cohort of U.S. adults. *New England Journal of Medicine* 348(17): 1625–1638.

Cauley, J. A., et al. 2005. Longitudinal study of changes in hip bone mineral density in Caucasian and African American women. *Journal of the American Geriatrics Society* 53(2): 183–189.

Centers for Disease Control and Prevention. 2005. Racial/ethnic and socioeconomic disparities in multiple risk factors for heart disease and stroke, United States, 2003. *Morbidity and Mortality Weekly Report* 54(5): 113–117.

Centers for Disease Control and Prevention. 1999. Achievements in public health, 1900–1999: Tobacco use, United States. *Morbidity and Mortality Weekly Report* 48(43): 986–993.

Centers for Disease Control and Prevention. 2004. REACH 2010 surveillance for health status in minority communities. *MMWR Surveillance Summaries* 53(SS-6).

Centers for Disease Control and Prevention, Division of Nutrition and Physical Activity. 1999. *Promoting Physical Activity: A Guide for Community Action.* Champaign, Ill.: Human Kinetics.

Glanz, K., F. M. Lewis, and B. K. Rimer, eds. 2002. *Health Behavior and Health Education: Theory, Research, and Practice,* 3rd ed. San Francisco: Jossey-Bass.

Institute of Medicine. 2001. *Exploring the Biological Contributions to Human Health: Does Sex Matter?* Washington, D.C.: National Academy Press.

International Human Genome Sequencing Consortium. 2004. Finishing the euchromatic sequence of the human genome. *Nature* 431: 931–945.

Jemal, A., et al. 2005. Cancer statistics, 2005. *CA: A Cancer Journal for Clinicians* 55(1): 10–30.

Kaiser Family Foundation. 2003. *Key Facts: Race, Ethnicity, and Medical Care.* Menlo Park, Calif.: Kaiser Family Foundation.

Martin, G., and J. Pear. 2003. *Behaviour Modification: What It Is and How to Do It,* 7th ed. Upper Saddle River, N.J.: Prentice Hall.

McClure, J. B. 2002. Are biomarkers useful treatment aids for promoting health behavior change? *American Journal of Preventive Medicine* 22(3): 200–207.

Mokdad, A. H., et al. 2003. Prevalence of obesity, diabetes, and obesity-related health risk factors, 2001. *Journal of the American Medical Association* 289(1): 76–79.

Mokdad, A. H., et al. 2004. Actual causes of death in the United States, 2000. *Journal of the American Medical Association* 291(10): 1238–1245.

Mokdad, A. H., et al. 2005. Correction: Actual causes of death in the United States, 2000. *Journal of the American Medical Association* 293(3): 293–294.

Muller, A. 2002. Education, income inequality, and mortality: A multiple regression analysis. *British Medical Journal* 324(7328): 23–25.

National Cancer Institute. 2004. *Cancer Facts: Cancer Clusters* (http://cis.nci.nih.gov/fact/3_58.htm; retrieved October 23, 2004).

National Center for Health Statistics. 2004. Health behaviors of adults: United States, 1999–2001. *Vital and Health Statistics* 10(219).

National Center for Health Statistics. 2004. *Health, United States, 2004, with Chartbook on Trends in the Health of Americans.* Hyattsville, Md.: National Center for Health Statistics.

Office of Hawaiian Affairs. 2002. *Native Hawaiian Databook June 2002* (http://oha.org/databook; retrieved October 21, 2004).

Slater, M. D., and D. E. Zimmerman. 2002. Characteristics of health-related Web sites identified by common Internet portals. *Journal of the American Medical Association* 288(3): 316–317.

Steenland, K., et al. 2003. Deaths due to injuries among employed adults: The effects of socioeconomic class. *Epidemiology* 14(1): 74–79.

U.S. Census Bureau. 2005. *We the People: Women and Men in the United States.* Washington, D.C.: U.S. Census Bureau.

U.S. Department of Health and Human Services. 2000. *Healthy People 2010,* 2nd ed. Washington, D.C.: DHHS.

World Health Organization. 2004. *Why Gender and Health?* (http://www.who.int/gender/genderandhealth/en; retrieved August 13, 2004).

2

Looking

AHEAD

After reading this chapter, you should be able to

- Explain what stress is and how people react to it—physically, emotionally, and behaviorally

- Describe the relationship between stress and disease

- List common sources of stress

- Describe techniques for preventing and managing stress

- Put together a step-by-step plan for successfully managing the stress in your life

Stress: The Constant Challenge

Test Your

Knowledge

1. Which of the following events can cause stress?
   a. taking out a loan
   b. failing a test
   c. graduating from college
   d. watching a hockey game

2. Moderate exercise can stimulate which of the following?
   a. analgesia (pain relief)
   b. birth of new brain cells
   c. relaxation

3. High levels of stress can impair memory and cause physical changes in the brain. True or false?

4. For which of the following disorders is stress a risk factor?
   a. diabetes
   b. arthritis
   c. premature menopause
   d. heart disease

5. About how many car crashes each year are caused by drowsy driving?
   a. 10,000
   b. 100,000
   c. 200,000

ANSWERS

1. ALL FOUR. Stress-producing factors can be pleasant or unpleasant and can include physical challenges and the achievement of personal goals as well as what would commonly be perceived as negative events.

2. ALL THREE. Regular exercise is linked to improvements in many dimensions of wellness.

3. TRUE. Low levels of stress may improve memory, but high stress levels impair learning and memory and, over the long term, may shrink an area of the brain called the hippocampus.

4. ALL FOUR. Stress—interacting with heredity, personality, social environment, and behavior—increases vulnerability to many health problems.

5. C. Among drivers age 18–29, 60% report driving while drowsy, and nearly 25% say they have fallen asleep at the wheel. Driving while drowsy is nearly as dangerous as driving while intoxicated.

Visit the *Core Concepts in Health* Online Learning Center (www.mhhe.com/insel10e) for study aids and many additional resources.

31

Everybody talks about stress. People say they're "overstressed" or "stressed out." They may blame stress for headaches or ulcers, and they may try to combat stress with aerobics classes—or drugs. But what is stress? And why is it important to manage it wisely?

Most people associate stress with negative events: the death of a close relative or friend, financial problems, or other unpleasant life changes that create nervous tension. But stress isn't merely nervous tension. And it isn't something to be avoided at all costs (Figure 2-1). In fact, only death brings complete freedom from stress. Before we explore more fully what stress is, consider this list of common stressful situations or events:

- Interviewing for a job
- Running in a race
- Being accepted to college
- Going out on a date
- Watching a basketball game
- Getting a promotion

Obviously, stress doesn't arise just from unpleasant situations. Stress can also be associated with physical challenges and the achievement of personal goals. Physical and psychological stress-producing factors can be pleasant or unpleasant. The actions you take in response to stress are influenced by your biological predispositions, past experiences, and current circumstances. Although you cannot change who you are or what you've been through in the past, you *can* modify your current behavior and seek out people, places, and experiences that will improve your ability to deal with stress. In other words, what is crucial is how you respond, whether in positive, life-enhancing ways or in negative, counterproductive ways.

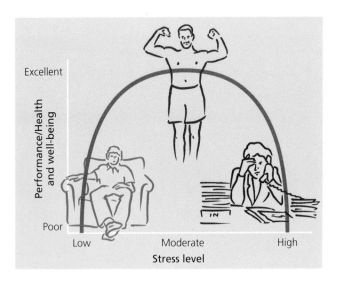

Figure 2-1   Stress level, performance, and well-being. A moderate level of stress challenges individuals in a way that promotes optimal performance and well-being. Too little stress, and people are not challenged enough to improve; too much stress, and the challenges become stressors that can impair physical and emotional health.

As a college student, you may be in one of the most stressful periods of your life (see the box "How High Is Your Stress Level?"). You may be on your own for the first time, or you may be juggling the demands of college with the responsibilities of a job, a family, or both. Financial pressures may be intense. Housing and transportation may be sources of additional hassles. You're also meeting new people, engaging in new activities, learning new information and skills, and setting a new course for your life. Good and bad, all these changes and challenges are likely to have a powerful effect on you, both physically and psychologically. Respond ineffectively to stress, and eventually it will take a toll on your sense of wellness. Learn effective responses, however, and you will enhance your health and gain a feeling of control over your life.

How do you know when your stress level is getting dangerously high? How can you develop techniques to cope positively with the stress that is part of your life? This chapter will help you discover answers to these questions.

WHAT IS STRESS?

Just what is stress, if such vastly different situations can cause it? In common usage, "stress" refers to two different things: situations that trigger physical and emotional reactions *and* the reactions themselves. In this text, we'll use the more precise term **stressor** for situations that trigger physical and emotional reactions and the term **stress response** for those reactions. A date and a final exam, then, are stressors; sweaty palms and a pounding heart are symptoms of the stress response. We'll use the term **stress** to describe the general physical and emotional state that accompanies the stress response. A person on a date or taking a final exam experiences stress.

Each individual's experience of stress depends on many factors, including the nature of the stressor and how the stressor is perceived. Responses to stressors include physical changes and emotional and behavioral responses.

Physical Responses to Stressors

Imagine that you are waiting to cross a street, perhaps daydreaming about a movie you saw last week. The light turns green and you step off the curb. Almost before you see it, you feel a car speeding toward you. With just a fraction of a second to spare, you leap safely out of harm's way. In that split second of danger and in the moments following it, you have experienced a predictable series of physical reactions. Your body has gone from a relaxed state to one prepared for physical action to cope with a threat to your life.

Two major control systems in your body are responsible for your physical response to stressors: the nervous system and the endocrine system. Through a variety of

Many symptoms of excess stress are easy to self-diagnose. To help determine how much stress you experience on a daily basis, answer the following questions:

1. How many of the symptoms of excess stress listed in the table below do you experience frequently?
2. Are you easily startled or irritated?
3. Are you increasingly forgetful?
4. Do you have trouble falling or staying asleep?
5. Do you continually worry about events in your future?
6. Do you feel as if you are constantly under pressure to produce?
7. Do you frequently use tobacco, alcohol, or other drugs to help you relax?
8. Do you often feel as if you have less energy than you need to finish the day?
9. Do you have recurrent stomachaches or headaches?
10. Is it difficult for you to find satisfaction in simple life pleasures?
11. Are you often disappointed in yourself and others?
12. Are you overly concerned with being liked or accepted by others?
13. Have you lost interest in intimacy or sex?
14. Are you concerned that you do not have enough money?

Experiencing some of the stress-related symptoms or answering yes to a few questions is normal. However, if you experience a large number of stress symptoms or you answered yes to a majority of the questions, you are likely experiencing a high level of stress. Take time out to develop effective stress-management techniques. Many coping strategies that can aid you in dealing with your college stressors are described in this chapter. Additionally, your school's counseling center can provide valuable support.

Symptoms of Excess Stress

Physical Symptoms	Emotional Symptoms	Behavioral Symptoms
Dry mouth	Anxiety or edginess	Crying
Excessive perspiration	Depression	Disrupted eating habits
Frequent illnesses	Fatigue	Disrupted sleeping habits
Gastrointestinal problems	Hypervigilance	Harsh treatment of others
Grinding of teeth	Impulsiveness	Increased use of tobacco, alcohol, or other drugs
Headaches	Inability to concentrate	Problems communicating
High blood pressure	Irritability	Sexual problems
Pounding heart	Trouble remembering things	Social isolation
Stiff neck or aching lower back		

rapid chemical reactions affecting almost every part of your body, you are primed to act quickly and appropriately in time of danger.

Actions of the Nervous System The nervous system consists primarily of the brain, spinal cord, and nerves. Part of the nervous system is under voluntary control: commanding your arm to reach for a chocolate, for instance. The part that is not under conscious supervision, such as what controls the digestion of the chocolate, is known as the **autonomic nervous system.** In addition to digestion, it controls heart rate, breathing, blood pressure, and hundreds of other functions you normally take for granted.

The autonomic nervous system consists of two divisions. The **parasympathetic division** is in control when you are relaxed; it aids in digesting food, storing energy, and promoting growth. In contrast, the **sympathetic division** is activated during arousal or when there is an emergency, such as severe pain, anger, or fear. Sympathetic nerves use the neurotransmitter **norepinephrine** to exert their actions on nearly every organ, sweat gland, blood

Terms VIW

stressor Any physical or psychological event or condition that produces stress.

stress response The physiological changes associated with stress.

stress The collective physiological and emotional responses to any stimulus that disturbs an individual's homeostasis.

autonomic nervous system The branch of the peripheral nervous system that, largely without conscious thought, controls basic body processes; consists of the sympathetic and parasympathetic divisions.

parasympathetic division A division of the autonomic system that moderates the excitatory effect of the sympathetic division, slowing metabolism and restoring energy supplies.

sympathetic division A division of the autonomic nervous system that reacts to danger or other challenges by almost instantly accelerating body processes.

norepinephrine A neurotransmitter released by the sympathetic nervous system onto target tissues to increase their function in the face of increased activity; when released in the brain, it causes arousal (increased attention, awareness, and alertness); also called *noradrenaline.*

vessel, and muscle to enable your body to handle an emergency. In general, it commands your body to stop storing energy and instead to mobilize all energy resources to respond to the crisis.

Actions of the Endocrine System

One important target of the sympathetic nervous system is the **endocrine system.** This system of glands, tissues, and cells helps control body functions by releasing **hormones** and other chemical messengers into the bloodstream. Chemicals released into the blood are relatively free to travel throughout the body. The sites of action for circulating stress hormones are determined by specialized receptors in target tissues. Thus, stress hormones will act only on those organs that have stress hormone receptors. Along with the nervous system, with which it closely interacts, the endocrine system helps prepare the body to respond to a stressor.

The Two Systems Together

How do both systems work together in an emergency? Let's go back to your close call with that car. Both reflexive and higher cognitive areas in your brain quickly make the decision that a large object traveling toward you at a high rate of speed is a threat and requires immediate action. A neurochemical message is

promptly sent to the **hypothalamus,** a hormonal control center in the brain, that its services are needed, and it releases a chemical wake-up call to the nearby **pituitary gland.** In turn, the pituitary gland releases **adrenocorticotropic hormone (ACTH)** into the bloodstream. When ACTH reaches the **adrenal glands,** located just above the kidneys, it stimulates them to release **cortisol** and other key hormones into the bloodstream. Simultaneously, sympathetic nerves instruct your adrenal glands to release the hormone **epinephrine,** or adrenaline, which in turn triggers a series of profound changes throughout your body (Figure 2-2). Your hearing and vision become more acute. Bronchi dilate to allow more air into your lungs. Your heart rate accelerates and blood pressure increases to ensure that your blood—and the oxygen, nutrients, and hormones it carries—will be rapidly distributed where needed. Your liver releases extra sugar into your bloodstream to provide an energy boost for your muscles and brain. Your digestion halts. You perspire more to cool your skin. **Endorphins** are released to relieve pain in case of injury. Blood cell production increases.

It was Sir Walter Cannon who first called these almost-instantaneous physical changes, collectively, the **fight-or-flight reaction.** These changes give you the heightened reflexes and strength you need to dodge the car or deal with other stressors. Although these physical changes may vary in intensity, the same basic set of physical reactions occurs in response to any type of stressor, positive or negative.

The Return to Homeostasis

Why doesn't your body remain in a hypervigilant state, perpetually ready for action? Why shouldn't your body always be prepared for a crisis? As you have probably guessed, it would be too exhausting. Your body actually resists dramatic changes. Whenever normal functioning is disrupted, such as during the fight-or-flight reaction, your body strives for **homeostasis,** a state in which blood pressure, heart rate, hormone levels, and other vital functions are maintained within a narrow range of normal.

Once a stressful situation ends, the parasympathetic division of your autonomic nervous system takes command and halts the reaction. It initiates the adjustments necessary to restore homeostasis. Your parasympathetic nervous system calms your body down, slowing a rapid heartbeat, drying sweaty palms, and returning breathing to normal. Gradually, your body resumes its normal "housekeeping" functions, such as digestion and temperature regulation. Damage that may have been sustained during the fight-or-flight reaction is repaired. The day after you narrowly dodge the car, you wake up feeling fine. In this way, your body can grow, repair itself, and acquire reserves of energy. When the next crisis comes, you'll be ready to respond—instantly—again.

The Fight-or-Flight Reaction in Modern Life

The fight-or-flight reaction is a part of our biological

Terms

endocrine system The system of glands, tissues, and cells that secrete hormones into the bloodstream to influence metabolism and other body processes.

hormone A chemical messenger produced in the body and transported by the bloodstream to target cells or organs for specific regulation of their activities.

hypothalamus A part of the brain that activates, controls, and integrates the autonomic mechanisms, endocrine activities, and many body functions.

pituitary gland The "master gland," closely linked with the hypothalamus, that controls other endocrine glands and secretes hormones that regulate growth, maturation, and reproduction.

adrenocorticotropic hormone (ACTH) A hormone, formed in the pituitary gland, that stimulates the outer layer of the adrenal gland to secrete its hormones.

adrenal glands Two glands, one lying atop each kidney, whose outer layer (cortex) produces steroid hormones such as cortisol and whose inner core (medulla) produces the hormones epinephrine and norepinephrine.

cortisol A steroid hormone secreted by the cortex (outer layer) of the adrenal gland; also called *hydrocortisone.*

epinephrine A hormone secreted by the medulla (inner core) of the adrenal gland that affects the functioning of organs involved in responding to a stressor; also called *adrenaline.*

endorphins Brain secretions that have pain-inhibiting effects.

fight-or-flight reaction A defense reaction that prepares an individual for conflict or escape by triggering hormonal, cardiovascular, metabolic, and other changes.

homeostasis A state of stability and consistency in an individual's physiological functioning.

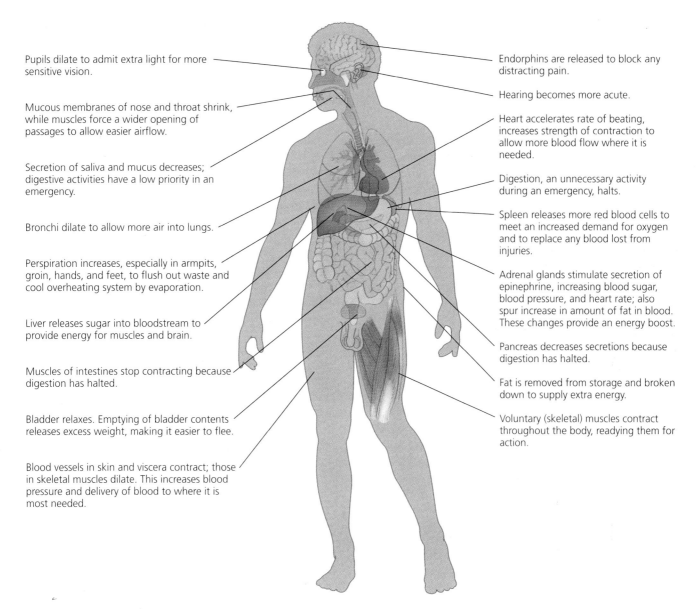

Pupils dilate to admit extra light for more sensitive vision.

Mucous membranes of nose and throat shrink, while muscles force a wider opening of passages to allow easier airflow.

Secretion of saliva and mucus decreases; digestive activities have a low priority in an emergency.

Bronchi dilate to allow more air into lungs.

Perspiration increases, especially in armpits, groin, hands, and feet, to flush out waste and cool overheating system by evaporation.

Liver releases sugar into bloodstream to provide energy for muscles and brain.

Muscles of intestines stop contracting because digestion has halted.

Bladder relaxes. Emptying of bladder contents releases excess weight, making it easier to flee.

Blood vessels in skin and viscera contract; those in skeletal muscles dilate. This increases blood pressure and delivery of blood to where it is most needed.

Endorphins are released to block any distracting pain.

Hearing becomes more acute.

Heart accelerates rate of beating, increases strength of contraction to allow more blood flow where it is needed.

Digestion, an unnecessary activity during an emergency, halts.

Spleen releases more red blood cells to meet an increased demand for oxygen and to replace any blood lost from injuries.

Adrenal glands stimulate secretion of epinephrine, increasing blood sugar, blood pressure, and heart rate; also spur increase in amount of fat in blood. These changes provide an energy boost.

Pancreas decreases secretions because digestion has halted.

Fat is removed from storage and broken down to supply extra energy.

Voluntary (skeletal) muscles contract throughout the body, readying them for action.

Figure 2-2 The fight-or-flight reaction. In response to a stressor, the autonomic nervous system and the endocrine system prepare the body to deal with an emergency.

heritage, a survival mechanism that has served humankind well. It enables our bodies to quickly prepare to escape from an injury or to engage in a physical battle. In modern life, however, the fight-or-flight reaction is often absurdly inappropriate. Many of the stressors we face in everyday life do not require a physical response—for example, an exam, a mess left by a roommate, or a red traffic light. Imagine that you are sitting quietly and then receive a letter saying that you have been denied a scholarship. You would probably quickly become more energized or alert, even irritated. You could feel a loss of appetite, and your respiration and heart rates would increase. Depending on the level of your response and state of physical fitness, you would feel other effects of sympathetic activation such as a slight throbbing in your upper extremities or temples, warmth in the face and neck region, and sweaty palms.

The fight-or-flight reaction prepares the body for physical action regardless of whether such action is a necessary or appropriate response to a particular stressor.

Emotional and Behavioral Responses to Stressors

The physical response to a stressor may vary in intensity from person to person and situation to situation, but we all experience a similar set of physical changes—the fight-or-flight reaction. However, there is a great deal of variation in how people view potential stressors and in how people respond to them. For example, you may feel confident about taking exams but be nervous about talking to people you don't know, whereas your roommate may love challenging social situations but be very nervous about taking tests. Many factors, some external and some internal, help explain these differences. Your cognitive appraisal of a potential stressor will influence how that particular stressor is viewed. Two factors that can reduce the magnitude of the stress response are successful prediction and the perception of having some control over the stressor. For instance, obtaining course syllabi at the beginning of the term allows you to predict the timing of major deadlines and exams. Having this predictive knowledge also allows you to exert some control over your study and recreation plans and can thus help reduce the stress caused by exams.

Cognitive appraisal is highly individual and strongly related to emotions. The facts of a situation—Who? What? Where? When?—typically are evaluated fairly consistently from person to person. Evaluation with respect to personal outcome, however, varies: What does this mean for me? Can I do anything about it? Will it improve or worsen? If an individual perceives a situation as exceeding her or his ability to cope, the result can be negative emotions and an inappropriate stress response. If, on the other hand, a person perceives a situation as a challenge that is within her or his ability to manage, more positive and appropriate responses are likely.

Effective and Ineffective Responses Our emotional and behavioral responses to stressors are as critical to our overall experience of stress as are our physical responses. Common emotional responses to stressors include anxiety, depression, fear, or exhilaration. Although emotional responses are determined in part by inborn personality, we often can moderate or learn to control them. Coping techniques are discussed later in the chapter.

Our behavioral responses—controlled by the **somatic nervous system,** which manages our conscious actions—are under our control. Effective behavioral responses can promote wellness and enable us to function at our best. Ineffective behavioral responses can impair wellness and can even become stressors themselves. Depending on the stressor involved, effective behavioral responses may include talking, laughing, exercising, meditating, learning time-management skills, or finding a more compatible roommate. Inappropriate behavioral responses include overeating, substance abuse, or expressing hostility toward others.

Let's consider the different emotional and behavioral responses of students, Amelia and David, to a common stressor: the first exam of the semester. Both students feel anxious as the exam is passed out. Amelia relaxes her muscles and starts by writing the answers she knows. On a second pass through the exam, she concentrates carefully on the wording of each question. Some material comes back to her, and she makes educated guesses on the remaining items. She spends the whole hour writing as much as she can and checking her answers. She leaves the room feeling calm, relaxed, and confident that she has done well on the exam.

David responds to his initial anxiety with more anxiety. He finds that he doesn't know some of the answers, and he becomes more worried. The more upset he gets, the less he can remember; and the more he blanks out, the more anxious he gets. He begins to imagine the consequences of failing the course and berates himself for not having studied more. David turns in his paper before the hour is up, without checking his answers or going back to the questions he skipped. He leaves feeling depressed and angry.

As you can see, although both Amelia and David experienced the physical stress response as the exam was passed out, their emotional and behavioral responses were quite different—and led to very different outcomes. What determines these differences? Emotional and behavioral responses to stressors depend on a complex set of factors that include personality, cultural background, gender, and past experiences.

Personality and Stress In any stressful situation, some people seem nervous and irritable whereas others are calm and composed. Why do people respond so differently to stressors? Scientists remain unsure about the precise causes of these and other behavioral differences among individuals, but they are beginning to identify the brain mechanisms that interact to produce complex emotions and thought processes. **Personality,** the sum of behavioral, cognitive, and emotional tendencies, clearly affects how an individual perceives and reacts to stressors. To investigate the links among personality, stress, and overall wellness, researchers have looked at different constellations of characteristics, or "personality types."

TYPE A, B, AND C PERSONALITIES In the 1960s, researchers began separating people into two basic personality types, Type A and Type B. Type A individuals tended to be more controlling, schedule driven, competitive, and even hostile. Type B individuals were less hurried, more contemplative, and more tolerant of others.

These personality designations received much attention as a result of the findings of Meyer Friedman and Ray Rosenman, who showed that Type A individuals were more likely to have heart disease (they studied middle-age Caucasian males almost exclusively). However, later studies show that most Type A individuals are quite healthy and perhaps even more successful at surviving heart disease than Type B individuals of the same age and

Terms

V iwx

somatic nervous system The branch of the peripheral nervous system that governs motor functions and sensory information; largely under our conscious control.

personality The sum of behavioral, cognitive, and emotional tendencies.

stage of disease; it may be that Type A people follow their medication and therapy schedules more exactly and tend to be more competitive against the disease. The only aspects of Type A personality that remain associated with a greater risk for heart disease in women and men of all ethnicities are anger, cynicism, and hostility (see Chapter 15 for more on the link between hostility and heart disease).

In terms of stress, Type A people may have a higher perceived stress level and greater coping difficulties, especially in social situations. They may react more explosively to stressors and become upset by events that others would consider only mild annoyances. Type B individuals, on the other hand, tend to be less frustrated by the flow of daily events and the actions of others.

Research into personality traits and cancer examined a Type C personality, characterized by difficulty expressing emotions, anger suppression, feelings of hopelessness and despair, and an exaggerated stress response to minor cognitive stressors. People who consistently show these traits have lower levels of immune cells important in fighting cancer as well as lower cancer survival rates. The heightened stress response associated with a Type C personality may be directly related to impaired immune function. Studies of Type A and C personalities suggest that it is beneficial to express your emotions but that consistent or exaggerated arousal or hostility toward others is unhealthy.

HARDINESS AND RESILIENCY Researchers have also looked at personality traits that seem to enable people to deal more successfully with stress. Psychologist Suzanne Kobasa examined "hardiness," a particular form of optimism. People with a hardy personality view potential stressors as challenges and opportunities for growth and learning, rather than as burdens. Hardy people tend to perceive fewer situations as stressful, and their reaction to stressors tends to be less intense. They are committed to their activities, have a sense of inner purpose, and feel at least partly in control of events in their lives.

Resiliency refers to personality traits associated with social and academic success in at-risk populations such as children from low-income families and people with mental or physical disabilities. Like hardy people, those with resiliency tend to set goals and face adversity through individual effort. The three basic types of resiliency center on how an individual responds to stress: nonreactive resiliency, in which a person does not react to stress; homeostatic resiliency, in which a person may react strongly but returns to baseline functioning fairly quickly; and positive growth resiliency, in which a person learns and grows. Resiliency is also associated with emotional intelligence and violence prevention.

People with a hardy or resilient personality typically have an internal locus of control. As described in Chapter 1, this means that they feel responsible for their own actions and in control of many of the events in their lives. This sense of control helps them cope with stress in a more positive way and put setbacks in proper perspective. Psychologist Martin Seligman coined the term "positive psychology," based on the idea that if young people are taught resiliency, hope, and optimism, they will be less susceptible to depression and will lead happier, more productive lives. People with an external locus of control—a belief that the events in their lives are controlled by outside factors—typically have more difficulties with stress. A person with an external locus of control may feel helpless in a stressful situation and believe it's pointless to make constructive attempts to deal with stressors.

Can a Person Develop a Stress-Resistant Personality? In addition to the models of personality presented here, researchers have developed more complex and encompassing models that look at other factors that influence behavioral and emotional responses to stressors. Visit the Online Learning Center for self-assessments relating to personality types and traits such as assertiveness.

Researchers have also looked at the extent to which temperament and personality are inherited. Basic emotional response patterns such as the tendency to seek out new experiences appear to have a strong hereditary component; the underlying factor may be genes that influence the activities of neurotransmitters like serotonin and dopamine. On the other hand, character traits such as the degree to which a person is self-directed appear much more closely linked to sociocultural factors than to heredity. It is important to note that the relationship between genes and behavior is extremely complex, so that even traits with a strong genetic component are profoundly influenced by environment and experience.

Is there anything people can do to change their personality and become more stress-resistant? It is unlikely that you can change your basic personality. However, you can change your typical behaviors and patterns of thinking and develop positive techniques for coping with stressors. Strategies for successful stress management are described later in the chapter. For starters, though, try a few of the following:

- Build greater social support through meaningful relationships.
- Take advantage of opportunities to participate in and contribute to your family and community in productive ways.
- Set slightly higher expectations for yourself with clear boundaries and expectations that are fair and consistent.
- Build life skills such as decision making, effective communication, and stress and conflict management.
- Do not try to control the outcome of every situation (for example, a team competition or a loved one's illness). Know your limitations and trust others.

Cultural Background Young adults from all over the world seek higher education at American colleges and universities. The vast majority of students come away from their undergraduate experience with a greater appreciation for other groups and cultures. However, when they are ignored, misunderstood, or disrespected, cultural differences in values, lifestyles, and what is considered to be acceptable behavior can be a source of stress and can lead to stereotyping, prejudice, discrimination, harassment, and even assault. The way you cope with stress and the way you interact with people of other cultures are influenced by the family and culture in which you were raised. Try to avoid the assumption that your way of life is the best or only way. If you take the time to learn about and from other cultures, you will become more aware of the potential strengths and weaknesses of your own culture. You will also reduce the likelihood of cultural differences becoming a source of stress for you.

Gender Like cultural background, our **gender role**— the activities, abilities, and behaviors our culture expects of us based on whether we're male or female—also affects our experience of stress. Some behavioral responses to stressors, such as crying or openly expressing anger, may be deemed more appropriate for one gender than the other. Strict adherence to gender roles can place limits on how a person responds to stress and can itself become a source of stress. Adherence to traditional gender roles can also affect the perception of a potential stressor. For example, if a man derives most of his sense of self-worth from his work, retirement may be a more stressful life change for him than for a woman whose self-image is based on several different roles.

Oxytocin, a hormone involved in social interaction and the regulation of mood, may underlie some of the gender differences in behavioral responses to stressors. Women produce more oxytocin than men do; and the hormone estrogen, which is more abundant in women, enhances its effects. Although both men do; and women experience the fight-or-flight physiological response to stress, women are more likely to respond behaviorally with a pattern of "tend-and-befriend"—nurturing friends and family and seeking social support and social contacts. Women are more likely to enhance their social networks in ways that reduce stress than to become aggressive or withdraw from difficult situations.

See the box "Women, Men, and Stress" for more on gender and stress.

Past Experiences Your past experiences significantly influence your response to stressors. For example, if you were unprepared for the first speech you gave in your speech class and performed poorly, you will probably experience greater anxiety in response to future assignments. If you had performed better, your confidence and sense of control would be greater, and you would probably

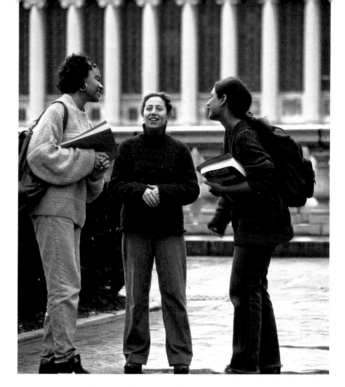

A person's emotional and behavioral responses to stressors depend on many different factors, including personality, gender, and cultural background. Research suggests that women are more likely than men to respond to stressors by seeking social support.

experience less stress with future speeches. Effective behavioral responses, in this case careful preparation and visualizing yourself giving a successful speech, can help overcome the effects of negative past experiences.

The Stress Experience as a Whole

Physical, emotional, and behavioral responses to stressors are intimately interrelated. The more intense the emotional response, the stronger the physical response. Effective behavioral responses can reduce stress; ineffective ones only worsen it. Sometimes people have such intense emotional responses and such ineffective or counterproductive behavioral responses to stressors that they need professional help with learning to cope. More often, however, people can learn to handle stressors on their own. Actions you can take to deal successfully with the stress in your life are described later in the chapter.

STRESS AND DISEASE

The role of stress in health and disease is complex, and much remains to be learned. However, evidence suggests that stress—interacting with a person's genetic predisposition, personality, social environment, and health-related behaviors—can increase vulnerability to numerous ailments. Several related theories have been proposed to explain the relationship between stress and disease.

Gender Matters

Special Stressors for Men and Women

Women are more likely than men to find themselves balancing multiple roles—student, employee, parent, spouse, caregiver to aging parents. Women who work outside of the home still do most of the housework, and time-related stress can be severe. All of these stressors can contribute to higher levels of stress-related health problems. Social forces can also undermine opportunities for women and cause stress. Women now make up more than half of the workforce but hold only 5% of the top leadership jobs. On average, women make less money than men with comparable jobs and are more likely to face sexual harassment. Disparity in domestic responsibilities, lack of integration into dominant organization coalitions, and even being considered excessively "nice" can all reduce the chances of being considered for leadership positions. The more women view themselves as fitting the traditional feminine gender stereotype, the less likely they are to report leadership aspirations.

Men who fit a traditional male gender role may feel the need to be active and in charge in all situations. They may have a communication style that is competitive and aggressive, causing stress in many interpersonal situations and limiting their ability to build social support networks. The responsibility to support a family may be felt very keenly among men with a traditional male gender role.

Physiological Differences and Stress

Due to hormonal differences, men are considered to be more biologically vulnerable to certain diseases. For example, because of a rise in circulating testosterone levels, from puberty onward, males have higher blood pressure than do age-matched females. Along with other risk factors, including fewer physician visits, the rise in testosterone produces greater wear and tear on the male circulatory system over time, leading to greater risk for cardiovascular disease. A part of the brain responsible for regulating fear and emotional balance, the amygdala, is very sensitive to testosterone. Thus, having more circulating testosterone may predispose men to see social situations as more threatening than a woman would see them, creating more frequent activation of the stress response.

Women, on the other hand, have higher levels of the hormone oxytocin and are more likely to respond to stressors by seeking social support. The tend-and-befriend coping response among women may give them a longevity advantage compared with men by decreasing the risk of stress-related disorders.

Gender and Stress Among College Students

Gender role development is a significant source of stress during college for both men and women, but there are gender differences in key stressors and coping strategies. College women are more likely than men to report having roommate conflicts and personal appearance issues. Men have more difficulty relating to and meeting other students, making friends, and dealing with peer pressure. College women report significantly higher emotional resources and ability to give and receive social support than do men. College men more frequently utilize physical coping resources than do women.

The General Adaptation Syndrome

Biologist Hans Selye, working in the 1930s and 1940s, was one of the first scientists to develop a comprehensive theory of stress and disease. Selye coined the term **general adaptation syndrome (GAS)** to describe what he believed was a universal and predictable response pattern to all stressors. He recognized that stressors could be pleasant, such as attending a party, or unpleasant, such as getting a flat tire or a bad grade. He called stress triggered by a pleasant stressor **eustress** and stress triggered by an unpleasant stressor **distress.** The sequence of physical responses associated with GAS is the same for both eustress and distress and occurs in three stages: alarm, resistance, and exhaustion (Figure 2-3).

Alarm   This stage includes the complex sequence of events brought on by the activation of the sympathetic nervous system and the endocrine system—the fight-or-flight reaction. During this stage, the body is more susceptible to disease or injury because it is geared up to deal with a crisis. A person in this phase may experience headaches, indigestion, anxiety, and disrupted sleeping and eating patterns.

Resistance   With continued stress, Selye theorized, the body developed a new level of homeostasis in which it was more resistant to disease and injury than it normally would be. During the resistance stage, a person can cope with normal life and added stress.

Exhaustion   As you might imagine, both the mobilization of forces during the alarm reaction and the maintenance of homeostasis during the resistance stage require a considerable amount of energy. If a stressor persists or if several stressors occur in succession, general exhaustion results. This is not the sort of exhaustion people complain

Terms

V ew

gender role A culturally expected pattern of behavior and attitudes determined by whether a person is male or female.

general adaptation syndrome (GAS) A pattern of stress responses consisting of three stages: alarm, resistance, and exhaustion.

eustress Stress resulting from a pleasant stressor.

distress Stress resulting from an unpleasant stressor.

Figure 2-3 The general adaptation syndrome. Selye observed a predictable sequence of responses to stress. During the alarm phase, a lower resistance to injury is evident. With continued stress, resistance to injury is actually enhanced. With prolonged exposure to repeated stressors, exhaustion sets in, with a return of low resistance levels seen during acute stress.

of after a long, busy day. It's a life-threatening type of physiological exhaustion characterized by symptoms such as distorted perceptions and disorganized thinking.

Allostatic Load

While Selye's model of GAS is still viewed as a key contribution to modern stress theory, some aspects of it are now discounted. For example, increased susceptibility to disease after repeated or prolonged stress is now thought to be due to the effects of the stress response itself rather than to a depletion of resources (Selye's exhaustion state). In particular, long-term overexposure to stress hormones such as cortisol has been linked with health problems. (High cortisol levels are associated with metabolic syndrome, a condition linked to increased risk of heart disease, diabetes, depression, and osteoporosis; metabolic syndrome is discussed further in Chapter 15.)

The long-term wear and tear of the stress response is called the *allostatic load.* An individual's allostatic load is dependent on many factors, including genetics, life experiences, and emotional and behavioral responses to stressors. A high allostatic load may be due to frequent stressors, poor adaptation to common stressors, an inability to shut down the stress response, or imbalances in the stress response of different body systems. A high allostatic load is linked with heart disease, hypertension, obesity, and reduced brain and immune system functioning. In other words, when your allostatic load exceeds your ability to cope, you are more likely to get sick.

Psychoneuroimmunology

One of the most fruitful areas of current research into the relationship between stress and disease is **psychoneuroimmunology (PNI).** PNI is the study of the interactions among the nervous system, the endocrine system, and the immune system. The underlying premise of PNI is that stress, through the actions of the nervous and endocrine systems, impairs the immune system and thereby affects health. But although there is strong evidence that stress-related suppression of the immune system can

increase vulnerability to disease in animals, the evidence in healthy humans is less clear. Even large stress-induced immune changes can have small clinical (medical) consequences because they are short term or because the immune system has redundant components and compensates for changes. In short, the immune system is remarkably flexible and capable of substantial change without compromising health. On the other hand, chronic stress in individuals predisposed to or experiencing disease may have more substantial consequences.

Researchers have discovered a complex network of nerve and chemical connections between the nervous and endocrine systems and the immune system. In general, increased levels of cortisol are linked to a decreased number of immune system cells, or lymphocytes (see Chapter 17 for more on the immune system). Epinephrine and norepinephrine appear to promote the release of lymphocytes but at the same time reduce their efficiency. Interestingly, scientists have identified hormone-like substances called neuropeptides that appear to translate stressful emotions into biochemical events, some of which impact the immune system, providing a physical link between emotions and immune function.

It is important to note that different types of stress may affect immunity in different ways. For instance, during acute stress (typically lasting between 5 and 100 minutes), white blood cells are selectively redistributed into the skin, where they contribute to enhancement of the immune response. During a stressful event sequence, such as loss of a loved one or a personal trauma and the events that follow, there are typically no overall significant immune changes. Chronic stressors such as caregiving or unemployment have negative effects on almost all functional measures of immunity. Chronic stress may cause prolonged secretion of cortisol and may accelerate the course of diseases that involve inflammation, including multiple sclerosis, heart disease, and type 2 diabetes.

Mood, personality, behavior, and immune functioning are intertwined. For example, people who are generally pessimistic may neglect the basics of health care, become passive when ill, and fail to engage in health-promoting behaviors. People who are depressed may reduce physical activity and social interaction, which may in turn affect the immune system and the cognitive appraisal of a stressor. Optimism, successful coping, and positive problem solving, on the other hand, may positively influence immunity. The pattern of interaction between the stress and immune responses allows for regulation of energy mobilization and redirection that is necessary to fight attackers both within and without.

Links Between Stress and Specific Conditions

Although much remains to be learned, it is clear that people who have unresolved chronic stress in their lives or who handle stressors poorly are at risk for a wide range of health problems. In the short term, the problem might be just a cold, a stiff neck, or a stomachache. Over the long term, the problems can be more severe—cardiovascular disease (CVD), high blood pressure, impaired immune function, or accelerated aging.

Cardiovascular Disease   During the stress response, heart rate increases and blood vessels constrict, causing blood pressure to rise. Chronic high blood pressure is a major cause of **atherosclerosis**, a disease in which blood vessels become damaged and caked with fatty deposits. These deposits can block arteries, causing heart attacks and strokes. The stress response can precipitate a heart attack in someone with underlying atherosclerosis. The stress response can also cause stress cardiomyopathy ("broken heart syndrome"), a condition that mimics a heart attack but doesn't actually damage the heart.

Certain types of emotional responses may increase a person's risk of CVD. So-called hot reactors, people who exhibit extreme increases in heart rate and blood pressure in response to emotional stressors, may face an increased risk of cardiovascular problems. As described earlier, people who tend to react to situations with anger and hostility are more likely to have heart attacks than are people with a less explosive, more trusting personality.

Stress has also been linked to some of the more recently identified risk factors for CVD. For example, inflammation is a key component of the damage to blood vessels that leads to heart attacks. Stress increases inflammation throughout the body. Stress-induced increases in inflammatory messenger molecules are also linked to elevated levels of homocysteine and c-reactive protein (CRP), two compounds that appear to be markers for CVD risk. Stress-related depression and anger are associated with elevated homocysteine levels, and job-related exhaustion is linked to high CRP levels in some people. Elevated CRP levels have also been implicated in insulin resistance and the development of diabetes, which is in turn a risk factor for CVD. It is clear that alleviation of stress can improve cardiovascular health. Refer to Chapter 15 for more on CVD.

Altered Functioning of the Immune System
Sometimes you seem to get sick when you can least afford it—during exam week, when you're going on vacation, or when you have a big job interview. As research in PNI suggests, this is more than mere coincidence. Some of the health problems linked to stress-related changes in immune function include the following:

- *Colds and other infections.* Stress can leave people more vulnerable to contracting a cold and less able to fight one off.

- *Asthma and allergies.* Stress is a trigger or aggravator of asthma, hives, eczema, and other allergies.

- *Cancer.* One function of the immune system is to recognize and destroy any abnormal cells produced in the body; left unchecked, such cells can develop into cancerous tumors. Stress does not cause cancer, but by compromising the immune system, it may increase a person's chance of developing cancer and decrease her or his chance of surviving it.

- *Chronic disease flare-ups.* Symptoms of diseases such as genital herpes and HIV infection may flare up during episodes of stress. In addition to decreasing the effectiveness of the immune system, stress may also distract people from their commitment to important disease-management behaviors such as eating a healthy diet, exercising, and taking medications.

Psychological Problems   The hormones and other chemicals released during the stress response cause emotional as well as physical changes (see the box "Stress and Your Brain"). Moreover, many stressors—a hurricane, for example, or the death of a loved one—are inherently anxiety-producing, depressing, or both. Stress has been found to contribute to psychological problems such as depression, panic attacks, anxiety, eating disorders, and post-traumatic stress disorder (PTSD). PTSD, which afflicts war veterans, rape and child abuse survivors, and others who have suffered or witnessed severe trauma, is characterized by nightmares, flashbacks, and a diminished capacity to experience or express emotion. (For more information, see Chapter 3.)

Other Health Problems   Many other health problems may be caused or worsened by uncontrolled stress, including the following:

- *Digestive problems.* Stress is associated with stomachaches, diarrhea, and constipation, and it may aggravate problems such as irritable bowel syndrome and ulcers.

- *Headaches.* Muscle contractions and changes in blood vessels associated with the stress response can cause tension headaches and trigger migraines (see the box "Headaches: A Common Symptom of Stress" on p. 43).

Terms

psychoneuroimmunology (PNI) The study of the interactions among the brain, the endocrine system, and the immune system.

atherosclerosis The buildup of fatty material in the lining of arteries that have become damaged from advancing age or high blood pressure; a leading cause of heart disease and stroke.

Like a computer that registers information in response to typing on a keyboard, your brain is able to respond to and store information about changes in your environment. Unlike a computer, your brain has the attribute of plasticity—it physically changes its structure and function in response to experience. Also unlike a computer, your brain is altered by psychological stress. Moderate stress enhances the ability to acquire information and remember daily events, while high levels of acute stress can impair learning. For example, people can often remember minute details following a fender bender but can't recall the events surrounding a

major car crash. Thus, it is good to be a little bit nervous before an exam—but not highly anxious.

The effects of stress on brain form and function are apparent in a structure called the hippocampus, which is involved in learning and memory. High levels of chronic stress cause brain cells (neurons) in the hippocampus to shrink in size or die, thus impairing learning and memory. Exciting new research in neuroscience has revealed that the hippocampus actually grows new neurons during adulthood. However, stress acts to reduce new cell birth in the hippocampus, reducing the replacement of lost

neurons. Together, these effects of stress result in fewer neurons and fewer connections between neurons in the hippocampus, thus decreasing the capacity for information processing. People who are depressed or who suffer from posttraumatic stress disorder have higher levels of stress hormones in their bloodstream and smaller hippocampi than others. Even in the absence of a serious disorder, it is thought that the accumulation of stress effects across the life span can contribute to brain aging. Thus, the way you cope with stress can affect the way your brain works both immediately and over the long term.

• *Insomnia and fatigue.* Chemical messengers produced during the fight-or-flight reaction promote alertness and ward off sleep. Sleep disruption in turn can produce fatigue and memory loss and, in the long run, can lead to more serious health problems.

• *Injuries.* Stress may distract people and cause them to become less vigilant about key injury prevention behaviors such as wearing a safety belt or bicycle helmet. On-the-job injuries, including repetitive-strain injury (RSI), are also linked to job stress.

• *Endocrine effects and pregnancy complications.* Menstrual irregularities and impotence are both associated with periods of unusual stress. The stress response is an integral part of menstruation and pregnancy, but women who experience significant additional stress before or during pregnancy may have an increased risk of delivering a premature or low-birth-weight infant. Certain stress-related factors may also affect the timing and experience of menopause. See Chapters 5 and 8 for more information on menstruation, pregnancy, and menopause.

• *Type 2 diabetes.* In the most common form of diabetes, glucose builds up in the bloodstream because the body doesn't produce enough insulin and/or the body's cells are insulin resistant. Cortisol stimulates the release of glucose from the liver and muscle cells into the bloodstream; chronic stress may contribute to the development of diabetes and exacerbate symptoms in those who already have it.

COMMON SOURCES OF STRESS

We are surrounded by stressors—at home, at school, on the job, and within ourselves. Being able to recognize

potential sources of stress is an important step in successfully managing the stress in our lives.

Major Life Changes

Any major change in your life that requires adjustment and accommodation can be a source of stress. Early adulthood and the college years are typically associated with many significant changes, such as moving out of the family home, establishing new relationships, setting educational and career goals, and developing a sense of identity and purpose. Even changes typically thought of as positive—graduation, job promotion, marriage—can be stressful. For older students, the collection of major life changes may be different but just as powerful—the challenge of balancing school, work, and family responsibilities; parenting teenagers; relationship stress; and providing care for aging parents.

Clusters of major life changes may be linked to the development of health problems in some people. Research indicates that some life changes, particularly those that are perceived negatively, can affect health. However, personality and coping skills are important moderating influences. People with a strong support network and a stress-resistant personality are less likely to become ill in response to major life changes than people with fewer internal and external resources.

Daily Hassles

Have you done any of the following in the past week?

• Misplaced your keys, wallet, or an assignment
• Had an argument with a troublesome neighbor, coworker, or customer

Are you among the more than 45 million Americans who have chronic, recurrent headaches? Headaches come in various types but are often grouped into three major categories: tension headaches, migraines, and cluster headaches. Other types of headaches have underlying organic causes, such as sinus congestion or infection.

Tension Headaches

Approximately 90% of all headaches are tension headaches, characterized by a dull, steady pain, usually on both sides of the head. It may feel as though a band of pressure is tightening around the head, and the pain may extend to the neck and shoulders. Acute tension headaches may last from hours to days, while chronic tension headaches may occur almost every day for months or even years. Psychological stress, poor posture, and immobility are the leading causes of tension headaches. There is no cure, but the pain can sometimes be relieved with over-the-counter painkillers and with therapies such as massage, relaxation, hot or cold showers, and rest.

If your headaches are frequent, keep a diary with details about the events surrounding each one. Are your headaches associated with late nights, academic deadlines, or long periods spent sitting at a computer? If you can identify the stressors that are consistently associated with your headaches, you can begin to gain more control over the situation. If you suffer persistent tension headaches, you should consult your physician.

Migraines

Migraines typically progress through a series of stages lasting from several minutes to several days. They may produce a variety of symptoms, including throbbing pain that starts on one side of the head and may spread; heightened sensitivity to light; visual disturbances such as flashing lights; nausea; and fatigue. About 70% of migraine sufferers are women, and migraine headaches may have a genetic component. Research suggests that people who get migraines may have abnormally excitable nerve cells in their brains. When triggered, these nerve cells send a wave of electrical activity throughout the brain, which in turn causes migraine symptoms. Potential triggers include menstruation, stress, fatigue, atmospheric changes, specific sounds or odors, and certain foods. The frequency of attacks varies from a few in a lifetime to several per week.

Keeping a headache journal can help a migraine sufferer identify headache triggers—the first step to avoiding them. In addition, many new treatments can help reduce the frequency, severity, and duration of migraines.

Cluster Headaches

Cluster headaches are extremely severe headaches that cause intense pain in and around one eye. They usually occur in clusters of one to three headaches each day over a period of weeks or months, alternating with periods of remission in which no headaches occur. About 90% of people with cluster headaches are male. There is no known cause or cure for cluster headaches, but a number of treatments are available. During cluster periods, it is important to refrain from smoking cigarettes and drinking alcohol, because these activities can trigger attacks.

For more on treating headaches, as well as warning signs for when a headache may signal a serious illness, refer to the self-care guide in Appendix B.

- Waited in a long line or been stuck in traffic or had another problem with transportation
- Worried about money
- Been upset about the weather

While major life changes are undoubtedly stressful, they seldom occur regularly. Psychologist Richard Lazarus has proposed that minor problems—life's daily hassles—can be an even greater source of stress because they occur much more often. People who perceive hassles negatively are likely to experience a moderate stress response every time they are faced with one. Over time, this can take a significant toll on health. Researchers have found that for some people daily hassles contribute to a general decrease in overall wellness. Remember, stress levels and coping abilities contribute to overall allostatic load.

College Stressors

College is a time of major life changes and abundant minor hassles. You will be learning new information and skills and making major decisions about your future. You may be away from home for the first time, or you may be adding extra responsibilities to a life already filled with job and family.

Academic Stressors Exams, grades, and choosing a major are among the many academic stressors faced by college students. In addition to an increased workload compared to that in high school, many students are unpleasantly surprised by the more rigorous evaluation of their work in college. Higher-quality efforts are expected of college students, so earning good grades takes more effort and dedication. Careful planning and preparation can help make academic stressors more predictable and manageable. Techniques for overcoming test anxiety, a common stress-related academic problem, are described in the Behavior Change Strategy at the end of the chapter.

Students close to graduation may find themselves faced with the need to plan for life after college—a potentially daunting task. Remember that you'll have many opportunities to change career paths in the future and that the training and life experience gained from one path can often be transferred to other endeavors.

Interpersonal Stressors   The college years often involve potential stressors such as establishing new relationships and balancing multiple roles—student, employee, friend, spouse, parent, and so on. You'll have the opportunity to meet new people and make new friends at the start of every term and in every new class and activity. Social engagements may be exhilarating for some and painful for others. Viewed as an exciting challenge or an odious necessity, interacting with others involves attention, on-the-spot decision making, and energy expenditure—and it's stressful. Be yourself, go with the flow, and try not to be overly concerned with being liked by everyone you meet.

Time-Related Pressures   Do you accept too many responsibilities or manage your time poorly? Time pressures are a problem for most students, but they may be particularly acute for those who also have job and family responsibilities. Most people do have enough time to fulfill all of their responsibilities but fail to manage their time or their priorities effectively. For these people, it's important to make a plan and *stick to it*. Strategies for effective time management are described in the next section.

Financial Concerns   As young adults leave home and become independent, financial responsibilities such as paying tuition, taking out loans, and managing living expenses are likely to arise. To complicate matters, tuition rates and competition for scholarships are at all-time highs, outpacing increases in family income. As college has become less affordable, more students are borrowing—and are borrowing more—to pay for college. Most students work full-time during the summer and part-time during the school year in order to meet their financial needs; some work full-time and support a family during the school year, creating additional time pressures. A student loan repayment looming over your head can also create substantial worries. A financial budget is as important as effective time management for successfully dealing with college stress. Create a financial plan for each upcoming month or term so you can put your mind more at ease and concentrate on your studies.

Stressors Among Nontraditional Students
Nontraditional students can be defined as individuals who, in addition to attending college, are married, a parent, a caretaker for an older family member, a full-time worker, and/or retraining for a new career. According to the National Center for Education Statistics, about 70% of undergraduates meet at least one of these criteria. Nontraditional students must often contend with the stress of increased responsibilities compared with traditional students, who are typically younger and have fewer demands

on their time. Interestingly, nontraditional students have been shown to have higher class attendance, less worry about academic performance, and greater enjoyment of homework; they are more likely to report concern about family responsibilities. Traditional students report being more concerned with social and peer relationships.

For nontraditional students, college enrollment stress can potentially disrupt family stability. Thus, more time and energy must be devoted to family concerns to offset this stress effect. Greater social support, especially from family and friends, is a stress buffer for married students and is related to better academic adjustment, personal and social adjustment, and commitment to college. However, married college students express greater marital distress than married couples not attending college. Married graduate students report more satisfaction with their educational programs but less satisfaction with their social and extracurricular activities, whereas commuting couples report less satisfaction with the time they are able to spend with their spouses compared with noncommuting couples. Time pressures may be especially severe for nontraditional students, so time-management strategies may be of particular importance.

Job-Related Stressors

More than one-third of Americans report that they always feel rushed, and nearly half say they would give up a day's pay for a day off. Tight schedules and overtime contribute to time-related pressures. Worries about job performance, salary, and job security are a source of stress for some people. Interactions with bosses, coworkers, and customers can also contribute to stress. High levels of job stress are also common for people who are left out of important decisions relating to their jobs. When workers are given the opportunity to shape how their jobs are performed, job satisfaction goes up and stress levels go down.

If job-related (or college-related) stress is severe or chronic, the result can be **burnout,** a state of physical, mental, and emotional exhaustion. Burnout occurs most often in highly motivated and driven individuals who feel that their work is not recognized or that they are not accomplishing their goals. People in the helping professions—teachers, social workers, caregivers, police officers, and so on—are also prone to burnout. For some who suffer from burnout, a vacation or leave of absence may be appropriate. For others, a reduced work schedule, better communication with superiors, or a change in job goals may be necessary. Improving time-management skills can also help.

Surveys indicate that as many as 40% of U.S. workers rate their jobs as "very or extremely stressful," and 25% say they are often or very often "burned out by their work." Problems at work are more strongly associated with health complaints than with any other life stressor—more so than even financial problems or family problems. Some 32.9 million working days are lost annually from people taking time

Term

VW   **burnout** A state of physical, mental, and emotional exhaustion.

Diverse Populations, Discrimination, and Stress

Dimensions of Diversity

Stress is universal, but within the United States, a nation defined by its diversity, some groups face unique stressors and have higher-than-average rates of stress-related physical and emotional problems. These groups include ethnic minorities and people with low incomes, disabilities, or atypical gender identities or sexual orientations. Many of the unique stressors that affect special populations stem from prejudice—biased, negative attitudes toward a group of people.

Discrimination occurs when people act according to their prejudices; it can be blatant or subtle. Blatant examples of discrimination are not common, but they are major stressors akin to significant life changes. Examples include a swastika painted on a Jewish studies house, the defacement of a sculpture honoring the achievements of a gay artist, and bullying of poor children because they wear the same clothes to school each day. Subtler acts may occur much more frequently. For example, an African American student in a mostly white college town feels that shopkeepers are keeping an eye on him; a male-to-female transgendered individual believes she has been "clocked" (discovered) and treated with less respect

by her professors and peers; a student using a wheelchair has difficulty with narrow aisles and high counters at local stores; and an obese executive is asked to purchase two seats on his business flights. Some of these social stressors are unique to certain groups, and it may be difficult for other people to understand how serious such stressors can be.

Recent immigrants to the United States must begin new lives in a new society; the stress associated with this process is called *acculturation stress*. Successful integration into a new society can occur in an open society where immigrants are free to retain any aspect of their cultural heritage and their native social customs and beliefs are valued. If there is great pressure to assimilate, minority immigrant groups may become disconnected from both their own culture and that of the host culture; marginalized groups can be targets of significant discrimination, even violence. Different immigrant groups experience variations in accultural stressors. For example, language barriers and limited formal education may make employment more difficult for some groups. In other groups, intense pressure is put on immigrant

children to do well in school and enter high-paying professions to boost the honor and position of the family; these high expectations can be a source of stress, guilt, and alienation from the family.

Minorities often face additional job- and school-related stressors because of stereotypes and discrimination. They make less money than whites in comparable jobs and with comparable levels of education, and they may find it more difficult to achieve leadership positions. Many ethnic minorities must develop basic skills that natives of the host nation take for granted; for example, learning to speak English, balancing ancestral and American cultures, and finding employment sufficient to pay for basic necessities. All these types of stressors can contribute to higher levels of stress-related health problems among minorities.

On a positive note, many people who experience hardship, disability, or prejudice develop effective, goal-directed coping skills and are successful at overcoming obstacles and managing the increased stress they face. Resiliency, hopeful expectations for the future, and spiritual wellness all support successful coping.

off because of illness. Mood and sleep disturbances, upset stomachs, headaches, and disturbed relationships with family and friends are examples of stress-related problems that are quick to develop, but the effects of job stress on chronic diseases are more difficult to see because chronic diseases take a long time to develop and can be influenced by many factors other than job stress. However, it is important to note that health care expenditures are nearly 50% greater for workers who report high levels of stress.

Job stress results from the interaction of the worker and the conditions of work. Employers are becoming more aware that unhealthy behaviors such as smoking and a sedentary lifestyle adversely affect the health and productivity of their employees and, ultimately, the bottom line. As a result, some employers are providing their employees with a variety of worksite-based health promotion and disease prevention programs, including stress-management programs. Worksite programs have been shown to improve employee health, increase productivity, and yield a significant return on investment for the employer. Check with your employer about what types of programs might be available and useful for you.

Social Stressors

Social networks that affect stress may be real or virtual; each type can help boost your ability to deal with the stress in your life or can itself become a stressor.

Real Social Networks Although social support is a key buffer against stress, your interactions with others can themselves be a source of stress. As mentioned earlier, the college years are often a time of great change in interpersonal relationships. The community and society in which you live can also be major sources of stress. Social stressors include prejudice and discrimination. You may feel stress as you try to relate to people of other ethnic or socioeconomic groups. As a member of a particular ethnic group, you may feel pressure to assimilate into mainstream society. If English is not your first language, you face the added burden of conducting many daily activities in a language with which you may not be completely comfortable. All of these pressures can become significant sources of stress. (See the box "Diverse Populations, Discrimination, and Stress" for more information.)

Mass violence occurs somewhat frequently in big cities—for example, when a deeply disturbed person gains access to guns or explosives. Certain areas of the country are also prone to natural disasters like hurricanes, flooding, and earthquakes. Less frequent in the United States are terrorist events such as those that occurred in Oklahoma in April 1995 or in Manhattan in February 1993 and September 2001. Not only do many people suffer direct physical harm during such events, but larger numbers of survivors, witnesses, and emergency personnel experience long-term psychological distress. While most recover, some develop post-traumatic stress disorder (PTSD), a more serious condition.

Cognitive, emotional, and behavioral reactions to trauma are highly variable, and it is normal for an individual to experience a variety of responses. Reactions may include disbelief and shock, fear, anger and resentment, anxiety about the future, difficulty concentrating or making decisions, mood swings, irritability, sadness and depression, panic, guilt, apathy, feelings of isolation or powerlessness, and many of the symptoms of excess stress (see the box on p. 33). Reactions may occur immediately or may be delayed until weeks or months after the event.

Signs of PTSD include reexperiencing the trauma in dreams and intrusive thoughts, feeling generally numb or detached from life, and feeling jumpy or hypervigilant. Following the September 11, 2001, attacks in New York, risk factors for PTSD included being a young adult (age 18–29), being female, having little social support, being close to the site of the attacks or involved in the rescue efforts, and watching a large amount of television coverage. The severity of a person's reaction is not necessarily proportional to the degree of objective loss; in some cases, for example, a person who watches events unfold in the media may experience a more negative or a longer-lasting reaction than someone more directly involved. See Chapter 3 for more on PTSD.

Taking positive steps can help you cope with difficult emotions. Consider the following strategies:

- Immediately after such an event, it is okay to break from your daily routine to evaluate your situation and mourn for others. It is important to share your experiences and feelings with empathetic listeners. Be a supportive listener yourself, and reassure children of their safety.

- Take a break from media coverage. Try to refrain from developing

nightmare scenarios for the future or generalizing the situation to all aspects of your life. Instead, find ways to help yourself and others. Donating money, blood, food, clothes, or time can ease difficult emotions and give you a greater sense of control. (In the aftermath of the September 11 attacks, such active coping strategies were shown to be related to lower rates of acute stress and PTSD.) For some people, forming political opinions provides a frame of reference through which to respond to terrorism, and voting can be a coping response because it is another way for people to exert some control over their futures.

- As time passes, maintain your schedule at home, school, and work. Continue to take care of your mind and body. Choose a healthy diet, exercise regularly, get plenty of sleep, and practice relaxation techniques. Try to avoid negative coping techniques such as using alcohol or other drugs.

Everyone copes with and recovers from tragedy differently. If you still feel overwhelmed by your emotions even weeks or months after the event, seek professional help.

Virtual Social Networks New technologies can potentially be time-savers because we don't have to go home or to the office to check our e-mail or phone messages, and we can call on a cell phone rather than jot down notes to pass on at a later time. Telecommuting can ease the time pressures on people who find it necessary to work from home, such as parents with young children or people with disabilities. However, increased electronic interactivity can also impinge on our personal space, waste time, and cause stress. For example, count the number of times you check for e-mail or voice messages and find that you have none, or the times you are interrupted by messages that are relatively meaningless. If your instructor or supervisor knows that you are not tied to a land line, he or she may expect a greater degree of communication and the ability to meet unusual deadlines. If you are experiencing information overload, learn to use multimedia devices wisely. Give out your phone number only when it is absolutely necessary. Schedule times when you completely sever your electronic ties. Consider the

financial savings that may arise from less frequent cell phone use.

Environmental Stressors

Claire loves the food at a certain restaurant, but she always feels "on edge" when eating there because of continuous loud background music. This is an example of an environmental stressor—some condition or event in the physical environment that causes stress. Environmental stressors include natural disasters, acts of violence, industrial accidents, and intrusive noises, smells, or sights. Like the loud music that bothers Claire, some environmental stressors are mere inconveniences that are easy to avoid. Others, such as pollen season for a hayfever sufferer or living next to a construction site, may be an unavoidable daily source of stress. For those who live in poor or violent neighborhoods or in a war-torn country, environmental stressors can be major life stressors (see the box "Coping After Terrorism, Mass Violence, or Natural Disasters").

Internal Stressors

Some stressors are found not in our interactions with our environment but within ourselves. We put pressure on ourselves to reach personal goals, and we continuously evaluate our progress and performance. Setting high goals and then striving to reach them can enhance self-esteem if the goals are reasonable. However, unrealistic expectations can be a significant source of stress and a serious blow to self-esteem. Other internal stressors are physical and emotional states such as illness and exhaustion; these can be both a cause and an effect of unmanaged stress.

TECHNIQUES FOR MANAGING STRESS

What can you do about all this stress? A great deal. By shoring up your social support systems; improving your communication skills; developing and maintaining healthy exercise, eating, and sleeping habits; and mastering simple techniques to identify and moderate individual stressors, you can learn to control the stress in your life—instead of allowing it to control you. The effort is well worth the time: People who manage stress effectively not only are healthier but also have more time to enjoy life and accomplish their goals.

Social Support

People need people. Sharing fears, frustrations, and joys not only makes life richer but also seems to contribute to the well-being of body and mind. Research supports this conclusion. One study of college students living in overcrowded apartments, for example, found that those with a strong social support system were less distressed by their cramped quarters than were the loners who navigated life's challenges on their own. Participation in a support group has been shown to improve the emotional health of cancer patients. Other studies have shown that married people live longer than single people and have lower death rates from a wide range of conditions. People with a strong social support system are also better able to withstand the stress of major life changes. The crucial common denominator in all these findings is meaningful connections with others.

Allow yourself time to nourish and maintain a network of people at home, at work, at school, or in your community that you can count on for emotional support, feedback, and nurturance. Consider becoming a volunteer to help build your social support system and enhance your spiritual wellness (see the section on spirituality later in the chapter). To evaluate your current social support system and to find strategies for strengthening your social ties, refer to the box "Healthy Connections" on page 48.

Exercise is a particularly effective antidote to stress.

Communication

Do you often find yourself angry at others? Some people express their anger directly by yelling or being aggressive; others express anger indirectly by excessively criticizing others or making cynical comments. A person who is angry with others often has difficulty forming and maintaining successful social relationships. Better communication skills can help: Learn to listen to others and to express your needs and desires nonaggressively. Increase your communication skills in order to decrease stress in your relationships—at school, at work, and at home.

At the other extreme, you may suppress your feelings and needs entirely. You may have trouble saying no and allow people to take advantage of you. Many businesses encourage employees to take assertiveness training workshops to help them overcome shyness and resistance to communicating their needs. Such communication skills are also valuable in social relationships. (For a fuller discussion of how to enhance communication and resolve interpersonal conflicts, see Chapters 3 and 4.)

Exercise

Exercise helps maintain a healthy body and mind and even stimulates the birth of new brain cells. Regular physical activity can reduce various aspects of stress as well. One recent study found that taking a long walk can help decrease anxiety and blood pressure. Another study found that just a brisk 10-minute walk leaves people feeling more relaxed and energetic for up to 2 hours. People who exercise regularly react with milder physical stress responses before, during, and after exposure to stressors. People who took three brisk 45-minute walks a week

Healthy Connections

Meaningful connections with others can play a key role in stress management and overall wellness. A sense of isolation can lead to chronic stress, which in turn can increase your susceptibility to temporary illnesses like colds and to chronic illnesses like heart disease. Although the mechanism isn't clear, social isolation can be as significant to mortality rates as factors like smoking, high blood pressure, and obesity.

There is no single best pattern of social support that works for everyone. However, research suggests that having a variety of types of relationships may be important for wellness. To help determine whether your social network measures up, answer true or false for each of the following statements.

T/F 1. If I needed an emergency loan of $100, there is someone I could get it from.

T/F 2. There is someone who takes pride in my accomplishments.

T/F 3. I often meet or talk with family or friends.

T/F 4. Most people I know think highly of me.

T/F 5. If I needed an early morning ride to the airport, there's no one I would feel comfortable asking to take me.

T/F 6. I feel there is no one with whom I can share my most private worries and fears.

T/F 7. Most of my friends are more successful making changes in their life than I am.

T/F 8. I would have a hard time finding someone to go with me on a day trip to the beach or country.

To calculate your score, add the number of true answers to questions 1–4 and the number of false answers to questions 5–8. If your score is 4 or more, you should have enough support to protect your health. If your score is 3 or less, you may need to reach out. There are a variety of things you can do to strengthen your social ties:

• *Foster friendships.* Keep in regular contact with your friends. Offer respect, trust, and acceptance, and provide help and support in times of need. Express appreciation for your friends.

• *Keep your family ties strong.* Stay in touch with the family members you feel close to. Participate in family activities and celebrations. If your family doesn't function well as a support system for its members, create a second "family" of people with whom you have built meaningful ties.

• *Get involved with a group.* Do volunteer work, take a class, attend a lecture series, join a religious group. These types of activities can give you a sense of security, a place to talk about your feelings or concerns, and a way to build new friendships. Choose activities that are meaningful to you and that include direct involvement with other people.

• *Build your communication skills.* The more you share your feelings with others, the closer the bonds between you will become. When others are speaking, be a considerate and attentive listener. (Chapters 3 and 4 include more information on effective communication.)

Individual relationships change over the course of your life, but it's never too late to build friendships or become more involved in your community. Your investment of time and energy in your social network will pay off—in a brighter outlook now, and in better health and well-being for the future.

SOURCE: Friends can be good medicine. 1998. As found in the *Mind/Body Newsletter* 7(1): 3–6. Center for the Advancement of Health; Quiz from Japenga, A. 1995. A Family of Friends. *Health*, November/December, 1994. Adapted with permission. Copyright © 2001 *Health*® magazine. For subscriptions please call 800-274-2522.

---

for 3 months reported that they perceived fewer daily hassles. Their sense of wellness also increased.

These findings are not surprising since, as stated earlier, the stress response mobilizes energy resources and readies the body for physical emergencies. If you experience stress and do not physically exert yourself, you are not completing the energy cycle. You may not be able to exercise while your daily stressors occur—during class, for example, or while sitting in a traffic jam—but you can be active later in the day. Physical activity allows you to expend the nervous energy you have built up and trains your body to more readily achieve homeostasis following future disturbances in normal functioning.

It's not hard to incorporate light to moderate exercise into your day. Walk to class or bike to the store instead of driving. Use the stairs instead of the elevator. Take a walk with a friend instead of getting a cup of coffee. Go bowling, play tennis, or roller-skate instead of seeing a movie.

Make a habit of taking a brisk after-dinner stroll. Plan hikes and easy bike outings for the weekends.

Consider taking a class in a kind of exercise you've always wanted to try, such as yoga, t'ai chi, square dancing, or fencing. The important thing is to find an activity that you enjoy, so it can become a habit and thereby an effective stress reducer. Chapter 13 presents guidelines for creating an exercise program to fit your individual needs and preferences.

Nutrition

A healthy diet will give you an energy bank to draw on whenever you experience stress. Eating wisely also will enhance your feelings of self-control and self-esteem. Learning the principles of sound nutrition is easy, and sensible eating habits rapidly become second nature when practiced regularly. (For more on sound nutrition, see Chapter 12.)

Mind/Body/Spirit

Avoiding or limiting caffeine is also important in stress management. Although one or two cups of coffee a day probably won't hurt you, caffeine is a mildly addictive stimulant that leaves some people jittery, irritable, and unable to sleep. Consuming caffeine during stressful situations can raise blood pressure and increase levels of cortisol. Tea, cola, some other soft drinks, chocolate, and more than a thousand over-the-counter drugs, including cold remedies, aspirin, and weight-loss preparations, also contain caffeine, sometimes in high doses.

Sleep

Lack of sleep can be both a cause and an effect of excess stress. Without sufficient sleep, our mental and physical processes steadily deteriorate. We get headaches, feel irritable, are unable to concentrate, forget things, and may be more susceptible to weight gain and illness. Levels of the stress hormones in the bloodstream vary throughout the day and are related to sleep patterns. Peak concentrations occur in the early morning, followed by a slow decline during the day and evening. Concentrations return to peak during the final stages of sleep and in the early morning hours. Acute sleep deprivation slows the daytime decline in stress hormones, so evening levels are higher than normal. A decrease in total sleep time also causes an increase in the release of stress hormones. Together, these changes may cause an increase in stress hormone levels throughout the day and may contribute to mental and physical deterioration. Fatigue and sleep deprivation are major factors in many fatal car, truck, and train crashes. Extreme sleep deprivation can lead to hallucinations and other psychotic symptoms as well as to a significant increase in heart attack risk.

Adequate sleep, on the other hand, improves mood, fosters feelings of competence and self-worth, and supports optimal mental and emotional functioning. If you are sleep-deprived, sleeping extra hours may significantly improve your daytime alertness and mental abilities. Sleep requirements vary considerably among individuals; some adults need only 5 hours of sleep, while others need 9 hours or more to feel fully refreshed and alert.

Sleep occurs in two phases: rapid eye movement (REM) and non-REM. Non-REM sleep consists of four stages of successively deeper sleep, during which blood pressure, heart rate, temperature, and breathing rate drop, growth hormone is released, and brain wave patterns become slow and even. REM sleep, during which dreams occur, is characterized by the rapid back-and-forth movement of the eyes under closed eyelids. Heart rate, blood pressure, and breathing rate increase; brain activity increases to levels equal to or greater than those during waking hours. Muscles in the limbs relax completely, causing temporary paralysis and preventing the sleeper from acting out her or his dreams. A sleeper goes through several cycles of non-REM and REM sleep each night. Stress hormone levels are low during deep sleep and increase during REM sleep. The increase in REM sleep duration with each sleep cycle may underlie the progressive increase in circulating stress hormones during the final stages of sleep.

Nearly everyone, at some time in life, has trouble falling asleep or staying asleep—a condition known as insomnia. The most common causes of insomnia are lifestyle factors, such as high caffeine or alcohol intake before bedtime; medical problems, such as a breathing disorder; and psychological stress. About 75% of people who suffer chronic insomnia report some stressful life event at the onset of their sleep problem. Due to the emotional stress that accompanies sleep disorders, stress-management techniques are often recommended. If you suffer from sleeping problems, try some of the strategies in the box "Overcoming Insomnia."

Time Management

A surprising number of the stressors in most people's lives relate to time. Many people never seem to have enough time, and they always seem to feel overwhelmed by the pace of their lives. Others have too much time on their hands and are often bored. Learning to manage your time successfully is crucial to coping with the stressors you face every day. Three common factors that negatively impact time management for college students are perfectionism, overcommitment, and procrastination.

Perfectionism is the need to constantly improve a project, situation, or personal trait. It is frequently based on a self-deprecating fear of failure or harsh judgment by friends or family. Student perfectionists often spend an inordinate amount of time rewriting papers, reorganizing notes, and rearranging their work space to the point that they sacrifice social interaction and sleep. Perfectionists will torture themselves for getting an A− instead of an A on a test rather than congratulate themselves on a job well done. They will appraise the situation negatively using "should" statements: "I should have studied an hour more each night," "I shouldn't have taken so much time off last weekend," and so on. There is no such thing as perfection, so perfectionists are striving for unreachable goals. This unfulfilled effort increases stress and compromises time spent on other academic projects and social functions that are integral to a fulfilling college experience. If perfectionism is a problem for you, try not to put so much pressure on yourself. Focus on doing your best rather than trying to be the best. College is not a competition; it is a setting for personal growth. Accept your limits and try not to expect so much of yourself or others.

Overcommitters are less concerned with the quality of their efforts. Instead, they take on project after project and activity after activity because they find it difficult to say no or to accurately assess their current workload. Being well-rounded is admirable, but there are only so many sports one can play, so many committees one can serve on, and so many social functions one can attend and still perform well academically. Overcommitters often feel they are missing

Overcoming Insomnia

Take Charge

Most people can overcome insomnia by discovering the cause of poor sleep and taking steps to remedy it. Insomnia that lasts for more than 6 months and interferes with daytime functioning requires consultation with a physician. Sleeping pills are not recommended for chronic insomnia because they can be habit-forming; they also lose their effectiveness over time.

If you're bothered by insomnia, here are some tips for getting a better night's sleep:

- Determine how much sleep you need to feel refreshed the next day, and don't sleep longer than that (but do make sure you get enough).

- Go to bed at the same time every night and, more important, get up at the same time every morning, 7 days a week, regardless of how much sleep you got. Don't nap during the day.

- Exercise every day, but not too close to bedtime. Your metabolism takes up to 6 hours to slow down after exercise.

- Avoid tobacco (nicotine is a stimulant), caffeine in the later part of the day, and alcohol before bedtime (it causes disturbed, fragmented sleep).

- Have a light snack before bedtime; you'll sleep better if you're not hungry.

- Use your bed only for sleep. Don't eat, read, study, or watch television in bed.

- Relax before bedtime with a warm bath (again, not too close to bedtime—allow about 2 hours for your metabolism to slow down afterward), a book, music, or relaxation exercises. Don't lie down in bed until you're sleepy.

- If you don't fall asleep in 15–20 minutes, or if you wake up and can't fall asleep again, get out of bed, leave the room if possible, and do something monotonous until you feel sleepy. Try distracting yourself with imagery instead of counting sheep; imagine yourself on a pleasant vacation or enjoying some beautiful scenery.

- Keep a clear perspective on your plight. Losing a night's sleep isn't the end of the world. Getting upset only makes it harder to fall asleep. Relax, and trust in your body's natural ability to drift off to sleep.

out when they say no to something, and they often don't fully experience many college activities because they don't take the time to immerse themselves in any one thing.

Procrastination—putting something off until later—is a problem for many people. People who put off key tasks and decisions may sabotage personal relationships, college life, careers, and health. Although reasons for procrastination vary, it often camouflages self-doubt, an unreasonable desire for perfection, or a reluctance to make changes. People who set impossibly high standards for themselves may actually protect their self-esteem by procrastinating; if they fail to complete a project, for example, their work will never be evaluated.

If procrastination or another time-related stressor is a problem for you, try some or all of the following strategies for managing your time more productively and creatively:

- *Set priorities.* Divide your tasks into three groups: essential, important, and trivial. Focus on the first two. Ignore the third.

- *Schedule tasks for peak efficiency.* You've undoubtedly noticed you're most productive at certain times of the day (or night). Schedule as many of your tasks for those hours as you can, and stick to your schedule.

- *Set realistic goals, and write them down.* Attainable goals spur you on. Impossible goals, by definition, cause frustration and failure. Fully commit yourself to achieving your goals by putting them in writing.

- *Budget enough time.* For each project you undertake, calculate how long it will take to complete. Then tack on

another 10–15%, or even 25%, as a buffer against mistakes, interruptions, or unanticipated problems.

- *Break down long-term goals into short-term ones.* Instead of waiting for or relying on large blocks of time, use short amounts of time to start a project or keep it moving. Say you have a 50-page report due and are about to panic. Divide the assignment into three tasks: research, outlining, and writing. Then budget enough time slots (of half an hour or an hour) to complete each task. Your steady progress will make you feel so much better that you'll be encouraged to continue.

- *Visualize the achievement of your goals.* By mentally rehearsing your performance of a task, you will be able to reach your goal more smoothly.

- *Keep track of the tasks you put off.* Analyze the reasons why you procrastinate. If the task is difficult or unpleasant, look for ways to make it easier or more fun. If you hate cleaning up your room, break the work into 10-minute tasks and do a little at a time. If you find the readings for one of your classes particularly difficult, choose an especially nice setting for your reading and then reward yourself each time you complete a section or chapter.

- *Consider doing your least favorite tasks first.* Once you have the most unpleasant tasks out of the way, you can have fun with the projects you enjoy more.

- *Consolidate tasks when possible.* For example, try walking to the store so that you run your errands and exercise in the same block of time.

- *Identify quick transitional tasks.* Keep a list of 5-minute tasks you can do while waiting or between other tasks, such as watering your plants, doing the dishes, or checking a homework assignment.

- *Delegate responsibility.* Asking for help when you have too much to do is no cop-out; it's good time management. Just don't delegate to others the jobs you know you should do yourself, such as researching a paper.

- *Say no when necessary.* If the demands made on you don't seem reasonable, say no—tactfully, but without guilt or apology.

- *Give yourself a break.* Allow time for play—free, unstructured time when you ignore the clock. Don't consider this a waste of time. Play renews you and enables you to work more efficiently.

- *Stop thinking or talking about what you're going to do, and just do it!* Sometimes the best solution for procrastination is to stop waiting for the right moment and just get started. You will probably find that things are not as bad as you feared, and your momentum will keep you going.

Strive for Greater Spirituality

Spirituality involves a high level of faith and commitment with respect to a well-defined worldview or belief system that gives a sense of meaning and purpose to existence. Spirituality also provides an ethical path to personal fulfillment that includes connectedness with self, others, and a higher power or larger reality. Overall, there appears to be a positive relationship between spirituality and adaptive coping, suggesting that aspects of spirituality and spiritual practices can play a significant role as a personal resource for coping. Spirituality can be enhanced through many activities, including participation in organized religion, spending time in nature or working on environmental issues, helping others, and engaging in personal spiritual practices such as prayer or meditation.

Despite the benefits of developing spiritual wellness, an ongoing survey of first-year college students found that the goal of succeeding financially has reached its highest point in 13 years, whereas the desire to "develop a meaningful philosophy of life" has dropped to its lowest point in the nearly 40-year history of the survey. On a more positive note, the same survey found high levels of volunteerism among college students. Through volunteering and engaging in personal spiritual practices, we may gain meaning, direction, purpose in life, and a greater sense of connectedness.

Confide in Yourself Through Writing

Confiding in others can help maintain physical and psychological health following a major life trauma. Keeping a diary is analogous to confiding in others, except that you are confiding in yourself. This form of coping with severe stress may be especially helpful for those who are shy or introverted and find it difficult to open up to others. Although writing about traumatic and stressful events may have a short-term negative effect on mood, over the long term, stress may be reduced and positive changes in health occur. A key to promoting beneficial results with respect to health and well-being through journaling is to write about one's emotional responses to a stressful event. Set aside a special time each day or week to journal your feelings about stressful events in your life.

Cognitive Techniques

Some stressors arise in our own minds. Ideas, beliefs, perceptions, and patterns of thinking can add to our stress level. Each of the techniques described below can help you change unhealthy thought patterns to ones that will help you cope with stress. As with any skill, mastering these techniques takes practice and patience.

Think and Act Constructively Worrying, someone once said, is like shoveling smoke. Think back to the worries you had last week. How many of them were needless? Think about things you *can* control. Try to stand aside from the problem, consider the positive steps you can take to solve it, and then carry them out. Remember, successful prediction of a stressful event is a major factor determining the magnitude of the stress response. In the evening, try to predict stressful events you might encounter the following day. Will you see someone who makes you feel uncomfortable? If so, decide now how you will interact with that person. Will you attend a class that doesn't hold your attention? Develop a strategy now that will help you maintain focus. Will you have to wait in line to register or buy tickets? If so, plan to pass the time by listening to music to relax or by catching up on some reading.

Take Control A situation often feels more stressful if you feel you're not in control of it. Time may seem to be slipping away before a big exam, for example. Unexpected obstacles may appear in your path, throwing you off course. When you feel your environment is controlling you instead of the other way around, take charge! Concentrate on what is possible to control, and set realistic goals. Be confident of your ability to succeed.

Problem-Solve Students with greater problem-solving abilities report greater adjustment to university life, higher motivation levels, lower stress levels while studying, and, on average, higher grades. When you find yourself stewing over a problem, take a moment to sit down with a piece of paper and go through a formal process of problem solving. Within a few minutes you can generate a plan. Try this approach:

1. Define the problem in one or two sentences.
2. Identify the causes of the problem.

Managing the many commitments of adult life—including work, school, and parenthood—can sometimes feel overwhelming and produce a great deal of stress. Time-management and problem-solving skills, including careful scheduling with a date book or handheld computer, can help people cope with busy days.

3. Consider alternative solutions; don't just stop with the most obvious one.

4. Weigh positive and negative consequences for each alternative.

5. Make a decision—choose a solution.

6. Make a list of what you will need to do to act on your decision.

7. Begin to carry out your list; if you're unable to do that, temporarily turn to other things.

8. Evaluate the outcome and revise your approach if necessary.

Modify Your Expectations   Expectations are exhausting and restricting. The fewer expectations you have, the more you can live spontaneously and joyfully. The more you expect from others, the more often you will feel let down. And trying to meet the expectations others have of you is often futile.

Maintain Positivity   If you catch your mind beating up on you—"Late for class again! You can't even cope with college! How do you expect to ever hold down a professional job?"—change your inner dialogue. Talk to

yourself as you would to a child you love: "You're a smart, capable person. You've solved other problems; you'll handle this one. Tomorrow you'll simply schedule things so you get to class with a few minutes to spare." (Chapter 3 has more information on self-talk.)

Cultivate Your Sense of Humor   When it comes to stress, laughter may be the best medicine. Even a fleeting smile produces changes in your autonomic nervous system that can lift your spirits. And a few minutes of belly laughing can be as invigorating as brisk exercise. Hearty laughter elevates your heart rate, aids digestion, eases pain, and triggers the release of endorphins and other pleasurable and stimulating chemicals in the brain. After a good laugh, your muscles go slack; your pulse and blood pressure dip below normal. You are relaxed. Cultivate the ability to laugh at yourself, and you'll have a handy and instantly effective stress reliever.

• Keep a humor journal. Write down funny things that you and others say, including unintentional slips of the tongue. Collect clever sayings that make you smile.

• Look at newspaper and magazine cartoons. Cut out those you find particularly funny and add them to your humor journal.

• Collect some funny props—clown noses, "arrow" headbands, Groucho glasses—that you can put on the next time you feel stressed or anxious. Or simply try making funny faces in front of a mirror.

• Watch funny films and television programs. In a study of college students, those who watched an episode of *Seinfeld* prior to giving an impromptu speech were less anxious and had a lower heart rate than those who didn't watch the program.

Weed Out Trivia   A major source of stress is trying to store too much data. Forget unimportant details (they will usually be self-evident) and organize important information. One technique you can try is to "chunk" the important material into categories. If your next exam covers three chapters from your textbook, consider each chapter a chunk of information. Then break down each chunk into its three or four most important features. Create a mental outline that allows you to trace your way from the most general category down to the most specific details. This technique can be applied to managing daily responsibilities as well. Break down your daily tasks into three or four categories, such as academics, family and friends, fitness, and daily living. For each, list the three most important items for the day. Items on the family and friends list might include caring for a child, calling home, and helping a classmate; your daily living items might be going to the dentist, buying gas, and shopping for dinner. Cross items off your mental outline as you complete them to free up memory and attention for the unexpected.

Live in the Present Do you clog your mind by reliving past events? Clinging to experiences and emotions, particularly unpleasant ones, can be a deadly business. Clear your mind of the old debris; let it go. Free yourself to enjoy life today.

Go with the Flow Remember that the branch that bends in the storm doesn't break. Try to flow with your life, accepting the things you can't change. Be forgiving of faults, your own and those of others. Instead of anticipating happiness at some indefinite point in the future, realize that pleasure is integral to being alive. You can create it every day of your life. View challenges as an opportunity to learn and grow. Be flexible. In this way, you can make stress work for you rather than against you, enhancing your overall wellness.

Relaxation Techniques

First identified and described by Herbert Benson of the Harvard Medical School, the **relaxation response** is a physiological state characterized by a feeling of warmth and quiet mental alertness. This is the opposite of the fight-or-flight reaction. When the relaxation response is triggered by a relaxation technique, heart rate, breathing, and metabolism slow down. Blood pressure and oxygen consumption decrease. At the same time, blood flow to the brain and skin increases, and brain waves shift from an alert beta rhythm to a relaxed alpha rhythm. Practiced regularly, relaxation techniques can counteract the debilitating effects of stress.

If you decide to try a relaxation technique, practice it daily until it becomes natural to you, and then use it whenever you feel the need. You may feel calmer and more refreshed after each session. If one technique doesn't seem to work well enough for you after you've given it a good try, try another one. You'll know you've mastered a deep relaxation technique when you start to see subtle changes in other areas of your life: You may notice you've been encountering fewer hassles, working more efficiently, or enjoying more free time. None of the techniques takes long to do—for instance, just a few minutes away from the TV should do the trick.

Progressive Relaxation Unlike most of the others, this simple method requires no imagination, willpower, or self-suggestion. You simply tense, and then relax, the muscles in your body, group by group. The technique, also known as deep muscle relaxation, helps you become aware of the muscle tension that occurs when you're under stress. When you consciously relax those muscles, other systems of the body get the message and ease up on the stress response.

Start, for example, with your right fist. Inhale as you tense it. Exhale as you relax it. Repeat. Next, contract and relax your right upper arm. Repeat. Do the same with your left arm. Then, beginning at your forehead and ending at your feet, contract and relax your other muscle groups. Repeat each contraction at least once, breathing in as you tense, breathing out as you relax. To speed up the process, tense and relax more muscles at one time—both arms simultaneously, for instance. With practice, you'll be able to relax very quickly and effectively by clenching and releasing only your fists.

Visualization Also known as using imagery, **visualization** lets you daydream without guilt. Athletes find that the technique enhances sports performance, and visualization is even part of the curriculum at U.S. Olympic training camps. You can use visualization to help you relax, change your habits, or perform well—whether on an exam, a stage, or a playing field.

Next time you feel stressed, close your eyes. Imagine yourself floating on a cloud, sitting on a mountaintop, or lying in a meadow. What do you see and hear? Is it cold out? Or damp? What do you smell? What do you taste? Involve all your senses. Your body will respond as if your imagery were real. An alternative: Close your eyes and imagine a deep purple light filling your body. Now change the color into a soothing gold. As the color lightens, so should your distress.

Visualization can also be used to rehearse for an upcoming event and enhance performance. By experiencing an event ahead of time in your mind, you can practice coping with any difficulties that may arise. Think positively, and you can "psych yourself up" for a successful experience.

Meditation The need to periodically stop our incessant mental chatter is so great that, from ancient times, hundreds of forms of **meditation** have developed in cultures all over the world. Meditation is a way of telling the mind to be quiet for a while. Because meditation has been at the core of many Eastern religions and philosophies, it has acquired an "Eastern" mystique that has caused some people to shy away from it. Yet meditation requires no special knowledge or background. Whatever philosophical, religious, or emotional reasons may be given for

Terms Vⁱⁱw

relaxation response A physiological state characterized by a feeling of warmth and quiet mental alertness.

visualization A technique for promoting relaxation or improving performance that involves creating or re-creating vivid mental pictures of a place or an experience; also called *imagery*.

meditation A technique for quieting the mind by focusing on a particular word, object (such as a candle flame), or process (such as breathing).

Dr. Herbert Benson developed a simple, practical technique for eliciting the relaxation response.

The Basic Technique

1. Pick a word, phrase, or object to focus on. If you like, you can choose a word or phrase that has a deep meaning for you, but any word or phrase will work. Some meditators prefer to focus on their breathing.

2. Take a comfortable position in a quiet environment, and close your eyes if you're not focusing on an object.

3. Relax your muscles.

4. Breathe slowly and naturally. If you're using a focus word or phrase, silently repeat it each time you exhale. If you're using an object, focus on it as you breathe.

5. Keep a passive attitude. Disregard thoughts that drift in.

6. Continue for 10–20 minutes, once or twice a day.

7. After you've finished, sit quietly for a few minutes with your eyes first closed and then open. Then stand up.

Suggestions

- Allow relaxation to occur at its own pace; don't try to force it. Don't be surprised if you can't tune out your mind for more than a few seconds at a time; it's not a reason for anger or frustration. The more you ignore the intrusions, the easier doing so will become.

- If you want to time your session, peek at a watch or clock occasionally, but don't set a jarring alarm.

- The technique works best on an empty stomach, before a meal or about 2 hours after eating. Avoid times of day when you're tired—unless you want to fall asleep.

- Although you'll feel refreshed even after the first session, it may take a month or more to get noticeable results. Be patient. Eventually the relaxation response will become so natural that it will occur spontaneously, or on demand, when you sit quietly for a few moments.

---

meditation, its power derives from its ability to elicit the relaxation response.

Meditation helps you tune out the world temporarily, removing you from both internal and external sources of stress. It allows you to transcend past conditioning, fixed expectations, and the trivial pursuits of the psyche; it clears out the mental smog. The "thinker" takes time out to become the "observer"—calmly attentive, without analyzing, judging, comparing, or rationalizing. Regular practice of this quiet awareness will subtly carry over into your daily life, encouraging physical and emotional balance no matter what confronts you. For a step-by-step description of a basic meditation technique, see the box "Meditation and the Relaxation Response."

Another form of meditation, known as *mindfulness meditation*, involves paying attention to physical sensations, perceptions, thoughts, and imagery. Instead of focusing on a word or object to quiet the mind, you observe thoughts that do occur without evaluating or judging them. Development of this ability requires regular practice but may eventually result in a more objective view of one's perceptions. It is believed that a greater understanding of one's moment-to-moment thought processes (mindful awareness) provides a richer and more vital sense of life and improves coping. Studies also suggest that people who rate high in mindfulness are less anxious and better able to deal with stress; among people with specific health problems, mindfulness can provide substantial benefits.

Deep Breathing Your breathing pattern is closely tied to your stress level. Deep, slow breathing is associ-

ated with relaxation. Rapid, shallow, often irregular breathing occurs during the stress response. With practice, you can learn to slow and quiet your breathing pattern, thereby also quieting your mind and relaxing your body. Breathing techniques can be used for on-the-spot tension relief as well as for long-term stress reduction.

The primary goal of many breathing exercises is to change your breathing pattern from chest breathing to diaphragmatic ("belly") breathing. During the day, most adults breathe by expanding their chest and raising their shoulders rather than by expanding their abdomen. This pattern of chest breathing is associated with stress, a sedentary lifestyle, restrictive clothing, and cultural preferences for a large chest and a small waist. Diaphragmatic breathing, which involves free expansion of the diaphragm and lower abdomen, is the pattern of breathing characteristic of children and sleeping adults. (The diaphragm is a sheet of muscle and connective tissue that divides the chest and abdominal cavities.) Diaphragmatic breathing is slower and deeper than chest breathing. For instructions on how to perform diaphragmatic breathing, refer to the box "Breathing for Relaxation."

Hatha Yoga *Yoga* is an ancient Sanskrit word referring to the union of mind, body, and soul. The development and practice of yoga are rooted in the Hindu philosophy of spiritual enlightenment. The founders of yoga developed a system of physical postures, called *asanas*, designed to cleanse the body of toxins, calm and clear the mind, bring energy into the body, and raise the level of consciousness.

Breathing for Relaxation

Diaphragmatic Breathing

1. Lie on your back with your body relaxed.

2. Place one hand on your chest and one on your abdomen. (You will use your hands to monitor the depth and location of your breathing.)

3. Inhale slowly and deeply through your nose into your abdomen. Your abdomen should push up as far as is comfortable. Your chest should expand only a little and only in conjunction with the movement of your abdomen.

4. Exhale gently through your mouth.

5. Continue diaphragmatic breathing for about 5–10 minutes per session. Focus on the sound and feel of your breathing.

Breathing In Relaxation, Breathing Out Tension

1. Assume a comfortable position, lying on your back or sitting in a chair.

2. Inhale slowly and deeply into your abdomen. Imagine the inhaled, warm air flowing to all parts of your body. Say to yourself, "Breathe in relaxation."

3. Exhale from your abdomen. Imagine tension flowing out of your body. Say to yourself, "Breathe out tension."

4. Pause before you inhale.

5. Continue for 5–10 minutes or until no tension remains in your body.

Chest Expansion

1. Sit in a comfortable chair, or stand.

2. Inhale slowly and deeply into your abdomen as you raise your arms out to the sides. Pull your shoulders and arms back and lift your chin slightly so that your chest opens up.

3. Exhale gradually as you lower your arms and chin, and return to the starting position.

4. Repeat 5–10 times or until your breathing is deep and regular and your body feels relaxed and energized.

Quick Tension Release

1. Inhale into your abdomen slowly and deeply as you count slowly to four.

2. Exhale slowly as you again count slowly to four. As you exhale, concentrate on relaxing your face, neck, shoulders, and chest.

3. Repeat several times. With each exhalation, feel more tension leaving your body.

SOURCES: Stop stress with a deep breath. 1996. *Health,* October, 53; Breathing for health and relaxation. 1995. *Mental Medicine Update* 4(2): 3–6; When you're stressed, catch your breath. 1995. *Mayo Clinic Health Letter;* December, 5.

Hatha yoga, the most common yoga style practiced in the United States, emphasizes physical balance and breathing control. It integrates components of flexibility, muscular strength and endurance, and muscle relaxation; it also sometimes serves as a preliminary to meditation.

A session of hatha yoga typically involves a series of *asanas,* held for a few seconds to several minutes, that stretch and relax different parts of the body. The emphasis is on breathing, stretching, and balance. There are hundreds of *asanas,* and they must be performed correctly in order to be beneficial. For this reason, qualified instruction is recommended, particularly for beginners. Regardless of whether you accept the philosophy and symbolism of different *asanas,* the practice of yoga can induce the relaxation response as well as develop body awareness, flexibility, and muscular strength and endurance.

Taijiquan A martial art that developed in China, taijiquan (or "tai chi") is a system of self-defense that incorporates philosophical concepts from Taoism and Confucianism. An important part of this philosophy is *chi,* an energy force that surrounds and permeates all things. In addition to serving as a means of self-defense, taijiquan aims to bring the body into balance and harmony with this universal energy in order to promote health and spiritual growth. It teaches practitioners to remain calm and centered, to conserve and concentrate energy, and to harmonize with fear. Taijiquan seeks to manipulate force by becoming part of it—"going with the flow," so to speak.

Taijiquan is considered the gentlest of the martial arts. Instead of using quick and powerful movements, taijiquan consists of a series of slow, fluid, elegant movements, which reinforce the idea of moving *with* rather than *against* the stressors of everyday life. The practice of taijiquan promotes relaxation and concentration as well as the development of body awareness, balance, muscular strength, and flexibility. It usually takes some time and practice to reap the stress-management benefits of taijiquan, and, as with yoga, it's best to begin with some qualified instruction.

Listening to Music Listening to music is another method of inducing relaxation. It has been shown to influence pulse, blood pressure, and the electrical activity of muscles. Studies of newborns and hospitalized stroke patients have shown that listening to soothing, lyrical music can lessen depression, anxiety, and stress levels. Exposure to rhythmic music has been shown to help people with

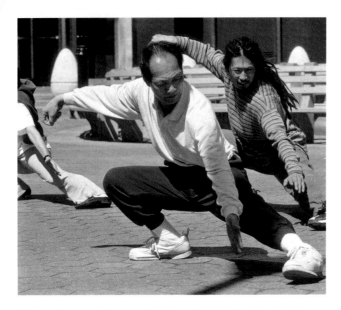

Taijiquan is among the many techniques for inducing the relaxation response. In addition to helping these men manage stress, regular practice of taijiquan will also improve their balance and increase their muscular strength and flexibility.

Parkinson's disease and other physical disabilities walk more steadily. Music therapy, which can involve both listening to music and creating music, has also been shown to be helpful in pain management, including lessening the need for anesthesia during labor. Although the effects of music are just beginning to be investigated, researchers have found that exposure to soothing music leads to reduced levels of the stress hormone cortisol and causes changes in the electrical activity in the brain.

To experience the stress-management benefits of music yourself, set aside a time to listen. Choose music that you enjoy and that makes you feel relaxed. To learn more about formal music therapy, contact the American Music Therapy Association (www.amta.org).

Biofeedback   Using **biofeedback** helps people reduce the stress response by enabling them to become more aware of their level of physiological arousal. It involves mechanical monitoring of some measure of the physiological stress response, such as perspiration, heart rate, skin temperature, or muscle tension. A person receives feedback about his or her condition through the use of sound (a tone or music), light, or a meter or dial. For example, as heart rate increases, the tone becomes louder; as it decreases, the tone softens. Through trial and error, people can learn to reduce their physiological stress response through conscious control.

Term

V∙W

biofeedback A technique in which monitoring devices are used to help a person become conscious of unconscious body processes, such as body temperature or blood pressure, in order to exert some control over them.

The point of biofeedback training is to teach how relaxation feels, how to induce relaxation, and how to transfer this skill to daily life (without the use of electronic equipment). In addition to monitoring equipment, biofeedback usually also requires the initial help of a therapist, stress counselor, or technician.

Other relaxation techniques include massage, hypnosis and self-hypnosis, and autogenic training. To learn more about these and other techniques for inducing the relaxation response, refer to For More Information at the end of the chapter.

Counterproductive Coping Strategies

College is a time when you'll learn to adapt to new and challenging situations and gain skills that will last a lifetime. It is also a time when many people develop habits, in response to stress, that are counterproductive and unhealthy and that may also last well beyond graduation.

Tobacco Use   Many young adults who never smoked in high school—and who rebuked their parents for tobacco use—smoke their first cigarette in college, usually at a party or bar or in a dorm with friends. Cigarettes and other tobacco products contain nicotine, a chemical that enhances the actions of neurotransmitters. Many smokers report that smoking helps them to cope with stress by providing a feeling of relaxation, giving them something to do with their hands in social situations, or breaking up monotony and routine. Nicotine can make you feel relaxed and even increase your ability to concentrate, but it is highly addictive and nicotine dependence itself is considered a psychological disorder. Cigarette smoke also contains many other substances that are harmful to your lungs and circulatory system and that cause heart disease, stroke, lung cancer, and emphysema. These negative consequences far outweigh any beneficial effects, and tobacco use should be avoided. The easiest thing to do is to not start. See Chapter 11 for more on the health effects of tobacco use and for tips on how to quit.

Use of Alcohol and Other Drugs   No college experience is complete without a party or two. Letting loose, dancing, laughing, and interacting with others—all are part of college parties and all can be very effective short-term coping strategies. However, partying in college is usually associated with drinking alcohol. Keg parties and drinking games can be fun, but they contribute to binge drinking and other forms of alcohol abuse. Like nicotine, alcohol is addictive, and many alcoholics find it hard to relax without a drink. Having a few drinks might make you feel temporarily at ease, and drinking until you're intoxicated may help you forget your current stressors. However, using alcohol to deal with stress places you at risk for all the short-term and long-term problems associated with alcohol abuse. It also does nothing to address the actual causes of stress in your life. Although moderate alcohol consumption may have potential health benefits for some people, many college students have patterns of drinking that detract from wellness. For more on the responsible use of alcohol, refer to Chapter 10.

Using other psychoactive drugs to cope with stress is also usually counterproductive:

- Caffeine raises cortisol levels and blood pressure and can make you feel more stressed; caffeine also disrupts sleep. Other stimulants, such as amphetamine, are used by some people in an attempt to cope with stress or sleepiness, making stress a risk factor for stimulant use. Stimulant drugs can activate the stress response, and they affect the same areas of the brain that are involved in regulating the stress response. It is unwise to tamper continually with brain systems so intimately associated with the stress response.

- Marijuana use is relatively common among college students, who report that they smoke marijuana in an effort to induce relaxation and for "mind expansion." Use of marijuana causes a brief period of euphoria and decreased short-term memory and attentional abilities. Physiological effects clearly show that marijuana use doesn't cause relaxation; in fact, some neurochemicals in marijuana act to enhance the stress response, and getting high on a regular basis can elicit panic attacks. To compound this, withdrawal from marijuana may also be associated with an increase in circulating stress hormones.

- Opioids such as morphine and heroin can mimic the effects of your body's natural painkillers and act to reduce anxiety. However, tolerance to opioids develops quickly, and many users become dependent. What starts as a quick fix for anxiety may rapidly become a life-altering addiction.

In general, it's not a good idea to alter your body chemistry with drugs in order to cope with stress. In moderation, substances such as caffeine and alcohol appear to have some positive attributes—but their use has many pitfalls and does not directly address the causes of stress in your life. Try some of the other coping strategies mentioned in this chapter instead. Use your natural ability to adapt.

Unhealthy Eating Habits   The nutrients in the food you eat provide energy and the substances needed to maintain your body. However, eating is also psychologically rewarding. We use food to end long days, to celebrate special events, and to enjoy the company of friends. The feelings of satiation and sedation that follow eating produce a relaxed state. However, regular use of eating as a means of coping with stress may lead to unhealthy eating habits.

Certain foods and supplements are sometimes thought to fight stress. Carbohydrates may reduce the stress response by promoting activity of the parasympathetic nervous system; however, a high-carbohydrate diet can lead to

excessive weight gain in sedentary people and is not recommended as a strategy for coping with stressors. In addition, some evidence suggests that greater ingestion of carbohydrates, simple sugars, and fatty foods may actually be a predisposing factor for psychological distress. Many dietary supplements are marketed for stress reduction, but supplements are not required to meet the same standards as medications in terms of safety, effectiveness, and manufacturing (see Chapters 12 and 21).

Binge eating is defined as eating a large quantity of food in a discrete period of time, accompanied by a sense of lack of control over eating. Binge eating may serve as an avoidance coping strategy and a temporary escape. However, the loss of control over eating is associated with negative emotional states, and binge eating is a risky behavior associated with weight gain and serious eating disorders. A good strategy to avoid unhealthy binge-eating habits is to make sure you eat breakfast and lunch in the first half of your day—rather than waiting until the evening to consume a real meal. Eating early in the day increases your metabolism and gives you the energy to engage in all your activities. In addition, early meals will decrease feelings of hunger later in the day. See Chapters 12 and 14 for more on a healthy diet and on eating disorders.

CREATING A PERSONAL PLAN FOR MANAGING STRESS

What are the most important sources of stress in your life? Are you coping successfully with these stressors? No single strategy or program for managing stress will work for everyone, but you can use the principles of behavior management described in Chapter 1 to tailor a plan specifically to your needs. The most important starting point for a successful stress-management plan is to learn to listen to your body. When you learn to recognize the stress response and the emotions and thoughts that accompany it, you'll be in a position to take charge of that crucial moment and handle it in a healthy way.

Identifying Stressors

Before you can learn to manage the stressors in your life, you have to identify them. A strategy many experts recommend is keeping a stress journal for a week or two. Keep a log of your daily activities, and assign a rating to your stress level for every hour. Each time you feel or express a stress response, record the time and the circumstances in your journal. Note what you were doing at the time, what you were thinking or feeling, and the outcome of your response.

After keeping your journal for a few weeks, you should be able to identify your key stressors and spot patterns in how you respond to them. Take note of the people, places, events, and patterns of thought and behavior that cause you the most stress. You may notice, for example, that mornings are usually the most stressful part of your day. Or you may discover that when you're angry at your roommate, you're apt to respond with behaviors that only make matters worse. Once you've outlined the general pattern of stress in your life, you may want to focus on a particularly problematic stressor or on an inappropriate behavioral response you've identified. Keep a stress log for another week or two that focuses just on the early morning hours, for example, or just on your arguments with your roommate. The more information you gather, the easier it will be to develop effective strategies for coping with the stressors in your life. Use the situations in which your stress level has dissipated as positive reinforcement that you have the ability to adapt to your stressors. Rise to the challenge of those events that continue to cause you stress. Keeping a journal allows you to be a bit more analytical about what produces the most stress in your life and fills in where your conscious memory fails you.

Designing Your Plan

Earlier in this chapter, you learned about many different techniques for combating stress. Now that you've identified the key stressors in your life, it's time to choose the techniques that will work best for you and create an action plan for change. Finding a buddy to work with you can make the process more fun and increase your chances of success. Some experts recommend drawing up a formal contract with yourself.

Whether or not you complete a contract, it's important to design rewards into your plan. You might treat yourself to a special breakfast in a favorite restaurant on the weekend (as long as you eat a nutritious breakfast every weekday morning). If you practice your relaxation techniques faithfully, you might reward yourself with a long bath or an hour of pleasure reading at the end of the day. It's also important to evaluate your plan regularly and redesign it as your needs change. Under times of increased stress, for example, you might want to focus on good eating, exercise, and relaxation habits. Over time, your new stress-management skills will become almost automatic. You'll feel better, accomplish more, and reduce your risk of disease.

Getting Help

If the techniques discussed so far don't provide you with enough relief from the stress in your life, you might want to read more about specific areas you wish to work on, consult a peer counselor, join a support group, or participate in a few psychotherapy sessions. Excellent self-help guides can be found in bookstores or the library. Additional resources are listed in the For More Information section at the end of the chapter.

Your student health center or student affairs office can tell you whether your campus has a peer counseling program. Such programs are usually staffed by volunteer students with special training that emphasizes maintaining confidentiality. Peer counselors can guide you to other campus or community resources or can simply provide understanding.

Support groups are typically organized around a particular issue or problem. In your area, you might find a support group for first-year students; for reentering students; for single parents; for students of your ethnicity, religion, or national origin; for people with eating disorders; or for rape survivors. The number of such groups has increased in recent years as more and more people discover how therapeutic it can be to talk with others who share the same situation.

Short-term psychotherapy can also be tremendously helpful in dealing with stress-related problems. Your student health center may offer psychotherapy on a sliding-fee scale; the county mental health center in your area may do the same. If you belong to any type of religious organization, check to see whether pastoral counseling is available. Your physician can refer you to psychotherapists in your community. Not all therapists are right for all people, so be prepared to have initial sessions with several. Choose the one you feel most comfortable with.

Tips for Today

Some stress is unavoidable in life. How you respond to it is what determines whether you become stressed out or maintain your serenity. For the stress you can't avoid, develop a range of stress-management techniques and strategies.

Right now you can

- Sit in a comfortable chair and practice deep breathing for 5–10 minutes.

- Visualize a relaxing, peaceful place and imagine yourself experiencing it as vividly as possible; you might "feel" a gentle breeze on your skin or "hear" the soothing sound of a waterfall. Stay there as long as you can.

- Stand up and do some stretching exercises, such as gently rolling your head from side to side, stretching your arms out in front of your body and over your head, and slowly bending over and letting your arms hang toward the floor.

- Get out your date book and schedule what you'll be doing the rest of today and tomorrow. Pencil in a short walk and a conversation with a friend. Plan to go to bed 15 minutes earlier than usual.

SUMMARY

- When confronted with a stressor, the body undergoes a set of physical changes known as the fight-or-flight reaction. The sympathetic nervous system and endocrine system act on many targets in the body to prepare it for action.

- Emotional and behavioral responses to stressors vary among individuals. Ineffective responses increase stress but can be moderated or changed.

- Factors that influence emotional and behavioral responses to stressors include personality, cultural background, gender, and past experiences.

- The general adaptation syndrome (GAS) has three stages: alarm, resistance, and exhaustion.

- A high allostatic load characterized by prolonged or repeated exposure to stress hormones can increase a person's risk of health problems.

- Psychoneuroimmunology (PNI) looks at how the physiological changes of the stress response affect the immune system and thereby increase the risk of illness.

- Health problems linked to stress include CVD, colds and other infections, asthma and allergies, cancer, flare-ups of chronic diseases, psychological problems, digestive problems, headaches, insomnia, and injuries.

- A cluster of major life events that require adjustment and accommodation can lead to increased stress and an increased risk of health problems. Minor daily hassles increase stress if they are perceived negatively.

- Sources of stress associated with college may be academic, interpersonal, time-related, or financial pressures.

- Job-related stress is common, particularly for employees who have little control over decisions relating to their jobs. If stress is severe or prolonged, burnout may occur.

- New and changing relationships, prejudice, and discrimination are examples of interpersonal and social stressors.

- Social support systems help buffer people against the effects of stress and make illness less likely. Good communication skills foster healthy relationships.

- Exercise, nutrition, sleep, and time management are wellness behaviors that reduce stress and increase energy.

- Cognitive techniques for managing stress involve developing new and healthy patterns of thinking, such as practicing problem solving, monitoring self-talk, and cultivating a sense of humor.

- The relaxation response is the opposite of the fight-or-flight reaction. Techniques that trigger it, including progressive relaxation, imagery, meditation, and deep breathing, counteract the effects of chronic stress. Counterproductive coping strategies include smoking, drinking, and unhealthy eating.

- A successful individualized plan for coping with stress begins with the use of a stress journal or log to identify and study stressors and inappropriate behavioral responses. Completing a contract and recruiting a buddy can help your stress-management plan succeed.

- Additional help in dealing with stress is available from self-help books, peer counseling, support groups, and psychotherapy.

Take Action

1. **Interview friends or family members.** Choose someone who seems to deal particularly well with stress. Interview that person about his or her methods for managing stress. What strategies does he or she use? What can you learn from that person that can be applied to your own life?

2. **Check out local services.** Investigate the services available in your community—such as peer counseling, support groups, and time-management classes—to help people deal with stress. If possible, visit or gather information on one or more of them. Write a description and evaluation of their services, including your personal reactions.

3. **Try a stress-management technique.** Reread the techniques described in this chapter, and choose one to try

for a week. After a trial period, evaluate the effectiveness of the strategy you chose. Did your stress level decrease during the week? Were you better able to deal with daily hassles and any more severe stressors that you encountered?

4. **Reach out to others by becoming a volunteer.** Whether or not you realize it, you likely have more physical, emotional, and intellectual resources than you need. Transfer some of these resources to people who would benefit greatly from just a few hours of your time and effort. In doing so, you may find that you also benefit in terms of greater self-esteem and appreciation for your own support system and the opportunities you have for a positive future. Look for an opportunity to volunteer to help others in your community.

For More Information

Books

Blonna, R. 2005. *Coping with Stress in a Changing World.* 3rd ed. New York: McGraw-Hill. *A comprehensive guide to stress management that includes separate chapters on college stressors and spirituality.*

Kabat-Zinn, J. 2005. *Coming to Our Senses: Healing Ourselves and the World Through Mindfulness.* New York: Hyperion. *Explores the connections among mindfulness, health, and our physical and spiritual well-being.*

Pennebaker, J. W. 2004. *Writing to Heal: A Guided Journal for Recovering from Trauma and Emotional Upheaval.* Oakland,

Calif.: New Harbinger Press. *Provides information about using journaling to cope with stress.*

Sapolsky, R. M. 2004. *Why Zebras Don't Get Ulcers.* 3rd ed. New York: Owl Books. *Describes the links between stress and disease in addition to strategies for stress management.*

Organizations and Web Sites

American Psychological Association. Provides information on stress management and psychological disorders.
  800-374-2721; 800-964-2000 (referrals)
  http://www.apa.org; http://helping.apa.org

Dealing with Test Anxiety

Are you a person who doesn't perform as well as you should on tests? Do you find that anxiety interferes with your ability to study effectively before the test and to think clearly in the test situation? If so, you may be experiencing test anxiety. Two methods that have proven effective in helping people deal with test anxiety are systematic desensitization and success rehearsal.

Systematic Desensitization

Systematic desensitization is based on the premise that you can't feel anxiety and be relaxed at the same time.

Phase I: Constructing an Anxiety Hierarchy Begin the first phase by thinking of ten or more situations related to your fear, such as hearing the announcement of the test date in class, studying for the test, sitting in the classroom waiting for the test to begin, reading the test questions, and so on. Write each situation on an index card, using a brief phrase to describe it on one side of the card. On the other side, list several realistic details or prompts that will help you vividly imagine yourself actually experiencing the situation. For example, if the situation is "hearing that 50% of the final grade will be based on the two exams," the prompts might include details such as "sitting in the big lecture auditorium in Baily Hall," "taking notes in my blue notebook," and "listening to Professor Smith's voice."

Next, arrange your cards in order, from least-tense to most-tense situation. Rate each situation to reflect the amount of anxiety you feel when you encounter it in real life, to confirm your anxiety hierarchy. Assign ratings on a scale of 0–100, and make sure the distances between items are fairly small and about equal. When you're sure your anxiety hierarchy is a true reflection of your feelings, number the cards.

Phase II: Learning and Practicing Muscle Relaxation The second phase of the program involves learning to relax your muscles and to recognize when they are relaxed (see the description of progressive relaxation in this chapter). As you become proficient at this technique, you'll be able to go to a deeply relaxed state within just a few minutes. When you can do this, go on to the next phase of the program.

Phase III: Implementing the Desensitization Program Use the quiet place where you practiced your relaxation exercises. Sit comfortably and place your stack of numbered cards within reach. Take several minutes to relax completely, and then look at the first card, reading both the brief phrase and the descriptive prompts. Close your eyes and imagine yourself in that situation for about 10 seconds. Then put the card down and relax completely for about 30 seconds. Look at the card again, imagine the situation for 10 seconds, and relax again for 30 seconds.

At this point, evaluate your current level of anxiety about the situation on the card in terms of the rating scale you devised earlier. If your anxiety level is 10 or below, relax for 2 minutes and go on to the second card. If it's higher than 10, repeat the routine with the same card until the anxiety decreases. If you have difficulty with a particular item, go back to the previous item; then try it again. If you still can't visualize it without anxiety, try to construct three new items with smaller steps between them and insert them before the troublesome item. You should be able to move through one to four items per session. Sessions can be conducted from twice a day to twice a week and should last no longer than 20 minutes. It's helpful to graph your progress in a way that has meaning for you.

After you have successfully completed your program, you should be desensitized to the real-life situations that previously caused anxiety. If you find that you do experience some anxiety in the real situations, take 30 seconds or a minute to relax completely, just as you did when you were practicing.

Success Rehearsal

To practice this variation on systematic desensitization, take your hierarchy of anxiety-producing situations and vividly imagine yourself successfully dealing with each one. Create a detailed scenario for each situation, and use your imagination to experience genuine feelings of confidence. Recognize your negative thoughts ("I'll be so nervous I won't be able to think straight") and replace them with positive ones ("Anxiety will keep me alert so I can do a good job"). Proceed one step at a time, thinking as you go of strategies for success that you can later implement. These might include the following:

- Before the test, find out everything you can about it—its format, the material to be covered, the grading criteria. Ask the instructor for practice materials. Study in advance; don't just cram the night before. Avoid all-nighters.

- Devise a study plan. This might include forming a study group with one or more classmates or outlining what you will study, when, where, and for how long. Generate your own questions and answer them.

- In the actual test situation, sit away from possible distractions, listen carefully to instructions, and ask for clarification if you don't understand a direction.

- During the test, answer the easiest questions first. If you don't know an answer and there is no penalty for incorrect answers, guess. If there are several questions you have difficulty answering, review the ones you have already handled. Figure out approximately how much time you have to cover each question.

- For math problems, try to estimate the answer before doing the precise calculations.

- For true-false questions, look for qualifiers such as *always* and *never.* Such questions are likely to be false.

- For essay questions, look for key words in the question that indicate what the instructor is looking for in the answer. Develop a brief outline of your answer, sketching out what you will cover. Stick to your outline, and keep track of the time you're spending on your answer. Don't get caught with unanswered questions when time is up.

- Remain calm and focused throughout the test. Don't let negative thoughts rattle you. Avoid worrying about past performance, how others are doing, or the negative consequences of a poor test grade. If you start to become nervous, take some deep breaths and relax your muscles completely for a minute or so.

The best way to counter test anxiety is with successful test-taking experiences. The more times you succeed, the more your test anxiety will recede. If you find that these methods aren't sufficient to get your anxiety under control, you may want to seek professional help.

Association for Applied Psychophysiology and Biofeedback. Provides information about biofeedback and referrals to certified biofeedback practitioners.

866-477-8892

http://www.aapb.org

Harvard Mind-Body Medical Institute. Provides information about stress-management and relaxation techniques.

http://www.mbmi.org

Interactive Budgeting Worksheet. An interactive calculator designed to help students balance income and expenses.

http://www.ed.gov/offices/OSFAP/DirectLoan/BudgetCalc/budget.html

Medical Basis for Stress. Includes information on recognizing stress and on the physiological basis of stress, self-assessments for stress levels, and techniques for managing stress.

http://www.teachhealth.com

National Institute for Occupational Safety and Health (NIOSH). Provides information and links on job stress.

http://www.cdc.gov/niosh/topics/stress

National Institute of Mental Health (NIMH). Publishes informative brochures about stress and stress management as well as other aspects of mental health.

866-615-6464

http://www.nimh.nih.gov

National Sleep Foundation. Provides information about sleep and how to overcome sleep problems such as insomnia and jet lag.

http://www.sleepfoundation.org

Student Counseling Virtual Pamphlet Collection. Links to online pamphlets from student counseling centers at colleges and universities across the country; topics include stress, sleep, and time management.

http://counseling.uchicago.edu/vpc

See also the listings for Chapters 1 and 3.

Selected Bibliography

American Psychological Association. 2005. *Learning to Deal with Stress* (http://helping.apa.org/articles/article.php?id=71; retrieved February 17, 2005).

American Psychological Association. 2005. *Managing Traumatic Stress: Tips for Recovering from Natural Disasters* (http://helping.apa.org/articles/article.php?id=69; retrieved February 17, 2005).

Baker, S. R. 2003. A prospective longitudinal investigation of social problem-solving appraisals on adjustment to university, stress, health, and academic motivation and performance. *Personality and Individual Differences* 35(3): 569–591.

Bhattacharya, G., and S. L. Schoppelrey. 2004. Preimmigration beliefs of life success, postimmigration experiences, and acculturative stress: South Asian immigrants in the United States. *Journal of Immigrant Health* 6(2): 83–92.

Bouchard T. J. Jr., and M. McGue. 2003. Genetic and environmental influences on human psychological differences. *Journal of Neurobiology* 54(1): 4–45.

Constantine, M. G., S. Okazaki, and S. O. Utsey. 2004. Self-concealment, social self-efficacy, acculturative stress, and depression in African, Asian, and Latin American international college students. *American Journal of Orthopsychiatry* 74(3): 230–241.

Cooper, A. E. 2003. An investigation of the relationships among spirituality, prayer and meditation, and aspects of stress and coping. *Dissertation Abstracts International: Section B: The Sciences and Engineering* 64(3-B): 1484.

Grossman, P., et al. 2004. Mindfulness-based stress reduction and health benefits: A meta analysis. *Journal of Psychosomatic Research* 57(1): 35–43.

La Civita, L. K. 2004. An examination of emotional intelligence factors: Their relationship to academic achievement and the implications for retention of the at-risk community college student. *Dissertation Abstracts International: Section A: Humanities and Social Sciences* 64(8-A): 2778.

Lane, J. D., et al. 2002. Caffeine affects cardiovascular and neuroendocrine activation at work and home. *Psychosomatic Medicine* 64(4): 595–603.

Liverant, G. I., S. G. Hofmann, and B. T. Litz. 2004. Coping and anxiety in college students after the September 11th terrorist attacks. *Anxiety, Stress and Coping: An International Journal* 17(2): 127–139.

Longest, M. Q. 2003. Non-reactive, homeostatic, and positive resiliency: Relationships and predictors. *Dissertation Abstracts International: Section B: The Sciences and Engineering* 64(2-B).

Meehan, D.-C.-M., and C. Negy. 2003. Undergraduate students' adaptation to college: Does being married make a difference? *Journal of College Student Development* 44: 670–689.

Meier-Ewert, H. K., et al. 2004. Effect of sleep loss on C-reactive protein, an inflammatory marker of cardiovascular risk. *Journal of the American College of Cardiology* 43: 678–683.

Melamed, S., et al. 2004. Association of fear of terror with low-grade inflammation among apparently healthy employed adults. *Psychosomatic Medicine* 66(4): 484–491.

National Mental Health Association. 2001. *Coping with Disaster: Tips for College Students* (http://www.nmha.org/reassurance/collegetips.cfm).

Pickering, T. G. 2003. Effects of stress and behavioral interventions in hypertension—Men are from Mars, women are from Venus: Stress, pets, and oxytocin. *Journal of Clinical Hypertension* 5(1): 86–8.

Ridley, M. 2003. *Nature Via Nurture.* New York: HarperCollins.

Sax, L. J., et al. 2004. *The American Freshman: National Norms for Fall 2003.* Los Angeles: UCLA Higher Education Research Institute.

Schlenger, W. E., et al. 2002. Psychological reactions to terrorist attacks. Findings from the National Study of Americans' Reactions to September 11. *Journal of the American Medical Association* 288(5): 581–588.

Schminke, M., et al. 2003. Back to the future: A classical consideration of the impact of technology on human resources management. In *Advances in Human Performance and Cognitive Engineering Research,* Vol. 3 (pp. 187–205), ed. D. Stone. Amsterdam: Elsevier Science/JAI Press.

Schwarze, N. J., J. M. Oliver, and P. J. Handal. 2003. Binge eating as related to negative self-awareness, depression, and avoidance coping in undergraduates. *Journal of College Student Development* 44(5): 644–652.

Segerstrom, S. C., and G. E. Miller. 2004. Psychological stress and the human immune system: A meta-analytic study of 30 years of inquiry. *Psychological Bulletin* 130: 601–630.

Smyth, J., and R. Helm. 2003. Focused expressive writing as self-help for stress and trauma. *Journal of Clinical Psychology* 59(2): 227–235.

Steptoe, A., et al. 2003. Influence of socioeconomic status and job control on plasma fibrinogen responses to acute mental stress. *Psychosomatic Medicine* 65(1): 137–144.

Steptoe, A., et al. 2004. Loneliness and neuroendocrine, cardiovascular, and inflammatory stress responses in middle-aged men and women. *Psychoneuroendocrinology* 29(5): 593–611.

Vorona, R. D., et al. 2005. Overweight and obese patients in a primary care population report less sleep than patients with a normal body mass index. *Archives of Internal Medicine* 165(1): 25–30.

Wetter, D. W., et al. 2004. Prevalence and predictors of transitions in smoking behavior among college students. *Health Psychology* 23(2): 168–177.

Wisner, K. L. 2004. Sex and psychiatry in the next 5 years. *Journal of Clinical Psychiatry* 65(4): 462–463.

Wittstein, I. S., et al. 2005. Neurohumoral features of myocardial stunning due to sudden emotional stress. *New England Journal of Medicine* 352(6): 539–548.

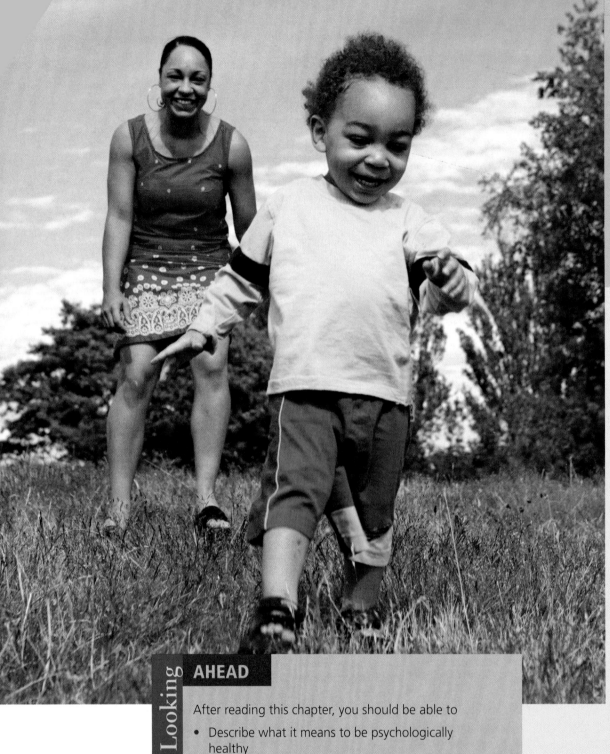

3

After reading this chapter, you should be able to

- Describe what it means to be psychologically healthy

- Explain how to develop and maintain a positive self-concept and healthy self-esteem

- Discuss the importance to psychological health of an optimistic outlook, good communication skills, and constructive approaches to dealing with loneliness and anger

- Describe common psychological disorders and list the warning signs of suicide

- Explain the different approaches and types of help available for psychological problems

Psychological Health

1. **Normality is a key component of psychological health.**
   True or false?

2. **Trying to think rationally about what bothers you won't get you very far, because psychological problems usually are due to emotions, not thinking.**
   True or false?

3. **About how many Americans have a diagnosable psychological disorder during the course of a year?**
   a. 5%
   b. 10%
   c. 20%

4. **People with enough willpower can force themselves to snap out of their depression.**
   True or false?

5. **A person who attempts suicide but survives did not really intend to die.**
   True or false?

ANSWERS

1. FALSE. Normality simply means being close to average, and having unusual ideas or attitudes doesn't mean that a person is mentally ill. The fact that people's ideas are varied makes life interesting and helps people respond in creative ways to life's challenges.

2. FALSE. Research has shown that getting people to adopt more realistic attitudes and beliefs about themselves and others can alleviate depression.

3. C. Other than substance-abuse problems, the most common types of disorders are simple phobias and depression. The majority of people with psychological disorders do not receive appropriate treatment.

4. FALSE. Depression, a disorder strongly linked to brain chemistry, can overcome whatever willpower a person has and make it impossible for her or him to make rational decisions—or any decisions at all.

5. FALSE. A person may intend to die but miscalculate the type or amount of drug needed or how to successfully carry out some other method of suicide.

Visit the *Core Concepts in Health* Online Learning Center (www.mhhe.com/insel10e) for study aids and many additional resources.

63

What exactly is psychological health? Many people over the centuries have expressed opinions about the nature of psychological (or mental) health. Some even claim that there is no such thing, that psychological health is just a myth. We disagree. We think there is such a thing as psychological health just as there is physical health—and the two are closely interrelated. Just as your body can work well or poorly, giving you pleasure or pain, your mind can also work well or poorly, resulting in happiness or unhappiness. Psychological health is a crucial component of overall wellness. (We are using "mental health" and "psychological health" interchangeably; the latter is the more current term, but it hasn't replaced "mental health" yet.)

If you feel pain and unhappiness rather than pleasure and happiness or if you sense that you could be functioning at a higher level, there may be ways you can help yourself—either on your own or with the aid of a professional. This chapter will explain how.

WHAT PSYCHOLOGICAL HEALTH IS NOT

Psychological health is not the same as psychological **normality.** Being mentally normal simply means being close to average. You can define normal body temperature because a few degrees above or below this temperature means physical sickness. But your ideas and attitudes can vary tremendously without your losing efficiency or feeling emotional distress. And psychological diversity is valuable; living in a society of people with varied ideas and lifestyles makes life interesting and challenging.

Conforming to social demands is not necessarily a mark of psychological health. If you don't question what's going on around you, you're not fulfilling your potential as a thinking, questioning human being. For example, our society admires the framers of the U.S. Constitution and the abolitionists who rebelled against injustices. If conformity signified mental health, then political dissent would indicate mental illness by definition (and we have seen that definition used by dictators). If such a definition were valid, Galileo would have been mad for insisting that the earth revolved around the sun.

Never seeking help for personal problems does not prove you are psychologically healthy, any more than seeking help proves you are mentally ill. Unhappy people may not want to seek professional help because they don't want to reveal their problems to others, may fear what their friends might think, or may not know whom to ask for help. People who are severely disturbed psychologically or emotionally may not even realize they need help, or they may become so suspicious of other people that they can only be treated without their consent.

We cannot say people are "mentally ill" or "mentally healthy" on the basis of symptoms alone. Life constantly presents problems. Time and life inevitably alter the environment as well as our minds and bodies, and changes present problems. The symptom of anxiety, for example, can help us face a problem and solve it before it gets too big. Someone who shows no anxiety may be refusing to recognize problems or do anything about them. A person who is anxious for good reason is likely to be judged more psychologically healthy in the long run than someone who is inappropriately calm.

Finally, we cannot judge psychological health from the way people look. All too often, a person who seems to be OK and even happy suddenly takes his or her own life. Usually such people lack close friends who might have known of their desperation. At an early age, we learn to conceal and lie. We may believe that our complaints put unfair demands on others. While suffering in silence can sometimes be a virtue, it can also impede getting help.

DEFINING PSYCHOLOGICAL HEALTH

It is even harder to say what psychological health *is* than what it is *not.* Psychological health can be defined either negatively as the absence of sickness or positively as the presence of wellness. The narrower, negative definition has several advantages: It concentrates attention on the worst problems and on the people most in need, and it tends to avoid value judgments about the best way to lead our lives. However, if we consider everyone to be mentally healthy who is not severely mentally disturbed, we end up ignoring common problems that can be addressed.

A positive definition—psychological health as the presence of wellness—is a more ambitious outlook, one that encourages us to fulfill our own potential. Freedom from disorders is only one factor in psychological wellness. During the 1960s, Abraham Maslow eloquently described an ideal of mental health in his book *Toward a Psychology of Being.* He was convinced that psychologists were too preoccupied with people who had failed in some way. He also disliked the way psychologists tried to reduce human striving to physiological needs or drives.

According to Maslow, there is a *hierarchy of needs,* listed here in order of decreasing urgency: physiological needs, safety, being loved, maintaining self-esteem, and self-actualization (Figure 3-1). When urgent needs like the need for food, water, shelter, sleep, and safety are satisfied, less urgent needs take priority. Most of us are well fed and feel reasonably safe, so we are driven by higher motives. Maslow's conclusions were based on his study of a group of visibly successful people who seemed to have lived, or be living, at their fullest, including Abraham Lincoln, Henry David Thoreau, Ludwig van Beethoven, Eleanor Roosevelt, and Albert Einstein, as well as some of his own friends and acquaintances. He stated that these people had achieved **self-actualization;**

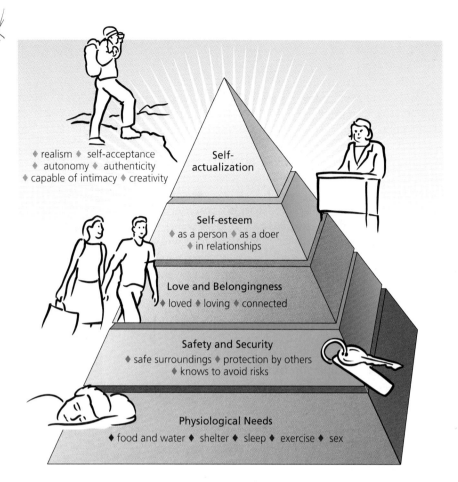

Figure 3-1 Maslow's hierarchy of needs.
People focus first on the needs at the bottom of the hierarchy because unless basic physiological needs are fulfilled, other needs have little meaning. Once urgent needs are satisfied, people can focus on higher motives. Those who make it to the top of the needs hierarchy achieve self-actualization—they have grown to fulfill much of their human potential and are able to act and make choices unfettered by unfulfilled needs at lower levels. SOURCE: Maslow, A. 1970. *Motivation and Personality,* 2nd ed. New York: Harper & Row.

Pyramid labels, top to bottom:

◆ realism ◆ self-acceptance ◆ autonomy ◆ authenticity ◆ capable of intimacy ◆ creativity
Self-actualization

Self-esteem
◆ as a person ◆ as a doer ◆ in relationships

Love and Belongingness
◆ loved ◆ loving ◆ connected

Safety and Security
◆ safe surroundings ◆ protection by others ◆ knows to avoid risks

Physiological Needs
◆ food and water ◆ shelter ◆ sleep ◆ exercise ◆ sex

he thought they had fulfilled a good measure of their human potential and suggested that self-actualized people all share certain qualities.

Realism

Self-actualized people are able to deal with the world as it is and not demand that it be otherwise. If you are realistic, you know the difference between what is and what you want. You also know what you can change and what you cannot. Unrealistic people often spend a great deal of time and energy trying to force the world and other people into their ideal picture. Realistic people accept evidence that contradicts what they want to believe, and if it is important evidence they modify their beliefs.

Acceptance

Psychologically healthy people can largely accept themselves and others. Self-acceptance means having a positive **self-concept,** or *self-image,* or appropriately high **self-esteem.** Such people have a positive but realistic mental image of themselves and positive feelings about who they are, what they are capable of, and what roles they play. People who feel good about themselves are likely to live up to their positive self-image and enjoy successes that in turn reinforce these good feelings. A good self-concept is

based on a realistic view of personal worth—it does not mean being egocentric or "stuck on yourself."

Being able to tolerate our own imperfections and still feel positive about ourselves helps us tolerate the imperfections of others. Psychologically healthy people tend to be optimistic about what they can expect from other people until experience proves their optimism to be unrealistic. Acceptance means being willing to interact with people who are imperfect and unlikely to change.

Autonomy

Psychologically healthy people are able to direct themselves, acting independently of their social environment. **Autonomy** is more than freedom from physical control

Terms

normality The psychological characteristics attributed to the majority of people in a population at a given time.

self-actualization The highest level of growth in Maslow's hierarchy.

self-concept The ideas, feelings, and perceptions one has about oneself; also called *self-image.*

self-esteem Satisfaction and confidence in oneself; the valuing of oneself as a person.

autonomy Independence; the sense of being self-directed.

by something outside the self. Many people, for example, shrink from expressing their feelings because they fear disapproval and rejection. They respond only to what they feel as outside pressure. Such behavior is **other-directed.** In contrast, **inner-directed** people find guidance from within, from their own values and feelings. They are not afraid to be themselves. Psychologically free people act because they choose to, not because they are driven or pressured. They have an internal locus of control and a high level of self-efficacy (see Chapter 1).

Autonomy can give healthy people certain childlike qualities. Very small children have a quality of being "real." They respond in a genuine, spontaneous way to whatever happens, without pretenses. Being genuine means not having to plan words or actions to get approval or make an impression. It means being aware of feelings and being willing to express them—being unself-consciously oneself. This quality is sometimes called **authenticity**; such people are *authentic,* the "real thing."

A Capacity for Intimacy

Healthy people are capable of physical and emotional intimacy. They can expose their feelings and thoughts to other people. They are open to the pleasure of intimate physical contact and to the risks and satisfactions of being close to others in a caring, sensitive way. Intimate physical contact may mean "good sex," but it also means something more—intense awareness of both your partner and yourself in which contact becomes communication. Chapters 4 and 5 discuss intimacy in more detail.

Creativity

Psychologically healthy people are creative and have a continuing fresh appreciation for what goes on around them. They are not necessarily great poets, artists, or musicians, but they do live their everyday lives in creative ways: "A first-rate soup is more creative than a second-rate painting." Creative people seem to see more and to be open to new experiences; they don't fear the unknown or need to minimize or avoid uncertainty.

How did Maslow's group achieve their exemplary psychological health, and (more important) how can *we* attain it? Maslow himself did not answer that question, but it undoubtedly helps to have been treated with respect,

Self-actualized people respond in a genuine, spontaneous way to what happens around them. They are capable of maintaining close interpersonal relationships.

love, and understanding as a child, to have experienced stability, and to have achieved a sense of mastery. As adults, since we cannot redo the past, we must concentrate on meeting current challenges in ways that will lead to long-term mental wellness. We must not consider ourselves failures if we do not become self-actualized in every way or at every moment. Self-actualization is an ideal to strive for even if we never or only occasionally attain it to the fullest degree.

MEETING LIFE'S CHALLENGES

Life is full of challenges—large and small. Everyone, regardless of heredity and family influences, must learn to cope successfully with new situations and new people. For emotional and mental wellness, each of us must continue to grow psychologically, developing new and more sophisticated coping mechanisms to suit our current lives. We must develop an adult identity that enhances our self-esteem and autonomy. We must also learn to communicate honestly, handle anger and loneliness appropriately, and avoid being defensive.

Growing Up Psychologically

How we respond to the challenges of life influences the development of our personality and identity. Psychologist Erik Erikson proposed that development proceeds through

Terms

V͜W

other-directed Guided in behavior by the values and expectations of others.

inner-directed Guided in behavior by an inner set of rules and values.

authenticity Genuineness.

Table 3-1 Erikson's Stages of Development

Age	Conflict	Important People	Task
Birth–1 year	Trust vs. mistrust	Mother or other primary caregiver	In being fed and comforted, developing the trust that others will respond to your needs
1–3 years	Autonomy vs. shame and self-doubt	Parents	In toilet training, locomotion, and exploration, learning self-control without losing the capacity for assertiveness
3–6 years	Initiative vs. guilt	Family	In playful talking and locomotion, developing a conscience based on parental prohibitions that is not too inhibiting
6–12 years	Industry vs. inferiority	Neighborhood and school	In school and playing with peers, learning the value of accomplishment and perseverance without feeling inadequate
Adolescence	Identity vs. identity confusion	Peers	Developing a stable sense of who you are—your needs, abilities, interpersonal style, and values
Young adulthood	Intimacy vs. isolation	Close friends, sex partners	Learning to live and share intimately with others, often in sexual relationships
Middle adulthood	Generativity vs. self-absorption	Work associates, children, community	Doing things for others, including parenting and civic activities
Older adulthood	Integrity vs. despair	Humankind	Affirming the value of life and its ideals

SOURCE: Erikson, E. 1963. *Childhood and Society.* New York: Norton.

a series of eight stages, extending throughout the life span. Each stage is characterized by a major crisis or turning point, a time of increased vulnerability as well as increased potential for psychological growth (Table 3-1).

The successful mastery of one stage is a basis for mastering the next, so early failures can have repercussions in later life. Fortunately, life provides ongoing opportunities for mastering these tasks. For example, although the development of trust begins in infancy, it is refined as we grow older. We learn to trust people outside our immediate family and to limit our trust by identifying people who are untrustworthy.

Developing an Adult Identity A primary task beginning in adolescence is the development of an adult identity: a unified sense of self, characterized by attitudes, beliefs, and ways of acting that are genuinely one's own. People with adult identities know who they are, what they are capable of, what roles they play, and their place among their peers. They have a sense of their own uniqueness but also appreciate what they have in common with others. They view themselves realistically and can assess their strengths and weaknesses without relying on the opinions of others. Achieving an identity also means that one can form intimate relationships with others while maintaining a strong sense of self.

Our identities evolve as we interact with the world and make choices about what we'd like to do and whom we'd like to model ourselves after. Developing an adult identity is particularly challenging in a heterogeneous, secular, and relatively affluent society like ours, in which many roles are possible, many choices are tolerated, and ample time is allowed for experimenting and making up one's mind.

Early identities are often modeled after parents—or the opposite of parents, in rebellion against what they represent. Later, peers, rock stars, sports heroes, and religious figures are added to the list of possible models. In high school and college, people often join cliques that assert a certain identity—the "jocks," the "brains," the "slackers." Although much of an identity is internal—a way of viewing oneself and the world—it can include things such as styles of talking and dressing, ornaments like earrings, and particular hairstyles.

Early identities are rarely permanent. A student who works for good grades and approval from parents and teachers one year can turn into a dropout devoted to hard rock and wild parties a year later. At some point, however, most of us adopt a more stable, individual identity that ties together the experiences of childhood and the expectations and aspirations of adulthood. Erikson's theory does not suggest that suddenly one day we assume our final identity and never change after that. Life is more interesting for people who continue to evolve into more distinct individuals, rather than being rigidly controlled by their pasts. Identity reflects a lifelong process, and it changes as a person develops new relationships and roles.

Developing an adult identity is an important part of psychological wellness. Without a personal identity, we begin to feel confused about who we are; Erikson called this situation an *identity crisis*. Until we have "found ourselves," we cannot have much self-esteem, because a self is not firmly in place.

How far have you gotten in developing your adult identity? Write down a list of characteristics you think a friend who knows you well would use to describe you. Rank them from the most to the least important. Your list might include elements such as gender, socioeconomic status, ethnic and/or religious identification, choice of college or major, parents' occupations, interests and talents, attitudes toward drugs and alcohol, style of dress, the kinds of people with whom you typically associate, your expected role in society, and aspects of your personality. Which elements of your identity do you feel are permanent, and which do you think may change over time? Are there any characteristics missing from your list that you'd like to add?

Another aid to developing an adult identity is to identify possible role models. Whom do you admire and want to be like? Which characteristics of that person do you want to emulate? How did that person acquire those characteristics, and how could you follow in her or his footsteps? Some role models might be willing to be mentors to you, spending time with you and sharing their wisdom.

Developing Intimacy Erikson's developmental stages don't end with establishing an adult identity. Learning to live intimately with others and finding a productive role for yourself in society are other tasks of adulthood—to be able to love and work.

People with established identities can form intimate relationships and sexual unions characterized by sharing, open communication, long-term commitment, and love. Those who lack a firm sense of self may have difficulty establishing relationships because they feel overwhelmed by closeness and the needs of another person. As a result, they experience only short-term, superficial relationships with others and may remain isolated. As described in Chapter 2, a lack of social support can affect getting both physical and psychological help. (Chapter 4 has more information about intimate relationships.)

Developing Values and Purpose in Your Life
Erikson assigned his last two stages, generativity versus self-absorption and integrity versus despair, to middle adulthood and older adulthood. But these stages are concerned with values and purpose in life, issues that need to be addressed by young people and reexamined throughout life. Values are criteria for judging what is good and bad; they underlie our moral decisions and behavior. The first morality of the young child is to consider "good" to mean what brings immediate and tangible rewards, and "bad," whatever results in punishment. An older child will explain right and wrong in terms of authority figures and rules. But the final stage of moral development, one that

not everyone attains, is being able to conceive of right and wrong in more abstract terms such as justice and virtue.

As adults we need to assess how far we have evolved morally and what values we actually have adopted, either explicitly or implicitly. Without an awareness of our personal values, our lives may be hurriedly driven forward by immediate desires and the passing demands of others. But are we doing things according to our principles? What are we striving for with our actions? Living according to values means considering your options carefully before making a choice, choosing between options without succumbing to outside pressures that oppose your values, and making a choice and acting on it rather than doing nothing. Your actions and how you justify them proclaim to others what you stand for.

A practical exercise for clarifying your values and goals is to write a draft of your obituary for a local newspaper. How would you like to be remembered? What would you like to have achieved? What will you have done to meet those goals? This obituary should not be a glorification, but an honest, realistic appraisal. End it by summarizing in a few sentences what was most important about your life. In reading what you have written, ask yourself, "How will I have to change to be the person I want to be?"

For more on developing meaning and purpose in your life, see the box "Paths to Spiritual Wellness." Visit the Online Learning Center for self-assessments that can help you identify your goals and values and suggest ways to boost your spiritual wellness.

Achieving Healthy Self-Esteem

Having a healthy level of self-esteem means regarding your self, which includes all aspects of your identity, as good, competent, and worthy of love. It is a critical component of wellness.

Developing a Positive Self-Concept Ideally, a positive self-concept begins in childhood, based on experiences both within the family and outside it. Children need to develop a sense of being loved and being able to give love and to accomplish their goals. If they feel rejected or neglected by their parents, they may fail to develop feelings of self-worth. They may grow to have a negative concept of themselves.

Another component of self-concept is integration. An integrated self-concept is one that you have made for yourself—not someone else's image of you or a mask that doesn't quite fit. Important building blocks of self-concept are the personality characteristics and mannerisms of parents, which children may adopt without realizing it. Later, they may be surprised to find themselves acting like one of their parents. Eventually, such building blocks should be reshaped and integrated into a new, individual personality.

A further aspect of self-concept is stability. Stability depends on the integration of the self and its freedom

Mind/Body/Spirit

Spiritual wellness means different things to different people. For many, it involves developing a set of guiding beliefs, principles, or values that give meaning and purpose to life. It helps people achieve a sense of wholeness within themselves and in their relationships with others. Spiritual wellness influences people on an individual level, as well as on a community level, where it can bond people together through compassion, love, forgiveness, and self-sacrifice. For some, spirituality includes a belief in a higher power. Regardless of how it is defined, the development of spiritual wellness is critical for overall health and well-being. Its development is closely tied to the other components of wellness, particularly psychological health.

There are many paths to spiritual wellness. One of the most common in our society is organized religion. Some people object to the notion that organized religion can contribute to psychological health and overall wellness, asserting that it reinforces people's tendency to deny real difficulties and to accept what can and should be changed. Freud criticized religion as wishful thinking; Marx called it an opiate to make the poor accept social injustice. However, many elements of religious belief and practice can promote psychological health.

Organized religion usually involves its members in a community where social and material support is available. Religious organizations offer a social network to those who might otherwise be isolated. The major religions provide paths for transforming the self in ways that can lead to greater happiness and serenity and reduce feelings of anxiety and hopelessness. In Christianity, salvation follows turning away from the selfish ego to God's sovereignty and grace, where a joy is found that frees the believer from anxious self-concern and despair. Islam is the word for a kind of self-surrender leading to peace with God. Buddhism teaches how to detach oneself from selfish desire, leading to compassion for the suffering of others and freedom from fear-engendering illusions. Judaism emphasizes the social and ethical redemption the Jewish community can experience if it follows the laws of God. Religions teach specific techniques for achieving these transformations of the self: prayer, both in groups and in private; meditation; the performance of rituals and ceremonies symbolizing religious truths; and good works and service to others. Christianity's faith and works are perhaps analogous to the cognitive and behavioral components of a program of behavior change.

Spiritual wellness does not require participation in organized religion. Many people find meaning and purpose in other ways. By spending time in nature or working on environmental issues, people can experience continuity with the natural world. Spiritual wellness can come through helping others in one's community or by promoting human rights, peace and harmony among people, and opportunities for human development on a global level. (The spiritual, psychological, and physical wellness benefits of helping others are discussed further in Chapter 19.) Other people develop spiritual wellness through art or through their personal relationships.

The search for meaning and purpose in life is reflected in Erikson's later stages of development. Particularly in the second half of life, people seem to have an urge to view their activities and consciousness from a transcendent perspective. Perhaps it is the approach of death that makes older people tend to take less interest in material possessions and to devote more time to interpersonal and altruistic pursuits. At every age, however, people seem to feel better if they have beliefs about the ultimate purpose of life and their own place in the universe.

from contradictions. People who have gotten mixed messages about themselves from parents and friends may have contradictory self-images, which defy integration and make them vulnerable to shifting levels of self-esteem. At times they regard themselves as entirely good, capable, and lovable—an ideal self—and at other times they see themselves as entirely bad, incompetent, and unworthy of love. While at the first pole, they may develop such an inflated ego that they totally ignore other people's needs and see others only as instruments for fulfilling their own desires. At the other pole, they may feel so small and weak that they run for protection to someone who seems powerful and caring. At neither extreme do such people see themselves or others realistically, and their relationships with other people are filled with misunderstandings and ultimately with conflict.

The concepts we have about ourselves and others are an important part of our personalities. And all the components of our self-concept profoundly influence our interpersonal relationships.

Meeting Challenges to Self-Esteem As an adult, you sometimes run into situations that challenge your self-concept: People you care about may tell you they don't love you or feel loved by you, or your attempts to accomplish a goal may end in failure. You can react to such challenges in several ways. The best approach is to acknowledge that something has gone wrong and try again, adjusting your goals to your abilities without radically revising your self-concept. Less productive responses are denying that anything went wrong and blaming someone else. These attitudes may preserve your self-concept temporarily, but in the long run they keep you from meeting the challenge. The worst reaction is to develop a lasting negative self-concept in which you feel bad, unloved, and ineffective—in other words, to become demoralized. Instead of coping, the

A positive self-concept begins in infancy. Knowing that he's loved and valued by his parents gives this baby a solid basis for lifelong psychological health.

demoralized person gives up, reinforcing the negative self-concept and setting in motion a cycle of bad self-concept and failure. In people who are genetically predisposed to depression, demoralization can progress to additional symptoms, discussed later in the chapter.

NOTICE YOUR PATTERNS OF THINKING One method for fighting demoralization is to recognize and test your negative thoughts and assumptions about yourself and others. The first step is to note exactly when an unpleasant emotion—feeling worthless, wanting to give up, feeling depressed—occurs or gets worse, to identify the events or daydreams that trigger that emotion, and to observe whatever thoughts come into your head just before or during the emotional experience. It is helpful to keep a daily journal about such events.

Consider the example of Jennifer, a student who went to the college counseling center because she'd been feeling "down" lately. Her social life had not been going well, and she had begun to think she was a boring, uninteresting person. Asked to keep a daily journal, she wrote that she felt let down and discouraged when a date who promised to meet

her at 7:30 P.M. was 15 minutes late. She had these thoughts: "He's not going to come. It's my fault. He has more important things to do. Maybe he's with someone else. He doesn't like me. Nobody likes me because I don't have anything interesting to say. What if he had a car accident?"

People who are demoralized tend to use all-or-nothing thinking. They overgeneralize from negative events. They overlook the positive and jump to negative conclusions, minimizing their own successes and magnifying the successes of others. They take responsibility for unfortunate situations that are not their fault. The minute Jennifer's date was late, she jumped to the conclusion that he was not coming and blamed herself for it. From that point she jumped to more negative conclusions and more unfounded overgeneralizations. Patterns of thinking that make events seem worse than they are in reality are called **cognitive distortions.**

DEVELOP REALISTIC SELF-TALK Jennifer needs to develop more rational responses. For Jennifer, more rational thinking could be "He's a little late so I'll reread the study questions." If he still hasn't come after 30 minutes, she might call him to see if something is holding him up, without jumping to any conclusions about the meaning of his lateness.

In your own fight against demoralization, it may be hard to figure out a rational response until hours or days after the event that upset you. But once you get used to noticing the way your mind works, you may be able to catch yourself thinking negatively and change the thought process before it goes too far.

This approach is not the same as positive thinking—substituting a positive thought for a negative one. Instead, you simply try to make your thoughts as logical and accurate as possible. If Jennifer continues to think she's boring, she should try to collect evidence to prove or disprove that. If she has exaggerated her dullness, as do many demoralized people, her investigations may prove her wrong. For example, she might ask her friends their candid opinions about her personality, and she can observe whether people seem interested in continuing a conversation with her.

Demoralized people can be so tenacious about their negative beliefs that they make them come true in a self-fulfilling prophecy. Jennifer might conclude that she is so boring no one will like her anyway, so she may as well not bother to be involved in what's going on around her. This behavior could help her negative belief become a reality. For additional tips on how to change distorted, negative ways of thinking, see the box "Realistic Self-Talk."

Being Less Defensive

Sometimes our wishes come into conflict with people around us or with our conscience, and we become frustrated and anxious. If we cannot resolve the conflict by changing the external situation, we try to resolve the

Terms

V\|w
cognitive distortion A pattern of thinking that makes events seem worse than they are.

defense mechanism A mental mechanism for coping with conflict or anxiety.

Take Charge

Realistic Self-Talk

Do your patterns of thinking make events seem worse than they truly are? Do negative beliefs about yourself become self-fulfilling prophecies? Substituting realistic self-talk for negative self-talk can help you build and maintain self-esteem and cope better with the challenges in your life. Here are some examples of common types of distorted, negative self-talk, along with suggestions for more accurate and rational responses.

Cognitive Distortion	Negative Self-Talk	Realistic Self-Talk
Focusing on negatives	School is so discouraging—nothing but one hassle after another.	School is pretty challenging and has its difficulties, but there certainly are rewards. It's really a mixture of good and bad.
Expecting the worst	Why would my boss want to meet with me this afternoon if not to fire me?	I wonder why my boss wants to meet with me. I guess I'll just have to wait and see.
Overgeneralizing	(After getting a poor grade on a paper) Just as I thought—I'm incompetent at everything.	I'll start working on the next paper earlier. That way, if I run into problems, I'll have time to consult with the TA.
Minimizing	I won the speech contest, but none of the other speakers was very good. I wouldn't have done as well against stiffer competition.	It may not have been the best speech I'll ever give, but it was good enough to win the contest. I'm really improving as a speaker.
Blaming others	I wouldn't have eaten so much last night if my friends hadn't insisted on going to that restaurant.	I overdid it last night. Next time I'll make different choices.
Expecting perfection	I should have scored 100% on this test. I can't believe I missed that one problem through a careless mistake.	Too bad I missed one problem through carelessness, but overall I did very well on this test. Next time I'll be more careful.
Believing you're the cause of everything	Sarah seems so depressed today. I wish I hadn't had that argument with her yesterday; it must have really upset her.	I wish I had handled the argument better, and in the future I'll try to. But I don't know if Sarah's behavior is related to what I said or even if she's depressed. In any case, I'm not responsible for how Sarah feels or acts; only she can take responsibility for that.
Thinking in black and white	I've got to score 10 points in the game today. Otherwise, I don't belong on the team.	I'm a good player or else I wouldn't be on the team. I'll play my best—that's all I can do.
Magnifying events	They went to a movie without me. I thought we were friends, but I guess I was wrong.	I'm disappointed they didn't ask me to the movie, but it doesn't mean our friendship is over. It's not that big a deal.

SOURCE: Adapted from Schafer, W. 1995. *Stress Management for Wellness*, 3rd ed. Copyright © 1996. Reprinted with permission of Wadsworth, a division of Thomson Learning: www.thomsonrights.com. Fax 800-730-2215.

conflict internally by rearranging our thoughts and feelings. Some standard **defense mechanisms** are listed in Table 3-2 on page 72. The drawback of many of these coping mechanisms is that although they succeed temporarily, they are dead-ends that make finding ultimate solutions much harder. Some mechanisms, such as substitution and humor, can be very useful for coping, as long as they don't keep us from being who we want to be.

Recognizing your favorite defense mechanisms can be difficult, because they've probably become habits, occurring unconsciously. But we each have some inkling about how our mind operates. By remembering the details of conflict situations you have been in, you may be able to figure out which defense mechanisms you used in successful or unsuccessful attempts to cope. Try to look at yourself as an objective, outside observer would and analyze your thoughts and behavior in a psychologically stressful situation from the past. Having insight into what strategies you typically use can lead to new, less defensive and more effective ways of coping in the future.

Being Optimistic

Optimism and pessimism are abstract concepts that might seem to have more to do with philosophy than with psychological health. However, many psychologists believe that pessimism is not just a symptom of everyday depression but an important root cause as well. Pessimists not only expect repeated failure and rejection but also perversely accept it as deserved. Pessimists do not see themselves as capable of

Table 3-2	**Defense and Coping Mechanisms**	
Mechanism	**Description**	**Example**
Projection	Reacting to unacceptable inner impulses as if they were from outside the self	A student who dislikes his roommate feels that the roommate dislikes him.
Repression	Expelling from awareness an unpleasant feeling, idea, or memory	The child of an alcoholic, neglectful father remembers him as a giving, loving person.
Denial	Refusing to acknowledge to yourself what you really know to be true	A person believes that smoking cigarettes won't harm her because she's young and healthy.
Passive-aggressive behavior	Expressing hostility toward someone by being covertly uncooperative or passive	A person tells a coworker, with whom she competes for project assignments, that she'll help him with a report but then never follows through.
Displacement	Shifting one's feelings about a person to another person	A student who is angry with one of his professors returns home and yells at one of his housemates.
Rationalization	Giving a false, acceptable reason when the real reason is unacceptable	A shy young man decides not to attend a dorm party, telling himself he'd be bored.
Substitution	Deliberately replacing a frustrating goal with one that is more attainable	A student having a difficult time passing courses in chemistry decides to change his major from biology to economics.
Humor	Finding something funny in unpleasant situations	A student whose bicycle has been stolen thinks how surprised the thief will be when he or she starts downhill and discovers the brakes don't work.

success, and they irrationally dismiss any evidence of their own accomplishments. This negative point of view is learned, typically at a young age from parents and other authority figures. But as an optimist would tell you, that means it also has the potential to be unlearned.

Psychologist Martin Seligman points out that we are more used to refuting negative statements, such as "The problem is going to last forever and ruin everything, and it's all my fault," when they come from a jealous rival rather than from our own mind. But refuting such negative self-statements is exactly what a pessimist must learn to do in order to avoid chronic unhappiness. Pessimists must first recognize and then dispute the false, negative predictions they generate about themselves. Seligman points out that learning to be optimistic is easier and more lasting than, for example, learning to eat less. Unlike refusing foods you love, disputing your own negative thoughts is fun—because doing so makes you feel better immediately.

Maintaining Honest Communication

Another important area of psychological functioning is communicating honestly with others. It can be very frustrating for us and for people around us if we cannot express what we want and feel. Others can hardly respond to our needs if they don't know what those needs are. We must recognize what we want to communicate and then express it clearly. For example, how do you feel about going to the party instead of to the movie? Do you care if your roommate talks on the phone late into the night? Some people know what they want others to do but don't state it clearly because they fear denial of the request, which they interpret as personal rejection. Such people might benefit from **assertiveness** training: learning to insist on their rights and to bargain for what they want. Assertiveness includes being able to say no or yes depending on the situation.

Because expressing feelings has become so central to popular psychology, many misconceptions have arisen. Neither "sharing" feelings with everyone on every occasion nor making important decisions based on feelings alone is a legitimate psychological health goal. But communicating your feelings appropriately and clearly is important. For example, if you tell people you feel sad, they may have various reactions. If they feel closer to you, they may express an intimate thought of their own. Or they may feel guilty because they think you're implying they have caused your sadness. They may even be angry because they feel obligated to help cheer you up.

Depending on your intention and your prediction of how a statement will be taken, you may or may not wish to make it. For example, if you say you feel like staying home tonight, you may also be implying something different. You could really be saying "Don't bother me" or opening a negotiation about what you would be willing to do that evening, given the right event or incentive.

Term

V̇i̇w **assertiveness** Expression that is forceful but not hostile.

Good communication means expressing yourself clearly. You don't need any special psychological jargon to communicate effectively. (For tips, see the box "Guidelines for Effective Communication" in Chapter 4, p. 104.)

Dealing with Loneliness

The right balance between being alone and being with others is often hard to achieve. Some people are motivated to socialize by a fear of being alone—not the best reason to spend time with others. If you discover how to be happy by yourself, you'll be better able to cope with periods when you're forced to be alone—for example, when you've just broken off a romantic relationship, when you've moved to a new town, or when your usual friends are away on vacation.

Unhappiness with being alone may come from interpreting it as a sign of rejection—that others are not interested in spending time with you. Before you conclude that, be sure that you give others a real chance to get to know you. Examine your patterns of thinking: You may harbor unrealistic expectations about other people—for example, that everyone you meet must like you and, if they don't, you must be terribly flawed. You might also consider the possibility that you expect too much from new acquaintances and, sensing this, they start to draw back, triggering your feelings of rejection. Not everyone you meet is a suitable and willing person for a close or intimate relationship. Feeling pressure to have such a relationship may lead you to take up with someone whose interests and needs are remote from yours or whose need to be cared for leaves you with little time of your own. You will have traded loneliness for potentially worse problems.

Loneliness is a passive feeling state. If you decide that you're not spending enough time with people, take action to change the situation. College life provides many opportunities to meet people. In addition to classes and dorms, there are organizations of all kinds—hiking clubs, religious groups, advocacy groups, and so on—that offer a chance to meet others who share your interests. If you're shy, you may have to push yourself to join such groups. Look for something you've enjoyed in the past or in which you have a genuine interest. If your loneliness is the result of missing absent friends, remember that communication at a distance is cheaper and easier than ever before. For many people, e-mail and cell phones offer more immediate and satisfying contact than letters for keeping up with people in their lives.

Dealing with Anger

Popular wisdom has said that you should express your anger rather than suppress it. Letting out your anger was thought to be beneficial for both psychological and physical health. However, recent studies have questioned this idea by showing that people who are overtly hostile seem to be at higher risk for heart attacks. Furthermore, angry words or actions won't contribute to psychological

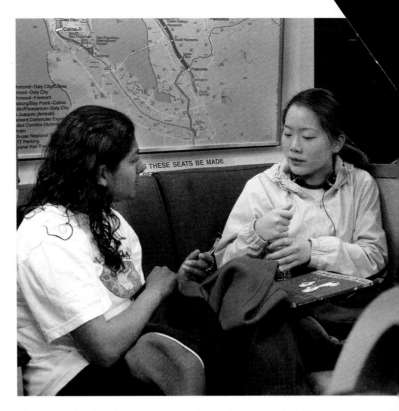

Communication is an important element in any interpersonal relationship. As these women express their thoughts and feelings to each other and listen attentively in response, they enhance their relationship, which in turn supports their psychological well-being.

wellness if they damage important personal or professional relationships or produce feelings of guilt or loss of control. Perhaps the best way to resolve this contradiction is to look at the expression of anger in each situation and distinguish between a gratuitous expression of anger and a reasonable level of self-assertiveness.

At one extreme are people who never express anger or any opinion that might offend others, even when their own rights and needs are being jeopardized. They may find themselves in unhealthy relationships, which they can neither change nor escape from. They may be chronically deprived of satisfaction at work and at home. If you have trouble expressing your anger, you might explore training in assertiveness and appropriate expressions of anger to help you learn to express your needs, desires, and opinions constructively.

At the other extreme are people whose anger is explosive or misdirected. Explosive anger, or rage, like a child's tantrum, renders individuals temporarily unable to think straight or to act in their own best interest. In the long term, frequent expressions of rage can increase the risk of heart disease (see Chapter 15).

Managing Your Own Anger If you feel explosive anger coming on, consider the following two strategies to head it off. First, try to *reframe* what you're thinking at that moment. You'll be less angry at another person if there is a possibility that his or her behavior was not intentionally directed against you. Did the man who cut into your lane on the freeway do it deliberately to spite you, or did he simply fail to see you? Look for possible mitigating factors that would make you less likely to blame him: Maybe he's late for a job interview and preoccupied with worries. If you're angry because you've just been criticized, avoid mentally replaying scenes from the past when you received similar unjust criticisms. Think about what is happening now, and try to act differently than in the past—less defensively and more analytically. What is it about me that makes it easy for this person to get my goat? Why am I taking it personally? Why am I acting like a jerk just because she did?

Second, until you're able to change your thinking, try to *distract* yourself. Use the old trick of counting to 10 before you respond, or start concentrating on your breathing. If needed, take a longer cooling-off period by leaving the situation until your anger has subsided. This does not mean that you should permanently avoid the issues and people who make you angry. When you've had a chance to think more clearly about the matter, return to it.

Dealing with Anger in Other People Anger can be infectious and disruptive to cooperation and communication. If someone you're with becomes very angry, respond "asymmetrically" by reacting not with anger but with calm. Try to validate the other person by acknowledging that he or she has some reason to be angry. This does not mean apologizing, if you don't think you're to blame, or accepting verbal abuse, which is always inappropriate. Try to focus on solving the problem by allowing the individual to explain why he or she is so angry and what can be done to alleviate the situation. Finally, if the person cannot be calmed, it may be best to disengage, at least temporarily. After a time-out, a rational problem-solving approach may become more successful.

PSYCHOLOGICAL DISORDERS

All of us have felt anxious at times, and in dealing with the anxiety we may have avoided doing something that we wanted to do or should have done. Most of us have had periods of feeling down when we became pessimistic, less energetic, and less able to enjoy life. Many of us have been bothered at times by irrational thoughts or odd feelings. Such feelings and thoughts can be normal responses to the ordinary challenges of life, but when emotions or irrational thoughts start to interfere with daily activities and rob us of our peace of mind, they can be considered symptoms of a psychological disorder.

Psychological disorders are generally the result of many factors. Genetic differences, which underlie differences in how the brain processes information and experience, are known to play an important role, especially in bipolar disorder and schizophrenia. However, exactly which genes are involved, and how they alter the structure and chemistry of the brain, is still under study. Learning and life events are important, too: Identical twins often don't have the same psychological disorders in spite of having identical genes. Some people have been exposed to more traumatic events than others, leading either to greater vulnerability to future traumas or, conversely, the development of better coping skills. Furthermore, what your parents, peers, and others have taught you strongly influences your level of self-esteem and how you deal with frightening or depressing life events (see the box "Ethnicity, Culture, and Psychological Disorders").

In this section, we'll take a closer look at some of the more common psychological disorders, including anxiety disorders, mood disorders, and schizophrenia. (Table 3-3 on p. 76 shows the likelihood of these disorders occurring during your lifetime and during the past year.) Elsewhere in this book you can learn about other disorders: sexual disorders in Chapter 5, disorders associated with drug and alcohol abuse in Chapters 9 and 10, eating disorders in Chapter 14, and Alzheimer's disease in Chapter 19.

Anxiety Disorders

Fear is a basic and useful emotion. Its value for our ancestors' survival cannot be overestimated; for modern humans, it provides motivation for self-protection and for learning to cope with new or potentially dangerous environmental or social situations. Only when fear is out of proportion to real danger can it be considered a problem. **Anxiety** is another word for fear, especially a feeling of fear that is not in response to any definite threat. Only when anxiety is experienced almost daily or in life situations that recur and cannot be avoided can anxiety be called a disorder. This section provides brief descriptions of the major types of anxiety disorders.

Simple Phobia The most common and most understandable anxiety disorder, **simple,** or **specific, phobia** is a fear of something definite like lightning or a particular animal or location. Examples of commonly feared animals are snakes, spiders, and dogs; frightening locations are often high places or enclosed spaces. Sometimes, but

---

Terms

V̌w

anxiety A feeling of fear that is not directed toward any definite threat.

simple (specific) phobia A persistent and excessive fear of a specific object, activity, or situation.

social phobia An excessive fear of performing in public; speaking in public is the most common example.

panic disorder A syndrome of severe anxiety attacks accompanied by physical symptoms.

Psychological disorders differ in incidence and symptoms across cultures and ethnic groups around the world. This variability is usually attributable to cultural differences—factors such as how symptoms are interpreted and communicated, whether treatment is sought, and whether a social stigma is attached to a particular symptom or disorder. Cultural differences relating to acculturation, ethnic identity, coping styles, social support, racism, and spirituality can increase the risk for, or provide protection from, psychological disorders.

Expression of Symptoms

People from different cultures or groups may manifest or describe symptoms differently. Consider the following examples:

- In Japan, where showing respect and consideration for others is highly valued, people with social phobia may be more distressed about the imagined harm to others by their social clumsiness than at their own embarrassment.

- Older African Americans may express depression in atypical ways—for example, denying depression by taking on a multitude of extra tasks.

- Somatization, the indirect reporting of psychological distress through nonspecific physical symptoms, occurs across ethnic groups but is more prevalent among some, including African Americans, Puerto Ricans, and Chinese Americans.

- Schizophrenia may manifest with different delusions depending on the local culture.

Attitudes Toward Symptoms, Diseases, and Treatment

An important cultural factor is whether a group regards symptoms of a psychological disorder as a social, moral, or health problem. It is relatively easy for Americans of northern European descent to regard an emotional problem as psychological in nature and to therefore accept a psychological treatment like therapy. For other groups, symptoms of psychological distress may be viewed as a spiritual problem, best dealt with by seeking guidance from religious figures.

Attitudes about disease influence whether patients will comply with professional treatment. For example, researchers looking at multiethnic clinics found that Southeast Asians were more likely than other groups to have no detectable blood levels of their prescribed antidepressant medication. The explanation for this, based on cultural norms, is that the patients' respect for the authority of the physician made them reluctant to admit that they did not agree with the doctor's recommendations and had not followed them.

People from some groups may have little hesitation about communicating intimate, personal problems to professional care providers. However, for others, particularly men and members of certain ethnic groups, loss of emotional control may be seen as a weakness. For all groups, culturally competent care is important to avoid misdiagnosis and inappropriate or ineffective treatment.

Genetic/Biological Risk Factors

Biology can also play a role in the differences seen among patients of different ethnic groups. There is accumulating evidence that genetic differences between ethnic groups can explain some differences in drug metabolism. For example, psychotropic drugs are broken down in the body by a specific enzyme known as CYP2C19. Reduction of the activity of this enzyme is caused by two mutations, one of which appears to be found only in Asian populations. People in whom the action of this enzyme is reduced are called poor metabolizers, who as a result are very sensitive to medications that are broken down by it. The percentage of poor metabolizers among Asians is about 20%; among Latinos, about 5%; and among whites, 3%. Asian patients thus tend to have more adverse reactions to the doses of drugs standardized principally on white patients in the United States.

SOURCES: Kleinman, A. 2004. Culture and depression. *New England Journal of Medicine* 351(10): 951–953; Kirmayer, L. J. 2001. Cultural variations in the clinical presentation of depression and anxiety: Implications for diagnosis and treatment. *Journal of Clinical Psychiatry* 62 (Suppl. 13): 22–28; Lin, K. M. 2001. Biological differences in depression and anxiety across races and ethnic groups. *Journal of Clinical Psychiatry* 62 (Suppl. 13): 13–19; Baker, F. M. 2001. Diagnosing depression in African Americans. *Community Mental Health Journal* 37(1): 31–38; U.S. Department of Health and Human Services. 2001. *Mental Health: Culture, Race, and Ethnicity—A Supplement to Mental Health: A Report of the Surgeon General.* Rockville, Md.: U.S. Department of Health and Human Services.

not always, these fears originate in bad experiences, such as being bitten by a snake. A special kind of simple phobia is fear of blood, injections, or seeing injured people. These fears usually come from a tendency to faint or become nauseated in such situations.

Social Phobia People with **social phobia** fear humiliation or embarrassment while being observed by others. Fear of speaking in public is perhaps the most common phobia of this kind. Extremely shy people can have social fears that extend to almost all social situations (see the box "Shyness" on p. 77). People with these kinds of fears may not continue in school as far as they could and may restrict themselves to lower-paying jobs where they do not have to come into contact with new people.

Panic Disorder People with **panic disorder** experience sudden unexpected surges in anxiety, accompanied by symptoms such as rapid and strong heartbeat, shortness of breath, loss of physical equilibrium, and a feeling of losing mental control. Such attacks usually begin in one's early twenties and can lead to a fear of being in crowds or closed places or of driving or flying. Sufferers fear that a panic attack will occur in a situation from which

Table 3-3 Prevalence of Selected Psychological Disorders Among Americans

	Men		Women	
Disorder	Lifetime Prevalence (%)	Past Year Prevalence (%)	Lifetime Prevalence (%)	Past Year Prevalence (%)
Anxiety disorders				
Simple phobia	6.7	4.4	15.7	13.2
Social phobia	11.1	6.6	15.5	9.1
Panic disorder	2.0	1.3	5.0	3.2
Generalized anxiety disorder	3.6	2.0	6.6	4.3
Obsessive-compulsive disorder	1.7	0.5	2.8	0.8
Post-traumatic stress disorder	5.0	1.5	10.4	3.5
Mood disorders				
Major depressive episode	12.0	5.5	20.4	7.7
Manic episode	1.6	1.4	1.7	1.3
Schizophrenia and related disorders	1.0	0.8	0.5	0.4

SOURCES: Kessler, R. C., et al. 2003. The epidemiology of major depressive disorder: Results from the National Comorbidity Survey Replication (NCS-R). *Journal of the American Medical Association* 289(23): 3095–3105. U.S. Department of Health and Human Services. 1999. *Mental Health: A Report of the Surgeon General.* Rockville, Md.: DHHS; Weissman, M. M. 1998. Cross-national epidemiology of obsessive-compulsive disorder. *CNS Spectrums* 3(5 Suppl. 1): 6–9; Kessler, R. C., et al. 1995. Posttraumatic stress disorder in the National Comorbidity Survey. *Archives of General Psychiatry* 52(12): 1048–1060; Kessler, R. C., et al. 1994; Lifetime and 12-month prevalence of DSM-III-R psychiatric disorders in the United States. *Archives of General Psychiatry* 51(1): 8–19.

escape is difficult (such as while in an elevator), where the attack could be incapacitating and result in a dangerous or embarrassing loss of control (such as while driving a car or shopping), or where no medical help would be available if needed (such as when a person is alone away from home). Fears such as these lead to avoidance of situations that might cause trouble. The fears and avoidance may spread to a large variety of situations until a person is virtually housebound, a condition called **agoraphobia.** People with

panic disorder can often function normally in feared situations if someone they trust accompanies them.

Generalized Anxiety Disorder   A basic reaction to future threats is to worry about them. **Generalized anxiety disorder (GAD)** is a diagnosis given to people whose worries have taken on a life of their own, pushing out other thoughts and refusing banishment by any effort of will. The topics of the worrying are ordinary concerns: Will I be able to pass the exam next Friday? Where will I get money to get my car fixed? Is my boyfriend really interested in me? Furthermore, the worrying is not completely unjustified—after all, thinking about problems can result in solving them. But this kind of thinking seems to just go around in circles, and the more you try to stop it, the more you feel at its mercy. The end result is a persistent feeling of nervousness, often accompanied by depression, which impairs one's ability to enjoy life and to get things done.

Obsessive-Compulsive Disorder   The diagnosis of **obsessive-compulsive disorder (OCD)** is given to people with obsessions or compulsions or both. **Obsessions** are recurrent, unwanted thoughts or impulses. Unlike the worries of GAD, they are not ordinary concerns but improbable fears such as of suddenly committing an antisocial act or of having been contaminated by germs. For example, a parent may have an impulse to kill a beloved child, or a person may brood over whether he or she got HIV from a handshake. **Compulsions** are repetitive, difficult-to-resist actions usually associated with

Terms

agoraphobia An anxiety disorder characterized by fear of being alone away from help and avoidance of many different places and situations; in extreme cases, a fear of leaving home. From the Greek for "fear of the public market."

generalized anxiety disorder (GAD) An anxiety disorder characterized by excessive, uncontrollable worry about all kinds of things and anxiety in many situations.

obsessive-compulsive disorder (OCD) An anxiety disorder characterized by uncontrollable, recurring thoughts and the performing of senseless rituals.

obsession A recurrent, irrational, unwanted thought or impulse.

compulsion An irrational, repetitive, forced action, usually associated with an obsession.

post-traumatic stress disorder (PTSD) An anxiety disorder characterized by reliving traumatic events through dreams, flashbacks, and hallucinations.

Shyness

Shyness is a form of social anxiety, a fear of what others will think of one's behavior or appearance. Physical signs include a rapid heartbeat, a nervous stomach, sweating, cold and clammy hands, blushing, dry mouth, a lump in the throat, and trembling muscles. Shy people are often excessively self-critical, and they engage in very negative self-talk. The accompanying feelings of self-consciousness, embarrassment, and unworthiness can be overwhelming.

To avoid situations that make them anxious, shy people may refrain from making eye contact or speaking up in public. They may shun social gatherings. They may avoid college courses or job promotions that demand more interpersonal interaction or public speaking. Shyness is not the same thing as being introverted. Introverts prefer solitude to society. Shy people often long to be more outgoing, but their own negative thoughts prevent them from enjoying the social interaction they desire. The consequences of severe shyness can include social isolation, loneliness, and lost personal and professional opportunities. Very shy people also have higher than average rates of other anxiety and mood disorders and of substance abuse.

Shyness is very common, with 40–50% of Americans describing themselves as shy. However, only about 7–13% of adults are so shy that their condition interferes seriously with work, school, daily life, or interpersonal relationships. Shyness is often hidden, and most shy people manage to appear reasonably outgoing, even though they suffer the physical and emotional symptoms of their anxiety. Many shy people do better in structured rather than spontaneous settings.

What causes people to be shy? Research indicates that for some the trait may be partly inherited. But for shyness, as for many health concerns, biology is not destiny. Many shy children outgrow their shyness, just as others acquire it later in life. Clearly, other factors are involved. The type of attachment between a child and his or her caregiver is important, as are parenting styles. Shyness is more common in cultures where children's failures are attributed to their own actions but successes are attributed to other people or events. People's experiences during critical developmental transitions, such as starting school and entering adolescence, have also been linked to shyness. For adults, the precipitating factor may be an event such as divorce or the loss of a job.

Recent surveys indicate that shyness rates may be rising in the United States. With the advent of technologies such as ATM machines, video games, voice mail, faxes, and e-mail, the opportunities for face-to-face interaction are diminishing. Electronic media can be a wonderful way for shy people to communicate, but they can also allow them to hide from all social interaction. In fact, one study found that greater use of the Internet was associated with a decline in participants' communication with family members, a reduction in the size of their social circles, and an increase in levels of depression and loneliness. It remains to be seen whether the first generation to have cradle-to-grave access to home computers, faxes, and the Internet will experience higher rates of shyness.

Shyness is often undiagnosed, but help is available. Shyness classes, assertiveness training groups, and public speaking clinics are available (see the Behavior Change Strategy at the end of the chapter). For the seriously shy, effective treatments include cognitive-behavioral therapy and antidepressant drugs.

If you're shy, try to remember that shyness is widespread and that there are worse fates. Some degree of shyness has an upside. Shy people tend to be gentle, supportive, kind, and sensitive; they are often exceptional listeners. People who think carefully before they speak or act are less likely to hurt the feelings of others. Shyness may also facilitate cooperation. For any group or society to function well, a variety of roles is required, and there is a place for quieter, more reflective individuals.

SOURCES: Furmark, T. 2002. Social phobia. *Acta Psychiatrica Scandinavica* 105(2): 84–93; Carducci, B. J. 1999. *Shyness: A Bold New Approach.* New York: Perennial; Kraut, R., et al. 1998. Internet paradox: A social technology that reduces social involvement and psychological well-being? *American Psychologist* 53(9): 1017–1031.

obsessions. A common compulsion is hand washing, associated with an obsessive fear of contamination by dirt. Other compulsions are counting and repeatedly checking whether something has been done—for example, whether a door has been locked or a stove turned off. People with OCD feel anxious, out of control, and embarrassed. Their rituals can occupy much of their time and make them inefficient at work and difficult to live with.

Post-Traumatic Stress Disorder People who suffer from **post-traumatic stress disorder (PTSD)** are reacting to severely traumatic events (events that produce a sense of terror and helplessness) such as physical violence to oneself or loved ones. Trauma occurs in personal assaults (rape, military combat), natural disasters (floods, earthquakes), and tragedies like fires and airplane or car crashes. Symptoms include reexperiencing the trauma in dreams and in intrusive memories, trying to avoid anything associated with the trauma, and numbing of feelings. Sleep disturbances and other symptoms of anxiety and depression also commonly occur. Such symptoms can last months or even years. PTSD symptoms often decrease substantially within 3 months, but in up to one-third of PTSD cases, the individual does not fully recover. Recovery may be slower in those who have previously experienced trauma or who suffer from ongoing psychological problems.

The terrorist attacks on September 11, 2001, brought PTSD into the spotlight. Among those affected were

You should get evaluated by a professional if you've had five or more of the following symptoms for more than 2 weeks or if any of these symptoms causes such a big change that you can't keep up your usual routine.

When You're Depressed

_____ You feel sad or cry a lot, and it doesn't go away.

_____ You feel guilty for no reason; you feel you're no good; you've lost your confidence.

_____ Life seems meaningless, or you think nothing good is ever going to happen again.

_____ You have a negative attitude a lot of the time, or it seems as if you have no feelings.

_____ You don't feel like doing a lot of the things you used to like—music, sports, being with friends, going out, and so on—and you want to be left alone most of the time.

_____ It's hard to make up your mind. You forget lots of things, and it's hard to concentrate.

_____ You get irritated often. Little things make you lose your temper; you overreact.

_____ Your sleep pattern changes: You start sleeping a lot more or you have trouble falling asleep at night; or you wake up really early most mornings and can't get back to sleep.

_____ Your eating pattern changes: You've lost your appetite or you eat a lot more.

_____ You feel restless and tired most of the time.

_____ You think about death or feel as if you're dying or have thoughts about committing suicide.

When You're Manic

_____ You feel high as a kite, like you're "on top of the world."

_____ You get unrealistic ideas about the great things you can do— things that you really can't do.

_____ Thoughts go racing through your head, you jump from one subject to another, and you talk a lot.

_____ You're a nonstop party, constantly running around.

_____ You do too many wild or risky things—with driving, with spending money, with sex, and so on.

_____ You're so "up" that you don't need much sleep.

_____ You're rebellious or irritable and can't get along at home or school or with your friends.

If you are concerned about depression in yourself or a friend, or if you are thinking about hurting or killing yourself, talk to someone about it and get help immediately. There are many sources of help: a good friend; an academic or resident adviser; the staff at the student health or counseling center; a professor, coach, or adviser; a local suicide or emergency hotline (get the phone number from the operator or directory) or the 911 operator; or a hospital emergency room.

SOURCE: National Institute of Mental Health. 1999. *Let's Talk About Depression* (http://www.nimh.nih.gov/publicat/letstalk.cfm; retrieved August 31, 2000).

survivors, rescue workers, passersby, residents of Manhattan in general, and, to some extent, television viewers around the world who saw countless repeated images of the devastation. Rates of PTSD symptoms were highest among people living near the World Trade Center; however, relatively few residents sought professional help for their symptoms. The general rule for treating PTSD in the immediate aftermath of a traumatic event has been to allow the victim to cope with what happened and to heal by avoiding thinking about it. However, if symptoms persist for weeks or months, and if daily functioning and interpersonal relationships are disrupted, then professional help is indicated.

Treating Anxiety Disorders Therapies for anxiety disorders range from medication to psychological interventions concentrating on a person's thoughts and behavior. As we will discuss later, different models of human nature lead to different ideas of appropriate treatment. Both drug treatments and cognitive-behavioral therapies have proved effective in panic disorder, obsessive-compulsive disorder, and generalized anxiety disorder. Simple phobias are best treated without drugs.

Mood Disorders

We all experience ups and downs in our mood in response to daily events. These temporary mood changes typically don't affect our overall emotional state or level of wellness. A person with a mood disorder, however, experiences emotional disturbances that are intense and persistent enough to affect normal functioning. The two most common mood disorders are depression and bipolar disorder.

Depression The most common mood disorder, **depression** has forms and degrees. It usually involves demoralization and can include the following:

• A feeling of sadness and hopelessness

• Loss of pleasure in doing usual activities

• Poor appetite and weight loss

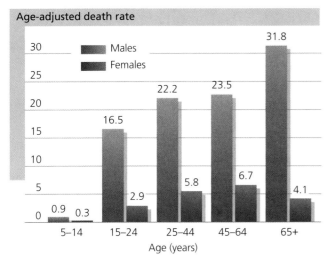

(a) Suicide rate by age and gender

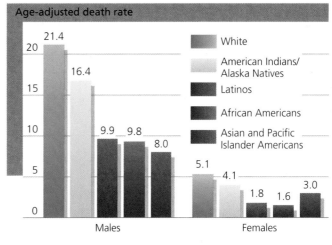

(b) Suicide rate by ethnicity and gender (all ages)

VITAL STATISTICS

Figure 3-2 Rates of suicide in the United States.   The rate of suicide varies by gender, age, and ethnicity. Rates are higher among men than women at all ages and are higher among whites compared to other groups. White men over age 65 have the highest rates of suicide.
SOURCE: National Center for Health Statistics. 2004. *Health, United States, 2004.* Hyattsville, Md.: National Center for Health Statistics.

- Insomnia or disturbed sleep
- Restlessness or, alternatively, fatigue
- Thoughts of worthlessness and guilt
- Trouble concentrating or making decisions
- Thoughts of death or suicide

Not all these features are present in every depressive episode. Sometimes instead of poor appetite and insomnia, the opposite occurs—eating too much and sleeping too long. Amazingly, people can have most of the symptoms of depression without feeling sad or hopeless or in a depressed mood, although they usually do experience a loss of interest or pleasure in things (see the box "Are You Suffering from a Mood Disorder?").

In major depression, symptoms are often severe; a diagnosis of *dysthymic disorder* may be applied to people who experience persistent symptoms of mild or moderate depression for two years or longer. In some cases, depression is a clear-cut reaction to specific events, such as the loss of a loved one or failing in school or work, whereas in other cases no trigger event is obvious. When there is an obvious external trigger, depression may be termed "exogenous." If the trigger is internal, depression is characterized as "endogenous."

RECOGNIZING THE WARNING SIGNS OF SUICIDE   One of the principal dangers of severe depression is suicide. Although a suicide attempt can occur unpredictably and unaccompanied by depression, the chances are greater if

symptoms are numerous and severe. Additional warning signs of suicide include the following:

- Expressing the wish to be dead or revealing contemplated methods
- Increasing social withdrawal and isolation
- A sudden, inexplicable lightening of mood (which can mean the person has finally decided to commit suicide)

Certain risk factors increase the likelihood of suicide:

- A history of previous attempts
- A suicide by a family member or friend
- Readily available means, such as guns or pills
- A history of substance abuse or eating disorders
- Serious medical problems

In the United States, men have much higher suicide rates than women, and whites and Native Americans have higher rates than other groups; white men over age 65 have the highest suicide rate (Figure 3-2). Women attempt three times as many suicides as men, yet men succeed at more than three times the rate of women (see the

Term

depression A mood disorder characterized by loss of interest, sadness, hopelessness, loss of appetite, disturbed sleep, and other physical symptoms.

The common belief that females are more emotional than males has both a positive and a negative side. On the one hand, women are thought to express positive emotions more clearly than men, especially those related to sympathy and caring. On the other hand, they are thought to be more prone to negative emotions such as depression and worry—an association supported in epidemiological studies of anxiety and mood disorders. One of the defining characteristics of a psychiatric disorder is that it interferes with daily activities and the ability to live a happy life. Thus, the higher incidence of anxiety and mood disorders in women is convincing evidence that they are more likely to suffer from emotional distress than are men.

Anxiety Disorders

Panic disorder is more than twice as common in women as in men, whereas obsessive-compulsive disorder occurs in men and women at about the same rate. In population surveys, social anxiety disorder is more common in women than in men, but men are more likely to seek treatment for it—perhaps because men are more likely to find it a barrier to success in white-collar jobs. In some surveys, PTSD is more common in women, but the incidence of PTSD depends on the incidence of traumatic events, which varies in different environments. Men are more often exposed to military combat, and women to rape. Trauma from motor vehicles crashes is a fairly common cause of PTSD in both sexes.

Depression and Suicide

Over their lifetimes, about 20% of women and 12% of men have serious depression. When women are depressed, they are more likely than men to experience guilt, anxiety, increased appetite and weight gain, and increased sleep. When women take antidepressants, they may need a lower dose than men; at the same dosage, blood levels of medication tend to be higher in women. An issue for women who may become pregnant is whether antidepressants can harm a fetus or newborn. The best evidence indicates that the most frequently prescribed types of antidepressants do not cause birth defects, although some studies have reported withdrawal symptoms in some newborns whose mothers used certain antidepressants.

Although suicidal behavior is strongly associated with depression, and depression is more prevalent in women, in the United States, many more men than women commit suicide. Until age 9, boys and girls have the same suicide rates; from 10 to 14 the boys' rate is twice as high; from 15 to 19, four times as high; and from 20 to 24, six times as high. Overall, about three times as many women as men attempt suicide, but women's attempts are less likely to be lethal. In the United States, 60% of male suicides involve firearms.

Factors Underlying Gender Differences

Why women have more problems with anxiety and depression than men is a matter of debate. Some experts think much of the difference is due to reporting bias: Women are more willing to admit to experiencing negative emotions, being stressed, or having difficulty coping. Women may also be more likely to seek treatment at a given level of symptoms.

Other experts point to biologically based sex differences, particularly in the level and action of hormones. Greater anxiety and depression in women compared with men is most pronounced between puberty and menopause, when female hormones are most active. However, this period of life is also the time in which women's social roles and expectations may be the most different from those of men. Women may put more emphasis on relationships in determining self-esteem, so the deterioration of a relationship is a cause of depression that can hit women harder than men. In addition, culturally determined gender roles are more likely to place women in situations where they have less control over key life decisions, and lack of autonomy is associated with depression.

The higher suicide rate among young men may relate to gender norms and expectations that men assert independence and physical prowess—sometimes expressed in risky, dangerous, and potentially self-destructive behavior. Such behavior, often involving drugs and alcohol and resulting in motor vehicle crashes, occurs more often in young people who later commit suicide. Even when suicidal intention is never expressed, suicidal impulses are often suspected of contributing to sudden deaths in this age group.

SOURCES: Sanz, E. J., et al. 2005. Selective serotonin reuptake inhibitors in pregnant women and neonatal withdrawal syndrome. *Lancet* 365(9458): 482–487. Kessler, R. C. 2003. Epidemiology of women and depression. *Journal of Affective Disorders* 74: 5–13; World Health Organization. 2002. *Gender and Mental Health.* Geneva: World Health Organization; Pigott, T. A. 1999. Gender differences in the epidemiology and treatment of anxiety disorders. *Journal of Clinical Psychiatry* 60 (Suppl. 18): 4–15; Langhinrichsen-Rohling, J., et al. 1998. Gender differences in the suicide-related behaviors of adolescents and young adults. *Sex Roles: A Journal of Research* 39(11–12): 839–854.

box "Depression, Anxiety, and Gender"). Worldwide, someone commits suicide every 40 seconds.

HELPING YOURSELF OR A FRIEND If you are severely depressed or know someone who is, expert help from a mental health professional is essential. Don't try to do it all yourself. If you suspect one of your friends is suicidally depressed, try to get him or her to see a professional.

Don't be afraid to discuss the possibility of suicide with people you fear are suicidal. You won't give them an idea they haven't already thought of (see the box "Myths About Suicide"). Asking direct questions is the best way to determine whether someone seriously intends to commit suicide. Encourage your friend to talk and to take positive steps to improve his or her situation. If you feel there is an immediate danger of suicide, ensure that the person is not

Myths About Suicide

Myth People who really intend to kill themselves do not let anyone know about it.
Fact This belief can be an excuse for doing nothing when someone says he or she might commit suicide. In fact, most people who eventually commit suicide *have* talked about doing it.

Myth People who made a suicide attempt but survived did not really intend to die.
Fact This may be true for certain people, but people who seriously want to end their life may fail because they misjudge what it takes. Even a pharmacist may misjudge the lethal dose of a drug.

Myth People who succeed in suicide really wanted to die.

Fact We cannot be sure of that either. Some people are only trying to make a dramatic gesture or plea for help but miscalculate.

Myth People who really want to kill themselves will do it regardless of any attempts to prevent them.
Fact Few people are single-minded about suicide even at the moment of attempting it. People who are quite determined to take their life today may change their mind completely tomorrow.

Myth Suicide is proof of mental illness.
Fact Many suicides are committed by people who do not meet ordinary criteria for mental illness, although people with depression, schizophrenia, and other

psychological disorders have a much higher than average suicide rate.

Myth People inherit suicidal tendencies.
Fact Certain kinds of depression that lead to suicide do have a genetic component. But many examples of suicide running in a family can be explained by factors such as psychologically identifying with a family member who committed suicide, often a parent.

Myth All suicides are irrational.
Fact By some standards all suicides may seem "irrational." But many people find it at least understandable that someone might want to commit suicide, for example, when approaching the end of a terminal illness or when facing a long prison term.

---

left alone, especially when he or she is emotionally upset and more likely to act impulsively. If you must leave your friend alone, have your friend promise not to do anything to harm himself or herself without first calling you. Get qualified help as soon as possible.

If your friend refuses help, you might try to contact your friend's relatives and tell them that you are worried. If the depressed person is a college student, you may need to let someone in your health service or college administration know your concerns. Finally, most communities have emergency help available, often in the form of a hotline telephone counseling service run by a suicide prevention agency (check the yellow pages).

TREATING DEPRESSION Although treatments are highly effective, only about 35% of people who suffer from depression currently seek treatment. Treatment for depression depends on its severity and on whether the depressed person is suicidal. The best initial treatment for moderate to severe depression is probably a combination of drug therapy and some kind of psychotherapy. Uppers such as amphetamines are not good antidepressants; much better are newer prescription antidepressants, although they may take several weeks to begin working. Therefore, when suicidal impulses are strong, hospitalization for a week or so may be necessary.

Antidepressants work by affecting the activity of key neurotransmitters in the brain, including serotonin (Figure 3-3). The over-the-counter herb St. John's wort may also affect serotonin levels, but because it is a dietary supplement it is not subject to the same type of testing and regulation as prescription medications

(see the box "Alternative Remedies for Depression" for more information). Anyone who may be suffering from depression should seek a medical evaluation rather than self-treating with supplements.

Electroconvulsive therapy (ECT) is effective for severe depression when other approaches have failed. In ECT, an epileptic-like seizure is induced by an electrical impulse transmitted through electrodes placed on the head. Patients are given an anesthetic and a muscle relaxant to reduce anxiety and prevent injuries associated with seizures. A typical course of ECT includes three treatments per week for 2 to 4 weeks.

One type of depression is treated in a unique way—by having sufferers sit with eyes open in front of a bright light source for an hour or so early every morning. These patients have **seasonal affective disorder (SAD)**, in which depression worsens during winter months as the number of hours of daylight diminishes and then improves with the lengthening of daylight in the spring and summer. Seasonal depression is more common among people who live at higher latitudes, where there are fewer hours of light in winter. Light therapy may work by extending the perceived

Terms

electroconvulsive therapy (ECT) The use of electric shock to induce brief, generalized seizures; used in the treatment of selected psychological disorders.

seasonal affective disorder (SAD) A mood disorder characterized by seasonal depression, usually occurring in winter, when there is less daylight.

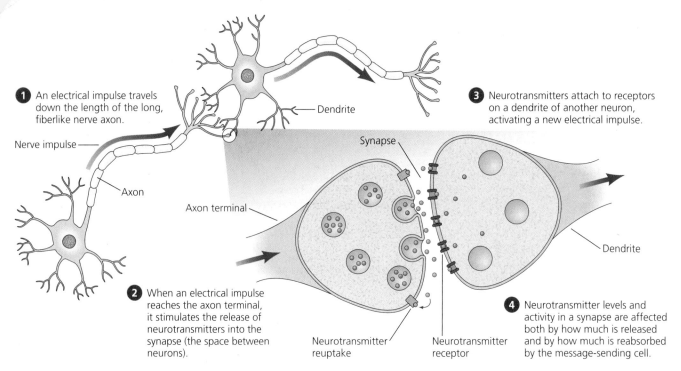

① An electrical impulse travels down the length of the long, fiberlike nerve axon.

Nerve impulse

Axon

② When an electrical impulse reaches the axon terminal, it stimulates the release of neurotransmitters into the synapse (the space between neurons).

Dendrite

Synapse

Axon terminal

Neurotransmitter reuptake

Neurotransmitter receptor

③ Neurotransmitters attach to receptors on a dendrite of another neuron, activating a new electrical impulse.

Dendrite

④ Neurotransmitter levels and activity in a synapse are affected both by how much is released and by how much is reabsorbed by the message-sending cell.

Figure 3-3   Nerve cell communication. Nerve cells (neurons) communicate through a combination of electrical impulses and chemical messages. Neurotransmitters such as serotonin and norepinephrine alter the overall responsiveness of the brain and are responsible for mood, level of attentiveness, and other psychological states. Many psychological disorders are related to problems with neurotransmitters and their receptors, and drug treatments frequently target them. For example, the antidepressant drug Prozac increases levels of serotonin by slowing the resorption (re-uptake) of serotonin.

length of the day and thus convincing the brain that it is summertime even during the winter months.

Mania and Bipolar Disorder   People who experience **mania,** a less common feature of mood disorders, are restless, have a lot of energy, need little sleep, and often talk nonstop. They may devote themselves to fantastic projects and spend more money than they can afford. Many manic people swing between manic and depressive states, a syndrome called **bipolar disorder** because of the two opposite poles of mood. Tranquilizers are used to treat individual manic episodes, while special drugs such as the salt lithium carbonate taken daily can prevent future mood swings.

Gender Differences   One of the mysteries about mood disorders is the gender gap in the incidence of depression. Although equal numbers of men and women suffer from bipolar disorder, women are nearly twice as likely as men to be clinically depressed. The Gender Matters box in this chapter discusses these differences further.

Schizophrenia

Schizophrenia can be severe and debilitating or quite mild and hardly noticeable. Although people are capable of diagnosing their own depression, they usually don't diagnose their own schizophrenia, because they often can't

see that anything is wrong. This disorder is not rare; in fact, 1 in every 100 people has a schizophrenic episode sometime in his or her lifetime, most commonly starting in adolescence. However, because people who are directly or indirectly affected do not like to talk about schizophrenia, its frequency is not generally appreciated. In addition, schizophrenic people tend to withdraw from society when they are ill, another factor making it seem rarer than it is.

Scientists are uncertain about the exact causes of schizophrenia. Researchers have identified possible chemical and structural differences in the brains of people with the disorder as well as several genes that appear to increase risk. Schizophrenia is likely caused by a combination of genes and environmental factors that occur during pregnancy and development. For example, children born to older fathers have higher rates of schizophrenia, as do children with prenatal exposure to certain infections or medications.

Some general characteristics of schizophrenia include the following:

- *Disorganized thoughts.* Thoughts may be expressed in a vague or confusing way.
- *Inappropriate emotions.* Emotions may be either absent or strong but inappropriate.
- *Delusions.* People with delusions—firmly held false beliefs—may think that their minds are controlled by outside forces, that people can read their minds,

Mainstream therapies for depression include medications accepted as safe and effective by government regulatory agencies, certain psychotherapies, and light therapy in the case of seasonal affective disorder. Yet, in surveys, 20% of people in the United States who suffer from depression report using unconventional therapies such as acupuncture, body movement therapy, homeopathy, qigong, faith healing, or herbs or other "natural" substances. With the exception of one herb, St. John's wort (*Hypericum perforatum*), these therapies have not been shown to be effective in double-blind placebo-controlled trials. Such trials are the only scientific way to show that a treatment has healing power beyond that of a **placebo.** (See Chapter 21 for more on different types of medical research studies.)

St. John's wort, a flowering plant that grows as a weed in the United States, has been reputed to have curative properties since the time of Hippocrates in ancient Greece. Modern pharmacological studies confirm that its active ingredients produce a number of biochemical and physiological changes in animals, although it's still unclear exactly how these changes might affect depression. Data from a number of studies suggest that St. John's wort could benefit people with mild to moderate depression, but concerns have been raised about the adequacy of those trials. Recently, two carefully designed trials were conducted on St. John's wort. In one, 375 mild to moderately depressed patients were randomly assigned to receive either a placebo or an extract of St. John's wort; the extract was statistically more effective than the placebo and did not have more side effects. In the other trial, 340 depressed patients were given either St. John's wort, a placebo, or sertraline, a prescription antidepressant. In that study, St. John's wort was no more effective than the placebo—but neither was sertraline. Because many other studies have shown sertraline to have better results than a placebo, this result casts doubt as to whether the study methods were sensitive enough to detect an antidepressant effect. In any case, consumers are left without a definitive answer on the effectiveness of St. John's wort.

An advantage of St. John's wort is that it causes fewer adverse effects than conventional antidepressants. In data from three studies including about 600 depressed patients, the herb produced no more adverse effects than did the placebo. There was no evidence of sedation, gastrointestinal disturbances, or other side effects associated with other antidepressants. However, the safety of St. John's wort in pregnancy has not been established, and it may interact with, and reduce the effectiveness of, certain medications, including oral contraceptives and some medications for treating heart disease, depression, HIV infections, and seizures.

One reason for the popularity of an herb for depression is that it doesn't require a prescription or any kind of contact with a physician or a therapist; for those who are not members of a generous health care plan, an herbal remedy may also be less expensive than a prescription antidepressant. On the other hand, people suffering from depression *should* seek professional advice and not try to get along entirely with self-diagnosis and self-help. If you are depressed enough to contemplate taking St. John's wort, you need to make an appointment to talk to a professional about your depression.

Bear in mind that St. John's wort does not work for everyone, and no expert advocates it for severe depression. Also, because herbal products are classified as dietary supplements, they are not scrutinized by the regulatory agencies that oversee prescription drugs. Thus, consumers have no guarantee that the product contains the herbs and dosages listed on the label (see Chapters 12 and 21 for more on dietary supplements).

SOURCES: Trautmann-Sponsel, R. D., and A. Dienel. 2004. Safety of Hypericum extract in mildly to moderately depressed outpatients: A review based on data from three randomized, placebo-controlled trials. *Journal of Affective Disorders* 82(2): 303–307; Lecrubier, Y., et al. 2002. Efficacy of St. John's wort extract WS 5570 in major depression: A double-blind, placebo-controlled trial. *American Journal of Psychiatry* 159: 1361–1366; Hypericum Depression Trial Study Group. 2002. Effect of *Hypericum perforatum* (St. John's wort) in major depressive disorder: A randomized controlled trial. *Journal of the American Medical Association* 287: 1807–1814; Shelton, R. C., et al. 2001. Effectiveness of St. John's Wort in major depression. *Journal of the American Medical Association* 285 (15): 1978–1986.

that they are great personages like Jesus Christ or the president of the United States, or that they are being persecuted by a group such as the CIA.

- *Auditory hallucinations.* Schizophrenic people may hear voices when no one is present.

- *Deteriorating social and work functioning.* Social withdrawal and increasingly poor performance at school or work may be so gradual that they are hardly noticed at first.

None of these characteristics is invariably present. Some schizophrenic people are quite logical except on the subject of their delusions. Others show disorganized thoughts but no delusions or hallucinations.

Terms

V w

mania A mood disorder characterized by excessive elation, irritability, talkativeness, inflated self-esteem, and expansiveness.

bipolar disorder A mental illness characterized by alternating periods of depression and mania.

schizophrenia A psychological disorder that involves a disturbance in thinking and in perceiving reality.

placebo A chemically inactive substance that a patient believes is an effective medical therapy for his or her condition. To help evaluate a therapy, medical researchers compare the effects of a particular therapy with the effects of a placebo. The "placebo effect" occurs when a patient responds to a placebo as if it were an active drug.

A schizophrenic person needs help from a mental health professional. Suicide is a risk in schizophrenia, and expert treatment can reduce that risk and minimize the social consequences of the illness by shortening the period when symptoms are active. The key element in treatment is regular medication. At times medication is like insulin for diabetes—it makes the difference between being able to function or not. Sometimes hospitalization is temporarily required to relieve family and friends.

MODELS OF HUMAN NATURE AND THERAPEUTIC CHANGE

It is not surprising that beings as complicated as we humans cannot be satisfactorily encompassed by a single perspective. In fact, at least four different perspectives—biological, behavioral, cognitive, and psychodynamic—can be applied to human problems such as the psychological disorders discussed in this chapter. Each perspective has a distinct view of human nature, and from those views of human nature come distinct therapeutic approaches.

The Biological Model

The biological model emphasizes that the mind's activity depends entirely on an organic structure, the brain, whose composition is genetically determined. The activity of neurons, mediated by complex chemical reactions, gives rise to our most complex thoughts, our most ardent desires, and our most pathological behavior. Of course, no one can assert that environment and learning have no influence. Even if the brain is nothing but a supercomputer, it still has to be programmed by experience.

Biological researchers have investigated all of the psychological disorders we have discussed and have found genetic influences on anxiety and depression that cannot be accounted for by environment and learning. The fact that drugs can make anxiety and depression worse or better is evidence that chemicals in the brain influence our moods. Magnetic resonance imaging of the brain shows that the structure of the brain is slightly different in people with schizophrenia.

Pharmacological Therapy The most important kind of therapy inspired by the biological model is pharmacological therapy. A list of some of the popular medications currently used for treating psychological disorders follows. All require a prescription from a psychiatrist or other medical doctor. All have received approval from the U.S. Food and Drug Administration (FDA) as being safe and more effective than a placebo. However, as with all pharmacological therapies, these drugs may cause side effects. For example, the side effects of widely used antidepressants range from diminished appetite to loss of

Pharmacological therapy (medication) is a common form of treatment for many psychological disorders. Medications can be very effective, but they do have risks and side effects, and they do not work for all patients.

sexual pleasure. In addition, an individual may have to try several drugs before finding one that is effective and has acceptable side effects.

1. *Antidepressants:* One group is called the selective serotonin reuptake inhibitors (SSRIs) because of one of their mechanisms of action; this group includes Prozac (fluoxetine), Paxil (paroxetine), Zoloft (sertraline), Luvox (fluvoxamine), Celexa (citalopram), and Lexapro (escitalopram). Another group is called the tricyclics after their chemical structure; it includes Aventyl (nortriptyline) and Elavil (amitriptyline). Nardil (phenelzine) is a monoamine oxidase inhibitor. Antidepressants that do not fit into these groups include Effexor (venlafaxine), Welbutrin (buproprion), Serzone (nefazodone), and Remeron (mirtazapine). Surprisingly, these antidepressants are as effective in treating panic disorder and certain kinds of chronic anxiety as they are in treating depression, and they may also alleviate the symptoms of obsessive-compulsive disorder.

2. *Mood stabilizers:* Lithium carbonate and Depakote (valproic acid) are the most important mood stabilizers. They are taken to prevent mood swings that occur in bipolar disorder and certain kinds of schizophrenia.

3. *Antipsychotics:* Older antipsychotics include Haldol (haloperidol) and Prolixin (fluphenazine); newer

antipsychotics (sometimes called "atypical") are Clozaril (clozapine), Zyprexa (olanzapine), Risperdal (risperidone), and Seroquel (quetiapine). The drugs reduce hallucinations and disordered thinking in people with schizophrenia, bipolar disorder, and delirium, and they have a calming effect on agitated patients.

4. *Anxiolytics (antianxiety agents) and hypnotics (sleeping pills):* One of the largest and most prescribed classes of anxiolytics is the benzodiazepines, a group of drugs that includes Valium (diazepam), Librium (chlordiazepoxide), Xanax (alprazolam), and Ativan (lorazepam); Dalmane (flurazepam), Restoril (temazepam), and Halcion (triazolam) are benzodiazepines marketed as sleeping aids. Newer hypnotics are Sonata (zaleplon) and Ambien (zolpidem).

5. *Stimulants:* Ritalin (methylphenidate) and Dexedrine (dextroamphetamine) are most commonly used for **attention-deficit/hyperactivity disorder (ADHD)** in children, and for excessive daytime sleepiness in adults.

Issues in the Use of Pharmacological Therapy

The discovery that many psychological disorders have a biological basis in disordered brain chemistry has led to a revolution in the treatment of many disorders, particularly depression. The new view of depression as based in brain chemistry has also lessened the stigma attached to the condition, leading more people to seek treatment, and antidepressants are now among the most widely prescribed drugs in the United States. The development of effective drugs has provided relief for many people, but the wide use of antidepressants has also raised many questions (see the box "Antidepressant Use in Young People" on p. 86).

Given the ability of antidepressants to affect brain chemistry and control symptoms, what role does psychotherapy have in treating depression? Research indicates that for mild cases of depression psychotherapy and antidepressants are about equally effective. For major depression, combined therapy is significantly more effective than either type of treatment alone. Some mental health professionals worry that health insurance companies, in an effort to save money, will favor drug therapy over psychotherapy for all patients. Psychotherapy may be particularly important for people whose condition has a strong psychosocial component. Therapy can help provide insight into factors that precipitated the depression, such as high levels of stress, a history of abuse, unresolved grief, or relationship problems. A therapist can also provide guidance in changing patterns of thinking and behavior that contribute to the problem.

What about the use of antidepressants to treat unwanted personality traits in psychologically healthy people? Anecdotal evidence suggests that Prozac and related drugs may help shy or pessimistic people become more outgoing and optimistic, for example. The potential use of antidepressants in this way has sparked ethical debate. Is some degree of vulnerability, anxiety, and sadness an essential part of being human? If antidepressants diminish or eliminate these feelings, will they rob people of the emotional experiences they need to grow and be creative? By masking mental pain, will they interfere with people's connection to reality and to their own emotional experience and expression? This ethical debate extends beyond the question of therapeutic benefits of antidepressants and other pharmacological treatments for psychological disorders.

The Behavioral Model

The behavioral model focuses on what people do—their overt behavior—rather than on brain structures and chemistry or on thoughts and consciousness. This model regards psychological problems as "maladaptive behavior" or bad habits. When and how a person learned bad behavior is less important than what makes it continue in the present. Behaviorists analyze behavior in terms of **stimulus, response,** and **reinforcement.** The essence of behavior therapy is to discover what reinforcements keep an undesirable behavior going and then to try to alter those reinforcements. For example, if people who fear speaking in class (the stimulus) remove themselves from that situation (the response), they experience immediate relief, which acts as reinforcement for future avoidance and escape.

To change their behavior, fearful people are taught to practice **exposure**—to deliberately and repeatedly enter the feared situation and remain in it until their fear begins to abate. Clients are often asked to keep a daily behavior journal to monitor the target behavior and the events that precede and follow it. A student who is afraid to speak in class might begin his behavioral therapy program by keeping a diary listing each time he makes a contribution to a classroom discussion, how long he speaks, and his anxiety levels before, during, and after speaking. He would then develop

Terms

V|w

attention-deficit/hyperactivity disorder (ADHD) A disorder characterized by persistent, pervasive problems with inattention and/or hyperactivity to a degree that is not considered appropriate for a child's developmental stage and that causes significant difficulties in school, work, or relationships.

stimulus Anything that causes a response.

response A reaction to a stimulus.

reinforcement Increasing the future probability of a response by following it with a reward.

exposure A therapeutic technique for treating fear in which the subject learns to come into direct contact with a feared situation.

On September 14, 2004, an FDA advisory committee voted in favor of recommending a warning label for antidepressant drugs on the basis of evidence that their use increases the risk of suicidal thinking and behavior in children and adolescents. The committee based its conclusions on published and unpublished data from trials sponsored by pharmaceutical companies. Controversy immediately followed: Parents wondered why it had taken so long to come to this conclusion, because most of the data had been around for years. Had drug companies ignored indications that their best-selling drugs were not safe? Had physicians deceived themselves and patients' families into thinking that drug treatments worked better than they really did?

Effectiveness

Drug treatment for depression is considered part of a success story in which people take seriously symptoms of depression and hints of suicidal thinking in children and teens. Over the past decade, the suicide rate among adolescents has fallen. Many factors have likely contributed to the decline, including stricter gun laws that make it harder for young people to gain access to guns. Drug treatment has also been considered a key factor in the decline in suicide rates.

To date, only one drug—fluoxetine (Prozac)—has been approved for use specifically in children and teens. Studies have found that fluoxetine causes a greater improvement than a placebo, but the combination of drug therapy and cognitive-behavioral therapy is more beneficial than either treatment alone. The placebo effect, in which people improve while taking pills containing inactive compounds, is significant in studies of depression and can exceed 30%—meaning almost a third of people receiving a placebo experience an improvement in their symptoms.

Many antidepressants other than fluoxetine, especially other SSRIs, are also prescribed to young people, but these other drugs haven't been shown to be effective for that age group. Unpublished research data indicates that some SSRIs are *not* effective in children and teens or are only slightly more effective than a placebo. These findings underscore the need for the publication of all research findings—not just positive ones—so that physicians and patients can make informed decisions about the risks and benefits of drug therapy.

Safety

All medications have potential risks and side effects. The problem associated with SSRIs that caused the FDA to act is the possibility that they increase the risk of suicide in some young people, particularly in the period immediately following the start of medication use. When study results were pooled, researchers found that in the short term, about 2–3% of users have an increased risk of suicidal thoughts and actions beyond the risk inherent from depression itself.

Researchers aren't exactly sure what causes this effect. Antidepressants are not immediately effective, and one theory is that SSRIs reverse the lethargy associated with depression more quickly than they relieve the depression itself, giving users the energy to contemplate suicide in the interim. It is thought that antidepressants work differently on the developing brains of young people than on the brains of adults, so there may be as yet unidentified effects.

Many questions remain unanswered. For example, does the increased risk of suicide associated with SSRI use persist over time? Are there factors that would help physicians identify patients at special risk from medication use? Are certain antidepressants safer or more dangerous than others? Does the risk extend into other age groups?

In October 2004, the FDA published a draft medication guide about using antidepressants in children and teens. It emphasizes that young people who take antidepressants should be monitored closely, especially when starting a new medication or changing the dosage of a drug. Depression is a serious illness that can increase the risk of suicide, and mental health professionals and patients must balance the risks of doing nothing against the potential risks and benefits of different types of treatments.

SOURCES: Food and Drug Administration. 2004. *FDA Proposed Medication Guide: About Using Antidepressants in Children or Teenagers* (http://www.fda.gov/cder/drug/antidepressants/SSRIMedicationGuide.htm; retrieved November 5, 2004); Newman, T. B. 2004. Treating depression in children: A black-box warning for antidressants in children? *New England Journal of Medicine* 351(16): 1595–1598; Brent, D. A. 2004. Treating depression in children: Antidepressants and pediatric depression—the risk of doing nothing. *New England Journal of Medicine* 351(16): 1598–1601; Treatment for Adolescents with Depression Study (TADS) Team. 2004. Fluoxetine, cognitive-behavioral therapy, and their combination for adolescents with depression. *Journal of the American Medical Association* 292(7): 807–820.

concrete but realistic goals for increasing his speaking frequency and contract with himself to reward his successes by spending more time in activities he finds enjoyable.

Although exposure to the real situation works best, exposure in one's imagination or through the virtual reality of computer simulation can also be effective. For example, in the case of someone afraid of flying, an imagined scenario would likely be vivid enough to elicit the fear necessary to practice exposure techniques. The Behavior Change Strategy at the end of Chapter 2 provides a model program for reducing test anxiety; refer to Chapter 1 for general strategies for behavior change.

The Cognitive Model

The cognitive model emphasizes the effect of ideas on behavior and feeling. According to this model, behavior results from complicated attitudes, expectations, and motives rather than from simple, immediate reinforcements. When behavioral therapies such as exposure work, it is because they change the way a person thinks about the feared situation and his or her ability to cope with it.

According to one cognitive theory, recurring false ideas produce feelings such as anxiety and depression. Identifying and exposing these ideas as false should relieve the painful emotion. For example, people who are anxious are thinking, "Something bad is going to happen and I won't be able to handle it." The therapist challenges such ideas in three ways: showing that there isn't enough evidence for the idea, suggesting different ways of looking at the situation, and showing that no disaster is going to occur. The therapist does not just state his or her position but encourages clients to examine the logic of their own ideas and then to test their truth.

For example, a student afraid of speaking in class may harbor thoughts such as "If I begin to speak, I'll say something stupid; if I say something stupid, the teacher and my classmates will lose respect for me; then I'll get a low grade, my classmates will avoid me, and life will be hell." In cognitive therapy, these ideas will be examined critically. If the student prepares, will he or she really sound stupid? Does every sentence said have to be exactly correct and beautifully delivered, or is that an unrealistic expectation? Will classmates' opinions be completely transformed by one presentation? Do classmates even care that much? And why does the student care so much about what *they* think? People in cognitive therapy are taught to notice their unrealistic thoughts and to substitute more realistic ones, and they are advised to repeatedly test their assumptions.

The Psychodynamic Model

The psychodynamic model also emphasizes thoughts, but it asserts that false ideas cannot be fought directly because they are fed by other, unconscious, ideas and impulses. Symptoms are not isolated pieces of behavior but results of a complex system of secret wishes, emotions, and fantasies hidden by active defenses that keep them unconscious (see Table 3-2). The role of the past in shaping the present is often emphasized in psychodynamic therapy. By having the client speak as freely as possible in front of the therapist, the therapist can help the client achieve some insight into the reasons for his or her apparently irrational and self-defeating thoughts and actions. In essence, a trustworthy therapist helps clients become more honest with themselves. One contemporary version of this approach, interpersonal therapy, focuses on the relationship between the person and others. The therapist takes an active role in helping the client to understand and overcome self-isolation and to develop interpersonal skills.

Newer therapies referred to variously as humanistic, existential, or experiential are like psychodynamic therapies in encouraging self-awareness, but they focus more on the present and future than the past. Clients are encouraged to get in touch with their subjective experience (the here and now). The therapist acts as a guide to self-

Gradually exposing a person to a feared object or situation can help overcome phobias. Use of virtual reality goggles allows this individual to simulate a realistic public speaking situation without having to worry about the presence of an actual audience.

exploration and as a facilitator for expanding the client's inherent human potential.

Evaluating the Models

Ignoring theoretical conflicts among psychological models, therapists have recently developed pragmatic *cognitive-behavioral therapies* that combine effective elements of both models in a single package. For example, the package for treating social anxiety emphasizes exposure as well as changing problematic patterns of thinking. Combined therapies have also been developed for panic disorder, obsessive-compulsive disorder, generalized anxiety disorder, and depression. These packages, involving ten or more individual or group sessions with a therapist and homework between sessions, have been shown to produce significant improvement.

Drug therapy and cognitive-behavioral therapies are also sometimes combined, especially in the case of depression. For anxiety disorders, both kinds of therapy are equally effective, but the effects of drug therapy last only as long as the drug is being taken, while cognitive-behavioral therapies produce longer-term improvement. For schizophrenia, drug therapy is a must, but a continuing relationship with therapists who give support and advice is also indispensable.

Psychodynamic therapies have been attacked as ineffective and endless. Of course, effectiveness is hard to demonstrate for therapies that do not focus on specific symptoms. But common sense tells us that being able to open yourself up and discuss your problems with a supportive but objective person who focuses on you and lets you speak freely can enhance your sense of self and reduce feelings of confusion and despair.

GETTING HELP

Knowing when self-help or professional help is required for mental health problems is usually not as difficult as knowing how to start or which professional to choose.

Self-Help

If you have a personal problem to solve, a smart way to begin is by finding out what you can do on your own. Some problems are specifically addressed in this book. Behavioral and some cognitive approaches are especially useful for helping yourself. They all involve becoming more aware of self-defeating actions and ideas and combating them in some way: by being more assertive; by communicating honestly; by raising your self-esteem by counteracting thoughts, people, and actions that undermine it; and by confronting, rather than avoiding, the things you fear. Get more information by seeing what books are available in the psychology or self-help sections of libraries and bookstores. But be selective. Watch out for self-help books making fantastic claims that deviate from mainstream approaches.

Some people find it helpful to express their feelings in a journal. Grappling with a painful experience in this way provides an emotional release and can help you develop more constructive ways of dealing with similar situations in the future. Research indicates that using a journal this way can improve physical as well as emotional wellness.

For some people, religious belief and practice may promote psychological health. Religious organizations provide a social network and a supportive community, and religious practices, such as prayer and meditation, offer a path for personal change and transformation.

Peer Counseling and Support Groups

Sharing your concerns with others is another helpful way of dealing with psychological health challenges. Just being able to share what's troubling you with an accepting, empathetic person can bring relief. Comparing notes with people who have problems similar to yours can give you new ideas about coping.

Many colleges offer peer counseling through a health center or through the psychology or education department. Peer counseling is usually done by volunteer students who have received special training that emphasizes confidentiality. Peer counselors may steer you toward an appropriate campus or community resource or simply offer a sympathetic ear.

Many self-help groups work on the principle of bringing together people with similar problems to share their experiences and support one another. Support groups are typically organized around a specific problem, such as eating disorders or substance abuse. Self-help groups may be listed in the phone book or the campus newspaper.

Professional Help

Sometimes self-help or talking to nonprofessionals is not enough. More objective, more expert, or more discreet help is needed. Many people have trouble accepting the need for professional help, and often those who most need help are the most unwilling to get it. You may someday find yourself having to overcome your own reluctance, or that of a friend, about seeking help.

Determining the Need for Professional Help

In some cases, professional help is optional. Some people are interested in improving their psychological health in a general way by going into individual or

Group therapy is just one of many different approaches to psychological counseling. If you have concerns you would like to discuss with a mental health professional, shop around to find the approach that works for you.

Choosing and Evaluating Mental Health Professionals

College students are usually in a good position to find convenient, affordable mental health care. Larger schools typically have both health services that employ psychiatrists and psychologists and counseling centers staffed by professionals and student peer counselors. Resources in the community may include a school of medicine, a hospital, and a variety of professionals who work independently. Although independent practitioners are listed in the telephone book, it's a good idea to get recommendations from physicians, clergy, friends who have been in therapy, or community agencies rather than pick a name at random.

Financial considerations are also important. Find out how much different services will cost and what your health insurance will cover. If you're not adequately covered by a health plan, don't let that stop you from getting help; investigate low-cost alternatives. City, county, and state governments often support mental health clinics for those who can afford to pay little or nothing for treatment. Some on-campus services may be free or offered at very little cost.

The cost of treatment is linked to how many therapy sessions will be needed, which in turn depends on the type of therapy and the nature of the problem. Psychological therapies focusing on specific problems may require eight or ten sessions at weekly intervals. Therapies aiming for psychological awareness and personality change can last months or years.

Deciding whether a therapist is right for you will require meeting the therapist in person. Before or during your first meeting, find out about the therapist's background and training:

- Does she or he have a degree from an appropriate professional school and a state license to practice?

- Has she or he had experience treating people with problems similar to yours?

- How much will therapy cost?

You have a right to know the answers to these questions and should not hesitate to ask them. After your initial meeting, evaluate your impressions:

- Does the therapist seem like a warm, intelligent person who would be able to help you and interested in doing so?

- Are you comfortable with the personality, values, and beliefs of the therapist?

- Is he or she willing to talk about the techniques in use? Do these techniques make sense to you?

If you answer yes to these questions, this therapist may be satisfactory for you. If you feel uncomfortable—and you're not in need of emergency care—it's worthwhile to set up one-time consultations with one or two others before you make up your mind. Take the time to find someone who feels right for you.

Later in your treatment, evaluate your progress:

- Are you being helped by the treatment?

- If you are displeased, is it because you aren't making progress, or because therapy is raising difficult, painful issues you don't want to deal with?

- Can you express dissatisfaction to your therapist? Such feedback can improve your treatment.

If you're convinced your therapy isn't working or is harmful, thank your therapist for her or his efforts, and find another.

---

group therapy to learn more about themselves and how to interact with others. Clearly, seeking professional help for these reasons is a matter of individual choice. Interpersonal friction among family members or between partners often falls in the middle between necessary and optional. Successful help with such problems can mean the difference between a painful divorce and a satisfying relationship.

It's sometimes difficult to determine whether someone needs professional help, but it is important to be aware of behaviors that may indicate a serious problem. Following are some strong indications that you or someone you know needs professional help:

- If depression, anxiety, or other emotional problems begin to interfere seriously with school or work performance or in getting along with others

- If suicide is attempted or is seriously considered (refer to the warning signs earlier in the chapter)

- If symptoms such as hallucinations, delusions, incoherent speech, or loss of memory occur

- If alcohol or drugs are used to the extent that they impair normal functioning during much of the week, if finding or taking drugs occupies much of the week, or if reducing their dosage leads to psychological or physiological withdrawal symptoms

Choosing a Mental Health Professional

Mental health workers belong to several different professions and have different roles. Psychiatrists are medical doctors. They are experts in deciding whether a medical disease lies behind psychological symptoms, and they are usually involved in treatment if medication or hospitalization is required. Clinical psychologists typically hold a Ph.D. degree; they are often experts in behavioral and cognitive therapies. Other mental health workers include social workers, licensed counselors, and clergy with special training in pastoral counseling. In hospitals and clinics, various mental health professionals may join together in treatment teams. For more on finding appropriate help, see the box "Choosing and Evaluating Mental Health Professionals."

Life inevitably brings change and challenge—they are a part of growth and development. Most of life's psychological challenges can be met with self-help and everyday skills—introspection and insight, honest communication, support from family and friends. Sometimes a psychological problem poses a greater challenge than we can handle on our own; for these situations, professional help is available.

Right now you can

- Consider the areas in your life where you can be creative (one of the qualities associated with self-actualization), whether in music, art, Web page design, party planning, or whatever you truly enjoy. With the knowledge that allowing your creative side to flourish is a valuable use of your time, plan a way to spend an hour or more on this activity this week.

- Sit down and write 100 positive adjectives that describe you (friendly, loyal, athletic, smart, musical, sensitive, and so on). If you can't think of 100 right now, write as many as you can and keep thinking about it over the next day or two until you reach 100.

- Take a serious look at how you've been feeling the past few weeks. If you have any feelings that are especially difficult to deal with, begin to think about how you can get help with them. Consider consulting the self-help section at the bookstore, talking to a trustworthy friend or peer counselor, or making an appointment with a staff person at the campus counseling center.

- Look at the list of defense mechanisms in Table 3-2. Do you recognize one you've used recently? Review the situation in your mind to see if there's a way you could have coped with it differently.

SUMMARY

- Psychological health encompasses more than a single particular state of normality. Psychological diversity is valuable among groups of people.

- Defining psychological health as the presence of wellness means that to be healthy you must strive to fulfill your potential.

- Maslow's definition of psychological health centered on self-actualization, the highest level in his hierarchy of needs. Self-actualized people have high self-esteem and are realistic, inner-directed, authentic, capable of emotional intimacy, and creative.

- Crucial parts of psychological wellness include developing an adult identity, establishing intimate relationships, and developing values and purpose in life.

- A sense of self-esteem develops during childhood as a result of giving and receiving love and learning to accomplish goals. Self-concept is challenged every day; healthy people adjust their goals to their abilities.

- Using defense mechanisms to cope with problems can make finding solutions harder. Analyzing thoughts and behavior can help people develop less defensive and more effective ways of coping.

- A pessimistic outlook can be damaging; it can be overcome by developing more realistic self-talk.

- Honest communication requires recognizing what needs to be said and saying it clearly. Assertiveness enables people to insist on their rights and to participate in the give-and-take of good communication.

- People may be lonely if they haven't developed ways to be happy on their own or if they interpret being alone as a sign of rejection. Lonely people can take action to expand their social contacts.

- Dealing successfully with anger involves distinguishing between a reasonable level of assertiveness and gratuitous expressions of anger, heading off rage by reframing thoughts and distracting oneself, and responding to the anger of others with an asymmetrical, problem-solving orientation.

- People with psychological disorders have symptoms severe enough to interfere with daily living.

- Anxiety is a fear that is not directed toward any definite threat. Anxiety disorders include simple phobias, social phobias, panic disorder, generalized anxiety disorder, obsessive-compulsive disorder, and post-traumatic stress disorder.

- Depression is a common mood disorder; loss of interest or pleasure in things seems to be its most universal symptom. Severe depression carries a high risk of suicide, and suicidally depressed people need professional help.

- Symptoms of mania include exalted moods with unrealistically high self-esteem, little need for sleep, and rapid speech. Mood swings between mania and depression characterize bipolar disorder.

- Schizophrenia is characterized by disorganized thoughts, inappropriate emotions, delusions, auditory hallucinations, and deteriorating social and work performance.

- The biological model emphasizes that the mind's activity depends on the brain, whose composition is genetically determined. Therapy based on the biological model is primarily pharmacological.

- The behavioral model focuses on overt behavior and treats psychological problems as bad habits. Behavior change is the focus of therapy.

- The cognitive model considers how ideas affect behavior and feelings; behavior results from complicated attitudes, expectations, and motives, not just from simple reinforcements. Cognitive therapy focuses on changing a person's thinking.

- The psychodynamic model asserts that false ideas are fed by unconscious ideas and cannot be addressed directly. Treatment is based on psychotherapy.

- Help is available in a variety of forms, including self-help, peer counseling, support groups, and therapy with a mental health professional. For serious problems, professional help may be the most appropriate.

Behavior Change Strategy

Shyness is often the result of both high anxiety levels and lack of key social skills. To help overcome shyness, you need to learn to manage your fear of social situations and to develop social skills such as appropriate eye contact, initiating topics in conversations, and maintaining the flow of conversations by asking questions and making appropriate responses. As described in the chapter, repeated *exposure* to the source of one's fear—in this case, social situations—is the best method for reducing anxiety. When you practice new behaviors, they gradually become easier and you experience less anxiety. A counterproductive strategy is avoiding situations that make you anxious. Although this approach works in the short term—you eliminate your anxiety because you escape the situation—it keeps you from meeting new people and having new experiences. Another counterproductive strategy is self-medicating with alcohol or drugs. Being under their influence actually prevents you from learning new social skills and new ways to handle your anxiety.

To reduce your anxiety in social situations, try some of the following strategies:

• Remember that physical stress reactions are short-term responses to fear. Don't dwell on them—remind yourself that they will pass, and they will.

• Refocus your attention away from the stress reaction you're experiencing and toward the social task at hand. Your nervousness is much less visible than you think.

• Allow a warm-up period for new situations. Realize that you will feel more nervous at first, and take steps to relax and become more comfortable. Refer to the suggestions for deep breathing and other relaxation techniques in Chapter 2.

• If possible, take breaks during anxiety-producing situations. For example, if you're at a party, take a moment to visit the restroom or step outside. Alternate between speaking with good friends and striking up conversations with new acquaintances.

• Watch your interpretations; having a stress reaction doesn't mean that you don't belong in the group, that you're unattractive or unworthy, or that the situation is too much for you. Try thinking of yourself as excited or highly alert instead of anxious.

• Avoid cognitive distortions and practice realistic self-talk. Replace your self-critical thoughts with more supportive ones: "No one else is perfect, and I don't have to be either." "It would have been good if I had a funny story to tell, but the conversation was interesting anyway."

• Give yourself a reality check: Ask if you're really in a life-threatening situation (or just at a party), if the outcome you're imagining is really likely (or the worst thing that could possibly happen), or if you're the only one who feels nervous (or if many other people might feel the same way).

• Don't think of conversations as evaluations; remind yourself that you don't have to prove yourself with every social interaction. And remember that most people are thinking more about themselves than they are about you.

Starting and maintaining conversations can be difficult for shy people, who may feel overwhelmed by their physical stress reaction. If small talk is a problem for you, try the following strategies:

• Introduce yourself early in the conversation. If you tend to forget names, repeat your new acquaintance's name to help fix it in your mind ("Nice to meet you, Amelia").

• Ask questions, and look for shared topics of interest. Simple, open-ended questions like "How's your presentation coming along?" or "How do you know our host?" encourage others to carry the conversation for a while and help bring forth a variety of subjects.

• Take turns talking, and elaborate on your answers. Simple yes and no answers don't move the conversation along. Try to relate something in your life—a course you're taking or a hobby you have—to something in the other person's life. Match self-disclosure with self-disclosure.

• Have something to say. Expand your mind and become knowledgeable about current events and local or campus news. If you have specialized knowledge about a topic, practice discussing it in ways that both beginners and experts can understand and appreciate.

• If you get stuck for something to say, try giving a compliment ("Great presentation!" or "I love your earrings.") or performing a social grace (pass the chips or get someone a drink).

• Be an active listener. Reward the other person with your full attention and with regular responses. Make frequent eye contact and maintain a relaxed but alert posture. (See Chapter 4 for more on being an active listener.)

At first, your new behaviors will likely make you anxious. Don't give up—things *will* get easier. Create lots of opportunities to practice your new behaviors; your goal is to make them routine activities. For example, striking up a conversation with someone in a registration or movie line can help you practice your small-talk skills in a nonthreatening setting. Once you are comfortable doing that, you might try initiating brief conversations with classmates about academic topics—the upcoming midterm, for example, or an assignment. Following that, you might try something more challenging, such as discussing a more personal topic or meeting new people in a social setting.

Regular practice and stress-management skills are critical. Using these techniques, you can increase your social skills and confidence level at the same time that you decrease your anxiety. Eventually, you'll be able to sustain social interactions with comfort and enjoyment. If you find that social anxiety is a major problem for you and self-help techniques don't seem to work, consider looking into a shyness clinic or treatment program on your campus.

SOURCES: Carducci, B. J. 1999. *Shyness: A Bold New Approach.* New York: Perennial; University of Texas at Dallas, Student Counseling Center, 2000. *Overcoming Social Anxiety* (http://www.utdallas.edu/student/slife/counseling/anxiety.html; retrieved August 31, 2000).

Take Action

1. **Become a peer counselor.** Many colleges and communities have peer counseling programs, hotline services (for both general problems and specific issues such as rape, suicide, and drug abuse), and other kinds of emergency counseling services. Some programs are staffed by trained volunteers. Investigate such programs in your school (through the health clinic or student services) or community (look in the yellow pages), and consider volunteering for one of them. The training and experience can help you understand both yourself and others.

2. **Consider assertiveness training.** Being assertive rather than passive or aggressive is a valuable skill that everyone can learn. To improve your ability to assert yourself appropriately, sign up for a workshop or class in assertiveness training on your campus or in your community.

3. **Support your spiritual side.** Turn off your phone, remove your watch, and spend some quiet time alone with your thoughts and feelings. Engage in an activity that contributes to your sense of spiritual well-being. Examples might include spending time in nature; experiencing art, architecture, or music; expressing your creativity; or engaging in a personal spiritual practice such as prayer, meditation, or yoga.

For More Information

Books

Antony, M. M. 2004. *10 Simple Solutions to Shyness: How to Overcome Shyness, Social Anxiety & Fear of Public Speaking*. Oakland, Calif.: New Harbinger. *Practical suggestions for fears of interacting with people you don't know.*

Bourne, E. J., and L. Garano. 2003. *Coping with Anxiety: Simple Ways to Relieve Anxiety, Fear, and Worry*. Oakland, Calif.: New Harbinger. *Provides concrete suggestions for dealing with anxieties.*

Casey, N. 2001. *Unholy Ghost: Writers on Depression*. New York: William Morrow. *An eloquent collection of essays about depression.*

Flach, F. 2003. *Resilience: The Power to Bounce Back When the Going Gets Tough*. Rev. ed. Long Island City, N.Y.: Hatherleigh Press. *Provides practical suggestions for personal growth in the face of stress and change.*

Frances, A., and M. B. First. 1999. *Your Mental Health: A Layman's Guide to the Psychiatrist's Bible*. New York: Scribner. *A resource-packed reference with information on dozens of mental disorders; based on the APA's DSM-IV.*

Klein, D. F., and P. H. Wender. 2005. *Understanding Depression*. 2nd ed. New York: Oxford University Press. *Includes information on symptoms, diagnosis, and a variety of treatments.*

Miklowitz, D. J. 2002. *The Bipolar Disorder Survival Guide: What You and Your Family Need to Know*. New York: Guilford Press. *Covers the origins, symptoms, and treatments for bipolar (or manic-depressive) disorder.*

Nasar, S. 2001. *A Beautiful Mind: The Life of Mathematical Genius and Nobel Laureate John Nash*. Carmichael, Calif.: Touchstone Books. *The story of how schizophrenia affected the life of a renowned mathematician.*

Rubin-Deutsch, J. 2003. *Why Can't I Ever Be Good Enough? Escaping the Limits of Your Childhood Roles*. Oakland, Calif.: New Harbinger. *Presents strategies for transforming unhealthy patterns of thought and interaction from childhood into more healthy adult roles.*

Wolpert, L. 2000. *Malignant Sadness: The Anatomy of Depression*. New York: Free Press. *A look at the nature of depression, with information for people with the disorder and their families.*

Organizations, Hotlines, and Web Sites

American Association of Suicidology. Provides information about suicide and resources for people in crisis.
http://www.suicidology.org

American Psychiatric Association (APA). Provides public information by pamphlet or online about a variety of topics, including depression, anxiety, eating disorders, and psychiatric medications.
888-357-7924; 703-907-7300
http://www.psych.org

American Psychological Association Consumer HelpCenter. Provides information about common challenges to psychological health and about how to obtain professional help.
800-964-2000
http://helping.apa.org

Anxiety Disorders Association of America (ADAA). Provides information and resources related to anxiety disorders, including listings of support groups.
http://www.adaa.org

Depression and Bipolar Support Alliance (DBSA). Provides educational materials and information about support groups and other resources.
800-826-3632
http://www.dbsalliance.org

Internet Mental Health. An encyclopedia of mental health information, including medical diagnostic criteria.
http://www.mentalhealth.com

NAMI (National Alliance for the Mentally Ill). Provides information and support for people who are affected by mental illness.
800-950-NAMI (Help Line)
http://www.nami.org

National Hopeline Network. 24-hour hotline for people who are thinking about suicide or know someone who is; calls are routed to local crisis centers.
800-SUICIDE

National Institute of Mental Health (NIMH). Provides helpful information about anxiety, depression, eating disorders, and other challenges to psychological health.
866-615-6464; 301-443-4513
http://www.nimh.nih.gov

National Mental Health Association. Provides consumer information on a variety of issues, including how to find help.
800-969-NMHA
http://www.nmha.org

National Mental Health Information Center. A one-stop source for information and resources relating to mental health.
800-789-2647
http://www.mentalhealth.org

Psych Central: Dr. John Grohol's Mental Health Page. A guide to psychology, support, and mental health issues, resources, and people on the Internet.

http://psychcentral.com

Student Counseling Virtual Pamphlet Collection. Provides links to more than 400 pamphlets produced by different student counseling centers; topics range from depression and anxiety to time management and assertiveness.

http://counseling.uchicago.edu/vpc

Surgeon General: Reports. Provides the text of reports from the U.S. Surgeon General, including the 1999 report on mental health and the 2001 supplement to the report that focuses on culture and ethnicity.

http://www.surgeongeneral.gov/library/reports.htm

World Health Organization: 2001 World Health Report. Focuses on mental health as a major cause of disability in both developed and developing countries.

http://www.who.int/whr/2001/en

The following sites include interactive online assessments for various psychological problems:

Depression-screening.org: http://www.depression-screening.org

Freedom from Fear: http://www.freedomfromfear.com

Selected Bibliography

American Psychiatric Association. 2000. *Diagnostic and Statistical Manual of Mental Disorders,* 4th ed., Text Revision *(DSM-IV-TR).* Washington, D.C.: American Psychiatric Association Press.

Benton, S. A., et al. 2003. Changes in counseling center client problems across 13 years. *Professional Psychology: Research and Practice* 34(1): 66–72.

Biederman, J., et al. 2001. Further evidence of association between behavioral inhibition and social anxiety in children. *American Journal of Psychiatry* 158(10): 1673–1679.

Boscarino, J. A., R. E. Adams, and C. R. Figley. 2004. Mental health service use 1-year after the World Trade Center disaster: Implications for mental health care. *Annals of General Hospital Psychiatry* 5: 346–358.

Brenes, G. A., et al. 2002. Do optimism and pessimism predict physical functioning? *Journal of Behavioral Medicine* 25(3): 219–231.

Cutler, J. L., et al. 2004. Comparing cognitive behavior therapy, interpersonal psychotherapy, and psychodynamic psychotherapy. *American Journal of Psychiatry* 161(9): 1567–1573.

Danner, D. D., D. A. Snowdon, and W. W. Friesen. 2001. Positive emotions in early life and longevity: Findings from the nun study. *Journal of Personality and Social Psychology* 80(5): 804–813.

Dervic, K., et al. 2004. Religious affiliation and suicide attempt. *American Journal of Psychiatry* 161(12): 2303–2308.

Food and Drug Administration. 2005. Safeguards for children taking antidepressants strengthened, *FDA Consumer,* January/February.

Gunnell, D., P. K. Magnusson, and F. Rasmussen. 2005. Low intelligence test scores in 18-year-old men and risk of suicide: Cohort study. *British Medical Journal* 330(7484): 167.

Hershel, J., J. A. Kaye, and S. S. Jick. 2004. Antidepressants and the risk of suicidal behaviors. *Journal of the American Medical Association* 292(3): 338–343.

Kendler, K. S., J. Myers, and C. A. Prescott. 2005. Sex differences in the relationship between social support and risk for major depression: A longitudinal study of opposite-sex twin pairs. *American Journal of Psychiatry* 162(2): 250–256.

Koh, K. B., C. H. Kim, and J. K. Park. 2002. Predominance of anger in depressive disorders compared with anxiety disorders and somatoform disorders. *Journal of Clinical Psychiatry* 63(6): 488–492.

Lewis, C. 2003. The lowdown on depression. *FDA Consumer,* January/February.

Licinio, J., and M. L. Wong. 2005. Opinion: Depression, antidepressants and suicidality: A critical appraisal. *Nature Reviews: Drug Discovery* 4(2): 165–171.

Maruta, T., et al. 2000. Optimists vs. pessimists: Survival rate among medical patients over a 30-year period. *Mayo Clinic Proceedings* 75(2): 140–143.

Messias, E., et al. 2004. Summer birth and deficit schizophrenia: A pooled analysis from 6 countries. *Archives of General Psychiatry* 61(10): 985–989.

Miller, M., D. Azrael, and D. Hemenway. 2002. Household firearm ownership and suicide rates in the United States. *Epidemiology* 13(5): 517–524.

Mufson, L., et al. 2004. A randomized effectiveness trial of interpersonal psychotherapy for depressed adolescents. *Archives of General Psychiatry* 61(6): 577–584.

Nathan, P. F., and J. M. Gorman, eds. 2002. *A Guide to Treatments That Work,* 2nd ed. Oxford: Oxford University Press.

Pampallona, S., et al. 2004. Combined pharmacotherapy and psychological treatment for depression: A systematic review. *Archives of General Psychiatry* 61(7): 714–719.

Pini, S., et al. 2001. Insight into illness in schizophrenia, schizo-affective disorder, and mood disorders with psychotic features. *American Journal of Psychiatry* 158(1): 122–125.

Qin, P., E. Agerbo, and P. M. Bo. 2002. Suicide risk in relation to family history of completed suicide and psychiatric disorders. *Lancet* 360(9340): 1126.

Rothwell, J. D. 2004. *In the Company of Others: An Introduction to Communication,* 2nd ed. New York: McGraw-Hill.

Schatzberg, A. F., J. O. Cole, and C. DeBattista. 2002. *Manual of Clinical Psychopharmacology,* 4th ed. Washington, D.C.: American Psychiatric Association.

Shedd, O. L., et al. 2004. The World Trade Center attack: Increased frequency of defibrillator shocks for ventricular arrhythmias in patients living remotely from New York City. *Journal of the American College of Cardiology* 44(6): 1265–1267.

Sheldon, K. M., and L. Houser-Marko. 2001. Self-concordance, goal attainment, and the pursuit of happiness: Can there be an upward spiral? *Journal of Personality and Social Psychology* 80(1): 152–165.

Simeon, D., et al. 2003. Peritraumatic reactions associated with the World Trade Center disaster. *American Journal of Psychiatry* 160(9): 1702–1705.

Simon, O. R., et al. 2002. Characteristics of impulsive suicide attempts and attempters. *Suicide and Life-Threatening Behavior* 32(1 Suppl): 49–59.

Snow, V., S. Lascher, and C. Mottur-Pilson. 2000. Pharmacological treatment of acute major depression and dysthymia. *Annals of Internal Medicine* 132(9): 738–742.

Stahl, S. M. 2002. *Essential Psychopharmacology of Antipsychotics and Mood Stabilizers.* Cambridge: Cambridge University Press.

Swanson, J. W., et al. 2002. The social-environmental context of violent behavior in persons treated for severe mental illness. *American Journal of Public Health* 92(9): 1523–1531.

Szegedi, A., et al. 2005. Acute treatment of moderate to severe depression with hypericum extract WS 5570 (St John's wort): Randomised controlled double blind non-inferiority trial versus paroxetine. *British Medical Journal,* February 11 epub.

Tsai, S. Y., et al. 2002. Risk factors for completed suicide in bipolar disorder. *Journal of Clinical Psychiatry* 63(6): 469–476.

Vaillant, G. E. 1977. *Adaptation to Life.* Boston: Little, Brown.

Walsh, B. T., et al. 2002. Placebo response in studies of major depression. *Journal of the American Medical Association* 287(14): 1840–1847.

Walsh, E., and T. Fahy. 2002. Violence in society. *British Medical Journal* 325(7363): 507–508.

World Health Organization. 2002. *World Report on Violence and Health.* Geneva: World Health Organization.

Zhang, X., et al. 2005. Loss-of-function mutation in tryptophan hydroxylase-2 identified in unipolar major depression. *Neuron* 45(1): 11–16.

4

Looking AHEAD

After reading this chapter, you should be able to

- Explain the qualities that help people develop intimate relationships

- Describe different types of love relationships and the stages they often go through

- Describe common challenges of forming and maintaining intimate relationships

- Explain some elements of healthy and productive communication

- Discuss relationship options available to adults today

- List some characteristics of successful families and some potential problems families face

- Explain some of the joys and challenges of being a parent

Intimate Relationships and Communication

Knowledge

1. **Couples who live together before marriage are less likely to get divorced than those who don't.**
   True or false?

2. **Most people are good judges of how friends and intimates will feel in response to inconsiderate behaviors such as being late or failing to return a borrowed item.**
   True or false?

3. **About what percentage of single American adults with Internet access have visited sites where singles meet?**
   a. 5%
   b. 10%
   c. 20%
   d. 30%

4. **Married people tend to be healthier and to live longer than unmarried people.**
   True or false?

5. **The love that lesbians and gay men experience is similar in quality to that experienced by heterosexuals.**
   True or false?

6. **What percentage of American households with children conform to the traditional model of wage-earning father and stay-at-home mother?**
   a. 5%
   b. 15%
   c. 30%

ANSWERS

1. FALSE. Studies have found that couples who cohabit before they get married are more likely to divorce than those who don't cohabit.

2. FALSE. Many people underestimate the negative reactions of others to their own inconsiderate behavior; this is particularly true of people who tend to repress their own negative feelings. Sensitivity to others' needs and feelings is key to maintaining healthy relationships.

3. D. About 28% of singles have visited dating sites, and about 10% have signed up. By 2006, it is estimated that 5.2 million single Americans will have posted online personal ads.

4. TRUE. One explanation is that marriage encourages healthy behaviors, and surveys have found that married people are more likely to wear safety belts, be physically active, and not smoke.

5. TRUE. Like heterosexual relationships, gay and lesbian partnerships provide intimacy, passion, and security. Most gay men and lesbians experience at least one long-term relationship with a single partner.

6. B. Dual-career couples now represent almost half of the U.S. labor force.

Visit the *Core Concepts in Health* Online Learning Center (www.mhhe.com/insel10e) for study aids and many additional resources.

95

Human beings need social relationships; we cannot thrive as solitary creatures. Nor could the human species survive if adults didn't cherish and support each other, if we didn't form strong mutual attachments with our infants, and if we didn't create families in which to raise children. Simply put, people need people.

Although people are held together in relationships by a variety of factors, the foundation of many relationships is love. Love in its many forms—romantic, passionate, platonic, parental—is the wellspring from which much of life's meaning and delight flows. In our culture, it binds us together as partners, parents, children, and friends. People devote tremendous energy to seeking mates, nurturing intimate relationships, keeping up friendships, maintaining marriages—all for the pleasure of loving and being loved.

Many human needs are satisfied in intimate relationships: the need for approval and affirmation, for companionship, for meaningful ties and a sense of belonging, for sexual satisfaction. Many of society's needs are fulfilled by relationships, too—most notably, the need to nurture and socialize children. Overall, healthy intimate relationships are an important contributor to the well-being of both individuals and society.

DEVELOPING INTIMATE RELATIONSHIPS

People who develop successful intimate relationships believe in themselves and in the people around them. They are willing to give of themselves—to share their ideas, feelings, time, needs—and to accept what others want to give them.

Self-Concept and Self-Esteem

The principal element that we all bring to our relationships is our *selves*. To have successful relationships, we must first accept and feel good about ourselves. A positive self-concept and a healthy level of self-esteem help us love and respect others. How and where do we acquire a positive sense of self?

As discussed in Chapter 3, the roots of our identity and sense of self can be found in childhood, in the relationships we had with our parents and other family members. As adults, we probably have a sense that we're basically lovable, worthwhile people and that we can trust others if, as babies and children, we felt loved, valued, and

respected; if adults responded to our needs in a reasonably appropriate way; and if they gave us the freedom to explore and develop a sense of being separate individuals.

Our personal identity isn't fixed or frozen. According to psychologist Erik Erikson, it continues to develop as we encounter and resolve various crises at each stage of life. The fundamental tasks of early childhood are the development of trust during infancy and of autonomy during toddlerhood. From these experiences and interactions we construct our first ideas about who we are. (For a more detailed discussion of Erikson's developmental theory, see Chapter 3.)

Another thing we learn in early childhood is **gender role**—the activities, abilities, and characteristics our culture deems appropriate for us based on whether we're male or female. In our society, men have traditionally been expected to work and provide for their families; to be aggressive, competitive, and power-oriented; and to use thinking and logic to solve problems. Women have been expected to take care of home and children; to be cooperative, supportive, and nurturing; and to approach life emotionally and intuitively. Although much more egalitarian gender roles are emerging in our society, the stereotypes we absorb in childhood tend to be deeply ingrained.

Our ways of relating to others may also be rooted in childhood. Some researchers have suggested that our adult styles of loving may be based on the style of **attachment** we established in infancy with our mother, father, or other primary caregiver. According to this view, people who are secure in their intimate relationships probably had a secure, trusting, mutually satisfying attachment to their mother, father, or other parenting figure. As adults, they find it relatively easy to get close to others. They don't worry about being abandoned or having someone get too close to them. They feel that other people like them and are generally well intentioned.

People who are clinging and dependent in their relationships may have had an "anxious/ambivalent" attachment, in which a parent's inconsistent responses made them unsure that their needs would be met. As adults, they worry about whether their partners really love them and will stay with them. They tend to feel that others don't want to get as close as they do. They want to merge completely with another person, which sometimes scares others away.

People who seem to run from relationships may have had an "anxious/avoidant" attachment, in which a parent's inappropriate responses made them want to escape from his or her sphere of influence. As adults, they feel uncomfortable being close to others. They're distrustful and fearful of becoming dependent. Their partners usually want more intimacy than they do.

Even if people's earliest experiences and relationships were less than ideal, however, they can still establish satisfying relationships in adulthood. People can be resilient and flexible. They have the capacity to change their

Terms

VViW

gender role A culturally expected pattern of behavior and attitudes determined by whether a person is male or female.

attachment The emotional tie between an infant and his or her caregiver or between two people in an intimate relationship.

ideas, beliefs, and behavior patterns. They can learn ways to raise their self-esteem; they can become more trusting, accepting, and appreciative of others; and they can acquire the communication and conflict-resolution skills for maintaining successful relationships. Although it helps to have a good start in life, it may be even more important to begin again, right from where you are.

Friendship

The first relationships we form outside the family are friendships. With members of either the same or the other sex, friendships give people the opportunity to share themselves and discover others. The friendships we form in childhood are important in our development; through them we learn about tolerance, sharing, and trust.

Friendships usually include most or all of the following characteristics:

- *Companionship.* Friends are relaxed and happy in each other's company. They typically have common values and interests and make plans to spend time together.

- *Respect.* Friends have a basic respect for each other's humanity and individuality. Good friends respect each other's feelings and opinions and work to resolve their differences without demeaning or insulting each other. They also show their respect by being honest with each other (see the box "Being a Good Friend" on p. 98).

- *Acceptance.* Friends accept each other—"warts and all." They feel free to be themselves and express their feelings spontaneously without fear of ridicule or criticism.

- *Help.* Sharing time, energy, and even material goods is important to friendship. Friends know they can rely on each other in times of need. They feel they can ask for help when the going gets tough.

- *Trust.* Friends are secure in the knowledge that they will not intentionally hurt each other. They feel safe confiding in each other.

- *Loyalty.* Friends can count on each other. They stand up for each other in both word and deed.

- *Mutuality.* Friends retain their individual identities, but close friendships are characterized by a sense of mutuality—"what affects you affects me." Friends share the ups and downs in each other's lives.

- *Reciprocity.* Friendships are reciprocal. There is give-and-take between friends and the feeling that both share joys and burdens more or less equally over time.

Intimate partnerships are like friendships in many ways, but they have additional characteristics. These relationships usually include sexual desire and expression, a greater demand for exclusiveness, and deeper levels of caring.

Close relationships without a sexual component are more common than those with sexual activity. Friendship satisfies our need for affection, affirmation, sharing, and companionship.

Friendships are usually considered both stabler and longer lasting than intimate partnerships. Friends are often more accepting and less critical than lovers, probably because their expectations are different. Like love relationships, friendships bind society together, providing people with emotional support and buffering them from stress.

Love, Sex, and Intimacy

Love is one of the most basic and profound human emotions. It is a powerful force in all our intimate relationships. Love encompasses opposites: affection and anger, excitement and boredom, stability and change, bonds and freedom. Love does not give us perfect happiness, but it does give our lives meaning.

In many kinds of adult relationships, love is closely intertwined with sexuality. In the past, marriage was considered the only acceptable context for sexual activities, but for many people today sex is legitimized by love. Many couples, both heterosexual and homosexual, live together in committed relationships. We now use personal standards rather than social norms to make decisions about sex. This trend toward personal responsibility results in an even greater emphasis on love than in the past.

Being a Good Friend

How to Make Friends

- Find people with interests similar to your own. Join a club, participate in sports, do volunteer work, or join a discussion group to meet people with common interests.

- Be a good listener. Take a genuine interest in people. Solicit their opinions, and take time to listen to their problems and ideas.

- Take risks. If you meet someone interesting, ask him or her to join you for a meal or an event you would both enjoy.

How to Be a Good Friend

- Be trustworthy. Honor all confidences, and don't talk about your friend behind his or her back.

- Tell your friend about yourself. Self-disclosure—letting your friend know about your real concerns and joys—signals trust.

- Be supportive and kind. Be there when your friend is going through a rough time. Don't criticize your friend or offer unsolicited advice.

- Develop your capacity for intimacy. Intimate relationships are genuine, spontaneous, and caring.

- Don't expect perfection. Like any relationship, your friendship may go through difficult times. Talk through conflicts as they arise.

For most people, love, sex, and commitment are closely linked ideals in intimate relationships. Love reflects the positive factors that draw people together and sustain them in a relationship. It includes trust, caring, respect, loyalty, interest in the other, and concern for the other's well-being. Sex brings excitement and passion to the relationship. It intensifies the relationship and adds fascination and pleasure. Commitment, the determination to continue, reflects the stable factors that help maintain the relationship. Responsibility, reliability, and faithfulness are characteristics of commitment. Although love, sex, and commitment are related, they are not necessarily connected. One can exist without the others. Despite the various "faces" of love, sex, and commitment, most of us long for a special relationship that contains them all.

Other elements can be identified as features of love, such as euphoria, preoccupation with the loved one, idealization of the loved one, and so on, but these tend to be temporary. These characteristics may include **infatuation,** which will fade or deepen into something more substantial. As relationships progress, the central aspects of love and commitment take on more importance.

Another way of looking at love has been proposed by psychologist Robert Sternberg. He sees love as being composed of intimacy, passion, and commitment (Figure 4-1). Intimacy refers to the feelings of warmth and closeness we have with someone we love. Passion refers to romance, attraction, and sexuality. Commitment refers to both the short-term decision that you love someone and the long-term commitment to be in the relationship.

According to Sternberg, these three elements can be enlarged, diminished, or combined in different ways. Each combination gives a different kind of love:

- *Liking* (intimacy only): Love between friends.
- *Infatuation* (passion only): An idealizing, obsessive, all-consuming love, characterized by a high degree of physical and emotional arousal; often unrequited; "love at first sight."
- *Romantic* (intimacy and passion): Love in which commitment may develop over time.
- *Fatuous* (passion and commitment): Deceptive love, the "whirlwind affair"; as passion fades, all that's left is commitment, but without time and intimacy, it's a poor foundation for an enduring relationship.
- *Empty* (commitment only): Dutiful love; also a poor foundation for a relationship.

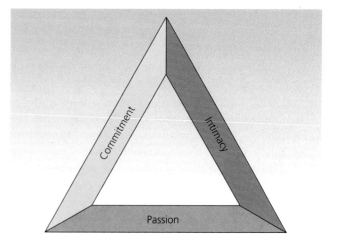

Figure 4-1 The love triangle. SOURCE: Sternberg, R., and M. Barnes. 1988. *The Psychology of Love.* New Haven: Yale University Press, p. 37. Copyright © 1998. Reprinted with permission.

Term

V w

infatuation An idealizing, obsessive attraction, characterized by a high degree of physical arousal.

- *Companionate* (intimacy and commitment): Essentially a committed friendship; often begins as romantic love, but as passion diminishes and intimacy increases, it is transformed into companionate love.
- *Consummate* (all three elements): The love that dreams are made of; difficult to sustain.

Men and women tend to have different views of the relationship between love (or intimacy) and sex (or passion). Numerous studies have found that men can separate love from sex rather easily, although many men find that their most erotic sexual experiences occur in the context of a love relationship. Women generally view sex from the point of view of a relationship. Some people believe you can have satisfying sex without love—with friends, acquaintances, or strangers. Although sex with love is an important norm in our culture, it is frequently disregarded in practice, as the high incidence of extrarelational affairs attests.

The Pleasure and Pain of Love The experience of intense love has confused and tormented lovers throughout history. They live in a tumultuous state of excitement, subject to wildly fluctuating feelings of joy and despair. They lose their appetite, can't sleep, and can think of nothing but the loved one. Is this happiness? Misery? Or both?

The contradictory nature of passionate love can be understood by recognizing that human emotions have two components: physiological arousal and an emotional explanation for the arousal. (For a discussion of the biochemical and hormonal processes involved in arousal, see the description of the stress response in Chapter 2.) Love is just one of many emotions accompanied by physiological arousal; numerous unpleasant ones can also generate arousal, such as fear, rejection, frustration, and challenge. Although experiences like attraction and sexual desire are pleasant, extreme excitement is similar to fear and is unpleasant. For this reason, passionate love may be too intense to enjoy. Over time, the physical intensity and excitement tend to diminish. When this happens, pleasure may actually increase.

The Transformation of Love All human relationships change over time, and love relationships are no exception. At first, love is likely to be characterized by high levels of passion and rapidly increasing intimacy. After a while, passion decreases as we become habituated to it and to the person. Generally, increasing the time spent together does not increase arousal.

Sometimes intimacy continues to grow at a deeper, less conscious level; at other times, the couple may drift apart. Commitment isn't necessarily diminished or altered by time. It grows more slowly and is maintained as long as we judge the relationship to be successful. If the relationship begins to deteriorate, the level of commitment usually decreases.

The disappearance of romance or passionate love is often experienced as a crisis in a relationship. If a more lasting love fails to emerge, the relationship will likely break up, and each person will search for another who will once again ignite his or her passion. Love does not necessarily have to be intensely passionate. When intensity diminishes, partners often discover a more enduring love. They can now move from absorption in each other to a relationship that includes external goals and projects, friends, and family. In this kind of intimate, more secure love, satisfaction comes not just from the relationship itself but also from achieving other creative goals, such as work or child rearing. The key to successful relationships is in transforming passion into an intimate love, based on closeness, caring, and the promise of a shared future. Only with the passage of time can love mature and deepen, allowing us to truly grow both psychologically and spiritually.

Challenges in Relationships

Many people believe that love naturally makes an intimate relationship easy to begin and maintain, but, in fact, obstacles and challenges often occur. Even in the best of circumstances, there are times when a loving relationship will be tested. Individuals bring to a relationship diverse needs and wants, some of which emerge only at times of change or stress. Common relationship challenges relate to self-disclosure, commitment, expectations, competitiveness, and jealousy.

Honesty and Openness Everyone looks for honesty and openness in an intimate relationship. However, especially at the beginning of a relationship, partners tend to engage in a certain amount of pretense in an effort to present themselves in the best possible manner. It's usually best to be yourself from the start to give both you and your potential partner a chance to find out if you are comfortable with each other's beliefs, interests, and lifestyles.

Getting close to another person by sharing thoughts and feelings is emotionally risky, but it is necessary for a relationship to deepen. Take your time, and self-disclose at a slow but steady rate—one that doesn't make you feel too vulnerable or your partner too uncomfortable. Over time, you and your partner will learn more about each other and feel more comfortable sharing. In fact, intimate familiarity with your partner's life is a key characteristic of successful long-term relationships (see the box "Love Maps Questionnaire").

Unequal or Premature Commitment Sometimes one person in an intimate partnership becomes more serious about the relationship than the other partner. In this situation, it can be very difficult to maintain a friendship without hurting the other person. Sometimes a couple makes a premature commitment, and then one of the partners has second thoughts and wants to break off the relationship. Sometimes both partners begin to

Chapter 4 Intimate Relationships and Communication

Assess Yourself

Love Maps Questionnaire

Emotionally intelligent couples have richly detailed "love maps"—they know about each other's history, major goals and beliefs, and day-to-day struggles. To assess the quality of your current love maps, answer each of the following questions with "true" or "false."

1. I can name my partner's best friends.
2. I can tell you what stresses my partner is currently facing.
3. I know the names of some of the people who have been irritating my partner lately.
4. I can tell you some of my partner's life dreams.
5. I am very familiar with my partner's religious beliefs and ideas.
6. I can tell you about my partner's basic philosophy of life.
7. I can list the relatives my partner likes the least.
8. I know my partner's favorite music.
9. I can list my partner's three favorite movies.
10. My partner is familiar with my current stresses.
11. I know the three most special times in my partner's life.
12. I can tell you the most stressful thing that happened to my partner as a child.
13. I can list my partner's major aspirations and hopes in life.
14. I know my partner's major current worries.
15. My partner knows who my friends are.
16. I know what my partner would want to do if he or she suddenly won the lottery.
17. I can tell you in detail my first impressions of my partner.
18. Periodically, I ask my partner about his or her world right now.
19. I feel that my partner knows me pretty well.
20. My partner is familiar with my hopes and aspirations.

Scoring: Give yourself one point for each "true" answer.

10 or above: This is an area of strength in your relationship. You have a fairly detailed map of your partner's everyday life, hopes, fears, and dreams. If you maintain this level of knowledge and understanding of each other, you'll be well equipped to handle any problem areas that crop up in your relationship.

Below 10: Your relationship could stand some improvement in this area. By taking the time to learn more about your partner now, you'll find that your relationship becomes stronger.

SOURCE: Gottman, J. M., and N. Silver. 1999. *The Seven Principles for Making Marriage Work.* New York: Three Rivers Press, pp. 50–51. Reprinted with permission.

---

realize that something is wrong, but each is afraid to tell the other. Most such problems can be dealt with only by honest and sensitive communication.

Unrealistic Expectations Each partner brings hopes and expectations to a relationship, some of which may be unrealistic, unfair, and, ultimately, very damaging to the relationship. For example, if you believe that love will eliminate all of your problems, you may start to blame your partner for anything that goes wrong in your life. Other common expectations that can hurt a relationship include the following:

- *Expecting your partner to change.* There are probably some things about your partner that you like more than others. It's OK to discuss them with your partner; however, it's unfair to demand that your partner change to meet all of your expectations. Accept the differences you see between your ideal and the reality.

- *Assuming that your partner has all the same opinions, priorities, interests, and goals as you.* You may share many things with your partner, but don't assume that you think the same about everything—or that you have to in order for the relationship to succeed. Agreement on key issues is important, but differences can enhance a relationship as long as partners understand and respect each other's points of view.

- *Believing that a relationship will fulfill all of your personal, financial, intellectual, and social needs.* Expecting a relationship to fulfill all your needs places too much pressure on your partner and on your relationship, and it will inevitably lead to disappointment. For your own well-being, it's important to maintain some degree of autonomy and self-sufficiency.

Competitiveness American social norms encourage a certain amount of healthy competition between intimate partners and friends. Games and competitive sports add flavor to the bonding process—as long as the focus is on fun. If one partner always feels the strong need to compete and win, it can detract from the sense of connectedness, interdependence, equality, and mutuality between partners. The same can be said for a perfectionistic need to be right in every instance—to "win" every argument.

Even if you're convinced you're right, a loving relationship won't work if you get everything your own way—it's just not fair. If competitiveness is a problem for you, ask yourself if your need to win is more important than your partner's feelings or the future of your relationship. Try engaging in noncompetitive activities or in an activity where you are a beginner and your partner excels. Accept that your partner may hold different views on issues than you do—and that those views may be just as valid and important to your partner as your own views are to you.

Strategies for Enhancing Support in Relationships

Take Charge

- *Be aware of the importance of support.* Time and energy spent on support will help both you and your partner deal with stress and create a positive atmosphere that will help when differences or conflicts do occur.

- *Learn to ask for help from your partner.* Try different ways of asking for help and support from your partner and make note of which approaches work best for your relationship.

- *Help your partner the way she or he would like to be helped.* Some people prefer empathy and emotional support, whereas others like more practical help with problems.

- *Avoid negativity, especially when being asked for help.* Asking for help puts a person in a vulnerable position. If your partner asks for your aid, be gracious and supportive; don't use phrases like "I told you so" or "You should have just. . . ." Otherwise, your partner may learn not to ask for your help or support at all.

- *Make positive attributions.* If you're unsure about the reasons for your partner's behavior, give her or him the benefit of the doubt. For example, if your partner arrives for a date 30 minutes late and in a bad mood, assume it's because she or he had a bad day rather than attributing it to a character flaw or relationship problem. Offer appropriate support.

- *Help yourself.* Develop coping strategies for times your partner won't be available. These might include things you can do for yourself, such as going for a walk, or other people you can turn to for support.

- *Keep relationship problems separate.* Avoid bringing up relationship problems when you are offering or asking for help.

- *Avoid giving advice.* Immediately offering advice when asked for help implies that you are smarter or more capable than your partner at solving your partner's difficulty. Begin by providing emotional support and validating your partner's feelings. Then, if asked, help brainstorm solutions.

SOURCE: Plante, T., and K. Sullivan. 2000. *Getting Together and Staying Together: The Stanford Course on Intimate Relationships.* Bloomington, Ind.: 1stBooks Library, now Author House. Reprinted with permission of the author.

Balancing Time Spent Together and Apart

You may enjoy time together with your partner, but you may also want to spend time alone or with other friends. If time apart is interpreted as rejection or lack of commitment, it can damage a relationship. It's important to talk with your partner about what time apart means and to share your feelings about what you expect from the relationship in terms of time together. Consider your partner's feelings carefully, and try to reach a compromise that satisfies both of you.

Differences in expectations about time spent together can mirror differences in ideas about emotional closeness. Any romantic relationship involves giving up some degree of autonomy in order to develop an identity as a couple. It's important to remember that every individual is unique and has different needs for distance and closeness in a relationship. As described earlier in the chapter, attachment styles developed early in life can affect people's level of comfort in close relationships. In addition, traditional gender roles tend to teach women to be caretakers of relationships and men to be independent and self-reliant.

Jealousy Jealousy is the angry, painful response to a partner's real, imagined, or likely involvement with a third person. Some people think that the existence of jealousy proves the existence of love, but jealousy is actually a more accurate yardstick for measuring insecurity or possessiveness. In its irrational and extreme forms, jealousy can destroy a relationship by its insistent demands and attempts at control. Jealousy is a factor in precipitating violence in dating relationships among both high school and college students, and abusive spouses often use jealousy to justify their violence. (Problems with control and violence in relationships are discusssed in Chapter 23.) People with a healthy level of self-esteem are less likely to feel jealous. When jealousy occurs in a relationship, it's important for the partners to communicate clearly with each other about their feelings.

Successful Relationships

A true intimate relationship is characterized by a conscious sense of connectedness to another person. It emerges after a period of deep sharing, and it reflects a warm, caring, and trusting concern between partners. Successful relationships result in a heightened sense of self-worth for both partners.

What steps can you take to build a successful relationship? To meet the relationship challenges described in this section, good communication and conflict-resolution skills are critical. You need to be able to communicate your needs and wants clearly, listen to your partner, negotiate, and compromise. These skills are described in detail in the next section of the chapter.

Another key to successful relationships is the ability to ask for and give support. Partners need to know that they can count on each other during difficult times. If you are having trouble getting or giving the support that you or your partner needs, try some of the suggestions in the box "Strategies for Enhancing Support in Relationships."

Unhealthy Relationships

Many of the strategies in this chapter suggest ways to make a relationship healthier and to enjoy greater intimacy. Equally important, however, is being able to recognize when a relationship is unhealthy. Relatively extreme examples of unhealthy relationships are those that are physically or emotionally abusive or that involve codependency; strategies for recognizing and addressing these problems are presented in Chapters 23 and 9, respectively.

Even relationships that are not abusive or codependent may still be unhealthy. Psychologist and relationship expert John Gottman suggests that if your relationship lacks love and respect and places little value on the time you and your partner have spent together, it may be time to get professional help or to end the partnership. Further, if your relationship is characterized by communication styles that include criticism, contempt, defensiveness, and withdrawal—despite real efforts to repair these destructive patterns—the relationship may not be salvageable. Consider these questions: Do you and your partner have more negative than positive experiences and interactions? Are there old hurts that you or your partner cannot forgive? Do you feel disrespected or unloved? Do you find it hard to feel positive feelings of affection for your partner? Does it feel as if your relationship has been a waste of time? Spiritual leaders suggest that relationships are unhealthy when you feel that your sense of spontaneity, your potential for inner growth and joy, and your connection to your spiritual life is deadened. There are negative physical and mental consequences of being in an unhappy relationship; and although breaking up is painful and difficult, it is ultimately better than living in a toxic relationship.

Ending a Relationship

Even when a couple starts out with the best of intentions, an intimate relationship may not last. The couple may have been mismatched to begin with, or the relationship may have failed to thrive and the partners then turned elsewhere for satisfaction. Some breakups occur quickly following direct action by one or both partners, but many others occur over an extended period during which partners repeatedly consider both breaking up and reconciling.

Ending an intimate relationship is usually difficult and painful. Both partners may feel attacked and abandoned, but feelings of distress are likely to be more acute for the rejected partner. If you are involved in a breakup, following these guidelines may help make the ending easier:

- *Give the relationship a fair chance before breaking up.* If it's still not working, you'll know you did everything you could.

- *Be fair and honest.* If you're the one who is initiating the breakup, don't try to make your partner feel responsible.

- *Be tactful and compassionate.* You can leave the relationship without deliberately damaging your partner's self-esteem. Emphasize your mutual incompatibility, and admit your own contributions to the problem.

- *If you are the rejected person, give yourself time to resolve your anger and pain.* Mobilize your coping resources, including social support and other stress-management techniques. You may go through a process of mourning the relationship, experiencing disbelief, anger, sadness, and finally acceptance. Remember that there are actually many people with whom you can potentially have an intimate relationship.

- *Recognize the value in the experience.* You honor the feelings that you shared with your partner by validating the relationship as a worthwhile experience. Ending a close relationship can teach you valuable lessons about your needs, preferences, strengths, and weaknesses. Use your insights to increase your chance of success in your next relationship.

Use the recovery period following a breakup for self-renewal. Redirect more of your attention to yourself, and reconnect with people and areas of your life that may have been neglected as a result of the relationship. Time will help heal the pain of the loss of the relationship.

COMMUNICATION

The key to developing and maintaining any type of intimate relationship is good communication. Most of the time, we don't actually think about communicating; we simply talk and behave naturally. But when problems arise—when we feel others don't understand us or when someone accuses us of not listening—we become aware of our limitations or, more commonly, what we think are other people's limitations. Miscommunication creates frustration and distances us from our friends and partners.

Nonverbal Communication

As much as 65% of face-to-face communication is nonverbal. Even when we're silent, we're communicating. We send messages when we look at someone or look away, lean forward or sit back, smile or frown. Especially important forms of nonverbal communication are touch, eye contact, and proximity. If someone we're talking to touches our hand or arm, looks into our eyes, and leans toward us when we talk, we get the message that the person is interested in us and cares about what we're saying. If a person keeps looking around the room while we're talking or takes a step backward, we get the impression the person is uninterested or wants to end the conversation.

The ability to interpret nonverbal messages correctly is important to the success of relationships. It's also important, when sending messages, to make sure our body language agrees with our words. When our verbal and nonverbal messages don't correspond, we send a mixed message.

Communication Skills

Three keys to good communication in relationships are self-disclosure, listening, and feedback.

- *Self-disclosure* involves revealing personal information that we ordinarily wouldn't reveal because of the risk involved. It usually increases feelings of closeness and moves the relationship to a deeper level of intimacy. Friends often disclose the most to each other, sharing feelings, experiences, hopes, and disappointments; married couples sometimes share less because they think they already know everything there is to know about each other.

- *Listening,* the second key of good communication, is a rare skill. Good listening skills require that we spend more time and energy trying to fully understand another person's "story" and less time judging, evaluating, blaming, advising, analyzing, or trying to control. Empathy, warmth, respect, and genuineness are qualities of skillful listeners. Attentive listening encourages friends or partners to share more and, in turn, to be attentive listeners. To connect with other people and develop real emotional intimacy, listening is essential.

- *Feedback,* a constructive response to another's self-disclosure, is the third key to good communication. Giving positive feedback means acknowledging that the friend's or partner's feelings are valid—no matter how upsetting or troubling—and offering self-disclosure in response. If, for example, your partner discloses unhappiness about your relationship, it is more constructive to say that you're concerned or saddened by that and want to hear more about it than to get angry, to blame, to try to inflict pain, or to withdraw. Self-disclosure and feedback can open the door to change, whereas other responses block communication and change. (For tips on improving your skills, see the box "Guidelines for Effective Communication." on p. 104)

Gender and Communication

Some of the difficulties people encounter in relationships can be traced to common gender differences in communication. Many authorities believe that, because of the way they've been raised, men and women generally approach conversation and communication differently. According to this view, men tend to use conversation in a *competitive* way, perhaps hoping to establish dominance in relationships. When male conversations are over, men often find themselves in a one-up or a one-down position.

Conflict is an inevitable part of any intimate relationship. Couples need to develop constructive ways of resolving conflicts in order to maintain a healthy relationship.

Women tend to use conversation in a more *affiliative* way, perhaps hoping to establish friendships. They negotiate various degrees of closeness, seeking to give and receive support. Men tend to talk more—though without disclosing more—and listen less. Women tend to use good listening skills such as eye contact, frequent nodding, focused attention, and asking relevant questions.

Although these are generalized patterns, they can translate into problems in specific conversations. Even when a man and a woman are talking about the same subject, their unconscious goals may be very different. The woman may be looking for understanding and closeness, while the man may be trying to demonstrate his competence by giving advice and solving problems. Both styles are valid; the problem comes when differences in style result in poor communication and misunderstanding. See the box "Gender and Communication" on page 105 for more information.

Sometimes communication is not the problem in a relationship—the partners understand each other all too well. The problem is that they're unable or unwilling to change or compromise. Although good communication can't salvage a bad relationship, it does enable couples to see their differences and make more informed decisions.

Conflict and Conflict Resolution

Conflict is natural in intimate relationships. No matter how close two people become, they still remain separate individuals with their own needs, desires, past experiences, and ways of seeing the world. In fact, the closer the

Guidelines for Effective Communication

Getting Started

- When you want to have a serious discussion with your partner, find an appropriate time and place. Choose a block of time when you will not be interrupted or rushed and a place that is private.

- Face your partner and maintain eye contact. Use nonverbal feedback to show that you are interested and involved in the communication process.

Being an Effective Speaker

- State your concern or issue as clearly as you can.

- Use "I" statements—statements about how *you* feel—rather than statements beginning with "You," which tell another person how you think he or she feels. When you use "I" statements, you are taking responsibility for your feelings. "You" statements are often blaming or accusatory and will probably get a defensive or resentful response. The statement "I feel unloved," for example, sends a clearer, less blaming message than the statement "You don't love me."

- Focus on a specific behavior rather than on the whole person. Be specific about the behavior you like or don't like. Avoid generalizations beginning with "You always" or "You never." Such statements make people feel defensive.

- Make constructive requests. Opening your request with "I would like" keeps the focus on your needs rather than your partner's supposed deficiencies.

- Avoid blaming, accusing, and belittling. Even if you are right, you have little to gain by putting your partner down. Studies have shown that when people feel criticized or attacked, they are less able to think rationally or solve problems constructively.

- Ask for action ahead of time, not after the fact. Tell your partner what you would like to have happen in the future; don't wait for him or her to blow it and then express anger or disappointment.

Being an Effective Listener

- Provide appropriate nonverbal feedback (nodding, smiling, making eye contact, and so on).

- Don't interrupt.

- Develop the skill of reflective listening. Don't judge, evaluate, analyze, or offer solutions (unless asked to do so). Your partner may just need to have you there in order to sort out feelings. By jumping in right away to "fix" the problem, you may actually be cutting off communication.

- Don't give unsolicited advice. Giving advice implies that you know more about what a person needs to do than he or she does; therefore, it often evokes anger or resentment.

- Clarify your understanding of what your partner is saying by restating it in your own words and asking if your understanding is correct. "I think you're saying that you would feel uncomfortable having dinner with my parents and that you'd prefer to meet them in a more casual setting. Is that right?" This type of specific feedback prevents misunderstandings and helps validate the speaker's feelings and message.

- Be sure you are really listening, not off somewhere in your mind rehearsing your reply. Try to tune in to your partner's feelings as well as the words.

- Let your partner know that you value what he or she is saying and want to understand. Respect for the other person is the cornerstone of effective communication.

---

relationship, the more differences and the more opportunities for conflict there will be. Conflict itself isn't dangerous to a relationship; in fact, it may indicate that the relationship is growing. But if it isn't handled in a constructive way, it will damage—and ultimately destroy—the relationship. Consider the following guidelines, but keep in mind that different couples communicate in different ways around conflict. See the box "Relationship Styles and Conflict Resolution" for more information on these different patterns.

Conflict is often accompanied by anger—a natural emotion, but one that can be difficult to handle. If we express anger, we run the risk of creating distrust, fear, and distance; if we act it out without thinking things through, we can cause the conflict to escalate; if we suppress anger, it turns into resentment and hostility. The best way to handle anger in a relationship is to recognize it as a symptom of something that requires at-

tention and needs to be changed. When angry, partners should back off until they calm down and then come back to the issue later and try to resolve it rationally. Negotiation will help dissipate the anger so the conflict can be resolved.

Although the sources of conflict for couples change over time, they primarily revolve around the basic tasks of living together: dividing the housework, handling money, spending time together, and so on. Sexual interaction is also a source of disagreement for many couples.

Although there are numerous theories on and approaches to conflict resolution, some basic strategies are generally useful in successfully negotiating with a partner:

1. *Clarify the issue.* Take responsibility for thinking through your feelings and discovering what's really bothering you. Agree that one partner will speak first and have

Take Charge

Gender Matters

Women and men view and approach relationships differently. One manifestation of these differences that tends to create difficulty in intimate relationships and communication is that women are generally more comfortable with emotion than are men. This difference has been traced in part to socialization and in part to biology.

From an early age, parents, teachers, and society send different messages to girls and boys regarding emotion. Boys learn to suppress and bury their feelings, especially fear and other emotions that make them feel vulnerable. Girls are encouraged to express and talk about their feelings. These differences are further reinforced by peer groups. Gender segregation is already apparent in preschool and increases throughout middle childhood for most children. Boys and girls spend most of their time with peers of the same gender, and their communication styles are very different. For example, when conflict arises, girls tend to care more about preserving their relationships, and boys care more about maintaining the game they were playing.

In addition to socialization differences, research now shows that men have a more intense physiological response to certain emotions. In discussions around conflict, a man's blood pressure and heart rate rise higher and remain elevated longer. Part of the reason may be that a man's internal dialogue repeats upsetting thoughts (for example, "How could she say that? I can't take this!"). When anyone is physiologically or emotionally overwhelmed ("flooded"), productive communication is impossible.

A common pattern that arises between men and women is called "confront-withdraw." A woman approaches her male partner because she is upset and wants to talk about it. The man tries to calm her down, provides solutions he sees as rational, and/or withdraws. This response may make his partner even more upset and demanding, which causes the man to further shut down. Given what we know about gender differences, we might understand the man's response as one of self-protection, because he is entering territory that is both unknown and physically unpleasant. In order to enjoy intimacy, however, men and women must work to better understand one another and develop a more compatible communication style.

Advice for Men

- When your partner raises an emotional topic, be aware of uncomfortable feelings and the desire to retreat.

- Do not run away (physically or emotionally)! Telling her to "calm down" will likely create the opposite response.

- Find a way to stay connected. This is the only way to deescalate the conflict.

- Empathize: Listen to what she is saying, and even if you disagree, communicate to her that you understand how she is feeling and where she is coming from. Often when a person feels genuinely heard, that is enough.

- Try not to think of her comments as personal attacks; instead, continue to empathize.

- You may need to calm yourself. Try taking long deep breaths, telling yourself that your partner needs to air her feelings, and remembering that she, too, wants the conflict to end.

- In some cases, a 20-minute break—during which you soothe yourself rather than think upsetting thoughts—can be helpful.

Advice for Women

- Try to be calm when approaching conflict; practice similar relaxation techniques to those described in "Advice for Men."

- Try to speak in ways that will not provoke defensiveness; complain rather than criticize, be specific, and use "I" statements.

- Try not to be critical of your partner's responses or his attempts to communicate.

- Be aware if he is withdrawing, and, if appropriate, help him to relax by using methods you have discussed previously. For example, reassure him that you love him, and put the argument in perspective. Be careful not to be condescending about this.

SOURCE: Gottman, J. 1994. *Why Marriages Succeed or Fail . . . and How You Can Make Yours Last.* New York: Simon & Schuster.

the chance to speak fully while the other listens. Then reverse the roles. Try to understand the other partner's position fully by repeating what you've heard and asking questions to clarify or elicit more information. Agree to talk only about the topic at hand and not get distracted by other issues. Sum up what your partner has said.

2. *Find out what each person wants.* Ask your partner to express his or her desires. Don't assume you know what your partner wants and speak for him or her. Clarify and summarize.

3. *Identify various alternatives for getting each person what he or she wants.* Practice brainstorming to generate a variety of options.

4. *Decide how to negotiate.* Work out some agreements or plans for change; for example, one partner will do one task and the other will do another task, or one partner will do a task in exchange for something he or she wants. Be willing to compromise, and avoid trying to "win." Find a solution that satisfies both partners.

5. *Solidify the agreements.* Go over the plan verbally and write it down, if necessary, to ensure that you both understand and agree to it.

6. *Review and renegotiate.* Decide on a time frame for trying out the new plan, and set a time to discuss how it's working. Make adjustments as needed.

According to relationship expert John Gottman, how partners work through conflict is more important in a relationship than sharing the same views or interests. There is no single right way to resolve disagreements or communicate around conflict, and not all stable and successful relationships look the same. Gottman identified three types of stable relationships, characterized primarily by their approach to dealing with conflict. He found that what is most important is not *which* type you fit into, but that you and your partner are the *same* type. By finding a style that works best for you and your partner, you are less likely to end up with a relationship characterized by criticism, contempt, defensiveness, and stonewalling—four types of communication that ultimately lead to a relationship's demise. You will instead have many more positive interactions than negative ones, helping to keep your relationship alive and healthy.

Most healthy relationships fall into one of the following three general patterns. Which one best describes you? Which one feels most comfortable for you? Which one is your ideal type of relationship? Is your partner the same type?

- *Validating couples* compromise often. When problems arise, they work them out calmly until a resolution develops that satisfies both partners. Validating couples are good at communicating and calm and respectful even when talking about areas of conflict; they "choose their battles" wisely. They are very skilled at listening, summarizing, and understanding their partner's position and feelings, even in an argument. Partners are very connected with each other—they share their time, possessions, and personal space easily; they are affectionate and open; and they value their togetherness and shared goals and values over their own.

- *Volatile couples* have passionate conflicts (and reconciliations), and they fight frequently, even over minor issues. They have very heated arguments in which both are intensely involved (one often trying to persuade the other of her or his position) but then passionately make up; in the end, they are able to resolve their conflict. The intensity of their arguments is equaled by the passion and excitement of their positive interactions. They openly and honestly express both their positive and negative thoughts and feelings. They see themselves as equals, and they value their independence. (Volatility does not indicate an unhealthy relationship unless communication is characterized by disrespect, power imbalance, conflict that does not lead to resolution, and/or abuse.)

- *Conflict avoiding couples* "agree to disagree" and do not often address their conflicts directly. In arguments, partners state their side (with little persuading of the other) and then drop the issue, agreeing that they disagree but also that it is not important enough to continue exploring. They feel that their areas of commonality and shared values make their areas of conflict insignificant in the big picture. They focus on the positive and make light of (minimize) or ignore their differences rather than resolving them. They value having separate space and independence; their lives tend to be peaceful. This type of communication style may cause a problem if a conflict arises that needs resolution; also, there is risk that one or both partners may end up feeling that their partner does not know them.

Not everyone fits neatly into one of these types; in fact, many couples find a blend of styles works best for them. All styles are equally stable—as long as both partners are in agreement about which one works best for them as a couple, and as long as the style supports positive interactions in the vast majority of instances. Finding a style that is comfortable for both partners is not always easy, but it is important for creating a relationship that will last.

For more information on this and/or how to more fully assess your relationship, see Gottman, J. 1994. *Why Marriages Succeed or Fail . . . and How You Can Make Yours Last.* New York: Simon & Schuster.

To resolve conflicts, partners have to feel safe in voicing disagreements. They have to trust that the discussion won't get out of control, that they won't be abandoned by the other, and that the partner won't take advantage of their vulnerability. Partners should follow some basic ground rules when they argue, such as avoiding ultimatums, resisting the urge to give the silent treatment, refusing to "hit below the belt," and not using sex to smooth over disagreements.

When you do argue, maintain a spirit of goodwill and avoid being harshly critical or contemptuous. Remember—you care about your partner and want things to work out. See the disagreement as a difficulty that the two of you have together rather than as something your partner does to you. Finish any serious discussions on a positive note by expressing your respect and affection for your partner and your appreciation for having been listened to. If you and your partner find that you argue again and again over the same issue, it may be better to stop trying to resolve that problem and instead come to accept the differences between you.

PAIRING AND SINGLEHOOD

Although most people eventually marry or commit to a partner, everyone spends some time as a single person, and nearly all make some attempt, consciously or unconsciously, to find a partner. Intimate relationships are as important for singles as for couples.

For many college students today, group activities have replaced dating as a way to meet and get to know potential partners.

Choosing a Partner

Most men and women select partners for long-term relationships through a fairly predictable process, although they may not be consciously aware of it. Most people pair with someone who lives in the same geographic area and who is similar in ethnic and socioeconomic background, educational level, lifestyle, physical attractiveness, and other traits. In simple terms, people select partners like themselves.

First attraction is based on easily observable characteristics: looks, dress, social status, and reciprocated interest. Once the euphoria of romantic love winds down, personality traits and behaviors become more significant factors in how the partners view each other. Through sharing and self-disclosure, they gradually gain a deeper knowledge of each other. The emphasis shifts to basic values, such as religious beliefs, political affiliation, sexual attitudes, and future aspirations regarding career, family, and children. At some point, they decide whether the relationship feels viable and is worthy of their continued commitment. If they are compatible, many people gradually discover deeper, more enduring forms of love.

Some suggest that perhaps the most important question for potential mates is, How much do we have in common? Although differences add interest to a relationship, similarities increase the chances of a relationship's success. If there are major differences, partners should ask first, How accepting of differences are we? and then, How well do we communicate? Acceptance and communication skills go a long way toward making a relationship work, no matter how different the partners. Areas in which differences can affect the relationship include values, religion, ethnicity, attitudes toward sexuality and gender roles, socioeconomic status, familiarity with the other's culture, and interactions with the extended family (see the box "Interfaith and Intrafaith Partnerships").

Dating

Every culture has certain rituals for pairing and finding mates. Parent-arranged marriages, still the norm in many cultures, are often very stable and permanent. Although the American cultural norm is personal choice in courtship and mate selection, the popularity of dating services (complete with personality tests and videotapes of prospects) and online matchmaking suggests that many people do want help finding a suitable partner (see the box "Online Relationships" on p. 109).

Most Americans—whether single, divorced or widowed, heterosexual or gay, younger or older—find romantic partners through some form of dating. They narrow the field through a process of getting to know each other. Dating often revolves around a mutually enjoyable activity, such as seeing a movie or having dinner. Traditionally, in the male-female dating pattern, the man took the lead, initiating the date, while the woman waited to be called. In this pattern, casual dating might evolve into steady or exclusive dating, then engagement, and finally marriage.

For many young people today, traditional dating has given way to a more casual form of getting together in groups. Greater equality between the sexes is at the root of this change. People go out in groups, rather than strictly as couples, and each person pays his or her way. A man and woman may begin to spend more time together, but often in the group context. If sexual involvement develops, it is more likely to be based on friendship, respect, and common interests than on expectations related to gender roles. In this model, mate selection may progress from getting together to living together to marriage.

Living Together

According to the U.S. Bureau of the Census, about 4 million heterosexual couples and an estimated 1.5 million gay and lesbian couples are currently living together.

Chapter 4   Intimate Relationships and Communication

The movie *My Big Fat Greek Wedding* achieved popularity not only because of its entertaining portrayal of the issues surrounding interfaith marriage but also because so many people could relate to it. Interfaith marriage is common among Americans; for example, about 50% of Jews and 25% of Roman Catholics marry a partner of a different faith. There are many types of interfaith partnerships, including partners from (1) two completely different religions, (2) two religions with similar roots, (3) two divisions of the same religion, or (4) two denominations from the same religious division. The latter two are often called intrafaith partnerships.

Marrying someone of a different faith can broaden the partners' worldview and enrich their lives; however, it can also be a potential stressor and a challenge to a relationship. Depending on how religious you and your partner are, the impact of being an interfaith couple will differ. There is no specifically correct way to address religious diversity in a partnership, but the following are some potential approaches.

Withdrawal: In some couples, both partners withdraw from their respective religions. Religious differences may be minimized, but the withdrawal may not last. If a partner was observant prior to the relationship, it is likely that she or he will want to become actively involved again. This often occurs with a significant life event such as the birth of a child or death of a parent.

Conversion: In many intrafaith couples, one partner converts to the religion of the other. Religious differences are decreased, but problems can occur if the partner who converts develops resentment, has difficulties with her or his family of origin, misses the old religion, or experiences feelings of guilt or betrayal.

Compromise: Some couples convert together to a new religion, possibly to a religion or denomination at a "midpoint" between their two religions. The couple may find a happy medium that is satisfying to both. However, both may experience the problems associated with conversion. (If this option applies to you, visit www.selectsmart.com for a fun way to begin the discussion.)

Multifaith: Some couples join both religions—formally or informally. They may alternate places of worship weekly or make other creative arrangements. The advantage of this pattern is that both partners maintain their religions and learn more about each other. Problems may arise if the religions have conflicting values or practices.

Ecumenical: In some relationships, partners merge their religions. They may combine the "best" of each or observe only the areas where the religions intersect. They may get the best of both worlds and/or discover that their religions have more in common than they thought. In some cases, however, the original religious institutions may condemn compromise.

Diversity: In some couples, each partner chooses to follow his or her own religion. If both partners are very religious, they do not then have to give up an important part of their lives. However, some partners consider this approach undesirable because it means more time spent apart.

Do Nothing: Some couples find no need to address religious differences because neither partner is observant or committed to a religion to an extent that it is a relationship challenge. They address specific issues if and when they arise.

Sometimes couples handle their religious differences without a problem until they have children. At this point, decisions may need to be made regarding (1) whether (and where) to baptize, christen, or circumcise a child, (2) who to choose as godparents or extended guardians, (3) whether or how to provide religious education for the child. It is also important in interfaith or intrafaith relationships to be aware that stressors may arise in wedding planning, as the families, communities, and religious institutions may have very different views of what to include in a wedding ceremony.

To maintain a successful partnership, couples should communicate about religious issues before getting married and, if applicable, before having children. Discuss the importance of your respective religions and your religious needs. Consider ways that you can honor each other's religious traditions. Learn to discuss issues relating to religion and spirituality in ways to bring you closer together.

SOURCES: Robinson, B. A. 2003. *Inter-Faith Marriages: Overview* (http://www.religioustolerance.org/ifm_menu.htm; retrieved November 4, 2004); Robinson, B. A. 1999. *How Inter-Faith and Intra-Faith Couples Handle Religious Differences* (http://www.religioustolerance.org/ifm_diff.htm; retrieved November 4, 2004).

Living together, or **cohabitation,** is one of the most rapid and dramatic social changes that has ever occurred in our society. It seems to be gaining acceptance as part of the normal mate-selection process. By age 30, about half of all men and women will have cohabited. Several factors are involved in this change, including greater acceptance of premarital sex, increased availability of contraceptives, the tendency for people to wait longer before getting married, and a larger pool of single and divorced individuals.

Cohabitation is more popular among younger people than older, although a significant number of older couples live together without marrying to avoid losing a source of income, such as Social Security benefits, should they

Term

cohabitation Living together in a sexual relationship without being married.

More and more people today are looking to the Internet to find friends and partners, and an estimated 22 million singles have tried online dating. Communicating with others in cyberspace allows people to be themselves in a relaxed atmosphere, to try out other personas, and to confide in others in a private and less vulnerable way. The Internet can also serve as "training wheels" for those who wish to develop their social skills.

The Internet is a good tool for locating people who share your hobbies and interests—whether music, rock climbing, *Avenue Q,* or computer games. You may or may not end up meeting in person, but if your goal is to communicate with someone about a common interest, e-mail, newsgroups, listservs, blogs (online journals), and chat rooms are all good options. You may be surprised how many people share your passions and interests! (The Online Learning Center has basic guidelines about finding and using these Internet resources.)

People looking for intimate partners are also using the Internet more than ever before. For those out of college, living in big cities, not interested in bar scenes, and/or looking to expand beyond their local network of friends, the Internet provides a rich resource for making connections. Many find that there is a sense of safety and comfort, along with efficiency, associated with online dating. It is easy to put yourself out there without too much investment—you can get to know someone from the comfort of your own home, the pace is up to you, and you can end the relationship at any time. With millions of singles using dating forums that allow them to outline exactly what they are seeking, the Internet can increase a person's chance of finding a good match.

There are drawbacks to meeting partners online, however. People can misrepresent themselves, pretending to be very different—older or younger or even of a different sex—than they really are. Investing time and emotional resources in an unrealistic romance can be painful. There have also been a few instances in which online romances have become dangerous or even deadly (see Chapter 23 for information on cyberstalking).

Because people have greater freedom to reveal only the best parts of themselves, users should also be aware of a greater tendency to idealize online partners—setting themselves up for later disappointment. If you find that your online friend seems more perfect than anyone you have ever met in person, consider that a warning sign. Looking for partners online can become like shopping—the choices available to you may increase your tendency to search for perfection or find fault quickly, thereby keeping you from giving people a chance. Remember what is most important to you and keep your expectations realistic.

When choosing partners online, you are also reducing an important and powerful source of information: chemistry and in-person intuition. Much of our communication is transmitted through body language and tone, which are not available online and cannot be fully captured even by Web cams. You will therefore need to trust your feelings regarding the process of the relationship. Are you revealing more than the other person? Is there a balance in the amount of time spent talking by each of you? Is the other person respecting your boundaries? Just as in real-life dating, online relationships require you to use common sense and to trust your instincts.

If you decide to pursue an online relationship, here are some strategies that can help you maximize your experience and keep you safe:

- To increase your chances of meeting people interested in you as a person, avoid sexually orientated Web sites.

- Know what you are looking for as well as what you have to offer someone else. If you are looking for a relationship, make that fact clear. Find out the other person's situation and intentions (recently out of a long-term relationship or marriage, looking for a serious relationship or just for a distraction, etc.).

- To start, you can answer someone else's ad, letting them know what you found interesting about their post. Or you can write an ad of your own—something unique that represents some of your interests and personality. Read others' ads to become inspired, have a friend help you write yours, and/or visit the Web site's guide for creating ads. An ad doesn't have to be "perfect" or represent all of you.

- Many Web sites have a place to put a photo, and if you are serious about the pursuit of a partner, you may find that you get many more responses when you post a photo. Know, however, that your photo can then be downloaded by anyone. If this does not feel comfortable, remember that it isn't necessary and that you can always choose to add one later.

- Until you know enough about a cyberfriend, don't give out personal information, including your real full name, school, or place of employment. Consider setting up a second e-mail account for sending and receiving dating-related e-mails.

- Take the relationship at a pace that feels comfortable for you, and don't feel you need to answer every e-mail the day you receive it. Reveal personal information only as it feels right for you.

- If someone does not answer your e-mail or show up for an appointment, try not to take it personally. There are many reasons why a person may not pursue the connection.

- Before deciding whether to meet an online friend in person, schedule a phone conversation or a series of phone conversations.

- Don't agree to meet someone face-to-face unless you feel completely comfortable about it. Always meet initially in a very public place—a museum, a coffee shop, or a restaurant. Bring along a friend to further increase your safety, or let a friend know where you will be.

Finally, take care that your pursuit of online relationships does not interfere with your other interpersonal relationships and social activities. There can be an addictive element to online dating that can become unhealthy. Don't use the Internet to escape from real-life problems or important personal issues, such as healing from the loss of a prior relationship. As described in Chapter 3, extensive use of the Internet is associated with greater loneliness, less communication with family members, and fewer social contacts. It is easy not to speak to real people all day and then retreat to your comfort zone and connect in cyberspace. Don't forget to stay interactive in the real world. To maximize your emotional and interpersonal wellness, use the Internet to widen your circle of friends, not shrink it.

marry. Living together provides many of the benefits of marriage: companionship; a setting for an enjoyable and meaningful relationship; the opportunity to develop greater intimacy through learning, compromising, and sharing; a satisfying sex life; and a way to save on living costs.

Living together has certain advantages over marriage. For one thing, it can give the partners a greater sense of autonomy. Not bound by the social rules and expectations that are part of the institution of marriage, partners may find it easier to keep their identity and more of their independence. Cohabitation doesn't incur the same obligations as marriage. If things don't work out, the partners may find it easier to leave a relationship that hasn't been legally sanctioned.

But living together has some liabilities, too. In most cases, the legal protections of marriage are absent, such as health insurance benefits and property and inheritance rights. These considerations can be particularly serious if the couple has children, from either former relationships or the current partnership. Since social acceptance of cohabitation is not universal, couples may feel family pressure to marry or otherwise change their living arrangements, especially if they have young children. The general trend, however, is toward legitimizing nonmarital partnerships; for example, some employers and communities now extend benefits to unmarried domestic partners.

Although many people choose cohabitation as a kind of trial marriage, unmarried partnerships tend to be less stable than marriages. In a survey of women age 15–44 who had cohabited, fewer than half were still living—married (37%) or unmarried (10%)—with their first live-in partner, 34% had dissolved the relationship prior to marriage, and 21% had married and then divorced their partner. There is little evidence that cohabitation before marriage leads to happier or longer-lasting marriages; in fact, some studies have found slightly less marital satisfaction and slightly higher divorce rates among couples who had previously cohabited. Researchers speculate that people who have cohabited might have higher

Greater openness has made gay men and lesbians more visible than they used to be, although they still constitute a minority of the population. Most gay men and lesbians have experienced at least one long-term relationship with a single partner.

expectations for marriage or might be less likely to adapt well to traditional marital roles.

Same-Sex Partnerships

Regardless of **sexual orientation**, most people look for love in a close, satisfying, committed relationship. A person whose sexual orientation is lesbian, gay, or bisexual (LGB) may be involved in a **homosexual** (same-sex) relationship. Same-sex couples have many similarities with **heterosexual** couples (those who seek members of the opposite sex). According to one study, most gay men and lesbians have experienced at least one long-term relationship with a single partner. Like any intimate relationship, same-sex partnerships provide intimacy, passion, and security.

One difference between heterosexual and homosexual couples is that same-sex partnerships tend to be more egalitarian (equal) and less organized around traditional gender roles. Same-sex couples put greater emphasis on partnership than on role assignment. Domestic tasks are shared or split, and both partners usually support themselves financially.

Another difference between heterosexual and homosexual relationships is that same-sex partners often have to deal with societal hostility or ambivalence toward their relationship, in contrast to the societal approval and rights given to heterosexual couples (see the box "Same-Sex Marriage and Civil Unions"). *Homophobia*, fear or hatred of homosexuals, can be obvious, as in the case of violence or

Terms

Viw

sexual orientation A consistent pattern of emotional and sexual attraction based on biological sex; it exists along a continuum that ranges from exclusive heterosexuality (attraction to people of the other sex) through bisexuality (attraction to people of both sexes) to exclusive homosexuality (attraction to people of one's own sex).

homosexual Emotional and sexual attraction to people of one's own sex.

heterosexual Emotional and sexual attraction to people of the other sex.

The push for legal recognition of same-sex partnerships began decades ago, but it was brought to the forefront of public debate beginning in the 1990s. Marriage is often viewed primarily as a social or religious institution, but it is in fact an institution defined by state and federal statutes that confer legal and economic rights and responsibilities. According to the U.S. General Accountability Office, there are more than 1000 federal laws in which a distinction is based on marriage. Marital status affects Social Security, federal tax status, Medicaid eligibility, inheritance, medical decision making and hospital visitation, child custody, and many other benefits.

In 2000, Vermont became the first state to offer the option of civil union to couples for whom legal marriage is not an option. A civil union is a legal status parallel to marriage—but it is valid only within the issuing state. Currently, the only state in which a same-sex couple can legally marry is Massachusetts, where officials began granting marriage licenses to same-sex couples in May 2004. San Francisco also began issuing licenses to same-sex couples in early 2004, but the California Supreme Court eventually ruled that the city had bypassed state law, and the court voided the more than 4000 same-sex marriages performed there. (Internationally, the Netherlands, Belgium, and certain provinces in Canada have legalized same-sex marriage; many other European countries offer civil unions.)

In the cases of Vermont and Massachusetts, state supreme courts ruled that under the states' constitutions, same-sex couples are entitled to the same benefits and protections as married couples. San Francisco officials acted based on their interpretation of the California state constitution's prohibition against discrimination, and the legal case over that constitutional question is still pending.

Other states and the federal government have passed laws and amendments to ban same-sex marriage. A federal law called the Defense of Marriage Act (DOMA), signed by President Clinton in 1996, defines marriage as the legal union between one man and one woman and refuses federal recognition of same-sex marriages. It also allows states to refuse to recognize same-sex marriages and civil unions performed in other states or countries. (Such action might otherwise be in violation of the U.S. Constitution's provision that each state will give "full faith and credit" to the laws of other states.) As of November 2004, more than 40 states had enacted their own mini-DOMAs and/or passed state constitutional amendments banning same-sex marriage and, in some cases, civil unions.

In 2004, President Bush endorsed an amendment to the U.S. Constitution, the "Federal Marriage Amendment," that would permanently ban same-sex marriage and prevent expected future legal challenges to federal and state DOMAs. Under the proposed amendment, states would still be allowed to grant civil unions. The amendment was defeated in Congress in fall 2004, but future action on it is likely.

What cases are made for and against civil union and same-sex marriage? Opponents put forth numerous arguments, including that the purpose of marriage is to procreate, that the Bible forbids same-sex unions, that homosexuals are seeking special rights, that it's bad for children and families, and that the majority of the population opposes such unions. The primary argument, however, is that same-sex marriage undermines the sanctity and validity of marriage as it is traditionally understood and thus undermines society.

Rules and restrictions on who can marry preserve the value of the institution of marriage, according to this view. The underlying assumption of this position is that homosexual behavior is a choice and that people can change their orientation, though the process may be difficult.

Proponents of civil unions and same-sex marriage believe that sexual orientation is outside the control of the individual and results from genetic and environmental factors that create an unchangeable orientation. The issue of same-sex union is then seen as one of basic civil rights, in which a group is being denied rights—to publicly express their commitment to one another, to provide security for their children, and to receive the legal and economic benefits afforded to married heterosexual couples—on the basis of something as unalterable as skin color.

To the argument that marriage has a traditional meaning in our society, proponents respond that, on the contrary, marriage is an evolving institution that changes as society changes. Prior to 1967, marriage between whites and African Americans was prohibited in parts of the United States; before the Civil War, African Americans were not allowed to marry at all. These and other trends, according to this view, are leading people to broaden their definition of marriage and to see same-sex marriage as just another variation.

Both opponents and proponents of same-sex marriage point out that marriage is healthy for both men and women and is the main social institution promoting family values; both sides see this assertion as supportive of their position. What remains to be seen is how society in general is going to view same-sex marriage in the future—as a furthering of American values or as an attack on them.

discrimination, or more subtle, such as how same-sex couples are portrayed in the media. Additional stress on a same-sex partnership may occur if an LGB individual is a member of a family or ethnic group that isn't entirely accepting of her or his sexual orientation. Bisexual individuals involved in heterosexual relationships may feel shame or guilt around the acceptance and privileges afforded to them by their heterosexual relationship. Due to the impact of societal disapproval, community resources and support may be more important for same-sex couples as a source of identity and social support than they are for heterosexuals. Many communities offer support groups for same-sex partners and families to help them build social networks and a sense of pride and acceptance.

Although many challenges for same-sex partnerships are common to all relationships, some issues are unique to LGB partnerships. Because men are not socialized to communicate about interpersonal and emotional issues, communication problems may be particularly common or acute in gay relationships. Some researchers suggest that the process of female socialization, with its emphasis on creating and maintaining intimacy, makes lesbian relationships more likely to be characterized by fusion, enmeshment, and a blurring of boundaries. Problems may also arise when one member of a same-sex relationship has come out, or publicly identified as LGB, earlier than the other; consequently, the more experienced individual may wonder and worry whether the partner's sexual orientation is transient. The less experienced member of the relationship may feel threatened by the partner's level of "outness" or involvement in the LGB community. If same-sex couples decide to seek counseling, it is important to find a therapist who is an ally to the LGB community and who has training and experience working with LGB couples.

See Chapter 5 for more information on sexual orientation, gender identity, and sexual behavior.

Singlehood

Despite the prevalence and popularity of marriage, a significant proportion of adults in our society are unmarried—more than 98 million single individuals. They are a diverse group, encompassing young people who have not married yet but plan to in the future, people who are living together (gay or heterosexual), divorced and widowed people, and those who would like to marry but haven't found a mate. The category includes people who are single both by choice and by chance. The largest group of unmarried adults have never been married (Figure 4-2).

Several factors contribute to the growing number of single people. One is the changing view of singlehood, which is increasingly being viewed as a legitimate alternative to marriage. Education and career are delaying the age at which young people are marrying. The median age for marriage is now 26.8 years for men and 25.1 years for women. More young people are living with their parents as they complete their education, seek jobs, or strive for financial independence. Many other single people live together without being married. Gay people who would marry their partners if they were legally permitted to do so are counted among the single population. High divorce rates mean more singles, and people who have experienced divorce in their families may have more negative attitudes about marriage and more positive attitudes about singlehood.

Being single doesn't mean not having close relationships, however. Single people may date, enjoy active and fulfilling social lives, and have a variety of sexual

Men

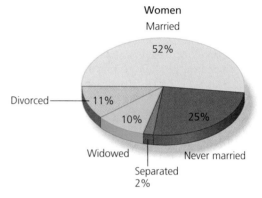

Women

VITAL STATISTICS

Figure 4-2 Marital status of the U.S. population age 15 years and older. SOURCE: U.S. Bureau of the Census. 2004. *Marital Status of People 15 Years and Over* (http://www.census.gov/population/www/socdemo/hh-fam/cps2003.html; retrieved November 5, 2004).

experiences and relationships. Other advantages of being single include more opportunities for personal and career development without concern for family obligations and more freedom and control in making life choices. Disadvantages include loneliness and a lack of companionship, as well as economic hardships (mainly for single women). Single men and women alike experience some discrimination and often are pressured to get married.

Nearly everyone has at least one episode of being single in adult life, whether prior to marriage, between marriages, following divorce or the death of a spouse, or for the entire adult life span. How enjoyable and valuable this single time is depends on several factors, including how deliberately the person has chosen it; how satisfied the person is with his or her social relationships, standard of living, and job; how comfortable the person feels when alone; and how resourceful and energetic the person is about creating an interesting and fulfilling life.

MARRIAGE

About 95% of all Americans marry at some time in their life. Marriage continues to remain popular because it satisfies several basic needs. There are many important

Mind/Body/Spirit

Research studies consistently underscore the importance of strengthening your family and social ties to help maintain emotional and physical wellness. Living alone, or simply feeling alone, can have a negative effect on both your state of mind and your physical health. Married people, on average, live longer than unmarried people—whether single, divorced, or widowed—and they score higher on measures of mental health. Those who are married have a lower prevalence of headaches, low-back pain, inactivity, and psychological distress. Research has consistently shown that married people report being happier than unmarried people, a finding that has been replicated in 42 nations worldwide. Findings suggest that there is something intrinsically beneficial about the long-term commitment that marriage represents.

People with strong social ties are less likely to become ill and tend to recover more quickly if they do. The benefits of intimate relationships have been demonstrated for a range of conditions: People with strong social support are less likely to catch colds. They recover better from heart attacks and live longer with heart disease. Among men with prostate can-

cer, those who are married live significantly longer than those who are single, divorced, or widowed. Women in satisfying marriages are less likely to develop risk factors associated with cardiovascular diseases than unmarried women or women in unhappy marriages. Research has demonstrated that a happy marriage is the best protection from sickness and premature death.

What is it about social relationships that support wellness? Some studies suggest that part of the answer is that people who get married are happier people long before they get married. But regarding physical health, friends and partners may encourage and reinforce healthy habits, such as exercising, eating right, and seeing a physician when needed. In times of illness, a loving partner can provide both practical help (sometimes financial) and emotional support. Feeling loved, esteemed, and valued brings comfort at a time of vulnerability, reduces anxiety, and mitigates the damaging effects of stress and risks of social isolation.

Although good relationships may help the sick get better, bad relationships may have the opposite effect. The impact of relationship quality on the

course of illness may be partly explained by effects of the immune system: A study of married couples whose fighting went beyond normal conflict and into criticism and name-calling found them to have weaker immune responses than couples whose arguments were more civil. (The immune effects were particularly strong among the wives, leading some researchers to postulate that women may be more aware of and affected by relationship problems.) New research shows that high marital stress is linked with risky lifestyle choices and behaviors and nonadherence to medical regimens. Similarly, unhappy marriages are associated with risk factors for heart disease, such as depression, hostility, and anger.

Marriage, of course, isn't the only support system available. Whether married, in a committed partnership, or single, if you have supportive people in your life, you are likely to enjoy better physical and emotional health than if you feel isolated and alone. So when you start planning lifestyle changes to improve your health and well-being, don't forget to nurture your relationships with family and friends. Relationships are powerful medicine.

social, moral, economic, and political aspects of marriage, all of which have changed over the years. In the past, people married mainly for practical reasons, such as raising children or forming an economic unit. Today, people marry more for personal, emotional reasons. This shift places a greater burden on marriage to fulfill certain expectations that are sometimes unreasonably high. People may assume that all their emotional needs will be met by their partner; they may think that fascination and passion will always remain at high levels; they may simply expect to "live happily ever after." When people enter marriage with such preconceptions, it may be harder for them to appreciate the benefits that marriage really offers.

Benefits of Marriage

The primary functions and benefits of marriage are those of any intimate relationship: affection, personal affirmation, companionship, sexual fulfillment, and emotional growth. Marriage also provides a setting in which to raise children, although an increasing number of couples

choose to remain childless, and people can also choose to raise children without being married. Marriage is also important for providing for the future. By committing themselves to the relationship, people establish themselves with lifelong companions as well as some insurance for their later years (see the box "Are Intimate Relationships Good for Your Health?").

Issues in Marriage

Although we might like to believe otherwise, love is not enough to make a successful marriage. Couples have to be strong and successful in their relationship before getting married, because relationship problems will be magnified rather than solved by marriage. The following relationship characteristics appear to be the best predictors of a happy marriage:

• The partners have realistic expectations about their relationship.

• Each feels good about the personality of the other.

- They communicate well.
- They have effective ways of resolving conflicts.
- They agree on religious/ethical values.
- They have an egalitarian role relationship.
- They have a good balance of individual versus joint interests and leisure activities.

Once married, couples must face many adjustment tasks. In addition to providing each other with emotional support, they have to negotiate and establish marital roles, establish domestic and career priorities, handle their finances, make sexual adjustments, manage boundaries and relationships with their extended family, and participate in the larger community.

Marital roles and responsibilities have undergone profound changes in recent years. Many couples no longer accept traditional role assumptions, such as that the husband is solely responsible for supporting the family and the wife is solely responsible for domestic work. Today, many husbands share domestic tasks, and many wives work outside the home. In fact, over 50% of married women are in the labor force, including women with babies under 1 year of age. Although women still take most of the responsibility for home and children even when they work and although men still suffer more job-related stress and health problems than women do, the trend is toward an equalization of responsibilities.

The Role of Commitment

Coping with all these challenges requires that couples be committed to remaining in the relationship through its inevitable ups and downs. They will need to be tolerant of each other's imperfections and keep their perspective and sense of humor. Commitment is based on conscious choice rather than on feelings, which, by their very nature, are transitory. Commitment is a promise of a shared future, a promise to be together, come what may. Committed partners put effort and energy into the relationship, no matter how they feel. They take time to attend to their partner, give compliments, and deal with conflict when necessary.

Commitment has become an important concept in recent years. We talk about people who are afraid of commitment or of "making a commitment" to a person or a relationship. To many people, commitment is a more important goal than living together or marriage.

Separation and Divorce

People marrying today have a 50–55% chance of divorcing. The high rate of divorce in the United States reflects our extremely high expectations for emotional fulfillment and satisfaction in marriage. It also indicates that we no longer believe in the permanence of marriage.

The process of divorce usually begins with an emotional separation. Often one partner is unhappy and looks beyond the relationship for other forms of validation. Dissatisfaction increases until the unhappy partner decides he or she can no longer stay. Physical separation follows, although it may take some time for the relationship to be over emotionally.

Except for the death of a spouse or family member, divorce is the greatest stress-producing event in life. Both men and women experience turmoil, depression, and lowered self-esteem during and after divorce. People experience separation distress and loneliness for about a year and then begin a recovery period of 1–3 years. During this time they gradually construct a postdivorce identity, along with a new pattern of life. Most people are surprised by how long it takes to recover from divorce. Children are especially vulnerable to the trauma of divorce, and sometimes counseling is appropriate to help them adjust to the changes in their lives. However, recent research has found that children who spend substantial time with both parents are usually better adjusted than those in sole custody arrangements and as well adjusted as their peers from intact families.

Despite the distress of separation and divorce, the negative effects are usually balanced sooner or later by the possibility of finding a more suitable partner, constructing a new life, and developing new aspects of the self. About 75% of all people who divorce remarry, often within 5 years. One result of the high divorce and remarriage rate is a growing number of stepfamilies (discussed in the next section).

FAMILY LIFE

American families are very different today than they were even a few decades ago. Currently, about half of all families are based on a first marriage; almost one-third are headed by a single parent; the remainder are remarriages or involve some other arrangement. Despite the tremendous variation apparent in American families, certain patterns can still be discerned.

For many young adults, the family life cycle begins with marriage. This first stage, when newlyweds are learning how to live together, ends abruptly when they have a baby. New parents have a new set of responsibilities, and their roles change profoundly and irreversibly—no more spontaneous outings to see a movie or leisurely Sunday mornings sipping coffee and browsing through the newspaper. The third member of the family, the new infant, demands around-the-clock attention.

Becoming a Parent

Few new parents have any preparation for the job of parenting, yet they have to assume that role literally overnight. They have to learn quickly how to hold a baby, how to change it, how to feed it, how to interpret its cries. No wonder the birth of the first child is one of the most stressful transitions for any couple.

Even couples with an egalitarian relationship before their first child is born find that their marital roles become more traditional with the arrival of the new baby. The father becomes the primary provider and protector, and the mother becomes the primary nurturer. Most research indicates that mothers have to make greater changes in their lives than fathers do. Although men today spend more time caring for their infants than ever before, women still take the ultimate responsibility for seeing that the baby is fed, clean, and comfortable. In addition, women are usually the ones who make job changes; they may quit working or reduce their hours in order to stay home with the baby for several months or more, or they may try to juggle the multiple roles of mother, homemaker, and employer/employee and feel guilty that they never have enough time to do justice to any of these roles.

Not surprisingly, marital satisfaction often declines after the birth of the first child. The wife who has stopped working may feel she is cut off from the world; the wife who is trying to fulfill duties both at home and on the job may feel overburdened and resentful. The husband may have a hard time adjusting to having to share his wife's love and attention with the baby.

But marital dissatisfaction after the baby is born is not inevitable. Couples who successfully weather the stresses of a new baby seem to have these three characteristics in common:

1. They had developed a strong relationship before the baby was born.

2. They had planned to have the child and want it very much.

3. They communicate well about their feelings and expectations.

Parenting

Sometimes being a parent is a source of unparalleled pleasure and pride—the first smile (at you), the first word, the first home run. But at other times parenting can seem like an overwhelming responsibility. How can you be sure you're not making some mistake that will stunt your child's physical, psychological, or emotional growth?

Parenting Styles   Most parents worry about their ability to raise a healthy, responsible, and well-adjusted child. Some had parents who were good role models, whereas others want to do things differently than their own parents did. Parents may wonder about the long-term impact of each decision they make on their child's well-being and personality. According to parenting ex-

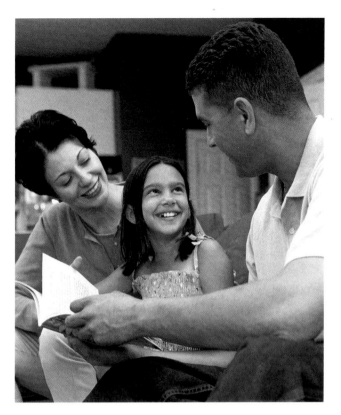

Setting clear boundaries, holding children to high expectations, and responding with warmth to children's needs are all positive parenting strategies.

perts, no one action or decision (within limits) will determine a child's personality or development; instead, what is most important is the *parenting style*, or overall approach to parenting.

Research by Diana Baumrind and others has revealed four general styles of parenting. The four styles vary primarily in parental demandingness and responsiveness. Demandingness encompasses the use of discipline and supervision, the expectation that children act responsibly and maturely, and the direct response to disobedience. Responsiveness refers to a parent's warmth and his or her intent to facilitate independence and self-confidence in a child by being supportive, connected, and understanding of the child's needs. Most parents use a blend of the four general styles but tend toward one style.

AUTHORITARIAN   Authoritarian parents are high in demandingness and low in responsiveness. They give orders and expect them to be obeyed, giving very little warmth or consideration to their children's special needs. They maintain a structured environment where the rules are explicit and set without input or discussion with the child. Children of authoritarian parents rate low on social competence, self-esteem, intellectual curiosity, spontaneity, and initiative. They perform fairly well in school and do not exhibit a lot of problem behavior; however, they have higher levels of depression.

AUTHORITATIVE Authoritative parents are high in both demandingness and responsiveness. They set clear boundaries and expectations, but they are also loving, supportive, and attuned to their children's needs. They are firm in their decisions but allow for a give-and-take in discussions with the intent of fostering independent thinking. Both authoritarian and authoritative parents hold their children to high expectations. The difference is that authoritarian parents expect their children to follow their commands without question or comment and authoritative parents are more likely to explain their reasoning and allow children to express themselves. Research consistently shows that children of authoritative parents are the best adjusted and rate particularly high in social competence.

PERMISSIVE (OR INDULGENT) Permissive parents are high in responsiveness and low in demandingness. They do not expect their children to act maturely but instead allow them to follow their own impulses. They are very warm, patient, and accepting, and they are focused on not stifling their child's innate creativity. They use little discipline and are often nontraditional. Children of permissive parents have difficulty with impulse-control, are immature, perform more poorly in school, have more problem behaviors, and take less responsibility for their actions. They also have higher self-esteem, better social skills, and lower levels of depression.

UNINVOLVED Uninvolved parents are low in both demandingness and responsiveness. They require little from their children and respond with little attention, frequency, or effort. In extreme cases, this style might reach the level of child neglect. Research has found that children of uninvolved parents perform worse in all areas measured compared with children of parents using the other styles.

Research across all ethnic groups has found that authoritative parenting has distinct advantages for children and that uninvolved parenting leads to the worst outcomes.

Children's Temperaments Different children inherently elicit different responses from parents and, therefore, affect parental styles. For example, a parent may put different demands on an aggressive child than a shy child. Every child has a tendency toward certain moods and a style of reacting—a temperament—that is apparent from infancy and often lasts into adulthood. Research has identified three basic temperament types;

most children show aspects of different temperaments but tend toward one

- *Easy children* are happy, content, and have regular sleeping and eating habits. They are adaptable and not easily upset.
- *Difficult children* are fussy, fearful in new situations or with strangers, and have irregular sleeping and feeding habits. They are easily upset and often hard to soothe.
- *Slow-to-warm-up children* are somewhat fussy and tend to react negatively or fearfully to new people or situations; however, they slowly warm up and adapt positively.

A match between parental style and child temperament is ideal. Difficulties tend to arise when there is a mismatch in temperaments/styles and the parent is not versed in parenting skills. For example, a parent who expects quick action in response to a command may not be a good match for a slow-to-respond child. Parents should be attuned to their child's distinct style and do their best to support the child.

Parenting and the Family Life Cycle Being a responsive and demanding parent is beneficial for children. Providing a balance of firm limits and clear structure along with high levels of warmth, nurturance, and respect for the child's own special needs and temperament as well as her or his growing independence is the best predictor for raising a healthy child. The important thing is to keep seeking ways to promote satisfaction for all family members—including the parents! It is also important for parents to develop and maintain confidence in their parenting skills, their common sense—and, above all, their love for their children.

At each stage of the family life cycle, the relationship between parents and children changes. And with those changes come new challenges. The parents' primary responsibility to a small, helpless baby is to ensure its physical well-being around the clock. As babies grow into toddlers and begin to crawl and walk and talk, they begin to be able to take care of some of their own physical needs. For parents, the challenge at this stage is to strike a balance between giving children the freedom to explore and setting limits that will keep the children safe and secure. As children grow toward adolescence, parents need to give them increasing independence and gradually be willing to let them risk success or failure on their own.

Marital satisfaction for most couples tends to decline somewhat while the children are in school. Reasons include the financial and emotional pressures of a growing family and the increased job and community responsibilities of parents in their thirties, forties, and fifties. Once the last child has left home, marital satisfaction

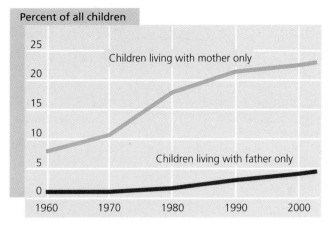

Percent of all children

25

Children living with mother only

20

15

10

5

Children living with father only

0

1960 1970 1980 1990 2000

VITAL STATISTICS

Figure 4-3 The growth of single-parent families in the United States. Since 1960, the number of children living in single-parent families has risen from about 9% to nearly 28%. Although the majority of these children live with their mother, a growing number of single-parent households are headed by fathers. SOURCE: U.S. Bureau of the Census. 2004. *Household Relationship and Living Arrangement of Children Under 18 Years* (http://www.census.gov/population/www/socdemo/hh-fam/cps2003.html; retrieved November 5, 2004).

usually increases because the couple have time to enjoy each other once more.

Single Parents

Chances are that you know a number of families who haven't followed the traditional family life cycle, or perhaps you're a member of such a family yourself. According to the U.S. Bureau of the Census, about 28% of all children under 18 live with only one parent (Figure 4-3). Today the family life cycle for many women is marriage, motherhood, divorce, single parenthood, remarriage, and widowhood.

In some single-parent families, the traditional family life cycle is reversed and the baby comes before the marriage. In these families, the single parent is usually a teenage mother; she may very well be African American or Latina, and she may never get married or may not marry for several years. In 2003, about 55% of all African American children were living with single parents, as were 30% of Latino children. In single-parent families that are the result of divorce, the mother usually has custody of the children, but about 20% of single-parent families are headed by fathers. About 7.5% of children under 18 live with one or both grandparents.

Economic difficulties are the primary problem for single mothers, especially for unmarried mothers who have not finished high school and have difficulty finding work. Divorced mothers usually experience a sharp drop in income the first few years on their own, but if they have job skills or education they usually can eventually support themselves and their children adequately. Other

problems for single mothers are the often-conflicting demands of playing both father and mother and the difficulty of satisfying their own needs for adult companionship and affection.

Financial pressures are also a complaint of single fathers, but they do not experience them to the extent that single mothers do. Because they are likely to have less practice than mothers in juggling parental and professional roles, they may worry that they do not spend enough time with their children. Because single fatherhood is not as common as single motherhood, however, the men who choose it are likely to be stable, established, and strongly motivated to be with their children.

Research about the effect on children of growing up in a single-parent family is inconclusive. Evidence seems to indicate that these children tend to have less success in school and in their careers than children from two-parent families, but these effects may be associated more strongly with low educational attainment of the single parent than with the absence of the second parent. Two-parent families are not necessarily better if one of the parents spends little time relating to the children or is physically or emotionally abusive.

Stepfamilies

Single parenthood is usually a transitional stage: About three out of four divorced women and about four out of five divorced men will ultimately remarry. Rates are lower for widowed men and women, but overall, almost half the marriages in the United States are remarriages for the husband, the wife, or both. If either partner brings children from a previous marriage into the new family unit, a stepfamily (or "blended family") is formed.

Stepfamilies are significantly different from primary families and should not be expected to duplicate the emotions and relationships of a primary family. Research has shown that healthy stepfamilies are less cohesive and more adaptable than healthy primary families; they have a greater capacity to allow for individual differences and accept that biologically related family members will have emotionally closer relationships. Stepfamilies gradually gain more of a sense of being a family as they build a history of shared daily experiences and major life events.

Successful Families

Family life can be extremely challenging. A strong family is not a family without problems; it's a family that copes successfully with stress and crisis (see the box "Strategies of Strong Families" on p. 118). Many families move through life without a clear direction. Successful families are intentionally more connected—members share experiences and meanings.

An excellent way to build strong family ties is to develop family rituals and routines—organized, repeated

Life is full of challenges; the key to life in a strong family is to work together to meet those challenges. The following are strategies used by strong families for dealing with life's difficulties:

- *Look for something positive in difficult situations.* No matter how difficult, most problems teach us something about ourselves and others that we can draw on in future situations.

- *Pull together.* Think of the problem not as one family member's difficulty but as a challenge for the family as a whole.

- *Get help outside the family.* Call on extended family members, supportive friends, neighbors, colleagues, church or synagogue members, and community professionals.

- *Create open channels of communication.* Challenges cannot be met when communication shuts down.

- *Keep things in perspective.* "These things, too, shall pass."

- *Adopt new roles in a flexible manner.* Crises often demand that individuals learn new approaches to life and take on different responsibilities.

- *Focus to minimize fragmentation.* Look at the big picture. Focusing on the details rather than the essentials can make people edgy, even hysterical.

- *Give up on worry, or put it in a box.* Worrying itself usually causes more misery than the problem at hand. Sometimes it's best to stuff the worry down or to resolve to worry 10 minutes a day and then forget about it. The mind simply has to rest.

- *Eat well, exercise, love each other, and get adequate sleep.* We often forget that we are biological beings. Like kindergartners, we need a good lunch and time to play. We need to have our hair stroked, we need a good hug, and we need a good nap.

- *Create a life full of meaning and purpose.* We all face severe crises in life. These challenges are simply unavoidable. Sometimes it helps to focus on others, to offer service to the community. Giving of ourselves brings a richness and dignity to our lives, in spite of the troubles we endure.

- *Actively meet challenges head-on.* Life's disasters do not go away when we look in another direction.

- *Go with the flow to some degree.* Sometimes we are relatively powerless in the face of a crisis. Simply saying to ourselves that things will get better with time can be useful.

- *Be prepared in advance for life's challenges.* Healthy family relationships are like an ample bank balance: If our relational accounts are in order, we will be able to weather life's most difficult storms—together.

SOURCE: Olson, D. H., and J. DeFrain. 2006. *Marriages and Families: Intimacy, Diversity, and Strengths,* 5th ed. New York: McGraw-Hill.

---

activities that have meaning for family members. Research has clearly shown that family routines and rituals are highly beneficial for couples, children, and families. Families with regular routines and rituals have healthier children, more satisfying marriages, and stronger family relationships. Some of the most common routines identified in research studies are dinnertime, a regular bedtime, and household chores; common rituals include birthdays, Christmas and other holidays, and Sunday activities. Family routines may even serve as protective factors, balancing out potential risk factors associated with single parent families and families with divorce and remarriage. You may want to consider incorporating a regular family mealtime into your family routine, as it allows parents and children to develop closer relationships and leads to better parenting, healthier children, and better school performance.

Although there is tremendous variation in American families, researchers have proposed that six major qualities or themes appear in strong families:

1. *Commitment.* The family is very important to its members; sexual fidelity between partners is included in commitment.

2. *Appreciation.* Family members care about one another and express their appreciation. The home is a positive place for family members.

3. *Communication.* Family members spend time listening to one another and enjoying one another's company. They talk about disagreements and attempt to solve problems.

4. *Time together.* Family members do things together, often simple activities that don't cost money.

5. *Spiritual wellness.* The family promotes sharing, love, and compassion for other human beings.

6. *Coping with stress and crisis.* When faced with illness, death, marital conflict, or other crises, family members pull together, seek help, and use other coping strategies to meet the challenge.

It may surprise some people that members of strong families are often seen at counseling centers. They know that the smartest thing to do in some situations is to get help. Many resources are available for individuals and families seeking counseling; people can turn to physicians, clergy, marriage and family counselors, psychologists, or other trained professionals.

Families—and intimate relationships of all kinds—are essential to our overall wellness. A fulfilling life nearly always involves other people. Whether we're single or married, young or old, heterosexual or gay, we continue to need meaningful relationships throughout life.

SUMMARY

- Healthy intimate relationships are an important component of the well-being of both individuals and society. Many intimate relationships are held together by love.

- Successful relationships begin with a positive sense of self and reasonably high self-esteem. Personal identity, gender roles, and styles of attachment are all rooted in childhood experiences.

- The characteristics of friendship include companionship, respect, acceptance, help, trust, loyalty, and reciprocity.

- Love, sex, and commitment are closely linked ideals in intimate relationships. Love includes trust, caring, respect, and loyalty. Sex brings excitement, fascination, and passion to the relationship.

- Sternberg sees love as composed of intimacy, passion, and commitment. He defines seven types of love based on various combinations of these elements, ranging from friendship to consummate love.

- Common challenges in relationships relate to issues of self-disclosure, commitment, expectations, competitiveness, balancing time spent together and apart, and jealousy. Partners in successful relationships have strong communication skills and support each other in difficult times.

- The keys to good communication in relationships are self-disclosure, listening, and feedback.

- Cultural differences in how men and women have learned to communicate can create misunderstandings and frustration in relationships.

- Conflict is inevitable in intimate relationships; partners need to have constructive ways to negotiate their differences.

- People usually choose partners like themselves. If partners are very different, acceptance and good communication skills are necessary to maintain the relationship.

- Most Americans find partners through dating or getting together in groups. Cohabitation is a growing social pattern that allows partners to get to know each other intimately without being married.

- Gay and lesbian partnerships are similar to heterosexual partnerships, with some differences. Partners often don't conform to traditional gender roles, and they may experience hostility or ambivalence rather than approval toward their partnership from society.

- Singlehood is a growing option in our society. Advantages include greater variety in sex partners and more freedom in making life decisions; disadvantages include loneliness and possible economic hardship, especially for single women.

- Marriage fulfills many functions for individuals and society. It can provide people with affection, affirmation, and sexual fulfillment; a context for child rearing; and the promise of lifelong companionship.

- Love isn't enough to ensure a successful marriage. Partners have to be realistic, feel good about each other, have communication and conflict-resolution skills, share values, and have a balance of individual and joint interests.

- Commitment helps maintain a relationship over time and through difficult changes.

- When problems can't be worked out, people often separate and divorce. Divorce is traumatic for all involved, especially children, but the negative effects are usually balanced in time by positive ones.

- Four general parenting styles are authoritarian, authoritative, permissive, and uninvolved; the authoritative style is usually associated with the best outcomes.

- At each stage of the family life cycle, relationships change. Marital satisfaction may be lower during the child-rearing years and higher later.

- Many families today are single-parent families. Problems for single parents include economic difficulties, conflicting demands, and time pressures.

- Stepfamilies are formed when single, divorced, or widowed people remarry and create new family units. Stepfamilies gradually gain more of a sense of being a family as they build a history of shared experiences.

- Important qualities of successful families include commitment to the family, appreciation of family members, communication, time spent together, spiritual wellness, and effective methods of dealing with stress.

Take Action

1. **Survey your friends.** Take an informal survey among your friends of what they find attractive in a member of the other sex and what they look for in a romantic partner. Are there substantial differences between people's responses? Do men and women look for different things?

2. **Find out how times have changed.** Ask your parents what their experiences of dating and courtship were like. How are they different from your experiences? What do your parents think of current customs?

3. **Reach out to others in your community.** Consider volunteering in your community to help promote successful families. Investigate opportunities such as youth-mentoring organizations like Big Brothers Big Sisters. Positive one-on-one relationships with youth have significant positive effects on you, the child you mentor, and the community as a whole.

For More Information

For resources in your area, check your campus directory for a counseling center or peer counseling program, or check the agencies listed in the Mental Health section of the phone book.

Books

Brooks, J. B. 2004. *The Process of Parenting,* 6th ed. New York: McGraw-Hill. *Demonstrates how parents and caregivers can translate their love and concern for children into effective parenting behavior.*

DeGenova, M. K., and F. P. Rice. 2005. *Intimate Relationships, Marriages, and Families,* 6th ed. New York: McGraw-Hill. *A comprehensive introduction to relationships.*

Gottman, J., and J. Declaire. 2002. *The Relationship Cure: A Five-Step Guide to Strengthening Your Marriage, Family, and Friendships.* New York: Three Rivers Press. *Provides research-based tools for improving communication and relationships.*

Olson, D., and J. DeFrain. 2006. *Marriages and Families: Intimacy, Diversity, and Strengths,* 5th ed. New York: McGraw-Hill. *A comprehensive introduction to relationships and families.*

Plante, T., and K. Sullivan. 2000. *Getting Together and Staying Together: The Stanford Course on Intimate Relationships.* Bloomington, Ind.: 1stBooks Library. *Provides a concise and practical approach to intimate relationships based on both clinical practice and scientific research.*

Schroeder, E. 2005. *Taking Sides: Clashing Views on Controversial Issues in Family and Personal Relationships.* New York: McGraw-Hill. *Presents a balanced look at issues such as same-sex marriage, male-female communication, the role of fathers, divorce, and child support.*

Sternberg, R. J. 2000. *Cupid's Arrow: The Course of Love Through Time.* New York: Cambridge University Press. *A review of Sternberg's triangular theory of love, with self-help advice.*

Tannen, D. 2001. *You Just Don't Understand: Women and Men in Conversation.* New York: Perennial Currents. *Provides information about gender differences in communication and how to overcome them.*

Organizations and Web Sites

American Association for Marriage and Family Therapy. Provides information on a variety of relationship issues and referrals to therapists.
http://www.aamft.org

Association for Couples in Marriage Enrichment (ACME). An organization that promotes activities to strengthen marriage; a resource for books, tapes, and other materials.
800-634-8325
http://www.bettermarriages.org

Family Education Network. Provides information about education, safety, health, and other family-related issues.
http://www.familyeducation.com

Go Ask Alice. Professional and peer educators provide answers to questions on many topics relating to interpersonal relationships and communication.
http://www.goaskalice.columbia.edu

Gottman Institute. Includes tips and suggestions for relationships and parenting, including an online relationships quiz.
http://www.gottman.com

Life Innovations. Provides materials for premarital counseling and marital enrichment.
800-331-1661
http://www.lifeinnovation.com

Online NewsHour: The Battle Over Same-Sex Marriage. Includes background information as well as debate among people representing different stands on the issue.
http://www.pbs.org/newshour/bb/law/gay_marriage

Parents Without Partners (PWP). Provides educational programs, literature, and support groups for single parents and their children. Search the online directory for a referral to a local chapter.
http://www.parentswithoutpartners.org

Student Counseling Virtual Pamphlet Collection. Provides links to pamphlets produced by different student counseling centers; topics include relationships, sexual orientation, and assertiveness.
http://counseling.uchicago.edu/vpc

United States Census Bureau. Provides current statistics on births, marriages, and living arrangements.
http://www.census.gov

Whole Family Center. Provides information on all types of family relationships; the site includes an online magazine and examples of real-life dramas for teens, couples, and parents.
http://www.wholefamily.com

Yahoo/Lesbians, Gays, and Bisexuals. A Web site and search engine that contains many links to information and support for lesbians and gays.
http://dir.yahoo.com/society_and_culture/cultures_and_groups

See also the listings for Chapters 3 and 8.

Selected Bibliography

Associated Press. 2004. *Voters in 11 States Reject Gay Marriage* (http://www.nytimes.com/aponline/national/AP-ELN-Gay-Marriage.html; retrieved November 3, 2004).

Batalova, J. A., and P. N. Cohen. 2002. Premarital cohabitation and housework: Couples in cross-national perspective. *Journal of Marriage and the Family* 64(3): 743–755.

Bauserman, R. 2002. Child adjustment in joint-custody versus sole-custody arrangements: A meta-analytic review. *Journal of Family Psychology* 16(1): 91–102.

Bookwala, J. 2005. The role of marital quality in physical health during the mature years. *Journal of Aging and Health* 17(1): 85–104.

Centers for Disease Control and Prevention. 2004. Marital status and health: United States, 1999–2002. *Advance Data from Vital and Health Statistics*, No. 351.

Cohan, C. L., and S. Kleinbaum. 2002. Toward a greater understanding of the cohabitation effect: Premarital cohabitation and marital communication. *Journal of Marriage and the Family* 64(1): 180–192.

Columbia University Health Education Program. 2002. *Go Ask Alice: Looking for Love Online* (http://www.goaskalice.columbia.edu/1185.html; retrieved February 17, 2003).

Darling, N. 1999. *Parenting Style and Its Correlates* (http://www.athealth.com/Practitioner/ceduc/parentingstyles.html; retrieved November 3, 2004).

Denton, W. H., et al. 2001. Cardiovascular reactivity and initiate/avoid patterns of marital communication: A test of Gottman's psychophysiologic model of marital interaction. *Journal of Behavioral Medicine* 24(5): 401–421.

Eng, P. M., et al. 2002. Social ties and change in social ties in relation to subsequent total and cause-specific mortality and coronary heart disease incidence in men. *American Journal of Epidemiology* 155(8): 700–709.

Fiese, B. H., et al. 2002. A review of 50 years of research on naturally occurring family routines and rituals: Cause for celebration? *Journal of Family Psychology* 16(4): 381–390.

Gallo, L. C., et al. 2003. Marital status and quality in middle-aged women: Associations with levels and trajectories of cardiovascular risk factors. *Health Psychology* 22(5): 453–463.

Goodman, R. F., and A. Gurian. 2001. *Parenting Styles/Children's Temperaments: The Match* (http://www.Aboutourkids.org; retrieved October 14, 2004).

Gottman, J. 1994. *Why marriages succeed or fail . . . and how you can make yours last.* New York: Simon & Schuster.

Harris, C. R. 2002. Sexual and romantic jealousy in heterosexual and homosexual adults. *Psychological Science* 13(1): 7–12.

Heller, P. E., and B. Wood. 2000. The influence of religious and ethnic differences on marital intimacy: Intermarriage versus intramarriage. *Journal of Marital and Family Therapy* 26(2): 241–252.

Human Rights Campaign. 2004. *Statewide Marriage Laws* (http://www.hrc.org; retrieved November 3, 2004).

Kaplan, M., and J. E. Maddux. 2002. Goals and marital satisfaction: Perceived support for personal goals and collective efficacy for collective goals. *Journal of Social and Clinical Psychology* 21(2): 157–164.

Lucas, R. E. 2003. Reexaming adaptation and the set point model of happiness: Reactions to changes in marital status. *Journal of Personality and Social Psychology* 84(3): 537–539.

Marech, R. 2005. The battle over same-sex marriage: One year later both sides claim victory, but courts will decide. *San Francisco Chronicle*, February 12.

McKinney, L. C., and L. S. Newman. 2002. Anticipating responses to one's own misdeeds: Repressive coping and the prediction of others' reactions to inconsiderate behavior. *Journal of Social and Clinical Psychology* 21(4): 427–440.

Medical memo: Marital stress and the heart. 2004. *Harvard Men's Health Watch*, May.

Mookadam, F., and H. M. Arthur. 2004. Social support and its relationship to morbidity and mortality after acute myocardial infarction: Systematic overview. *Archives of Internal Medicine* 164(14): 1514–1518.

Murray, S. L., et al. 2002. When rejection stings: How self-esteem constrains relationship-enhancement processes. *Journal of Personality and Social Psychology* 83(3): 556–573.

Murray, S. L., et al. 2003. Once hurt, twice hurtful: How perceived regard regulates daily marital interactions. *Journal of Personality and Social Psychology* 84(1): 126–147.

Najib, A., et al. 2004. Regional brain activity in women grieving a romantic relationship breakup. *American Journal of Psychiatry* 161(12): 2245–2256.

National Center for Health Statistics. 2002. *Cohabitation, Marriage, Divorce, and Remarriage in the United States.* Vital and Health Statistics, Series 23, Number 22.

Olson, D., and J. DeFrain. 2006. *Marriages and Families,* 5th ed. New York: McGraw-Hill.

Online NewsHour. 2004. *The Battle Over Same-Sex Marriage: Expert Debate* (http://www.bs.org/newshour/bb/law/gay_marriage/q3.html; retrieved November 1, 2004).

Pedersen, W. C., et al. 2002. Evolved sex differences in the number of partners desired? *Psychological Science* 13(2): 157–161.

Plante, T., and K. Sullivan. 2000. *Getting Together and Staying Together: The Stanford Course on Intimate Relationships.* Bloomington, Ind.: 1stBooks Library.

Strong, B., et al. 2005. *Human Sexuality: Diversity in Contemporary America,* 5th ed. New York: McGraw-Hill.

Suler, J. 1997. *The Final Showdown Between In-Person and Cyberspace Relationships* (http://www1.rider.edu/users/suler/psycyber/showdown.html; retrieved August 28, 2000).

Tower, R. B., S. V. Kasl, and A. S. Darefsky. 2002. Types of marital closeness and mortality risk in older couples. *Psychosomatic Medicine* 64(4): 644–659.

Wainright, J. L., S. T. Russell, and C. J. Patterson. 2004. Psychosocial adjustment, school outcomes, and romantic relationships of adolescents with same-sex parents. *Child Development* 75(6): 1886–1898.

Whisman, M. A., L. A. Uebelacker, and L. M. Weinstock. 2004. Psychopathology and marital satisfaction: the importance of evaluating both partners. *Journal of Consulting and Clinical Psychology* 72(5): 830–838.

White, L., and J. G. Gilbreth. 2001. When children have two fathers: Effects of relationships with stepfathers and noncustodial fathers on adolescent outcomes. *Journal of Marriage and the Family* 63(1): 155–167.

Wu, Z., and R. Hart. 2002. The effects of marital and nonmarital union transition on health. *Journal of Marriage and the Family* 64(2): 420–432.

5

Looking **AHEAD**

After reading this chapter, you should be able to

- Describe the structure and function of the female and male sex organs

- Explain the changes in sexual functioning that occur across the life span

- Describe how the sex organs function during sexual activity and list common causes of sexual problems

- Outline the factors that influence sexual behavior and the various ways human sexuality can be expressed

- Describe guidelines for safe, responsible sexual behavior

Sex and Your Body

Knowledge

1. **Early in development, all embryos begin as female.**
   True or false?

2. **Which of the following is a risk factor for erectile dysfunction ("impotence")?**
   a. smoking
   b. overweight
   c. physical inactivity

3. **Calcium supplements may reduce symptoms of premenstrual syndrome (PMS) in some women.**
   True or false?

4. **Alcohol consumption by young people is associated with unplanned, unprotected sexual activity and higher rates of sexually transmitted diseases (STDs).**
   True or false?

5. **Women's motivations for having sex are usually to express love, whereas men's motives are usually physical.**
   True or false?

6. **About 10% (one in ten) of young people (age 10–17) who regularly use the Internet have encountered unwanted online pornography or been exposed to unwanted sexual solicitations or approaches through the Internet.**
   True or false?

ANSWERS

1. TRUE. Without the influence of sex hormones, all embryos would develop into females.

2. ALL THREE. 70–80% of cases of erectile dysfunction are thought to involve physical factors.

3. TRUE. Other self-help strategies for PMS include exercise, stress reduction, and a diet low in fat and rich in complex carbohydrates.

4. TRUE. Studies have shown that raising the drinking age and increasing the price of beer (through taxes) leads to a decrease in STD rates among young adults.

5. FALSE. Although this statement is often true for men and women under 40, after age 40, physical gratification becomes the more common motivation for women, while emotional expression becomes more important for men.

6. FALSE. About 24% (one in four) of young people have encountered unwanted online pornography, and 20% (one in five) have been exposed to unwanted sexual solicitations via the Internet.

Visit the *Core Concepts in Health* Online Learning Center (www.mhhe.com/insel10e) for study aids and many additional resources.

Humans are sexual beings. Sexual activity is the source of our most intense physical pleasures, a central ingredient in many of our intimate emotional relationships, and, of course, the key to the reproduction of our species.

Sexuality is more than just sexual behavior. It includes biological sex (being biologically male or female), gender (masculine and feminine behaviors), sexual anatomy and physiology, sexual functioning and practices, and social and sexual interactions with others. Our individual sense of identity is powerfully influenced by our sexuality. We think of ourselves in very fundamental ways as male or female; as heterosexual or homosexual; as single, attached, married, or divorced. Sexuality is a complex, interacting group of inborn, biological characteristics and acquired behaviors people learn in the course of growing up in a particular family, community, and society.

Sexuality arouses intense feelings, and communicating about it is highly emotionally charged. Because of its basic role in human life, sexual expression is usually regulated with restrictions and taboos—written and unwritten laws specifying which functions and behaviors are acceptable and "normal" and which are unacceptable and "abnormal." Young people growing up in the United States are bombarded with conflicting messages about sex from television, movies, magazines, and popular music. The mass media suggest that the average person is a sexual athlete who continually jumps in and out of bed without using contraception, producing offspring, or contracting disease. Although parents, educators, and other responsible adults present a more balanced picture, they may convey their own hidden messages as well. Ignorance, confusion, and fear are often the result.

Basic information about the body and about sexual functioning and behavior is vital to healthy adult life. Once we understand the facts, we have a better basis for evaluating the messages we get and for making informed, responsible choices about our sexual activities. If you have questions about aspects of your physical sexuality, this chapter will provide you with some answers.

SEXUAL ANATOMY

In spite of their different appearances, the sex organs of men and women arise from the same structures and fulfill similar functions. Each person has a pair of **gonads**; ovaries are the female gonads, and testes are the male gonads. The gonads produce **germ cells** and sex hormones. The germ cells are ova (eggs) in females and sperm in males. Ova and sperm are the basic units of reproduction; their union results in the creation of a new life.

Female Sex Organs

The external sex organs, or genitals, of the female are called the **vulva** (Figure 5-1a). The mons pubis, a rounded mass of fatty tissue over the pubic bone, becomes covered with hair during puberty (biological maturation). Below it are two paired folds of skin called the labia majora (major lips) and the labia minora (minor lips). Enclosed within are the clitoris, the opening of the urethra, and the opening of the vagina. The **clitoris** is highly sensitive to touch and plays an important role in female sexual arousal and orgasm. The clitoris, like the penis, consists of a shaft, glans, and spongy tissue that fills with blood during sexual excitement. The glans is the most sensitive part of the clitoris and is covered by the clitoral hood, or **prepuce**, which is formed from the upper portion of the labia minora.

The female urethra leads directly from the urinary bladder to its opening between the clitoris and the opening of the vagina; it conducts urine from the bladder to the outside of the body. Unlike the male urethra, it is independent of the genitals.

The vaginal opening is partially covered by the hymen. This membrane can be stretched or torn during athletic activity or when a woman has sexual intercourse for the first time. The idea that an intact hymen is the sign of a virgin is a myth. The **vagina** is the passage that leads to the internal reproductive organs (Figure 5-1b). It is the female structure for heterosexual sexual intercourse and also serves as the birth canal. Its soft, flexible walls are normally in contact with each other. A cylinder of muscles surrounds the vagina. During sexual excitement, the tension in these muscles increases and the walls of the vagina swell with blood.

Terms

V W

sexuality A dimension of personality shaped by biological, psychosocial, and cultural forces and concerning all aspects of sexual behavior.

gonads The primary reproductive organs that produce germ cells and sex hormones; the ovaries and testes.

germ cells Sperm and ova (eggs).

vulva The external female genitals, or sex organs.

clitoris The highly sensitive female genital structure.

prepuce The foreskin of the clitoris or penis.

vagina The passage leading from the female genitals to the internal reproductive organs; the birth canal.

cervix The end of the uterus opening toward the vagina.

uterus The hollow, thick-walled, muscular organ in which the fertilized egg develops; the womb.

ovary One of two female reproductive glands that produce ova (eggs) and sex hormones; ovaries are the female gonads.

penis The male genital structure consisting of spongy tissue that becomes engorged with blood during sexual excitement.

scrotum The loose sac of skin and muscle fibers that contains the testes.

testis One of two male gonads, the site of sperm production; plural, *testes*. Also called *testicle*.

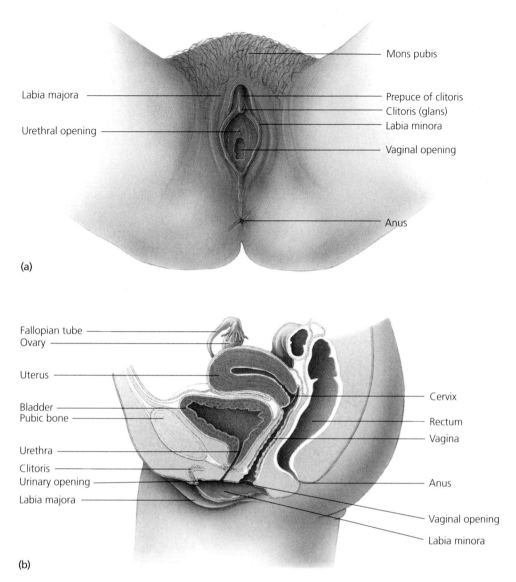

Labels on figure (a):
- Mons pubis
- Labia majora
- Prepuce of clitoris
- Clitoris (glans)
- Labia minora
- Urethral opening
- Vaginal opening
- Anus

(a)

Labels on figure (b):
- Fallopian tube
- Ovary
- Uterus
- Bladder
- Pubic bone
- Urethra
- Clitoris
- Urinary opening
- Labia majora
- Cervix
- Rectum
- Vagina
- Anus
- Vaginal opening
- Labia minora

(b)

Figure 5-1   The female sex organs.   (a) External structures; (b) internal structures.

Projecting into the upper part of the vagina is the **cervix,** the neck of the uterus. Inside the pear-shaped **uterus,** which slants forward above the bladder, the fertilized egg is implanted and grows into a *fetus.* A pair of *fallopian tubes* (or *oviducts*) extend from the top of the uterus. The end of each oviduct surrounds an **ovary** and guides the mature ovum down into the uterus after the egg bursts from its follicle on the surface of the ovary.

Male Sex Organs

A man's external sex organs, or genitals, are the penis and the scrotum (Figure 5-2a, p. 126). The **penis** consists of spongy tissue that becomes engorged with blood during sexual excitement, causing the organ to enlarge and become erect. The **scrotum** is a pouch that contains a pair of **testes.** The purpose of the scrotum is to maintain the

testes at a temperature approximately 5°F below that of the rest of the body—that is, at about 93.6°F. The process of sperm production is extremely heat-sensitive. In hot temperatures the muscles in the scrotum relax, and the testes move away from the heat of the body. This ability to regulate the temperature of the testes is important because elevated testicular temperature can interfere with normal sperm production.

Through the entire length of the penis runs the urethra, which can carry both urine and *semen,* the sperm-carrying fluid, to the opening at the tip of the glans (Figure 5-2b). Although urine and semen share a common passage, they are prevented from mixing together by muscles that control their entry into the urethra.

The testes contain tightly packed seminiferous tubules within which sperm are produced. These tubules end in a maze of ducts that flow into a single storage tube called

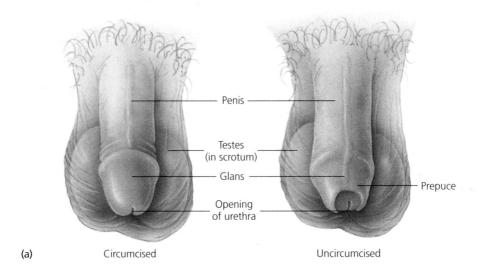

Penis

Testes
(in scrotum)

Glans

Prepuce

Opening
of urethra

(a)   Circumcised   Uncircumcised

Bladder

Pubic bone

Vas deferens

Corpus
spongiosum

Penis

Urethra

Opening of
urethra

(b)

Seminal vesicle

Rectum

Prostate

Cowper's gland

Anus

Epididymis

Testis

Scrotum

Figure 5-2 The male sex organs. (a) External structures; (b) internal structures.

the *epididymis,* on the surface of each testis. This tube leads to the *vas deferens,* a tube that rises into the abdominal cavity. Inside the prostate gland, the two vasa deferentia join the ducts of the two *seminal vesicles,* whose secretions provide nutrients to semen. The *prostate gland* produces some of the fluid in semen that nourishes and transports sperm. The tubes of the seminal vesicle and the vas deferens on each side lead to the *ejaculatory duct,* which joins the urethra. The *Cowper's glands* (bulbourethral glands) are two small structures flanking the urethra. During sexual arousal, these glands secrete a clear, mucuslike fluid that appears at the tip of the penis. The exact purpose of preejaculatory fluid is not known, but it is thought to help lubricate the urethra to facilitate

the passage of sperm. In some men, preejaculatory fluid may contain sperm, so withdrawal of the penis before ejaculation is not a reliable form of contraception.

Circumcision   The smooth, rounded tip of the penis is the highly sensitive **glans,** an important component in sexual arousal. The glans is partially covered by the foreskin, or prepuce, a retractable fold of skin that is removed by **circumcision** in about 60–70% of newborn males in the United States. Circumcision is performed for cultural, religious, and hygienic reasons, and rates of circumcision vary widely among different groups. Worldwide, the rate is about 20%. Most Europeans, Asians, South and Central Americans, and Africans do not perform circumcision;

Jews and Muslims are the major groups who circumcise for religious reasons.

The pros and cons of this simple procedure have been widely debated. Citing research findings, proponents argue that it promotes cleanliness and reduces the risk of urinary tract infections (UTIs) in newborns and the risk of sexually transmitted diseases (STDs), including HIV, later in life. STD education and the practice of abstinence or low-risk sexual behaviors have a far greater impact on the transmission of STDs than does circumcision. However, where safer sex practices are not adhered to, circumcision can have a protective effect. Recent studies done in Africa and India, where rates of HIV infection and AIDS are high, have clearly shown that circumcision has a protective effect against HIV infection.

Opponents of circumcision state that it is an unnecessary surgical procedure that causes pain and puts a baby at risk for complications. They also argue that, by removing the foreskin, circumcision exposes the glans of the penis to constant irritation by clothing, thereby reducing its sensitivity; research into this issue has been inconclusive. Two studies of adult men who underwent circumcision examined the claims of superior sexual sensitivity and satisfaction for uncircumcised males. In both studies, an increase in sexual activity and sexual satisfaction (less pain during intercourse) was reported following circumcision, but in the larger of the two studies, reduced erectile function and decreased penile sensitivity were also reported. It must be noted that in almost all cases the circumcision was done for medical reasons, such as an overly tight foreskin that may have inhibited sexual functioning to some degree before the surgery. The debate continues.

In part because the overall risk of infant UTIs is low, the American Academy of Pediatrics (AAP) takes the position (opposed by some physicians) that although circumcision has potential medical benefits, the research is not sufficient to recommend the procedure routinely. When circumcision is performed, the AAP recommends that painkilling medication be provided. Although the debate focuses on medical concerns, most parents make their decision based on social or cultural factors. Fathers tend to want their sons to look like them and their peers. Whether to circumcise is a decision each family must make individually.

HORMONES AND THE REPRODUCTIVE LIFE CYCLE

Many cultural and personal factors help shape the expression of your sexuality. But biology also plays an important role, particularly through the action of *hormones*, chemical messengers that are secreted directly into the bloodstream by the **endocrine glands.** The sex hormones produced by the ovaries or testes have a major influence on the development and function of the reproductive system throughout life. The sex hormones made by the testes are called **androgens,** the most important of which is *testosterone*. The female sex hormones, produced by the ovaries, belong to two groups: **estrogens** and **progestins,** the most important of which is *progesterone*. The cortex of the **adrenal glands** also produces androgens in both males and females.

The hormones produced by the testes, the ovaries, and the adrenal glands are regulated by the hormones of the **pituitary gland,** located at the base of the brain. This gland in turn is controlled by hormones produced by the **hypothalamus** in the brain. Sex hormones exert their primary developmental influences first in the embryo stage and later during adolescence.

Differentiation of the Embryo

The biological sex of an individual is determined by the fertilizing sperm at the time of conception. All human cells normally contain 23 pairs of chromosomes. In 22 of the pairs, the two partner chromosomes match. But in the twenty-third pair, the **sex chromosomes,** two configurations are possible. Individuals with two matching X chromosomes are female, and individuals with one X and one Y chromosome are male. Thus, at the time of conception, the genetic sex is established: Females are XX and males are XY (see the box "Sexual Differentiation, Hormones, and the Brain" on p. 128).

The genetic sex will dictate whether the undifferentiated gonads will become ovaries or testes. If a Y chromosome is present, the gonads will become testes; the testes

Terms

glans The rounded head of the penis or the clitoris.

circumcision Surgical removal of the foreskin of the penis.

endocrine glands Glands that produce hormones.

androgens Male sex hormones produced by the testes in males and by the adrenal glands in both sexes.

estrogens A class of female sex hormones, produced by the ovaries, that bring about sexual maturation at puberty and maintain reproductive functions.

progestins A class of female sex hormones, produced by the ovaries, that sustain reproductive functions.

adrenal glands Endocrine glands, located over the kidneys, that produce androgens (among other hormones).

pituitary gland An endocrine gland at the base of the brain that produces follicle-stimulating hormone (FSH) and luteinizing hormone (LH), among others.

hypothalamus A region of the brain above the pituitary gland whose hormones control the secretions of the pituitary; also involved in the nervous control of sexual functions.

sex chromosomes The X and Y chromosomes, which determine an individual's biological sex.

Males and females are different from each other in many ways, but we are also very similar. We develop from the same embryonic tissue, and for every female reproductive structure there is a male counterpart. The presence or absence of androgens determines how the sex organs develop. The entire process is known as sexual differentiation.

As described in the chapter, chromosomal or genetic sex is established at conception: A genetic female has two X chromosomes; a genetic male has one X and one Y chromosome. A single gene on the Y chromosome dictates that the undifferentiated gonads in a genetic male will develop into testes.

The testes in a male produce testosterone and other hormones that circulate throughout the body and bathe each cell. Testosterone induces the reproductive structures to become male sex organs; in the absence of testosterone, the reproductive structures develop into female sex organs. Each male and female reproductive structure develops from the same undifferentiated tissue, so every structure in one sex has its counterpart in the other. For example, the tissue that gives rise to the clitoris in females becomes the penis in males, and the tissue that gives rise to the labia majora in females becomes the scrotum in males. The appearance of the genitals is sometimes called gonadal sex.

Exposure to hormones affects more than just the reproductive organs; it also influences development of the brain. It has been demonstrated many times that males tend to perform better than females at tasks requiring spatial skills and females perform better than males on tests of verbal ability and verbal memory. If androgens are involved in this gender difference, we would expect genetic females exposed to androgens to do better at spatial skills and genetic males deprived of androgens to do worse—and this is exactly what we find.

In a condition known as androgen insensitivity syndrome, genetic males do not have cell receptors for male hormones and they develop physically as females—and their spatial skills are more like those of females than males. The converse occurs when genetic females are exposed before birth to excess male hormones. In a fascinating study of twins, it was found that opposite-sex female twins had a more masculine pattern of skills and behavior compared with same-sex female twins. In opposite-sex twins, the female twin is exposed in utero to some of the androgens produced by her male twin, and these androgens influence her brain organization and thus her spatial skills.

Each person is the product of biological events that act upon the cells in the body, including the brain. However, the physical and social environment then shapes this biological foundation to produce unique individuals. Some researchers point to the human past as a way to explain sex differences in language and visual-spatial skills. For example, the early division of labor with men as hunters and women as food gatherers, camp organizers, and child raisers may have selected for different skills based on gender, including visual-spatial skills in men and communication skills in women.

SOURCES: Cohen-Bendahan, C., et al. 2004. Prenatal exposure to testosterone and functional lateralization: A study in same-sex and opposite-sex twin girls. *Psychoneuroendocrinology* 29(7): 911–916; Sinisi, A., et al. 2003. Sexual differentiation. *Journal of Endocrinological Investigation* 26(3 Suppl.): 23–28; Joseph, R. 2000. The evolution of sex differences in language, sexuality, and visual-spatial skills. *Archives of Sexual Behavior* 29(1): 35–66.

will produce the male hormone **testosterone.** Testosterone circulates throughout the body and causes the undifferentiated reproductive structures to develop into male sex organs (penis, scrotum, and so on). If a Y chromosome is not present, there is no testosterone and the gonads become ovaries and the reproductive structures develop into female sex organs (clitoris, labia, and so on).

Female Sexual Maturation

Although humans are fully sexually differentiated at birth, the differences between males and females are accentuated at **puberty,** the period during which the reproductive system matures, secondary sex characteristics develop, and the bodies of males and females come to appear more distinctive. The changes of puberty are induced by testosterone in the male and estrogen and **progesterone** in the female.

Physical Changes The first sign of puberty in girls is breast development, followed by a rounding of the hips and buttocks. As the breasts develop, hair appears in the pubic region and later in the underarms. Shortly after the onset of breast development, girls show an increase in growth rate. Breast development usually begins between ages 8 and 13, and the time of rapid body growth occurs between ages 9 and 15. Estrogens and progestins from the ovaries, as well as androgens from the adrenal glands, are responsible for the female secondary sex characteristics, the physical changes that occur at puberty.

The Menstrual Cycle A major landmark of puberty for young women is the onset of the **menstrual cycle,** the monthly ovarian cycle that leads to menstruation (loss of blood and tissue lining the uterus) in the absence of pregnancy. The timing of *menarche,* or the first *menstrual period,* varies with several factors, including ethnicity, but it occurs at about the age of 12.1–12.7 years in the United States. It may also normally start several years earlier or later.

The menstrual cycle consists of four phases: (1) menses, (2) the estrogenic phase, (3) ovulation, and (4) the

The physical changes of puberty usually begin between the ages of 8 and 13 for girls and 10 and 14 for boys. Once they reach puberty, these adolescents are biologically adults, but it will take another 5–10 years for them to become adults in social and psychological terms.

progestational phase (Figure 5-3). The day of the onset of bleeding is considered to be day 1 of the cycle. For the purposes of our discussion, a cycle of 28 days will be used; however, normal cycles vary in length.

During menses, characterized by the menstrual flow, blood levels of hormones from the ovaries and the anterior pituitary gland are relatively low. This phase of the cycle usually lasts from day 1 to about day 5.

The estrogenic phase begins when the menstrual flow ceases and the anterior pituitary begins to produce increasing amounts of follicle-stimulating hormone (FSH) and luteinizing hormone (LH). Under the influence of FSH, an egg-containing ovarian *follicle* begins to mature, producing increasingly higher amounts of estrogens. Stimulated by estrogen, the *endometrium,* the uterine lining, thickens with large numbers of blood vessels and uterine glands.

A surge of a potent estrogen called *estradiol* from the follicle causes the anterior pituitary to release a large burst of LH and a smaller amount of FSH. The high concentration of LH stimulates the developing follicle to release its ovum. This event is known as *ovulation.* After ovulation, the follicle is transformed into the **corpus luteum,** which produces progesterone and estrogen. Ovulation usually occurs about 14 days prior to the onset of menstrual flow, a fact that can be used to predict the most fertile time during the menstrual cycle, useful in both fertility treatment and natural family planning methods (see Chapter 6).

During the progestational phase of the cycle, the amount of progesterone secreted from the corpus luteum increases and remains high until the onset of the next menses. Under the influence of estrogen and progesterone, the endometrium continues to develop, readying itself to receive and nourish a fertilized ovum. When pregnancy occurs, the fertilized egg produces the hormone human chorionic gonadotropin (HCG), which maintains the corpus luteum. Thus, levels of ovarian hormones remain high and the uterine lining is preserved, preventing menses.

If pregnancy does not occur, the corpus luteum degenerates, and estrogen and progesterone levels gradually fall. Below certain hormonal levels, the endometrium can no longer be maintained, and it begins to slough off, initiating menses. As the levels of ovarian hormones fall, a slight rise in LH and FSH occurs, and a new menstrual cycle begins.

MENSTRUAL PROBLEMS Menstruation is a normal biological process, but it may cause physical or psychological problems. *Dysmenorrhea* is characterized by cramps in the lower abdomen, backache, vomiting, nausea, a bloated feeling, diarrhea, and loss of appetite. Some of these symptoms can be attributed to uterine muscular contractions caused by chemicals called *prostaglandins.* Any drug that blocks the effects of prostaglandins, such as aspirin or

Terms

testosterone The most important androgen (male sex hormone); stimulates an embryo to develop into a male and induces the development of male secondary sex characteristics during puberty.

puberty The period of biological maturation during adolescence.

progesterone The most important progestin (female sex hormone); induces the development of female secondary sex characteristics during puberty, regulates the menstrual cycle, and sustains pregnancy.

menstrual cycle The monthly ovarian cycle, regulated by pituitary and ovarian hormones; in the absence of pregnancy, menstruation occurs.

corpus luteum The part of the ovarian follicle left after ovulation, which secretes estrogen and progesterone during the second half of the menstrual cycle.

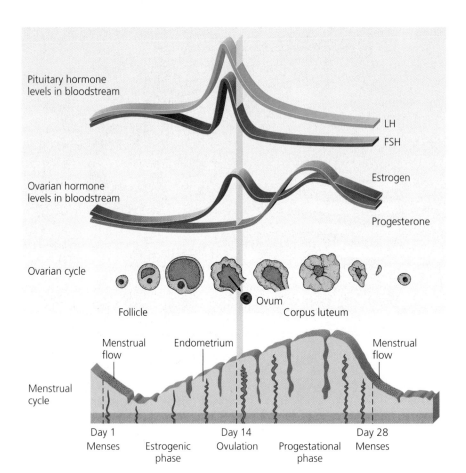

Pituitary hormone levels in bloodstream

LH

FSH

Ovarian hormone levels in bloodstream

Estrogen

Progesterone

Ovarian cycle

Ovum

Follicle   Corpus luteum

Menstrual flow   Endometrium   Menstrual flow

Menstrual cycle

Day 1
Menses

Estrogenic phase

Day 14
Ovulation

Progestational phase

Day 28
Menses

Figure 5-3 The menstrual cycle. The anterior pituitary releases FSH and LH, which stimulate the ovarian follicle to develop and release a mature egg. The ovarian follicle releases estrogen and progesterone, which stimulate the endometrium to continue to develop so that it will be ready to receive and nourish a fertilized egg. Unless pregnancy occurs, ovarian hormone levels fall and the endometrium sloughs off (menses).

ibuprofen, will usually alleviate some of the symptoms of dysmenorrhea.

Many women experience transient physical and emotional symptoms prior to the onset of their menstrual flow. Depending on their severity, these symptoms may be categorized along a continuum: **premenstrual tension, premenstrual syndrome (PMS),** and **premenstrual dysphoric disorder (PMDD).** Premenstrual tension symptoms are mild and may include negative mood changes and physical symptoms such as abdominal cramping and backache. More severe symptoms are classified as PMS; very severe symptoms that cause impairment in social functioning and work-related activities are classified as PMDD. All three conditions share a definite

pattern: Symptoms appear prior to the onset of menses and disappear within a few days after the start of menstruation. As many as 75% of women report some discomfort prior to the onset of menses, 20–50% of women experience PMS symptoms, and 3–10% meet the criteria for PMDD.

Symptoms associated with PMS and PMDD include physical changes such as breast tenderness, water retention (bloating), headache, and fatigue; insomnia or excessive sleep; appetite changes and food cravings; irritability, anger, and increased interpersonal conflict; mood swings; depression and sadness; anxiety and tearfulness; inability to concentrate; social withdrawal; and the sense that one is out of control or overwhelmed. The key to diagnosing PMS and PMDD is to keep a daily diary of symptoms over several menstrual cycles. PMDD is distinguished from PMS by the severity of symptoms, which in PMDD interfere significantly with work or school and with usual social activities and relationships.

Despite many research studies, the causes of PMS and PMDD are still unknown, and it is unclear why some women are more vulnerable than others. Research has focused on a variety of substances in the body that may fluctuate with the menstrual cycle, including progesterone, estrogen, prostaglandins, serotonin and other neurotransmitters, calcium, magnesium, and the naturally occurring opiate beta-endorphin. Most researchers

Terms

V**i**ew

premenstrual tension Mild physical and emotional changes associated with the time before the onset of menses; symptoms can include abdominal cramping and backache.

premenstrual syndrome (PMS) A disorder characterized by physical discomfort, psychological distress, and behavioral changes that begin after ovulation and cease when menstruation begins.

premenstrual dysphoric disorder (PMDD) Severe form of PMS, characterized by symptoms serious enough to interfere with work or school or with social activities and relationships.

Many dietary supplements have been promoted for relief of the symptoms of PMS; those described below are among the most commonly advocated compounds. Only one supplement, calcium, has been shown to provide relief in rigorous clinical studies; several others show promise, but more research is needed.

- *Calcium.* Blood calcium levels are lower during the premenstrual period, and careful research studies have shown calcium supplements to be effective at relieving symptoms of PMS. (A large study showed that 48% of women taking calcium experienced relief, compared to 30% taking a placebo. Although this rate is lower than that for women taking prescription medications such as SSRIs, calcium does offer relief for some women.) The amount of calcium taken by women in these studies, 1000–1200 mg per day, is within accepted safety limits for calcium intake and may also be beneficial for building and maintaining bone density (see Chapter 12 for more on recommended intakes of vitamins and minerals).

- *Magnesium.* Levels of magnesium in certain body cells are lower in women with PMS, and magnesium is involved in neurotransmitter activity. Some small studies have found magnesium to be effective in relieving PMS symptoms; however, a more recent study found that the only effect was a decrease in fluid retention. Magnesium supplements can cause side effects, including diarrhea, in some people and so should be used with caution.

- *Vitamin B-6.* Vitamin B-6 plays an important role in the synthesis of neurotransmitters, so researchers have proposed that taking supplements of vitamin B-6 may help reduce mood-related symptoms of PMS. Doses in the accepted range of 50–100 mg per day may produce a very mild benefit. Care should be taken, however, because long-term use of high doses of vitamin B-6 can cause permanent nerve damage.

- *Vitamin E.* Although the mechanism is unclear, one study found that vitamin E supplements may improve PMS symptoms. Further research is needed.

- *Carbohydrates.* Some women with PMS report craving carbohydrate-rich foods, a change in diet that may actually alleviate the mood-related symptoms of PMS. Increased intake of carbohydrates may increase blood levels of tryptophan, an amino acid the body uses to produce the neurotransmitter serotonin. Although some dietary supplements containing mixtures of carbohydrates have been marketed for PMS symptoms, it is unclear whether these are any more effective than changing the diet to include more carbohydrate-rich fruits, vegetables, and grains.

SOURCES: American Academy of Family Physicians. 2004. *PMS: What You Can Do to Ease Your Symptoms* (http://familydoctor.org/141.xml; retrieved November 8, 2004); Elliot, H. 2002. Premenstrual dysphoric disorder: A guide for the treating physician. *North Carolina Medical Journal* 63: 72–75; Bendich, A. 2000. Review: The potential for dietary supplements to reduce premenstrual syndrome (PMS) symptoms. *Journal of the American College of Nutrition* 19(1): 3–12.

feel that PMS is probably caused by a combination of hormonal, nutritional, and psychological factors.

Selective serotonin reuptake inhibitors (SSRIs), including Sarafem, Zoloft, Paxil, and Celexa, are the first-line treatment for PMDD. Until recently, women using SSRIs took the medication throughout the entire menstrual cycle, but it has now been shown that taking the medication during just the progestational phase of the cycle is similarly effective. Progestational phase use reduces the exposure to the drug and its associated side effects, and it lowers the cost of treatment. Antianxiety medications and progesterone have also been tested for progestational phase administration but show little positive effect in easing symptoms.

Other drug treatments include estrogen, certain oral contraceptives, diuretics to minimize water retention, and drugs such as aspirin, ibuprofen, and more potent prescription prostaglandin inhibitors that block the effects of prostaglandins. A number of vitamins, minerals, and other dietary supplements have also been studied for PMS relief; see the box "Dietary Supplements and PMS" for more information.

Certain lifestyle changes are often recommended to help prevent or minimize symptoms of PMS and PMDD. The following strategies provide relief for many women, and all of them can contribute to a healthy lifestyle at any time.

- *Limit salt intake.* Salt promotes water retention and bloating. Avoid salty foods.

- *Exercise.* Women who exercise experience fewer symptoms both before and after their menstrual periods.

- *Don't use alcohol or tobacco.* Alcohol and tobacco may aggravate certain symptoms of PMS and PMDD.

- *Eat a nutritious diet.* Choose a low-fat diet rich in complex carbohydrates from vegetables, fruits, and whole-grain breads, cereals, and pasta. Obtain an adequate calcium intake from calcium-rich foods and, if needed, supplements. Minimize your intake of sugar and caffeine, and avoid chocolate, which is rich in both.

- *Relax.* Stress reduction is always beneficial, and stressful events can trigger PMS symptoms. Try relaxation techniques during the premenstrual time.

If symptoms persist, keep a daily diary to track both the types of symptoms you experience and their severity. See your physician for an evaluation and to learn more about treatments that are available only with a prescription.

Male Sexual Maturation

Reproductive maturation of boys occurs about 2 years later than that of girls; it usually begins at about age 10 or 11. Physical changes include enlargement of the testes, development of pubic hair, growth of the penis, the onset of ejaculation (usually at about age 11 or 12), deepening of the voice, the appearance of facial hair, and a period of rapid growth.

Aging and Human Sexuality

Changes in hormone production and sexual functioning occur as we age. As a woman approaches age 50, her ovaries gradually cease to function and she enters **menopause,** the cessation of menstruation. For some women, the associated drop in hormone production causes symptoms that are troublesome. The most common physical symptom of menopause is hot flashes, sensations of warmth rising to the face from the upper chest, with or without perspiration and chills. Other symptoms include headaches, dizziness, palpitations, and joint pains. Osteoporosis—decreasing bone density—can develop, making older women more vulnerable to fractures. Some menopausal women become moody, even markedly depressed, and they may also experience fatigue, irritability, and forgetfulness.

To alleviate the symptoms of menopause and reduce the risk of heart disease and osteoporosis, millions of women have been prescribed hormone replacement therapy (HRT), a regimen of hormones that includes estrogen and progesterone. In the summer of 2002, an ongoing study of HRT involving more than 16,000 women was halted because the women taking HRT for long periods suffered more strokes, heart attacks, and blood clots and had a higher incidence of breast cancer than women in the study taking a placebo. The risks for such health problems were small but significant enough to halt the study. The positive findings from this study were a reduction in hip fractures and a reduced risk of colon cancer among the women taking HRT. As a result of these findings, women taking HRT were advised to consult their health care providers about their personal risks and benefits. (See Chapters 12, 15, and 19 for more information on osteoporosis, heart disease, and HRT.)

As a result of decreased estrogen production during menopause, the vaginal walls become thin, and lubrication in response to sexual arousal diminishes; sexual intercourse may become painful. Hormonal treatment or the use of lubricants during intercourse can minimize these problems.

In men, testosterone production gradually decreases with age. This drop is associated with a loss of energy, depressed mood, decreased sex drive, erectile dysfunction, decreased muscle mass and osteoporosis. Clinical

Although sexual physiology changes as people get older, many men and women readily adjust to these alterations. Sexual activity can continue throughout life for people like this healthy and vigorous older couple.

trials involving small sample sizes have shown that testosterone replacement therapy can improve many of these symptoms, but due to small sample sizes and length of the studies the risks of testosterone replacement therapy can't be assessed. As men get older, they depend more on direct physical stimulation for sexual arousal. They take longer to achieve an erection and find it more difficult to maintain; orgasmic contractions are less intense. Older men with erectile dysfunction are often prescribed medications such as Viagra or even more successful therapies that combine medication with a testosterone gel applied to the skin; see the section on sexual dysfunction later in the chapter for more information.

As women and men age, sexual activity can continue to be a source of pleasure and satisfaction for them. A recent survey found that nearly half of all Americans age 60 or older engage in sexual activity at least once a month.

SEXUAL FUNCTIONING

In this section, we discuss sexual physiology—how the sex organs function during sexual activity—and problems that can occur with sexual functioning. Sexual activity is based on stimulus and response. Erotic stimulation leads to sexual arousal (excitement), which may culminate in the intensely pleasurable experience of orgasm. But sexual activity should not be thought of only in terms of the sex organs. Responses to sexual stimulation involve not just the genitals but the entire body—and the mind as well.

Sexual Stimulation

Sexual excitement can come from many sources, both physical and psychological. Although physical stimuli have an obvious and direct effect, some people believe psychological stimuli—thoughts, fantasies, desires, perceptions—are even more powerfully erotic. Regardless of the source of erotic stimuli, all stimulation has a physical basis, which is given meaning by the brain.

Physical Stimulation Physical stimulation comes through the senses: We are aroused by things we see, hear, taste, smell, and feel. Most often, sexual stimuli come from other people, but they may also come from books, photographs, paintings, songs, films, or other sources.

The most obvious and effective physical stimulation is touching. Even though culturally defined practices vary and individual people have different preferences, most sexual encounters eventually involve some form of touching with hands, lips, and body surfaces. Kissing, caressing, fondling, and hugging are as much a part of sexual encounters as they are of expressing affection.

The most intense form of stimulation by touching involves the genitals. The clitoris and the glans of the penis are particularly sensitive to such stimulation. Other highly responsive areas include the vaginal opening, the nipples, the breasts, the insides of the thighs, the buttocks, the anal region, the scrotum, the lips, and the earlobes. Such sexually sensitive areas, or **erogenous zones**, are especially susceptible to sexual arousal for most people, most of the time. Often, though, what determines the response is not *what* is touched but how, for how long, and by whom. Under the right circumstances, touching any part of the body can cause sexual arousal.

Psychological Stimulation Sexual arousal also has an important psychological component, regardless of the nature of the physical stimulation. Fantasies, ideas, memories of past experiences, and mood can all generate sexual excitement. Erotic thoughts may be linked to an imagined person or situation or to a sexual experience from the past. Fantasies may involve activities a person doesn't actually wish to experience in reality, usually because they're dangerous, frightening, or forbidden.

Arousal is also powerfully influenced by emotions. How you feel about a person and how the person feels about you matter tremendously in how sexually responsive you are likely to be. Even the most direct forms of physical stimulation carry emotional overtones. Kissing, caressing, and fondling express affection and caring. The emotional charge they give to a sexual interaction is at least as significant to sexual arousal as the purely physical stimulation achieved by touching.

The Sexual Response Cycle

Noted sex researchers William Masters and Virginia Johnson were the first to describe in detail the human sexual response cycle. Men and women respond physiologically with a predictable set of reactions, regardless of the nature of the stimulation (Figure 5-4, p. 134).

Two physiological mechanisms explain most genital and bodily reactions during sexual arousal and orgasm. These mechanisms are vasocongestion and myotonia. **Vasocongestion** is the engorgement of tissues that results when more blood flows into an organ than is flowing out. Thus, the penis becomes erect on the same principle that makes a garden hose become stiff when the water is turned on. **Myotonia** is increased muscular tension, which culminates in rhythmical muscular contractions during orgasm.

Four phases characterize the sexual response cycle:

1. In the *excitement phase,* the penis becomes erect as its tissues become engorged with blood. The testes expand and are pulled upward within the scrotum. In women, the clitoris and the labia are similarly engorged with blood, and the vaginal walls become moist with lubricating fluid.

2. The *plateau phase* is an extension of the excitement phase. Reactions become more marked. In men, the penis becomes harder, and the testes become larger. In women, the lower part of the vagina swells, as its upper end expands and vaginal lubrication increases.

3. In the *orgasmic phase,* or **orgasm**, rhythmic contractions occur along the man's penis, urethra, prostate gland, seminal vesicles, and muscles in the pelvic and anal regions. These involuntary muscular contractions

Terms

menopause The cessation of menstruation, occurring gradually around age 50.

erogenous zone Any region of the body highly responsive to sexual stimulation.

vasocongestion The accumulation of blood in tissues and organs.

myotonia Increased muscular tension.

orgasm The discharge of accumulated sexual tension with characteristic genital and bodily manifestations and a subjective sensation of intense pleasure.

MALE

Vasocongestion of penis results in erection

Partial erection

Unstimulated state

Testes pull up

Skin of scrotum tenses, thickens, and elevates

Excitement

Cowper's gland secretion

Color of glans darkens

Prostate gland enlarges

Cowper's gland

Testes increase in size and are fully elevated

Scrotum thickens

Plateau

Penile contractions

Sperm and semen expelled by rhythmic contractions of urethra

Vas deferens contracts

Internal muscle of bladder contracts

Prostate gland contracts

Seminal vesicles contract

Rectal muscle contracts

Orgasm

Erection subsides

Unstimulated state

Scrotum thins, folds return

Testes return to normal size and position

Resolution

FEMALE

Pubic bone

Bladder

Uterus elevates

Vaginal lubrication appears

Clitoris enlarges

Labia minora swell

Labia majora

Excitement

Uterus elevates further

Upper part of vagina expands

Vaginal walls swell

Color of labia darkens

Plateau

Contractions in uterus

Rhythmic contractions in vagina

Rectal muscle contracts

Orgasm

Uterus lowers

Vagina returns to normal

Labia return to normal size and color

Resolution

Figure 5-4   Stages of the sexual response cycle.

lead to the ejaculation of **semen,** which consists of sperm cells from the testes and secretions from the prostate gland and seminal vesicles. In women, contractions occur in the lower part of the vagina and in the uterus, as well as in the pelvic region and the anus.

4. In the *resolution phase,* all the changes initiated during the excitement phase are reversed. Excess blood drains from tissues, the muscles in the region relax, and the genital structures return to their unstimulated state.

More general physical reactions accompany the genital changes in both men and women. Beginning with the excitement phase, nipples become erect, the woman's breasts begin to swell, and in both sexes the skin of the chest becomes flushed; these changes are more marked in women. The heart rate doubles by the plateau phase, and respiration becomes faster. During orgasm, breathing becomes irregular and the person may moan or cry out. A feeling of warmth leads to increased sweating during the resolution phase. Deep relaxation and a sense of well-being pervade the body and the mind.

Male and female reactions during the sexual response cycle differ somewhat. Generally, the male pattern is more uniform, whereas the female pattern is more varied. For instance, the female excitement phase may lead directly to orgasm, or orgasmic and plateau phases may be fused.

Male orgasm is marked by the ejaculation of semen. After ejaculation, men enter a *refractory period,* during which they cannot be restimulated to orgasm. Women do not have a refractory period, and immediate restimulation to orgasm is possible.

Sexual Problems

Both physical and psychological factors can interfere with sexual functioning. If you are in poor physical health or experiencing high levels of stress or anxiety, sexual functioning may be negatively affected. Difficulties may be caused by infection and other sexual health problems. Disturbances in sexual desire, performance, or satisfaction are referred to as **sexual dysfunctions.**

Common Sexual Health Problems   Some problems with sexual functioning are due to treatable or preventable infections or other sexual health problems. Conditions that affect women include the following:

• *Vaginitis,* inflammation of the vagina, is caused by a variety of organisms: *Candida* (yeast infection), *Trichomonas* (trichomoniasis), and the overgrowth of a variety of bacteria (bacterial vaginosis). Symptoms include vaginal discharge, vaginal irritation, and pain during intercourse. (See Chapters 17 and 18 for more on yeast infection, trichomoniasis, and bacterial vaginosis.)

• *Endometriosis* is the growth of endometrial tissue (tissue normally found lining the uterus) outside the uterus. It occurs most often in women of childbearing age, and pain in the lower abdomen and pelvis is the most common symptom. Painful premenstrual intercourse may occur. Endometriosis can cause serious problems if left untreated because the endometrial tissue can scar and partially or completely block the oviducts, causing infertility (difficulty conceiving) or sterility (the inability to conceive). Endometriosis is treated with hormone therapy and/or surgery.

• *Pelvic inflammatory disease (PID)* is an infection of the uterus, oviducts, or ovaries caused when microorganisms spread to these areas from the vagina. Approximately 50–75% of PID cases are caused by sexually transmitted organisms associated with diseases such as gonorrhea and chlamydia. PID can cause scarring of the oviducts, resulting in infertility or sterility. Symptoms include pain in the abdomen and pelvis, fever, and possibly pain during intercourse. (Sexually transmitted diseases are discussed in detail in Chapter 18.)

Sexual health problems that affect men include the following:

• *Prostatitis* is inflammation or infection of the prostate gland. Symptoms are fever, chills, pain in the genital region, frequent urination, and, in some cases, painful ejaculation. More common in men over 40, prostatitis is treated with antibiotics.

• *Testicular cancer* occurs most commonly in men in their twenties and thirties. A rare cancer, it has a very high cure rate if detected early. A testicular self-exam should be performed regularly (see Chapter 16).

Sexual Dysfunctions   The term *sexual dysfunction* encompasses disturbances in sexual desire, performance, or satisfaction. A wide variety of physical conditions and drugs may interfere with sexual functioning; psychological causes and problems in intimate relationships can be important factors in some cases. The same two mechanisms—vasocongestion and myotonia—that are the basis of the sexual response cycle are also at the root of the main forms of sexual disturbance: an inability to become aroused and problems experiencing orgasm.

COMMON SEXUAL DYSFUNCTIONS   Common sexual dysfunctions in men include **erectile dysfunction** (previously called impotence), the inability to have or maintain

Terms

Vw

semen Seminal fluid, consisting of sperm cells and secretions from the prostate gland and seminal vesicles.

sexual dysfunction A disturbance in sexual desire, performance, or satisfaction.

erectile dysfunction The inability to have or maintain an erection.

an erection sufficient for sexual intercourse; **premature ejaculation,** ejaculation before or just on penetration of the vagina or anus; and **retarded ejaculation,** the inability to ejaculate once an erection is achieved. Many men experience occasional difficulty achieving an erection or ejaculating because of excessive alcohol consumption, fatigue, or stress. In fact, it is estimated that 50% of American men experience occasional bouts of erectile dysfunction and retarded ejaculation.

Two sexual dysfunctions in women are **vaginismus,** in which the woman experiences painful involuntary muscular spasms when sexual intercourse is attempted, and **orgasmic dysfunction,** the inability to experience orgasm. Vaginismus is a conditioned reflex probably related to fear of intercourse. Orgasmic dysfunction has been the subject of a great deal of discussion over the years, as people debated the nature of the female orgasm and what constitutes dysfunction in women. Many women experience orgasm but not during intercourse, or they experience orgasm during intercourse only if the clitoris is directly stimulated at the same time. In general, the inability to experience orgasm under certain circumstances is a problem only if the woman considers it so.

TREATING SEXUAL DYSFUNCTION Most forms of sexual dysfunction are treatable. The first step is to have a thorough physical examination to identify any underlying medical condition that may be responsible for the problem. Heart disease and diabetes, for example, may cause erectile dysfunction; in fact, up to 80% of all erectile problems are thought to be due to physical factors, particularly vascular problems involving restriction of blood flow. Smoking affects blood vessels and blood flow in the penis and is an independent risk factor for erectile dysfunction. Drugs and medications, especially alcohol and medications used to treat high blood pressure, may also inhibit sexual response.

If physical problems continue to interfere with sexual response, many treatments are available, particularly for erectile dysfunction. In 1998, Viagra (sildenafil citrate),

the first-ever prescription pill for erectile dysfunction, was introduced; it quickly became the most successful new prescription drug in history. Since the introduction of Viagra, two other oral medications with actions similar to Viagra, Cialis (tadalafil) and Levitra (vardenafil), have been approved by the FDA. All three work by enhancing the effects of nitric oxide, a chemical that relaxes smooth muscles in the penis. This increases the amount of blood flow and allows a natural erection to occur in response to sexual stimulation. The medications are generally safe for healthy men, but they should not be used by men who have a high risk of heart attack or stroke. They are effective in only about 70% of users, and there are potential side effects, including headaches, indigestion, facial flushing, and back pain.

Recent research found that there has been a more than 300% increase in Viagra use by men between the ages of 18 and 45 since 1998—possibly due to use of the drug for recreational rather than medical purposes. Research suggests that medication may cut the refractory period in men who do not have erectile dysfunction; younger men may also be using it to cope with performance anxiety or the effects of other drugs. Although Viagra is not approved by the FDA for use by women, a growing number of women are trying the drug; research findings, however, are mixed as to whether Viagra can increase sex drive and satisfaction levels in women. Consumers should also note that as many as half of the Viagra pills sold on the Internet may be counterfeit.

Other treatments for erectile dysfunction in men are available. Prostaglandin E can be administered with a fine needle into the penis or placed into the tip of the penis as a tiny suppository about the size of a grain of rice; it works by relaxing the smooth muscles lining the blood vessels in the penis. For a small number of men with testosterone deficiency, hormone replacement therapy is an option. There are also vacuum devices that pull blood into the penis, and in cases where other treatments are unsuccessful, penile implants can be used.

If no physical problem is found, a sexual dysfunction may be psychosocial in origin. Psychosocial causes of dysfunction include troubled relationships, a lack of sexual skills, irrational attitudes and beliefs, anxiety, and psychosexual trauma, such as sexual abuse or rape. Many of these problems can be addressed by sex therapy methods that seek to modify the beliefs and behavior patterns that are interfering with satisfactory sexual relationships. A therapist may recommend books or films to help counter sexual myths and teach sexual skills. A therapist can also promote open discussion between partners and suggest specific activities or techniques. For example, premature ejaculation is often treated by the squeeze technique, in which the tip of the penis is squeezed when the man feels he is about to ejaculate.

Terms

V\|w

premature ejaculation Involuntary orgasm before or shortly after the penis enters the vagina or anus; ejaculation that takes place sooner than desired.

retarded ejaculation The inability to ejaculate when one wishes to during intercourse.

vaginismus Painful, involuntary muscular contractions in the vagina that occur when sexual intercourse is attempted.

orgasmic dysfunction The inability to experience orgasm.

masturbation Self-stimulation for the purpose of sexual arousal and orgasm.

gender identity A person's personal, internal sense of maleness or femaleness.

Women who seek treatment for orgasmic dysfunction often have not had the chance to learn through trial and error what types of stimulation will excite them and bring them to orgasm. Most sex therapists prefer to treat this problem with **masturbation** (genital self-stimulation). Women are taught about their own anatomy and sexual responses and then are encouraged to experiment with masturbation until they experience orgasm. Once they can masturbate to orgasm, they can transfer this learning to sexual intercourse with a partner. Substances being tested for the treatment of female sexual dysfunction include prostaglandin creams and testosterone patches. Another option is a device recently approved by the FDA that creates suction over the clitoris in order to increase blood flow and sensation.

Sexual problems are closely tied to emotional and psychological concerns and to a person's perceptions, beliefs, thoughts, values, and relationships with others.

SEXUAL BEHAVIOR

Many behaviors stem from sexual impulses, and sexual expression takes a variety of forms. Probably the most basic aspect of sexuality is reproduction, the process of producing offspring. As important as reproduction is, the intention of creating a child accounts for only a small measure of sexual activity; most people have sex for other reasons as well.

Sexual excitement and satisfaction are aspects of sexual behavior separate from reproduction. The intensely pleasurable sensations of arousal and orgasm are probably the strongest motivators for human sexual behavior. People are infinitely varied in the ways they seek to experience erotic pleasure. In this section, we examine how sexual behavior develops and take a closer look at different sexual behaviors.

The Development of Sexual Behavior

Sexual behavior is a product of many factors, including genetics, physiology, psychology, and social and cultural influences. Our behavior is shaped by the interplay of our biological predispositions and our learning experiences throughout life.

Gender Roles and Gender Identity
The term *gender* is usually used to refer to the state of being male or female; people often use the word *sex* to mean the same thing. Strictly speaking, *sex* refers only to being biologically male or female, while *gender* encompasses both your biological sex and your masculine or feminine behaviors. As mentioned in Chapter 4, your gender role is everything you do in your daily life that expresses your maleness or femaleness to others, including dress, speech patterns, and mannerisms. Your **gender identity** is your personal, inner sense of being male or female.

Biological sex, gender role, and gender identity are usually in agreement, but some people experience conflict among them. For example, a male who feels trapped in the body of a male and who wants to be a female may exhibit the gender role of a male, but his gender identity is that of a female. The umbrella term *transgender* is often used to describe any individual whose appearance, personal characteristics, or behavior differs from the social and cultural norms for males and females. Transgendered individuals include the following:

- Transsexual men and women, who feel their biological sex does not match their gender identity. Transsexuals may seek sex reassignment, which involves surgery to change the appearance of the genitals and hormonal treatments to induce secondary sex characteristics such as breasts or facial hair.

- Transvestites, who enjoy wearing clothing identified with the other gender. Cross-dressing covers a broad range of behaviors, from wearing one article of clothing of the other sex in a private location to wearing an entire outfit in public.

- Intersexed individuals, who were born with ambiguous genitals—neither fully female nor fully male—due to genetic or hormonal abnormalities. Intersexed individuals may or may not have undergone surgery as infants to assign them to a particular sex.

- Men or women, regardless of sexual orientation, whose appearance, characteristics, or behavior is perceived as gender-atypical in their society or culture.

BIOLOGICAL AND CULTURAL INFLUENCES Some gender characteristics are determined biologically, such as the genitals a person is born with and the secondary sex characteristics that develop at puberty. Others are defined by society and learned in the course of growing up. From birth, children are encouraged to behave in ways their culture deems appropriate for one sex or the other. In our society, parents usually give children gender-specific names, clothes, and toys, and children may model their own behavior after their same-sex parent. People are far more likely to tell a boy why the car is accelerating and a girl why the cookies aren't chewy. Family and friends create an environment that teaches the child how to act appropriately as a girl or a boy. Teachers, television, books, and even strangers model these gender roles.

Gender roles vary from one society to another and from one time to another. In the United States today, for example, many women shave their legs and wear makeup; in Muslim countries, women wear robes and veils that conceal their face and body. Each set of behaviors expresses some learned aspect of the female gender role in that society, and each set would be inappropriate in the other society. Standards of sexual attractiveness also vary from one culture to another.

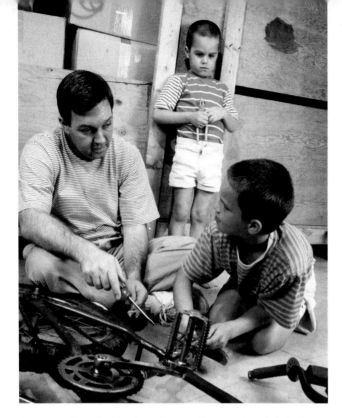

Our sense of gender identity and many of our gender-role behaviors are overwhelmingly influenced by cultural factors. This young boy is learning gender-specific behaviors by imitating his father.

An extreme example of how cultural traditions can affect gender roles and sexual activity is female genital mutilation, a procedure often called "female circumcision." In over 20 African countries, some parts of Asia and the Middle East, and immigrant communities elsewhere, female infants, children, or young women may undergo a procedure in which parts of the clitoris and labia are removed. In some procedures, only the hood of the clitoris is removed. In others, the entire clitoris, the labia minora, and parts of the labia majora are removed. The sides of the labia majora may be sewn together, leaving only a small opening for the passage of urine and menstrual blood. The effects of these painful procedures can include bleeding, infection, the inability to enjoy sex, and infertility.

The practice probably developed as a way of controlling women's sexuality and ensuring that a woman would be a virgin at the time of marriage. Upon marriage, the husband reopens the labia to allow intercourse and childbirth. It is interesting to note that surgery to remove all or part of the clitoris was practiced by physicians in the nineteenth century in both England and the United States, primarily as a "cure" for masturbation.

Many countries, including the United Kingdom, Sweden, and Belgium, now have laws against female genital mutilation, and the World Health Organization and other groups are trying to educate people about the negative medical consequences of the procedures.

GENDER-ROLE FLEXIBILITY Historically, gender roles have tended to highlight and emphasize the differences between males and females, but new gender roles are emerging in our society that reflect more of a mix of male and female characteristics and behaviors. This tendency toward *androgyny* greatly broadens the range of experiences available to both males and females. Androgynous adults are less stereotyped in their thinking; in how they look, dress, and act; in how they divide work in the home; in how they think about jobs and careers; and in how they express themselves sexually. Women in our society today are able, and even expected, to be much more assertive, competitive, ambitious, and powerful than they were allowed to be in the past; likewise, men can be more sensitive, articulate, nurturing, and emotionally expressive.

Gender, Sexuality, and the Mass Media Many of our ideas about sexuality and gender roles are shaped by the mass media. Television, movies, music, magazines, and advertisements are awash with sexual images. These images are usually of young, sexy people promising passionately fulfilling relationships. Women and men are often portrayed in traditional gender roles, with provocatively dressed women in need of protection interacting with aggressive and muscular men.

Media images of sexuality are often more influential than the family in shaping the sexual attitudes and behaviors of adolescents and college students. Yet these images are usually unrealistic and help perpetuate stereotypes of women and men in our society. The mass media rarely portray people negotiating safer sex or communicating seriously about other sexual issues.

Childhood Sexual Behavior The capacity to respond sexually is present at birth. Ultrasound studies suggest that boys experience erections in the uterus. After birth, both sexes have the capacity for orgasm, though many babies may not experience it. As people grow, many discover this capacity through self-exploration. Sexual behaviors gradually emerge in childhood; self-exploration and touching the genitals are common forms of play, observed among infants as young as 6 months. They gradually lead to more deliberate forms of masturbation, with or without orgasm.

Children often engage in sexual play with playmates by exploring each other's genitals. These activities are often part of games like "playing house" or "playing doctor." By age 12, 40% of boys have engaged in sex play; the peak exploration age for girls is 9, by which time 14% have had such experiences.

Adolescent Sexuality A person who has experienced puberty is biologically an adult. But in psychological and social terms, people take 5–10 more years to attain full adult status. This discrepancy between biological and social maturity creates considerable confusion

Mind/Body/Spirit

Sexual Decision Making

Choosing to have sex can change a relationship as well as an individual's life. In making decisions about sexual activity, you owe it to yourself and your partner to think and talk honestly about your choices. Consider the following issues:

- *Your background, beliefs, and goals.* What are your religious, moral, and/or personal values regarding relationships and sex? What are your priorities at this time, and how will a sexual relationship fit into your goals and plans for the future? Are you physically, emotionally, and financially ready to accept the potential consequences of the choices you make? How will you feel if you act in ways that are not consistent with your values and goals?

- *Your relationship with your partner.* How do you feel about your partner and your relationship? Do you respect and trust each other? Do you feel comfortable talking about sexual issues, and have you discussed contraception, pregnancy, and safer sex? How do you think having sex will affect your relationship and how you feel about yourself and your partner? What does having sex mean to each of you?

- *Your reasons for having sex.* Are you feeling pressured to have sex? Are you afraid of losing your partner if you say no? Are you too embarrassed, shy, or insecure to say no or discuss waiting? Are you being honest with yourself and your partner about your reasons for moving into a sexual relationship?

Personal decisions about sex should always be respected. You have the right to make your own choices and to do only what you feel comfortable with. When you make choices about sex based on self-respect, along with physical, emotional, and spiritual considerations, you'll be more likely to feel good about your decisions—now and in the future—and to enhance your health and well-being.

---

over what constitutes appropriate sexual behavior during adolescence.

Sexual fantasies and dreams become more common and explicit in adolescence than at earlier ages, often as an accompaniment to masturbation. Research has shown that about 80% of teenage boys and 55% of teenage girls masturbate more or less regularly. Once puberty is reached, orgasm in boys is accompanied by ejaculation. Teenage boys also experience **nocturnal emissions** ("wet dreams"). Some girls also have orgasmic dreams. In general, masturbation does not carry the social stigma and imagined perils of former times, but adolescents—and many adults as well—are often still embarrassed by it.

Sexual interaction during adolescence usually takes place between peers in the context of dating. Sexual intimacy is usually expressed in such relationships through petting and necking, which may involve kissing, caressing, and stimulating the breasts and genitals. These activities lead to arousal but may not culminate in orgasm.

Many American teenagers also engage in premarital sexual relations. Recent surveys indicate that the average age of first sexual intercourse is about 17.2 years for girls and 16.6 years for boys; among high school seniors, about 60% report that they have had sexual intercourse. Rates for premarital sex vary considerably from one group to another, however, based on ethnic, educational, socioeconomic, religious, geographic, and other factors. Engaging in sexual intercourse for the first time is affected by these same factors, plus psychological readiness, fear of consequences, being in love, going steady, peer pressure, and the need to act like an adult, gain popularity, or rebel. Some people thoughtfully weigh decisions, and others plunge recklessly. A mother's relationship with her daughter has been shown to influence the timing of first intercourse. Girls who perceive that their mother disapproves of their having sex are more likely to delay first intercourse.

Adolescent sexual behaviors are not confined to heterosexual relationships. Beginning in childhood, sex play involves members of one's own sex as well as of the other sex. Homosexual attractions, with or without sexual encounters, are likewise common in adolescence. For many these are youthful experiments and don't mean that participants will ultimately be homosexual. For a minority they may be a factor in adult sexual orientation. Most adult gay men and women trace their preferences to their early years.

Adult Sexuality Early adulthood is a time when people make important life choices—a time of increasing responsibility in terms of interpersonal relationships and family life (see the box "Sexual Decision Making"). In recent years, both in the United States and abroad, there has been a definite trend toward marriage at a later age than in past decades. And before marriage, more young adults are driven by an internal need to become sexually knowledgeable. Today, more people in their twenties believe that becoming sexually experienced rather than preserving virginity is an important prelude to selecting a mate. Take the quiz in the box "Your Sexual Attitudes" on page 140 to explore your own beliefs and opinions about sex.

Term	
nocturnal emissions Orgasm and ejaculation (wet dream) during sleep.	

Assess Yourself

For each statement, circle the response that most closely reflects your position.

	Agree	Not Sure	Disagree
1. Sex education encourages young people to have sex.	1	2	3
2. Homosexuality is a healthy, normal expression of sexuality.	3	2	1
3. Members of the other sex will think more highly of you if you remain mysterious.	1	2	3
4. It's better to wait until marriage to have sex.	1	2	3
5. Abortion should be a personal, private choice for a woman.	3	2	1
6. It's natural for men to have more sexual freedom than women do.	1	2	3
7. Condoms should not be made available to teenagers.	1	2	3
8. Access to pornography should not be restricted for adults.	3	2	1
9. A woman who is raped usually does something to provoke it.	1	2	3
10. Contraception is the woman's responsibility.	1	2	3
11. Feminism has had a positive influence on society.	3	2	1
12. Masturbation is a healthy expression of sexuality.	3	2	1
13. I have many friends of the other sex.	3	2	1
14. Prostitution should be legalized.	3	2	1
15. Women use sex for love; men use love for sex.	1	2	3
16. Our society is too sexually permissive.	1	2	3
17. The man should be the undisputed head of the household.	1	2	3
18. Having sex just for pleasure is OK.	3	2	1

Scoring

Add up the numbers you circled to obtain your overall score.

1–18   Traditional attitude about sexuality

19–36   Ambivalent or mixed attitude about sexuality

37–54   Open, progressive attitude about sexuality

A survey investigating women's and men's motivations for engaging in sexual activities found that motivations change with age (Figure 5-5). Younger men state that they engage in sex for physical reasons, whereas women of the same age state that they engage in sex for emotional reasons. As men and women get older, their motives change; men more often engage in sex for emotional reasons, and women more often for physical reasons. In the oldest age groups, women's and men's motives for sex are actually the reverse of those of the earliest age groups. In addition to age, factors such as ethnicity, educational attainment, and living arrangements also influence adult choices about sexuality; see the box "Are There Ethnic Differences in Sexual Decision Making and Behavior?" on page 142.

Adult sexuality can include any of the sexual behaviors and practices described in this chapter. In mature love relationships, people ideally can integrate all the aspects of intimacy—physical, sexual, emotional—so that sexuality is a deeply meaningful part of how they express love.

Sexuality in Illness and Disability   Any disease or disability that affects mobility, well-being, self-esteem, or body image has the potential to affect sexual expression. People with chronic diseases or disabilities often have special needs regarding their sexual behavior. They must also confront widespread myths that they are asexual. In our culture, only people conforming to a narrow standard of youth, attractiveness, and ability are seen as sexual beings. But sexuality is integral to all of us, regardless of our physical status.

The diagnosis of a chronic illness or the onset of a disability usually requires major adjustments in many areas of life, including sexuality. At first, sexual activity may take a low priority because of fear and the loss of self-esteem. Individuals and couples can learn to become creative about sexual expression and develop new approaches based on the limitations of the disability. Developing a positive body image is often a particularly important, and difficult, adjustment for people with physical illness or limitations.

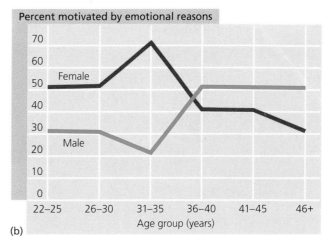

Figure 5-5   Motivations for engaging in sex by age and gender. (a) The physical motive. (b) The emotional motive.   SOURCES: Data from Laumann, E., et al. 1994. *The Social Organization of Sexuality: Sexual Practices in the United States.* Chicago: University of Chicago Press; Sprague, J., and D. Quadagno. 1989. Gender and sexual motivation. *Journal of Psychology and Human Sexuality* 2: 57–76.

Sexual Orientation

As discussed in Chapter 4, sexual orientation is a consistent pattern of emotional and sexual attraction based on biological sex. It exists along a continuum that ranges from exclusive heterosexuality (attraction to people of the other sex) through bisexuality (attraction to people of both sexes) to exclusive homosexuality (attraction to people of one's own sex). The terms *straight* and *gay* are often used to refer to heterosexuals and homosexuals, respectively, and female homosexuals are also referred to as lesbians.

Sexual orientation involves feelings and self-concept, and individuals may or may not express their sexual orientation in their behavior. In national surveys, about 2–6% of men identify themselves as homosexuals and about 1.5% of women identify themselves as lesbians. It is difficult to gauge the accuracy of these estimates because people may not tell the truth in surveys that probe very sensitive and private aspects of their lives.

Heterosexuality   The great majority of people are heterosexual. The heterosexual lifestyle usually includes all the behavior and relationship patterns described in Chapter 4: dating, engagement and/or living together, and marriage.

Homosexuality   Homosexuality exists in almost all cultures. Many homosexual couples form long-lasting close and stable ties. The lifestyle of homosexual people depends largely on whether they are open about their sexual orientation. Those who feel forced to be secretive may lead a double life, one public and one private. Those who have come out participate more actively in gay activities and organizations.

Some people are threatened or upset by homosexuality, perhaps because homosexuals are viewed as different or because no one is sure how sexual orientation develops.

The "gay liberation" movement of the 1970s and 1980s helped dispel some of the historical prejudice against gays and lesbians, but homosexuality still has not received widespread societal approval. In extreme cases, irrational fear or hatred of homosexuals—known as **homophobia**—causes people to discriminate against or even attack homosexuals.

The major difference between heterosexuals and homosexuals is in their choice of sex partners. Homosexual individuals are as varied and different from one another as are heterosexuals. Just like heterosexuals, lesbians and gay men may be in long-term, committed relationships or they may date different people. They have the same responsibilities and concerns as anyone else. They have job commitments, they raise children, and they seek to fulfill their potential in all areas of their lives. For homosexuals, bisexuals, and heterosexuals, sexual expression is but one facet of human experience.

Bisexuality   Some bisexual individuals are involved with partners of both sexes at the same time, whereas others may alternate between same-sex partners and partners of the other sex ("serial bisexuality"). HIV infection is a risk associated with bisexuality, particularly in cases where bisexual men don't disclose their sexual orientation to their female partners. The largest group of bisexuals are married men who have secret sexual involvements with men but who rarely have female sexual contacts outside marriage.

The Origins of Sexual Orientation   Many theories have been proposed to account for the development

Term

homophobia   Fear or hatred of homosexuals.

Dimensions of Diversity

Are There Ethnic Differences in Sexual Decision Making and Behavior?

What are some of the key influences on sexual behavior? Are there any trends related to ethnicity? In general, researchers have found that ethnicity contributes to differences in sexual behaviors—but that other variables are equally important. Thus, it is important to examine all the variables that might influence sexual behavior, including age, income, educational attainment, and living arrangements.

In a study comparing low-income women from different groups, there was one area in which ethnicity appeared to have an influence independent of other factors. When the women were asked who makes the decision about the timing and type of sexual activity, 80% of Latinas stated it was a mutual decision with their partner. White women were also likely to report mutual decision making (64%). African American women were less likely to report a mutual decision (47%) but more likely to report that they made the decision themselves (31%). Only 6% of Latinas and 13% of white women

reported that they made the decision as to the timing and type of sexual activity with their partners.

A mix of sexual behaviors was identified. Vaginal intercourse was the most common behavior among all the participants in the study, followed by oral sex and then anal sex. African American women were less likely to engage in oral sex (26%) compared with white women (58%) and Latinas (56%). Among women with high educational attainment, rates of oral sex went up for white women and down for African American women. Rates of oral sex were also lower for older African American women and Latinas.

African American women in the survey reported more sexual partners in the past 6 months compared with white women and Latinas. However, women of all ethnicities who were not living with a partner were more likely to report multiple sexual partners, and fewer African American women in this study were living with a partner. Thus, living arrangement was a

more important factor than ethnicity in influencing the number of sexual partners.

Ethnic differences also exist in sexual issues among college students. A recent study found that African American and Latino students reported higher levels of unwanted noncondom use compared with white students. Unwanted noncondom use refers to a situation in which an individual intends to use condoms with her or his partner but then does not because of the influence of the partner. These findings warrant further study because African Americans and Latinos are disproportionately represented among new cases of HIV infection in the United States.

SOURCES: Smith, L. 2003. Partner influence on noncondom use: Gender and ethnic differences. *Journal of Sex Research* 40(4): 346–350; Quadagno, D., et al. 1998. Ethnic differences in sexual decisions and sexual behaviors. *Archive of Sexual Behavior* 27(1): 57–75; Bogart, L., H. Cecil, and S. Pinkerton. 2000. Hispanic adults' beliefs, attitudes and intentions regarding the female condom. *Journal of Behavioral Medicine* 23(2): 181–206.

of sexual orientation. Biological theories have focused on genetic and hormonal influences. One study found structural differences between homosexual and heterosexual men in the brain region that controls sexual behavior. It remains unclear, however, whether this anatomical variation represents a cause or a result of sexual orientation. Another possible influence is differing levels of prenatal hormones, which may affect fetal brain development.

Evidence for a genetic basis for sexual orientation was provided by a recent study of 108 sets of female twins in which at least one twin was a lesbian. Researchers found that among the identical twins, both twins were lesbians in 48% of the cases; among nonidentical twins, both twins were lesbians in 16% of the cases. Among adopted girls with a lesbian sister, only 6% of the adoptive siblings were homosexual. Although these results may suggest a genetic component to sexual orientation, other influences must also operate because not all identical twins share the same orientation. There is no evidence that sexual orientation is determined solely by biological or genetic factors.

Many psychological theories have also been proposed. Researchers have looked at how much contact children have with members of the two sexes, at the types of relationships children have with their parents, and at family dynamics. Early negative experiences with heterosexuality or positive experiences with homosexuality have also been proposed as possible influences. The significant

growth of single-parent families over the past 40 years has not been accompanied by large shifts in sexual orientation among Americans, so it is unlikely that family dynamics or early learning experiences are strong factors in determining sexual orientation.

Most scientists today agree that sexual orientation is most likely the result of the complex interaction of biological, psychological, and social factors, possibly different in the case of each individual.

Varieties of Human Sexual Behavior

Most people express their sexuality in a variety of ways. Some sexual behaviors are aimed at self-stimulation only, such as masturbation, whereas other practices involve interaction with others in behaviors such as kissing and intercourse. Some people choose not to express their sexuality and practice celibacy instead.

Celibacy Continuous abstention from sexual activities, termed **celibacy,** can be a conscious and deliberate choice, or it can be necessitated by circumstances. Health considerations and religious and moral beliefs may lead some people to celibacy, particularly until marriage or until an acceptable partner appears. A disadvantage of the celibate life is that it may lack physical contact and affection.

Human sexuality is not just a matter of bodies responding to each other. This couple's physical experiences together will be powerfully affected by their emotions, ideas, and values and by the quality of their relationship.

tioned earlier, some body areas, the erogenous zones, are much more sensitive to touch as a sexual stimulus than others. Touching can convey a variety of messages, including affection, comfort, and a desire for further sexual contact.

During arousal, many men and women manually and orally stimulate each other by touching, stroking, and caressing their partner's genitals. Men and women vary greatly in their preferences for the type, pacing, and vigor of such **foreplay.** Working out the details to accommodate each other's pleasure is a key to enjoying these activities. Direct communication about preferences can enhance sexual pleasure and protect both partners from physical and psychological discomfort.

Oral-Genital Stimulation   Cunnilingus (the stimulation of the female genitals with the lips and tongue) and **fellatio** (the stimulation of the penis with the mouth) are quite common practices. Although prevalence varies in different populations, 70–90% of men and women report that they have engaged in oral sex. Oral sex may be practiced either as part of foreplay or as a sex act culminating in orgasm. Like all acts of sexual expression between two people, oral sex requires the cooperation and consent of both partners. If they disagree about its acceptability, they need to discuss their feelings and try to reach a mutually pleasing solution.

Anal Intercourse   About 10% of heterosexuals and 50% of homosexual males regularly practice anal stimulation and penetration by the penis or a finger. The receiver does not usually reach orgasm from anal intercourse, though men usually experience orgasm while penetrating. Many people have strongly negative attitudes toward anal sex because they consider it unclean, unnatural, or unappealing. Because the anus is composed of delicate tissues that tear easily under such pressure, anal intercourse is one of the riskiest of sexual behaviors associated with the transmission of HIV and the bacteria that cause gonorrhea and syphilis. The use of condoms is highly recommended for anyone engaging in anal sex. Special care and precaution should be exercised if anal sex is practiced—cleanliness, lubrication, and gentle entry at the very least. Anything that is inserted into the anus should not subsequently be put into the vagina unless it has been thoroughly washed. Bacteria normally present in the anus can cause vaginal infections.

Many people use the related term *abstinence* to refer to avoidance of just one sexual activity—intercourse. The use of abstinence to prevent pregnancy and sexually transmitted diseases is discussed in Chapters 6 and 18.

Autoeroticism and Masturbation   The most common form of **autoeroticism** is **erotic fantasy,** creating imaginary experiences that range from fleeting thoughts to elaborate scenarios. Fantasies may be replays of past sexual experiences or fabrications based on unfulfilled wishes or taken from books, drawings, or photographs.

Masturbation involves manually stimulating the genitals, rubbing them against objects (such as a pillow), or using stimulating devices such as vibrators. Although commonly associated with adolescence, masturbation is practiced by many throughout adult life. It may be used as a substitute for sexual intercourse or as part of sexual activity with a partner. Masturbation gives a person control over the pace, time, and method of sexual release and pleasure. On average, two out of three college students masturbate a few times a week, others do it more or less frequently, and some don't do it at all.

Touching and Foreplay   Tactile stimulation, or touching, is integral to sexual experiences, whether in the form of massage, kissing, fondling, or holding. Our entire body surface is a sensory organ, and touching almost anywhere can enhance intimacy and sexual arousal. As men-

Terms

Vw

celibacy Continuous abstention from sexual activity.

autoeroticism Behavior aimed at sexual self-stimulation.

erotic fantasy Sexually arousing thoughts and daydreams.

foreplay Kissing, touching, and any form of oral or genital contact that stimulates people toward intercourse.

cunnilingus Oral stimulation of the female genitals.

fellatio Oral stimulation of the penis.

Sexual Intercourse For most adults, most of the time, **sexual intercourse** is the ultimate sexual experience. Men and women engage in coitus—make love—to fulfill both sexual and psychological needs. The most common heterosexual practice is the man inserting his erect penis into the woman's dilated and lubricated vagina after sufficient arousal.

Much has been written on how to enhance pleasure through various coital techniques, positions, and practices. For a woman, the key factor in physical readiness for coitus is adequate vaginal lubrication, and in psychological readiness, being aroused and receptive. For a man, the setting and the partner must arouse him to attain and maintain an erection. Personal preferences vary, but most people prefer a safe, private setting. Candlelight and music, for example, can enhance the mood of the occasion. Psychological factors and the quality of the relationship are more important to overall sexual satisfaction than sophisticated or exotic sexual techniques.

Atypical and Problematic Sexual Behaviors

In American culture, many kinds of sexual behavior are accepted. However, some types of sexual expression are considered harmful; they may be against the law or classified as mental disorders, or both. Because sexual behavior occurs on a continuum, it is sometimes difficult to differentiate a behavior that is simply atypical from one that is harmful. When attempting to evaluate an unusual sexual behavior, experts consider the issues of consent between partners and whether physical or psychological harm is done to the individual or to others.

Sexual fantasies and behaviors that are consensual—agreed on by adult partners—but that are not statistically typical of American sexual behaviors are known as **atypical sexual behaviors.** An example of an atypical sexual behavior is the consensual use of sex toys. Behaviors classified as mental disorders, or **paraphilias,** are characterized by recurring, intense sexual fantasies and urges that involve nonhuman objects, the suffering or humiliation of oneself or one's partner, or children or other nonconsenting individuals. Examples are peeping into strangers' homes, making obscene phone calls, and having sexual contact with children. The effects of paraphilic behavior on others range from minor upset to serious physical and long-term psychological harm.

The use of force and coercion in sexual relationships is one of the most serious problems in human interactions. The most extreme manifestation of **sexual coercion**—forcing a person to submit to another's sexual desires—is rape, but sexual coercion occurs in many subtler forms, such as sexual harassment. Sexual coercion—including rape, the sexual abuse of children, and sexual harassment—is discussed in detail in Chapter 23.

Commercial Sex

Conflicting feelings about sexuality are apparent in the attitudes of Americans toward commercial sex: prostitution and sexually oriented materials such as videos, magazines, and books. Our society condemns sexually explicit material and prostitution, but it also provides their customers.

Pornography Derived from the Greek word meaning "the writing of prostitutes," **pornography** is now often defined as obscene literature, art, or movies. A major problem in identifying pornographic material is that different people and communities have different opinions about what is obscene. Differing definitions of obscenity have led to many legal battles over potentially pornographic materials. Currently, the sale and rental of pornographic materials is restricted so that only adults can legally obtain them; materials depicting children in sexual contexts are illegal in any format or setting.

The appearance of thousands of sexually oriented Web sites has expanded the number of people with access to pornographic materials and has made enforcing pornography laws more difficult. People who might have hesitated to buy magazines or rent videos in person can now access sexually explicit material privately and anonymously (see the box "Cybersex"). Of special concern is the increased availability of illegal materials, such as child pornography, that previously could be acquired only with great difficulty and at great legal risk. Web sites that sell pornography take in more than $1 billion each year, and there are many online newsgroups where visitors exchange materials for free. Adult Web sites typically have the warning "You must be 18 to enter," but these warnings are not effective if users can simply click a button to verify their age. More effective are screening software programs that can be installed on individual computers; these programs block access to adults-only Web sites and newsgroups. Other strategies to keep minors from accessing pornography online include subscription-based adult verification services and credit card requirements.

Terms

Vw

sexual intercourse Sexual relations involving genital union; also called *coitus,* and also known as making love.

atypical sexual behavior Consensual sexual behavior that is not statistically typical within a population.

paraphilia A mental disorder characterized by recurring, intense sexual fantasies and urges that involve nonhuman objects, the suffering or humiliation of oneself or one's partner, or children or other nonconsenting individuals.

sexual coercion The use of physical or psychological force or intimidation to make a person submit to sexual demands.

pornography The explicit or obscene depiction of sexual activities in pictures, writing, or other material.

prostitution The exchange of sexual services for money.

About 15% of all Internet users report visiting sexual Internet sites, and sex is the most frequently searched-for topic. Most sexual sites feature pornographic images and/or sexually oriented chat rooms. A survey of nearly 10,000 users of sexual Internet sites found that about the same number of men and women visit sexual sites; men are more likely to visit sites with visual images, while women are more likely to visit chat rooms. People in chat rooms may engage in a range of behaviors, from mild flirtation with a group of chatroom visitors to private, real-time discussions of explicit sexual activities with another Internet user.

Cybersex or "virtual sex" can be defined as erotic interaction between individuals whose bodies never come in contact with each other. This is the type of "sex" that occurs in cyberspace, the space provided by human communication where the body is absent. Many cybersex participants report feeling some degree of sexual excitement; some masturbate while viewing erotic images online or engaging in sexual chat. Typical reasons given by cybersex users are that it allows them to break away from daily routines, explore fantasies, relieve stress, and spice up their sex life. In cyberspace we can make ourselves glamorous, beautiful or handsome, rich, educated individuals with a full social life. It is a fantasy world that anyone with a computer can enter.

Research into cybersex has identified some potential benefits of easily available online sexual material. The anonymous nature of the Internet gives people a sense of freedom and allows them to try out different identities and to seek sexual fulfillment in ways that they would not feel comfortable with in real life. They may feel freer to talk openly about their sexual concerns or fantasies. A great deal of factual information about sexual behavior, contraception, and STDs is available for people who might not otherwise access such information; sexually oriented products such as condoms are also easily obtainable. Online sexual information may facilitate candid discussions between partners. In addition, the Internet provides opportunities for social contact and support among people with special concerns who might otherwise feel isolated.

However, cybersex can cause problems for some people. Surveys indicate that about 5–8% of people who use the Internet for sex spend more than 11 hours per week online, with some people spending more than 50 hours per week online for sexual pursuits. This group is much more likely to report problems with work or interpersonal relationships than are people who spend lesser amounts of time online (see Chapter 9 for more on compulsive and addictive behaviors). For people who already feel isolated and lonely, cybersex may increase their social isolation as they spend more time online and less time reaching out to others in person. Online sexual encounters may offer the illusion of intimacy, but they do not have all the complexities or all the benefits of long-term, real-world intimate relationships. Online behaviors that are thought to have the potential to become excessive, addictive, obsessive, and/or compulsive include using online pornography for masturbation, engaging in online relationships, and using the Internet for sexually related crimes such as harassment or cyberstalking.

For people involved in committed relationships, cybersex may be viewed as emotional infidelity and a threat to the relationship. People are likely to feel betrayed if they discover their partner has secretly been investing time and energy in online sexual interaction with others. In addition, the availability of certain types of sexual materials may reinforce abusive or problematic behaviors. For example, people have used the Internet to obtain child pornography and to contact young people and solicit meetings.

As described in Chapter 4, some people use the Internet to look for intimate partners whom they can meet face-to-face. Although online interaction has some special advantages for meeting people, including the opportunity to focus on interests and values before physical appearance, there are also potential dangers. Refer to Chapter 4 for more on the potential benefits and costs of looking for intimate partnerships online.

SOURCES: Whitty, M. 2003. Cyberflirting: Playing at love on the Internet. *Theory and Psychology* 13(3): 339–357; Goodson, P., D. McCormick, and A. Evans. 2001. Searching for sexually explicit materials on the Internet: An exploratory study of college students' behaviors and attitudes. *Archives of Sexual Behavior* 30(2): 101–118; Griffiths, M. 2001. Sex on the Internet: Observations and implications for Internet sex addiction. *Journal of Sex Research* 38: 333–342; *Sexual Addiction and Compulsivity.* 2000. Volume 7 (issue devoted to the topic of sex on the Internet).

Many people distinguish between "soft porn" and "hard porn" materials. Soft porn, often marketed for couples, typically includes an apparently loving couple having sex in a relaxed setting. There is mutual kissing and touching, and both partners are shown as having a positive experience. In hard porn, there is usually little mutual touching, and only the male appears to enjoy the experience. Hard porn sometimes explicitly depicts sexual violence and exploitation. Hard porn materials tend to be the focus of more criticism than soft porn materials.

Much of the debate about pornography focuses on whether it is harmful. Some people argue that adults who want to view pornographic materials in the privacy of their own homes should be allowed to do so. Others feel that the exposure to explicit sexual material can lead to delinquent or criminal behavior, such as rape or the sexual abuse of children. Currently, there is no reliable evidence that pornography by itself leads to violence or paraphilic behavior, and debate is likely to continue.

Prostitution   The exchange of sexual services for money is **prostitution**. Prostitutes may be men, women, or children, and the buyer of a prostitute's services is nearly always a man. Except in parts of Nevada, prostitution is illegal in the United States.

Sex with a prostitute provides the customer with sexual release without commitment, the expectation of intimacy, or fear of rejection. Some men patronize prostitutes

Take Charge

To talk with your partner about sexuality, follow the general suggestions for effective communication given in Chapter 4. Getting started may be the most difficult part. Some people feel more comfortable if they begin by talking about talking—that is, initiating a discussion about why people are so uncomfortable talking about sexuality. Talking about sexual histories—how partners first learned about sex or how family and cultural background influenced sexual values and attitudes—is another way to get started. Reading about sex can also be a good beginning: Partners can read an article or book and then discuss their reactions.

Be honest about what you feel and what you want from your partner. Cultural and personal obstacles to discussing sexual subjects can be difficult to overcome, but self-disclosure is important for successful relationships. Research indicates that when one partner openly discusses attitudes and feelings, the other partner is more likely to do the same. If your partner seems hesitant to open up, try asking open-ended or either/or questions: "Where do you like to be touched?" or "Would you like to talk about this now or wait until later?"

If something is bothering you about your sexual relationship, choose a good time to initiate a discussion with your partner. Be specific and direct but also tactful. Focus on what you actually observe, rather than on what you think the behavior means.

"You didn't touch or hug me when your friends were around" is an observation. "You're ashamed of me around your friends" is an inference about your partner's feelings. Try focusing on a specific behavior that concerns you rather than on the person as a whole—your partner can change behaviors but not his or her entire personality. For example, you could say "I'd like you to take a few minutes away from studying to kiss me" instead of "You're so caught up in your work, you never have time for me."

If you are going to make a statement that your partner may interpret as criticism, try mixing it with something positive: "I love spending time with you, but I feel annoyed when you. . . ." Similarly, if your partner says something that upsets you, don't lash back. An aggressive response may make you feel better in the short run, but it will not help the communication process or the quality of the relationship.

If you want to say no to some sexual activity, say no unequivocally. Don't send mixed messages. If you are afraid of hurting your partner's feelings, offer an alternative if it's appropriate: "I am uncomfortable with that. How about . . .?"

If you're in love, you may think that the sexual aspects of a relationship will work out magically without discussion. However, partners who never talk about sex deny themselves the opportunity to increase their closeness and improve their relationship.

---

to have sex with a different type of partner than usual or to engage in a type of sex their usual partner will not permit. Most customers are white, middle-class, middle-aged, and married. Although they come from a wide variety of backgrounds, prostitutes are usually motivated to join the profession because of money.

AIDS is a major concern for prostitutes and their customers. Many prostitutes are injecting drug users or are involved with men who are. The rate of HIV infection among prostitutes varies widely, but in some parts of the country it is as high as 25–50%.

Responsible Sexual Behavior

Healthy sexuality is an important part of adult life. It can be a source of pleasurable experiences and emotions and an important part of intimate partnerships. But sexual behavior also carries many responsibilities, and you need to make choices about your sexuality that contribute to your well-being and that of your partner.

Open, Honest Communication Each partner needs to clearly indicate what sexual involvement means to him or her. Does it mean love, fun, a permanent commitment, or something else? The intentions of both partners should be clear. For strategies on how to talk about sexual issues with your partner, refer to the box "Communicating About Sexuality."

Agreed-On Sexual Activities No one should pressure or coerce a partner. Sexual behaviors should be consistent with the sexual values, preferences, and comfort level of both partners. Everyone has the right to refuse sexual activity at any time.

Sexual Privacy Intimate relationships involving sexual activity are based on trust, and that trust can be violated if partners reveal private information about the relationship to others. Sexual privacy also involves respecting other people—not engaging in activities in the presence of others that would make them uncomfortable. The question of how to handle bringing a partner back to a shared dorm room is something that many college students must address. Roommates should be respectful of one another and discuss the situation in advance to avoid embarrassing encounters.

Using Contraception If pregnancy is not desired, contraception should be used during sexual intercourse. Both partners need to take responsibility for protecting against unwanted pregnancy. Partners should discuss contraception before sexual involvement begins. (See Chapter 6 for more information on contraception.)

Safer Sex Both partners should be aware of and practice safer sex to guard against sexually transmitted diseases (STDs). The U.S. Surgeon General stated in his

Sexual activity has many potential consequences, including pregnancy, disease, and emotional changes in the relationship. Responsible sexual behavior includes discussing these consequences openly and honestly.

Wellness includes understanding and enjoying your own sexuality. This means understanding your sexual anatomy, physiology, and functioning; your sexual orientation; and the various ways of expressing your sexuality and of interacting sexually with others. A healthy sexual life is built on acceptance of yourself and good communication with your partner.

Right now you can

• Make a decision to deal with any sexual question or problem that you've been avoiding. Unless you're sure it's not a physical problem, begin by making an appointment with your physician.

• Take a few moments to reflect on and articulate to yourself exactly what your beliefs are about sexual relationships at this point in your life. Consider your values, emotions, plans, and resources; also consider whether you are acting in accordance with your beliefs.

• If you are in a sexual relationship, think about how you and your partner communicate about sex. If there's something you want to discuss, plan how you will broach the subject. Refer to the box "Communicating About Sexuality" for ideas on how to begin.

• If you are in a sexual relationship, ask yourself whether you are acting responsibly and in the best interest of yourself and your partner 100% of the time. For example, do you always respect each other's wishes and limits when it comes to sexual activity? Do you always avoid mixing sex and alcohol or drugs? If the answer to these or any similar questions is no, resolve to change that behavior.

2001 *Call to Action to Promote Sexual Health and Responsible Sexual Behavior* that the United States faces a significant challenge to the sexual health of its people due to the high levels of STDs. Many sexual behaviors carry the risk of STDs, including HIV infection. Partners should be honest about their health and any medical conditions and work out a plan for protection. Behaviors that carry no risk of HIV infection are those that don't involve the exchange of body fluids (blood, semen, and vaginal secretions). Anyone who is not in a mutually monogamous relationship with an uninfected partner and who wishes to have sex should always use a condom. (For more information on STDs and safer sex practices, see Chapter 18.)

Sober Sex   The use of alcohol or drugs in sexual situations increases the risk of unplanned, unprotected sexual activity. This is particularly true of young adults, many of whom engage in episodes of binge drinking during social events. The link between intoxication and unsafe sex is illustrated by a recent study that found that states with higher drinking ages and higher beer taxes have lower rates of STDs. Alcohol and drugs impair judgment and should not be used in association with sexual activity.

Taking Responsibility for Consequences   Individuals should be aware of the physical and emotional consequences of their sexual behavior and accept responsibility for them. Consequences include pregnancy, STDs, and emotional changes in the relationship between partners.

SUMMARY

• The female external sex organs are called the vulva; the clitoris plays an important role in sexual arousal and orgasm. The vagina leads to the internal sex organs, including the uterus, oviducts, and ovaries.

• The male external sex organs are the penis and the scrotum; the glans of the penis is an important site of sexual arousal. Internal sexual structures include the testes, vasa deferentia, seminal vesicles, and prostate gland.

• The fertilizing sperm determines the sex of the individual. Specialized genes on the Y chromosome initiate the process of male sexual differentiation in the embryo.

• Hormones initiate the changes that occur during puberty: The reproductive system matures, secondary sex characteristics develop, and the bodies of males and females become more distinctive.

• The menstrual cycle consists of four phases: menses, the estrogenic phase, ovulation, and the progestational phase.

• The ovaries gradually cease to function as women approach age 50 and enter menopause. The pattern of male sexual responses changes with age, and testosterone production gradually decreases.

- Sexual activity is based on stimulus and response. Stimulation may be physical or psychological.

- Vasocongestion and myotonia are the primary physiological mechanisms of sexual arousal.

- The sexual response cycle has four stages: excitement, plateau, orgasm, and resolution.

- Physical and psychological problems can both interfere with sexual functioning. A treatment for sexual dysfunction first addresses any underlying medical conditions and then looks at psychosocial problems.

- Some gender characteristics are determined biologically, and others are defined by society. Children learn traits and behaviors traditionally deemed appropriate for one sex or the other.

- The ability to respond sexually is present at birth. Sexual behaviors emerging in childhood include self-exploration, perhaps leading to masturbation.

- Although puberty defines biological adulthood, people take 5–10 more years to reach social maturity. Sexual fantasies and dreams and nocturnal emissions characterize adolescent sexuality.

- A person's sexual orientation can be heterosexual, homosexual, or bisexual. Possible influences include genetics, hormonal factors, and early childhood experiences.

- Human sexual behaviors include celibacy, erotic fantasy, masturbation, touching, cunnilingus, fellatio, anal intercourse, and coitus.

- To evaluate whether an atypical sexual behavior is problematic, experts consider the issues of consent between partners and whether the behavior results in physical or psychological harm.

- Pornography and prostitution are examples of the commercialization of sex; sexual stimulation is exchanged for money.

- Responsible sexuality includes open, honest communication; agreed-on sexual activities; sexual privacy; using contraception; safer sex practices; sober sex; and taking responsibility for consequences.

Take Action

1. **Learn more:** Many reputable self-help books about sexual functioning are available in libraries and bookstores. If you're not satisfied with your level of knowledge and understanding, consider consulting some other sources.

2. **Evaluate your relationship:** If you have an intimate sexual relationship with a regular partner, think honestly about what is satisfying about it and what you would like to change. Is there anything you want to discuss with your partner but have been afraid to bring up? Take a chance, and talk with your partner about it.

For More Information

Books

Carlson, K. J., S. A. Eisenstat, and T. Ziporyn. 2004. *The New Harvard Guide to Women's Health*. Cambridge, Mass.: Belknap Press; Simon, H. B. 2004. *The Harvard Medical School Guide to Men's Health: Lessons from the Harvard Men's Health Studies*. New York: Free Press. *These books provide research-based information about a wide variety of health issues, including sexuality, contraception, and sexually transmitted diseases.*

Colapinto, J. 2000. *As Nature Made Him: The Boy Who Was Raised as a Girl*. New York: HarperCollins. *Tells the fascinating story of a boy who, following a botched circumcision, is raised as a girl until the age of 14, at which time he chooses to live life as a male; offers interesting perspectives on the nature vs. nurture controversy surrounding gender identity.*

Halbreich, U. 2003. New advances in premenstrual syndromes (PMS/PMDD). *Psychoneuroendocrinology* Special Issue vol. 28(Suppl 3). *An entire issue devoted to all aspects of PMS and PMDD, including symptoms, treatments, and possible causes.*

Marcus, E. 1999. *Is It a Choice? Answers to 300 of the Most Frequently Asked Questions About Gays and Lesbian People*. San Francisco: Harper. *Candid and informative information on coming out, family roles, and politics.*

Strong, B., et al. 2005. *Human Sexuality: Diversity in Contemporary America*, 5th ed. New York: McGraw-Hill. *A comprehensive introduction to human sexuality.*

Taverner, W. J. 2006. *Taking Sides: Clashing Views on Controversial Issues in Human Sexuality*, 9th ed. New York: McGraw-Hill. *Includes pro and con position statements on sexuality issues relating to biology, behavior, and legal and social issues.*

Vliet, E. L. 2002. *Screaming to Be Heard: Hormonal Connections Women Suspect and Doctors Still Ignore*. New York: M. Evans and Company. *Despite an overly dramatic title, this book provides current and unbiased coverage of all aspects of menopause.*

Organizations and Web Sites

American Association of Sex Educators, Counselors, and Therapists (AASECT). Certifies sex educators, counselors, and therapists and provides listings of local therapists dealing with sexual problems.
   http://www.aasect.org

Center for Young Women's Health. Includes information about topics such as menstruation, gynecological exams, eating disorders, body piercing, and sexual health.
   http://www.youngwomenshealth.org

Dr. Drew. Provides answers to frequently asked questions about sexuality and relationships, geared toward young adults.
   http://www.drDrew.com

Go Ask Alice. Professional and peer educators provide answers to questions on many topics relating to sexuality.
   http://www.goaskalice.columbia.edu

The Kinsey Institute for Research in Sex, Gender, and Reproduction. One of the oldest and most respected institutions doing research on sexuality.

http://www.indiana.edu/~kinsey

Male Health Center. A commercial site that provides a variety of information on male sexual health topics.

http://www.malehealthcenter.com

New York University Sexual Disorders Screening. Provides interactive online screening tests for common sexual disorders.

http://www.med.nyu.edu/psych/screens/disorder_male.html (men)

http://www.med.nyu.edu/psych/screens/disorder_women .html (women)

North American Menopause Society (NAMS). Provides general information about menopause and lists of local support groups and menopause clinicians; Web site includes a helpful section with answers to frequently asked questions.

http://www.menopause.org

San Jose Marital and Sexuality Centre. Provides articles on issues relating to cybersex and an online sexual compulsion assessment.

http://www.sex-centre.com

Sexuality Information and Education Council of the United States (SIECUS). Provides information on many aspects of sexuality and has an extensive library and numerous publications.

http://www.siecus.org

Talking with Kids. Provides advice for parents about talking with children about difficult issues, including sex, relationships, and STDs.

http://www.talkingwithkids.org

U.S. Food and Drug Administration/Consumer Drug Information. Provides information and cautions about the use of drugs to treat sexual dysfunction in men.

http://www.fda.gov/cder/consumerinfo/

See also the listings for Chapters 4, 6–8, and 18.

Selected Bibliography

Agot, K. E., et al. 2004. Risk of HIV-1 in rural Kenya: A comparison of circumcised and uncircumcised men. *Epidemiology* 15(2): 157–163.

American College of Obstetricians and Gynecologists. 2003. *Premenstrual Syndrome.* Washington, D.C.: American College of Obstetricians and Gynecologists.

American Psychological Association. 2005. *Answers to Your Questions About Sexual Orientation and Homosexuality* (http://www.apa.org/publinfo/answers.html; retrieved February 22, 2005).

Aversa, A., et al. 2000. Effects of sildenafil (Viagra) administration on seminal parameters and post-ejaculatory refractory time in normal males. *Human Reproduction* 15(1): 131–140.

Centers for Disease Control and Prevention. 2004. Teenagers in the United States: Sexual activity, contraceptive use, and childbearing, 2002. *Vital and Health Statistics* 23(24).

Centers for Disease Control and Prevention. 2000. Alcohol policy and sexually transmitted disease rates—United States, 1981–1995. *Morbidity and Mortality Weekly Report* 49(16): 346–349.

Currah, P., and S. Minter. 2000. *Transgender Equality: A Handbook for Activists and Policymakers.* Washington, D.C.: National Gay and Lesbian Task Force.

Delate, T., V. Simmons, and B. Motheral. 2004. Patterns of use of sildenafil among commercially insured adults in the United States, 1998–2002. *International Journal of Impotence Research* 16: 313–318.

Diseker, R., et al. 2000. Circumcision and STD in the United States: Cross-sectional and cohort analyses. *Sexually Transmitted Infections* 76: 474–479.

Fink, K., C. Carson, and R. DeVellis. 2002. Adult circumcision outcomes study: Effect on erectile function, penile sensitivity, sexual activity and satisfaction. *Journal of Urology* 167: 2113–2116.

Food and Drug Administration. 2003. *Menopause and Hormones* (http://www.fda.gov/womens/menopause/mht-FS.html; retrieved February 23, 2005).

Food and Drug Administration. 2000. *FDA Clears New Female Sexual Therapy Device* (http://www.fda.gov/bbs/topics/ANSWERS/ANS01012.html; retrieved September 6, 2000).

Freeman, E. W. 2004. Luteal phase administration of agents for the treatment of premenstrual dysphoric disorder. *CNS Drugs* 18(7): 453–468.

Gades, N. M., et al. 2005. Association between smoking and erectile dysfunction: A population-based study. *American Journal of Epidemiology* 161(4): 346–351.

Grady-Weliky, T. A. 2003. Clinical practice. Premenstrual dysphoric disorder. *New England Journal of Medicine* 348(5): 433–438.

Griffiths, M. 2001. Sex on the Internet: Observations and implications for Internet sex addiction. *Journal of Sex Research* 38: 3333–3342.

Hershberger, S. L., and N. L. Segal. 2004. The cognitive, behavioral, and personality profiles of male monozygotic triplet set discordant for sexual orientation. *Archives of Sexual Behavior* 33(5): 497–514.

Hijazi, R. A., and G. R. Cunningham. 2004. Andropause: Is androgen replacement therapy indicated for the aging male? *Annual Review of Medicine* 56: 117–137.

Hutcheson, J. C. 2004. Male neonatal circumcision: Indications, controversies and complications. *Urologic Clinics of North America* 31(3): 461–471.

Laumann, E. O., et al. 2005. Sexual problems among women and men aged 40–80 y: Prevalence and correlates identified in the Global Study of Sexual Attitudes and Behaviors. *International Journal of Impotence Research* 17(1): 39–57.

Leiblum, S. R. 2001. Critical overview of the new consensus-based definitions and classification of female sexual dysfunction. *Journal of Sex and Marital Therapy* 27(2): 159–167.

Nelson, C. P., et al. 2005. The increasing incidence of newborn circumcision: Data from the nationwide inpatient sample. *Journal of Urology* 173(3): 978–981.

Otis, M., and W. Skinner. 2004. An exploratory study of differences in views of factors affecting sexual orientation for a sample of lesbians and gay men. *Psychological Reports* 94(3 Pt 2): 1173–1179.

Pills for erectile dysfunction: Now there are three. 2004. *Harvard Men's Health Watch*, April.

Sommer, F., and U. Engelmann. 2004. Future options for combination therapy in the management of erectile dysfunction in older men. *Drugs and Aging* 21(9): 555–564.

Strong, B., et al. 2005. *Human Sexuality: Diversity in Contemporary America,* 5th ed. New York: McGraw-Hill.

U.S. Surgeon General. 2001. *The Surgeon General's Call to Action to Promote Sexual Health and Responsible Sexual Behavior* (http://www.surgeongeneral.gov/library/sexualhealth/call.htm; retrieved October 10, 2002).

Wang, L., et al. 2004. Stress and dysmenorrhoea: A population based prospective study. *Occupational and Environmental Medicine* 61(12): 1021–1026.

World Health Organization. 2000. *Fact Sheet: Female Genital Mutilation* (http://www.who.int/mediacentre/factsheets/fs241/en; retrieved June 14, 2000).

Wu, T., P. Mendola, and G. M. Buck. 2002. Ethnic differences in the presence of secondary sex characteristics and menarche among U.S. girls: The Third National Health and Nutrition Examination Survey, 1988–1994. *Pediatrics* 110(4): 752–757.

6

plan B
(LEVONORGESTREL)

Vaginal
Contraceptive
Film

FEMALE
CONDOM

Looking **AHEAD**

After reading this chapter, you should be able to

- Explain how contraceptives work and how to interpret information about a contraceptive method's effectiveness, risks, and benefits

- List the most popular contraceptives, and discuss their advantages, disadvantages, and effectiveness

- Discuss issues related to contraception, including nonmarital sexual relationships, gender differences, sex education for teenagers, and communication between partners

- Choose a method of contraception based on the needs of the user and the safety and effectiveness of the method

Contraception

Knowledge

1. **Which of the following contraceptive methods offers the best protection against pregnancy? Which offers the best protection against sexually transmitted diseases?**
   a. oral contraceptives
   b. injectable contraceptives
   c. male condoms
   d. diaphragm with spermicidal foam

2. **Oral contraceptive users typically gain a significant amount of weight.**
   True or false?

3. **Hand lotion, Vaseline (petroleum jelly), and baby oil are good choices for condom lubricants.**
   True or false?

4. **About one in ten young people (age 15–24) reports having had unprotected sex because of the use of alcohol or other drugs.**
   True or false?

5. **What percentage of women say they can't trust men to take responsibility for contraception?**
   a. 25%
   b. 50%
   c. 75%

ANSWERS

1. B AND C. Injectable contraceptives are the most effective at preventing pregnancy; male condoms are the most effective against sexually transmitted diseases.

2. FALSE. Oral contraceptive use is not associated with significant, if any, weight gain; if there is an effect, it is small and may be due to short-term fluid retention.

3. FALSE. Only water-based lubricants such as K-Y Jelly should be used as condom lubricants. Any product that contains mineral oil can cause latex condoms to disintegrate, beginning within 60 seconds of its being applied.

4. FALSE. The figure is about one in four. Mixing alcohol, drugs, and sex substantially increases the risk of unprotected sexual activity, unintended pregnancy, and STDs.

5. C. In the same survey, 66% of men agreed with this assessment.

WW Visit the *Core Concepts in Health* Online Learning Center (www.mhhe.com/insel10e) for study aids and many additional resources.

151

In her lifetime, the ovaries of an average woman release over 400 eggs, one a month for about 35 years. Each egg is capable of developing into a human embryo if fertilized by one of the millions of sperm a man produces in every ejaculate. Furthermore, unlike most other mammals, humans are capable of sexual activity at any time of the month or year. These facts help explain why people have always had a compelling interest in controlling fertility and in preventing unwanted pregnancies. Historical writings dating back to the fourth century B.C. mention the use of douches, sponges, and crude methods of abortion. Other materials mentioned as potential contraceptives include lemon juice, parsley, seaweed, olive oil, camphor, and opium. Although not fully understood at the time, the underlying principle of these trial-and-error methods was the same as that of today's **contraceptives:** preventing **conception** by blocking the female's egg from uniting with the male's sperm, thereby preventing pregnancy.

Modern contraceptive methods are much more predictable and effective than in the past, and people in developed countries now have many options when it comes to making decisions about their sexual and contraceptive behavior. Worldwide, however, the situation is quite different. People in many countries have little access to contraceptive information and supplies. It is estimated that nearly 30% of all pregnancies worldwide are unplanned or unwanted, and unintended pregnancies are associated with higher rates of complications and deaths. (The statistical consequences of contraceptive decisions are shown in Table 6-1, but the risks are not spread equally across all countries. For example, 98% of deaths from complications of childbirth occur in developing countries.)

In addition to the primary purpose of preventing pregnancy, many types of contraception play an important role in protecting against **sexually transmitted diseases (STDs).** Being informed about the realities and risks and making responsible decisions about sexual and contraceptive behavior are crucial components of lifelong wellness. But because such decisions are emotional, complex, and difficult, people tend to avoid them or to deal with them ineffectively.

Although biological, social, and media pressures often encourage sexual activity at ever-younger ages, few forces in the United States support a factual, realistic discussion of the importance of either postponing sexual intercourse or using contraception when intercourse is chosen. Our present superficial approaches to education are clearly ineffective: The United States has one of the highest teen pregnancy rates of all developed nations. Because many of the changing roles of women are severely compromised by unplanned child rearing and because the option of abortion is becoming more restricted, the problem is even worse than the numbers show.

This chapter provides basic information on the various contraceptive methods, including their advantages and

VITAL STATISTICS

Table 6-1	Worldwide Sexual Behavior and Its Consequences	
		Estimated Daily Occurrence
Cases of curable STDs		930,000
Pregnancies		575,000
Births		365,000
Abortions		130,000
Cases of HIV infection		13,000
Deaths—from AIDS		8,000
—from childbirth complications		1,500
—from STDs (excluding AIDS)		500
—from unsafe abortions		200

SOURCES: United Nations Population Fund; Joint United Nations Programme on HIV/AIDS; World Health Organization.

disadvantages; STDs are discussed in Chapter 18. The issues raised should encourage you to think about your own beliefs and attitudes about sexual behavior and contraception and to discuss them with others. Among the most important choices of your life will be deciding what type of sexual involvement is best for you and when you are ready for a sexual relationship; equally critical is the commitment to always protect yourself against unwanted pregnancy and STDs.

PRINCIPLES OF CONTRACEPTION

A variety of effective approaches in preventing conception are based on different principles of birth control. **Barrier methods** work by physically blocking the sperm from reaching the egg. Diaphragms, condoms, and several other methods are based on this principle. *Hormonal methods,* such as oral contraceptives (birth control pills), alter the biochemistry of the woman's body, preventing **ovulation** (the release of the egg) and producing changes that make it more difficult for the sperm to reach the egg if ovulation does occur. So-called *natural methods* of contraception are based on the fact that egg and sperm have to be present at the same time if fertilization is to occur. Finally, *surgical methods*—female and male sterilization—more or less permanently prevent transport of the sperm or eggs to the site of conception.

All contraceptive methods have advantages and disadvantages that make them appropriate for some people but not for others or the best choice at one period of life but not at another. Factors that affect the choice of method include effectiveness, convenience, cost, reversibility, side effects and risks, and protection against STDs. Later in this chapter, we help you sort through these factors to decide

Myth Taking borrowed birth control pills for a few days before having sexual relations gives reliable protection against pregnancy.

Fact Instructions for taking birth control pills must be followed carefully to provide effective contraception. With most pills, this means starting them with a menstrual period and then taking one every day.

Myth Pregnancy never occurs when unprotected intercourse takes place just before or just after a menstrual period.

Fact Menstrual cycles may be irregular, and ovulation may occur at unpredictable times.

Myth During sexual relations, sperm enter the vagina only during ejaculation and never before.

Fact The small amounts of fluid secreted before ejaculation may contain sperm. This is why withdrawing the penis from the vagina just prior to ejaculation is not an effective method of contraception.

Myth If semen is deposited just outside the vaginal entrance, pregnancy cannot occur.

Fact Although sperm usually live about 72 hours within the woman's body, they can live up to 6 or 7 days and are capable of traveling through the vagina and up into the uterus and oviducts.

Myth Douching immediately after sexual relations can prevent sperm from reaching and fertilizing an egg.

Fact During ejaculation (within the vagina), some sperm begin to enter the cervix and uterus. Because these sperm are no longer in the vagina, it is impossible to remove them by douching after sexual relations. Douching may actually push the sperm up farther.

Myth A woman who is breastfeeding does not have to use any contraceptive method to prevent pregnancy.

Fact Frequent and regular breastfeeding may at times prevent ovulation, but not consistently and reliably. Ovulation and pregnancy may occur before the first period after delivering a baby.

Myth Women can't become pregnant the first time they have intercourse.

Fact *Any time* intercourse without protection takes place, sperm may unite with an egg to begin a pregnancy. There is nothing unique about first intercourse that prevents this.

Myth Taking a "rest" from the pill periodically is necessary for safety.

Fact There are no known medical benefits from taking a prolonged break from OC use; the risks and benefits of ongoing pill use should be evaluated for each individual. Pregnancy commonly occurs when one method of contraception is stopped and not effectively replaced by another method.

Myth Pregnancy is impossible if partners have sex while standing up.

Fact Sperm can travel and reach the ovum regardless of body position.

---

on the method that's best for you. (See the box "Myths About Contraception" to make sure you're not basing your current choices on common misinformation.)

Effectiveness, one of the factors listed above, requires further explanation. Contraceptive effectiveness is partly determined by the reliability of the method itself—the failure rate if it were always used exactly as directed ("perfect use"). Effectiveness is also determined by characteristics of the user, including fertility of the individual, frequency of intercourse, and, more important, how consistently and correctly the method is used. This "typical use" **contraceptive failure rate** is based on studies that directly measure the percentage of women experiencing an unintended pregnancy in the first year of contraceptive use. For example, the 8% failure rate of oral contraceptives means 8 out of 100 typical users will become pregnant in the first year. This failure rate is likely to be lower for women who are consistently careful in following instructions and higher for those who are frequently careless; the "perfect use" failure rate is 0.3%. Similarly, the 16% failure rate of typical diaphragm use can be decreased or increased significantly by how correct and consistent the woman is in using the device.

Another measure of effectiveness is the **continuation rate**—the percentage of people who continue to use the method after a specified period of time. This measure is important because many unintended pregnancies occur when a method is stopped and not immediately replaced with another. Thus, a contraceptive with a high continuation rate would be more effective at preventing pregnancy than one with a low continuation rate.

We turn now to a description of the various contraceptive methods, discussing first those that are reversible and then those that are permanent.

Terms

contraceptive Any agent that can prevent conception; condoms, diaphragms, intrauterine devices, and oral contraceptives are examples.

conception The fusion of ovum and sperm, resulting in a fertilized egg, or zygote.

sexually transmitted disease (STD) Any of several contagious diseases contracted through intimate sexual contact.

barrier method A contraceptive that acts as a physical barrier, blocking the sperm from uniting with the egg.

ovulation The release of the egg (ovum) from the ovaries.

contraceptive failure rate The percentage of women using a particular contraceptive method who experience an unintended pregnancy in the first year of use.

continuation rate The percentage of women who continue to use a particular contraceptive after a specified period of time.

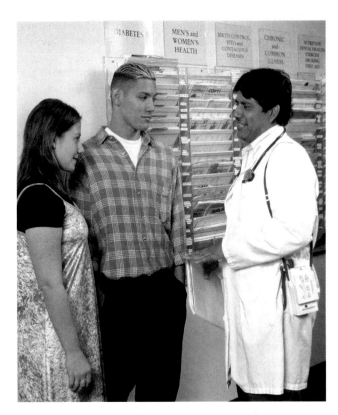

To be effective, contraceptives should be chosen thoughtfully and used correctly. A careful explanation by a health care professional will help this couple choose a method that is right for them.

REVERSIBLE CONTRACEPTION

Reversibility is an extremely important consideration for young adults when they choose a contraceptive method, because most people either plan to have children or at least want to keep their options open until they're older. In this section we discuss the reversible contraceptives, beginning with the hormonal methods, then moving to the barrier methods, and finally covering the natural methods.

Oral Contraceptives: The Pill

A century ago or more, a researcher made a key observation: Ovulation does not occur during pregnancy. Further research brought to light the hormonal mechanism: During pregnancy, the corpus luteum secretes progesterone and estrogen in amounts high enough to suppress ovulation. (Refer to Chapter 5 for a complete discussion of the hormonal control of the menstrual cycle.) **Oral contraceptives (OCs),** or birth control pills, prevent ovulation by mimicking the hormonal activity of the corpus luteum. The active ingredients in OCs are estrogen and progestins, laboratory-made compounds that are closely related to progesterone.

In addition to preventing ovulation, the birth control pill has other backup contraceptive effects. It inhibits the

movement of sperm by thickening the cervical mucus, alters the rate of ovum transport by means of its hormonal effects on the oviducts, and may prevent implantation by changing the lining of the uterus, in the unlikely event that a fertilized ovum reaches that area.

The most common type of OC is the combination pill. Each 1-month packet contains 3 weeks of pills that combine varying types and amounts of estrogen and progestin. Most packets also include a 1-week supply of inactive pills to be taken following the hormone pills; others simply instruct the woman to take no pills at all for 1 week before starting the next cycle. During the week in which no hormones are taken, a light menstrual period occurs. Many different types of combination pills are available today, and if minor problems occur with one brand, a woman can switch to another.

A newer option that became available in 2003 is the extended-cycle OC Seasonale. With Seasonale, a woman takes active pills for 84 consecutive days, followed by inactive pills for a week; this pattern reduces the number of menstrual periods from 13 per year to just 4 per year. However, spotting and slight bleeding are quite common, especially during the first months of use.

Another, much less common, type of OC is the minipill, a small dose of a synthetic progesterone taken every day of the month. Because the minipill contains no estrogen, it has fewer side effects and health risks, but it is associated with more irregular bleeding patterns.

A woman is usually advised to start the first cycle of pills with a menstrual period to increase effectiveness and eliminate the possibility of unsuspected pregnancy. She must take each month's pills completely and according to instructions. Taking a few pills just prior to having sexual intercourse will not provide effective contraception.

Hormonal adjustments that occur during the first cycle or two may cause slight bleeding between periods. This spotting is considered normal. Full effectiveness cannot be guaranteed during the first week because maximal levels of hormones haven't yet been reached. A backup method is recommended during the first week and any subsequent cycle in which the woman forgets to take any pills.

Since its approval by the FDA in 1960, the pill has remained a popular contraceptive in the United States. OC use declined temporarily in the late 1970s following publicity regarding possible increased risks of heart attack and stroke. However, these risks have been substantially reduced by the use of lower-dosage pills (those with 50 micrograms or less of estrogen) and the identification of women at higher risk for complications. Today, OCs are the most widely used form of contraception among unmarried women and are second only to sterilization among married women.

Advantages The main advantage of the oral contraceptive is its high degree of effectiveness in preventing pregnancy. Nearly all unplanned pregnancies result because the pills were not taken as directed. The pill is relatively simple to use and does not require any interruptions that could hinder sexual spontaneity. Most women also enjoy the predictable regularity of periods, as well as the decrease in cramps and blood loss. For young women, the reversibility of the pill is especially important; **fertility**—the ability to reproduce—returns after the pill is discontinued (although not always immediately).

Medical advantages include a decreased incidence of benign breast disease, iron-deficiency anemia, pelvic inflammatory disease (PID), ectopic pregnancy, colon and rectal cancer, endometrial cancer (of the lining of the uterus), and ovarian cancer. Women who have never used the pill are twice as likely to develop endometrial or ovarian cancer as those who have taken it for at least 5 years.

Disadvantages Although oral contraceptives do lower the risk of PID, they do not protect against HIV infection or other STDs in the lower reproductive tract. OCs have been associated with increased cervical chlamydia. Regular condom use is recommended for an OC user, unless she is in a long-term, mutually monogamous relationship with an uninfected partner.

The hormones in birth control pills influence all tissues of the body, and they can lead to a variety of minor disturbances. Symptoms of early pregnancy—morning nausea and swollen breasts, for example—may appear during the first few months of OC use. They usually disappear by the fourth cycle. Other side effects include depression, nervousness, changes in sex drive, dizziness, generalized headaches, migraine, bleeding between periods, and changes in the lining of the walls of the vagina, with an increase in clear or white vaginal discharge. Chloasma, or "mask of pregnancy," sometimes occurs, causing brown "giant freckles" to appear on the face. Acne may develop or worsen, but, in most women, using the pill causes acne to clear up, and it is sometimes prescribed for that purpose.

Serious side effects have been reported in a small number of women. These include blood clots, stroke, and heart attack, concentrated mostly in older women who smoke or have a history of circulatory disease. Recent studies have shown no increased risk of stroke or heart attack for healthy, young, nonsmoking women on lower-dosage pills. OC users may be slightly more prone to high blood pressure, blood clots in the legs and arms, and benign liver tumors that may rupture and bleed. OC use is associated with little, if any, increase in breast cancer and a slight increase in cervical cancer; however, earlier detection and other variables such as number of sexual partners may account for much of this increase. The link between OC use and cervical cancer appears to pertain primarily to women infected with human papillomavirus, an STD. Most adverse effects of OCs disappear after pill use is discontinued, and studies show no long-term effect on mortality.

Birth control pills are not recommended for women with a history of blood clots, heart disease or stroke, any

form of cancer or liver tumor, or impaired liver function. Women with certain other health conditions or behaviors, including migraines, high blood pressure, cigarette smoking, and sickle-cell disease, require close monitoring.

In trying to decide whether to use oral contraceptives, each woman needs to weigh the benefits against the risks. To make an informed decision, she should seek the help of a health care professional in evaluating the known risk variables that apply to her (see the box "Obtaining a Contraceptive from a Health Clinic or Physician" on p. 156). A woman can take several steps to decrease her risk from OC use:

1. Request a low-dosage pill.
2. Stop smoking.
3. Follow the dosage carefully and consistently.
4. Be alert to preliminary danger signals, which can be remembered with the word ACHES:

   Abdominal pain (severe)

   Chest pain (severe), cough, shortness of breath or sharp pain on breathing in

   Headaches (severe), dizziness, weakness, or numbness, especially if one-sided

   Eye problems (vision loss or blurring) and/or speech problems

   Severe leg pain (calf or thigh)

5. Have regular checkups to monitor blood pressure, weight, and urine, and have an annual examination of the thyroid, breasts, abdomen, and pelvis.
6. Have regular **Pap tests** to check for early cervical changes. Because OC use may temporarily increase some women's susceptibility to the STDs chlamydia and gonorrhea, regular screening for those diseases is also recommended, especially when condoms aren't being used.

For most women, the known, directly associated risk of death from taking birth control pills is much lower than the risk of death from pregnancy (Table 6-2, p. 157).

Effectiveness Oral contraceptive effectiveness varies substantially because it depends so much on individual factors. If taken exactly as directed, the failure rate is extremely low (0.3%). However, among average users, lapses

---

Terms

oral contraceptive (OC) Any of various hormone compounds (estrogen and progestins) in pill form that prevent conception by preventing ovulation.

fertility The ability to reproduce.

Pap test A scraping of cells from the cervix for examination under a microscope to detect cancer.

Critical Consumer

If you are a woman who is considering a method of contraception that requires a prescription or professional fitting or insertion, you'll need to go to a health clinic or a physician to get it. Many of the female methods—including the hormonal methods, IUDs, and the diaphragm and cervical cap—require at least an initial professional visit. The thought of visiting a physician's office or health clinic to discuss and obtain contraception makes many people nervous. Keep in mind that the people in the office are health care professionals who will not pass moral judgment on you. They are dedicated to meeting your health care needs. Knowing what to expect can help you get more from your visit.

Before Your Visit

You can prepare for a more successful visit by doing the following:

1. Pull together your personal and family medical history. Make sure it's accurate and up-to-date.

2. Review the section in this chapter titled "Which Contraceptive Method Is Right for You?" Carefully consider each topic, and discuss it with your partner if that would be helpful.

3. Write down any questions you have. Clarify in your own mind what you need to find out about your contraceptive options.

4. If you have questions about sexually transmitted diseases or other aspects of sexuality, write those down, too.

5. If you like, plan to have your partner, a friend, or a family member accompany you to your appointment.

During Your Visit

When you arrive, you'll probably be asked to fill out forms covering your background and medical history. A physician or staff member will then review the various contraceptive methods with you and answer your questions. She or he can help you evaluate the key factors affecting your choice of method, including health risks, lifestyle factors, cost, and protection against STDs. You may have blood and urine samples taken for lab tests.

The Physical Exam

Your physical exam will probably include a check of your breasts, external genitals, and abdomen, plus a Pap test and possible screening for certain STDs. The exam will help ensure that you can safely use the method you have chosen, as well as protect your overall health. If this is your first pelvic exam and/or you feel nervous or uncomfortable, tell the clinician, and ask her or him to explain each step of the examination.

For the pelvic exam, you will be asked to lie on your back on an examination table, with your feet in metal stirrups and your knees bent. The exam doesn't usually hurt. An instrument called a speculum will be inserted into the vagina to hold it open so the clinician can look at the cervix and vaginal walls. For the Pap test, the clinician will scrape some cells from the cervix and place them on a glass slide. These cells will be analyzed for any signs of cancer. You may feel a slight pressure while the cells are collected. The clinician will also check your internal organs by placing two gloved fingers into the vagina and the other hand on the lower abdomen. He or she will palpate (examine by touching) the uterus and ovaries to check for any abnormalities.

If you're getting a diaphragm or a cervical cap, you will be fitted for it at this time. The clinician will probably try different sizes to find the best fit and then will show you how to insert and remove it.

Following Your Exam

After your exam, a health care worker will either provide you with your contraceptive, arrange for a further appointment (if necessary), or give you a prescription. Make sure you know exactly how to use the method you've chosen. Written instructions and information may be available. Be sure you have a phone number you can call if you have questions later.

---

such as forgetting to take a pill do occur, and a typical first-year failure rate is 8%. The continuation rate for OCs also varies; the average rate is 68% after 1 year.

Contraceptive Skin Patch

A contraceptive skin patch, OrthoEvra, was approved by the FDA in 2001. When applied to the skin, the thin, 1¾-inch square patch slowly releases an estrogen and a progestin into the bloodstream. The contraceptive patch prevents pregnancy in the same way as combination OCs, following a similar schedule. Each patch is worn continuously for 1 week and is replaced on the same day of the week for 3 consecutive weeks. The fourth week is patch-free, allowing a woman to have her menstrual period.

The patch can be worn on the upper outer arm, abdomen, buttocks, or upper torso (excluding the breasts); it is designed to stick to skin even during bathing or swimming. If a patch should fall off for more than a day, the FDA advises starting a new 4-week cycle of patches and using a backup method of contraception for the first week. In studies of the device, the patch detached and had to be replaced in fewer than 3% of cases.

Advantages With both perfect and typical use, the patch is as effective as OCs in preventing pregnancy. Compliance seems to be higher with the patch than with OCs, probably because the patch requires weekly instead of daily action. Medical benefits are likely to be comparable to those of OCs.

Table 6-2 — Contraceptive Risks

Contraceptive Method	Risk of Death in Any Given Year
Oral contraceptives	
Nonsmoker	1 in 66,700
Age less than 35	1 in 200,000
Age 35–44	1 in 28,600
Heavy smoker (25 or more cigarettes/day)	1 in 1,700
Age less than 35	1 in 5,300
Age 35–44	1 in 700
IUDs	1 in 10,000,000
Barrier methods, spermicides	none
Fertility awareness methods, withdrawal	none
Sterilization	
Laparoscopic tubal ligation	1 in 38,500
Hysterectomy	1 in 1,600
Vasectomy	1 in 1,000,000
Pregnancy and childbirth	1 in 10,000

SOURCE: Hatcher, R. A., et al. 2004. *Contraceptive Technology*, 18th rev. ed. New York: Ardent Media. Reprinted by permission of Ardent Media, Inc.

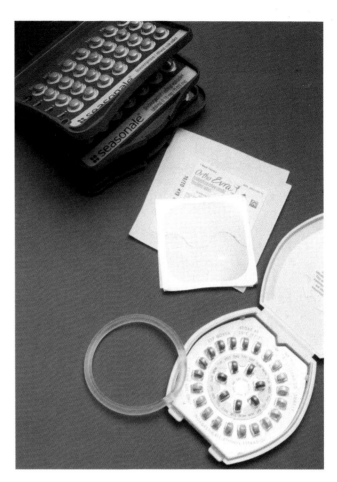

Reversible hormonal contraceptives are available in several forms. To maintain hormone levels in the blood, oral contraceptives are taken daily, the contraceptive patch is replaced weekly, and the vaginal ring is left in place for 3 weeks.

Disadvantages With patch use, additional measures must be taken for protection against STDs. Minor side effects are similar to those of OCs, although breast discomfort may be more common in patch users. Some women also experience skin irritation around the patch. More serious complications and precautions are thought to be similar to those of OCs, including an increased risk of side effects among women who smoke.

Effectiveness With perfect use, the failure rate is very low (0.3%) in the first year of use. The typical failure rate is 8%. The product appears to be less effective when used by women weighing more than 198 pounds.

Vaginal Contraceptive Ring

The NuvaRing, approved by the FDA in October 2001, is a vaginal ring that resembles the rim of a diaphragm and is molded with a mixture of progestin and estrogen. The 2-inch ring slowly releases hormones and maintains blood hormone levels comparable to those found with OC use; it prevents pregnancy in the same way as OCs. A woman inserts the ring anytime during the first 5 days of her menstrual period and leaves it in place for 3 weeks. During the fourth week, which is ring-free, her next menstrual period occurs. A new ring is then inserted.

Backup contraception must be used for the first 7 days of the first ring use or if the ring has been removed for more than 3 hours during use. The device is usually not felt during intercourse, and removal is not recommended; however, if it is removed for less than 3 hours, no backup is needed. A diaphragm is not recommended as a backup contraceptive with the NuvaRing because the ring may interfere with the placement of a diaphragm.

Advantages The NuvaRing offers 1 month of protection with no daily or weekly action required. It does not require a fitting by a clinician, and exact placement in the vagina is not critical as it is with a diaphragm. Medical benefits are probably similar to those of OCs.

Disadvantages The NuvaRing gives no protection against STDs. Side effects are roughly comparable to those seen with OC use, except for a lower incidence of nausea and vomiting. Other side effects may include vaginal discharge, vaginitis, and vaginal irritation. Medical risks also are similar to those found with OC use.

Effectiveness As with the pill and patch, the perfect use failure rate is 0.3% and the typical use failure rate is 8%.

Contraceptive Implants

Contraceptive implants are placed under the skin and deliver a small but steady dose of hormones over a period of several years. Implants have been used for more than 25 years in various countries, including several in Europe, South America, Asia, and Scandinavia. In 1990, the Norplant contraceptive implant became available in the United States. Norplant consists of six flexible, matchstick-size capsules that contain progestin, a synthetic progesterone. The capsules are placed under the skin, usually on the inside of a woman's upper arm in a fan-shaped configuration. The progestin in Norplant has several contraceptive effects: Hormonal shifts may inhibit ovulation and affect development of the uterine lining, thickening of cervical mucus inhibits the movement of sperm, and transport of the egg through the fallopian tubes may be slowed.

The use of Norplant by American women dropped substantially after its first few years of availability because of ongoing lawsuits and related complaints, and Norplant is no longer being distributed. Current users can leave the implants in place for the full 5 years, however. Other types of contraceptive implants are available in other countries and may soon be available in the United States; these include a single capsule device, Implanon, and the two-capsule Norplant 2. In studies, these implants have been easier to insert and remove than the six-capsule Norplant. Contraceptive implants are best suited for women who wish to have continuous and long-term protection against pregnancy.

Advantages Norplant implants are highly effective. After insertion of the implants, no further action is required for up to 5 years of protection; at the same time, contraceptive effects are quickly reversed upon removal. Because Norplant, unlike the combination pill, contains no estrogen, it carries a lower risk of certain side effects, such as blood clots and other cardiovascular complications. In addition, the progestin is released at a steady rate, in smaller quantities than are found in oral contraceptives. The thickened cervical mucus resulting from Norplant use has a protective effect against PID.

Disadvantages Like the pill, Norplant gives no protection against HIV infection and STDs in the lower reproductive tract. Although the implants are barely visible, their appearance may bother some women. Only specially trained practitioners can insert or remove the implants, and removal is sometimes difficult.

The most common side effects of contraceptive implants are menstrual irregularities, including longer menstrual periods, spotting between periods, or having no bleeding at all. The menstrual cycle usually becomes more regular after 1 year of use. Less common side effects include headaches, weight gain, breast tenderness, nausea, acne, and mood swings. Cautions and more serious health concerns are similar to those associated with oral contraceptives but are less common.

Effectiveness Typical failure rates are very low (0.05%) in the first year, increasing slowly with each additional year of use. The cumulative failure rate of Norplant at the end of 5 years is about 1.9%.

Injectable Contraceptives

Hormonal contraceptive injections were developed in the 1960s and are currently being used in at least 80 countries throughout the world. The first injectable contraceptive approved for use in the United States was Depo-Provera, which uses long-acting progestins. Injected into the arm or buttocks, Depo-Provera is usually given every 12 weeks, although it actually provides effective contraception for a few weeks beyond that. As another progestin-only contraceptive, it prevents pregnancy in the same ways as Norplant.

Lunelle, an injectable containing both estrogen and progestin, was approved for use in the United States in 2000. Lunelle injections are given every month rather than every 3 months as with Depo-Provera. Lunelle prevents pregnancy in the same way as OCs. (Lunelle became unavailable in 2002 following a voluntary recall and manufacturing hold; for its current status, check with your health care provider.)

Advantages Injectable contraceptives are highly effective and require little action on the part of the user. Because the injections leave no trace and involve no ongoing supplies, injectables allow women almost total privacy in their decision to use contraception. Like Norplant, Depo-Provera has no estrogen-related side effects; it requires only periodic injections rather than the minor surgical procedures of implant insertion and removal. Lunelle, which does contain estrogen, has many of the same benefits as oral contraceptives and may be preferred by women who do not want to take a pill every day.

Disadvantages Injectable contraceptives provide no protection against HIV infection and STDs in the lower reproductive tract. A woman must visit a health care facility every month (Lunelle) or every 3 months (Depo-Provera) to receive the injections. The side effects of Depo-Provera are similar to those of Norplant; menstrual irregularities are the most common, and after 1 year of using Depo-Provera many women have no menstrual bleeding at all. Lunelle causes less menstrual irregularity than Depo-Provera. Weight gain is a common side effect of both Depo-Provera and Lunelle. After discontinuing the use of Depo-Provera, women may experience temporary infertility for up to 12 months; with Lunelle, fertility usually returns within 2 to 3 months of the last injection.

Reasons for not using Depo-Provera are similar to those for not using Norplant; contraindications for Lunelle are similar to those for OCs. Although early animal studies indicated that Depo-Provera increases the risk of breast and other cancers, the FDA has concluded that worldwide studies and years of human use have shown the risk of cancer in humans to be minimal or nonexistent. Extended use of Depo-Provera is associated with decreased bone density, a risk factor for osteoporosis (see Chapter 12); women are advised to use Depo-Provera as a long-term contraceptive (longer than 2 years, for example) only if other methods are inadequate. Studies have found that bone density rebounds when use of Depo-Provera stops.

Effectiveness   Perfect use failure rates are 0.3% for Depo-Provera and 0.5% for Lunelle. With typical use, failure rates increase to 3% for both types of injectables in the first year of use. The 1-year continuation rate for both Depo-Provera and Lunelle is about 56%.

Emergency Contraception

Emergency contraception refers to postcoital methods— those used after unprotected sexual intercourse. An emergency contraceptive may be appropriate if a regularly used method has failed (for example, if a condom breaks) or if unprotected sex has occurred. Emergency contraceptives are designed only for emergency use and should not be relied on as a regular method.

The most frequently used emergency contraceptive is a two-dose regimen of certain oral contraceptives. Researchers are still uncertain precisely how OCs work as emergency contraceptives. Opponents of their use argue that if they act by preventing implantation of a fertilized egg, they may actually be **abortifacients**; however, recent evidence indicates that prevention of implantation is not their primary mode of action. Postcoital pills appear to work primarily by inhibiting or delaying ovulation and by altering the transport of sperm and/or eggs.

Two products specifically designed for emergency contraception have been approved by the FDA for use in the United States—Plan B and Preven. Plan B contains two progestin-only pills that may be taken together or in separate doses; efficacy and side effects are similar for the two regimens. The first dose should be taken as soon as possible within 120 hours after inadequately protected sex. If the doses are split, the second dose is usually taken 12 hours after the first and may be taken more than 120 hours after unprotected sex.

In 2004, the manufacturer of Preven stopped making the product, but existing stocks can still be used. The Preven kit contains two pills, both containing estrogen and progestin. The first dose should be taken as soon as possible within 72 hours of unprotected intercourse; the second dose is taken 12 hours later. The most common side effects are nausea, vomiting, and breast tenderness.

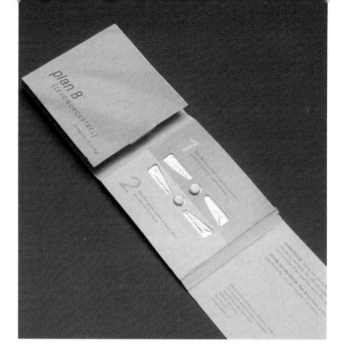

Emergency hormonal contraceptives can reduce the risk of pregnancy by nearly 90% if taken within 72 hours of unprotected intercourse. The most commonly used regimens for emergency contraception involve taking two doses of hormones about 12 hours apart.

Plan B is more effective than Preven and causes less nausea and vomiting; if taken within 24 hours after intercourse, Plan B may prevent as many as 95% of expected pregnancies. Overall, Plan B reduces pregnancy risk by about 89%, and Preven, by about 74%. Both are most effective if initiated in the first 12 hours.

Emergency contraceptive pills are available without a prescription in many European countries, and several U.S. states allow pharmacists to dispense emergency contraceptive packets directly, without a physician prescription (California, Washington, Alaska, New Mexico, Maine, and Hawaii, as of 2005). The benefit of easier access is to shorten the time between inadequately protected sex and use of the pills, thereby increasing their effectiveness. Some clinicians advise women to keep a prescription for, or a packet of, emergency contraceptives on hand. Research has found that ready access to emergency contraception does *not* lead to an increase in unprotected intercourse, unintended pregnancies, or STDs.

In May 2004, an FDA expert advisory panel voted to approve Plan B as an over-the-counter (OTC) medication. However, in an unusual move, the FDA rejected the panel's recommendation, citing concern that young teens could not take the drug safely without a physician's guidance. The American College of Obstetricians and Gynecologists and other organizations responded that all scientific questions about the safety and use of Plan B have been

Term

abortifacient An agent or substance that induces abortion.

resolved and political considerations had influenced the FDA's decision; check the FDA Web site for further updates on Plan B's status.

Emergency contraceptives are available by prescription in all states, but not all physicians, hospitals, and/or pharmacies prescribe or provide emergency contraceptive pills, even in cases of sexual assault. So-called refusal or conscience clauses, originally designed to allow physicians to refuse to perform abortions because of personal moral or religions objections, are being applied to a wider range of health care activities and participants. Thus, for example, physicians may refuse to discuss or prescribe emergency contraceptives, and pharmacists may refuse to fill prescriptions for them—or even for standard OCs. Call the Emergency Contraception Hotline (888-NOT-2-LATE) for more information about access.

Intrauterine devices, discussed in the next section, can also be used for emergency contraception: If inserted within 5 days of unprotected intercourse, they are even more effective than OCs. However, because their use is more complicated, they are not used nearly as frequently. In addition, mifepristone, the "abortion pill," is being studied as another possible option (see Chapter 7 for more on mifepristone).

The Intrauterine Device (IUD)

The **intrauterine device (IUD)** is a small plastic device placed in the uterus as a contraceptive. At the height of its popularity in the early 1970s, about 10% of all women using contraceptives in the United States had an IUD. But in the late 1970s IUD use began to decline, mostly as a result of publicity about the increased risk of serious infections associated with the popular Dalkon Shield and its withdrawal from the market. Two IUDs are now available in the United States: the Copper T-380A (also known as the ParaGard), which gives protection for up to 10 years, and the Levonorgestral IUD (Mirena), approved in 2000, which releases small amounts of progestin and is effective for up to 5 years.

Researchers do not know exactly how IUDs prevent pregnancy. Current evidence suggests that they work primarily by preventing fertilization. IUDs may cause biochemical changes in the uterus and affect the movement of sperm and eggs; although less likely, they may also interfere with implantation of fertilized eggs. Mirena slowly releases very small amounts of hormones, which impedes fertilization or implantation.

An IUD must be inserted and removed by a trained professional. It can be inserted at any time during the menstrual cycle, as long as the woman is not pregnant. The device is threaded into a sterile inserter, which is introduced through the cervix; a plunger pushes the IUD into the uterus. The threads protruding from the cervix are trimmed so that only 1–1½ inches remain in the upper vagina (Figure 6-1).

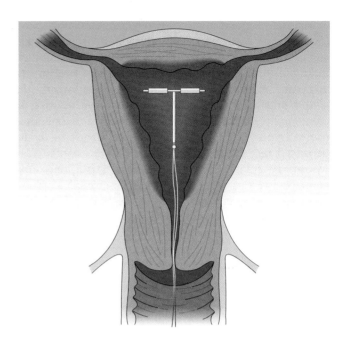

Figure 6-1   An IUD (Copper T-380A) properly positioned in the uterus. The attached threads that protrude from the cervix into the upper vagina allow the woman to check to make sure that the IUD is in place.

Advantages   Intrauterine devices are highly reliable and are simple and convenient to use, requiring no attention except for a periodic check of the string position. They do not require the woman to anticipate or interrupt sexual activity. Usually IUDs have only localized side effects, and in the absence of complications they are considered a fully reversible contraceptive. In most cases, fertility is restored as soon as the IUD is removed. The long-term expense of using an IUD is low.

Disadvantages   Most side effects of IUD use are limited to the genital tract. Heavy menstrual flow and bleeding and spotting between periods may occur, although with Mirena menstrual periods tend to become shorter and lighter over time. Another side effect is pain, particularly uterine cramps and backache, which seem to occur most often in women who have never been pregnant. Spontaneous expulsion of the IUD happens to 5–6% of women within the first year, most commonly during the first months after insertion. The older the woman is and the more children she has had, the less likely she is to expel the device. In about 1 of 1000 insertions, the IUD punctures the wall of the uterus and may migrate into the abdominal cavity.

A serious but rare complication of IUD use is pelvic inflammatory disease (PID). Most pelvic infections among IUD users are relatively mild and can be treated successfully with antibiotics. However, early and adequate treatment is critical—a lingering infection can lead to tubal scarring and subsequent infertility.

Some physicians advise against the use of IUDs by young women who have never been pregnant because of the increased incidence of side effects in this group and the risk of infection with the possibility of subsequent infertility. IUDs are not recommended for women of any age who have a history of pelvic infection or who are at high risk for STDs. They are also unsuitable for women with suspected pregnancy, large tumors of the uterus or other anatomical abnormalities, irregular or unexplained bleeding, a history of ectopic pregnancy, or rheumatic heart disease. No evidence has been found linking IUD use to cancer. IUDs offer no protection against STDs.

Early IUD danger signals are abdominal pain, fever, chills, foul-smelling vaginal discharge, irregular menstrual periods, and other unusual vaginal bleeding. A change in string length should also be noted. An annual checkup is important and should include a Pap test and a blood check for anemia if menstrual flow has increased.

Effectiveness The typical failure rate of IUDs during the first year of use is 0.8% for the ParaGard and 0.1% for Mirena. Effectiveness can be increased by periodically checking to see that the device is in place and by using a backup method for the first few months after IUD insertion. If pregnancy occurs, the IUD should be removed to safeguard the health of the woman and to maintain the pregnancy. The continuation rate of IUDs is about 80% after 1 year of use.

Male Condoms

The **male condom** is a thin sheath designed to cover the penis during sexual intercourse. Most brands available in the United States are made of latex, although condoms made of polyurethane are also now available. Condoms prevent sperm from entering the vagina and provide protection against disease. Condoms are the most widely used barrier method and the third most popular of all contraceptive methods used in the United States, after the pill and female sterilization.

Condom sales have increased dramatically in recent years, primarily because they are the only method that provides substantial protection against HIV infection as well as some protection against other STDs. At least one-third of all male condoms are bought by women. This figure will probably increase as more women become aware of the serious risks associated with STDs and assume the right to insist on condom use. Women are more likely to contract an STD from an infected partner than men are. Women also face additional health risks from STDs, including cervical cancer, PID, ectopic pregnancy (which is potentially life-threatening), and infertility.

The man or his partner must put the condom on the penis before it is inserted into the vagina, because the small amounts of fluid that may be secreted unnoticed prior to **ejaculation** often contain sperm capable of causing pregnancy. The rolled-up condom is placed over the head of the erect penis and unrolled down to the base of the penis,

Condoms come in a variety of sizes, textures, and colors; some brands have a reservoir tip designed to collect semen. Used consistently and correctly, condoms provide the most reliable protection available against HIV infection for sexually active people.

leaving a half-inch space (without air) at the tip to collect semen (Figure 6-2, p. 162). Some brands of condoms have a reservoir tip designed for this purpose. Uncircumcised men must first pull back the foreskin of the penis. Partners must be careful not to damage the condom with fingernails, rings, or other rough objects.

Prelubricated condoms are available containing the **spermicide** nonoxynol-9, the same agent found in many of the contraceptive creams that women use. However, there is no evidence that spermicidal condoms are more effective than condoms without spermicide, even though they cost more. Furthermore, these condoms have been associated with urinary tract infections in women and, if they cause tissue irritation, an increased risk of HIV transmission.

If desired, users can lubricate their own condoms with contraceptive foam, creams, or jelly. If vaginal irritation

Terms

intrauterine device (IUD) A plastic device inserted into the uterus as a contraceptive.

male condom A sheath, usually made of thin latex (synthetic rubber), that covers the penis during sexual intercourse; used for contraception and to prevent STDs.

ejaculation An abrupt discharge of semen from the penis after sexual stimulation.

spermicide A chemical agent that kills sperm.

Figure 6-2 Use of the male condom. (a) Place the rolled-up condom over the head of the erect penis. Hold the top half-inch of the condom (with air squeezed out) to leave room for semen. (b) While holding the tip, unroll the condom onto the penis. Gently smooth out any air bubbles. (c) Unroll the condom down to the base of the penis. (d) To avoid spilling semen after ejaculation, hold the condom around the base of the penis as the penis is withdrawn. Remove the condom away from your partner, taking care not to spill any semen.

occurs with these products, water-based preparations such as K-Y Jelly can be used. Any products that contain mineral or vegetable oil—including baby oil, many lotions, regular Vaseline petroleum jelly, cooking oils (corn oil, Crisco, butter, and so on), and some vaginal lubricants and anti-fungal or anti-itch creams—should never be used with latex condoms; they can cause latex to begin to disintegrate within 60 seconds, thus greatly increasing the chance of condom breakage. (Polyurethane is not affected by oil-based products.)

When the man loses his erection after ejaculating, the condom loses its tight fit. To avoid spilling semen, the condom must be held around the base of the penis as the penis is withdrawn. If any semen is spilled on the vulva, sperm may find their way to the uterus.

Advantages   Condoms are easy to purchase and are available without prescription or medical supervision (see the box "Buying and Using Over-the-Counter Contraceptives"). Simple to use, they provide for greater male participation in contraception. Their effects are immediately and completely reversible. In addition to being free of medical side effects (other than occasional allergic reactions), latex condoms help protect against STDs. Con-

doms made of polyurethane are appropriate for people who are allergic to latex. However, they are more likely to slip or break than latex condoms, and therefore may give less protection against STDs and pregnancy. (Lambskin condoms permit the passage of HIV and other disease-causing organisms, so they can be used only for pregnancy prevention, not the prevention of STDs.) Except for abstinence, correct and consistent use of latex male condoms offers the most reliable available protection against the transmission of HIV.

Disadvantages   The two most common complaints about condoms are that they diminish sensation and interfere with spontaneity. Although some people find these drawbacks serious, others consider them only minor disadvantages. Many couples learn to creatively integrate condom use into their sexual practices. Indeed, it can be a way to improve communication and share responsibility in a relationship.

Effectiveness   In actual use, the failure rate of condoms varies considerably. First-year rates among typical users average about 15%. At least some pregnancies happen because the condom is carelessly removed after ejaculation. Some may also occur because of breakage or slippage, which may happen 1–2 times in every 100 instances of use for latex condoms and up to 10 times in every 100 instances for polyurethane condoms. Breakage is more common among inexperienced users. Other contributing factors include poorly fitting condoms, insufficient lubrication, excessively vigorous sex, and improper storage (because heat destroys rubber, latex condoms should not be stored for long periods in a wallet or a car's glove compartment). To help ensure quality, condoms should not be used past their expiration date or more than 5 years past their date of manufacture (2 years for those with spermicide). It is important to note, however, that most condom failures are due to inconsistent or improper use, not problems with condom quality.

If a condom breaks or is carelessly removed, the risk of pregnancy can be reduced somewhat by the immediate use of a vaginal spermicide. Some clinicians recommend keeping emergency contraceptive pills on hand. If the emergency contraceptive Plan B is taken within 1 hour of inadequately protected sex, the failure rate is only about 0.14%. The most common cause of pregnancy with condom users is "taking a chance"—that is, occasionally not using a condom at all—or waiting to use it until after preejaculate fluid (which may contain some sperm) has already entered the vagina.

Female Condoms

A female condom is a latex or polyurethane pouch that a woman or her partner inserts into her vagina. Although the female condom is preferred in certain situations

Critical Consumer

You can buy several types of contraceptives without a prescription. These have several advantages—they are readily accessible and relatively inexpensive, they are moderately effective at preventing pregnancy, and some offer some protection against HIV infection and other STDs. But like all methods, over-the-counter contraceptives work only if they are used correctly. The following guidelines can help you maximize the effectiveness of your method of choice.

Male Condoms

- *Buy latex condoms.* If you're allergic to latex, use a polyurethane condom or wear a lambskin condom under a latex one. Lambskin condoms provide no STD protection; polyurethane condoms may provide less protection against pregnancy and STDs than latex condoms do, but more studies are needed.

- *Buy and use condoms while they are fresh.* Packages have an expiration date or a manufacturing date. Don't use a condom after the expiration date or more than 5 years after the manufacturing date (2 years if it contains spermicide).

- *Try different styles and sizes.* Male condoms come in a variety of textures, colors, shapes, lubricants, and sizes. Shop around until you find a brand that's right for you. Condom widths and lengths vary by about 10–20%. A condom that is too tight may be uncomfortable and more likely to break; one that is too loose may slip off.

- *Use "thinner" condoms with caution.* Condoms advertised as "thinner" are often no thinner than others, and those that really are the thinnest tend to break more easily.

- *Don't remove the condom from an individual sealed wrapper until you're ready to use it.* Open the packet carefully. Don't use a condom if it's gummy, dried out, or discolored. Keep extra condoms on hand.

- *Store condoms correctly.* Don't leave condoms in extreme heat or cold, and don't carry them in a pocket wallet.

- *Use only water-based lubricants.* Never use oil-based lubricants like Vaseline or hand lotion, as they may cause a latex condom to break. Avoid oil-based vaginal products.

- *Use male condoms correctly* (see Figure 6-2). Use a new condom every time you have intercourse. Misuse is by far the leading reason that condoms fail.

- *Use emergency contraceptive pills if a condom slips or breaks.*

Female Condoms

- *Make sure your condom comes with the necessary supplies and information.* The Reality female condom comes individually wrapped. With your condom, you should receive a leaflet containing instructions and a small bottle of additional lubricant.

- *Buy and use female condoms while they are fresh.* Check the expiration dates on the condom packet and the lubricant bottle.

- *Buy several condoms.* Buy one or more for practice before using one during sex. Have a backup in case you have a problem with insertion or use.

- *Read the leaflet instructions carefully.* Practice inserting the condom and checking that it's in the proper position.

- *Use the female condom correctly.* Make sure the penis is inserted into the pouch and that the outer ring is not pushed into the vagina. Add lubricant around the outer ring if needed.

- *Use emergency contraception pills if a condom slips or breaks.*

Contraceptive Sponges

- *Buy and use contraceptive sponges when they are fresh.* Check the expiration date on each package.

- *Read and follow the package instructions carefully.* Moisten the sponge with water and place high in the vagina.

- *Use each sponge only once.* The sponge may be left in place for up to 24 hours without the addition of spermicide for repeated intercourse.

Spermicides

- *Try different types of spermicides.* You may find one type easier or more convenient to use. Foams come in aerosol cans and are similar to shaving cream in consistency. Foams are thicker than creams, which are thicker than jellies. Foams, creams, and jellies usually require applicators; spermicidal suppositories and films do not.

- *Read and follow the package directions carefully.* Cans of foam must be shaken before use. Jellies and creams are often inserted with an applicator just outside the entrance to the cervix. Suppositories and film must be placed with a finger.

- *Pay close attention to the timing of use.* Follow the package instructions for inserting the spermicide at the appropriate time before intercourse actually occurs. Spermicides have a fairly narrow window of effectiveness. Be sure to also allow the recommended amount of time for suppositories and films to dissolve.

- *Use an additional full dose for each additional act of intercourse.*

- *Leave the spermicide in place for 8 hours after the last act of intercourse.*

- *Consider using spermicides with another form of birth control.* These include a condom, diaphragm, or cervical cap. Combined use provides greater protection against pregnancy.

Emergency Contraceptive Pills

Researchers estimate that 51,000 abortions were prevented by use of emergency contraception in 2000, and the FDA is considering changing the status of emergency contraceptive pills from prescription to over-the-counter. Several states allow women to obtain the pills from a pharmacist without a prescription. If emergency contraceptive pills become more widely available over the counter, it will be important for users to follow the instructions carefully.

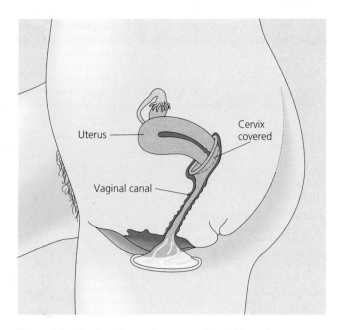

Figure 6-3 The female condom properly positioned.

because it requires less participation on the part of the male partner, its overall popularity remains far below that of the male condom.

The female condom currently available is a disposable device that comes in one size and consists of a soft, loose-fitting polyurethane sheath with two flexible rings (Figure 6-3). The ring at the closed end is inserted into the vagina and placed at the cervix much like a diaphragm. The ring at the open end remains outside the vagina. The walls of the condom protect the inside of the vagina.

The directions that accompany the condom should be followed closely. It can be inserted up to 8 hours before intercourse and should be used with the supplied lubricant or a spermicide to prevent penile irritation. As with male condoms, users need to take care not to tear the condom during insertion or removal. Following intercourse, the woman should remove the condom immediately, before standing up. By twisting and squeezing the outer ring, she can prevent the spilling of semen. A new condom should be used for each act of sexual intercourse. A female condom should not be used with a male condom because when the two are used together slippage is more likely to occur.

Advantages For many women, the greatest advantage of the female condom is the control it gives them over contraception and STD prevention. (Partner cooperation is still important, however.) Female condoms can be inserted before sexual activity and are thus less disruptive than male condoms. Because the outer part of the condom covers the area around the vaginal opening as well as the base of the penis during intercourse, it offers potentially better protection against genital warts or herpes. The polyurethane pouch can be used by people who are allergic to latex. And because polyurethane is thin and pliable, there is little loss of sensation. When used correctly, the female condom should theoretically provide protection against HIV transmission and STDs comparable to that of the latex male condom. However, in research involving typical users, the female condom was less effective in preventing both pregnancy and STDs. With careful instruction and practice, effectiveness can be improved.

Disadvantages As with the traditional condom, interference with spontaneity is likely to be a common complaint. The outer ring, which hangs visibly outside the vagina, may be bothersome during foreplay; if so, couples may choose to put the device in just before intercourse. During coitus, both partners must take care that the penis is inserted into the pouch, not outside it, and that the device does not slip inside the vagina. For many couples, initial awkwardness and difficulty are largely eliminated after a few weeks' use. Female condoms, like male condoms, are made for one-time use. A single female condom costs about four times as much as a single male condom.

Effectiveness The typical first-year failure rate of the female condom is 21%. For women who follow instructions carefully and consistently, the failure rate is considerably lower. Although the female condom rarely breaks during use, slippage occurs in nearly one in ten users. The risk of being exposed to semen is higher if the relationship is new or short-term, if intercourse is very active, and if there is a large disparity between vagina and penis sizes.

The Diaphragm with Spermicide

Before oral contraceptives were introduced, about 25% of all American couples who used any form of contraception relied on the **diaphragm.** Many former diaphragm users have been won over to the pill or to IUDs, but the diaphragm continues to offer advantages that are important to some couples.

The diaphragm is a dome-shaped cup of thin rubber stretched over a collapsible metal ring. When correctly used with spermicidal cream or jelly, the diaphragm covers the cervix, blocking sperm from entering the uterus.

A diaphragm can be obtained only by prescription. Because of individual anatomical differences, a diaphragm must be carefully fitted by a trained clinician to ensure both comfort and effectiveness. The fitting should be checked with each routine annual medical examination, as well as after childbirth, abortion, or a weight change of more than 10 pounds.

The woman spreads spermicidal jelly or cream on the diaphragm before inserting it and checking its placement (Figure 6-4). If more than 6 hours elapse between the time of insertion and the time of intercourse, additional spermicide must be applied. The diaphragm must be left in place for at least 6 hours after the last act of coitus to give the spermicide enough time to kill all the sperm.

Figure 6-4 Use of the diaphragm. Wash your hands with soap and water before inserting the diaphragm. It can be inserted while squatting, lying down, or standing with one foot raised. (a) Place about a tablespoon of spermicidal jelly or cream in the concave side of the diaphragm, and spread it around the inside of the diaphragm and around the rim. (b) Squeeze the diaphragm into a long, narrow shape between the thumb and forefinger. Insert it into the vagina, and push it up along the back wall of the vagina as far as it will go. (c) Check its position to make sure the cervix is completely covered and that the front rim of the diaphragm is tucked behind the pubic bone.

To remove the diaphragm, the woman simply hooks the front rim down from the pubic bone with one finger and pulls it out. She should wash it with mild soap and water, rinse it, pat it dry, and then examine it for holes or cracks. Defects would most likely develop near the rim and can be spotted by looking at the diaphragm in front of a bright light. After inspecting the diaphragm, she should dust it with cornstarch (*not* talcum powder, which may damage it and irritate the vagina) and store it in its case.

Advantages   Diaphragm use is less intrusive than male condom use because a diaphragm can be inserted up to 6 hours before intercourse. Its use can be limited to times of sexual activity only, and it allows for immediate and total reversibility. The diaphragm is free of medical side effects (other than rare allergic reactions). When used along with spermicidal jelly or cream, it offers significant protection against gonorrhea and possibly chlamydia, STDs that are transmitted only by semen and for which the cervix is the sole site of entry. Diaphragm use can also protect the cervix from semen infected with the human papillomavirus, which has been implicated as an important factor in cellular changes in the cervix that can lead to cancer. However, the diaphragm is unlikely to protect against STDs that can be transmitted through vaginal or vulvar surfaces (in addition to the cervix), including HIV infection, genital herpes, and syphilis.

Disadvantages   Diaphragms must always be used with a spermicide, so a woman must keep both of these somewhat bulky supplies with her whenever she anticipates sexual activity. Diaphragms require extra attention, since they must be cleaned and stored with care to preserve their effectiveness. Some women cannot wear a diaphragm because of their vaginal or uterine anatomy. In other women, diaphragm use can cause an increase in bladder infections and may need to be discontinued if repeated infections occur. It has also been associated with a slightly increased risk of **toxic shock syndrome (TSS)**, an occasionally fatal bacterial infection. To diminish the risk of TSS, a woman should wash her hands carefully with soap and water before inserting or removing the diaphragm, should not use the diaphragm during menstruation or in the presence of an abnormal vaginal discharge, and should never leave the device in place for more than 24 hours.

Terms

diaphragm A contraceptive device consisting of a flexible, dome-shaped cup that covers the cervix and prevents sperm from entering the uterus.

toxic shock syndrome (TSS) A bacterial disease usually associated with tampon use; can also occur in men; symptoms include weakness, cold and clammy hands, fever, nausea, and headache. TSS can progress to life-threatening complications, including very low blood pressure (shock) and kidney and liver failure.

Effectiveness The effectiveness of the diaphragm mainly depends on whether it is used properly. In actual practice, women rarely use it correctly every time they have intercourse. Typical failure rates are 16% during the first year of use. The main causes of failure are incorrect insertion, inconsistent use, and inaccurate fitting. Sometimes, too, the vaginal walls expand during sexual stimulation, causing the diaphragm to be dislodged. If a diaphragm slips during intercourse, a woman may choose to use emergency contraception.

Lea's Shield

Lea's Shield, a one-size-fits-all diaphragm-like device, was approved by the FDA in 2002 and is now available by prescription. Made of silicone rubber, it can be used by people allergic to latex, and it is not damaged by petroleum-based products. The shield has a valve allowing the flow of air and fluids from the cervix as well as a loop that aids in insertion and removal. The device may be inserted at any time prior to intercourse, but should be left in place for 8 hours after last intercourse; it can be worn for up to 48 hours. Like the diaphragm, it must be used with spermicide. Studies completed thus far have reported advantages, disadvantages, and failure rates similar to those of the diaphragm.

The Cervical Cap

The **cervical cap**, another barrier device, is a thimble-shaped rubber or plastic cup that fits snugly over the cervix and is held in place by suction. The cap comes in various sizes and must be fitted by a trained clinician. It is used in a manner similar to that of the diaphragm, with a small amount of spermicide being placed in the cup before each insertion.

Advantages Advantages of the cervical cap are similar to those associated with diaphragm use and include partial STD protection. It is an alternative for women who cannot use a diaphragm because of anatomical reasons or recurrent urinary tract infections. Because the cap fits tightly, it does not require a fresh dose of spermicide with repeated intercourse. It may be left in place for up to 48 hours (compared with 24 hours for the diaphragm).

Disadvantages Along with most of the disadvantages associated with the diaphragm, difficulty with insertion and removal is more common for cervical cap users. In addition, some studies have indicated that women who use the cap rather than the diaphragm initially have a higher rate of abnormal Pap test results. In most cases, these are due to inflammation or infections of the cervix, conditions that are easily treatable. As a safety precaution, the FDA requires that the cap be prescribed only for women with normal Pap tests and that a repeat Pap test

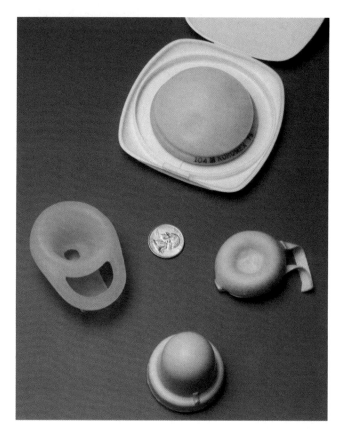

The diaphragm (top), Lea's Shield (left), and cervical cap (bottom) work by covering the mouth of the cervix, blocking sperm from entering the cervix; all require a prescription. The sponge (right), which is available without a prescription or fitting, acts as a barrier, a spermicide, and a seminal fluid absorbent.

be done after 3 months of use to confirm that no changes have occurred. Because there may be a slightly increased risk of TSS with prolonged use, the cap should not be left in place for more than 48 hours.

Effectiveness Studies indicate that for women who have never had children, cervical cap failure rate is about 16%, similar to that of the diaphragm. For women who have given birth, the failure rate goes up to about 32%.

The Contraceptive Sponge

The **sponge** was sold in the United States between 1983 and 1995, at which time the original manufacturer decided to withdraw the contraceptive rather than bring its manufacturing plant up to FDA standards. The safety or effectiveness of the sponge itself was never in question, and FDA approval of the product was never rescinded. A new company bought the rights to the sponge and reintroduced it in Canada in 2003; the FDA approved the return of the sponge to the U.S. market in 2005.

The sponge is a round, absorbent device about 2 inches in diameter with a polyester loop on one side (for removal) and a concave dimple on the other side, which helps it fit snugly over the cervix. The sponge is made of polyurethane and is presaturated with the same spermicide that is used in contraceptive creams and foams. The spermicide is activated when moistened with a small amount of water just before insertion. The sponge, which can be used only once, acts as a barrier, as a spermicide, and as a seminal fluid absorbent.

Advantages The sponge offers advantages similar to those of the diaphragm and cervical cap, including partial protection against some STDs. In addition, sponges can be obtained without a prescription or professional fitting, and they may be safely left in place for 24 hours without the addition of spermicide for repeated intercourse.

Disadvantages Reported disadvantages include difficulty with removal and an unpleasant odor if left in place for more than 18 hours. Allergic reactions, such as irritation of the vagina, are more common with the sponge than with other spermicide products, probably because the overall dose contained in each sponge is significantly higher than that used with other methods. (It contains 1 gram of spermicide compared with the 60–100 mg present in one application of other spermicidal products.) If irritation of the vaginal lining does occur, the risk of yeast infections and STDs (including HIV) may increase. Because the sponge has also been associated with toxic shock syndrome, the same precautions must be taken as described for diaphragm use. A sponge user should be especially alert for symptoms of TSS when the sponge has been difficult to remove or was not removed intact. It is not known how much spermicide is absorbed through the vaginal walls with this device or what the possible effects are of recurring, extended exposure.

Effectiveness The typical effectiveness of the sponge is slightly lower than that of the diaphragm (20% failure rate during the first year of use) for women who have never experienced childbirth. For women who have had a child, however, sponge effectiveness is significantly lower than diaphragm effectiveness. One possible explanation is that its size may be insufficient to adequately cover the cervix after childbirth. To ensure effectiveness, the user should carefully check the expiration date on each sponge, as shelf life is limited.

Vaginal Spermicides

Spermicidal compounds developed for use with a diaphragm have been adapted for use without a diaphragm by combining them with a bulky base. Foams, creams, jellies, suppositories, and films are all available. Foam is sold in an aerosol bottle or a metal container with an applicator that fits on the nozzle. Creams and jellies are sold in tubes with an applicator that can be screwed onto the opening of the tube (Figure 6-5).

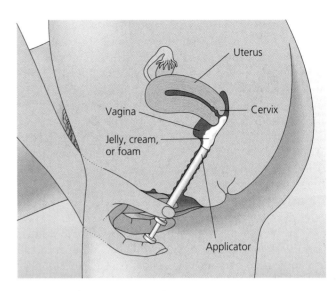

Figure 6-5   The application of spermicide.

Foams, creams, and jellies must be placed deep in the vagina near the cervical entrance and must be inserted no more than 30 minutes before intercourse. After an hour, their effectiveness is drastically reduced, and a new dose must be inserted. Another application is also required before each repeated act of coitus. If the woman wants to **douche,** she should wait for at least 6 hours after the last intercourse to make sure that there has been time for the spermicide to kill all the sperm; douching is not recommended, however, because it can irritate vaginal tissue and increase the risk of various infections.

The spermicidal suppository is small and easily inserted like a tampon. Because body heat is needed to dissolve and activate the suppository, it is important to wait at least 15 minutes after insertion before having intercourse. The suppository's spermicidal effects are limited in time, and coitus should take place within 1 hour of insertion. A new suppository is required for every act of intercourse.

The Vaginal Contraceptive Film (VCF)® is a paper-thin 2-inch square of film that contains spermicide. It is folded over one or two fingers and placed high in the vagina, as close to the cervix as possible. In about 15 minutes the film dissolves into a spermicidal gel that is effective for up to 1 hour. A new film must be inserted for each act of intercourse.

Terms

cervical cap A thimble-shaped cup that fits over the cervix, to be used with spermicide.

sponge A contraceptive device about 2 inches in diameter that fits over the cervix and acts as a barrier, spermicide, and seminal fluid absorbent.

douche To apply a stream of water or other solutions to a body part or cavity such as the vagina; not a contraceptive technique.

Advantages The use of vaginal spermicides is relatively simple and can be limited to times of sexual activity. They are readily available in most drugstores and do not require a prescription or a pelvic examination. Spermicides allow for complete and immediate reversibility, and the only medical side effects are occasional allergic reactions. Vaginal spermicides may provide limited protection against some STDs but should never be used instead of condoms for reliable protection, especially when there is any risk of HIV infection.

Disadvantages When used alone, vaginal spermicides must be inserted shortly before intercourse, so their use may be seen as an annoying disruption. Some women find the slight increase in vaginal fluids after spermicide use unpleasant. Spermicides can alter the balance of bacteria in the vagina. Because this may increase the occurrence of yeast infections and urinary tract infections, women who are especially prone to these infections may want to avoid spermicides. Also, this method does not protect against gonorrhea, chlamydia, or HIV. Overuse of spermicides can irritate vaginal tissues; if this occurs, the risk of HIV transmission may actually increase.

Effectiveness The reported effectiveness rates of vaginal spermicides vary widely, depending partly on how consistently and carefully instructions are followed. The typical failure rate is about 29% during the first year of use. Of the various types of spermicides, foam is probably the most effective, because its effervescent mass forms a denser and more evenly distributed barrier to the cervical opening. Creams and jellies provide only minimal protection unless used with a diaphragm or cervical cap. Spermicide use is generally recommended only in combination with other barrier methods or as a backup to other contraceptives.

✳ Abstinence, Fertility Awareness, and Withdrawal

Millions of people throughout the world do not use any of the contraceptive methods we have described, either because of religious conviction or cultural prohibitions or because of poverty or lack of information and supplies. If they use any method at all, they are likely to use one of the following relatively "natural" methods of attempting to prevent conception.

Terms

abstinence Avoidance of sexual intercourse; a method of contraception.

fertility awareness method (FAM) A method of preventing conception based on avoiding intercourse during the fertile phase of a woman's cycle.

Abstinence The decision not to engage in sexual intercourse for a chosen period of time, or **abstinence**, has been practiced throughout history for a variety of reasons. Until relatively recently, many people abstained because they had no other contraceptive measures. Today, few American women rely on periodic abstinence as a contraceptive method. For those who do, other methods may simply seem unsuitable. Concern about possible side effects, STDs, and unwanted pregnancy may be factors. For others, the most important reason for choosing abstinence is a moral one, based on cultural or religious beliefs or strongly held personal values (see the box "Sexual Decision Making" on p. 139). Individuals may feel that sexual intercourse is appropriate only for married couples or for people in serious, committed relationships. Abstinence may also be considered the wisest choice in terms of an individual's emotional needs. A period of abstinence may be useful as a time to focus energies on other aspects of interpersonal or personal growth.

Anyone can practice abstinence at any time, including people who are not yet sexually active, those who are beginning a relationship with a new partner, and those who are not currently in a relationship. Couples may choose abstinence to allow time for their relationship to grow. A period of abstinence allows partners to get to know each other better and to develop trust and respect for each other. Many couples who do choose to abstain from sexual intercourse in the traditional sense turn to other mutually satisfying alternatives. When open communication between partners exists, many new avenues may be explored. These may include dancing, massage, hugging, kissing, petting, mutual masturbation, and oral-genital sex. (Note: Some of these activities carry a risk of STD transmission; see Chapter 18 for more information.) Sexual feelings and intimacy may be expressed and satisfied through a wide range of activities.

The Fertility Awareness Method The basis for the **fertility awareness method (FAM)** is abstinence from coitus during the fertile phase of a woman's menstrual cycle. Ordinarily only one egg is released by the ovaries each month, and it lives about 24 hours unless it is fertilized. Sperm deposited in the vagina may be capable of fertilizing an egg for up to 6–7 days, so conception can theoretically occur only during 8 days of any cycle. Predicting which 8 days is difficult. It is done by either the calendar method or the temperature method. Information on cyclical changes of the cervical mucus can also help determine the time of ovulation.

The *calendar method* is based on the knowledge that the average woman releases an egg 14–16 days before her next period begins. Few women menstruate with complete regularity, so a record of the menstrual cycle must be kept for 12 months, during which time some other method of contraception must be used. The first day of each period is counted as day 1. To determine the first

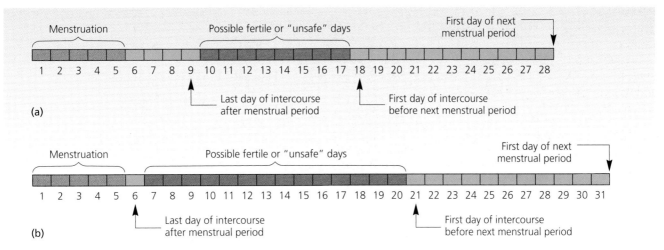

Figure 6-6 The fertility awareness method of contraception. This chart shows the safe and unsafe days for (a) a woman with a regular 28-day cycle and (b) a woman with an irregular cycle ranging from 25 to 31 days.

fertile, or "unsafe," day of the cycle, subtract 18 from the number of days in the shortest cycle (Figure 6-6). To determine the last unsafe day of the cycle, subtract 11 from the number of days in the longest cycle.

A variation of the calendar method known as the Standard Days Method (SDM) can be used by women with regular menstrual cycles between 26 and 32 days long. Couples must avoid unprotected intercourse on days 8 through 19 of the woman's cycle. Some women who use SDM use a string of color-coded beads known as Cycle-Beads™ to track their fertile days.

The *temperature method* is based on the knowledge that a woman's body temperature drops slightly just before ovulation and rises slightly after ovulation. A woman using the temperature method records her basal (resting) body temperature (BBT) every morning before getting out of bed and before eating or drinking anything. Once the temperature pattern is apparent (usually after about 3 months), the unsafe period for intercourse can be calculated as the interval from day 5 (day 1 is the first day of the period) until 3 days after the rise in BBT. To arrive at a shorter unsafe period, some women combine the calendar and temperature methods, calculating the first unsafe day from the shortest cycle of the calendar chart and the last unsafe day as the third day after a rise in BBT.

The *mucus method* (or Billings method) is based on changes in the cervical secretions throughout the menstrual cycle. During the estrogenic phase, cervical mucus increases and is clear and slippery. At the time of ovulation, some women can detect a slight change in the texture of the mucus and find that it is more likely to form an elastic thread when stretched between thumb and finger. After ovulation, these secretions become cloudy and sticky and decrease in quantity. Infertile, safe days are likely to occur during the relatively dry days

just before and after menstruation. These additional clues have been found to be helpful by some couples who rely on the fertility awareness method. One problem that may interfere with this method is that vaginal infections or vaginal products or medication can also alter the cervical mucus.

FAM is not recommended for women who have very irregular cycles—about 15% of all menstruating women. Any woman for whom pregnancy would be a serious problem should not rely on FAM alone, because the failure rate is high—approximately 25% during the first year of use. FAM offers no protection against STDs.

Withdrawal   In withdrawal, or coitus interruptus, the male removes his penis from the vagina just before he ejaculates. Withdrawal has a relatively high failure rate because the male has to overcome a powerful biological urge. In addition, because preejaculatory fluid may contain viable sperm, pregnancy can occur even if the man withdraws prior to ejaculation. Sexual pleasure is often affected because the man must remain in control and the sexual experience of both partners is interrupted.

Failure rates for typical use are about 27% in the first year. Men who are less experienced with sexual intercourse and withdrawal or who have difficulty in foretelling when ejaculation will occur have higher failure rates. Withdrawal does not protect against STDs.

Combining Methods

Couples can choose to combine the preceding methods in a variety of ways, both to add STD protection and/or to increase contraceptive effectiveness. For example, condoms are strongly recommended along with OCs whenever there is a risk of STDs (Table 6-3, p. 170). Foam may be added to condom use to increase protection against

Table 6-3 Contraceptive Methods and STD Protection

Method	Level of Protection
Hormonal methods	Do not protect against HIV or STDs in lower reproductive tract; increase risk of cervical chlamydia; provide some protection against PID.
IUD	Does not protect against STDs; associated with PID in first month after insertion.
Latex or polyurethane male condom	Best method for protection against STDs (if used correctly); does not protect against infections from lesions that are not covered by the condom. (Lambskin condoms do not protect against STDs.)
Female condom	Theoretically should reduce the risk of STDs, but research results are not yet available.
Diaphragm, sponge, or cervical cap	Protects against cervical infections and PID. Research results regarding HIV protection are contradictory, but diaphragms, sponges, and cervical caps are not as effective as male condoms and should not be relied on for protection.
Spermicide	Modestly reduces the risk of some vaginal and cervical STDs; does not reduce the risk of HIV, chlamydia, or gonorrhea. If vaginal irritation occurs, infection risk may increase.
FAM	Does not protect against STDs.
Sterilization	Does not protect against STDs.
Abstinence	Complete protection against STDs (as long as all activities that involve the exchange of body fluids are avoided).

Abstinence or sex with a mutually monogamous, uninfected partner is the surest way to protect yourself against HIV and other STDs. Barring this, correct and consistent use of latex male condoms provides the best protection against STDs.

both STDs and pregnancy. For many couples, and especially for women, the added benefits far outweigh the extra effort and expense.

Table 6-4 summarizes the effectiveness of available contraceptive methods.

PERMANENT CONTRACEPTION: STERILIZATION

Sterilization is permanent, and it is highly effective at preventing pregnancy. For these reasons, it is becoming an increasingly popular method of contraception. At present it is the most commonly used method both in the United States and in the world. It is especially popular among couples who have been married 10 or more years, as well as couples who have had all the children they intend to have. Sterilization provides no protection against STDs.

An important consideration in choosing sterilization is that, in most cases, it cannot be reversed and should be considered permanent. Although the chances of restoring fertility are being increased by modern surgical techniques, such operations are costly, and pregnancy can never be guaranteed. Some couples choosing male sterilization store sperm as a way of extending the option of childbearing.

Some studies indicate that male sterilization is preferable to female sterilization for a variety of reasons. The overall cost of a female procedure is about four times that of a male procedure, and women are much more likely than men to experience both minor and major complications following the operation. Furthermore, feelings of regret seem to be somewhat more prevalent in women than in men after sterilization. Men seeking vasectomies are typically white, married, relatively affluent and well educated, and privately insured.

Although some physicians will perform surgery for sterilization on request, most require a thorough discussion with both partners before the operation. Most physicians also recommend that people who have religious conflicts, psychological problems related to sex, or unstable marriages not be sterilized. Young couples who might later change their minds are also frequently advised not to undergo sterilization.

Terms

sterilization Surgically altering the reproductive system to prevent pregnancy. Vasectomy is the procedure in males; tubal sterilization or hysterectomy is the procedure in females.

vasectomy The surgical severing of the ducts that carry sperm to the ejaculatory duct.

vasa deferentia The two ducts that carry sperm to the ejaculatory duct; singular, vas deferens.

Table 6-4	Contraceptive Effectiveness	
	Percentage of Women Experiencing an Unintended Pregnancy in the First Year of Use	
Method	**Typical Use**	**Perfect Use**
Mirena IUD	0.1	0.1
Male sterilization (vasectomy)	0.15	0.1
Female sterilization	0.5	0.5
ParaGard (Copper T-380A)	0.8	0.6
Lunelle injections	3	0.05
Depo-Provera injections	3	0.3
Oral contraceptives	8	0.3
OrthoEvra patch	8	0.3
NuvaRing	8	0.3
Male condom (latex or polyurethane)	15	2
Diaphragm with spermicide	16	6
Cervical cap with spermicide*	16	9
Sponge*	16	9
Female condom	21	5
Fertility awareness method	25	
Calendar alone		9
Combination of FAM methods		2
Withdrawal	27	4
Spermicides (alone)	29	18
Chance (no method)	85	85

*For women who have given birth, the rates of unintended pregnancy increase to 32% for typical use and 26% for perfect use for the cervical cap and to 32% for typical use and 20% for perfect use for the sponge.

SOURCE: Hatcher, R. A., et al. 2004. *Contraceptive Technology*, 18th rev. ed. New York: Ardent Media. Reprinted by permission of Ardent Media, Inc.

Male Sterilization: Vasectomy

The procedure for male sterilization, **vasectomy**, involves severing the **vasa deferentia**, two tiny ducts that transport sperm from the testes to the seminal vesicles (see Figure 5-2). The testes continue to produce sperm, but the sperm are absorbed into the body. Because the testes contribute only about 10% of the total seminal fluid, the actual quantity of ejaculate is only slightly reduced. Hormone production from the testes continues with very little change, and secondary sex characteristics are not altered.

Vasectomy is ordinarily performed in a physician's office and takes about 30 minutes. A local anesthetic is injected

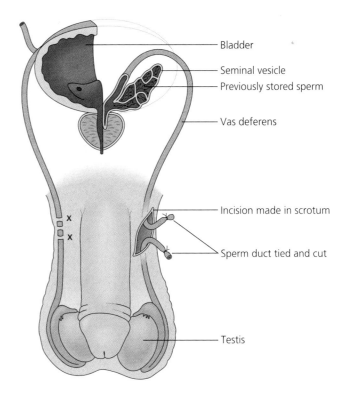

Figure 6-7 Vasectomy. This surgical procedure involves severing the vasa deferentia, thereby preventing sperm from being transported and ejaculated.

into the skin of the scrotum near the vasa. Small incisions are made at the upper end of the scrotum where it joins the body, and the vas deferens on each side is exposed, severed, and tied off or sealed by electrocautery. A plastic clamp (Vasclip) the size of a grain of rice was approved by the FDA in 2003 and may become more popular as more physicians become trained and experienced in its use; although also permanent, the use of the clip may cause less tissue damage and pain following surgery. The incisions are then closed with sutures, and a small dressing is applied (Figure 6-7). Pain and swelling are usually slight and can be relieved with ice compresses, aspirin, and the use of a scrotal support. Bleeding and infection occasionally develop but are usually easily treated. Fewer complications occur with an alternative procedure involving a midline puncture rather than incisions; this "no-scalpel" technique is used in about 30% of vasectomies performed in the United States. After either procedure, most men are ready to return to work in 2 days.

Men can have sex again as soon as they feel no further discomfort, usually after about a week. Another method of contraception must be used for the next 20 ejaculations or 3 months after vasectomy, however, because sperm produced before the operation may still be present in the semen. Microscopic examination of a semen sample can confirm that sperm are no longer present in the ejaculate.

Vasectomy is highly effective. In a small number of cases, a severed vas rejoins itself, so some physicians advise yearly examination of a semen sample. The overall

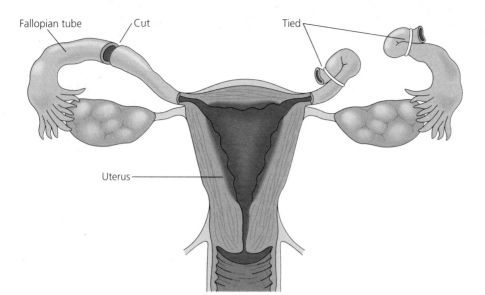

Fallopian tube — Cut — Tied

Uterus —

Figure 6-8 Tubal sterilization. This procedure involves severing or blocking the fallopian tubes, thereby preventing eggs from traveling from the ovaries to the uterus. It is a more complex procedure than vasectomy.

failure rate for vasectomy is 0.15%. No strong links have been found between vasectomy and chronic diseases, and the bulk of the evidence now indicates that men with vasectomies are not at increased risk for heart disease, prostate cancer, or testicular cancer.

Although some surgeons report pregnancy rates of about 80% for partners of men who have their vasectomies reversed within 10 years of the original procedure, most studies report figures in the 50% range. In at least half of all men who have had vasectomies, the process of absorbing sperm (instead of ejaculating it) results in antisperm antibodies that may interfere with later fertility. Other factors, such as length of time between the vasectomy and the reversal surgery, may also be important predictors of reversal success.

Female Sterilization

The most common method of female sterilization involves severing, or in some manner blocking, the oviducts, thereby preventing the egg from reaching the uterus and the sperm from entering the fallopian tubes (see Figure 5-1). Ovulation and menstruation continue, but the unfertilized eggs are released into the abdominal cavity and absorbed. Although progesterone levels in the blood may decline slightly, hormone production by the ovaries and secondary sex characteristics are generally not affected.

Tubal sterilization is most commonly performed by a method called **laparoscopy.** A laparoscope, a tube containing a small light, is inserted through a small

abdominal incision, and the surgeon looks through it to locate the fallopian tubes. Instruments are passed either through the laparoscope or through a second small incision, and the two fallopian tubes are sealed off with ties or staples or by electrocautery (Figure 6-8). General anesthesia is usually used. The operation takes about 15 minutes, and women can usually leave the hospital 2–4 hours after surgery. Tubal sterilization can also be performed shortly after a vaginal delivery, or in the case of cesarean section immediately after the uterine incision is repaired.

Although tubal sterilization is somewhat riskier than vasectomy, with a rate of minor complications of about 6–11%, it is the more common procedure (see the box "Contraceptive Use Among American Women"). Potential problems include bowel injury, wound infection, and bleeding. Serious complications are rare, and the death rate is low.

The failure rate for tubal sterilization is about 0.5%. When pregnancies do occur, an increased percentage of them are ectopic. Some complaints of long-term abdominal discomfort and menstrual irregularity following tubal sterilization have been reported, but recent studies have not found any association between them. Because reversibility rates are low and the procedure is costly, female sterilization should be considered permanent.

A new female sterilization device was approved by the FDA in 2002. The Essure System consists of tiny spring-like metallic implants that are inserted through the vagina, into the fallopian tubes, using a special catheter. Within several months, scar tissue forms over the implants, blocking the tubes. A backup method may be used until a test shows that the tubes are occluded. Placement of the device doesn't require an incision or general anesthesia, and recovery time is quicker than that following tubal sterilization. Only clinicians with specialized training and equipment can perform this procedure, and in some cases a second procedure is required.

Terms

V W

tubal sterilization Severing or in some manner blocking the oviducts, preventing eggs from reaching the uterus.

laparoscopy Examining the internal organs by inserting a tube containing a small light through an abdominal incision.

Dimensions of Diversity

Contraceptive Use Among American Women

About 62 million women in the United States are in their childbearing years (15–44) and thus face decisions about contraception. Overall, about 62% of American women use some form of contraception, and most of the remaining 38% are either sterile, pregnant or trying to become pregnant, or not sexually active. Only 7% of American women are fertile, sexually active, and not seeking pregnancy *and* not using contraceptives; this small group accounts for almost half of the 3 million unintended pregnancies that occur each year. The unintended pregnancies that occur among contraceptive users are usually the result of inconsistent or incorrect use of methods. For example, one-third of barrier method users report not using their method every time they have intercourse.

Oral contraceptives and female sterilization are the two most popular methods among American women (see figure). However, choice of contraceptive method and consistency of use vary with age, marital status, and other factors:

• *Age:* Sterilization is much more common among older women, particularly those who are over 35 years of age and/or who have had children. Older women are also much more likely to use reversible methods consistently—they are least likely to miss pills and most

likely to use barrier methods during every act of intercourse. Young women between ages 15 and 17 who use OCs are more likely by far to miss pills than women in any other age group.

• *Marital status:* Women who are or were married have much higher rates of sterilization than women who have never been married. Those who have never been married have high rates of OC and condom usage.

• *Ethnicity:* Overall rates of contraceptive use and use of OCs are highest among white women. Female sterilization, implants, and injectables are more often used by African American women and Latinas, and IUD use is highest among Latinas. Condom use is highest among Asian American women and similar across other ethnic groups. Male sterilization is much more common among white men than among men of other ethnic groups.

• *Socioeconomic status and educational attainment:* Low socioeconomic status and low educational attainment are associated with high rates of female sterilization and low rates of pill and condom use. However, women who are poor or have low educational attainment and who do use OCs have higher rates of consistent use than women who are wealthier or have more education. About 20% of women

age 15–44 lack adequate health insurance, increasing the cost and difficulty of obtaining contraceptives.

Some trends in contraceptive use may also reflect the differing priorities and experiences of women and men. For example, female sterilization is more expensive and carries greater health risks than male sterilization—yet it is more than twice as common. (Worldwide, female sterilization is more than four times as common as male sterilization.) This pattern may reflect culturally defined gender roles and the fact that women are more directly affected by unintended pregnancy. In surveys, women rate pregnancy prevention as the single most important factor when choosing a contraceptive method; in contrast, men rate STD prevention as equally important.

SOURCES: Alan Guttmacher Institute. 2005. *Facts in Brief: Contraceptive Use.* New York: Alan Guttmacher Institute; Alan Guttmacher Institute. 2004. *Issues in Brief: Preventing Unintended Pregnancy in the U.S.* (http://www.agi-usa.org/pubs/ib2004no3.html; retrieved August 23, 2004); National Center for Health Statistics. 2004. Use of contraception and use of family planning services in the United States: 1982–2002. *Advance Data from Vital and Health Statistics,* No. 350. Grady, W. R., D. H. Klepinger, and A. Nelson-Wally. 1999. Contraceptive characteristics: The perceptions and priorities of men and women. *Family Planning Perspectives* 31(4): 168–175.

Women not using contraception (38.1% of U.S. women)

- Sterile for noncontraceptive reasons or with sterile male partner (3.1%)
- Sexually active (7.4%)
- Pregnant, post-partum, or seeking pregnancy (9.5%)
- Not sexually active (18.1%)
- Other (0.6%)
- IUDs (1.3%)
- Implant, one-month injectable, or patch (0.8%)
- Diaphragm (0.2%)

Method reported by women using contraception (61.9% of U.S. women)

- Female sterilization (16.7%)
- Oral contraceptives (18.9%)
- Condoms (11.1%)
- Male sterilization (5.7%)
- Withdrawal (2.5%)
- 3-month injectable (3.3%)
- Fertility awareness method (0.9%)

Contraceptive use among American women age 15–44 years.

Many people have a difficult time talking about contraception with a potential sex partner. How should you bring it up? And whose responsibility is it, anyway? Talking about the subject may be embarrassing at first, but imagine the possible consequences of *not* talking about it. An unintended pregnancy or a sexually transmitted disease could profoundly affect you for the rest of your life. Talking about contraception is one way of showing that you care about yourself, your partner, and your future.

Before you talk with your partner, explore your own thoughts and feelings. Find out the facts about different methods of contraception, and decide which one you think would be most appropriate for you. If you're nervous about having this discussion with your partner, it may help to practice with a friend.

Pick a good time to bring up the subject. Don't wait until you've started to have sex. A time when you're both feeling comfortable and relaxed will maximize your chances of having

a good discussion. Tell your partner what you know about contraception and how you feel about using it, and talk about what steps you both need to take to get and use a method you can live with. Listen to what your partner has to say, and try to understand his or her point of view. You may need to have more than one discussion, and it may take some time for both of you to feel comfortable with the subject. *But don't have sex until this issue is resolved.*

If you want your partner to be involved but he or she isn't interested in talking about contraception, or if he or she leaves all the responsibility for it up to you, consider whether this is really a person you want to be sexually involved with. If you decide to go ahead with the involvement, you may want to enlist the support of a friend, family member, or health care worker to help you make and implement decisions about the essential issue of contraception.

Hysterectomy, removal of the uterus, is the preferred method of sterilization for only a small number of women, usually those with preexisting menstrual problems. Because of the risks involved, hysterectomy is not recommended unless the woman has disease or damage of the uterus and future surgery appears inevitable.

ISSUES IN CONTRACEPTION

The subject of contraception is closely tied to several issues that are currently receiving much attention in the United States, such as premarital sexual relations, gender differences, and sexuality education for teens.

When Is It OK to Begin Having Sexual Relations?

Answers to that question strongly affect a society's approach to contraception. Opinions on the appropriate age or time to begin having sex often determine one's views on sexuality education and contraception accessibility. Americans have a wide range of opinions on this issue: only after marriage; when 18 years or older; when in a loving, stable relationship; when the partners have completed their education and/or could support a child; whenever both partners feel ready and are using protection against pregnancy and STDs.

Opinions about appropriate sexual behavior shift from one decade to another. Although attitudes became more

liberal during the 1960s and 1970s, people started having more restrictive views in the 1980s and 1990s. Today, the most common reasons for disapproving of sex are the risk of exposure to STDs, the risk of pregnancy, and moral or religious beliefs. According to recent data, most of today's young Americans are somewhat permissive regarding premarital sex. Although many approve of sexual relations for couples who are seriously dating or engaged to be married, they are less accepting of sexual intercourse on a first date or at the casual dating stage.

Closely related to the issue of beginning sexual relations is a more personal question: What would you consider the ideal amount of previous sexual experience for you and your partner? Again, opinions vary, especially in terms of what is desirable for men and for women. Limited experience is still more commonly deemed desirable for women, whereas being "sexually experienced" is often valued more highly for men.

As more women consider careers for themselves and therefore often delay childbearing and even marriage, the likelihood of sexual activity and the critical need for pregnancy and STD prevention only increase. As a result, making decisions about sexual activity and contraception becomes even more important to those starting college or a career. Unfortunately, however, many individuals in this age group—even those who protect their health in all other areas of their life—end up taking high risks in their sexual behavior. Ambivalence and a lack of communication about who will "take charge" are common and are partly due to the denial of, and hypocrisy about, sexual behavior that exists in our society. (For guidelines on improving your own communication, see the box "Talking with a Partner About Contraception.") Alcohol and drug use are also strongly linked to risky sexual behavior.

Term

V W   hysterectomy Total or partial surgical removal of the uterus.

Even the best of the present methods of contraception have drawbacks, and the search continues for the ideal method—more effective, safer, cheaper, easier to use, more readily available, easily reversible, and acceptable to more people. Many new methods are widely used in other countries long before they become available in the United States. This delay is partly due to higher costs of safety testing in the United States, greater liability risks for manufacturers, and lower levels of government funding for contraceptive research.

Despite delays, the past decade has seen several new methods approved and marketed in the United States, a trend that is likely to continue. The options expected to become available in the near future are variations of current methods: new combinations of hormones in OCs, implants, injectables, rings, and emergency contraceptives; new designs for IUDs and condoms; and new spermicides and microbicides that are effective in destroying viruses and bacteria as well as sperm. Some of the other methods being studied are described below.

New Ways of Delivering Hormones

As described in the discussion of contraceptive implants, several *new types of implants* are being developed, including Implanon and Norplant 2. A kit for an *at-home version of the Lunelle injectable contraceptive* is also under development;

this kit would allow women to self-administer the injections, eliminating the need for monthly clinic visits.

Similar to Norplant, *biodegradable implants* are placed under the skin and deliver small doses of hormones over a long period of time. Unlike Norplant, the capsules dissolve over time, eliminating the need for surgical removal. *Injectable microspheres,* tiny clusters of molecules filled with hormones, also dissolve as they deliver a steady dose of hormones over many months.

New Barrier Methods

FemCap, made of silicone, is a prescription barrier contraceptive shaped like a sailor's hat with a dome that covers the cervix. It is designed to fit more comfortably and to dislodge less frequently than conventional cervical caps. New prototypes of the female condom and the vaginal sponge may also become available.

Hormonal Contraceptives for Men

Male and female hormones can interfere with sperm development in the male, just as they suppress ovulation in the female. One promising contraceptive under study combines a daily pill or implant containing a progestin with a testosterone pellet implanted under the skin and replaced every 12 weeks. This combination has been shown to reduce sperm production to zero, although some men report side effects similar to those women may

experience when taking OCs: headaches, acne, and increased appetite.

Contraceptive Immunization

Immunity to fertility has occasionally (though rarely) occurred as a result of a man's being unintentionally sensitized to his own sperm cells. He then produces antibodies that inactivate sperm as if they were disease organisms. In theory, a woman could be purposely sensitized against her own egg cells or against her partner's sperm cells. Another immunocontraceptive under study targets just the zona pellucida (ZP), the protein covering of the egg cell. Immunization against ZP would temporarily block sperm from penetrating the egg without affecting normal egg development. Concerns that the antibodies may cross-react with untargeted hormones in the body have slowed research in this area.

Reversible Sterilization

Present methods of sterilization in both men and women are reversible 50–70% of the time. Several new techniques are being studied in the hope that restoring fertility can be made easier and more predictable. These techniques include injecting liquid silicone into the fallopian tubes, where it solidifies and forms a plug, and placing various types of clips and plugs on the vasa to totally block sperm flow. These plugs or clips could then be removed if an individual wanted to restore fertility.

Contraception and Gender Differences

A second issue, one all couples must confront, is the differing significance of contraception to women and men. The consequences of not using contraception are markedly different for men and women. In past years, women have accepted the primary responsibility of contraception, along with related side effects and health risks, partly because of the wider spectrum of methods available to them and partly because women have greater personal investment in preventing pregnancy and childbearing. Men still have very few contraceptive options, with condoms being the only reversible method currently available (see the box "Future Methods of Contraception"). Recently, however, men's participation has become critical, since condom use is central to safer sex even when OCs or other methods are being used by women.

Although dependent primarily on the cooperation of the man, condom use and the prevention of STDs have potentially greater consequences for the woman. Whereas men may suffer only local and short-term effects from the most common diseases (not including HIV infection), women face an increased risk of serious long-term effects, such as cervical cancer and/or pelvic infection with associated infertility, from these same prevalent STDs. In addition, women are more likely than men to contract HIV from an infected partner. In other words, although dependent on the male, condom use is clearly a more important issue for women. The female condom may offer a helpful alternative, but the cooperation of the male partner is still needed to ensure correct use.

The experience of an unintended pregnancy is very different for the two involved partners. Although men do

What can be done to increase men's involvement in contraception? Around the world, experts are trying diverse approaches:

• Develop programs and campaigns that stress the importance of information, counseling, and medical care relating to sexual and reproductive matters from adolescence on. Men are less likely than women to seek regular checkups, but regular care for men would benefit men in their own right and both men and women as individuals, couples, and families.

• Recruit and train male health workers, who can be important advocates and role models for healthful behaviors. Expand educational material and clinical programs that focus on male contraception and reproductive health.

• Focus on men as obstacles to women's contraceptive use and as an untapped group of potential users. Educate men about the ways in which stereotypical views of male or female sexuality can inhibit good reproductive health for both men and women. Stress the importance of shared responsibility.

• Develop educational and clinical programs specifically targeted at young men. Men in their early 20s are most likely to engage in risky sexual behaviors and to have adverse reproductive health outcomes. Surveys indicate that most men use a condom the first time they have intercourse, but condom use subsequently declines—and there is much greater reliance on female contraceptive methods.

What can individuals do? Men can increase their participation in contraception in the following ways:

• Initiate and support communication regarding contraception and STD protection.

• Buy and use condoms whenever appropriate.

• Help pay contraceptive costs.

• Be available for shared responsibility in the resolution of an unintended pregnancy, should one occur.

SOURCES: United Nations Population Fund. 2004. *The State of World Population Report 2004.* New York: UNFPA; Alan Guttmacher Institute. 2004. *In Their Own Right: Addressing the Sexual and Reproductive Health of American Men.* New York: Alan Guttmacher Institute; Armstrong, B. 2003. The young men's clinic: Addressing men's reproductive health and responsibilities. *Perspectives on Sexual and Reproductive Health* 35(5): 220–225.

---

suffer emotional stress from such an unexpected occurrence (and sometimes share financial and/or custodial responsibilities), women are much more intimately affected, obviously by the biological process of pregnancy itself as well as the outcome: abortion, adoption, or parenting. In addition, our societal attitudes are more severely punitive toward the woman and place much greater responsibility and blame on her when an unintended pregnancy occurs. Fortunately, there is growing interest in the roles and responsibilities of men in family planning (see the box "Men's Involvement in Contraception").

Sexuality and Contraception Education for Teenagers

A third controversial issue is sexuality education and pregnancy prevention programs for teenagers. Again, opinion in the United States is sharply divided. Certain groups are concerned that more sexuality education and especially the availability of contraceptives will lead to more sexual activity and promiscuity. They maintain that greater access to improved contraception was a key factor contributing to the sexual revolution in the 1960s and that the ensuing liberal sexual attitudes have been generally more destructive than helpful. They point to an increase in divorce, a rise in STDs, and a general relaxing of standards of morality as related negative effects.

Many in this group urge that sexuality education be handled in the home, where parents can instill moral values, including premarital abstinence. According to some in this group, young people should primarily be taught to "just say no." They see most public education about contraception, especially facilities that make supplies available, as only increasing the problem.

Other groups argue that encouraging the public availability of contraceptive information and supplies does not necessarily result in an increase in promiscuous sexual behavior, pointing to the fact that many young teenagers are already pregnant when they first visit a health care facility. These groups assert that parents are not effectively dealing with the issues and that a broader, coordinated approach involving public institutions, including schools, is needed, along with parental input. Many current programs focus on postponing sexual involvement but also emphasize contraceptive use for individuals who are sexually active. Increased availability of contraceptive information and methods is considered a necessary and realistic part of this approach.

During the 1990s, U.S. teenage pregnancy and birth rates dropped to record low levels, but they remain significantly higher than rates in other developed countries. The teen pregnancy rate in the United States is nearly twice that in Canada and Great Britain, for example, and approximately 4 times that in France, 5 times that in Germany, and 9 times that in the Netherlands. The teen abortion rate in the United States is nearly 8 times higher than in Germany, 7 times higher than in the Netherlands, and 3 times higher than in France. The rate of gonorrhea

How old should people be when they become sexually active? The answer depends on the personal values, beliefs, and experiences of the individuals involved.

among U.S. teens is more than 50 times higher than the rate in the Netherlands or France; rates of HIV infection, syphilis, and chlamydia among teens are also much higher in the United States. Levels of sexual activity and age at first intercourse do not differ significantly in these countries but that sexually active U.S. teens are less likely to use any contraceptive method and particularly less likely to use one of the more effective hormonal methods.

Reports by the Alan Guttmacher Institute and Advocates for Youth have noted some attitudes and programs in other developed countries that may help explain their lower teen pregnancy rates:

• Childbearing is strongly regarded as adult behavior, to be considered when young people have completed their education, are in stable relationships, and are financially independent from their parents. This attitude is weaker and varies across regions and groups in the United States.

• Young people who are sexually active are expected to protect themselves and their partners from pregnancy and STDs, and state or public schools typically provide comprehensive information about prevention. More than one-third of U.S. school districts currently provide abstinence-only sexuality education.

• In many European countries, governments support large, long-term public education campaigns promoting responsible sexual behavior. These campaigns are direct and humorous, focus on safety and pleasure, and utilize many outlets, including the Internet, television, films, radio, and billboards.

• Young people in other developed countries typically have easier access to contraceptives and reproductive

health services than do young people in the United States. Contraceptives are typically free or are inexpensive through national health insurance. U.S. teens may encounter logistical, financial, or legal barriers to contraceptive access. Some states have or are considering parental notification laws that would apply to minors seeking prescription contraceptives at family planning clinics. Surveys indicate that such laws are likely to increase the number of teens using no contraception or less effective over-the-counter contraceptives.

Sexuality and contraceptive education remains a volatile issue. Studies show that sexually active students who receive comprehensive sexuality education are more likely to use contraceptives and that those who are not sexually active are not encouraged to initiate having sex. Abstinence-only school programs, on the other hand, do not appear to reduce the number of teens who are having sex. Although a great deal of focus has been placed on HIV and STDs prevention, the nearly 1 million U.S. teenage pregnancies that occur each year are a serious public health problem and warrant much greater national attention.

WHICH CONTRACEPTIVE METHOD IS RIGHT FOR YOU?

The process of choosing and using a contraceptive method can be complex and varies from one couple to another. Each person must consider many variables in deciding which method is most acceptable and appropriate for her or him. Key considerations include those listed here:

1. *Health risks.* Is there anything in your personal or family medical history that would affect your choice of method? For each method you consider, what are the potential health risks that apply to you? For example, IUDs are not recommended for young women without children because of an increased risk of pelvic infection and subsequent infertility. Hormonal methods should be used only after a clinical evaluation of your medical history. Other methods have only minor and local side effects. Talk with your physician about the potential health effects of different methods for you.

2. *The implications of an unplanned pregnancy.* How would an unplanned pregnancy affect you and your future? What are your feelings regarding the options— abortion, adoption, or raising a child? If effectiveness is of critical importance to you, carefully consider the ways the effectiveness of each method can be improved. Abstinence is 100% effective, if maintained. If used correctly, hormonal methods offer very good protection against pregnancy. Barrier methods can be combined with spermicides to improve their effectiveness.

3. *STD risk.* How likely are you to be exposed to any sexually transmitted diseases? Have you and your

If you are sexually active, you need to use the contraceptive method that will work best for you. A number of factors may be involved in your decision. The following questions will help you sort out these factors and choose an appropriate method. Answer yes (Y) or no (N) for each statement as it applies to you and, if appropriate, your partner.

_____ 1. I like sexual spontaneity and don't want to be bothered with contraception at the time of sexual intercourse.

_____ 2. I need a contraceptive immediately.

_____ 3. It is very important that I do not become pregnant now.

_____ 4. I want a contraceptive method that will protect me and my partner against sexually transmitted diseases.

_____ 5. I prefer a contraceptive method that requires the cooperation and involvement of both partners.

_____ 6. I have sexual intercourse frequently.

_____ 7. I have sexual intercourse infrequently.

_____ 8. I am forgetful or have a variable daily routine.

_____ 9. I have more than one sex partner.

_____ 10. I have heavy periods with cramps.

_____ 11. I prefer a method that requires little or no action or bother on my part.

_____ 12. I am a nursing mother.

_____ 13. I want the option of conceiving immediately after discontinuing contraception.

_____ 14. I want a contraceptive method with few or no side effects.

If you answered yes to the statements whose numbers are listed in the left-hand columns below, the method in the right-hand columns might be a good choice for you.

1, 3, 6, 10, 11, 12*	Oral contraceptives	2, 5, 7, 8, 12, 13, 14	Vaginal spermicides and sponge
1, 3, 6, 8, 10, 11	Contraceptive patch, vaginal ring	5, 7, 12, 13, 14	Diaphragm and spermicide, cervical cap
1, 3, 6, 8, 10, 11, 12*	Contraceptive injectables	5, 7, 13, 14	FAM and withdrawal
1, 3, 6, 8, 11, 12, 13	IUD		
2, 4, 5, 7, 8, 9, 12, 13, 14	Condoms (male and female)		

12*Progestin-only hormonal contraceptives (the minipill and Depo-Provera injections) are safe for use by nursing mothers; contraceptives that include estrogen are not usually recommended.

Your answers may indicate that more than one method would be appropriate for you. To help narrow your choices, circle the numbers of the statements that are *most* important for you. Before you make a final choice, talk with your partner(s) and your physician. Consider your own lifestyle and preferences, as well as the features of each method (effectiveness, side effects, costs, and so on). For maximum protection against pregnancy and STDs, you might want to consider combining two methods. It's also a good idea to be prepared for change; the method that seems right for you now may be inappropriate if your circumstances become different.

partner been screened for STDs recently? Have you openly and honestly discussed your past sexual behavior? Condom use is of critical importance whenever any risk of STDs is present. This is especially true when you are not in an exclusive, long-term relationship or when you are taking the pill, because cervical changes that occur during hormone use may increase vulnerability to certain diseases. Abstinence or activities that don't involve intercourse or any other exchange of body fluids can be a satisfactory alternative for some people.

4. *Convenience and comfort level.* How do your partner and you view each of the methods? Which would you most likely use consistently? The hormonal methods are generally ranked high in this category, unless there are negative side effects and health risks or forgetting to take pills is a problem for you. Some people think condom use disrupts spontaneity and lowers penile sensitivity. (Creative approaches to condom use and improved quality can decrease these concerns.) The diaphragm, cervical cap, contraceptive sponge, female condom, and spermicides can be inserted before intercourse begins but are still considered a significant inconvenience by some.

5. *Type of relationship.* How easy is it for you to talk with your partner about contraception? How willing is

he or she to be involved? Barrier methods require more motivation and sense of responsibility from *each* partner than hormonal methods do. When the method depends on the cooperation of one's partner, assertiveness is necessary, no matter how difficult. This is especially true in new relationships, when condom use is most important. When sexual activity is infrequent, a barrier method may make more sense than an IUD or one of the hormonal methods.

6. *Ease and cost of obtaining and maintaining each method.* If a physical exam and clinic follow-up are required, how readily accessible is this to you? Can you and your partner afford the associated expenses of the method? Investigate the costs of different methods. Find out if your insurance covers any of the costs.

7. *Religious or philosophical beliefs.* Are any of the methods unacceptable to you because of your personal beliefs? For some, abstinence and/or FAM may be the only permissible contraceptive methods.

Whatever your needs, circumstances, or beliefs, *do* make a choice about contraception. Not choosing anything is the one method known *not* to work. (To help make a choice that's right for you, take the quiz in the box "Which Contraceptive Method Is Right for You and Your Partner?") This is an area in which taking charge of your health has immediate and profound implications for your future. The method you choose today won't necessarily be the one you'll want to use your whole life or even next year. But it should be one that works for you right now.

SUMMARY

- Barrier methods of contraception physically prevent sperm from reaching the egg; hormonal methods are designed to prevent ovulation, fertilization, and/or implantation; and surgical methods permanently block the movement of sperm or eggs to the site of conception.

- The choice of contraceptive method depends on effectiveness, convenience, cost, reversibility, side effects and risk factors, and protection against STDs. The concept of effectiveness includes failure rate and continuation rate.

- Hormonal methods may include a combination of estrogen and progestins or progesterone alone. Hormones may be delivered via pills, patch, vaginal ring, implants, or injections.

- Hormonal methods prevent ovulation, inhibit the movement of sperm, and affect the uterine lining so that implantation is prevented.

- The most commonly used emergency contraceptives are two-dose regimens of OCs. In some states, pharmacists can now dispense these pills without a prescription.

- How IUDs work is not clearly understood; they may cause biochemical changes in the uterus, affect movement of sperm and eggs, or interfere with the implantation of the egg in the uterus.

- Male condoms are simple to use, immediately reversible, and provide STD protection; female condoms are available but are more difficult to use.

- The diaphragm, Lea's Shield, cervical cap, and contraceptive sponge cover the cervix and block sperm from entering; all are used with or contain spermicide.

- Vaginal spermicides come in the form of foams, creams, jellies, suppositories, and film.

- So-called natural methods include abstinence, withdrawal, and fertility awareness method (FAM); the latter is based on avoiding intercourse during the fertile phase of a woman's menstrual cycle.

- Combining methods can increase contraceptive effectiveness and help protect against STDs.

- Vasectomy—male sterilization—involves severing the vasa deferentia. Female sterilization involves severing or blocking the oviducts so that the egg cannot reach the uterus.

- Key issues in contraception include decisions about when it is OK to have sex, gender differences in the significance of contraception to women and men, and sexuality education and contraception accessibility for teens.

- Issues to be considered in choosing a contraceptive include the individual health risks of each method, the implications of an unplanned pregnancy, STD risk, convenience and comfort level, type of relationship, the cost and ease of obtaining and maintaining each method, and religious or philosophical beliefs.

1.   **Visit a health care provider:** Make an appointment with a physician or other health care provider to review the health risks of different contraceptive methods as they apply to you. For each method, determine whether any risk factors associated with its use apply to you or your partner.

2.   **Visit a drugstore:** Visit a local drugstore and make a list of the contraceptives sold there, along with their prices. Next, investigate the costs of prescription contraceptive methods by contacting your physician, medical clinic, and/or pharmacy. Estimate the annual cost of regular use for each method, and rank the methods from most to least expensive.

3.   **Develop a public service campaign:** Devise a public service campaign that will encourage men to become more involved in contraception. Your campaign might use techniques such as TV and print advertisements, radio announcements, and posters. Look at other public service campaigns and advertisements for ideas. What sorts of images do you think would be motivational? What sort of tone and message do you think would be most effective?

For More Information

Books

Guillebaud, J. 2004. *Contraception Today.* New York: Martin Dunitz. *Although written for clinicians, also serves as a good reference book for nonprofessionals seeking information on contraceptives.*

Hatcher, R. A., et al. 2004. *Contraceptive Technology,* 18th ed. New York: Ardent Media. *A reliable source of up-to-date information on contraception.*

Hatcher, R. A., et al. 2004. *A Pocket Guide to Managing Contraception, 2004–2005.* Tiger, Ga.: Bridging the Gap Foundation. *An easy-to-use, reliable source of contraceptive information.*

Hatcher, R. A., et al. 2005. *Safely Sexual,* 2nd ed. New York: Ardent Media. *Realistic recommendations on the prevention of unplanned pregnancy, as well as HIV infection and other STDs.*

Tone, A. 2001. *Devices and Desires: Men, Women, and the Commercialization of Contraception in the United States.* New York: Hill & Wang. *An engaging history of contraception in America.*

V W Organizations, Hotlines, and Web Sites

The Alan Guttmacher Institute. A nonprofit institute for reproductive health research, policy analysis, and public education.
   212-248-1111
   http://www.agi-usa.org

Ann Rose's Ultimate Birth Control Links Page. A Web site with information on methods of birth control and decision-making strategies.
   http://www.ultimatebirthcontrol.com

Association of Reproductive Health Professionals. Offers educational materials about family planning, contraception, and other reproductive health issues; the Web site includes an interactive questionnaire to help people choose contraceptive methods.
   202-466-3825
   http://www.arhp.org

Emergency Contraception Hotline. Provides information and referrals.
   888-NOT-2-LATE

Emergency Contraception Web Site. Provides extensive information about emergency contraception; sponsored by the Office of Population Research at Princeton University.
   http://www.not-2-late.com

It's Your Sex Life. Provides information about sexuality, relationships, contraceptives, and STDs; geared toward teenagers and young adults.
   http://www.itsyoursexlife.com

Kaiser Family Foundation: Women's Health Policy: Contraception. Provides information and reports focused on how policies impact reproductive health care and access to contraceptives.
   http://www.kff.org/womenshealth/contraception.cfm

Managing Contraception. Provides brief descriptions and tips for using many forms of contraception.
   http://www.managingcontraception.com

Planned Parenthood Federation of America. Provides information on family planning, contraception, and abortion and provides counseling services.
   800-230-PLAN
   http://www.plannedparenthood.org

Reproductive Health Online (Reproline). Presents information on contraceptive methods currently available and those under study for future use.
   http://www.reproline.jhu.edu

The following are some of the many organizations focusing on family planning and reproductive health issues worldwide:

Family Health International
   http://www.fhi.org

Global Reproductive Health Forum at Harvard
   http://www.hsph.harvard.edu/Organizations/healthnet

International Planned Parenthood Federation
   http://www.ippf.org

Safe Motherhood
   http://www.safemotherhood.org

United Nations Population Fund
   http://www.unfpa.org

WHO World Health Day 2005: Make Every Mother and Child Count
   http://www.who.int/world-health-day/2005/en

See also the listings for Chapters 5, 7, 8, and 18.

Althuis, M. D., et al. 2003. Hormonal content and potency of oral contraceptives and breast cancer risk among young women. *British Journal of Cancer* 88(1): 50–57.

Baldasti, E., B. Wimmer-Puchinger, and K. Loschke. 2003. Acceptability of the long-term contraceptive levonorgestrel-releasing intrauterine system (Mirena): A 3-year follow-up study. *Contraception* 67(2): 87–91.

Barone, M. A., et al. 2004. Characteristics of men receiving vasectomies in the United States, 1998–1999. *Perspectives on Sexual and Reproductive Health* 36(1): 27–33.

Bennett, S. E., and N. P. Assefi. 2005. School-based teenage pregnancy prevention programs: A systematic review of randomized controlled trials. *Journal of Adolescent Health* 36(1): 72–81.

Berenson, A. B., et al. 2004. Effects of hormonal contraception on bone mineral density after 24 months of use. *Obstetrics and Gynecology* 103(5 Pt 1): 899–906.

Burkman, R., et al. 2004. Safety concerns and health benefits associated with oral contraception. *American Journal of Obstetrics and Gynecology* 190(4 Suppl): 5–22.

Burkman, R. T., 2004. The transdermal contraceptive system. *American Journal of Obstetrics and Gynecology* 190(4 Suppl): S49–53.

Cates, W., and M. J. Steiner. 2002. Dual protection against unintended pregnancy and sexually transmitted infections: What is the best contraceptive approach? *Sexually Transmitted Diseases* 29(3): 168–174.

Chan, W. S., et al. 2004. Risk of stroke in women exposed to low-dose oral contraceptives: A critical evaluation of the evidence. *Archives of Internal Medicine* 164(7): 741–747.

Consistent condom use is key to prevention. 2002. *International Family Planning Perspectives* 28(2): 57.

Cooper, M. L. 2002. Alcohol use and risky sexual behavior among college students and youth: Evaluating the evidence. *Journal of Studies on Alcohol* 63(2): 101–117.

Cox, B., et al. 2002. Vasectomy and risk of prostate cancer. *Journal of the American Medical Association* 287(23): 3110–3115.

Delves, P. J., et al. 2002. Antifertility vaccines. *Trends in Immunology* 23(4): 213–219.

Gallo, M. F., et al. 2004. Combination estrogen-progestin contraceptives and body weight: Systematic review of randomized controlled trials. *Obstetrics and Gynecology* 103(2): 359–373.

Gold, M. A., et al. 2004. The effects of advance provision of emergency contraception on adolescent women's sexual and contraceptive behaviors. *Journal of Pediatric and Adolescent Gynecology* 17(2): 87–96.

Harper, C. C., et al. 2004. Tolerability of levonorgestrel emergency contraception in adolescents. *American Journal of Obstetrics and Gynecology* 191(4): 1158–1163.

Hatcher, R. A., et al. 2004. *Contraceptive Technology*, 18th ed. New York: Ardent Media.

Henzl, M. R., and M. L. Polan. 2004. Avoiding menstruation: A review of health and lifestyle issues. *Journal of Reproductive Medicine* 49(3): 162–174.

Herndon, E. J., and M. Zieman. 2004. New contraceptive options. *American Family Physician* 69(4): 853–860.

Hubacher, D. 2002. The checkered history and bright future of intrauterine contraception in the United States. *Perspectives on Sexual and Reproductive Health* 34(2): 98–103.

International Medical Advisory Panel. 2004. IMAP statement on emergency contraception. *International Planned Parenthood Federation Medical Bulletin* 38(1): 1–3.

Johansson, E. D. 2004. Future developments in hormonal contraception. *American Journal of Obstetrics and Gynecology* 190(4 Suppl): 69–71.

Johansson, E. D., and R. Sitruk-Ware. 2004. New delivery systems in contraception: Vaginal rings. *American Journal of Obstetrics and Gynecology* 190(4 Suppl): 54–59.

Jones, R. K., et al. 2005. Adolescents' reports of parental knowledge of adolescents' use of sexual health services and their reactions to mandated parental notification for prescription contraception. *Journal of the American Medical Association* 293(3): 340–348.

Jones, R. K., J. E. Darroch, and S. K. Henshaw. 2002. Contraceptive use among U.S. women having abortions in 2000–2001. *Perspectives on Sexual and Reproductive Health* 34(6): 294–303.

Kaiser Family Foundation. 2004. *Fact Sheet: Emergency Contraceptive Pill.* Menlo Park, Calif.: Kaiser Family Foundation.

Kaufman, M. 2004. Experts not behind reversal on Plan B: FDA bowed to politics, critics say. *San Francisco Chronicle*, 18 June, A4.

Kulczycki, A., et al. 2004. The acceptability of the female and male condom: A randomized crossover trial. *Perspectives on Sexual and Reproductive Health* 36(3): 114–119.

Lane, T. 2003. High proportions of college men using condoms report errors and problems. *Perspectives on Sexual and Reproductive Health* 35(1).

Litt, I. F. 2005. Placing emergency contraception in the hands of women. *Journal of the American Medical Association* 293(1): 98–99.

Maher, J. E., et al. 2004. Acceptability of the vaginal diaphragm among current users. *Perspectives on Sexual and Reproductive Health* 36(2): 64–71.

Marchbanks, P. A., et al. 2002. Oral contraceptives and the risk of breast cancer. *New England Journal of Medicine* 346(26): 2025–2032.

Moodley, J. 2004. Combined oral contraceptives and cervical cancer. *Current Opinions in Obstetrics and Gynecology* 16(1): 27–29.

Raine, T. R., et al. 2005. Direct access to emergency contraception through pharmacies and effect on unintended pregnancy and STIs. *Journal of the American Medical Association* 293(1): 54–62.

Roddy, R. E., et al. 2002. Effect of nonoxynol-9 on urogenital gonorrhea and chlamydial infection: A randomized controlled trial. *Journal of the American Medical Association* 287(9): 1117–1122.

Rodrigues, I., F. Grou, and J. Joly. 2001. Effectiveness of emergency contraceptive pills between 72 and 120 hours after unprotected sexual intercourse. *American Journal of Obstetrics and Gynecology* 184(4): 531–537.

Schildkraut, J. M., et al. 2002. Impact of progestin and estrogen potency in oral contraceptives on ovarian cancer risk. *Journal of the National Cancer Institute* 94(1): 32–38.

Scholes, D., et al. 2005. Change in bone mineral density among adolescent women using and discontinuing depot medroxyprogesterone acetate contraception. *Archives of Pediatrics and Adolescent Medicine* 159(2): 139–44.

Shafii, T., et al. 2004. Is condom use habit forming? Condom use at sexual debut and subsequent condom use. *Sexually Transmitted Diseases* 31(6): 366–372.

Sonfield, A. 2004. New refusal clauses shatter balance between provider "conscience," patient needs. *The Guttmacher Report on Public Policy* 7(3).

Spitzer, W. O., et al. 2002. Myocardial infarction and third generation oral contraceptives: Aggregation of recent studies. *Human Reproduction* 17(9): 2307–2314.

Tanne, J. H. 2005. Abstinence only programmes do not change sexual behaviour, Texas study shows. *British Medical Journal* 330(7487): 326.

Trussell, J., et al. 2004. The role of emergency contraception. *American Journal of Obstetrics and Gynecology* 190(4 Suppl): 30–38.

Walsh, T. L., et al. 2003. Evaluation of the efficacy of a nonlatex condom: Results for a randomized, controlled clinical trial. *Perspectives on Sexual and Reproductive Health* 35(2): 79–86.

7

Looking AHEAD

After reading this chapter, you should be able to

- Describe the history and current legal status of abortion in the United States

- Explain the current debate over abortion, including the main points of the pro-choice and pro-life points of view

- Describe the methods of abortion available in the United States

- List possible physical and psychological effects of abortion

- Discuss the decision-making process a woman and her partner may go through when facing an unintended pregnancy

Abortion

1. **About what percentage of abortions in the United States take place in the first 12 weeks of pregnancy?**
   a. 60%
   b. 70%
   c. 80%
   d. 90%

2. **A majority of Americans are in favor of the right to a legal abortion in some circumstances.**
   True or false?

3. **About how many American women have an abortion in any given year?**
   a. 1 in 1000
   b. 1 in 100
   c. 1 in 50

4. **About 25% of all pregnancies in the United States are unintended, and about 25% of unintended pregnancies are terminated by abortion.**
   True or false?

5. **Abortion rates have risen considerably in European countries where medical abortion is widely available.**
   True or false?

ANSWERS

1. D. About 90% of all abortions take place in the first 12 weeks of pregnancy; nearly 60% take place in the first 8 weeks.

2. TRUE. Current polls indicate that about 24% of Americans favor the right to legal abortion in all circumstances, and an additional 56% favor the right in some circumstances. About 19% of Americans think that abortion should be illegal in all circumstances.

3. C. At current rates, about 40% of American women will have had at least one abortion by the time they are 45 years old.

4. FALSE. About half of all pregnancies in the United States are unintended, and about half of these are terminated by abortion.

5. FALSE. A recent study of abortion rates in France, Great Britain, and Sweden showed no increase in overall abortion rates despite the increasing use of abortion-inducing drugs such as mifepristone (RU-486).

Visit the *Core Concepts in Health* Online Learning Center (www.mhhe.com/insel10e) for study aids and many additional resources.

183

In the United States today, few issues are as complex and emotion-filled as abortion. Although most public attention has focused on legal definitions and restrictions, the most difficult aspects of abortion actually take place at a much more personal level. Because the majority of women having abortions are young, many college students have had some type of direct exposure to these more personal experiences of abortion. They are in a key position to understand and address the contributing factors as well as the broad effects of unintended pregnancies and abortion. Instead of simply attempting to legislate certain behaviors, they can choose to grapple with the complex human factors that go into the prevention as well as the "treatment" of unintended pregnancy. This chapter will provide basic information on abortion, including the current focuses of controversy. We hope it will act as a springboard for you to form your own views and, more important, personal plans for constructive action.

THE ABORTION ISSUE

The discussion that follows presents various perspectives on abortion. The word **abortion**, by strict definition, means the expulsion of an embryo or fetus from the uterus before it is sufficiently developed to survive. As commonly used, however, *abortion* refers only to those expulsions that are artificially induced by mechanical means or drugs, and *miscarriage* is generally used for a spontaneous abortion, one that occurs naturally with no causal intervention. In this chapter, *abortion* will mean a deliberately induced expulsion.

The History of Abortion in the United States

For more than two centuries, abortion policy in the United States followed English common law, which made the practice a crime only when performed after "quickening" (fetal movement that begins at about 20 weeks). There was little public objection to this policy until the early 1800s, when an anti-abortion movement began, led primarily by physicians who questioned the doctrine of quickening and who objected to the growing practice of abortion by untrained persons (in part because it weakened their control of medical services).

This anti-abortion drive gained minimal attention until the mid-1800s, when newspaper advertisements for

abortion preparations became common and concern grew that women were using abortion as a means of birth control (and perhaps to cover up extramarital activity). There was much discussion about the corruption of morality among women in the United States, and by the 1900s abortion was illegal in every state. These anti-abortion laws stayed in effect until the 1960s, when courts began to invalidate them on the grounds of constitutional vagueness and violation of the right to privacy (see the box "Timeline of Selected Key Abortion Decisions and Legislation").

Current Legal Status

In 1973, the U.S. Supreme Court made abortion legal in the landmark case of *Roe v. Wade*. To replace the restrictions most states still imposed at that time, the justices devised new standards to govern abortion decisions. They divided pregnancy into three parts, or trimesters, giving a pregnant woman less choice about abortion as she advances toward full term. In the first trimester, the abortion decision must be left to the judgment of the pregnant woman and her physician. During the second trimester, similar rights remain but a state may regulate factors that protect the health of the woman, such as type of facility where an abortion may be performed. In the third trimester, when the fetus is viable (capable of survival outside of the uterus), a state may regulate and even bar all abortions except those considered necessary to preserve the mother's life or health.

Since 1973, repeated campaigns have been waged to overturn the *Roe v. Wade* decision and to ban abortion altogether. Although abortion remains legal throughout the United States, rulings by the Supreme Court in 1989 (*Webster v. Reproductive Health Services*) and 1992 (*Planned Parenthood of Southeastern Pennsylvania v. Casey*) allow states to regulate abortion throughout pregnancy as long as an "undue burden" is not imposed on women seeking the procedure. As a result, states have passed a variety of laws that have had the effect of reducing women's access to abortion. These laws include bans on the use of public funding, employees, and facilities for abortion services; mandatory counseling and waiting periods; insurance prohibitions; and requirements for parental consent for minors.

In addition to state abortion restrictions, the U.S. Congress has barred the use of federal Medicaid funds to pay for abortions, except when a woman's life is in danger or in cases of rape or incest. Currently, only 15 states provide nonfederal public money to assist some poor women seeking medically necessary abortions. Concerns have been raised that a two-tiered system has been created—one for women with means and another for those without. The overall abortion rate declined 11% between 1994 and 2000, but the rate among women of low socioeconomic status rose during this period. Women below

Term

VIW **abortion** The expulsion or removal of an embryo or fetus from the uterus.

1700s to mid-1800s Abortion is generally legal throughout the United States.

Mid-1800s to mid-1900s Abortion becomes illegal in all 50 states, with certain exceptions that vary by state (for example, to save the life of the mother). The federal Comstock Act of 1873 makes it illegal to distribute or possess information about, or devices or medications for, contraception or abortion.

1965 *Griswold v. Connecticut:* The Supreme Court overturns a law prohibiting use of contraceptives by married couples, stating that it violates the right of marital privacy guaranteed in the Bill of Rights.

1967–1973 Some states rewrite their abortion laws, including four states that repeal abortion bans.

1972 *Eisenstadt v. Baird:* The Supreme Court overturns a law banning distribution of contraceptives to unmarried adults, stating that the ban violates the equal protection clause of the constitution.

1973 *Roe v. Wade:* The Supreme Court strikes down a Texas law banning abortion and rules that abortion is encompassed within the constitutional right to privacy. The court divides pregnancy into three trimesters and states that during the first trimester, decisions about abortion should be left up to the woman and her physician. After the first trimester, states may regulate abortion in ways related to maternal health; once the fetus is viable, states

may regulate or ban abortion except when abortion is necessary to preserve the life or health of the mother.

1976 *Planned Parenthood of Central Missouri v. Danforth:* The Supreme Court rules against a statute that requires married women to obtain their spouse's approval before having an abortion and requires minors to obtain written parental consent.

1980 *Harris v. McRae:* The Supreme Court upholds restrictions on Medicaid funding for abortions except as needed to protect the life of the mother or in other special circumstances.

1986 *Thornburgh v. American College of Obstetricians and Gynecologists:* The Supreme Court strikes down a law requiring any woman seeking an abortion to receive a state-scripted lecture from her physician about potential risks and possible alternatives.

1989 *Webster v. Reproductive Health Services:* The Supreme Court upholds a state law prohibiting the use of public facilities for abortions that are not medically necessary and requiring physicians to do viability testing on fetuses of more than 20 weeks' gestation.

1991 *Rust v. Sullivan:* The Supreme Court rules that clinics receiving federal Title X (family planning) funding can be prohibited from counseling, referring, or providing information about abortions.

1992 *Planned Parenthood of Southeastern Pennsylvania v. Casey:* The Supreme Court upholds the *Roe* decision but allows states to restrict abortion access as long as the restrictions do not impose

an undue burden on women seeking abortions. It upholds a provision requiring minors to obtain consent from one parent or a judge (judicial bypass) to obtain an abortion.

1994 Congress passes the Freedom of Access to Clinics Act, making it a crime to injure, intimidate, or interfere through threats, force, or physical obstruction with a woman's right to obtain reproductive health services, including abortion.

2000 The FDA approves mifepristone (RU-486), the abortion pill.

2000 *Stenberg v. Carhart:* The Supreme Court finds a law banning partial-birth abortion unconstitutional because it lacks an exception for the health of the mother and imposes an undue burden on women seeking abortions.

2003 Congress passes and President Bush signs the Partial Birth Abortion Ban Act with no exception to the ban in cases of risk to a woman's health.

2004 The Partial Birth Abortion Ban Act is declared unconstitutional by federal judges in San Francisco, New York, and Lincoln, Nebraska; the decisions are expected to be appealed to the Supreme Court.

SOURCES: Cornell University Legal Information Institute. 2004. *U.S. Supreme Court Decisions* (http://supct.law.cornell.edu/supct/; retrieved November 15, 2004), CBS News. 2004. *Abortion Timeline* (http://www.cbsnews.com/htdocs/abortion/timeline.html; retrieved November 15, 2004); National Public Radio. 2003. *History of the Abortion Debate: Timeline of Significant Supreme Court Decisions* (http://www.npr.org/news/specials/roevwade/timeline.html; retrieved November 15, 2004).

the federal poverty threshold have an abortion rate more than four times higher than higher income women.

Opponents of abortion, unsuccessful so far in their efforts to see *Roe v. Wade* overturned or a constitutional amendment passed to outlaw abortion, have recently focused on specific methods of abortion. For example, many states and the U.S. Congress have passed legislation outlawing a particular method of late-term abortion referred to by abortion opponents as "partial birth abortion." (*Partial birth abortion* is a nonmedical term for a rarely used abortion method discussed later in this chapter.) However, a Nebraska ban on partial birth abortion was struck down in a 5 to 4 decision by the Supreme Court in June 2000 (*Stenberg v. Carhart*). A similar federal ban (the Partial Birth Abortion Act of 2003) was declared unconstitutional by three federal judges, but additional legislative and legal action on this issue is likely.

Voting for political candidates with well-defined views on abortion is one way individuals can influence the legal status of abortion in the United States.

Legal and legislative efforts have also targeted medications that can be used to induce abortion. The drug mifepristone (RU-486) was used extensively for years in other countries to perform nonsurgical early abortions before being approved for use in the United States. Mifepristone is discussed in detail later in the chapter.

Both pro-choice and pro-life groups are likely to remain active, seeking to advance their positions both by promoting legislation and by supporting political candidates who share their views.

Moral Considerations

Along with the legal debates are ongoing arguments between pro-life and pro-choice groups regarding the ethics of abortion (see the two "The Opposing Views" boxes). Central to the pro-life position is the belief that the fertilized egg must be valued as a human being from the moment of conception and that abortion at any time is equivalent to murder. This group holds that any woman who has sexual intercourse knows that pregnancy is a possibility, and should she willingly have intercourse and get pregnant, she is morally obligated to carry the pregnancy through. Pro-life followers encourage adoption for women who feel they are unable to raise the child and point out how many couples are seeking babies for adoption. Pro-life individuals do not consider the availability of legal abortion as essential to women's well-being but view it instead as having an overall destructive effect on our traditional morals and values.

In contrast, the pro-choice viewpoint holds that distinctions must be made between the stages of fetal development and that preserving the fetus early in pregnancy (or *gestation*) is not always the ultimate moral concern.

Members of this group maintain that women must have the freedom to decide whether and when to have children; they argue that pregnancy can result from contraceptive failure or other factors out of a woman's control. (All contraceptive methods except abstinence have the potential for failure.) When pregnancy does occur, pro-choice individuals believe that the most moral decision possible must be determined according to each situation and that, in some cases, greater injustice would result if abortion were not an option. If legal abortions were not available, pro-choice supporters say, "back-alley shops" and do-it-yourself techniques, with their many health risks, as well as the births of unplanned children, would again grow in number. Others argue that discrimination in health care would result, since wealthy women could more easily make the travel arrangements necessary for a legal abortion elsewhere.

Some people strongly identify exclusively with either the pro-life or the pro-choice stance, but many have moral beliefs that are blurred, less defined, and in some cases a mixture of the two. Many people instinctively feel that the fetus gains increasing human value as a pregnancy advances. In this view, early abortion, especially before the 8th week, is acceptable, whereas later abortion, when the fetus appears more like an infant, is unacceptable. Although the most vocal groups in the abortion debate tend to paint a black-and-white picture, the majority of Americans view abortion as a complex issue without any easy answers.

Public Opinion

In general, U.S. public opinion on abortion seems to change depending on the specific situation. Many individuals approve of legal abortion as an option when destructive health or welfare consequences could result from continuing pregnancy, but they do not advocate abortion as a simple way out of an inconvenient situation. Overall, most adults in the United States continue to approve of legal abortion and are opposed to overturning the basic right to abortion established in *Roe v. Wade* (Figure 7-1, p. 189). But the amount of public support varies considerably depending on the circumstances surrounding the abortion request (Table 7-1, p. 190).

For example, people who feel that abortion should be available in early pregnancy often question at which stage in later pregnancy the fetus's rights should take precedence over the woman's rights. The 1973 U.S. Supreme Court decision considered viability the key criterion in establishing the point beyond which a woman's right to choose abortion becomes markedly restricted. In 1973, viability was generally considered to be about 26–28 weeks. Today it is about 24 weeks, with isolated cases of survival at 23 weeks. Although neonatal intensive care units continue to advance technologically, most

In Focus

The Opposing Views: Pro-Choice

Nancy Keenan

Pro-choice is not pro-abortion. Pro-choice is pro-freedom, pro-family and pro-children. Pro-choice is about the right to make the most personal private decisions without intrusion from the government. Pro-choice is about the lives, health, and well being of women; it is about the right to decide whether and when to have children. No other issue has more impact on women's ability to chart the course of their own lives.

No matter how strong the outer protection of love, marriage, income and stability, each pregnancy comes down to a separate judgment for each woman. No one wants an abortion. For many women the decision of whether or not to have an abortion is wrapped in questions of morality, religion, and ethics. But no matter how the decision is made, a woman's right to make this decision should be guaranteed.

Yet anti-choice politicians would reduce a real woman's real dilemma into a black and white line in a law book or a court ruling. They would reduce her and her future to the margins of her own situation. They would strip her of her own power and her own body. The situation of that woman affects us all, the loss of her rights means the loss of everyone's rights—male or female—whether we could ever imagine ourselves in that situation or not.

Standing up for a woman's right to choose does not mean ignoring the implications of that decision. Indeed, we must rededicate ourselves to making sure that as few women as possible face that choice.

Reducing the need for abortions should be everyone's goal, no matter which side of the debate they are on. We should all agree that the best approach is to make abortion less necessary by promoting access to birth control—including emergency contraception—and comprehensive, age appropriate, sex education that combines information about abstinence with other ways to prevent unintended pregnancy. The result of chipping away these basic preventative steps is more unintended pregnancies and more abortions.

More than thirty years after *Roe v. Wade,* the pro-choice movement is still fighting to protect and defend a woman's constitutional right to choose. Unlike the other rights we expect as Americans, this is not one we can take for granted. In 1973 the question before the Supreme Court in *Roe* was: Who should make the deeply personal decision about pregnancy and childbirth? The answer: the woman. In their decision the Supreme Court upheld the belief of pro-choice Americans that decisions about a woman's reproductive health are a personal and private matter, one that should be between a woman, her doctor, her family, and her god—not the government.

Young Americans have grown up in an environment of freedom and limitless possibility. However, this freedom is systematically being chipped away at by politicians in Washington, DC and numerous state capitals. Opponents of choice are trying not only to take away the right to choose an abortion but have launched an attack against birth control as well. They are urging pharmacists to stop filling birth control prescriptions—even for married women, even when they need the pills not only for contraception but to treat other medical conditions as well. The FDA ignored recommendations from scientists, doctors, and its own advisory panel and denied women access to Plan-B, an emergency contraception that if taken within 72 hours could prevent half of all unintended pregnancies and therefore prevent many abortions. It is decisions like these that place ideology over science that jeopardize women's health. All women deserve access to a full range of reproductive health care, including contraception, healthy childbearing, adoption, and abortion.

Pro-choice means trusting women, not politicians, to make personal, private decisions. It means respecting a zone of privacy and the autonomy of the individual. Being pro-choice means valuing women's health and the Constitutional right that protects it. And respecting the values of Americans' views on the topic compels us to give women the tools they need to make abortion rarer.

Nancy Keenan is president of NARAL Pro-Choice America, www.ProChoiceAmerica.org. Reprinted with permission.

---

experts feel that viability cannot be expected beyond this limit.

Other individuals associate fetal rights not with viability but with earlier developmental characteristics such as the onset of heartbeat, brain size, and nervous system maturity. Still others believe that the moment of conception is the only critical point to consider. For them, all other developmental stages are irrelevant to the abortion debate. As can be seen from such wide variation of opinion, objective measures of humanness and clear-cut guidelines regarding fetal rights are elusive, and decisions remain ambiguous.

Although opinions vary as to whether, or when, abortion rights should be tightly regulated by law, most people agree that abortions done later in pregnancy present more difficulties in personal, medical, philosophical, and social terms. Of all abortions done after the 12th week of gestation, about 30% are performed on teenagers. Possible explanations include teenagers' ignorance, denial, fear, and lack of supportive family or friends, as well as state regulatory hurdles faced by teenagers. Other typical recipients of late abortions include low-income women, who may have more difficulty finding suitable facilities as well as necessary funds, and women nearing menopause who fail to recognize a delayed period as pregnancy. Another small group of women who may seek late abortion includes those who have learned through genetic tests that the fetus has a specific abnormality.

J. C. Willke, M.D.

In considering abortion, the first question to ask is: What is this that grows within the woman? Is this human life? Or when will it be? If it's not human life, then a case can be made to permit abortion. If, however, this being is fully human, sexed, alive, complete, and intact from the first-cell stage, then a second human life exists and we have a collision of the rights of two humans.

So, first, let's ask: Is this human life? The answer lies in books on biology, embryology, and fetology. In these sciences there is no disagreement on the facts of when human life begins. At the union of sperm and ovum there exists a living, single-celled, complete human organism. It is already male or female, is alive and growing, and is human, as the 46 human chromosomes in the cell's nucleus mark this microscopic being as a member of the human family. This is arguably the most complicated cell in the entire world; it contains more information than could be contained in all of NASA's computers. As this single-celled human organism divides and subdivides, each cell in turn contains progressively less information, is more specialized.

At 1 week of life, this embryonic human attaches to the nutrient lining of the woman's womb and soon sends into her body a hormonal message that stops her period. About 4 days after the time when the woman's period would have begun, the embryo's heart begins to beat. At 40 days, brain waves can be recorded. By 10 weeks, the structure of the body is completely formed. By 3 months, all organ systems are functioning. To deny that fully human life begins at fertilization is to deny the known facts of fetal development and biological science.

Some argue that life existed in the sperm and ovum and will exist in the future. True, but we are not asking about generic life, but rather about this one unique individual's human life, which begins at fertilization and ends at death.

Some would measure the beginning of human life with a theologic yardstick,

speaking of soul, God, and creation. In a secular state, however, we cannot use a theologic belief to define when human life begins for the purpose of making laws that either protect or allow the destruction of that life.

Others use various philosophical definitions of when the fullness of humanness exists, such as when cognition and self-consciousness are possible, when love is exchanged, when a being is declared to be "humanized" or "socialized," or when certain biological mileposts are reached. Though these definitions are arrived at by intellectual processes, they cannot be scientifically proven. Open to disagreement among people of good will, these definitions are also beliefs. We should not impose either religious or philosophical beliefs upon others in our culture. If one defines human life from the facts of natural science, then human life, complete and intact, begins at fertilization. That is a fact that we must face and work with.

Because this is human life from the very moment of conception, the issues touching that life are those of civil rights and human rights and the laws protecting those rights.

Let's ask a second question: Should there be equal protection under the law for all living humans? Or should the law discriminate fatally against entire classes of humans, in this case against those still living in the womb?

Interestingly enough, our nation faced a similar situation once before—slavery. In 1857, the Supreme Court ruled in the Dred Scott case that black people were not legal persons before the law. They were the property of the slave owner, who could buy, sell, or even kill them. Abolitionists' protests were countered: "Now look, you find slavery morally offensive? Well, you don't have to own a slave. But don't force your morality on the owner, for he has the constitutional right to choose to own a slave." In 1973, the Court did it again. In *Roe v. Wade,* also by a 7 to 2 margin, it ruled that unborn

people were not legal persons. They were the property of the owner (the mother), who could keep or kill. Pro-lifers objected, to hear the same response. "Look, you find abortion morally offensive. Well, you don't have to have one. But don't force your morality on the owner (the woman), for she now has the constitutional right to choose, to kill."

The *Dred Scott* decision discriminated by skin color; *Roe v. Wade* discriminates by place of residence: still living in the womb. Each is a civil rights outrage.

A woman has a right to her own body, but to say that the little passenger residing within her is a part of her body is to utter a biological absurdity.

But she does not want this child? Since when does anyone's right to live depend upon someone else wanting them? Killing the unwanted is a monstrous evil.

A woman's issue? Women make up the overwhelming majority in the pro-life movement, and opinion polls consistently show more opposition to abortion from females than from males.

So, should a woman have the right to choose? I have a right to free speech, but not to shout "fire" in a theater. A person's right to anything stops when it injures or kills another living human.

No one should minimize the problems of pregnant women. With adequate counseling, informed consent, and the involvement of parents, husbands, and friends, we can help solve most of their problems—but sadly, never all of them. The pivotal question is: Should any civilized nation give to one citizen the absolute legal right to kill another to solve that first person's personal problem? I think not. We must give women far more help, both privately and publicly, than is available today. But we simply cannot continue to solve their personal problems by allowing the ghastly violence of killing tiny, innocent humans.

J. C. Wilke, M. D. is president of the Life Issues Institute and The International Right to Life Federation. Reprinted by permission.

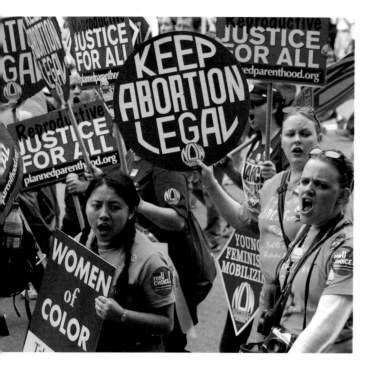

Pro-choice groups believe that the decision to end or continue a pregnancy is a personal matter that should be left up to the individual.

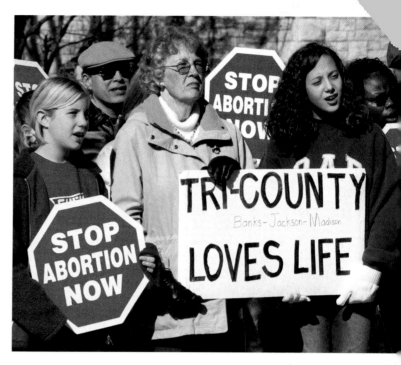

Pro-life groups oppose abortion on the basis of their belief that life begins at the moment of conception.

Personal Considerations

For the pregnant woman who is considering abortion, the usual legal and moral arguments may sound meaningless as she attempts to weigh the many short- and long-term ramifications for all lives directly concerned. If she chooses abortion, can she accept that decision in terms of her own religious and moral beliefs? What are her long-range feelings likely to be regarding this decision? What are her partner's feelings regarding abortion, and how will she deal with his response? Does she have a supportive relative or friend who will help her through this time of emotional adjustment? Which medical facility offering abortions would be most suitable for her? What about transportation and costs? (Figures 7-2 and 7-3 present statistical information about women who choose abortion.)

For the woman who decides against abortion and chooses instead to continue the pregnancy, there are other questions. If she decides to raise the child herself, will she

W VITAL STATISTICS

Figure 7-1 Public opinion about abortion.
The graph represents responses to this question: Do you think abortions should be legal under any circumstances, legal only under certain circumstances, or illegal in all circumstances? SOURCE: Gallup Organization. 2004. *Gallup Poll Tuesday Briefing: Abortion* (http://www.gallup.com/content/print.aspx?ci=1574; retrieved September 7, 2004).

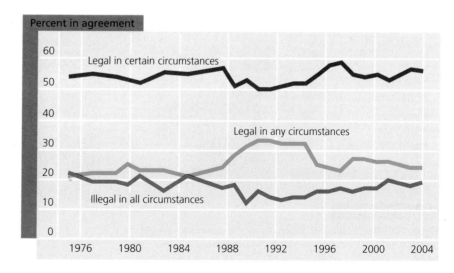

Table 7-1 | Views on Abortion

1. Should abortion be legal in the following circumstances?

	Yes
The woman's life is endangered.	85%
The woman's physical health is endangered.	77%
The pregnancy was caused by rape or incest.	76%
The woman's mental health is endangered.	63%
There is evidence that the baby is physically or mentally impaired.	56%
The woman or family cannot afford to raise the child.	35%

2. Should abortion be legal during the following stages of pregnancy?

	Yes
In the first 3 months	66%
In the second 3 months	25%
In the last 3 months	10%

SOURCE: Gallup Organization. 2004. *Gallup Poll Tuesday Briefing: Abortion* (http://www.gallup.com/content/print.aspx?ci=1576; retrieved September 7, 2004).

have the resources to do it well? Is a supportive, lasting relationship with her partner likely? If not, how does she feel about being a single parent? Are family members available to help with the many demands of child rearing? If she is young, what will be the effects on her own growth? Will she be able to continue with her educational and personal goals? What about the ongoing financial responsibilities?

If the pregnant woman considers adoption, she will have to try to predict what her emotional responses will be throughout the full-term pregnancy and the adoption process. What are her long-range feelings likely to be? What is the best setting for her during her pregnancy? How can she best maintain continuity with the rest of her life and her long-term goals? What type of adoption would be most appropriate? (The box "The Adoption Option" addresses some of these questions.)

Current Trends

Clearly, all responses to unintended pregnancy can be difficult, including abortion and especially late abortion. Fortunately, with the increased accessibility to legalized abortion following the mid-1970s, the rate of late abortions

Figure 7-2   Distribution of abortions by the woman's age and by the weeks of gestation.   SOURCE: Centers for Disease Control and Prevention. 2004. Abortion surveillance—United States, 2001. *Morbidity and Mortality Weekly Report Surveillance Summaries* 53 (SS-9).

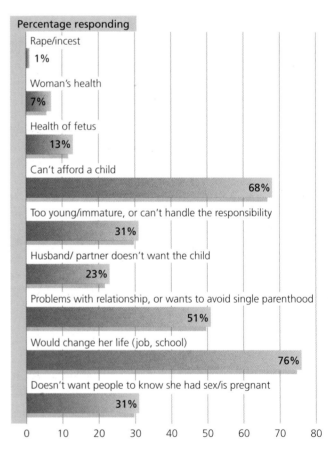

Figure 7-3   The reasons women choose abortions.   The respondents in this study were allowed to give more than one answer.
SOURCE: Data from the Alan Guttmacher Institute.

One of the options available to a woman facing an unplanned pregnancy is adoption. Between 1952 and 1972, nearly 9% of unmarried pregnant women gave their children up for adoption; currently, however, only about 2% of women choose to place a child for adoption. This decline is probably due to a variety of factors, including increased rates of contraceptive use and an easing of the social stigma of single parenthood. The drop in adoption rates in the 1970s probably reflected an increase in the abortion rate following the 1973 legalization of abortion; however, since 1990 adoption rates have remained steady, while the abortion rate has declined, indicating that women are not choosing abortion over adoption. Women who place their children for adoption tend to come from higher socio-economic backgrounds and to have higher levels of educational attainment than those who choose to keep their babies or have an abortion. They are also likely to have greater educational and vocational goals for themselves than those who keep their children. Often, women who choose adoption come from supportive families who assist them throughout the experience.

If you are pregnant and considering adoption, make sure you explore all possibilities before you make a final choice. The decision to go through an unwanted pregnancy and then give the baby to another family is difficult and takes tremendous love, maturity, and courage. Adoption is permanent: The adoptive parents will raise your child and have legal authority for his or her welfare. Think about your life now and in the future as you weigh alternatives. There are many people who can help you consider your options, including your partner, friends, family members, or a professional counselor at a crisis pregnancy center, a family planning clinic, or a family services, social services, or adoption agency. A counselor should always treat you with respect and be willing to discuss all your options with you—keeping the baby, having an abortion, or arranging an adoption. If you aren't comfortable with a particular counselor, find a different one.

There are two types of adoptions, confidential and open. In confidential adoption, the birth parents and the adoptive parents never know each other. Adoptive parents will be given any information, such as medical information, that they would need to help take care of the child. A later meeting between the child and birth parents is possible in confidential adoption, however, if the birth parents leave information with the agency or lawyer who handled the adoption and/or in a national adoption registry.

In an open adoption, the birth parents and adoptive parents know something about each other. There are different levels of openness, ranging from reading a brief description of prospective adoptive parents to meeting them and sharing full information. Birth parents may also be able to arrange to stay in touch with the family over the years, by visiting, calling, or writing. Some women feel that an open adoption enables them to keep in touch with a baby they will always love; others feel that this would be too difficult and decide against contact with the adoptive family.

In all states, you can work with a licensed child-placing (adoption) agency. In most, you can also work directly with an adopting couple or their attorney; this is called a private or independent adoption. Prospective adoptive parents can be located through personal ads, a physician, adoptive parent support groups, national matching services, and family members and friends. To find an agency or lawyer who will arrange the type of adoption you want, ask about their rules and procedures. For example, will you receive financial help and counseling? Will you be able to have the amount of information about the adoptive parents and the amount of contact with the baby that you want? If your baby is a child of color and it is important to you that the adoptive parents are of the same ethnic or racial background, ask if the agency or attorney has such families approved and waiting for placement. Some agencies specialize in finding families for children of color.

You will also need to consider the reaction and rights of the birth father. A woman can choose to have an abortion without the consent or knowledge of the father, but once the baby is born, the father has certain rights. These rights vary from state to state, but, at a minimum, most states require that the birth father be notified of the adoption. In some states, the birth father may be able to take the child even if the mother prefers that the child go to an adoptive family.

As with abortion, there are emotional and physical risks associated with pregnancy, childbirth, and adoption. Throughout the adoption process, make sure that you have the help you need and that you carefully consider all your options. Deciding how to handle an unplanned pregnancy is important, and you have the power to make your own decisions.

SOURCES: National Adoption Information Clearinghouse. 2000. *Are You Pregnant and Thinking About Adoption?* (http://naic.acf.hhs.gov/pubs/f_pregna.cfm; retrieved November 16, 2004); National Adoption Information Clearinghouse. 2000. *Placing Children for Adoption* (http://naic.acf.hhs.gov/pubs/s_place.cfm; retrieved November 16, 2004).

dropped steadily, until fewer than 2% of all abortions were performed at more than 20 weeks and fewer than 12% at more than 12 weeks by the 1990s. The overall abortion *rate* rose during most of the 1970s, leveled off around 1980, and decreased in the 1990s (Figure 7-4, p. 192). As much as 43% of the decline in abortion between 1994 and 2000 may be attributable to the use of emergency contraception (see Chapter 6). Possible future influences on the number, rate, and timing of abortions in the United States include legal decisions, more widespread availability of emergency contraceptives, and the increasing use of medical abortion.

Since the 1989 *Webster* and 1992 *Casey* decisions, many states have imposed additional restrictions on

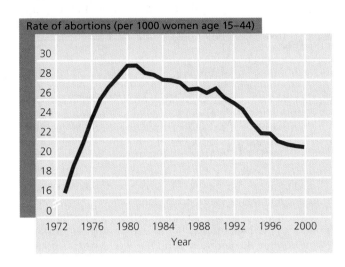

Figure 7-4 Number and rate of abortions in the United States. SOURCE: Finer, L. B., and S. K. Henshaw. 2003. Abortion incidence and services in the United States in 2000. *Perspectives on Sexual and Reproductive Health* 35(1): 6–15.

abortion. In 2004, 29 states required mandatory counseling, in 26 states followed by a waiting period; 34 states required parental consent or notification for minors; more than half of the states banned certain abortion procedures; and 35 states severely restricted the use of public funds for abortion. Overall, the number of state laws restricting abortion has more than quadrupled since 1995. Research into the effects of these restrictions has been mixed. Some studies indicate that parental consent and notification laws may result in minors traveling out of state to obtain abortions. Mandatory delay laws have been found to influence the number and timing of abortions. Further research is needed to establish whether these types of restrictions constitute an undue burden for women seeking abortions.

Adding to the legal restrictions is the growing scarcity of physicians willing to provide abortion services. Currently, 87% of all U.S. counties, 96% of nonmetropolitan counties, and about 57% of metropolitan areas have no abortion providers. It is unclear whether the approval of mifepristone for medical abortion will significantly affect these numbers. The diminishing number of providers is due in part to increased anti-abortion protests and violence, including arson, bombings, and the murders of several physicians and clinic workers. Women living in areas that have restrictive laws and few abortion providers may continue to obtain abortions, but they are likely to face significant increases in expense and time delays. If the constitutional right to abortion is to be maintained, these obstacles need to be carefully considered.

Unless accompanied by a greater effort at preventing unwanted pregnancy, legal changes alone will probably not dramatically reduce the number of abortions. At current rates, about 40% of American women will have had at least one abortion by the time they are 45 years old. Based on national research, the typical American woman having an abortion is age 20–30, has a previous birth, has never been married, is poor, lives in a metropolitan area, and is Christian. For a broader perspective, see the box "Abortion Around the World."

We hope the recent surge of public interest in sexual behavior, largely due to the fear of STDs, will lead to more open discussions of sexuality and contraception for individuals who choose to be sexually active. With more communication and a better understanding of one's personal need for intimacy and closeness, individuals and couples can perhaps make informed, responsible decisions about the best way to meet those needs. For those who choose to include sexual intercourse as part of their relationships, contraception should be made readily available and be correctly used (see Chapter 6). Other measures that might help decrease the demand for abortion include the following economic and social reforms: increased options for working women, more dual parenting, maternal/paternal leaves, improved child care facilities, and quality prenatal and postnatal care available for all people regardless of socioeconomic status.

METHODS OF ABORTION

Abortion methods can be divided into two categories: surgical and medical. Surgical abortion is by far the most common, accounting for about 98% of all abortions

As one would expect, the legal status, availability, and safety of abortion vary widely around the world. Of the approximately 46 million abortions performed each year worldwide, about 26 million are legal and 20 million illegal (see the figure).

- 25% of the world's people live in countries where laws ban abortion entirely or permit it only to save the life of a pregnant woman. In more than 100 countries, abortion is not permitted in cases of rape or incest.

- 14% of the world's people live in countries with somewhat less restrictive laws that permit abortion to protect a pregnant woman's physical or mental health.

- 61% of the world's people live in countries where abortion is permitted either for a wide range of reasons or without restriction as to reason. Many of these countries do have regulations or restrictions such as third-party authorizations, waiting periods, or mandatory counseling, and many place limits on gestational age and the types of facilities where abortions can be performed.

Even in countries where abortion is illegal, women still undergo abortions. In fact, many countries with strict anti-abortion laws have high rates of abortion and, because most procedures are carried out secretly in unsafe conditions, high rates of serious complications. Nearly all of the 70,000 abortion-related deaths each year occur in countries with strict abortion laws. Almost all occur in developing countries. Worldwide, nearly one in ten pregnancies ends in an *unsafe* abortion. In countries where abortion is legal, widely available at low cost, and performed under safe conditions, abortion rates are relatively low and serious complications rare. (Widespread availability of contraception is another factor associated with low rates of abortion.)

Legal status is not the sole determinant of the availability of safe abortion services, however. How the laws are interpreted and enforced can be just as critical. For example, in some countries that allow abortion for mental health reasons, the law is interpreted to allow the majority of women seeking abortions to obtain them; in other countries with comparable laws, few abortions are allowed. Enforcement also varies. For example, in Mozambique, where abortion is officially banned, women can obtain abortions on request at many hospitals, and abortion-related legal charges are rarely filed. In other countries, laws are strictly enforced, and both women who have abortions and abortion providers are prosecuted. It is estimated that two-thirds of women currently in prison in Nepal have been convicted of undergoing illegal abortions. Strict enforcement of anti-abortion laws tends to disproportionately affect poor women because wealthier women can pay to obtain discreet, safe abortions from private physicians, thus avoiding the more tightly regulated public hospitals.

The attitudes and beliefs of the medical community also influence the availability of abortion services. For example, in Nigeria, many physicians will perform abortions in spite of legal bans because the medical community believes in the need for safe abortion services. On the flip side, major medical associations in Poland and the Republic of Ireland have adopted guidelines that are stricter than their country's laws.

The number and location of abortion providers and the cost of abortion services also influence the true availability of abortion in a particular country, regardless of its actual legal status. Community and physician opposition to abortion has left parts of the United States, Austria, and Germany without abortion providers, despite the fact that abortion is legal in all three countries. In contrast, policies in Denmark go beyond just permitting safe abortion to ensuring that services are widely available: There, each county must have at least one hospital that has the capacity to perform abortions, and services are free.

SOURCES: World Health Organization. 2004. *Unsafe Abortion: Global and Regional Estimates of the Incidence of Unsafe Abortion and Associated Mortality in 2000.* Geneva: World Health Organization; Berer, M. 2000. Making abortions safe: A matter of good public health policy and practice. *Bulletin of the World Health Organization* 78(5): 580–592; Henshaw, S. K., S. Singh, and T. Hass. 1999. The incidence of abortion worldwide. *International Family Planning Perspectives* 25: S30–S38; Rahman, A., L. Katzive, and S. K. Henshaw. 1998. A global review of laws on induced abortion, 1985–1997. *International Family Planning Perspectives* 24(2): 56–64.

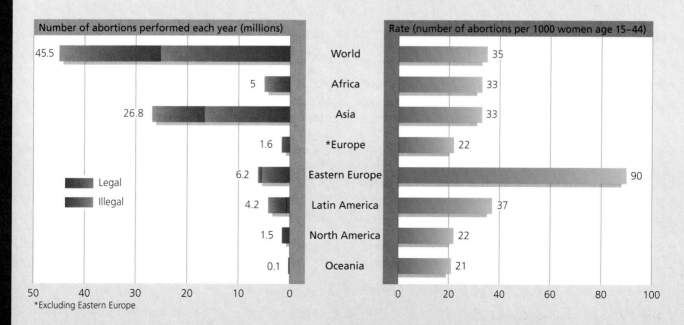

performed in the United States. Medical abortion, in which medications are used to induce abortion, may become more common following the approval in 2000 of mifepristone (RU-486, or Mifeprex). Emergency contraception—pills taken or IUDs inserted immediately after unprotected sexual intercourse—are generally not considered abortifacients (agents that produce abortion) from a medical viewpoint, because they act before implantation of the fertilized egg, if one is present (see Chapter 6). Therefore, these topics are not discussed here.

Suction Curettage

First developed in China in 1958, **suction curettage** (also called *vacuum aspiration*) is the most common method for abortions performed from the 6th to the 12th week of pregnancy. It is used in about 90% of all abortions performed in the United States. The procedure can be done quickly, usually on an outpatient basis, and the risk of complications is small.

A sedative may be given, along with a **local anesthetic.** A speculum is inserted into the vagina, and the cervix is cleansed with a surgical solution. The cervix is dilated and a suction curette, a specially designed hollow tube, is then inserted into the uterus (Figure 7-5). The curette is attached to the rubber tubing of an electric pump, and suction is applied. In 20–30 seconds, the uterus is emptied. Moderate cramping is common during evacuation. To ensure that no fragments of tissue are left in the uterus, the doctor usually scrapes the uterine lining with a metal curette, an instrument with a spoonlike tip. The entire suction curettage procedure takes only 5–10 minutes.

After a few hours in a recovering area, the woman can return home. She is usually instructed not to have intercourse or use tampons for several weeks after the abortion and to return for a 2-week postabortion examination. This follow-up exam is important to verify that

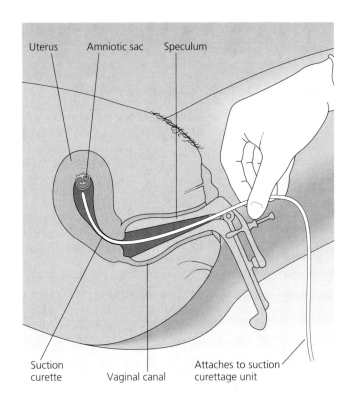

Figure 7-5 labels: Uterus | Amniotic sac | Speculum | Suction curette | Vaginal canal | Attaches to suction curettage unit

Figure 7-5   Suction curettage. This procedure takes 5–10 minutes and can be performed up to the 12th week of pregnancy.

the abortion was complete and that no signs of infection are present.

Manual Vacuum Aspiration

Accurate and easy-to-use home pregnancy tests have made it increasingly common for women to know they are pregnant at very early stages of gestation, just at the time of a missed period. If a pregnant woman seeking an abortion is only 4 or 5 weeks past the time of her last period, she is sometimes told to wait several weeks before having the procedure. This is because suction curettage is believed to be safer and more effective when performed at least 6 or 7 weeks after the last menstrual period. A relatively new option for women at the very earliest stages of pregnancy is a surgical procedure called **manual vacuum aspiration (MVA).** This method is not available in all clinics, but as more experience is gained with the procedure, MVA may become increasingly available to women who desire very early surgical abortion.

In MVA, the cervix is dilated, and a plastic tube attached to a handheld syringe is inserted through the cervix. The uterus is emptied with gentle suction provided by the syringe. Careful inspection of the aspirated material is critical to ensure that the gestational sac has been removed. Ultrasonography and follow-up pregnancy

Terms

Vïw

suction curettage Removal of the embryo or fetus by means of suction; also called *vacuum aspiration.*

local anesthetic A drug that blocks the nerves carrying pain sensations to the brain; in abortion and childbirth, the nerves running from the pelvic area to the brain are affected while the woman is left awake and alert.

manual vacuum aspiration (MVA) The vacuum aspiration of uterine contents shortly after a missed period using a handheld syringe.

dilation and evacuation (D & E) The method of abortion most commonly used between 13 and 24 weeks of pregnancy. Following dilation of the cervix, both vacuum aspiration and curettage instruments are used as needed.

testing are also used to make sure that the abortion is complete.

Abortion After the First Trimester

Only about 1 in 10 abortions is performed after the 12th week of pregnancy. The method most commonly used for abortion from 13 to 24 weeks of pregnancy is **dilation and evacuation (D & E)**. The cervix is opened using dilators, which gradually expand the cervix overnight while the woman is at home. The next day, the uterus is emptied using surgical instruments and the aspirating machine. The more advanced the pregnancy, the higher the incidence of complications.

Partial birth abortion is a nonmedical term for a particular type of D & E. In this procedure, the fetal limbs and body are delivered first and then the skull is collapsed to allow it to pass more easily through the cervix. This procedure is performed only rarely, but it can be useful in the presence of particular fetal anomalies such as severe hydrocephalus (a condition in which fluid collects around the brain, causing brain damage and an enlarged head). This procedure has been the target of abortion opponents.

Labor induction is another infrequently used method of late abortion. Prostaglandins, chemicals that cause uterine contractions, are used to induce labor, sometimes in conjunction with injections of salt or urea into the uterus. The delivery of the fetus usually occurs in 6–24 hours. The woman is hospitalized during this process. Fewer than 1% of abortions performed in the United States use the induction method.

Medical Abortion

Ending a pregnancy with medications rather than surgery is an option for women who are in the early phase of pregnancy. Medical abortion is generally used in very early pregnancy, within 49 days of the last menstrual period. The combination of drugs that is given causes the embryo and products of conception to be passed out through the vagina, as in a natural miscarriage. An ultrasound may be performed before giving the medication to make sure that the pregnancy dates are accurate, because complication rates for medical abortion are higher if the pregnancy is more advanced.

Advantages and Disadvantages of Medical Abortion
Medical abortion is generally safer than surgical abortion because it involves no anesthesia or surgical risks. Some women feel that medical abortion allows them to take more control of the procedure and gives them more privacy than a surgical abortion would. Medical abortion can also be done very early in pregnancy.

The major disadvantages of medical abortion are that the process takes days or even weeks to complete (early surgical abortion generally takes less than an hour and can be done under sedation) and that bleeding after the procedure is often heavier and lasts longer than with surgical abortion. A woman selecting medical abortion needs to be prepared for cramping and bleeding, which can sometimes be painful. This can occur at inconvenient times, so it is important to have help at home and to be able to leave work or school, if necessary. Medical abortion also generally requires more clinic visits (three) than surgical abortion. The cost to the patient is generally about the same.

Drugs Used for Medical Abortion
Mifepristone, misoprostol, and methotrexate are three widely used drugs for medical abortion. Mifepristone blocks the effect of progesterone that is produced by the ovaries after implantation of the fertilized egg. The loss of progesterone support causes the uterine lining and any fertilized egg to shed. Mifepristone is currently approved for use up to 49 days following the last menstrual period, but studies show that it can be effective up to 63 days following the last menstrual period. A woman takes a dose of mifepristone and follows it up two days later with a second drug, the prostaglandin analog misoprostol, which induces contractions. The two-drug regimen has a rate of completed abortion of about 92–95%; the success rate is highest early in pregnancy.

Side effects include nausea, vomiting, diarrhea, and abdominal pain. Vaginal bleeding is often more prolonged than with surgical abortion (9–16 days), but total blood loss is similar. In a few cases, bleeding is heavy, and a follow-up suction curettage is necessary to complete the abortion in a small percentage of women. This is generally done in the emergency room at the hospital, or at a clinic. With mifepristone and misoprostol, abortion can take anywhere from a few hours to several weeks; about 50% of abortions occur within 4 hours, and 75% within 24 hours. Two weeks after taking mifepristone, a woman must return to her health care provider for a follow-up visit to ensure that the abortion is complete.

Another drug, methotrexate, can also be used with prostaglandin for early medical abortion. Methotrexate has been approved by the FDA for cancer treatment since 1953 and is also commonly used to treat rheumatoid arthritis. Although not approved specifically for early abortion, it has been used for that purpose. Methotrexate stops the embryonic or fetal cells from dividing; it is followed by a dose of prostaglandin in a regimen similar to that for mifepristone. With this combination of drugs, 80–85% of women will abort within 2 weeks; up to 95% will abort within 30 days. Because mifepristone acts more quickly than methotrexate and is slightly more effective, it is likely that mifepristone will become the preferred medication for medical abortion.

COMPLICATIONS OF ABORTION

Along with questions regarding the actual procedure of abortion, many people have concerns about possible aftereffects. More information is gradually being gathered on this important subject.

Possible Physical Effects

The incidence of immediate problems following an abortion (infection, bleeding, trauma to the cervix or uterus, and incomplete abortion requiring repeat curettage) varies widely. The potential for problems is significantly reduced by a woman's good health, early timing of the abortion, use of the suction method, performance by a well-trained clinician, and the availability and use of prompt follow-up care.

Problems related to infection can be minimized through preabortion testing and treatment for gonorrhea, chlamydia, and other infections. Some clinicians routinely give antibiotics after an abortion, while others treat only those women who have a history or current symptoms of pelvic infection. Postabortion danger signs are

- Fever above 100°F
- Abdominal pain or swelling, cramping, or backache
- Abdominal tenderness (to pressure)
- Prolonged or heavy bleeding
- Foul-smelling vaginal discharge
- Vomiting or fainting
- Delay in resuming menstrual periods (6 weeks or more)

Some cramping and bleeding are an expected part of ending a pregnancy. In rare cases, life-threatening bleeding, infections, or other problems can occur following a miscarriage, surgical abortion, or medical abortion. Prompt medical attention should be sought if heavy bleeding, severe abdominal pain, or fever occurs. Excessive bleeding during or after an abortion is rare with early suction curettage. In later-stage pregnancies, the use of uterus-contracting medication significantly reduces the risk of bleeding. Some pain medications may increase bleeding, so patients should check with their physician about appropriate medications for postoperative pain.

Incomplete abortion means that some pregnancy tissue has remained in the uterus. With this condition, or when blood clots form in the uterus shortly after an abortion, severe cramping and signs of infection can occur, and a repeat suction curettage is usually needed. On rare occasions, a pregnancy may continue after an incomplete abortion. The recommended follow-up exam is important to establish that the abortion was complete.

Missed ectopic pregnancy is another potentially serious problem that can surface after an abortion. Surgical abortion techniques remove tissue from the uterus but will miss an ectopic pregnancy developing outside of the uterus. If an ectopic pregnancy goes untreated, the embryo can eventually become large enough to rupture the fallopian tube, causing potentially catastrophic bleeding. Tissue removed during an abortion is normally examined for evidence that the gestational sac or embryo has been removed. If there is any doubt, ultrasound and follow-up pregnancy testing can reveal whether an ectopic pregnancy is present.

Studies on long-term complications—subsequent infertility, spontaneous second abortions, premature delivery, and babies of low birth weight—have not revealed any major risks with the most common abortion methods. The risk of postabortion infertility seems to be very low, especially when any signs of infection are reported and treated promptly. There is also apparently no effect on the outcome of future pregnancies when an early suction curettage is performed with minimal cervical dilation; with later abortions and with repeated or multiple abortions, there is only a slight risk, if any. Studies of medical abortion have also shown no adverse effects on the outcome of a subsequent pregnancy. For Rh-negative women, dangerous sensitization (the buildup of antibodies) can be minimized by an injection of Rh-immune globulin given within 72 hours of the procedure.

A few studies have reported that women who have abortions have an increased risk of breast cancer. However, a well-designed study of 1.5 million Danish women found no connection between a woman's abortion history and her risk of breast cancer. A 2003 workshop convened by the National Cancer Institute and a 2004 analysis published in the journal *Lancet* also concluded that having an abortion or miscarriage does not increase a woman's subsequent risk of breast cancer.

The overall risk of death is low. Mortality rates have decreased substantially since abortion was legalized in 1973 (Table 7-2).

Possible Psychological Effects

After an exhaustive review completed in 1988, the then surgeon general, C. Everett Koop, concluded that the available evidence failed to demonstrate either a negative or a positive long-term impact of abortion on mental health. More recent research has resulted in the same general conclusion. The psychological side effects of abortion are less clearly defined than the physical ones. Responses vary and depend on the individual woman's psychological makeup, family background, current personal and social relationships, cultural attitudes, and many other factors. A woman who has specific goals with a somewhat structured life pattern may be able to incorporate her decision to have an abortion as the unequivocally best and acceptable course more easily than a woman who feels uncertain about her future.

Table 7-2	Abortion Risks

	Risk of Death in Any Given Year
Legal abortion	
Before 9 weeks	1 in 262,800
9–12 weeks	1 in 100,100
13–15 weeks	1 in 34,400
After 15 weeks	1 in 10,200
Illegal abortion	1 in 3,000
Pregnancy and childbirth	1 in 10,000

SOURCES: Hatcher, R. A., et al. 2004. *Contraceptive Technology,* 18th ed. New York: Ardent Media; Carlson, K. J., S. A. Eisenstat, and T. Ziporyn. 2004. *The New Harvard Guide to Women's Health.* Cambridge, Mass.: Harvard University Press.

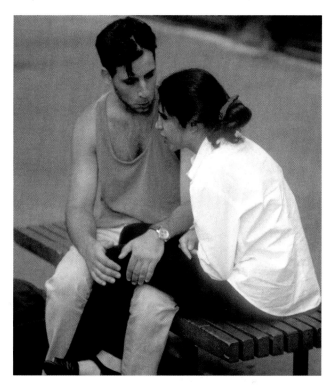

When an unintended pregnancy occurs, both partners can weigh important considerations and together choose an appropriate course of action.

Although many women experience great relief after an abortion and virtually no negative feelings, some go through a period of ambivalence. Along with relief, they often feel a mixture of other responses, such as guilt, regret, loss, sadness, and/or anger. When a woman feels she was pressured into sexual intercourse or into the abortion, she may feel bitter. If she had strongly believed abortion to be immoral, she may wonder if she is still a good person. Many of these feelings are strongest immediately after the abortion, when hormonal shifts are occurring; such feelings often pass quite rapidly. Others take time to resolve and fade only slowly. It is important for a woman to realize that a mixture of feelings is natural.

For a woman who does experience psychological or emotional effects after an abortion, talking with a close friend or family member can be very helpful. Supportive people can help her feel positive about herself and her decision. Although a legal and common procedure in the United States, abortion is still treated very secretively in most of our society, so it is easy for a woman to feel isolated and alone. Some women may specifically seek out other women who have had an abortion. Many clinical centers that offer abortions make such peer counseling available. Other women find they can identify with case histories in books written on abortion, which can help them deal with their own reactions. In a few cases, unresolved emotions may persist, and a woman should seek professional counseling.

DECISION MAKING AND UNINTENDED PREGNANCY

When faced with an unintended pregnancy, women differ greatly in their approach to decision making (see the box "Personal Decisions About Abortion"). Unprotected sexual intercourse may be followed immediately by a vague sense of anxiety. When symptoms of pregnancy appear, some women—especially young women—respond with denial, ascribing the delayed menstruation and other signs to other causes. Several days or weeks may elapse before the woman finally has the pregnancy confirmed (a major cause of late abortions). After a positive test, women often feel a mixture of anxiety, depression, guilt, and anger, sometimes tinged with some anticipation and delight. The actual decision making can vary widely. Some women calmly and resolutely make a choice within a very short time, while others, feeling panic and chaos, wrestle with the decision for several weeks. For some women, it is the first time in their lives that they feel unable to find the right answer and instead must settle for a best although difficult, solution.

The response of a woman's partner can have a significant influence on how she experiences an unintended pregnancy. Men's emotional reactions can vary considerably. Some withdraw and choose to remain completely detached; others simply press for the most expedient solution (usually abortion). Still others feel very emotionally involved and wish to play an active role in decision making. Partners can be very helpful, both in weighing important considerations and in actually helping with the chosen course of action. Some couples find that an abortion experience draws them closer

Susan

Susan was a first-year college student who was caught up in her new academic and social activities. Bill (another student) and she had been dating for about 3 months, when one evening she decided to take a chance and not use contraception because she had just finished her menstrual period. When her next period was 2 weeks overdue, she had a pregnancy test. It was positive.

From the moment she found out, Susan considered only one option: abortion. "I couldn't have raised a child," she said. "And I wouldn't bring a child into the world unless I could take the responsibility for it. I think it would be worse to ruin my future and a baby's life because of a mistake." When Bill first learned of the pregnancy, he became distant, but he did agree to help pay for the abortion. Soon, however, he withdrew completely and had no further contact with Susan.

The hardest time for Susan was before the abortion, when she found herself crying frequently. She talked a lot with a close girlfriend, who went with her to the clinic and stayed with her after the abortion. Like all women who have abortions, Susan needed comforting.

After the abortion, Susan felt very strongly that she had made the best decision, but she did occasionally wonder how she would feel in future years. After meeting a new boyfriend with whom she could talk openly, Susan felt more certain than ever that she had made the right choice.

Helen

Helen was attending a junior college and working part-time when she found out she was pregnant. She and Mike had met just a couple of months before the pregnancy. They both planned to become parents at some point in their lives, but this was earlier than either of them had expected. They discussed all the options, and they agreed that getting married and keeping their child was the only acceptable solution.

Helen gave up school for the time being, and Mike took on more hours at work to help pay for the additional expense of a child. Six months after they were married, their daughter was born. Helen and Mike say that it was at this period of their life that they really got to know each other. "Our apartment was so small, we couldn't help but learn everything about each other."

It's now 8 years later, and Helen and Mike have two children. Mike works full-time but hopes to return to school and complete his degree in the future. Helen works part-time and attends evening classes twice a week. They'd like to move to a larger apartment and to travel more, but they can't afford to. "We've given up a lot, and it's still a struggle. But we're a happy family, and we know that we made the right choice for us."

Anna

Anna was shocked when she found out she was pregnant. She was sure she wasn't ready to be a parent herself; she was too young and still hadn't sorted out what she wanted from life. But Anna also felt that having an abortion would be wrong. So she decided to have the baby and put it up for adoption. "I myself am adopted, so adoption seemed a natural choice, and the best one available to me."

Her boyfriend broke up with her when she told him. But her parents were supportive and helped arrange for her baby's placement in a good home. Anna knew she would have to give up her baby as soon as it was born, but during her pregnancy she developed a powerful bond with her child. Anna delivered her son and left the hospital 3 days later. "I had to just give the baby to the nurse and walk out. My parents and I cried. I spent nine months preparing for that moment, but it was still so painful."

After a year Anna still hurts, but she doesn't regret her decision. "Keeping him would have changed my life completely, and I knew I wasn't ready to be a mother. I couldn't have given my son the kind of life I want him to have." She's proud that she went through her pregnancy. As an adopted child herself, Anna felt she owed her son the same chance that her biological mother gave her.

together; for others, it's the last straw in an already unstable relationship.

Parents can also be helpful. However, if there are serious disagreements, a stressful situation can become even more difficult. Over half of the states have parental consent or notification requirements, although there are judicial bypass procedures in which a judge can decide either that a minor is mature and can give informed consent or that an abortion would be in her best interest.

No matter which of the available options to unintended pregnancy is chosen, a series of questions is likely to arise that must be addressed (see the section "Personal Considerations" earlier in the chapter). Although a prompt decision has critical advantages, careful deliberation is important. If there are strong feelings of uncertainty or ambivalence, hasty action should be avoided.

Having a supportive confidant, such as a partner, other close friend, or family member, can be very important in sorting out complex feelings. Along with listening and offering understanding and perspective, supportive people can help find suitable medical personnel and plan financial arrangements. Once a course of action has been chosen, a sense of moving ahead usually follows, and the next step toward resolution can be taken.

Abortion is a controversial and volatile issue in our society and a difficult choice for individuals. Legal, moral, personal, and medical considerations all enter into views and decisions about abortion. You may never have to face an unintended pregnancy, but you should know what choices you would have—abortion, adoption, parenthood—as well as where you stand on the issue.

Right now you can

- Take some time to examine your feelings about becoming a parent unexpectedly.

- Take time to consider your views on the morality of abortion. Refer to the boxes in this chapter for some thoughtful ideas about the subject.

- If you are sexually active, talk to your partner about abortion. Do you have similar views and feelings, or are they different? How would you resolve a conflict?

- If you are sexually active, reexamine your contraceptive method and make sure you have made the right choice. Remember that no method of contraception is 100% effective.

SUMMARY

- The common use of the word *abortion* refers only to artificially induced expulsion of the fetus.

- Until the mid-1800s, abortion in the United States was legal if it took place before the 20th week of pregnancy; more restrictive laws passed by the various states remained in effect until they began to be invalidated by courts in the 1960s.

- The 1973 *Roe v. Wade* Supreme Court case devised new standards to govern abortion decisions; based on the trimesters of pregnancy, it limited a woman's choices as her pregnancy advanced.

- Although the Supreme Court continued to uphold its 1973 decision, it gave states further power to regulate abortion in *Webster v. Reproductive Health Services* and *Planned Parenthood of Southeastern Pennsylvania v. Casey*.

- The controversy between pro-life and pro-choice viewpoints focuses on the issue of when life begins. Pro-life groups believe that a fertilized egg is a human life from the moment of conception and that any abortion is a murder. Pro-choice groups distinguish between stages of fetal development and argue that a woman should make the final decision regarding her pregnancy.

- Overall public opinion in the United States supports legal abortion in at least some circumstances and opposes overturning *Roe v. Wade*. Opinion changes according to individual situations.

- Most people agree that abortions performed late in pregnancy present personal, medical, philosophical, and social problems.

- The woman considering abortion must think about her own religious and moral beliefs, her long-range reactions, support from others, and the cost and availability of the procedure.

- In suction curettage, the preferred method of abortion from the 6th to the 12th week of pregnancy, an electric pump is used to remove the uterine contents; also, the physician scrapes the uterine lining with a metal curette.

- Manual vacuum aspiration is the aspiration of the uterine contents using suction provided by a handheld syringe.

- The most common abortion method after the first trimester is dilation and evacuation (D & E), in which the uterus is emptied using aspiration and surgical instruments. Labor induction is used much less frequently.

- Medical abortion is performed with a combination of drugs very early in pregnancy; drugs used include mifepristone, misoprostol, and methotrexate.

- Physical complications following abortion can be minimized by overall good patient health, early timing, use of the suction method, a well-trained physician, and follow-up care.

- Psychological aftereffects of abortion vary with the individual. Many women go through a period of ambivalence; the strongest feelings usually occur immediately after the abortion. Having a supportive partner, friend, and/or family member can be helpful.

- Women who face unintended pregnancy differ in the way they make decisions; some make their choice calmly and quickly, while others struggle for weeks. It is often a matter of finding the best, not necessarily the right, solution.

Take Action

1. **Conduct an opinion survey:** Survey your classmates about their position on the abortion issue. How many people consider themselves pro-choice and how many pro-life? How strong are their opinions? What, if anything, might cause them to change their minds? Do opinions seem to depend on age, gender, or any other factor?

2. **Check your contraceptive practices:** Now that you have information about abortion, reevaluate your contraceptive practices. If they aren't adequate to prevent unintended pregnancy, make any changes you consider necessary to protect yourself and your partner.

For More Information

Books

Baer, J. S., ed. 2002. *Historical and Multicultural Encyclopedia of Women's Reproductive Rights in the United States*. Westport, Conn.: Greenwood Publishing. *Includes background on the political, legal, scientific, and cultural issues relating to abortion.*

Harris, M. M., ed. 2004. *Abortion: An Eternal Social and Moral Issue*. Farmington Hills, Mich.: Thomson Gale. *A brief reference outlining legal, political, and ethical issues.*

National Abortion and Reproductive Rights Action League Foundation. 2005. *Who Decides? A State-by-State Review of Abortion and Reproductive Rights*. Washington, D.C.: NARAL Foundation. *An in-depth annual review of the legal status of reproductive rights in the United States.*

Pertman, Adam. 2001. *Adoption Nation: How the Adoption Revolution Is Transforming America*. New York: Basic Books. *Discusses legal, social, and emotional issues relevant to adoptive parents, birth parents, and adoptees.*

W̶W̶ Organizations and Web Sites

Abortion Law Homepage. Includes an overview of the background and state of U.S abortion law, including the text of major legal decisions.

    http://hometown.aol.com/abtrbng

Alan Guttmacher Institute. Publishes books and fact sheets on reproductive health issues; its journal, *The Guttmacher Report on Public policy*, provides timely analysis of national reproductive health policy debates.

    212-248-1111

    http://www.agi-usa.org

National Abortion and Reproductive Rights Action League. Provides information on the politics of the pro-choice movement. Also provides information on the abortion laws and politics in each state.

    202-973-3000

    http://www.naral.org

National Adoption Information Clearinghouse. Provides resources on all aspects of adoption.

    888-251-0075

    http://naic.acf.hhs.gov

National Right to Life Committee. Provides information on alternatives to abortion and the politics of the pro-life movement.

    202-626-8800

    http://www.nrlc.org

Planned Parenthood Federation of America. Provides information on family planning, contraception, and abortion and provides counseling services.

    800-230-PLAN

    http://www.plannedparenthood.org.

U.S. Food and Drug Administration: Mifepristone. Provides information on the testing, labeling, and use of mifepristone.

    http://www.fda.gov/cder/drug/infopage/mifepristone

See also the listings for Chapters 5, 6, and 8.

Selected Bibliography

Alan Guttmacher Institute. 2003. *Facts in Brief: Induced Abortion* (http://www.agi-usa.org/pubs/fb_induced_abortion.html; retrieved February 20, 2003).

Alan Guttmacher Institute. 2002. *European Experience Shows That It Takes Time for Medical Abortion to Be Widely Used* (http://www.guttmacher.org/pubs/archives/nr_340302.html; retrieved September 20, 2002).

Annas, G. J. 2001. Partial-birth abortion and the Supreme Court. *New England Journal of Medicine* 344(2): 152–156.

Ashok, P. W., et al. 2005. Patient preference in a randomized study comparing medical and surgical abortion at 10–13 weeks gestation. *Contraception* 71(2): 143–8.

Beral, V., et al. 2004. Breast cancer and abortion: Collaborative reanalysis of data from 53 epidemiological studies, including 83,000 women with breast cancer from 16 countries. *Lancet* 363(9414): 1007–1016.

Boonstra, H. 2002. Mifepristone in the United States: Status and future. *Guttmacher Report on Public Policy*, August.

Broen, A. N., et al. 2004. Psychological impact on women of miscarriage versus induced abortion: A 2-year follow-up study. *Psychosomatic Medicine* 66: 265–271.

Centers for Disease Control and Prevention. 2004. Abortion surveillance—United States, 2001. *Morbidity and Mortality Weekly Report* 53(SS-9).

Chen, A., et al. 2004. Mifepristone-induced early abortion and outcome of subsequent wanted pregnancy. *American Journal of Epidemiology* 160(2): 110–117.

Christin-Maitre, S., P. Bouchar, and I. Spitz. 2000. Drug therapy: Medical termination of pregnancy. *New England Journal of Medicine* 342(13): 946–956.

Daillard, C. 2004. Courts strike "partial-birth" abortion ban; decisions presage future debates. *Guttmacher Report on Public Policy* 7(4): 1–3, 14.

Ellertson, C. 1997. Mandatory parental involvement in minors' abortions: Effects of the laws in Minnesota, Missouri, and Indiana. *American Journal of Public Health* 87(8): 1367–1374.

Espey, E., et al. 2005. Abortion education in medical schools: a national survey. *American Journal of Obstetrics and Gynecology* 192(2): 640–3.

Finer, L. B., and S. K. Henshaw. 2003. Abortion incidence and services in the United States in 2000. *Perspectives on Sexual Reproductive Health* 35(1): 6–15.

Food and Drug Administration. 2004. *Medication Guide: Mifeprex* (http://www.fda.gov/cder/drug/infopage/mifepristone/medicationguide.htm; retrieved November 15, 2004).

Fox, M. C., M. D. Creinin, and B. Harwood. 2002. Mifepristone and vaginal misoprostol on the same day for abortion from 50 to 63 days' gestation. *Contraception* 66(4): 225–229.

Grimes, D. A. 2005. Risks of mifepristone abortion in context. *Contraception* 71(3): 161.

Henshaw, S. K., and L. B. Finer. 2003. The accessibility of abortion services in the United States, 2001. *Perspectives on Sexual Reproductive Health* 35(1): 16–24.

Jones, R. K., J. E. Darroch, and S. K. Henshaw. 2002. Patterns in the socio-economic characteristics of women obtaining abortions in 2000–2001. *Perspectives on Sexual and Reproductive Health* 34(5): 226–235.

Jones, R., and S. Henshaw. 2002. Mifepristone for early medical abortion: Experiences in France, Great Britain, and Sweden. *Perspectives on Sexual and Reproductive Health* 34(3): 154–161.

Kero, A., and A. Lalos. 2004. Reactions and reflections in men, 4 and 12 months post-abortion. *Journal of Psychosomatic Obstetrics and Gynaecology* 25(2): 135–143.

Melbye, M., et al. 1997. Induced abortion and the risk of breast cancer. *New England Journal of Medicine* 336(2): 81–85.

National Abortion and Reproductive Rights Action League. 2004. *Who Decides: A State-by-State Review of Abortion and Reproductive Rights* (http://www.naral.org; retrieved November 16, 2004).

National Cancer Institute. 2003. *Cancer Facts: Abortion, Miscarriage, and Breast Cancer Risk* (http://cis.nci.nih.gov/fact/3_75.htm; retrieved November 16, 2004).

Pruitt, S. L., and P. D. Mullen. 2005. Contraception or abortion? Inaccurate descriptions of emergency contraception in newspaper articles, 1992–2002. *Contraception* 71(1): 14–21.

Rorbye, D., M. Norgaard, and L. Nilas. 2005. Medical versus surgical abortion: Comparing satisfaction and potential confounders in a partly randomized study. *Human Reproduction* 20(3): 834–838.

Schaff, E. A., S. L. Fielding, and C. Westhoff. 2002. Randomized trial of oral versus vaginal misoprostol 2 days after mifepristone 200 mg for abortion up to 63 days of pregnancy. *Contraception* 66(4): 247–250.

Shannon, C. S., et al. 2005. Multicenter trial of a simplified mifepristone medical abortion regimen. *Obstetrics and Gynecology* 105(2): 345–351.

Wiebe, E., et al. 2004. A fatal case of *Clostridium sordellii* septic shock syndrome associated with medical abortion. *Obstetrics and Gynecology* 104(5 Pt 2): 1142–1144.

Wiebe, E. R. 2001. Misoprostol administration in medical abortion. A comparison of three regimens. *Journal of Reproductive Medicine* 46(2): 125–129.

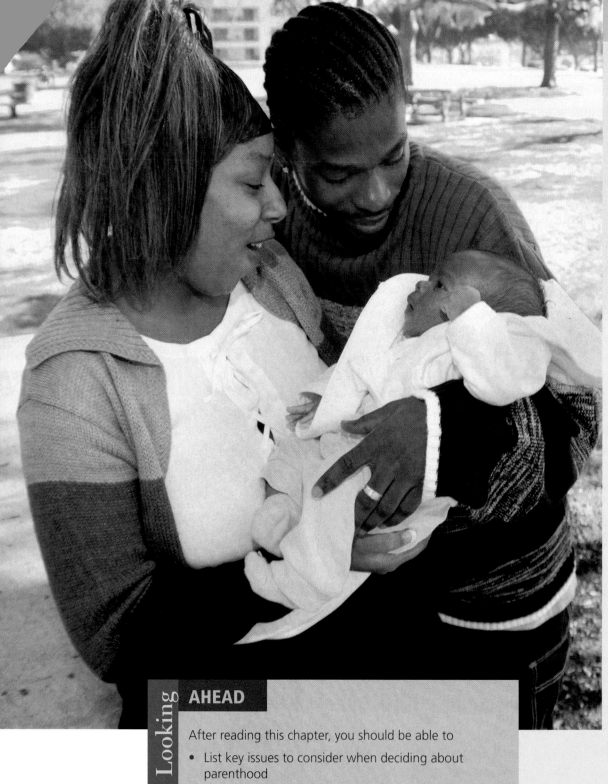

8

After reading this chapter, you should be able to

- List key issues to consider when deciding about parenthood

- Explain the process of conception, and describe the most common causes and treatments for infertility

- Describe the physical and emotional changes a pregnant woman typically experiences

- Discuss the stages of fetal development

- List the important components of good prenatal care

- Describe the process of labor and delivery

Pregnancy and Childbirth

1. **What is the approximate annual cost of raising a child born today?**
   a. $3500
   b. $6500
   c. $9500

2. **What is the leading cause of female infertility?**
   a. growths in the uterus
   b. exposure to radiation
   c. blocked fallopian tubes caused by STDs

3. **Before conception and in the early weeks of pregnancy, adequate intake of which of the following nutrients can reduce the risk of spina bifida and other neural tube defects?**
   a. iron
   b. folic acid
   c. calcium

4. **Cigarette smoking before or during pregnancy is linked to which of the following?**
   a. higher rates of infertility among men and women
   b. increased risk of low birth weight among infants
   c. decreased likelihood of having a male infant
   d. increased risk of attention-deficit/hyperactivity disorder among children exposed in utero

5. **The position in which babies sleep has a significant impact on their risk of dying from sudden infant death syndrome (SIDS).**
   True or false?

ANSWERS

1. C. On average, it costs about $9500 per year to raise a child; with inflation, this translates into about $235,000 to raise a child to age 18.

2. C. If left untreated, the STDs gonorrhea and chlamydia can lead to tubal scarring and blockage. Leading causes of male infertility include low sperm count and poor sperm motility, usually as a result of injury, infection, birth defects, or subjecting the testes to high temperatures. One recent study linked repeated use of laptop computers with increased scrotal temperature and potential effects on male fertility.

3. B. It is recommended that all reproductive-age women consume 400 µg of folic acid from fortified foods and/or supplements each day to reduce the risk of spina bifida and other neural tube defects.

4. ALL FOUR. Smoking has many negative effects on infants and on the reproductive systems of both men and women. The reduction in male births associated with smoking may result from problems with sperm quality, especially those sperm cells with a Y chromosome.

5. TRUE. The rate of SIDS in the United States has dropped over 40% since 1992, when an education campaign called "Back to Sleep" was implemented to teach parents and caregivers to put babies to bed on their backs instead of their stomachs.

WW Visit the *Core Concepts in Health* Online Learning Center (www.mhhe.com/insel10e) for study aids and many additional resources.

203

eciding whether to become a parent is one of the
most important decisions you will ever make.
Having a child changes your life forever, and deciding not to have children has equally far-reaching implications. Yet many people approach this momentous decision with only the vaguest notion of what is involved in pregnancy and childbirth. An estimated half of the approximately 4 million babies born every year in the United States are from unintentional pregnancies.

Today, with changing cultural expectations and increasingly sophisticated contraceptive technology, you have more choice about becoming a parent than people have ever had before. Until recently it was expected that virtually every married couple would have children. Now you can choose whether, when, and how you want to have a child. (The average age of first-time U.S. mothers has increased steadily since 1970 from 21.4 to 25.1 years.) And you don't have to be part of a married couple to have a child. About one-third of all U.S. births are to unmarried women.

Pregnancy is a relatively comfortable experience for most women, and the outcome is predictably happy. Yet problems occur for others. Some couples who have always planned for children may find that they are unable to conceive; others may face complications during pregnancy. Some problems are impossible to prevent, but you can make choices that minimize the risks and maximize the benefits for yourself, your partner, and your children.

Having a child is one of the most arduous, important, and rewarding enterprises that human beings undertake. The more you know about it—about conception and pregnancy, fetal development and prenatal care, childbirth and parenting—the more capable you will be of making intelligent, informed decisions about it. This chapter presents information you can use both now and later in your life to make the choices about pregnancy and childbirth that are right for you.

PREPARATION FOR PARENTHOOD

Before you decide whether or when to become a parent, you'll want to consider your suitability and readiness. If you make the decision to have a child, there are actions you can take before the pregnancy begins to help ensure a healthy outcome for all.

Deciding to Become a Parent

Many factors must be taken into account when you are considering parenthood. Following are some questions to ask yourself and some issues to consider when making this decision. Some issues are relevant to both men and women; others apply only to women.

• *Your physical health and your age.* Are you in reasonably good health? If not, can you improve your health by changing your lifestyle, perhaps by modifying your diet or giving up cigarettes, alcohol, or drugs? Are you overweight? Do you have physical conditions, such as diabetes or high blood pressure, that will require extra care and medical attention during pregnancy? Do you or your partner have a family history of genetic problems that a baby might inherit? Does your age place you or your baby at risk? (Teenagers and women over 35 have a higher incidence of some problems.) Improving your health before pregnancy (discussed in the next section) can help ensure a trouble-free pregnancy and a healthy baby.

• *Your financial circumstances.* Can you afford a child? Will your health insurance cover the costs of pregnancy, delivery, and medical attention for mother and baby before and after the birth, including physicians' fees and hospital costs? Supplies for the baby are expensive, too—diapers, bedding, cribs, strollers, car seats, clothing, food and medical supplies, and child care. Depending on a variety of factors, including age of child, number of children, family income, and region of residence, the annual cost of raising a child averages about $9500. With inflation, the cost of raising a child to age 18 averages about $235,000 per child for a middle-class family with two children. If one parent has quit his or her job to care for the child or is on parental leave, the family must live on one income.

• *Your relationship with your partner.* Are you in a stable relationship, and do both of you want a child? Are your views compatible on issues such as child-rearing goals, the distribution of responsibility for the child, and work and housework obligations?

• *Your educational, career, and child care plans.* Have you completed as much of your education as you want right now? Have you established yourself in a career, if that is something you want to do? Have you investigated parental leave and company-sponsored child care? Do you and your partner agree on child care arrangements, and does such child care exist in your community? Some experts advise against full-time child care for babies under 1 year, but studies have found no permanent adverse effects of early child care on child development. Some people consider the child care issue the most difficult in parenting.

• *Your emotional readiness for parenthood.* Do you have the emotional discipline and stamina to care for and nurture an infant? Are you prepared to have a helpless baby completely dependent on you all day and all night? Are you willing to change your lifestyle to provide the best conditions for a baby's development, both before and after birth?

• *Your social support system.* Do you have a network of family and friends who will help you with the baby? Are there community resources you can call on for additional assistance? A family's social support system is one

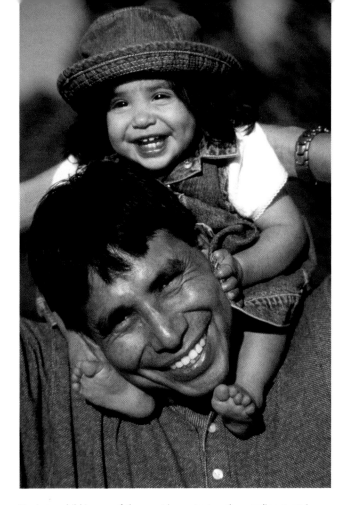

Having a child is one of the most important and rewarding experiences a person can undertake. Careful preparation can help maximize the benefits for both parents and children.

of the most important factors affecting its ability to adjust to a baby and cope with new responsibilities.

- *Your personal qualities, attitudes toward children, and aptitude for parenting.* Do you like infants, young children, and adolescents? Do you think time with children is time well spent? Do you feel good enough about yourself to love and respect others? Do you have safe ways of handling anger, frustration, and impatience?

- *Your philosophical or religious beliefs.* Some people question the value of bringing more people into an already overcrowded world. They feel that human beings have already fulfilled the biblical directive to be fruitful and multiply, and they choose not to have children.

Preconception Care

The birth of a healthy baby depends in part on the mother's overall wellness *before* conception. The U.S. Public Health Service recommends that all women receive health care to help them prepare for pregnancy. **Preconception care** should include an assessment of health risks, the promotion of healthy lifestyle behaviors, and any treatments necessary to reduce risk. Following are some of the

questions, tests, and treatments you and your partner may encounter during preconception care:

1.   Do you have any preexisting medical conditions, such as diabetes, epilepsy, asthma, high blood pressure, or anemia? There may be things you can do to improve the chances of a trouble-free pregnancy and a positive outcome.

2.   Are you taking any prescription or over-the-counter medications or dietary supplements? Some medications can harm the **fetus,** so you may need to change or discontinue their use to help ensure a healthy pregnancy.

3.   Have you had any prior problems with pregnancy and delivery, including miscarriage, premature birth, ectopic pregnancy, or delivery complications? Some problems are due to physical or hormonal difficulties that can be treated.

4.   Does your age place you at risk for infertility or health problems during pregnancy, or does it increase the likelihood that your baby may have a genetic or chromosomal disorder? Pregnant teenagers may need special nutritional counseling during pregnancy to meet the needs of their own growing body as well as the baby's. The incidence of Down syndrome increases with maternal age; genetic testing and counseling are often recommended for women age 35 and older. Older women may also find that it is harder to become pregnant.

5.   Do you smoke, drink, or take other drugs? These habits are dangerous for the baby, and a health care professional can recommend treatment programs. If you are a heavy consumer of caffeine, cutting back before and during pregnancy is recommended.

6.   Do you currently have any infections, or do you need any additional vaccinations? Women at risk for hepatitis B or not immunized against rubella (German measles) should be vaccinated. Women who have not had chicken pox (varicella) or been previously immunized can be tested to see if vaccination is indicated for them. Women not immune to parvovirus B19, which causes toxoplasmosis, or "fifth disease," a disease transmitted in contaminated food or by animals, especially cats, can find out how to prevent infection during pregnancy (both these diseases can cause miscarriage or complications in pregnancy and/or for the developing fetus). Testing for tuberculosis and certain STDs can ensure treatment prior to pregnancy. (See Chapters 17 and 18 for more information about STDs and other infectious diseases.)

Terms

V w

preconception care Health care in preparation for pregnancy.

fetus The developmental stage of a human from the 9th week after conception to the moment of birth.

7. Are you at risk for HIV infection (see Chapter 18)? If so, you should be tested before you or your partner becomes pregnant. Babies born to HIV-infected mothers can become infected.

8. Do you eat a balanced diet? Are you particularly underweight or overweight? Do you suffer from an eating disorder? Do you have special dietary habits, such as being a vegetarian? Nutritional counseling can help you create a plan for healthy eating, before and during pregnancy. Your physician may also prescribe multivitamins, particularly folic acid. The U.S. Public Health Service recommends that all women of childbearing age take extra folic acid because during the first few weeks of pregnancy it reduces the risk of neural tube defects such as spina bifida (see p. 220).

9. Were you a diethylstilbestrol (DES) baby? Daughters born to women who were given DES during pregnancy to prevent miscarriage—a common practice from the 1940s to the early 1970s—are at risk for a variety of problems with conception and pregnancy. DES daughters may need special monitoring and care to identify and treat problems as soon as they develop. (For more on DES, see Chapter 16.)

10. Do twins or multiple births run in your family? If so, this tendency may increase the likelihood of a multiple birth. Multiple births are also increased in mothers who are obese, older than 40, or using certain reproductive technologies to achieve pregnancy.

11. Do either you or your partner have a family history of any genetic disease? Have you or any family member had a child with a birth defect or mental impairment? Genetic testing and counseling can determine whether you are a carrier for a specific disease, what the effects of the disease would be, and whether a baby you conceive

can be tested prenatally. Members of certain ethnic groups are at higher risk for genetic disorders that are more prevalent within their groups than in the general population. For more information on these disorders, refer to the box "Ethnicity and Genetic Diseases."

Additional tests or changes in behavior may be recommended if you have recently traveled outside the United States; if you work with chemicals, radiation, or toxic substances; if you participate in physically demanding or hazardous activities or occupations; or if you face significant psychosocial risks, including homelessness, an unsafe home environment, or mental illness.

UNDERSTANDING FERTILITY

Conceiving a child is a highly complex process. Although many couples conceive readily, others can testify to the difficulties that can be encountered.

Conception

The process of **conception** involves the **fertilization** of an ovum (egg) from a woman by a sperm from a man (Figure 8-1). Every month during a woman's fertile years, her body prepares itself for conception and pregnancy. In one of her **ovaries** an egg ripens and is released from its **follicle**. The egg, about the size of a pinpoint, travels through an **oviduct**, or **fallopian tube**, to the **uterus** in 3–4 days. The **endometrium**, or lining of the uterus, has already thickened for the implantation of a **fertilized egg**, or *zygote*. If the egg is not fertilized, it lasts about 24 hours and then disintegrates. It is expelled along with the uterine lining during menstruation.

Sperm cells are produced in the man's **testes** and ejaculated from his penis into the woman's vagina during sexual intercourse (except in cases of artificial insemination or assisted reproduction; see p. 210). Sperm cells are much smaller than eggs. The typical ejaculate contains millions of sperm, but only a few complete the journey through the uterus and up the fallopian tube to the egg. Many sperm cells do not survive the acidic environment of the vagina. Once through the cervix and into the uterus, many sperm cells are diverted to the wrong oviduct or get stuck along the way. Of those that reach the egg, only one will penetrate its hard outer layer. As sperm approach the egg, they release enzymes that soften this outer layer. Enzymes from hundreds of sperm must be released in order for the egg's outer layer to soften enough to allow one sperm cell to penetrate. The first sperm cell that bumps into a spot that is soft enough can swim into the egg cell. It then merges with the nucleus of the egg, and fertilization occurs. The sperm's tail, its means of locomotion, gets stuck in the outer membrane and drops off, leaving the sperm head inside the egg. The egg then releases a chemical that makes it impenetrable by other sperm.

Terms

conception The fusion of ovum and sperm, resulting in a fertilized egg.

fertilization The initiation of biological reproduction: the union of the nucleus of an egg cell with the nucleus of a sperm cell.

ovary One of the two female reproductive organs that produce ova (eggs) and sex hormones.

follicle One of many saclike structures within the ovary in which eggs mature.

oviduct (fallopian tube) One of two passages through which eggs travel from the ovaries to the uterus; the site of fertilization.

uterus The hollow, thick-walled, muscular organ in which the fertilized egg develops; the womb.

endometrium The mucous membrane that forms the inner lining of the cavity of the uterus.

fertilized egg The egg after penetration by a sperm; a *zygote*.

testis One of two male reproductive organs; the testes are the site of sperm production.

Dimensions of Diversity

Ethnicity and Genetic Diseases

Genes carry the chemical instructions that determine the development of hundreds of individual traits, including disease risks, in every human being. Many traits and conditions involve multiple genes and environmental influences. However, some diseases can be traced to a mutation in a single gene.

Children inherit one set of genes from each parent. If only one copy of an abnormal gene is necessary to produce a disease, then it is termed a *dominant* gene. Diseases that are carried by dominant genes seldom skip a generation: Anyone who carries the gene will probably get the disease. If two copies of an abnormal gene (one from each parent) are necessary for a disease to occur, then the gene is called *recessive*. Many common diseases caused by recessive genes occur disproportionately in certain ethnic groups. Prospective parents who come from the same ethnic group can be tested for any recessive diseases found in that group. If both are carriers, each of their children will have about a 25% chance of developing the disease.

Learning all you can about diseases that affect members of your ethnic group can be a lifesaver. Not only can you learn about the risk to your children, but you may also discover there are things you can do to manage the disease and reduce its impact.

• *Sickle-cell disease* affects about 1 out of every 500 African Americans and 1 out of every 1200 Latinos. In this disease, the red blood cells, which carry oxygen to the body's tissues, change shape; the normal doughnut-shaped cells become sickle-shaped. These altered cells carry less oxygen and clog small blood vessels.

People who inherit one gene for sickle-cell disease (about 1 in 12 African Americans) experience only mild symptoms; those with two genes become severely, often fatally, ill. Interestingly, people who inherit one sickle-cell gene are far more resistant to malaria than are those without the gene, leading geneticists to conclude that the sickle-cell trait might have developed in tropical regions as an adaptation to the widespread presence of malaria.

If you are at risk for sickle-cell disease, you can

1. Get genetic counseling to help determine your family's genetic pattern and the degree of risk to you and your potential offspring

2. Take particular care to reduce stress and respond to minor infections, because red blood cells become

sickle-shaped during periods of stress on the body

3. Get regular checkups and appropriate treatment

• *Hemochromatosis* ("iron overload") affects about 1 in 250 Americans; most at risk are people of Northern European (especially Irish), Mediterranean, and Hispanic descent. In people with hemochromatosis, the body absorbs and stores up to ten times the normal amount of iron. Over time, iron deposits form in the joints, liver, heart, and pancreas. If untreated, hemochromatosis can cause organ failure and death.

Early symptoms are often vague, but early detection and treatment are necessary to prevent damage. If you have any family members with the disorder, get tested. Treatment involves reducing iron stores by removing blood from the body (a process also known as phlebotomy or "bloodletting").

• *Tay-Sachs disease,* another recessive disorder, occurs annually in approximately 1 out of every 1000 Jews of Eastern European ancestry. People with Tay-Sachs disease are unable to metabolize fat properly; as a result, the brain and other nerve tissues deteriorate. Affected children begin by showing weaknesses in their movements and eventually develop blindness and seizures. This disease is fatal, and death usually occurs by age 3 or 4.

If you are of Eastern European Jewish ancestry and are planning to have children, genetic counseling and blood testing will help you assess the chances that you and your mate will produce a child with Tay-Sachs disease.

• *Cystic fibrosis* occurs in 1 in every 2000 Caucasians per year; about 1 in 20 carries one copy of the cystic fibrosis gene. Because essential enzymes of the pancreas are deficient, nutrients are not properly absorbed. Thick mucus impairs functioning in the lungs and intestinal tracts of people with this disease. The disease is often fatal in early childhood, but medical treatments are increasingly effective in reducing symptoms and prolonging life. In some cases, symptoms do not appear until early adulthood.

If there is a history of cystic fibrosis in your family and you plan to have children, genetic tests and counseling can help in assessing the risk to your prospective offspring.

• *Thalassemia* is a blood disease found most often among Italians, Greeks, and, to a lesser extent, African Americans and Asians. When inherited from one parent, this form of anemia is mild; when two genes are present, the disease is severe and can cause fetal death. Children with this condition require repeated blood transfusions, eventually resulting in a damaging iron buildup. New medical interventions, such as genetic engineering, bone marrow transplants, and chemicals that bind with excess iron and remove it from the body, offer promise. Stem cell transplantation of cells obtained from the umbilical cord blood of an unaffected sibling or donor is already being used in some cases.

If you are at risk of carrying thalassemia, you can

1. Get regular checkups and monitor your health for symptoms

2. Learn symptom management

3. Get genetic counseling to assess the risk to your offspring

• *Lactose intolerance* is a less serious condition affecting about 30–50 million Americans, including a majority of Asian Americans, Native Americans, and African Americans. Although all people are dependent on milk in the early years, by about age 4 many lose the ability to absorb lactose, the chief nutrient in milk. This lactose intolerance results from an absence of lactase, an enzyme that permits the efficient digestion of milk. When lactose-intolerant people ingest more than 1 or 2 servings of milk or dairy products, they suffer from gas pains and diarrhea. Studies show that lactose intolerance is especially prevalent in cultures where milk is relatively unimportant after weaning, suggesting that evolutionary adaptation has played a role in its development.

If you suspect lactose intolerance, see your physician for a test. If you are lactose intolerant, use trial and error to determine how many servings of dairy products you can consume without symptoms. If you react to very small amounts of lactose, try lactose-reduced products or lactase drops or tablets.

Other health problems that have a hereditary component and that disproportionately affect certain ethnic groups include diabetes, osteoporosis, high blood pressure, alcoholism, and certain types of cancer. These links are discussed in later chapters.

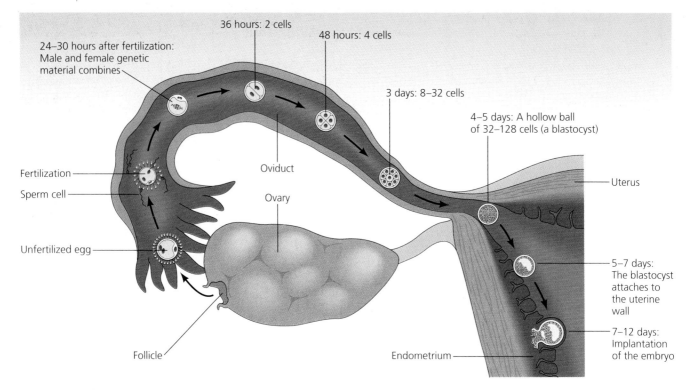

24–30 hours after fertilization: Male and female genetic material combines

36 hours: 2 cells

48 hours: 4 cells

3 days: 8–32 cells

4–5 days: A hollow ball of 32–128 cells (a blastocyst)

Oviduct

Ovary

Fertilization

Sperm cell

Unfertilized egg

Follicle

Uterus

5–7 days: The blastocyst attaches to the uterine wall

7–12 days: Implantation of the embryo

Endometrium

Figure 8-1   Fertilization and early development of the embryo. The unfertilized egg is released from an ovarian follicle into the oviduct, where it is fertilized by a sperm cell. As the fertilized egg moves through the oviduct toward the uterus, the genetic material from the egg and sperm combines, and the egg begins to divide. When the egg reaches the uterus, it is in the form of a hollow ball of cells called a blastocyst, which becomes implanted in the endometrium.

The ovum carries the hereditary characteristics of the mother and her ancestors; sperm cells carry the hereditary characteristics of the father and his ancestors. Each parent cell—egg or sperm—contains 23 chromosomes, each of which contains **genes**, packages of chemical instructions for the developing baby. Genes provide the blueprint for a unique individual (see the box "Creating a Family Health Tree").

As soon as fertilization occurs, the zygote starts to undergo the cell division that begins the growth process. It continues to divide as it travels through the oviduct to the uterus. Upon reaching the uterus, the cluster of cells, now called a *blastocyst*, becomes implanted in the endometrium.

The usual course of events is that one egg and one sperm unite to produce one fertilized egg and one baby. But if the ovaries release two (or more) eggs during ovulation and if both eggs are fertilized, twins will develop. These twins will be no more alike than siblings from different pregnancies, because each will have come from a different fertilized egg. Twins who develop this way are referred to as **fraternal twins**; they may be the same sex or different sexes. Twins can also develop from the division of a single fertilized egg into two cells that develop separately. Because these babies share all genetic material, they will be **identical twins**.

Infertility

Although the main concern for many women and men, especially if they are young and single, is how *not* to get pregnant, the reverse is true for millions of couples who have difficulty conceiving. **Infertility** is usually defined as the inability to conceive after trying for a year or more. It affects about 6 million couples—10% of the reproductive-age population of the United States. Over a million couples seek treatment for infertility each year. Although the focus is often on women, up to 40% of the factors contributing to infertility are male, and in about 15% of infertile couples, both partners have problems. Therefore, it is important that each individual be evaluated.

Terms

V w

gene The basic unit of heredity; a section of a chromosone containing chemical instructions for making a particular protein.

fraternal twins Twins who develop from separate fertilized eggs; not genetically identical.

identical twins Twins who develop from the division of a single zygote; genetically identical.

infertility The inability to conceive after trying for a year or more.

The genetic inheritance that each of us receives from our parents—and that our children receive from us—contains more than just physical characteristics, such as eye and hair color. Heredity also contributes to our risk of developing certain diseases and disorders. For certain uncommon illnesses such as hemophilia and sickle-cell disease, heredity is the primary cause; if your parents pass on the necessary genes, you'll get the disease. But heredity plays a subtler role in many other diseases, which are caused at least in part by environmental influences such as infection, cancer-causing chemicals, and physical inactivity. Although your genes alone will not produce those diseases, they can determine how susceptible you are. Researchers have found a genetic influence in many common disorders, including heart disease, diabetes, depression, asthma, alcoholism, and certain forms of cancer.

Knowing that a specific disease runs in your family can save your life. It allows you to watch for early warning signs and get screening tests more often than you otherwise would. Changing health habits, too, can be valuable for people with a family history of certain diseases. An individual with a family history of high cholesterol and early heart disease can increase physical activity and pay special attention to diet.

In general, the more relatives with a genetically transmitted disease and the closer they are to you, the greater your risk. However, nongenetic factors—such

as health habits—can also play a role. Signs of strong hereditary influence include early onset of the disease, appearance of the disease largely or exclusively on one side of the family, onset of the same disease at the same age in more than one relative, and developing the disease despite good health habits.

You can put together a simple family health tree by compiling a few key facts on your primary relatives: siblings, parents, aunts and uncles, and grandparents. Those facts include the date of birth, major diseases, health-related conditions and habits, and, for deceased relatives, the age at death as well as the cause. Because certain diseases are more common in particular ethnic groups, also record the ethnic background of each grandparent. Next, create a tree, using the example here as a guide. Then show your tree to a physician or genetic counselor, who can help you target the health behaviors and screening tests that are most important for you and help you determine whether genetic testing might be appropriate.

A Sample Family Health Tree and What It Means

The 55-year-old woman who prepared this family tree has a strong family history of osteoporosis on her mother's side. Based on this, her physician may suggest a bone density test to help gauge her risk and recommend bone-healthy lifestyle changes. She also has several close relatives on her father's side of the family

who had high cholesterol levels and had heart attacks at an early age. These risk factors significantly increase her chance of having a heart attack.

The woman has two aunts who died of breast cancer, but there are several reasons not to be overly concerned. Aunts are second-degree relatives, more distantly related to her than her mother or sister (first-degree relatives). In addition, they came from different sides of the family, and they developed the disease quite late in life. Given these factors, it is likely that these cases of breast cancer did not have a significant genetic origin.

Looking at her family history can help this woman make important decisions about behaviors such as moderate alcohol consumption, which may lower the risk of heart attack but which may also slightly increase the risk of breast cancer. Based on her family history, her physician may recommend bone density testing to determine her risk of dangerous fractures and recommend medication and a heart-healthy diet to reduce her unhealthy cholesterol level and overall heart attack risk.

SOURCES: From "Prepare for the Future: Know Your Ancestors" and "Creating a Family Health Tree" © 1999 by Consumers Union of U.S., Inc. Yonkers, NY 10703-1057, a nonprofit organization. Reprinted with permission from the September 1999 issue of *Consumer Reports on Health*® for educational purposes only. No commercial use or reproduction permitted. www.ConsumerReports.org.

Female Infertility   Female infertility usually results from one of two key causes—tubal blockage (40%) or failure to ovulate (40%). An additional 10% of cases of infertility are due to anatomical abnormalities, benign growths in the uterus, thyroid disease, and other uncommon conditions; the remaining 10% of cases are unexplained.

Blocked fallopian tubes are most commonly the result of *pelvic inflammatory disease (PID)*, a serious complication of several sexually transmitted diseases. Most cases of PID are associated with untreated cases of chlamydia or gonorrhea. More than 1.5 million cases of PID are treated each year, but physicians estimate that half may go untreated because of an absence of symptoms. Other causes of PID include infections associated with abortion and certain types of older IUDs. Tubal blockages can also be caused by prior surgery or by *endometriosis*, a condition in which endometrial (uterine) tissue grows outside of the uterus. This tissue responds to hormones and can cause pain, bleeding, scarring, and adhesions. Endometriosis is typically treated with hormonal therapy and surgery.

Age impacts fertility; beginning at around age 30, a woman's fertility naturally begins to decline. Age is probably the main factor in ovulation failure. Exposure to toxic chemicals or radiation also appears to reduce fertility, as does cigarette smoking.

Male Infertility   The leading causes of infertility among men are low sperm count, lack of sperm motility (the ability to move spontaneously), misshapen sperm, and blocked passageways between the testes and the urethra. Smoking may cause reduced sperm counts and abnormal sperm. The sons of mothers who took DES may have increased sperm abnormalities and fertility problems. Certain prescription and illegal drugs also affect the number of sperm. Large doses of marijuana, for example, cause lower sperm counts and suppress certain reproductive hormones. Other causes of sperm problems include injury to the testicles, infection (especially from mumps during adulthood), birth defects, and subjecting the testes to high temperatures.

Some studies indicate that sperm counts worldwide have dropped by as much as 50% over the past 30 years. Evidence suggests that toxic substances such as lead, chemical pollutants, and radiation are responsible for this decrease. Recent research has also focused on a class of chemicals known as *endocrine disrupters*—substances found widely in the environment that mimic or interfere with the body's hormones, thereby causing problems with reproduction and development. Examples of hormone mimics include dioxin, PCBs, DDT, and compounds used in some plastics. Animal studies have linked prenatal exposure to endocrine disrupters with feminized genitalia and other reproductive problems in male offspring. Scientists do not yet know, however, what effects endocrine disrupters may have on human health and fertility.

Treating Infertility   About 90% of infertile couples receive a physical diagnosis for their condition; for the remaining 10%, the cause of the infertility remains unexplained. Most cases of infertility are treated with conventional medical therapies: Surgery can repair oviducts, clear up endometriosis, and correct anatomical problems in both men and women. Fertility drugs can help women ovulate, although they carry the risk of causing multiple births. If these conventional treatments don't work, couples can turn to more advanced techniques (see below). However, most infertility treatments are expensive and emotionally draining, and their success is uncertain. Some infertile couples choose not to try to have children, whereas others turn to adoption. One measure you can take now to avoid infertility is to protect yourself against STDs and to treat promptly and completely any disease you do contract. Also, couples who are ready should consider trying to conceive prior to the woman's late 30s to decrease the probability of age-related infertility.

INTRAUTERINE INSEMINATION   Male infertility can sometimes be overcome by collecting and concentrating the man's sperm and introducing it by syringe into a woman's vagina or uterus, a procedure known as **artificial (intrauterine) insemination.** To increase the probability of success, the woman is often given fertility drugs to induce ovulation prior to the insemination procedure. The sperm can be provided by the woman's partner or, if there are severe problems with his sperm or he carries a serious genetic disorder, by a donor. Donor sperm are also used by single women and lesbian couples who wish to conceive using artificial insemination. The success rate is about 60%. There are about 30,000 births each year from intrauterine insemination.

IVF, GIFT, AND ZIFT   Three related techniques for overcoming infertility involve removing mature eggs from a woman's ovary. Fewer than 5% of infertile American couples who seek treatment try these techniques. In **in vitro fertilization (IVF)**, the harvested eggs are mixed with

Terms

V w

artificial (intrauterine) insemination The introduction of semen into the vagina by artificial means, usually by syringe.

in vitro fertilization (IVF) Combining egg and sperm outside of the body and inserting the fertilized egg into the uterus.

cloning Asexual reproduction in which offspring are genetically identical to one parent. DNA from the cell of one animal is transferred to an egg from which DNA has been removed; the egg is then placed in a surrogate and develops as though it were an embryo derived from two parents.

gamete intrafallopian transfer (GIFT) Surgically introducing eggs and sperm into the fallopian tube prior to fertilization.

zygote intrafallopian transfer (ZIFT) Surgically introducing a fertilized egg into the fallopian tube.

In the United States, more than 45,000 infants are born each year as a result of assisted reproductive technology (ART) techniques like IVF, GIFT, and ZIFT. Research into the areas of genetics and cloning promise even more breakthroughs for ART treatments. With these advances, however, come many medical, ethical, and legal questions. Below are a few of the most advanced techniques currently in use and under study.

Use of donor eggs, donor sperm, and/or donor embryos is fairly common in ART treatments. In some instances, this results in a child with a complex network of biological and legal parents. For example, in the case of IVF involving donor eggs and sperm and a surrogate mother, who are the legal parents of the child?

The use of donor eggs and embryos has also allowed women in their 50s to complete pregnancy and deliver a baby. The resulting offspring is no more genetically related to the woman than an adopted child would be. Use of ART in women of this age is controversial.

Intracytoplasmic sperm injection (ICSI), in which a single sperm is injected into a mature egg, was originally developed to overcome cases of severe male infertility; it is now used for a broader range of conditions. Concerns have been raised because some studies have linked ICSI to an increase in genetic defects in offspring. In addition, ICSI allows men who are infertile due to Y chromosome defects to have children, even though any sons they have will inherit the defect and also be infertile.

Cryopreservation of ovarian tissue and/or unfertilized eggs has been studied as a possible means of preserving fertility in women undergoing cancer therapy. In 2004, the first woman gave birth after having ovarian tissue removed and frozen prior to cancer chemotherapy and then reimplanted. This technique could potentially be used in women who choose to delay child bearing; and several controversial companies offer this technique to women in their 30s.

Freezing embryos is common in ART because multiple eggs are usually harvested and fertilized during IVF. If the initial IVF cycle is unsuccessful, the backup embryos can be used for additional attempts. Once ART treatment is completed, couples may choose to donate leftover embryos for use by another infertile couple or to have them destroyed. A more controversial potential use of extra embryos is for the creation of stem cell lines (see Chapter 19).

Preimplantation genetic diagnosis, in which embryos created through IVF undergo genetic analysis before implantation in the womb, was originally developed to help couples at risk for genetic diseases. It has now begun to be offered by some physicians for sex selection in couples who have no fertility problems. This is considered controversial because a particular gender isn't a disease that needs to be prevented, and there remains the difficult question of what becomes of the "wrong sex" embryos—freezing, donation, destruction, or use in research.

Injection of the cytoplasm (the material in a cell that surrounds the nucleus) from a younger woman's egg into an older woman's egg has begun to be used as a possible means of reducing genetic errors in the older woman's egg. These errors occur in so-called mitochondrial DNA, genetic material in the cytoplasm of the cell that is passed along unchanged to offspring.

Nuclear transfer, a technique related to cytoplasm injection, uses cloning technology—the transfer of the nucleus from an older woman's egg into an egg from a younger woman from which the nucleus has been removed. In cytoplasm injection and nuclear transfer, the offspring carry DNA from two women—nuclear DNA from one woman and mitochondrial DNA from a second woman—and so have three genetic "parents."

What about cloning? **Cloning** is different from any of the techniques discussed above because it is a form of asexual reproduction. A clone carries the genes of only one person, not two. However, as described above, the cloning technique of nuclear transfer could potentially be used in the treatment of infertility. Nuclear transfer could theoretically also be used to create a child that is the genetic offspring of two people of the same sex. In 2004, scientists announced that they had created a mouse from two unfertilized eggs.

sperm in a laboratory dish. If eggs are successfully fertilized, one or more of the resulting embryos are inserted into the woman's uterus. IVF is often used by women with blocked oviducts. In **gamete intrafallopian transfer (GIFT)**, eggs and sperm are surgically placed into the fallopian tubes prior to fertilization. In **zygote intrafallopian transfer (ZIFT)**, eggs are fertilized outside the woman's body and surgically introduced into the oviducts after they begin to divide. GIFT and ZIFT can be used by women who have at least one open fallopian tube. Variations on these three techniques are also becoming available (see the box "Reproductive Technology").

IVF, GIFT, and ZIFT do have drawbacks. Success rates vary from about 23% to 47%. They cost between $8000 and $12,000 per procedure and may require five or more cycles to produce one live birth. They also increase the chance of multiple births, which in turn increases the risk of premature birth and maternal complications, including pregnancy-related hypertension and diabetes.

SURROGATE MOTHERHOOD Surrogate motherhood is a controversial approach to infertility. This practice involves a contract between an infertile couple and a fertile woman who agrees to carry a fetus. The surrogate mother agrees to be artificially inseminated by the father's sperm or to undergo IVF with the couple's embryo, to carry the baby to term, and to give it to the couple at birth. In return, the couple pays her for her services. There are thought to be several hundred births to surrogate mothers each year in the United States. Some people think that surrogate motherhood is essentially an arrangement to sell a baby, and they worry about the psychological consequences for children who learn that their mothers "sold" them. Experience has shown, too, that some surrogate mothers have a very difficult time giving up the baby and are unwilling to fulfill the contract after the birth, causing emotional trauma for themselves and the couple.

Emotional Responses to Infertility Couples who seek treatment for infertility have often already confronted the possibility of not being able to become biological parents. Many infertile couples feel they have lost control over a major area of their lives. They may lose perspective on the rest of their lives as they focus more and more on the reasons for their infertility and on treatment. Infertile couples may need to set their own limits on how much treatment they are willing to undergo. Support groups for infertile couples can provide help in this difficult situation, but there are few easy answers to infertility. If treatment is unsuccessful, couples must mourn the loss of the children they will never bear. They will need to make some kind of decision about their future—whether to pursue plans for adoption or another treatment or to adjust to childlessness and go on with their lives.

PREGNANCY

Pregnancy is usually discussed in terms of **trimesters**—three periods of about 3 months (or 13 weeks) each. During the first trimester, the mother experiences a few physical changes and some fairly common symptoms. During the second trimester, often the most peaceful time of pregnancy, the mother gains weight, looks noticeably pregnant, and may experience a general sense of well-being if she is happy about having a child. The third trimester is the hardest for the mother because she must breathe, digest, excrete, and circulate blood for herself and the growing fetus. The weight of the fetus, the pressure of its body on her organs, and its increased demands on her system cause discomfort and fatigue and may make the mother increasingly impatient to give birth.

Pregnancy Tests

The earliest tests for pregnancy are chemical tests designed to detect the presence of **human chorionic gonadotropin (HCG)**, a hormone produced by the implanted fertilized egg. These tests may be performed as early as 2 weeks after fertilization. Home pregnancy test kits, which are sold without a prescription in drugstores, include a small sample of red blood cells coated with HCG antibodies, to which the woman adds a small amount of her urine. If the concentration of HCG is great enough, it will clump together with the HCG antibodies, indicating that the woman is pregnant. Home pregnancy tests can be very reliable, but the instructions must be followed carefully. If a home test done at the time of a missed menstrual period is negative, retesting after

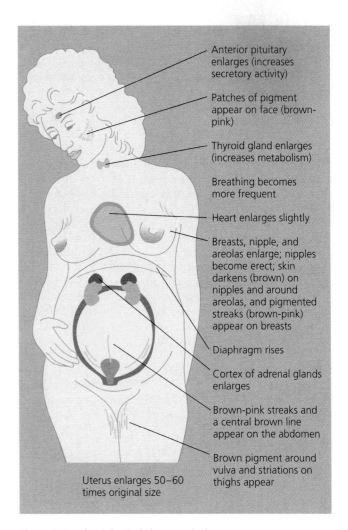

Figure 8-2 Physiological changes during pregnancy.

Labels in figure:
- Anterior pituitary enlarges (increases secretory activity)
- Patches of pigment appear on face (brown-pink)
- Thyroid gland enlarges (increases metabolism)
- Breathing becomes more frequent
- Heart enlarges slightly
- Breasts, nipple, and areolas enlarge; nipples become erect; skin darkens (brown) on nipples and around areolas, and pigmented streaks (brown-pink) appear on breasts
- Diaphragm rises
- Cortex of adrenal glands enlarges
- Brown-pink streaks and a central brown line appear on the abdomen
- Brown pigment around vulva and striations on thighs appear
- Uterus enlarges 50–60 times original size

another week is recommended. In the first day or two following a missed period, the concentration of HCG may be too low to be detected by the test.

Changes in the Woman's Body

Hormonal changes begin as soon as the egg is fertilized, and for the next 9 months the woman's body nourishes the fetus and adjusts to its growth. Let's take a closer look at the changes of early, middle, and late pregnancy (Figure 8-2).

Early Signs and Symptoms Early recognition of pregnancy is important, especially for women with physical problems and nutritional deficiencies. The following symptoms are not absolute indications of pregnancy, but they are reasons to visit a gynecologist:

- *A missed menstrual period.* If an egg has been fertilized and implanted in the uterine wall, the endometrium is retained to nourish the embryo. A woman who misses a period after having intercourse may be pregnant.

- *Slight bleeding.* Slight bleeding may follow implantation of the fertilized egg. Because this happens about the time a period is expected, the bleeding is sometimes mistaken for menstrual flow. It usually lasts only a few days.

- *Nausea.* About two-thirds of pregnant women feel nauseated, probably as a reaction to increased levels of progesterone and other hormones. Often called morning sickness, some women have it all day long. It frequently begins during the 3rd or 4th week and disappears by the 12th week. In some cases, it can last throughout a pregnancy.

- *Breast tenderness.* Some women experience breast tenderness, swelling, and tingling, usually described as different from the tenderness experienced before menstruation.

- *Increased urination.* Increased frequency of urination can occur soon after the missed period.

- *Sleepiness, fatigue, and emotional upset.* These symptoms result from hormonal changes. Fatigue can be surprisingly overwhelming in the first trimester but usually improves significantly around the third month of pregnancy.

The first reliable physical signs of pregnancy can be distinguished about 4 weeks after a woman misses her menstrual period. A softening of the uterus just above the cervix, called *Hegar's sign,* and other changes in the cervix and pelvis are apparent during a pelvic examination. The labia minora and the cervix may take on a purple color rather than their usual pink hue.

Four weeks after a woman misses her menstrual period, she would be considered to be about 8 weeks pregnant because pregnancy is calculated from the time of a woman's last menstrual period rather than from the time of actual fertilization. (The timing of ovulation and fertilization is often difficult to determine.) Although a woman should see her physician to determine her due date, due dates can be approximated by subtracting 3 months from the date of the last menstrual period and then adding 7 days. For example, a woman whose last menstrual period began on September 20th would have a due date of about June 27th.

Continuing Changes in the Woman's Body

The most obvious changes during pregnancy occur in the reproductive organs. During the first 3 months, the uterus enlarges to about three times its nonpregnant size, but it still cannot be felt in the abdomen. By the 4th month, it is large enough to make the abdomen protrude. By the 7th or 8th month, the uterus pushes up into the rib cage, which makes breathing slightly more difficult. The breasts enlarge and are sensitive; by week 8, they may tingle or throb. The pigmented area around the nipple, the areola, darkens and broadens.

Other changes are going on as well. Early in pregnancy, the muscles and ligaments attached to bones begin to soften and stretch. The joints between the pelvic bones loosen and spread, making it easier to have a baby but harder to walk. The circulatory system becomes more efficient to accommodate the blood volume, which increases by 50%, and the heart pumps it more rapidly. Much of the increased blood flow goes to the uterus and placenta (the organ that exchanges nutrients and waste between mother and fetus). The mother's lungs also become more efficient, and her rib cage widens to permit her to inhale up to 40% more air. Much of the oxygen goes to the fetus. The kidneys become highly efficient, removing waste products from fetal circulation and producing large amounts of urine by midpregnancy.

Women of normal weight gain an average of 18-25% of their initial weight: 20–28 pounds for a woman weighing 110, 23–32 pounds for a woman weighing 128. Women who begin pregnancy underweight are advised to gain more; obese women are advised to gain less. About 60% of weight gained relates directly to the baby—about 6.8 pounds for the baby and 7.5 pounds for the placenta, amniotic fluid, heavier breasts and uterus—and 40% accumulates over the mother's entire body as fluid (blood, about 4 pounds) and fat (4–8 pounds). As the woman's skin stretches, small breaks may occur in the elastic fibers of the lower layer of skin, producing *stretch marks* on her abdomen, hips, breasts, or thighs. Increased pigment production darkens the skin in 90% of pregnant women, especially in places that have stretched.

Changes During the Later Stages of Pregnancy

By the end of the 6th month, the increased needs of the fetus place a burden on the mother's lungs, heart, and kidneys. Her back may ache from the pressure of the baby's weight and from having to throw her shoulders back to keep her balance while standing (Figure 8-3, p. 214). Her body retains more water, perhaps up to 3 extra quarts of fluid. Her legs, hands, ankles, or feet may swell, and she may be bothered by leg cramps, heartburn, or constipation. Despite discomfort, both her digestion and her metabolism are working at top efficiency.

The uterus prepares for childbirth with preliminary contractions, called **Braxton Hicks contractions.** Unlike true labor contractions, these are usually short, irregular, and painless. The mother may only be aware that at times her abdomen is hard to the touch. These contractions become more frequent and intense as the delivery date approaches.

Terms

trimester One of the three 3-month periods of pregnancy.

human chorionic gonadotropin (HCG) A hormone produced by the fertilized egg that can be detected in the urine or blood of the mother within a few weeks of conception.

Braxton Hicks contractions Uterine contractions that occur during the third trimester of pregnancy, preparing for labor.

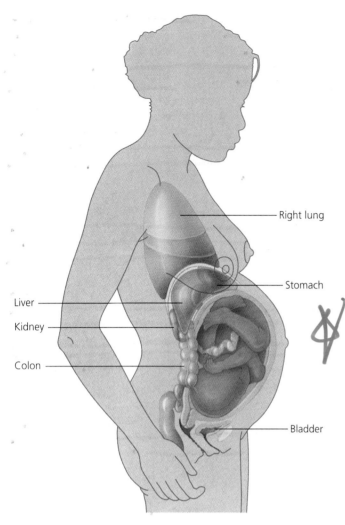

Figure 8-3   The woman and fetus during the third trimester of pregnancy. Pressure from the rapidly growing fetus on the mother's lungs, bladder, stomach, and other organs may cause shortness of breath, heartburn, and the need for frequent urination. The mother's uterus has expanded to 50–60 times its original size.

In the 9th month, the baby settles into the pelvic bones, usually head down, fitting snugly. This process, called **lightening**, allows the uterus to sink down about 2 inches, producing a visible change in the mother's profile. Pelvic pressure increases, and pressure on the diaphragm lightens. Breathing becomes easier; urination becomes more frequent. Sometimes, after a first pregnancy, the baby doesn't settle down into the pelvis until labor begins.

Emotional Responses to Pregnancy

A woman's feelings during pregnancy will depend on her circumstances—her self-image, how she feels about pregnancy and motherhood, whether the pregnancy was planned, what type of relationship she has with her partner, whether she has a secure home situation, and many other factors. A first pregnancy is especially important because it has traditionally symbolized the transition to maturity and is a major developmental milestone in the lives of mothers—and fathers as well (see the box "Pregnancy Tasks for Fathers").

Both partners may have fears about the approaching birth, their ability to be good parents, and the ways in which the baby will affect their own relationship. These concerns are normal, and sharing them can deepen and strengthen a relationship. For a woman without a partner or whose partner is not supportive, it's important that she find other sources of support, perhaps from friends, family members, or support groups. The relationships that parents-to-be have with their parents may also undergo changes. Impending parenthood may encourage them to assert their independence from their parents, but it may also enable them to identify with their parents' own experience of pregnancy, childbirth, and parenting.

Rapid changes in hormone levels can cause a pregnant woman to experience unpredictable emotions. A great part of pregnancy is beyond the woman's control—her changing appearance, her energy level, her variable moods—and some women need extra support and reassurance to keep on an even keel. Hormonal changes can also make women feel exhilarated and euphoric, although for some women such moods are temporary.

Like the physical changes that accompany pregnancy, emotional responses also change as the pregnancy develops. During the first trimester, the pregnant woman may fear that she may miscarry or that the child will not be normal. Education about pregnancy and childbirth and support from her partner, friends, relatives, and health care professionals are important antidotes to these fears. During the second trimester, the pregnant woman can feel the fetus move within her, and worries about miscarriages usually begin to diminish. She may look and feel radiantly happy and be delighted as her pregnancy begins to show. However, she may also worry that her increasing size makes her unattractive. Reassurance from her partner can ease these fears.

The third trimester is the time of greatest physical stress during the pregnancy. A woman may find that her physical abilities are limited by her size. Because some women feel physically awkward and sexually unattractive, they may experience periods of depression. But many also feel a great deal of happy excitement and anticipation. The fetus may already be looked on as a member of the family, and both parents may begin talking to the fetus and interacting with it by patting the mother's belly. The upcoming birth will probably be a focus for both the woman and her partner.

Fetal Development

Now that we've seen what happens to the mother's body during pregnancy, let's consider the development of the fetus (Figure 8-4, p. 216).

Fathers-to-be can play an important role in a happy and successful pregnancy.

Before the Pregnancy

• *Consider your lifestyle and health habits*. A healthy lifestyle can help boost fertility and improve pregnancy outcome. Being too thin or too heavy may lower a man's sperm count, as may marijuana use. Men who smoke and drink have a lower concentration of sperm and a lower percentage of active sperm. Exposure to chemicals on the job may also play a role in poor pregnancy outcomes.

• *Check your budget, financial situation, and insurance status*. What is the paternal leave policy at your place of employment? Do you have health insurance, life insurance, disability insurance, and a will? Do you (and your partner or child) qualify for special benefits such as Medicaid? Can you make a budget and stick to it? Try putting away extra money every month now—both to practice living on a tighter budget and to actually save up for the baby.

• *Get any necessary health checks and genetic counseling*. See the discussion of potential health concerns in the section on "Preconception Care." Testing for STDs may be recommended for some men; many STDs have no symptoms but can be potentially dangerous for the developing fetus, especially if the mother

contracts the infection during her pregnancy. Genetic screening and counseling may be recommended for couples at risk for a specific inherited disease.

During the Pregnancy

• *Help your partner stay healthy during the pregnancy*. If you smoke, quit; secondhand smoke is dangerous for the developing fetus. Support your partner by making other lifestyle changes and/or joining her in any changes she's making; for example, drink nonalcoholic beverages, take walks with her, get extra sleep.

• *Help around the home and with planning for the baby*. Help shop for necessary clothes and equipment, and help get your residence ready for a baby. Pregnancy is hard work, so providing extra help with household chores and errands can be an important element of support. (Due to the risk of infection by toxoplasmosis, one specific chore that should be avoided by pregnant women is handling cat litter; if you and your partner have a cat, emptying the litter box should be your job.)

• *Be involved*. Go to all the prenatal visits, birth preparation or education classes, hospital and nursery tours, and so on. Learn more about pregnancy, childbirth, and parenting by reading books, visiting Internet sites, and talking with others.

After the Baby Arrives

• *Help meet your baby's needs*. If your job allows, take parental leave to help with the new baby. Support the new mother by helping with baby care (feeding, diaper changes), laundry, shopping, and other chores. Take turns or join the mother when the baby needs care or feeding during the night; one survey found that more than half of fathers continue to sleep or pretend to be asleep when their babies cry during the night.

• *Support your partner, and reach out to others for help*. It is normal for a new mother to be tired and to experience mood changes, and some men also experience anxiety about their new role. Good communication between partners and help from supportive relatives and friends can help new parents adjust.

SOURCES: March of Dimes. 2004. *Just for Dad: Becoming a Dad* (http://www.modimes.org/pnhec/362_757.asp; retrieved September 8, 2004); Jensen, T. K., et al. 2004. Body mass index in relation to semen quality and reproductive hormones among 1,558 Danish men. *Fertility and Sterility* 82(4): 863–870; Martini, A. C., et al. 2004. Effects of alcohol and cigarette consumption on human seminal quality. *Fertility and Sterility* 82(2): 374–377; BBC News. 2004. *Dads "Sleep On" While Babies Cry* (http://news.bbc.co.uk/1/hi/health/3638756.stm; retrieved November 19, 2004).

The First Trimester   About 30 hours after the egg is fertilized, the cell divides, and this process of cell division repeats many times. As the cluster of cells drifts down the oviduct, several different kinds of cells emerge. The entire set of genetic instructions is passed to every cell, but each cell follows only certain instructions; if this were not the case, there would be no different organs or body parts. For example, all cells carry genes for hair color and eye color, but only the cells of the hair follicles and irises (of the eye) respond to that information.

On about the fourth day after fertilization, the cluster, now about 32–128 cells and hollow, arrives in the uterus; this is a **blastocyst.** On about the sixth or seventh day, the blastocyst attaches to the uterine wall, usually along the upper curve; over the next few days, it becomes firmly implanted and begins to draw nourishment from the endometrium, the uterine lining.

The blastocyst becomes an **embryo** by about the end of the 2nd week after fertilization. The inner cells of the blastocyst separate into three layers. One layer becomes inner body parts, the digestive and respiratory systems; the middle layer becomes muscle, bone, blood, kidneys, and sex glands; and the third layer becomes the skin, hair, and nervous tissue.

Terms

lightening A process in which the uterus sinks down because the baby's head settles into the pelvic area.

blastocyst A stage of development, days 6–14, when the cell cluster becomes the embryo and placenta.

embryo The stage of development between blastocyst and fetus; about weeks 2–8.

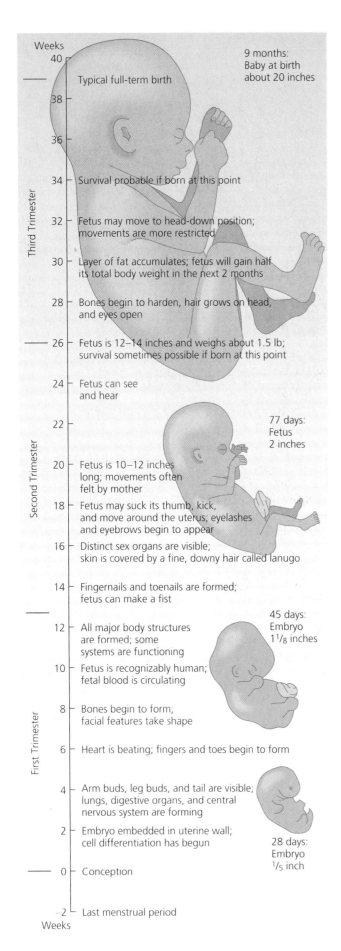

Weeks
40 — Typical full-term birth

9 months:
Baby at birth
about 20 inches

38

36

Third Trimester

34 — Survival probable if born at this point

32 — Fetus may move to head-down position; movements are more restricted

30 — Layer of fat accumulates; fetus will gain half its total body weight in the next 2 months

28 — Bones begin to harden, hair grows on head, and eyes open

26 — Fetus is 12–14 inches and weighs about 1.5 lb; survival sometimes possible if born at this point

24 — Fetus can see and hear

22

Second Trimester

77 days:
Fetus
2 inches

20 — Fetus is 10–12 inches long; movements often felt by mother

18 — Fetus may suck its thumb, kick, and move around the uterus; eyelashes and eyebrows begin to appear

16 — Distinct sex organs are visible; skin is covered by a fine, downy hair called lanugo

14 — Fingernails and toenails are formed; fetus can make a fist

45 days:
Embryo
1 1/8 inches

12 — All major body structures are formed; some systems are functioning

10 — Fetus is recognizably human; fetal blood is circulating

8 — Bones begin to form; facial features take shape

6 — Heart is beating; fingers and toes begin to form

First Trimester

4 — Arm buds, leg buds, and tail are visible; lungs, digestive organs, and central nervous system are forming

2 — Embryo embedded in uterine wall; cell differentiation has begun

28 days:
Embryo
1/5 inch

0 — Conception

−2 — Last menstrual period
Weeks

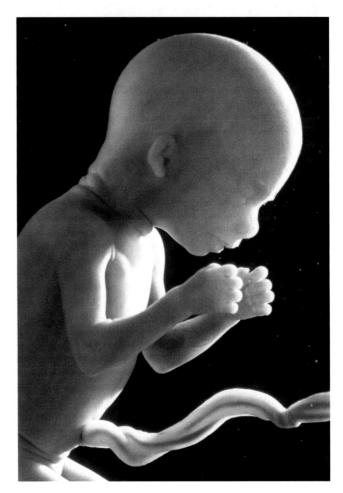

By the 4th month, the fetus is growing rapidly and is about 10 inches long. Weighing about 6 ounces, it moves vigorously in the uterus and can suck, frown, and turn its head.

The outermost shell of cells becomes the **placenta, umbilical cord,** and **amniotic sac** (Figure 8-5). A network of blood vessels called chorionic villi eventually forms the placenta. The human placenta is a two-way exchange of nutrients and waste materials between the mother and the fetus. The placenta brings oxygen and nutrients to the fetus and transports waste products out. The placenta does not provide a perfect barrier between the fetal circulation and the maternal circulation, however. Some blood cells are exchanged and certain substances, such as alcohol, pass freely from the maternal circulation through the placenta to the fetus.

The period between weeks 2 and 9 is a time of rapid differentiation and change. All the major body structures are formed during this time, including the heart, brain, liver, lungs, and sex organs; the eyes, nose, ears, arms, and legs also appear. Some organs begin to function—the heart begins to beat, and the liver starts producing blood

Figure 8-4   A chronology of milestones in prenatal development.

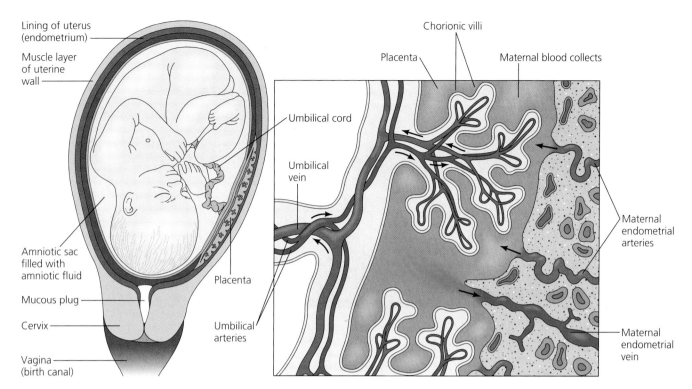

Figure 8-5 A cross-sectional view of the fetus in the uterus and an enlargement of the placenta.

*Labels in figure:*

Lining of uterus (endometrium)

Muscle layer of uterine wall

Amniotic sac filled with amniotic fluid

Mucous plug

Cervix

Vagina (birth canal)

Umbilical cord

Umbilical vein

Placenta

Umbilical arteries

Chorionic villi

Placenta

Maternal blood collects

Maternal endometrial arteries

Maternal endometrial vein

cells. Because body structures are forming, the developing organism is vulnerable to damage from environmental influences such as drugs and infections (discussed in detail in sections that follow).

By the end of the 2nd month, the brain sends out impulses that coordinate the functioning of other organs. The embryo is now a fetus, and most further changes will be in the size and refinement of working body parts. In the 3rd month, the fetus begins to be quite active. By the end of the first trimester, the fetus is about 4 inches long and weighs 1 ounce.

The Second Trimester   To grow during the second trimester, to about 14 inches and 1.5 pounds, the fetus must have large amounts of food, oxygen, and water, which come from the mother through the placenta. All body systems are operating, and the fetal heartbeat can be heard with a stethoscope. Fetal movements can be felt by the mother beginning in the 4th or 5th month. Against great odds, a fetus born prematurely at the end of the second trimester might survive.

The Third Trimester   The fetus gains most of its birth weight during the last 3 months. Some of the weight is fatty tissue under the skin that insulates the fetus and supplies food. The fetus must obtain large amounts of calcium, iron, and nitrogen from the food the mother eats. Some 85% of the calcium and iron she consumes goes into the fetal bloodstream.

Although the fetus may live if it is born during the 7th month, it needs the fat layer acquired in the 8th month and time for the organs, especially the respiratory and digestive organs, to develop. It also needs the immunity supplied by the antibodies in the mother's blood during the final 3 months. The antibodies protect the fetus against many of the diseases to which she has acquired immunity. These immunities wear off within 6 months after birth, but breast milk can help the baby further resist infections because it also contains maternal antibodies.

Diagnosing Fetal Abnormalities   Information about the health and sex of a fetus can be obtained prior to birth through prenatal testing. The most common tests now used are ultrasound, amniocentesis, chorionic villus sampling (CVS), and the triple marker screen.

Terms   V w

placenta The organ through which the fetus receives nourishment and empties waste via the mother's circulatory system; after birth, the placenta is expelled from the uterus.

umbilical cord The cord connecting the placenta and fetus, through which nutrients pass.

amniotic sac A membranous pouch enclosing and protecting the fetus, containing amniotic fluid.

Ultrasonography provides information about the position, size, and physical condition of a fetus in the uterus. This mother-to-be can see her baby move and perhaps tell its sex by watching it on the screen.

Ultrasonography (also called *ultrasound*) uses high-frequency sound waves to create a **sonogram,** or visual image, of the fetus in the uterus. Sonograms show the position of the fetus, its size and gestational age, and the presence of certain anatomical problems. Sonograms can sometimes be used to determine the sex of the fetus. Sonograms are considered safe for a pregnant woman and the fetus, but the FDA advises against "keepsake" sonograms performed for no medical purpose.

Amniocentesis involves the removal of fluid from the uterus with a long, thin needle inserted through the abdominal wall. It is usually performed between 14 and 18 weeks into the pregnancy, although earlier amniocentesis is becoming available at some centers. A genetic analysis of the fetal cells in the fluid can reveal the presence of chromosomal disorders, such as Down syndrome, and some genetic diseases, including Tay-Sachs disease. The sex of the fetus can also be determined. Most amniocentesis tests are performed on pregnant women over age 35, who have a greater risk of chromosomal abnormalities, or in cases where the fetus is known to be at risk for a

particular chromosomal or genetic defect. Amniocentesis carries a slight risk (a 0.3–0.7% chance of miscarriage).

A newer alternative is **chorionic villus sampling (CVS),** which can be performed earlier in pregnancy than amniocentesis, between weeks 10 and 12. This procedure involves removal through the cervix (by catheter) or abdomen (by needle) of a tiny section of chorionic villi, which contain fetal cells that then can be analyzed. CVS carries a slightly higher risk of miscarriage than does amniocentesis (0.5–1%).

The **triple marker screen (TMS)** is a maternal blood test that can be used to help identify fetuses with neural tube defects, Down syndrome, and other anomalies. Blood is taken from the mother at 16–19 weeks of pregnancy and analyzed for three hormone levels—human chorionic gonadotropin (HCG), unconjugated estriol, and alpha-fetoprotein (AFP). The three hormone levels are compared to appropriate standards, and the results are used to estimate the probability that the fetus has particular anomalies. TMS is a screening test rather than a diagnostic test; in the case of abnormal TMS results, parents may choose further testing such as ultrasonography or amniocentesis.

A new first trimester screening test for Down syndrome combines ultrasound evaluation of nuchal translucency (the thickness of the back of the fetus's neck) with maternal blood testing. This test can be done between the 10th and 14th week of pregnancy. If results indicate an increased risk of abnormality, further diagnostic studies such as amniocentesis can be done for confirmation.

Genetic counselors explain the results of the different tests so that parents can understand their implications. If a fetus is found to have a defect, it may be carried to term, aborted, or, in rare instances, treated while still in the uterus. Results of most current screening tests are not available until after week 12 of pregnancy; consequently,

Terms

V w

ultrasonography The use of high-frequency sound waves to view the fetus in the uterus; also known as *ultrasound.*

sonogram The visual image of the fetus produced by ultrasonography.

amniocentesis A process in which amniotic fluid is removed and analyzed to detect possible birth defects.

chorionic villus sampling (CVS) Surgical removal of a tiny section of chorionic villi to be analyzed for genetic defects.

triple marker screen (TMS) Measurement of alpha-fetoprotein, estriol, and human chorionic gonadotropin to assess risk of fetal anomalies.

Pregnancy is a time of great change for a pregnant woman, and these changes can increase her level of stress. High levels of stress can have the same adverse effects on a pregnant woman as they do on anyone else (see Chapter 2). However, recent research suggests that stress can also affect the course of pregnancy and the health of the fetus.

Researchers have linked high levels of stress to miscarriage, preterm labor, and low birth weight. In one study, women who reported high levels of job stress were found to have a risk of miscarriage two to three times higher than that of less-stressed women. Other studies have found that pregnant women who experience major life changes, traumatic experiences, or high levels of pregnancy-related anxiety are at greater risk for preterm labor and for having a low-birth-weight infant. Stress hormones may constrict blood flow to the placenta, depriving the fetus of the oxygen and nutrients needed for optimal growth and development. Stress hormones also play a role in triggering labor, so high hormone levels may also increase the risk of preterm labor. Stress may also affect the behavior of a pregnant woman; negative coping techniques such as use of tobacco, alcohol, and other drugs can adversely affect a developing fetus. On the flip side, social support during pregnancy has been linked to improved fetal growth and healthy birth weight.

The time in pregnancy in which stress is experienced may be important in determining its effects. A study of earthquake survivors found that women who were in their first trimester when the earthquake occurred were at increased risk for preterm labor; women further along in their pregnancies experienced no such increase in risk. Researchers hypothesize that hormones produced in the later stages of pregnancy may protect both mother and fetus from the effects of stress.

High levels of stress have also been linked to birth defects. Although the overall risk of birth defects is very low, women who experience severe emotional trauma around the time of conception or during the first trimester are more likely to have an infant with defects of the skull, spine, palate, or limbs. The relationship between stress and birth defects has been found to be significantly greater in women with lower levels of education, suggesting that chronic stressors and behaviors that go along with low educational attainment and low income may increase the impact of stressful life events on fetal development.

As described in the discussion of fetal programming, stress during pregnancy can have even longer-term effects. Stress leads to high maternal levels of the hormone cortisol; when maternal diet is also poor, more cortisol crosses the placenta and reaches the fetal brain. Prenatal exposure to high levels of cortisol may increase susceptibility to stress in adulthood and permanently raise blood pressure.

Researchers have studied the long-term effects of stress by looking at children of pregnant Dutch women who experienced high levels of physical and emotional stress during the "Hunger Winter" of 1944–1945, when the Nazis blockaded the western Netherlands. Fetuses exposed to the famine early in development were found to be at increased risk of central nervous system defects and, as adults, obesity and schizophrenia. Studies of English children born in areas of poverty in the early 1900s found links between poor prenatal conditions and high blood pressure and heart disease. Although most American women do not experience such extreme stressors during pregnancy, these studies reinforce the importance of adequate prenatal care, including stress management and social support.

---

if abortion is chosen, it is likely to involve one of the more medically complex and physically difficult methods (see Chapter 7). Researchers are searching for new fetal screening techniques that are less invasive and that can be done earlier in pregnancy.

Fetal Programming   Amniocentesis, CVS, and TMS look for chromosomal, genetic, and other anomalies that typically cause immediate problems. A new area of study known as fetal programming theory focuses on how conditions in the womb may influence the risk of adult diseases. For example, researchers have linked low birth weight to an increased risk of heart disease, high blood pressure, obesity, diabetes, and schizophrenia; high birth weight in female infants, however, has been linked to an increased risk of breast cancer in later life.

How might conditions during gestation affect the risk of adult diseases? A number of studies have looked at groups of people born in areas of poverty or at times of famine, when pregnant women were unable to obtain an adequate diet. The poor prenatal conditions that stunt the growth of a developing fetus and lead to low birth weight may also affect specific organs. For example, if energy is limited, resources may be directed toward the developing fetal brain and away from other organs, including the liver and kidneys. Later in life, a small liver may be unable to clear cholesterol from the bloodstream, thereby increasing cholesterol levels and raising the risk of heart disease; undersized kidneys may be less able to regulate blood pressure. The fetus may also respond to limited resources by developing a permanently thrifty metabolism that triggers increased appetite and fat storage—leading to a greater risk of adult obesity and diabetes. Stress, both physical and emotional, increases maternal levels of the hormone cortisol, which in turn may permanently affect an infant's system of blood pressure regulation (see the box "Stress and Pregnancy").

Hormones may also be involved in the link between high birth weight and increased risk of breast cancer. Growth factors that contribute to high birth weight include leptin, insulin, and estrogen. Exposure to high levels of these in the womb may alter developing breast tissue in such a way that, when exposed to estrogen later in life, breast cells may be more likely to become malignant.

Although fetal programming theory is not yet embraced by all scientists, these studies emphasize that everything that occurs during pregnancy can have an impact on the developing fetus. For pregnant women, adequate nutrition and stress management are vital for both their own health and the health of the fetus (see the next section on prenatal care). In the future, people may be able to use information about their birth weight and other indicators of gestational conditions just as they can now use family history and genetic information—to alert them to special health risks they may face and to give them the opportunity to respond appropriately to maximize their health and well-being.

The Importance of Prenatal Care

Adequate prenatal care—a nutritious diet, exercise, adequate rest, avoidance of drugs, and regular medical evaluation—is essential to the health of both mother and baby. The pregnant woman cannot help but be responsible for the condition of the baby she carries. Everything she eats, drinks, and does affects the fetus in some respect. The fetus gets its nutrients and oxygen from the mother's bloodstream and has its wastes removed the same way. Many harmful substances can also be passed to the fetus via the placenta and umbilical cord. For these reasons, a mother's caring for her own health during pregnancy is a lifelong investment in her child's health.

Regular Checkups In the woman's first visit to her obstetrician, she will be asked for a detailed medical history of herself and her family. The physician or midwife will note any hereditary conditions that may assume increased significance during pregnancy. The tendency to develop gestational diabetes (diabetes during pregnancy only), for example, can be inherited; appropriate treatment during pregnancy reduces the risk of serious harm.

The woman is given a complete physical exam and is informed about appropriate diet. She returns for regular checkups throughout the pregnancy, during which her blood pressure and weight gain are measured, her urine is analyzed, and the size and position of the fetus are monitored. Regular prenatal visits also give the mother a chance to discuss her concerns and assure herself that everything is proceeding normally. Physicians, midwives, health educators, and teachers of childbirth classes can provide the mother with invaluable information.

Blood Tests A blood sample is taken during the initial prenatal visit to determine blood type and detect possible anemia or Rh incompatibilities. The Rh factor is a blood protein. If an Rh-positive father and an Rh-negative mother conceive an Rh-positive baby, the baby's blood will be incompatible with the mother's. If some of the baby's blood enters the mother's bloodstream during delivery, she will

develop antibodies to it just as she would toward a virus. If she has subsequent Rh-positive babies, the antibodies in the mother's blood, passing through the placenta, will destroy the fetus's red blood cells, possibly leading to jaundice, anemia, mental retardation, or death. This condition is completely treatable with a serum called Rh-immune globulin, which destroys Rh-positive cells as they enter the mother's body and prevents her from forming antibodies to them. Rh-immune globulin is given to Rh-negative mothers in the third trimester and again after the birth if the baby is found to be Rh-positive. Blood may also be tested for evidence of hepatitis B, syphilis, rubella immunity, thyroid problems, and, with the mother's permission, HIV infection.

Prenatal Nutrition The saying that a pregnant woman needs to "eat for two" is true. A nutritious diet throughout pregnancy is essential for both the fetus and the mother. Not only does the baby get all its nutrients from the mother, but it also competes with her for nutrients not sufficiently available to meet both their needs. When a woman's diet is low in iron or calcium, the fetus receives most of it, and the mother may become deficient in the mineral. To meet the increased nutritional demands of her body, a pregnant woman shouldn't just eat more; she should make sure that her diet is nutritionally adequate (see the box "Healthy Eating During Pregnancy").

Adequate intake of the B vitamin folic acid before conception and in the early weeks of pregnancy has been shown to decrease the risk of neural tube defects, including spina bifida. It is recommended that any woman capable of becoming pregnant consume at least 400 μg (0.4 mg) of folic acid daily from fortified foods and/or supplements, in addition to folate from a varied diet. For women who have already had a pregnancy involving a fetus with a neural tube defect, the CDC recommends consulting with a physician about taking a much larger amount of folic acid (4 mg), starting 1 month before conception and continuing through the first trimester. Folate is found naturally in leafy green vegetables, legumes, citrus fruits, and most berries. Beginning in 1998, enriched grain products have been fortified with small amounts of folic acid; the incidence of neural tube defects has dropped by more than 25% since fortification began.

Avoiding Drugs and Other Environmental Hazards In addition to the food the mother eats, the drugs she takes and the chemicals she is exposed to affect the fetus. Everything the mother ingests may eventually reach the fetus in some proportion. Some drugs harm the fetus but not the mother because the fetus is in the process of developing and because the proper dose for the mother is a massive dose for the fetus.

During the first trimester, when the major body structures are rapidly forming, the fetus is extremely vulnerable to environmental factors such as viral infections, radiation, drugs, and other **teratogens**, any of which can cause

Take Charge

A healthy diet is a key part of prenatal care. To maintain her own health and help the fetus grow, a woman needs to consume about 250–500 extra calories per day during pregnancy. Breast-feeding an infant requires even more energy—about 500 or more extra calories per day.

Healthy Choices

To ensure a balanced intake of key nutrients, pregnant women should follow the U.S. Department of Agriculture's Food Guide, which is based on five basic food groups. For a moderately active pregnant woman consuming about 2400 calories per day, the daily recommended intake from each group is as follows:

- Fruits: 2 cups

- Vegetables: 3 cups total, including a mixture of legumes (dry beans and peas) and dark green, orange, or deep yellow, and starchy vegetables

- Grains: 8 ounce-equivalents, with 1 slice of bread or ½ cup of cooked grains being the equivalent of 1 ounce; half of daily grain servings should be whole grains

- Lean meat, poultry, fish, dry beans, eggs, and nuts: 6.5 ounces of lean meat or the equivalent

- Milk, yogurt, and cheese: 3 cups

Fats, oils, and sweets should be used sparingly according to total energy needs. Finally, it is also important to consume an adequate amount of fluids—the equivalent of about 11 cups of liquid from beverages and foods. See Chapter 12 for a more detailed discussed of the Food Guide.

Supplements

Some physicians may prescribe vitamin and mineral supplements for women who are pregnant or lactating or who are trying to get pregnant. Supplements may be for a particular nutrient, such as folic acid or iron, or may be a multivitamin and mineral supplement. It is important that a pregnant woman not supplement beyond her physician's advice because some vitamins and minerals are harmful if taken in excess. It is also important not to take herbal dietary supplements without consulting a physician; few dietary supplements have been tested for safety during pregnancy, and some have been shown to be dangerous.

Food Safety

Pregnant women should give special attention to food safety because foodborne pathogens can be particularly dangerous during pregnancy. Two such pathogens are *Listeria monocytogenes* and *Toxoplasma gondii*. *Listeria* is a bacterium most often found in undercooked or ready-to-eat meat, poultry, or seafood; soft cheeses; products made with unpasteurized milk; and unpasteurized juice. Listeriosis causes flulike symptoms in pregnant women; if the fetus is infected, the result can be miscarriage, premature birth, or birth defects.

T. gondii, a parasite carried by cats, can also contaminate food or soil. Toxoplasmosis is typically caused by eating undercooked meat or poultry or unwashed fruits and vegetables, cleaning a litter box, or handling contaminated soil. Toxoplasmosis causes few symptoms in pregnant women, but if passed to the fetus it may cause miscarriage or mental impairment.

To avoid foodborne illness, pregnant women should wash their hands thoroughly before preparing or eating food and after handling raw meats or using the bathroom. They should cook meat, poultry, and seafood thoroughly and reheat leftovers or ready-to-eat foods until steaming hot. Fruits and vegetables should be thoroughly washed under running water, and unpasteurized juices and milk should be avoided. Pregnant women may choose to avoid foods that are most likely to carry dangerous pathogens. (Interestingly, researchers have found that the types of foods that pregnant women with "morning sickness" tend to avoid—meat, fish, poultry, eggs, and strong-tasting vegetables—are those that have historically been most likely to carry dangerous microorganisms or natural toxins, suggesting that morning sickness may be a protective adaptation.)

One further food safety recommendation for pregnant women relates to fish. Most types of fish are good choices for a healthy diet, but a few types can be contaminated with mercury or industrial pollutants. The FDA advises pregnant women not to eat swordfish, shark, king mackerel, or tilefish and to limit overall fish consumption to 12 ounces per week. Pregnant women are also advised to check with their local health departments before consuming any game fish.

For a more detailed discussion of recommended food choices, serving sizes, and food safety guidelines, see Chapter 12.

---

congenital malformations, or birth defects. The most susceptible body parts are those growing most rapidly at the time of exposure. The rubella (German measles) virus, for example, can cause a congenital malformation of a delicate system such as the eyes or ears, leading to blindness or deafness, if exposure occurs during the first trimester, but it does no damage later in the pregnancy. Similarly, the drug thalidomide taken early in pregnancy prevents the formation of arms and legs in fetuses, but taken later, when limbs are already formed, it causes no damage. Other drugs can cause damage throughout prenatal development.

ALCOHOL Alcohol is a potent teratogen. Getting drunk just one time during pregnancy may be enough to cause brain damage in a fetus. A high level of alcohol consumption

Terms

teratogen An agent or influence that causes physical defects in a developing fetus.

congenital malformation A physical defect existing at the time of birth, either inherited or caused during gestation.

---

during pregnancy is associated with miscarriages, stillbirths, and, in live babies, **fetal alcohol syndrome (FAS).** A baby born with FAS is likely to suffer from a small head and body size, unusual facial characteristics, congenital heart defects, defective joints, mental impairment, and abnormal behavior patterns. The Centers for Disease Control and Prevention (CDC) estimate that about 1 out of every 1000 infants born in the United States has FAS. The rate is highest among those of low socioeconomic status, African Americans, and Native Americans. Researchers now doubt that any level of alcohol consumption is safe, and they recommend total abstinence during pregnancy (see Chapter 10).

TOBACCO Pregnant women who smoke should quit, and nonsmoking pregnant women should avoid places where people smoke. Smoking during pregnancy increases the risk of miscarriage, low birth weight, and infant death; it may also cause genetic damage. If nicotine levels in a mother's bloodstream are high, fetal breathing rate and movement become more rapid; the fetus may also metabolize cancer-causing by-products of tobacco. Infants of women who smoke during pregnancy have poorer lung function at birth, and exposure to secondhand smoke after birth increases a baby's susceptibility to pneumonia and bronchitis. If a mother who smokes breast-feeds, her infant will be exposed to tobacco chemicals through breast milk. See Chapter 11 for more on the effects of smoking.

CAFFEINE Caffeine, a powerful stimulant, should be used conservatively by pregnant women. It puts both mother and fetus under stress by raising the level of the hormone epinephrine. Caffeine also reduces the blood supply to the uterus. One study found that consuming the amount of caffeine in five or more cups of coffee a day doubled the risk of miscarriage. Coffee, colas, strong black tea, and chocolate are high in caffeine, as are over-the-counter medications such as Excedrin and NōDōz (see Chapter 9). A pregnant woman should limit her caffeine intake to no more than the equivalent of about two cups of coffee per day.

DRUGS AND CHEMICALS Some prescription drugs can also harm the fetus, so they should be used only under medical supervision. Accutane, a popular anti-acne drug, is thought to have been responsible for over 1000 cases of severe birth defects in the 1980s. Vitamins, aspirin, and other over-the-counter drugs should be used only under a physician's direction. Large doses of vitamin A, for example, can cause birth defects. Chemicals and pollutants can also pose a danger to the fetus. Mercury, from fish contaminated by industrial pollution, is known to cause physical deformities. Continuous exposure to lead, found in some paint products and in water from lead pipes, has been implicated as a cause of a variety of learning disorders. Any product containing chemicals—including chemical fertilizers, solvents, and pesticides—should be avoided or used with extreme caution.

STDs AND OTHER INFECTIONS Infections, including those that are sexually transmitted, are another serious problem for the fetus. The most common cause of life-threatening infections in newborns is Group B streptococcus (GBS), a type of bacterium that can cause pneumonia, meningitis, and blood infections. Many pregnant women carry GBS but do not become ill, so routine screening close to the time of delivery is recommended. A woman who carries GBS and who has certain other conditions, such as fever during labor, may be given intravenous antibiotics at the time of labor to reduce the risk of passing GBS to her baby.

If a mother contracts rubella during the first trimester, her child may be born with physical or mental disabilities. Immunization against measles must take place before pregnancy, because the immunization is harmful to the fetus. Syphilis can infect and kill a fetus; if the baby is born alive, it will have syphilis. Penicillin taken by the mother during pregnancy cures syphilis in both mother and fetus. Gonorrhea can infect the baby during delivery and cause blindness. Because gonorrhea is often asymptomatic, in many states the eyes of newborns are routinely treated with erythromycin ointment to destroy gonorrheal bacteria. All pregnant women should be tested for hepatitis B, a virus that can pass from the mother to the infant at birth. Infants of infected mothers can be immunized shortly after birth.

Herpes simplex can damage the baby's eyes and brain and cause death, and no cure has yet been discovered for it. Genital herpes can be transmitted to the baby during delivery if the mother's infection is in the active phase. If this is the case, the baby may be delivered by cesarean section. An initial outbreak of herpes can be dangerous if it occurs during pregnancy because the virus may pass through the placenta to the fetus. For this reason, it is important to know if the pregnant woman or her partner has a history of herpes. If the woman has not had herpes, but her partner has, she may be at increased risk for contracting the infection and having the initial outbreak during the pregnancy. In some situations, women may be tested to see if they have blood evidence of herpes infection. Once the baby is born, any caregiver who is experiencing a herpes outbreak should wash his or her hands often and not permit contact between hands or contaminated objects and the baby's mucous membranes (inside of eyes, mouth, nose, penis, vagina, vulva, and rectum).

The human immunodeficiency virus (HIV), which causes AIDS, can be passed to the fetus by an HIV-infected mother during pregnancy, labor and delivery, or

Term

V̄i̅w

fetal alcohol syndrome (FAS) A combination of birth defects caused by excessive alcohol consumption by the mother during pregnancy.

Table 8-1 Selected Environmental Factors Associated with Problems in a Fetus or Infant

Agent or Condition	Potential Effects
Accutane (acne medication)	Small head, mental impairment, deformed or absent ears, heart defects, cleft lip and palate
Alcohol	Unusual facial characteristics, small head, heart defects, mental impairment, defective joints
Chlamydia	Eye infections, pneumonia
Cigarette smoking	Miscarriage, stillbirth, low birth weight, respiratory problems, sudden infant death
Cocaine	Miscarriage, stillbirth, low birth weight, small head, defects of genital and urinary tracts
Cytomegalovirus (CMV)	Small head, mental impairment, blindness
Diabetes (insulin-dependent)	Malformations of the brain, spine, and heart
Gonorrhea	Eye infection leading to blindness if untreated
Herpes	Brain damage, death
HIV infection	Impaired immunity, death
Lead	Reduced IQ, learning disorders
Marijuana	Impaired fetal growth, increase in alcohol-related fetal damage
Mercury	Brain damage
Propecia (hair loss medication)	Abnormalities of the male sex organs
Radiation (high dose)	Small head, growth and mental impairment, multiple birth defects
Rubella (German measles)	Malformation of eyes or ears causing deafness or blindness; small head; mental impairment
Syphilis	Fetal death and miscarriage, prematurity, physical deformities
Tetracycline	Pigmentation of teeth, underdevelopment of enamel
Vitamin A (excess)	Miscarriage; defects of the head, brain, spine, and urinary tract

breastfeeding. Nationwide, more than 9000 children under age 13 have been diagnosed with AIDS, and many more are infected with HIV. The babies most at risk are those whose mothers inject drugs or are the sex partners of men who inject drugs. HIV testing is critical for any woman at risk for HIV, and some physicians recommend routine testing for all pregnant women. Antiviral drugs, given to an HIV-infected mother during pregnancy and delivery and to her newborn immediately following birth, reduce the rate of HIV transmission from mother to infant from 25% to 5% or less. Of course, women should also take all the necessary precautions against HIV infection during pregnancy. (See Chapter 18 for more on HIV and other STDs.)

Environmental factors affecting fetal or infant development are summarized in Table 8-1.

Prenatal Activity and Exercise Physical activity during pregnancy contributes to mental and physical wellness. Women can continue working at their jobs until late in their pregnancy, provided the work isn't so physically demanding that it jeopardizes their health. At the same time, pregnant women need more rest and sleep to maintain their own well-being and that of the fetus.

A moderate exercise program during pregnancy does not adversely affect pregnancy or birth; in fact, regular exercise appears to improve a woman's chance of an on-time

delivery. The amniotic sac protects the fetus, and normal activities will not harm it. A woman who exercised before becoming pregnant can often continue her program, with appropriate modifications to maintain her comfort and safety. A pregnant woman who hasn't been exercising and wants to start should first consult a physician. Regular cardiorespiratory endurance exercise is recommended. Walking, swimming, and stationary cycling are all good choices; more strenuous activities that could result in a fall, such as skiing, skating, or horseback riding, are best delayed until after the birth. Recommendations for exercising safely during pregnancy include the following:

- Exercise regularly (at least three times a week) rather than intermittently.

- After 20 weeks of pregnancy, avoid exercise that requires lying on your back. Research indicates that this position restricts blood flow to the uterus. Also avoid prolonged periods of motionless standing.

- Modify the intensity of your exercise according to how you feel. Stop exercising if you feel fatigued, and don't exercise to exhaustion. You may find that non–weight-bearing exercises such as swimming and cycling are more comfortable than weight-bearing activities in the later months of pregnancy; they also minimize the risk of injury.

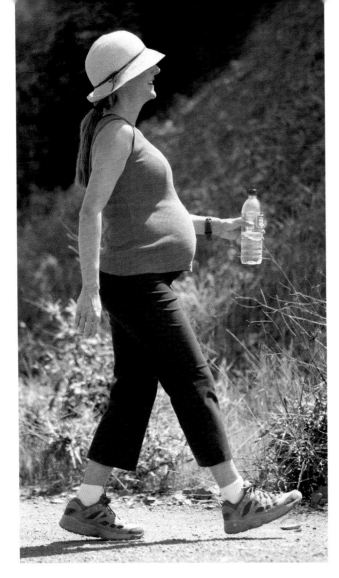

A woman's body changes drastically during pregnancy to accommodate and nourish the growing fetus. Prenatal exercise helps this woman stay healthy while her body works to sustain two lives.

- Avoid any type of exercise that has the potential for even mild abdominal trauma, and take care when performing any activity in which balance is important or in which losing balance would be dangerous. Pregnancy shifts your center of gravity.

- Avoid heat stress, particularly during the first trimester, by drinking an adequate amount of fluid, wearing appropriate clothing, and avoiding activity in hot and humid weather.

- If you experience any unusual symptoms, stop exercising and consult your physician. Warning signs include pain, vaginal bleeding, dizziness, rapid heartbeat, shortness of breath, and uterine contractions.

- Resume prepregnancy exercise routines gradually. Many of the changes of pregnancy persist for 4–6 weeks after delivery.

Kegel exercises, to strengthen the pelvic floor muscles, are also recommended for pregnant women. These exercises are performed by alternately contracting and releasing the muscles used to stop the flow of urine. Each contraction should be held for about 5 seconds. Kegel exercises should be done several times a day, for a total of about 50 repetitions daily.

Prenatal exercise classes are valuable because they teach exercises that tone the body muscles involved in birth, especially those of the abdomen, back, and legs. Toned-up muscles aid delivery and help the body regain its nonpregnant shape afterward.

Preparing for Birth   Childbirth classes are almost a routine part of the prenatal experience for both mothers and fathers these days. These classes typically teach the details of the birth process as well as relaxation techniques to help deal with the discomfort of labor and delivery. The mother learns and practices a variety of techniques so she will be able to choose what works best for her during labor when the time comes. The father typically acts as a coach, supporting his partner emotionally and helping her with her breathing and relaxing. He remains with her throughout labor and delivery, even when a cesarean section is performed. It can be an important and fulfilling time for the parents to be together.

Complications of Pregnancy and Pregnancy Loss

Pregnancy usually proceeds without major complications. Sometimes, however, complications may prevent full-term development of the fetus or affect the health of the infant at birth. As discussed earlier in the chapter, exposure to harmful substances, such as alcohol or drugs, can harm the fetus. Other complications are caused by physiological problems or genetic abnormalities.

Ectopic Pregnancy   In an **ectopic pregnancy,** the fertilized egg implants and begins to develop outside of the uterus, usually in an oviduct. Ectopic pregnancies usually occur because the fallopian tube is blocked, most often as a result of pelvic inflammatory disease; smoking also increases a woman's risk for ectopic pregnancy. The embryo may spontaneously abort, or the embryo and placenta may continue to expand until they rupture the oviduct. Sharp pain on one side of the abdomen or in the lower back, usually in about the 7th or 8th week, may signal an ectopic pregnancy, and there may be irregular bleeding. If bleeding from a rupture is severe, the woman may go into shock, characterized by low blood pressure, a fast pulse, weakness, and fainting. Surgical removal of the embryo and the oviduct may be necessary to save the mother's life, although microsurgery can sometimes be used to repair the damaged oviduct. If diagnosed early, before the oviduct ruptures, ectopic pregnancy can often be successfully treated without surgery with injections of methotrexate. The incidence of

Critical Consumer

Making a Birth Plan

A variety of birth situations can have positive physical and psychological outcomes. Parents should choose what is appropriate for their medical circumstances and what feels most comfortable to them. Prospective parents should discuss their preferences in the following areas with their physician or midwife:

1. Who will be present at the birth? The father? Friends? Children and other relatives? Will young siblings be allowed to visit the mother and new baby?

2. What type of room will the mother be in during labor, delivery, and recovery? How many times will she be moved?

3. What types of tables, beds, or birthing chairs are available? What type of environment can be created for the birth? Can specific music be played?

4. Will the mother receive any routine preparation, such as an enema, intravenous feeding, or shaving of the pubic area?

5. What is the policy regarding food and drink during labor? Will the mother have the option of walking around or taking a shower or bath during labor?

6. Under what circumstances does the physician or midwife administer drugs to induce or augment labor? The use of these drugs tends to change the course of labor and carries a small risk.

7. Is **electronic fetal monitoring (EFM)** typically used during labor? About 75% of all births are electronically monitored, but there is disagreement among medical authorities about the risks or benefits of EFM. The American College of Obstetricians and Gynecologists offers periodic monitoring using a stethoscope rather than EFM for low-risk pregnancies.

8. Under what circumstances will an **episiotomy,** an incision at the base of the vaginal opening, be performed? Are any steps taken to avoid it?

9. Under what circumstances will forceps or vacuum extraction be used? In some cases of fetal distress, the use of forceps or vacuum extraction may be necessary to save the infant's life, but some authorities believe these techniques are overused.

10. What types of medications are typically used during labor and delivery? Some form of anesthetic is usually administered during most hospital deliveries, as are hormones that intensify the contractions and shrink the uterus after delivery. Different types of anesthetics, including short-acting narcotics, regional nerve blocks, and local anesthetics, may be available; each has different effects on the mother and the fetus.

11. Under what conditions or circumstances does the physician perform a cesarean section? If prospective parents are concerned, they should research the cesarean frequency rates of different physicians before they make their final choice.

12. Who will "catch" the baby as she or he is born? Who will cut the umbilical cord?

13. What will be done to the baby immediately after birth? What kinds of tests and procedures will be done on the baby, and when?

14. How often will the baby be brought to the mother while they remain in the hospital or birthing center? Can the baby stay in the mother's room rather than in the nursery? This practice is known as **rooming-in.**

15. How will the baby be fed—by breast or bottle? Will feeding be on a schedule or on demand? Is there someone with breastfeeding experience available to answer questions if necessary?

the uterine contractions, the number of prior deliveries, and other factors. The length of labor is generally shorter for second and subsequent births.

The First Stage of Labor The first stage of labor averages 13 hours for a first birth, although there is a wide variation among women. It begins with cervical effacement and dilation and continues until the cervix is completely dilated (10 centimeters). Contractions usually last about 30 seconds and occur every 15–20 minutes at first, more often later. The prepared mother relaxes as much as possible during these contractions to allow labor to proceed without being blocked by tension. Early in the first stage, a small amount of bleeding may occur as a plug of slightly bloody mucus that blocked the opening of the cervix during pregnancy is expelled. In some women, the amniotic sac ruptures and the fluid rushes out; this is sometimes referred to as the "water breaking."

The last part of the first stage of labor, called **transition,** is characterized by strong and frequent contractions, much more intense than in the early stages of labor. Contractions may last 60–90 seconds and occur every 1–3 minutes. During transition the cervix opens completely, to a diameter of about 10 centimeters. The head of the fetus usually measures 9–10 centimeters; thus once the cervix has dilated completely, the head can pass through. Many women report that transition, which normally lasts about 30–60 minutes, is the most difficult part of labor.

The Second Stage of Labor The second stage of labor begins with complete cervical dilation and ends with the delivery of the baby. The baby is slowly pushed down, through the bones of the pelvic ring, past the cervix, and into the vagina, which it stretches open. The mother bears down with the contractions to help push

(a)

(b)

(c)

Figure 8-6 Birth: labor and delivery. (a) The first stage of labor; (b) the second stage of labor: delivery of the baby; (c) the third stage of labor: expulsion of the placenta.

the baby down and out. Some women find this the most difficult part of labor; others find that the contractions and bearing down bring a sense of relief. The baby's back bends, the head turns to fit through the narrowest parts of the passageway, and the soft bones of the baby's skull move together and overlap as it is squeezed through the pelvis. When the top of the head appears at the vaginal opening, the baby is said to be crowning.

As the head of the baby emerges, the physician or midwife will remove any mucus from the mouth and nose, wipe the baby's face, and check to ensure that the umbilical cord is not around the neck. With a few more contractions, the baby's shoulders and body emerge. As the baby is squeezed through the pelvis, cervix, and vagina, the fluid in the lungs is forced out by the pressure on the baby's chest. Once this pressure is released as the baby emerges from the vagina, the chest expands and the lungs fill with air for the first time. The baby will still be connected to the mother via the umbilical cord, which is not cut until it stops pulsating. The baby will appear wet and often is covered with a milky substance. The baby's head may be oddly shaped at first, due to the molding of the soft plates of bone during birth, but it usually takes on a more rounded appearance within 24 hours.

The Third Stage of Labor In the third stage of labor, the uterus continues to contract until the placenta is expelled. This stage usually takes 5–20 minutes. If the placenta does not come out on its own, the physician or midwife may exert gentle pressure on the abdomen to help with its delivery. It is important that the entire placenta be expelled; if part remains in the uterus, it may cause infection or bleeding. Breastfeeding soon after delivery helps control uterine bleeding because it stimulates the secretion of a hormone that makes the uterus contract; massaging the abdomen may also help.

In the meantime, the physical condition of the baby will be assessed with the **Apgar score**, a formalized system for assessing the baby's need for medical assistance during the first few minutes of life. Heart rate, respiration, color, reflexes, and muscle tone are individually rated with a score of 0–2, and a total score between 0 and 10 is given at 1 and 5 minutes after birth. A score of 7–10 at 5 minutes is considered normal. The baby is then usually wrapped securely in a blanket and returned to the mother, who may begin to nurse the baby right away.

Pain Relief During Labor and Delivery Women vary in how much pain they experience in childbirth. First babies are typically the most challenging to deliver, as the birth canal has never stretched to this extent before. It is recommended that women and their partners learn about labor and what kinds of choices are available for pain relief. Childbirth preparation courses are a good place to start, and communicating with one's obstetrician or midwife is essential to assess the approaches that will be available. Breathing and relaxation techniques such as Lamaze or Bradley have been used effectively, and they are often modified by the laboring women to be even more effective. Forms of hypnosis can also be used.

The most commonly employed medical intervention for pain relief is the epidural. This procedure involves placing a thin plastic catheter between the vertebrae in the lower back. Medication that reduces the transmission of pain signals to the brain is given through this catheter. Local anesthetic drugs are given in low concentration in order to minimize weakening of the leg muscles so that the mother can effectively push during the birth. The amount of medication given is quite low and does not accumulate in the baby or interfere with the baby's transition after birth. The mother is awake and is an active participant in the birth. Because the pain relief is often quite successful, this approach has become popular and is offered in many hospitals.

Women can also elect to have narcotics, such as fentanyl or demerol, given for pain relief during labor, but these medications usually provide less pain relief than the epidural and, if given shortly before the birth, can cause the baby to be less vigorous at birth. Local anesthesia is available for repair of any tear or episiotomy if the mother has not used an epidural for the labor.

Cesarean Deliveries   About 26% of the babies born in the United States are delivered by **cesarean section,** in which the baby is removed through a surgical incision in the abdominal wall and uterus. Cesarean sections are necessary when a baby cannot be delivered vaginally—for example, if the baby's head is bigger than the mother's pelvic girdle or if the baby is in an unusual position. If the mother has a serious health condition such as high blood pressure, a cesarean may be safer for her than labor and a vaginal delivery. Cesareans are more common among women who are overweight or have diabetes. Other reasons for cesarean delivery include abnormal or difficult labor, fetal distress, and the presence of a dangerous infection like herpes that can be passed to the baby during delivery. A growing number of cesareans are performed on low-risk mothers; researchers hope further analysis will help determine if the trend is due to patient choice, physician choice, or a combination of the two.

Repeat cesarean deliveries are also very common. About 85% of American women who have had one child by cesarean have subsequent children delivered the same way. Although the risk of complications from a vaginal delivery after a previous cesarean delivery is low, there is a small (1%) risk of serious complication to the mother and baby if the previous uterine scar opens during labor (uterine rupture). For this reason, women and their doctors may choose to deliver by elective repeat caesarean.

A cesarean section is major surgery and carries some risk, but it is relatively safe. A regional anesthetic such as a spinal or epidural anesthetic may be used so the woman can remain conscious during the operation. The father may be present.

The Postpartum Period

The **postpartum period,** a stage of about 3 months following childbirth, is a time of critical family adjustments. Parenthood—a job that goes on around the clock without relief—begins literally overnight, and the transition can cause considerable physical and emotional stress.

Following a vaginal delivery, mothers usually leave the hospital within 1–3 days (after a cesarean section, they usually stay 3–5 days). Uterine contractions will occur from time to time for several days after delivery, especially during nursing, as the uterus begins to return to its prebirth size. It usually takes 6–8 weeks for a woman's reproductive organs to return to their prebirth condition. She will have a bloody discharge called *lochia* for 3–6 weeks after the birth.

Within the first few days after birth, a baby will undergo screening for certain genetic conditions such as sickle cell disease; the mandated tests vary by state. The baby's head—if somewhat pointed following a vaginal delivery—will become more rounded within a few days. It takes about a week for the umbilical cord stump to shrivel and fall off. Regular infant check-ups for health screenings and immunizations usually begin when the infant is two weeks of age.

Currently, just over 60% of mothers breast-feed their infants for some period, up from about 10% in 1970. **Lactation,** the production of milk, begins about 3 days after childbirth. Prior to that time (sometimes as early as the second trimester), **colostrum** is secreted by the nipples. Colostrum contains antibodies that help protect the newborn from infectious diseases and is also high in protein.

The American Academy of Pediatrics recommends breastfeeding exclusively for 6 months, in combination with solid food until the baby is 1 year of age, and then for as long after that as a mother and baby desire. Currently, only 14% of U.S. mothers breastfeed exclusively for 6 months. Human milk is perfectly suited to the baby's nutritional needs and digestive capabilities, and it supplies the baby with antibodies. Breastfeeding decreases

---

Terms   Vw

Apgar score A formalized system for assessing a newborn's need for medical assistance.

cesarean section A surgical incision through the abdominal wall and uterus, performed to deliver a fetus.

postpartum period The period of about 3 months after delivering a baby.

lactation The production of milk.

colostrum A yellowish fluid secreted by the mammary glands around the time of childbirth until milk comes in, about the third day.

Breastfeeding can enhance the bond between mother and child. The American Academy of Pediatrics recommends breastfeeding exclusively for 6 months and then in combination with solid food until the baby is at least 1 year of age.

the incidence of infant ear infections, allergies, anemia, diarrhea, and bacterial meningitis; breastfed babies are less likely to be overweight when they reach preschool age. One study has even suggested that children who are breastfed do better in school and score higher on standardized tests. Breastfeeding is also beneficial to the mother: It stimulates contractions that help the uterus return to normal more rapidly, contributes to postpregnancy weight loss, and may reduce the risk of ovarian cancer, breast cancer, and postmenopausal hip fracture. Nursing also provides a sense of closeness and emotional well-being for mother and child. For women who want to breast-feed but who have problems, help is available from support groups, books, or a lactation consultant.

Term

V**i**w

postpartum depression An emotional low that may be experienced by the mother following childbirth.

For some women, physical problems such as tenderness or infection of the nipples can make breastfeeding difficult. If a woman has an illness or requires drug treatment, she may have to bottle-feed her baby because drugs and infectious agents may show up in breast milk. Breastfeeding can be restrictive, making it especially difficult for working mothers. Employers rarely provide nursing breaks, so bottlefeeding or the use of a breast pump (to express milk for use while the mother is away from her infant) may be the only practical alternatives. Bottlefeeding makes it easier to tell how much milk an infant is taking in, and bottlefed infants tend to sleep longer. Bottlefeeding also allows the father or other caregiver to share in the nurturing process. Both breastfeeding and bottlefeeding can be part of loving, secure parent-child relationships.

When a mother doesn't nurse, menstruation usually begins within about 10 weeks. Breastfeeding can prevent the return of menstruation for 6 months or longer because the hormone prolactin, which aids milk production, suppresses hormones vital to the development of mature eggs. However, ovulation—and pregnancy—can occur before menstruation returns, so breastfeeding is not a highly reliable contraceptive method; if a woman wishes to avoid pregnancy, she should use a more reliable method. If the mother becomes pregnant while still nursing, she needs to make sure that she is receiving adequate nutrition, because the energy requirement for both breastfeeding and gestating is immense. With proper counseling, breastfeeding can continue until near delivery.

Many women experience fluctuating emotions during the postpartum period as hormone levels change. The physical stress of labor, as well as dehydration, blood loss, and other physical factors, contributes to lowering the woman's stamina. About 50–80% of new mothers experience "baby blues," characterized by episodes of sadness, weeping, anxiety, headache, sleep disturbances, and irritability. A mother may feel lonely and anxious about caring for her infant. About 10% of new mothers experience **postpartum depression,** a more disabling syndrome characterized by despondency, mood swings, guilt, and occasional hostility. Rest, sharing feelings and concerns with others, and relying on supportive relatives and friends for assistance are usually helpful in dealing with mild cases of the baby blues or postpartum depression, which generally lasts only a few weeks. If the depression is serious, professional treatment may be needed. Some men also seem to get a form of postpartum depression, characterized by anxiety about their changing role and feelings of inadequacy. Both mothers and fathers need time to adjust to their new roles as parents.

Another feature of the postpartum period is the development of attachment—the strong emotional tie that grows between the baby and the adult who cares for the baby. Parents can foster secure attachment relationships in the early weeks and months by responding sensitively to the baby's true needs. Parents who respond appropriately to the baby's signals of gazing, looking away, smiling, and crying establish feelings of trust in their child. They feed the baby when she's hungry, for example; respond when she cries; interact with her when she gazes, smiles, or babbles; and stop stimulating her when she frowns or looks away. A secure attachment relationship helps the child develop and function well socially, emotionally, and mentally.

For most people, the arrival of a child provides a deep sense of joy and accomplishment. However, adjusting to parenthood requires effort and energy. Talking with friends and relatives about their experiences during the first few weeks or months with a baby can help prepare new parents for the period when the baby's needs may require all the energy that both parents have to expend. But the pleasures of nurturing a new baby are substantial, and many parents look back on this time as one of the most significant and joyful of their lives.

Having a child is one of life's most important events. It transforms people as individuals, as partners in a relationship, and as members of a family. Preparation for being a parent begins long before pregnancy; it includes healthy lifestyle choices in all the areas of wellness.

Right now you can

- Take some time to think about whether *you* want to have children; try to cut through the cultural, societal, family, and personal expectations that may stand in the way of your making the decision you really want to make.

- Think of one thing your mother or father did as a parent that you particularly disliked; if you become a parent, how can you keep from repeating that behavior with your children?

- Think of one thing your mother or father did as a parent that you particularly liked; if you become a parent, how can you make sure you do the same thing with your children?

- If you are sexually active, consider your sexual behavior and your contraceptive choice (or lack of one). Are you taking any chances that would jeopardize your future fertility or reproductive options? If so, resolve to change that behavior.

- If you smoke, start thinking about how to quit.

- If you are sedentary, start thinking about a form of moderate exercise that you can continue throughout your life, such as swimming or walking. Make a plan to begin the activity today or tomorrow.

SUMMARY

- Factors to consider when deciding if and when to have a child include physical health and age; financial circumstances; relationship with your partner; educational,

career, and child care plans; emotional readiness for parenthood; social support system; personal qualities, attitudes toward children, and aptitude for parenting; and philosophical or religious beliefs.

- Preconception care examines factors such as preexisting medical conditions, current medications, age of the mother, lifestyle behaviors, infections, nutritional status, and family history of genetic disease.

- Fertilization is a complex process culminating when a sperm penetrates the membrane of the egg released from the woman's ovary.

- Infertility affects about 10% of the reproductive-age population of the United States. The leading causes of infertility in women are blocked oviducts and ovulation disorders. Exposure to toxins, injury to the testicles, and infection can cause infertility in men.

- Early signs and symptoms of pregnancy include a missed menstrual period; slight bleeding; nausea; breast tenderness; increased urination; fatigue and emotional upset; and a softening of the uterus just above the cervix.

- During pregnancy, the uterus enlarges until it pushes up into the rib cage; the breasts enlarge and may secrete colostrum; the muscles and ligaments soften and stretch; and the circulatory system, lungs, and kidneys become more efficient.

- The fetal anatomy is almost completely formed in the first trimester and is refined in the second; during the third trimester, the fetus grows and gains most of its weight, storing nutrients in fatty tissues.

- Prenatal tests include ultrasound, amniocentesis, chorionic villus sampling, and triple marker screening.

- Health care during pregnancy includes a complete history and physical at the beginning, followed by regular checkups for blood pressure, weight gain, and size and position of the fetus.

- Important elements of prenatal care include good nutrition; avoiding drugs, alcohol, tobacco, infections, and other harmful environmental agents or conditions; regular physical activity; and childbirth classes.

- Pregnancy usually proceeds without major complications. Problems that can occur include ectopic pregnancy, spontaneous abortion, preeclampsia, and low birth weight. The loss of a fetus or infant is deeply felt by most parents, who need time to grieve and heal.

- Couples preparing for childbirth may have many options to choose from, including type of practitioner and facility.

- The first stage of labor begins with contractions that exert pressure on the cervix, causing effacement and dilation. The second stage begins with complete cervical dilation and ends when the baby emerges. The third stage of labor is expulsion of the placenta.

- During the postpartum period, the mother's body begins to return to its prepregnancy state, and she begins to breast-feed. Both mother and father must adjust to their new roles as parents, as they develop a strong emotional tie to their baby.

Take Action

1. **Listen to birth stories:** Interview your parents to find out what your birth was like. What were their personal preferences, and what were the cultural conditions like at the time? Find out as much as you can about hospital procedure, the use of anesthetics, length of hospital stay, and so on. Did your father have a role in your birth? If possible, also interview your grandparents or someone of their generation and someone who became a parent in the past few years. How were their experiences different from those of your parents'?

2. **Investigate childbirth facilities in your community.** If possible, visit the maternity wing of a hospital and an alternative birth center. What do you like about them, and what do you not like? What types of childbirth preparation classes do they offer? Which of these do you feel most comfortable with? Why?

For More Information

Books

Appelbaum, A., and S. Ilse. 2000. *Empty Arms: Coping After Miscarriage, Stillbirth, and Infant Death*, rev. ed. Maple Plain, Minn.: Wintergreen Press. *A sensitive guide to the experience of pregnancy loss.*

Milunsky, A. 2002. *Your Genetic Destiny: Know Your Genes, Secure Your Health, Save Your Life.* Cambridge, Mass.: Perseus. *Provides information on compiling a family health history, genetic counseling, genetic testing, and the causes and treatments of common genetic disorders.*

Ogle, A., and L. Mazzullo. 2002. *Prepare for a Healthy Conception.* New York: Ballantine. *Provides practical information about preconception care.*

Tsiaras, A., and B. Werth. 2002. *From Conception to Birth: A Life Unfolds.* New York: Doubleday. *The story of prenatal development and birth, told in text and in stunning photographs and medical imaging.*

Wisot, A. L., and D. R. Meldrum. 2004. *Conceptions & Misconceptions: The Informed Consumer's Guide Through the Maze of In Vitro Fertilization & Assisted Reproduction Techniques*, 2nd ed. Vancouver: Hartley and Marks. *A consumer-friendly explanation of assisted reproduction.*

The following are a few of the many excellent guides to conception, pregnancy, and birth:

American College of Obstetricians and Gynecologists. 2005. *Your Pregnancy and Birth*, 4th ed. Washington, D.C.: ACOG.

Curtis, G. B., and J. Schuler. 2003. *Your Pregnancy for the Father-to-Be.* Cambridge, Mass.: Perseus.

Lichtman, R., L. L. Simpson, and A. Rosenfield. 2005. *Dr. Guttmacher's Pregnancy, Birth & Family Planning*, updated ed. New York: New American Library.

Mayo Clinic. 2004. *Mayo Clinic Guide to a Healthy Pregnancy.* New York: HarperResource.

🖥 Organizations and Web Sites

American College of Obstetricians and Gynecologists (ACOG). Provides written materials relating to many aspects of preconception care, pregnancy, and childbirth.
202-638-5577
http://www.acog.org

The American Society for Reproductive Medicine. Provides up-to-date information on all aspects of infertility.
205-978-5000
http://www.asrm.org

Centers for Disease Control and Prevention, National Center on Birth Defects and Developmental Disabilities. Provides information about a variety of topics related to birth defects, including fetal alcohol syndrome and the importance of folic acid.
http://www.cdc.gov/ncbddd

Childbirth.Org. Contains medical information and personal stories about all phases of pregnancy and birth.
http://www.childbirth.org

Generational Health. Helps you create a family health tree online and provides information about detection and screening for any conditions that are common in your family history.
http://www.generationalhealth.com

Health Resources and Services Administration (HRSA): Maternal and Child Health. Provides publications, videos, and other resources relating to maternal, infant, and family health.
888-ASK-HRSA
http://www.ask.hrsa.gov/MCH.cfm

International Council on Infertility Information Dissemination. A Web site that includes information on current research and treatments for infertility.
http://www.inciid.org

La Leche League International. Provides advice and support for breastfeeding mothers.
800-LaLeche
http://www.lalecheleague.org

The March of Dimes. Provides public education materials on many pregnancy-related topics, including preconception care, genetic screening, diet and exercise, and the effects of smoking and drinking during pregnancy.
888-MODIMES; 914-428-7100
http://www.modimes.org

National Institute of Child Health and Human Development. Provides information about reproductive and genetic problems; sponsors the "Back to Sleep" campaign to fight SIDS.
800-505-CRIB (Back to Sleep hotline)
http://www.nichd.nih.gov

Resolve. Provides information, support, and referrals for people facing infertility.

888-623-0744 (National Helpline)

http://www.resolve.org

SHARE. Provides information, support, and referrals to parents who have experienced miscarriage, stillbirth, or infant death.

800-821-6819

The following sites include information, graphics, and video clips of fetal development:

Nova/Odyssey of Life

http://www.pbs.org/wgbh/nova/odyssey/clips

Visible Embryo

http://visembryo.com

Selected Bibliography

American Academy of Pediatrics Section on Breastfeeding. 2005. Breast-feeding and the use of human milk. *Pediatrics* 115(2): 496–506.

Andrade, S. E., et al. 2004. Prescription drug use in pregnancy. *American Journal of Obstetrics and Gynecology* 191(2): 398–407.

Bouyer, J., et al. 2003. Risk factors for ectopic pregnancy: A comprehensive analysis based on a large case-control, population-based study in France. *American Journal of Epidemiology* 157(3): 185–194.

Centers for Disease Control and Prevention. 2004. Assisted reproductive technology surveillance, United States, 2001. *MMWR Surveillance Summaries* 53(SS01): 1–20.

Centers for Disease Control and Prevention. 2004. Blood mercury levels in young children and childbearing-aged women. *Morbidity and Mortality Weekly Report* 53(43): 1018–1020.

Centers for Disease Control and Prevention. 2004. Spina bifida and anencephaly before and after folic acid mandate. *Morbidity and Mortality Weekly Report* 53(17): 362–365.

Centers for Disease Control and Prevention. 2004. Use of vitamins containing folic acid among women of childbearing age—United States, 2004. *Morbidity and Mortality Weekly Report* 53(36): 847–850.

Clapp, J. F., et al. 2002. Continuing regular exercise during pregnancy: Effect of exercise volume on fetoplacental growth. *American Journal of Obstetrics and Gynecology* 186(1): 142–147.

Clausen, T. D., et al. 2005. Poor pregnancy outcome in women with type 2 diabetes. *Diabetes Care* 28(2): 323–328.

Cole, L. A., et al. 2004. Accuracy of home pregnancy tests at the time of missed menses. *American Journal of Obstetrics and Gynecology* 190(1): 100–105.

Currie, J., and M. Rich. 2004. Fit and well: Maintaining women's participation in pre- and postnatal exercise. *ACSM's Health and Fitness Journal,* July/August.

Declercq, E., F. Menacker, and M. MacDorman. 2005. Rise in "no indicated risk" primary caesareans in the United States, 1991–2001: Cross sectional analysis. *British Medical Journal* 330(7482): 71–72.

de la Chica, R. A., et al. 2005. Chromosomal instability in amniocytes from fetuses of mothers who smoke. *Journal of the American Medical Association* 293(10): 1212–1222.

Dole, N., et al. 2003. Maternal stress and preterm birth. *American Journal of Epidemiology* 157(1): 14–24.

Ehrenberg, H. M., et al. 2004. The influence of obesity and diabetes on the risk of cesarean delivery. *American Journal of Obstetrics and Gynecology* 191(3): 969–974.

Forsum, E. 2004. Energy requirements during pregnancy: Old questions and new findings. *American Journal of Clinical Nutrition* 79(6): 933–934.

George, L., et al. 2002. Plasma folate levels and risk of spontaneous abortion. *Journal of the American Medical Association* 288(15): 1867–1873.

Godfrey, K. M., and D. J. Barker. 2000. Fetal nutrition and adult disease. *American Journal of Clinical Nutrition* 71(5 Suppl): 1344S–1352S.

Innes, K. E., et al. 2004. Association of a woman's own birth weight with her subsequent risk for pregnancy-induced hypertension. *American Journal of Epidemiology* 158(9): 861–870.

Jernstrom, H., et al. 2004. Breast-feeding and the risk of breast cancer in BRCA1 and BRCA2 mutation carriers. *Journal of the National Cancer Institute* 96(14): 1094–1098.

Jimenez-Chillaron, J. C., et al. 2005. Beta-cell secretory dysfunction in the pathogenesis of low birth weight-associated diabetes. *Diabetes* 54(3): 702–711.

Kalb, C. 2004. Brave new babies. *Newsweek,* 26 January.

Landon, M. B., et al. 2004. Maternal and perinatal outcomes associated with a trial of labor after prior cesarean delivery. *New England Journal of Medicine* 351(25): 2581–2589.

Leridon, H. 2004. Can assisted reproduction technology compensate for the natural decline in fertility with age? A model assessment. *Human Reproduction* 19(7): 1548–1553.

Levine, R. J., et al. 2005. Urinary placental growth factor and risk of preeclampsia. *Journal of the American Medical Association* 293(1): 77–85.

March of Dimes. 1999. *Stress and Pregnancy* (http://www.modimes.org/HealthLibrary2/FactSheets/Stress_and_Pregnancy.htm; retrieved September 25, 2000).

Martindale, D. 2004. Mickey has two moms. *Scientific American,* July.

McCormack, V. A., et al. 2005. Birth characteristics and *adult cancer incidence: Swedish cohort of over 11,000 men and women.* International Journal of Cancer, Feb 7 epub.

Morkved, S., et al. Pelvic floor muscle training during pregnancy to prevent urinary incontinence. *Obstetrics and Gynecology* 101(2): 313–319.

Mortaz, M., et al. 2001. Birth weight, subsequent growth, and cholesterol metabolism in children 8–12 years old born preterm. *Archives of Disease in Childhood* 84(3): 212–217.

Mortensen, E. L., et al. 2002. The association between duration of breast-feeding and adult intelligence. *Journal of the American Medical Association* 287(18): 2365–2371.

National Center for Health Statistics. 2005. Explaining the 2001–2 infant mortality increase. *National Vital Statistics Reports* 53(12).

Newman, R. B., et al. 2001. Occupational fatigue and preterm premature rupture of membranes. *American Journal of Obstetrics and Gynecology* 184(3): 438–446.

Rados, C. 2004. FDA cautions against ultrasound "keepsake" images. *FDA Consumer,* January/February.

Reddy, U. M., A. M Branum, and M. A. Klebanoff. 2005. Relationship of maternal body mass index and height to twinning. *Obstetrics and Gynecology* 105(3): 593–597.

Roseboom, T. J., et al. 2001. Maternal nutrition during gestation and blood pressure in later life. *Journal of Hypertension* 19(1): 29–34.

Russell, R. B., et al. 2003. The changing epidemiology of multiple births in the United States. *Obstetrics and Gynecology* 101(1): 129–135.

Sheynki, Y., et al. 2005. Increase in scrotal temperature in laptop computer users. *Human Reproduction* 20(2): 452–455.

Stoll, B. J., et al. 2004. Neurodevelopmental and growth impairment among extremely low-birth-weight infants with neonatal infection. *Journal of the American Medical Association* 292(19): 2357–2365.

Tough, S. C., et al. 2002. Delayed childbearing and its impact on population rate changes in lower birth weight, multiple birth, and preterm delivery. *Pediatrics* 109(3): 399–403.

Vahratian, A., et al. 2004. Multivitamin use and the risk of preterm birth. *American Journal of Epidemiology* 160(9): 886–892.

Voelker, R. 2005. The business of baby pictures: Controversy brews over "keepsake" fetal ultrasounds. *Journal of the American Medication Association* 293(1): 25–27.

9

After reading this chapter, you should be able to

- Define and discuss the concepts of addictive behavior, substance abuse, and substance dependence

- Explain factors contributing to drug use and dependence

- List the major categories of psychoactive drugs and describe their effects, methods of use, and potential for abuse and dependence

- Discuss social issues related to psychoactive drug use and its prevention and treatment

- Evaluate the role of drugs and other addictive behaviors in your life and identify your risk factors for abuse or dependence

The Use and Abuse of Psychoactive Drugs

Knowledge

1. **Addictions always involve drugs that cause physical withdrawal symptoms when the person stops taking them.**
   True or false?

2. **Which of the following is the most widely used illegal drug among college students?**
   a. cocaine
   b. hallucinogens
   c. marijuana
   d. heroin

3. **Caffeine use can produce physical dependence.**
   True or false?

4. **Which of the following drugs is most addictive?**
   a. marijuana
   b. nicotine
   c. Valium
   d. LSD

5. **About what percentage of street drugs contain the promised primary ingredient?**
   a. 50%
   b. 66%
   c. 75%

ANSWERS

1. FALSE. Both assertions in this statement are wrong. Addiction does not always involve a drug, but even when it does, withdrawing from that drug may not result in physical symptoms.

2. C. Marijuana ranks first, with hallucinogens a distant second. In surveys, the vast majority of college students (80%) report no drug use in the previous month.

3. TRUE. Regular users of caffeine develop physical tolerance, needing more caffeine to produce the same level of alertness. Many also experience withdrawal symptoms, such as headaches and irritability, when they decrease their intake.

4. B. Valium is also addictive, LSD and marijuana less so. Nicotine is believed to be the most highly addictive psychoactive drug.

5. A. This figure is even lower for drugs that are difficult to obtain or manufacture. Street drugs may be sold in unsafe dosages and are typically mixed ("cut") with cheaper and often more hazardous substances.

VIW Visit the *Core Concepts in Health* Online Learning Center (www.mhhe.com/insel10e) for study aids and many additional resources.

235

The use of **drugs** for both medical and social purposes is widespread in American society (Table 9-1). Many people believe that every problem, no matter how large or small, has or should have a chemical solution. For fatigue, many turn to caffeine; for insomnia, sleeping pills; for anxiety or boredom, alcohol or other recreational drugs. Advertisements, social pressures, and the human desire for quick solutions to life's difficult problems all contribute to the prevailing attitude that drugs can ease all pain. Unfortunately, using drugs can—and often does—have serious consequences.

The most serious consequences are abuse and addiction. The drugs most often associated with abuse are **psychoactive drugs**—those that alter a person's experiences or consciousness. In the short term, psychoactive drugs can cause **intoxication,** a state in which sometimes unpredictable physical and emotional changes occur. A person who is intoxicated may experience potentially serious changes in physical functioning, and his or her emotions and judgment may be affected in ways that lead to uncharacteristic and unsafe behavior. In the long term, recurrent drug use can have profound physical, emotional, and social effects.

This chapter introduces the general concept of addictive behavior and then focuses on the major classes of psychoactive drugs: their short- and long-term effects, their potential for abuse and addiction, and other issues related to their use. Alcohol and nicotine—two of the most widely used psychoactive drugs and those that have the greatest negative impact on wellness in terms of disease, injury, and death—are treated in detail in Chapters 10 and 11.

ADDICTIVE BEHAVIOR

Although addiction is most often associated with drug use, many experts now extend the concept of addiction to other behaviors. **Addictive behaviors** are habits that have gotten out of control, with resulting negative effects on a person's health. Looking at the nature of addiction and a range of addictive behaviors can help us understand similar behaviors when they involve drugs.

Terms

V!W

drug Any chemical other than food intended to affect the structure or function of the body.

psychoactive drug A drug that can alter a person's consciousness or experience.

intoxication The state of being mentally affected by a chemical (literally, a state of being poisoned).

addictive behavior Any habit that has gotten out of control, resulting in a negative effect on one's health.

W!W VITAL STATISTICS

Table 9-1	Nonmedical Drug Use Among Americans

	Percentage Using Substance in the Past 30 Days	
	College Students (age 18–22)	All Americans (age 12 and older)
Any illicit drug	21.4	8.2
Tobacco (all forms)	36.4	29.8
Cigarettes	31.4	25.4
Smokeless tobacco	3.8	3.3
Cigars	10.5	5.4
Pipe tobacco	0.9	0.7
Alcohol	64.9	50.1
Binge alcohol use	43.5	22.6
Marijuana/hashish	18.4	6.2
Cocaine	2.1	1.0
Crack	0.0	0.3
Heroin	0.0	0.1
Hallucinogens	1.8	0.4
LSD	0.4	0.1
Ecstasy	0.6	0.2
Inhalants	0.6	0.2
Psychotherapeutics*	5.8	2.7
Pain relievers	4.4	2.0
Tranquilizers	1.3	0.8
Stimulants	1.3	0.5
Methamphetamine	0.1	0.3
Sedatives	0.1	0.1

*Nonmedical use of prescription-type pain relievers, tranquilizers, stimulants, or sedatives.

SOURCE: Office of Applied Studies, Substance Abuse and Mental Health Services Administration. 2004. *National Survey on Drug Use and Health* (http://oas.samhsa.gov/nhsda.htm; retrieved December 6, 2004).

What Is Addiction?

The word *addiction* tends to be a highly charged one for most people. We may jokingly say we're addicted to fudge swirl ice cream or our morning jog, but most of us think of true addiction as a habitual and uncontrollable behavior, usually involving the use of a drug. Some people think of addiction as a moral flaw or a personal weakness. Others think addictions arise from certain personality traits, genetic factors, or socioeconomic influences. Views on the causes of addictions have an impact on our attitudes toward people with addictive disorders, as well as on the approaches to treatment.

Historically, the term *addiction* was applied only when the habitual use of a drug produced chemical changes in the user's body. One such change is physical tolerance, in which the body adapts to a drug so that the initial dose no longer produces the original emotional or psychological effects. This process, caused by chemical changes, means the user has to take larger and larger doses of the drug to achieve the same high. (Tolerance will be discussed in greater detail later in the chapter.) The concept of addiction as a disease process, one based in brain chemistry, rather than a moral failing, has led to many advances in the understanding and treatment of drug addiction.

Some scientists think that other behaviors may share some of the chemistry of drug addiction. They suggest that activities like gambling, eating, exercising, and sex trigger the release of brain chemicals that cause a pleasurable rush in much the same way that psychoactive drugs do. The brain's own chemicals thus become the "drug" that can cause addiction. These theorists suggest that drug addiction and addiction to other pleasurable behaviors have a common mechanism in the brain. In this view, addiction is partly the result of our own natural wiring.

However, and very important, the view that addiction is based in our brain chemistry does *not* imply that an individual bears no responsibility for his or her addictive behavior. Many experts believe that it is inaccurate and counterproductive to think of all bad habits and excessive behaviors as diseases. They point to other factors, especially lifestyle and personality traits, that play key roles in the development of addictive behaviors. Before we consider what those factors are, let's first look in more detail at what constitutes addictive behavior.

Characteristics of Addictive Behavior

It is often difficult to distinguish between a healthy habit and one that has become an addiction. Experts have identified some general characteristics typically associated with addictive behaviors:

- *Reinforcement.* Addictive behaviors are physically and/or psychologically reinforcing. Some aspect of the behavior produces pleasurable physical and/or emotional states or relieves negative ones.

- *Compulsion or craving.* The individual feels a strong compulsion—a compelling need—to engage in the behavior, often accompanied by obsessive planning for the next opportunity to perform it.

- *Loss of control.* The individual loses control over the behavior and cannot block the impulse to engage in it. He or she may deny that the behavior is problematic or may have tried but failed to control it.

- *Escalation.* Addiction often involves a pattern of escalation, in which more and more of a particular substance or activity is required to produce its desired effects. This escalation typically means that a person must give an increasing amount of his or her time, attention, and resources to the behavior.

- *Negative consequences.* The behavior continues despite serious negative consequences, such as

problems with academic or job performance, personal relationships, and health; legal or financial troubles are also typical.

The Development of Addiction

There is no single cause of addiction. Instead, characteristics of an individual person, of the environment in which the person lives, and of the substance or behavior he or she abuses combine in an addictive behavior. Although addictive behaviors share many common characteristics, the importance of these different factors varies from one case to another, even when the addiction is to the same substance or behavior.

We all engage in activities that are potentially addictive. Some of these activities can be part of a wellness lifestyle if they are done appropriately and in moderation, but if a behavior starts to be excessive, it may become an addiction. An addiction often starts when a person does something he or she thinks will bring pleasure or help avoid pain. The activity may be drinking a beer, going on the Internet, playing the lottery, or going shopping. If it works, and the behavior does bring pleasure or alleviates pain, the person is likely to repeat it. He or she becomes increasingly dependent on the behavior, and tolerance may develop—that is, the person needs more of the behavior to feel the same effect. Eventually, the behavior becomes a central focus of the person's life, and there is a deterioration in other areas, such as school performance or relationships. The behavior no longer brings pleasure, but it is necessary to avoid the pain of going without it. What started as a seemingly innocent way of feeling good can become a prison.

Many common behaviors are potentially addictive, but most people who engage in them do not develop problems. The reason, again, lies in the combination of factors that are involved in the development of addiction, including personality, lifestyle, heredity, the social and physical environment, and the nature of the substance or behavior in question. For a behavior to become an addiction, these diverse factors must come together in a certain way. For example, nicotine, the psychoactive drug in tobacco, has a very high potential for physical addiction; but a person who doesn't choose to try cigarettes, perhaps because of family influence or a tendency to develop asthma, will never develop nicotine addiction.

Characteristics of People with Addictions

The causes and course of an addiction are extremely varied, but people with addictions do seem to share some characteristics. Many use the substance or activity as a substitute for other, healthier, coping strategies. People vary in their ability to manage their lives, and those who have the most trouble dealing with stress and painful emotions may be more susceptible to addiction.

Some people may have a genetic predisposition to addiction to a particular substance; such predispositions may involve variations in brain chemistry. People with addictive disorders usually have a distinct preference for a particular addictive behavior. They also often have problems with impulse control and self-regulation and tend to be risk takers.

Examples of Addictive Behaviors

The use and abuse of psychoactive drugs is explored in detail later in the chapter. In this section, we examine some behaviors that are not related to drugs and that can become addictive for some people.

Compulsive or Pathological Gambling   Many people gamble casually by putting a dollar in the office football pool, buying a lottery ticket, or going to the races. But some become compulsive gamblers, unable to resist or control the urge to gamble, even in the face of financial and personal ruin. Most compulsive gamblers say they are seeking excitement even more than money. Increasingly larger bets are necessary to produce the desired level of excitement. A series of losses can lead to a perceived need to keep placing bets to win back the money. When financial resources become strained, the person may lie or steal to pay off debts. The consequences of compulsive gambling are not just financial; the suicide rate of compulsive gamblers is 20 times higher than that of the general population.

Compulsive gamblers may gamble to relieve negative feelings and become restless and irritable when they are unable to gamble. As with many addictive behaviors, compulsive gambling may begin or flare up in times of stress. The earlier a person starts to gamble, the more likely he or she is to become a pathological gambler. Gambling is often linked to other risky behaviors, and many compulsive gamblers also have drug and alcohol abuse problems.

The American Psychiatric Association (APA) recognizes pathological gambling as a mental disorder and lists ten characteristic behaviors, including preoccupation with gambling, unsuccessful efforts to cut back or quit, using gambling to escape problems, and lying to family members to conceal the extent of involvement with gambling. Compulsive gambling shares many of these behaviors with other addictions, including drug use. An estimated 1.1 million adolescents and 1.9 million adults in the United States may be compulsive gamblers. These numbers may increase due to the spread of legalized gambling, both on the Internet and on American Indian tribal reservations.

In a recent survey of more than 10,000 students from more than 100 colleges, 42% of students reported having gambled at least once in the past year, and about 3% reported gambling at least once a week. Rates were

Most people who gamble do so casually and occasionally, but for a few the habit spins out of control and becomes the central focus of their life. The availability of gambling on the Internet makes it even more difficult for pathological gamblers to control their compulsion.

significantly higher among men than women. Other characteristics associated with gambling among college students included more time watching TV, more time using a computer nonacademically, less time studying, lower grades, participation in intercollegiate athletics, and alcohol use and binge drinking.

Sex and Love Addiction   More controversial is the notion of addiction to sex or love. Some researchers believe that the initial rush of arousal and erotic or romantic chemistry produces an effect in the brain comparable to that of taking amphetamines or morphine. After a time, the brain becomes desensitized, and the addict must then seek his or her next rush by pursuing a new partner. According to this view, cheating on a partner, having many partners, and sexually victimizing others are behaviors parallel to drug-seeking behavior. Behaviors associated with so-called sex addicts include an extreme preoccupation with sex, a compulsion to have sex repeatedly within a short period of time, spending a great deal of time and energy looking for partners or engaging in sex, using sex as a means of relieving painful feelings, and suffering negative emotional, personal, and professional consequences as a result of sexual activities.

Some experts are reluctant to call compulsive sexual activity a true addiction. However, even therapists who challenge the concept of sex addiction recognize that some people become overly preoccupied with sex, cannot seem to control their sex drive, and act in potentially harmful ways in order to obtain satisfaction. This pattern of sexual behavior does seem to meet the criteria for addictive behaviors discussed earlier.

Compulsive Spending or Shopping Nearly everyone splurges at the mall or goes into debt once in a while. But a compulsive spender repeatedly gives in to the impulse to buy much more than he or she needs or can afford. For the compulsive shopper, spending may serve to relieve painful feelings such as depression or anxiety, or it may produce positive emotions such as excitement or happiness. Compulsive spenders usually buy luxury items rather than daily necessities. Men tend to buy cars, exercise equipment, and sporting gear; women tend to buy clothes, jewelry, and perfume. Some experts link compulsive shopping with neglect or abuse during childhood; it also seems to be associated with eating disorders, depression, and bipolar disorder. Some compulsive shoppers are helped by antidepressant medications.

Compulsive shoppers are usually significantly distressed by their behavior and its social, personal, and financial consequences. Characteristics of out-of-control spending include shopping in order to "feel better," using money or time that had been set aside for other purposes, hiding spending from others, and spending so much that the shopper goes into debt or engages in illegal activities such as shoplifting or writing bad checks. Like other addictive behaviors, compulsive shopping is characterized by a loss of control over the behavior and significant negative consequences.

Internet Addiction Some recent research has indicated that surfing the World Wide Web can also be addictive. In order to spend more time online, Internet addicts skip important social, school, or recreational activities, thereby damaging personal relationships and jeopardizing academic and job performance. Despite the negative consequences they are experiencing, they don't feel able to stop. The Internet addicts identified in one study averaged 38 online hours per week. Internet addicts may feel uncomfortable or be moody when they are not online. They may be preoccupied with getting back online and may stay there longer than they intend. As with other addictive behaviors described here, online addicts may be using their behavior to alleviate stress or avoid painful emotions.

Activities by Internet addicts may take many forms, some of which, such as e-mail and chat rooms, are specific to the online format. However, widespread access to the Internet may expose many more people to other potentially addictive behaviors, including gambling, shopping, and sex. The Internet is convenient, easily accessible, and affordable; it is also anonymous, so people who might have hesitated to gamble or make expensive purchases in public may feel less inhibited when these activities can take place privately. There are thousands of online gambling sites and millions of online stores that allow people to gamble or shop from their homes at all times of the day or night; in addition, sites featuring online auctions or stock trading offer activities that are very similar to gambling. As described in Chapter 5, easy access to sexually oriented Web sites can lead to cybersex addiction for some people. It remains to be seen whether increasing access to the Internet among Americans will lead to more problems with many types of addictive behaviors.

Other behaviors that can become addictive include eating, watching TV, and working. Any substance or activity that becomes the focus of a person's life at the expense of other needs and interests can be damaging to health.

We turn now to the substances most commonly associated with addiction: psychoactive drugs.

DRUG USE, ABUSE, AND DEPENDENCE

Drugs are chemicals other than food that are intended to affect the structure or function of the body. They include prescription medicines such as antibiotics and antidepressants; nonprescription, or over-the-counter (OTC), substances such as alcohol, tobacco, and caffeine products; and illegal substances such as LSD and heroin. The use of drugs is not a new phenomenon in society; in fact, drug use has a long history.

The Drug Tradition

Using drugs to alter consciousness is an ancient and universal pursuit. People have used alcohol for celebration and intoxication for thousands of years. People in all parts of the world have discovered and exploited the psychoactive properties of various local plants, such as the coca plant in South America and the opium poppy in the Middle East and Far East.

Beginning in the nineteenth century, chemists were successful in extracting the active chemicals from medicinal plants, such as morphine from the opium poppy and cocaine from the coca leaf. This was the beginning of modern *pharmacy,* the art of compounding drugs, and of *pharmacology,* the science and study of drugs. From this point on, a variety of drugs began to be produced, including codeine, LSD, methamphetamine, and heroin (Figure 9-1).

Initially, the manufacture and sale of these new drugs were not regulated. Pure morphine or cocaine could be purchased by mail order, and the makers of patent medicines and tonics included potentially addictive drugs in their products without informing the consumer of either the ingredients or the dangers. The earliest version of the soft drink Coca-Cola contained cocaine, which accounted for the lift it provided.

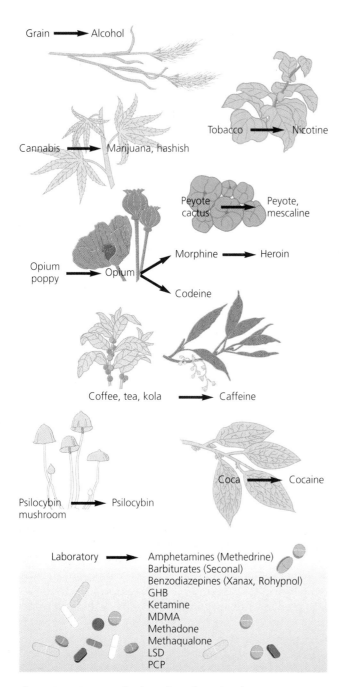

Grain ——→ Alcohol

Cannabis ——→ Marijuana, hashish

Tobacco ——→ Nicotine

Peyote cactus ——→ Peyote, mescaline

Opium poppy ——→ Opium ——→ Morphine ——→ Heroin
Opium ——→ Codeine

Coffee, tea, kola ——→ Caffeine

Coca ——→ Cocaine

Psilocybin mushroom ——→ Psilocybin

Laboratory ——→ Amphetamines (Methedrine)
Barbiturates (Seconal)
Benzodiazepines (Xanax, Rohypnol)
GHB
Ketamine
MDMA
Methadone
Methaqualone
LSD
PCP

Figure 9-1   Sources of selected psychoactive drugs.

Drug addiction among middle-class Europeans and North Americans was more common by 1900 than at any time before or since. Concerns about drug addiction and the need to regulate drug sales and manufacture led in the early 1900s to the passage of U.S. federal drug laws. Middle-class use of the regulated drugs dropped, and drug use became restricted to, and increasingly identified with, criminal subcultures.

Nonmedical (recreational) drug use expanded in the general U.S. population during the 1960s and 1970s, reaching a peak in 1979. Drug use rates then declined until the early to mid-1990s, when drug use rates began to rise in certain age groups. Although it is appropriate for us to be concerned about these increases, no one should lose sight of the fact that the vast majority of young people still do not use marijuana or other illicit drugs.

Drug Abuse and Dependence

The APA's *Diagnostic and Statistical Manual of Mental Disorders* is the authoritative reference for defining all sorts of behavioral disorders, including those related to drugs. The APA has chosen not to use the term *addiction*, in part because it is so broad and has so many connotations. Instead, the APA refers to two forms of substance (drug) disorders: substance abuse and substance dependence. Both are maladaptive patterns of substance use that lead to significant impairment or distress. Although the APA's definitions are more precise and more directly related to drug use, they clearly encompass the general characteristics of addictive behavior described in the last section.

Drug Abuse   As defined by the APA, **substance abuse** involves one or more of the following:

- Recurrent drug use, resulting in a failure to fulfill major responsibilities at work, school, or home
- Recurrent drug use in situations in which it is physically hazardous, such as before or while driving a car
- Recurrent drug-related legal problems
- Continued drug use despite persistent social or interpersonal problems caused or exacerbated by the effects of the drug

The pattern of use may be constant or intermittent, and **physical dependence** may or may not be present. For example, a person who smokes marijuana once a week and cuts classes because he or she is high is abusing marijuana, even though he or she is not physically dependent.

Drug Dependence   **Substance dependence** is a more complex disorder and is what many people associate with the idea of addiction. The seven specific criteria the APA uses to diagnose substance dependence are listed below. The first two are associated with physical dependence; the final five are associated with compulsive use. To be considered dependent, an individual must experience a cluster of three or more of these seven symptoms during a 12-month period.

1. *Developing tolerance to the substance.* When a person requires increased amounts of a substance to achieve the desired effect or notices a markedly diminished effect with continued use of the same amount, he or she has developed **tolerance.** For example, heavy heroin users may need to take ten times the amount they took at the beginning in order to achieve the desired effect; such a large dose would be lethal to a

nonuser. The degree to which tolerance develops varies widely depending on the drug.

2. *Experiencing withdrawal.* In an individual who has maintained prolonged, heavy use of a substance, a drop in its concentration within the body can result in unpleasant physical and cognitive **withdrawal** symptoms. The person is likely to take the substance to relieve or avoid those symptoms. Withdrawal symptoms are different for different drugs. For example, nausea, vomiting, and tremors are common for alcohol, opioids, and sedatives; for stimulants like amphetamines, cocaine, and caffeine, fatigue and irritability may occur. Other drugs have no significant withdrawal symptoms.

3. *Taking the substance in larger amounts or over a longer period than was originally intended.*

4. *Expressing a persistent desire to cut down or regulate substance use.* This desire is often accompanied by many unsuccessful efforts to reduce or discontinue use of the substance.

5. *Spending a great deal of time obtaining the substance, using the substance, or recovering from its effects.*

6. *Giving up or reducing important social, school, work, or recreational activities because of substance use.* A dependent person may withdraw from family activities and hobbies in order to use the substance in private or to spend more time with substance-using friends.

7. *Continuing to use the substance in spite of recognizing that it is contributing to a psychological or physical problem.* For example, a person might continue to use cocaine despite recognizing that she is suffering from cocaine-induced depression.

If a drug-dependent person experiences either tolerance or withdrawal, he or she is considered physically dependent. However, not everyone who experiences tolerance or withdrawal is drug dependent. For example, a hospital patient who is prescribed therapeutic doses of morphine to relieve pain may develop a tolerance to the drug and experience withdrawal symptoms when the prescription is discontinued. But without showing any signs of compulsive use, this individual would not be considered dependent. Dependence can occur without a physical component, based solely on compulsive use. For example, people with at least three symptoms of compulsive use of marijuana who show no signs of tolerance or withdrawal are suffering from substance dependence. In general, dependence problems that involve physical dependence carry a greater risk of immediate general medical problems and higher relapse rates.

Who Uses Drugs?

The use and abuse of drugs occur at all income and education levels, among all ethnic groups, and at all ages.

One reason for our society's concern with the casual or recreational use of illegal drugs is that it is not really possible to know when drug use will lead to abuse or dependence. Some casual users develop substance-related problems; others do not. Some psychoactive drugs are more likely than others to lead to dependence (Table 9-2), but some users of even heroin or cocaine do not meet the APA's criteria for substance dependence. However, people who begin to use drugs at very young ages have a greater risk for dependence and serious health consequences.

Although we can't accurately predict which drug users will become drug abusers, researchers have identified some characteristics that place young people at higher-than-average risk for *trying* illicit drugs. Being male is one risk factor: Although gender differences in drug use are gradually narrowing, males are still about twice as likely as females to abuse illicit drugs (see the box "Gender Differences in Drug Use and Abuse" on p. 243). An adolescent who has a poor self-image; lacks self-control; uses tobacco; has an eating disorder; is aggressive, impulsive, or moody; or suffers from attention-deficit/hyperactivity disorder (ADHD) may be at increased risk for trying drugs. A thrill-seeking or risk-taking personality is another factor. People who drive too fast or who don't wear safety belts may have this personality type, which is characterized by a sense of invincibility. Such people find it easy to dismiss warnings of danger, whether about drugs or safety belts—"That only happens to other people; it could never happen to me."

Belonging to a peer group or family that accepts or rewards drug use is a significant risk factor for trying illicit drugs. One survey of people in drug treatment found that 20% had used drugs with their parents, usually before age 18. Chaotic home environments, dysfunctional families, and parental abuse also increase risk. Children with no parental monitoring after school

Terms

substance abuse A maladaptive pattern of use of any substance that persists despite adverse social, psychological, or medical consequences. The pattern may be intermittent, with or without tolerance and physical dependence.

physical dependence The result of physiological adaptation that occurs in response to the frequent presence of a drug; typically associated with tolerance and withdrawal.

substance dependence A cluster of cognitive, behavioral, and physiological symptoms that occur in an individual who continues to use a substance despite suffering significant substance-related problems, leading to significant impairment or distress; also known as *addiction.*

tolerance Lower sensitivity to a drug so that a given dose no longer exerts the usual effect and larger doses are needed.

withdrawal Physical and psychological symptoms that follow the interrupted use of a drug on which a user is physically dependent; symptoms may be mild or life-threatening.

Table 9-2 — Psychoactive Drugs and Their Potential for Producing Dependence

Drug	Potential for Dependence — Physical	Potential for Dependence — Psychological
Nicotine	Very high	Very high
Heroin	Very high	Very high
Methamphetamine smoked ("ice")	Very high	Very high
Crack cocaine	Possible	Very high
Alcohol	High	High
Methaqualone	High	High
Barbiturates	High	Moderate
Amphetamine	Possible	High
Cocaine	Possible	High
Diazepam (Valium)	Low	High
PCP	Unknown	High
Chloral hydrate ("mickey")	Moderate	Moderate
Codeine	Moderate	Moderate
Marijuana/ hashish	Unknown	Moderate
Inhalants	Unknown	Moderate
Steroids	Possible	Possible
LSD	None	Unknown
MDMA (ecstasy)	Unknown	Unknown

SOURCES: National Clearinghouse for Alcohol and Drug Information. 2002. *Drugs of Abuse* (http://www.health.org/govpubs/rpo926; retrieved December 8, 2004); Beers, M. H., and R. Berkow, eds. 1999. *Merck Manual of Diagnosis and Therapy*, 17th ed. Rahway, N.J.: Merck; Food and Drug Administration. 1995. Nicotine in cigarettes and smokeless tobacco products is a drug and these products are nicotine delivery devices under the Federal Food, Drug, and Cosmetic Act. *Federal Register* 60(155): 41454–41459.

are more likely to try illicit drugs than those with regular adult supervision. Adolescent girls who date boys 2 or more years older than themselves are more likely to use drugs. Young people who live in disadvantaged areas are more likely to be offered drugs at a young age, increasing their risk of drug use. Especially at younger ages, the risk of using drugs is higher for people who come from a single-parent family, for those whose parents failed to complete high school, and for those who are uninterested in school and earn poor grades. However, drug use rates among middle-class youths with college-educated parents tend to catch up with, and in some cases outstrip, those of other groups by the time students reach the twelfth grade.

What about people who *don't* use drugs? As a group, nonusers also share some characteristics. Not surprisingly, people who perceive drug use as risky and who disapprove of it are less likely to use drugs than those who

believe otherwise. Drug use is also less common among people who have positive self-esteem and self-concept and who are assertive, independent thinkers who are not controlled by peer pressure. Self-control, social competence, optimism, academic achievement, and regular church attendance are also linked to lower rates of drug use (see the box "Spirituality and Drug Abuse" on p. 244).

Home environments are also influential: Coming from a strong family, one that has a clear policy on drug use, is another characteristic of people who don't use drugs. Young people who communicate openly with their parents and feel supported by them are also less likely to use drugs. Although parents may feel they have little effect on their children's drug-related attitudes and behaviors, evidence suggests that they can be a major influence. Some parents may wait too long to express a clear drug policy. Recent surveys indicate that attitudes about drugs and access and exposure to drugs change most dramatically between the ages of 12 and 13. Compared to a 12-year-old, a 13-year-old is about three times more likely to know teens who use and sell drugs and to know where and how to buy drugs. Yet nearly half of 13-year-olds report that their parents have never seriously discussed the dangers of illegal drugs with them.

Why Do People Use Drugs?

The answer to this question depends on both the user and the drug. Young people, especially those from middle-class backgrounds, are frequently drawn to drugs by the allure of the exciting and illegal. They may be curious, rebellious, or vulnerable to peer pressure. They may want to appear to be daring and to be part of the group. Young people may want to imitate adult models in their lives or in the movies. Most people who have taken illicit drugs have done so on an experimental basis, typically trying the drug one or more times but not continuing. The main factors in the initial choice of a drug are whether it is available and whether other people around are already using it.

Although some people use drugs because they have a desire to alter their mood or are seeking a spiritual experience, others are motivated primarily by a desire to escape boredom, anxiety, depression, feelings of worthlessness, or other distressing symptoms of psychological problems. They use drugs as a way to cope with the difficulties they are experiencing in life. The common practice in our society of seeking a drug solution to every problem is a factor in the widespread reliance on both illicit and prescription drugs.

For people living in poverty in the inner cities, many of these reasons for using drugs are magnified. The problems are more devastating, the need for escape more compelling. Furthermore, the buying and selling of drugs provide access to an unofficial, alternative economy that may seem like an opportunity for success.

Men are more likely than women to use, abuse, and be dependent on illicit drugs. Rates of use are similar in males and females age 12–17, but among those 18 and older, more men than women use drugs and have problems associated with drug use (see table). Men account for about 80% of arrests for drug abuse violations, 70% of admissions for treatment, and 65% of drug-related deaths.

There are also gender differences in why and how young people use drugs. Young males tend to use alcohol or drugs for sensation seeking or to enhance their social status, factors tied to culturally based gender roles. Young women tend to use drugs to improve mood, increase confidence, and reduce inhibitions. Boys are likelier to receive offers to use drugs in public settings, whereas girls are likelier to receive offers in a private place such as a friend's residence.

Despite overall lower rates of drug use, females may have unique biological vulnerabilities to certain drugs, and they may move more quickly from use to abuse. Major life transitions, including the physical and emotional changes associated with puberty, increase the risk of drug use and abuse for girls more so than for boys. Certain other drug abuse risk factors are also more common in female adolescents, including depression, low self-esteem, eating disorders, and a history of physical or sexual abuse.

Adolescent boys and girls share some protective factors relating to drug abuse, including positive family relationships and extracurricular activities; religious involvement is protective for both boys and girls but may be more protective for girls. Among older men and women, marriage, children, and employment are associated with lower rates of drug abuse and dependence. Rates of drug abuse and dependence among married adults are less than half of those among unmarried adults; similar patterns are seen when comparing adults who live with children versus those who do not live with children and adults who are employed versus those who are unemployed.

National Survey Results: Percent Reporting in Past Year

	Males	Females
Illicit drug use*	17.2	12.4
Age 12–17	21.7	21.9
Age 18–25	38.6	30.5
Age 26 and older	12.6	8.1
Drove under influence of illicit drug	6.6	2.8
Illicit drug abuse or dependence	3.7	2.1
Treatment for drug dependence	1.0	0.5

*Illicit drugs include marijuana/hashish, cocaine, heroin, hallucinogens, inhalants, and prescription-type psychotherapeutics used nonmedically.

SOURCES: Office of Applied Studies, Substance Abuse and Mental Health Services Administration. 2004. *The NSDUH Report: Gender Differences in Substance Dependence and Abuse*, October 29; Office of National Drug Control Policy. 2004. *Women and Drugs* (http://whitehousedrugpolicy.gov/drugfact/women/index.html; retrieved December 7, 2004); National Center on Addiction and Substance Abuse at Columbia University. 2003. *The Formative Years: Pathways to Substance Abuse Among Girls and Young Women Ages 8–22*. New York: National Center on Addiction and Substance Abuse.

Risk Factors for Dependence

Why do some people use psychoactive drugs without becoming dependent, whereas others aren't as lucky? The answer seems to be a combination of physical, psychological, and social factors. Research indicates that some people may be born with certain characteristics of brain chemistry or metabolism that make them more vulnerable to drug dependence. Other research suggests that people who were exposed to drugs while still in the womb may have an increased risk of abusing drugs themselves later in life.

Psychological risk factors for drug dependence include difficulty in controlling impulses and a strong need for excitement, stimulation, and immediate gratification. Feelings of rejection, hostility, aggression, anxiety, or depression are also associated with drug dependence. People may turn to drugs to blot out their emotional pain.

People with mental illnesses have a very high risk of substance dependence. Research shows that about one-third of people with psychological disorders also have a substance-dependence problem and about one-third of those have another mental disorder. People with two or more coexisting mental disorders are referred to as having **dual (co-occurring) disorders.** Diagnosis of psychological problems among people with substance dependence can be very difficult because drug intoxication and withdrawal can mimic the symptoms of a mental illness.

Term

dual (co-occurring) disorder The presence of two or more mental disorders simultaneously in the same person; for example, drug dependence and depression.

Spirituality and Drug Abuse

The use of alcohol and other drugs is intertwined with spirituality and religion. Some religions use drugs in the quest for spiritual transcendence: American Indian, Polynesian, African, and other indigenous religions have used psychoactive drugs such as peyote, khat, alcohol, and hashish for expanding consciousness and developing personal spirituality. For other religions, the use of psychoactive drugs is seen as a threat to spirituality. In Islam, for example, the consumption of alcohol and certain other drugs is strictly forbidden. Although there are diverse religious viewpoints on drug use, many religions infer some link between psychoactive drugs and spirituality.

In studies of American teens and adults, spiritual or religious involvement is generally associated with a lower risk of trying psychoactive drugs and, for those who do use drugs, a lower risk of heavy use and dependence. The mechanism for this protective effect is unclear; possibilities include the adoption of a strict code of behavior or set of principles that forbids drug use, the presence of a social support system for abstinence or moderation, and the promotion of a large, complex set of values that includes avoidance of drug use. The relationship between religious faith and avoidance of drug use appears to be even stronger in teens than in adults. One recent study found that teens who felt they had a personal relationship with the divine and/or who belonged to a more fundamentalist religious denomination were less likely to engage in substance use and abuse than other teens. Teens who attend 25 or more religious services per year are about half as likely to use illicit drugs compared with teens who attend services less frequently. Overall, people who spend time regularly engaging in spiritual practices such as prayer and transcendental meditation have lower rates of drug abuse.

People with current substance-abuse problems tend to have lower rates of religious affiliation and involvement and lower levels of spiritual wellness, characterized by a lack of a sense of meaning in life. One of the hallmarks of drug dependence is spending increasing amounts of time and energy obtaining and using drugs; such a pattern of behavior inevitably reduces the resources an individual puts toward developing physical, emotional, and spiritual wellness.

What about those seeking to break their dependence on drugs? Among people in treatment for substance abuse, higher levels of religious faith and spirituality may contribute to the recovery process. A study of people recovering from alcohol or other drug abuse found that spirituality and religiosity were associated with increased coping skills, greater optimism about life, greater resilience to stress, and greater perceived social support. If, for a particular individual, there is a spiritual aspect to his or her substance-abuse problem, then it is likely that spirituality may also play a role in recovery.

More research is needed to clarify the relationships among spirituality, religion, drug use, and recovery. One of the difficulties in conducting research in this area is the difficulty in defining and measuring spirituality and religious involvement. Spirituality is a complex part of human nature, involving behavior, belief, and experience. And although behaviors such as the spiritual practices of prayer or meditation can be measured, it is more difficult to determine what such practices mean to an individual and her or his overall sense of self.

SOURCES: Substance Abuse and Mental Health Network. 2004. Religious beliefs and substance use among youths. *NSDUH Report*, January; Plante, T. G., and D. A. Pardini. 2000. Religious denomination affiliation and psychological health: Results from a substance abuse population. Presented at the American Psychological Association Annual Convention, August 7; Miller, L., M. Davies, and S. Greenwald. 2000. Religiosity and substance use and abuse among adolescents in the national comorbidity survey. *Journal of the American Academy of Child and Adolescent Psychiatry* 39(9): 1190–1197; Miller, W. R. 1998. Researching the spiritual dimensions of alcohol and other drug problems. *Addiction* 93(7): 979–990.

Social factors that may influence drug dependence include growing up in a family in which a parent or sibling abused drugs, belonging to a peer group that emphasizes and encourages drug abuse, and living in poverty. Because they have easy access to drugs, health care professionals are also at a higher risk. To determine whether you are at risk, take the quiz in the box "Do You Have a Problem with Drugs?"

Other Risks of Drug Use

Dependence is not the only serious potential consequence of drug use.

Intoxication People who are under the influence of drugs—intoxicated—may act in uncharacteristic and unsafe ways because both their physical and mental functioning are impaired. They are more likely to be injured from a variety of causes, including falls, drowning, and automobile crashes; to engage in unsafe sex, increasing their risk for sexually transmitted diseases and unintended pregnancy; and to be involved in incidents of aggression and violence, including sexual assault.

Unintended Side Effects Psychoactive drugs have many physical and psychological effects beyond the alteration of consciousness. These effects range from nausea and constipation to paranoia, depression, and heart failure. Some drugs also carry the risk of potentially fatal overdose.

Unknown Drug Constituents There is no quality control in the illegal drug market, so the composition, dosage, and toxicity of street drugs is highly variable.

Answer yes (Y) or no (N) to the following questions:

_____ 1. Do you take the drug regularly?

_____ 2. Have you been taking the drug for a long time?

_____ 3. Do you always take the drug in certain situations or when you're with certain people?

_____ 4. Do you find it difficult to stop using the drug? Do you feel powerless to quit?

_____ 5. Have you tried repeatedly to cut down or control your use of the drug?

_____ 6. Do you need to take a larger dose of the drug in order to get the same high you're used to?

_____ 7. Do you feel specific symptoms if you cut back or stop using the drug?

_____ 8. Do you frequently take another psychoactive substance to relieve withdrawal symptoms?

_____ 9. Do you take the drug to feel "normal"?

_____ 10. Do you go to extreme lengths or put yourself in dangerous situations to get the drug?

_____ 11. Do you hide your drug use from others? Have you ever lied about what you're using or how much you use?

_____ 12. Do people close to you ask you about your drug use?

_____ 13. Are you spending more and more time with people who use the same drug as you?

_____ 14. Do you think about the drug when you're not high, figuring out ways to get it?

_____ 15. If you stop taking the drug, do you feel bad until you can take it again?

_____ 16. Does the drug interfere with your ability to study, work, or socialize?

_____ 17. Do you skip important school, work, social, or recreational activities in order to obtain or use the drug?

_____ 18. Do you continue to use the drug despite a physical or mental disorder or despite a significant problem that you know is made worse by drug use?

_____ 19. Have you developed a mental or physical condition or disorder because of prolonged drug use?

_____ 20. Have you done something dangerous or that you regret while under the influence of the drug?

The more times you answer yes, the more likely it is that you are developing a dependence on the drug. If your answers suggest dependence, talk to someone at your school health clinic or to your physician about taking care of the problem before it gets worse.

Studies of samples indicate that many street drugs don't contain their promised primary ingredient; in some cases, a drug may be present in unsafe dosages or mixed with other drugs to boost the effects. Careless manufacturing practices can result in the presence of toxic contaminants.

Risks Associated with Injection Drug Use

Heroin and related drugs are those most often injected, but cocaine, amphetamines, and other drugs, including steroids, may also be injected. Many injection drug users (IDUs) share or reuse needles, syringes, and other injection equipment, which can easily become contaminated with the user's blood. Small amounts of blood can carry enough human immunodeficiency virus (HIV) and hepatitis C virus (HCV) to be infectious, and injection drug use accounts for almost a third of all AIDS cases and half of all hepatitis C cases reported in the United States. It's estimated that about 15% of current IDUs are infected with HIV and as many as 80% may carry HCV (hepatitis and HIV/AIDS are discussed further in Chapters 17 and 18). Unsterile injection practices can cause skin and soft tissue infections, which can progress to gangrene and be fatal if untreated. Other risks include endocarditis (infection of the heart valves), tuberculosis, and tetanus.

The surest way to prevent diseases related to injection drug use is never to inject drugs. Those who do inject drugs should use a new needle and syringe with each injection and should use sterile water and other equipment to prepare drugs. Bleach or boiling water may kill some viruses and bacteria, but they are not foolproof sterilization methods. Many viruses can survive in a syringe for a month or more.

Syringe exchange programs (SEPs)—in which IDUs can turn in a used syringe and get back a new one free—have been advocated to help slow the spread of HIV and reduce the rates and cost of other health problems associated with injection drug use. Opponents of SEPs argue that supplying addicts with syringes gives them the message that illegal drug use is acceptable and could thus exacerbate the nation's drug problem. However, studies have shown that well-implemented SEPs do not increase the use of drugs, and most offer AIDS counseling and provide referrals to drug treatment programs. Getting people off drugs is clearly the best solution, but there are far more IDUs (an estimated 1.5 million in the United States) than treatment facilities can currently handle.

Legal Consequences   Many psychoactive drugs are illegal, so using them can result in large fines and/or imprisonment. The FBI reports nearly 1.7 million drug-related arrests each year. Possession of marijuana, heroin, or cocaine are the most commonly reported violations.

In the following sections of the chapter, you'll learn more about how drugs affect the body and how drug use and abuse affect individuals, families, and society as a whole.

HOW DRUGS AFFECT THE BODY

The psychoactive drugs discussed in this chapter have complex and variable effects, many of which can be traced to changes in brain chemistry. However, the same drug may affect different people differently or the same person in different ways under different circumstances. Beyond a fairly predictable general change in brain chemistry, the effects of a drug may vary depending on three general categories of factors: drug factors, user factors, and social factors.

Changes in Brain Chemistry

How can different drugs produce such different effects—making a person alert and wired or dull and sleepy? Psychoactive drugs produce most of their key effects by acting on brain chemistry in a characteristic fashion. Before any changes in brain chemistry can occur, however, molecules of the drug have to be carried to the brain through the bloodstream via a particular route of administration. A drug that is taken by mouth has to dissolve in the stomach, be absorbed into the bloodstream through the lining of the small intestine, and then pass through the liver, heart, and lungs before returning to the heart to be carried via arteries to the brain. A drug that is already dissolved and is injected directly into the bloodstream will reach the brain in much less time, and drugs that are inhaled and absorbed by the lungs travel to the brain even more rapidly. The more quickly a drug reaches the brain, the more likely the user is to become dependent.

Terms

pharmacological properties The overall effects of a drug on a person's behavior, psychology, and chemistry.

dose-response function The relationship between the amount of a drug taken and the intensity or type of the resulting effect.

time-action function The relationship between the time elapsed since a drug was taken and the intensity of its effect.

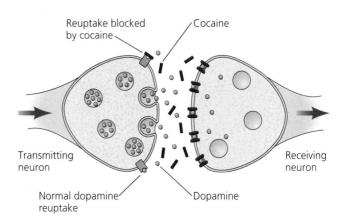

Figure 9-2   Effect of cocaine on brain chemistry.   Under normal circumstances, the amount of dopamine at a synapse is controlled in part by the re-uptake of dopamine by the transmitting neuron. Cocaine blocks the removal of dopamine from a synapse; the resulting buildup of dopamine causes continuous stimulation of the receiving neurons.

Once a psychoactive drug reaches the brain, it acts on one or more neurotransmitters, either increasing or decreasing their concentration and actions. Cocaine, for example, affects dopamine, a neurotransmitter thought to play a key role in the process of reinforcement—the brain's way of telling itself "That's good; do the same thing again." As described in Chapter 3, when a neurotransmitter is released by one neuron to signal another neuron, its level or concentration is controlled in part by the reuptake or resorption of the neurotransmitter by the releasing neuron. Cocaine inhibits the resorption of dopamine, thereby increasing the concentration of dopamine in the synapse and lengthening the time of its action (Figure 9-2). The euphoria produced by cocaine is thought to be a result of its effect on dopamine. Heroin, nicotine, alcohol, and amphetamines also affect dopamine levels through their effects on the brain.

The duration of a drug's effect depends on many factors and may range from 5 minutes (crack cocaine) to 12 or more hours (LSD). As drugs circulate through the body, they are metabolized by the liver and eventually excreted by the kidneys in urine. Small amounts may also be eliminated in other ways, including in sweat, in breast milk, and via the lungs.

Drug Factors

When different drugs or dosages produce different effects, the differences are usually caused by one or more of five different drug factors:

1.   The **pharmacological properties** of a drug are its overall effects on a person's body chemistry, behavior, and psychology. The pharmacological properties also include the amount of a drug required to exert various effects, the time course of these effects, and other characteristics, such as a drug's chemical composition.

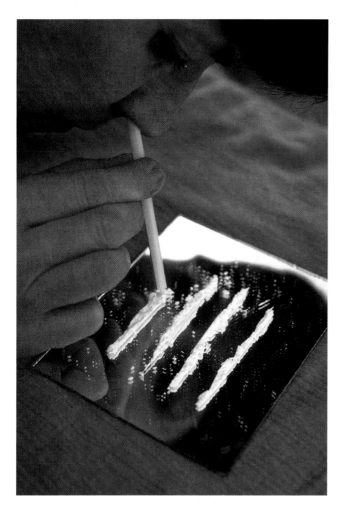

Method of use is one variable in the overall effect of a drug on the body. Sniffing, or snorting, cocaine produces effects in 2–3 minutes. With other methods, such as injecting it intravenously, inhaling vapors, or smoking crack, the effects of cocaine are felt within seconds.

4. The person's *drug use history* may influence the effects of a drug. A given amount of alcohol, for example, will generally affect a habitual drinker less than an occasional drinker. Tolerance to some drugs, such as LSD, builds rapidly. To experience the same effect, a user has to abstain from the drug for a period of time before that dosage will again exert its original effects.

5. The *method of use (or route of administration)* has a direct effect on how strong a response a drug produces. Methods of use include ingestion, inhalation, injection, and absorption through the skin or tissue linings. Drugs are usually injected in one of three ways: intravenously (IV, or mainlining), intramuscularly (IM), or subcutaneously (SC, or skin popping). If a drug is taken by a method that allows the drug to enter the bloodstream and reach the brain rapidly, the effects are usually stronger and the potential for dependence greater than when the method involves slower absorption. For example, injecting a drug intravenously produces stronger effects than swallowing the same drug. Inhaling a drug, such as when tobacco or crack cocaine is smoked, produces very rapid effects on the brain.

User Factors

The second category of factors that determine how a person will respond to a particular drug involves certain physical and psychological characteristics. Body mass is one variable. The effects of a certain dose of a drug on a 100-pound person will be twice as great as on a 200-pound person. Other variables include general health and genetic factors. For example, some people have an inherited ability to rapidly metabolize a cough suppressant called dextromethorphan, which also has psychoactive properties. These people must take a higher-than-normal dose to get a given cough-suppressant effect.

If a person's biochemical state is already altered by another drug, this too can make a difference. Some drugs intensify the effects of other drugs, as is the case with alcohol and sedatives. Some drugs block the effects of other drugs, such as when a tranquilizer is used to relieve anxiety caused by cocaine. Interactions between drugs, including many prescription and OTC medications, can be unpredictable and dangerous.

One physical condition that requires special precautions is pregnancy. It can be risky for a woman to use any drugs at all during pregnancy, including alcohol and common OTC preparations like cough medicine. The risks are greatest during the first trimester, when the fetus's body is rapidly forming and even small biochemical alterations in the mother can have a devastating effect on fetal development. Even later, the fetus is more susceptible than the mother to the adverse effects of any drugs she takes. The fetus may even become physically dependent on a drug being taken by the mother and suffer withdrawal symptoms after birth.

2. The **dose-response function** is the relationship between the amount of drug taken and the type and intensity of the resulting effect. Many psychological effects of drugs reach a plateau in the dose-response function, so that increasing the dose does not increase the effect any further. With LSD, for example, the maximum changes in perception occur at a certain dose, and no further changes in perception take place if higher doses are taken. However, all drugs have more than one effect, and the dose-response functions usually are different for different effects. This means that increasing the dose of any drug may begin to result in additional effects, which are likely to be increasingly unpleasant or dangerous at high doses.

3. The **time-action function** is the relationship between the time elapsed since a drug was taken and the intensity of its effect. The effects of a drug are greatest when concentrations of the drug in body tissues are changing fastest, especially if they are increasing.

Sometimes a person's response to a drug is strongly influenced by the user's expectations about how he or she will react (the psychological *set*). With large doses, the drug's chemical properties do seem to have the strongest effect on the user's response. But with small doses, psychological (and social) factors are often more important. When people strongly believe that a given drug will affect them a certain way, they are likely to experience those effects regardless of the drug's pharmacological properties. In one study, regular users of marijuana reported a moderate level of intoxication **(high)** after using a cigarette that smelled and tasted like marijuana but contained no THC, the active ingredient in marijuana. This is an example of the **placebo effect**—when a person receives an inert substance yet responds as if it were an active drug. (The placebo effect is discussed in more detail in Chapter 21.) In other studies, subjects who smoked low doses of real marijuana that they believed to be a placebo experienced no effects from the drug. Clearly, the user's expectations had a greater effect on the smokers than the drug itself.

Social Factors

The *setting* is the physical and social environment surrounding the drug use. If a person uses marijuana at home with trusted friends and pleasant music, the effects are likely to be different from the effects if the same dose is taken in an austere experimental laboratory with an impassive research technician. Similarly, the dose of alcohol that produces mild euphoria and stimulation at a noisy, active cocktail party might induce sleepiness and slight depression when taken at home while alone.

REPRESENTATIVE PSYCHOACTIVE DRUGS

What are the major psychoactive drugs, and how do they produce their effects? We discuss six different representative groups in this chapter: (1) opioids, (2) central nervous system depressants, (3) central nervous system stimulants, (4) marijuana and other cannabis products, (5) hallucinogens, and (6) inhalants (Figure 9-3). Some of these drugs are classified according to how they affect the body; others—the opioids and the cannabis products—are classified according to their chemical makeup. (For the sources of selected psychoactive drugs, see Figure 9-1.)

Opioids

Also called *narcotics,* **opioids** are natural or synthetic (laboratory-made) drugs that relieve pain, cause drowsiness, and induce **euphoria.** Especially in small doses, opioids have beneficial medical uses, including pain relief and cough suppression. Opium, morphine, heroin, methadone, codeine, hydrocodone, oxycodone, meperidine, and fentanyl are examples of drugs in this category. Opioids tend to reduce anxiety and produce lethargy, apathy, and an inability to concentrate. Opioid users become less active and less responsive to frustration, hunger, and sexual stimulation. These effects are more pronounced in novice users; with repeated use, many effects diminish.

Opioids are typically injected or absorbed into the body from the stomach, intestines, nasal membranes (from snorting or sniffing), or lungs (from smoking). Effects depend on the method of administration. If brain levels of the drug change rapidly, more immediate effects will result. Although the euphoria associated with opioids is an important factor in their abuse, many people experience a feeling of uneasiness when they first use these drugs. Users also often feel nauseated and vomit, and they may have other unpleasant sensations. Even so, the abuse of opioids often results in dependence. Tolerance can develop rapidly and be pronounced. Withdrawal symptoms include cramps, chills, sweating, nausea, tremors, irritability, and feelings of panic.

Rates of heroin use have always been low, but there are periodic episodes of increased use among some groups. Use among college students remains below 1%, but between 1991 and 2000 heroin use among high school seniors more than doubled, mostly due to increased rates of sniffing or smoking the drug. Although these users avoid the special disease risks of injection drug use, including HIV infection, dependence can readily result from sniffing and smoking heroin. In addition, the potentially high but variable purity of street heroin poses a risk of unintentional overdose. Symptoms of overdose include respiratory depression, coma, and constriction of the pupils; death can result.

Problems with abuse have recently been reported for oxycodone and hydrocodone, narcotics found in prescription pain relievers including OxyContin and Vicodin. When taken as prescribed in tablet form, these drugs treat moderate to severe chronic pain and do not typically lead to abuse. However, like other opioids, use of prescription painkillers can lead to abuse and dependence. Oxycodone

Terms

V̇Ẇ

high The subjectively pleasing effects of a drug, usually felt quite soon after the drug is taken.

placebo effect A response to an inert or innocuous medication given in place of an active drug.

opioid Any of several natural or synthetic drugs that relieve pain and cause drowsiness and/or euphoria; examples are opium, morphine, and heroin; also called *narcotic.*

euphoria An exaggerated feeling of well-being.

Category	Representative drugs	Street names	Appearance	Methods of use	Short-term effects
Opioids	Heroin	Dope, H, junk, brown sugar, smack	White/dark brown powder; dark tar or coal-like substance	Injected, smoked, snorted	Relief of anxiety and pain; euphoria; lethargy, apathy, drowsiness, confusion, inability to concentrate; nausea, constipation, respiratory depression
	Opium	Big O, black stuff, hop	Dark brown or black chunks	Swallowed, smoked	
	Morphine	M, Miss Emma, monkey, white stuff	White crystals, liquid solution	Injected, swallowed, smoked	
	Oxycodone, codeine, hydrocodone	Oxy, O.C., killer, Captain Cody, schoolboy, vike	Tablets, powder made from crushing tablets	Swallowed, injected, snorted	
Central nervous system depressants	Barbiturates	Barbs, reds, red birds, yellows, yellow jackets	Colored capsules	Swallowed, injected	Reduced anxiety, mood changes, lowered inhibitions, impaired muscle coordination, reduced pulse rate, drowsiness, loss of consciousness, respiratory depression
	Benzodiazepines (e.g., Valium, Xanax, Rohypnol)	Candy, downers, tranks, roofies, forget-me pill	Tablets	Swallowed, injected	
	Methaqualone	Ludes, quad, quay	Tablets	Injected, swallowed	
	Gamma hydroxy butyrate (GHB)	G, Georgia home boy, grievous bodily harm	Clear liquid, white powder	Swallowed	
Central nervous system stimulants	Amphetamine, methamphet-amine	Bennies, speed, black beauties, uppers, chalk, crank, crystal, ice, meth	Tablets, capsules, white powder, white crystals	Injected, swallowed, smoked, snorted	Increased heart rate, blood pressure, metabolism; increased mental alertness and energy; nervousness, insomnia, impulsive behavior; reduced appetite
	Cocaine, crack cocaine	Blow, C, candy, coke, flake, rock, toot	White powder, beige pellets or rocks	Injected, smoked, snorted	
	Ritalin	JIF, MPH, R-ball, Skippy	Tablets	Injected, swallowed, snorted	
Marijuana and other cannabis products	Marijuana	Dope, grass, joints, Mary Jane, reefer, skunk, weed	Dried leaves and stems	Smoked, swallowed	Euphoria, slowed thinking and reaction time, confusion, anxiety, impaired balance and coordination, increased heart rate
	Hashish	Hash, hemp, boom, gangster	Dark, resin-like compound formed into rocks or blocks	Smoked, swallowed	
Hallucinogens	LSD	Acid, boomers, blotter, yellow sunshines	Blotter paper, liquid, gelatin tabs, pills	Swallowed, absorbed through mouth tissues	Altered states of perception and feeling; nausea; increased heart rate, blood pressure; delirium; impaired motor function; numbness, weakness
	Mescaline (peyote)	Buttons, cactus, mesc	Brown buttons, liquid	Swallowed, smoked	
	Psilocybin	Shrooms, magic mushrooms	Dried mushrooms	Swallowed	
	Ketamine	K, special K, cat valium, vitamin K	Clear liquid, white or beige powder	Injected, snorted, smoked	
	PCP	Angel dust, hog, love boat, peace pill	White to brown powder, tablets	Injected, swallowed, smoked, snorted	
	MDMA (ecstasy)	X, peace, clarity, Adam	Tablets	Swallowed	
Inhalants	Solvents, aerosols, nitrites, anesthetics	Laughing gas, poppers, snappers, whippets	Household products, sprays, glues, paint thinner, petroleum products	Inhaled through nose or mouth	Stimulation, loss of inhibition, slurred speech, loss of motor coordination, loss of consciousness

Figure 9-3 Commonly abused drugs and their effects SOURCES: National Institute on Drug Abuse. 2004. *Commonly Abused Drugs* (http://www.drugabuse.gov/DrugPages/DrugsofAbuse.html; retrieved December 9, 2004); U.S. Drug Enforcement Agency. 2004. *Photo Library* (http://www.usdoj.gov:80/dea/photo_library.html; retrieved December 9, 2004); U.S. Drug Enforcement Agency. 2004. *Drug Briefs and Backgrounds* (http://www.usdoj.gov:80/dea/concern/concern.htm; retrieved December 9, 2004).

and hydrocodone can be abused orally; the long-acting form of oxycodone is also sometimes crushed and snorted or dissolved and injected, providing a powerful heroin-like high. When taken in large doses or combined with other drugs, oxycodone and hydrocodone can cause fatal respiratory depression; withdrawal symptoms are similar to those for heroin.

Central Nervous System Depressants

Central nervous system **depressants,** also known as **sedative-hypnotics,** slow down the overall activity of the **central nervous system (CNS).** The result can range from mild **sedation** to death, depending on the various factors involved—which drug is used, how it's taken, how tolerant the user is, and so on. CNS depressants include alcohol (discussed in Chapter 10), barbiturates, and other sedatives.

Types The various types of barbiturates are similar in chemical composition and action, but they differ in how quickly and how long they act. Drug users call barbiturates downers or downs and refer to specific brands by names that describe the color and design of the capsules: "reds" or "red devils" for Seconal, "yellows" or "yellow jackets" for Nembutal. People usually take barbiturates in capsules, but they may also inject them.

Antianxiety agents, also called sedatives or **tranquilizers,** include the benzodiazepines such as Xanax, Valium, Librium, clonazepam (Klonopin), and flunitrazepam (Rohypnol, also called roofies). Other CNS depressants include methaqualone (Quaalude), ethchlorvynol (Placidyl), chloral hydrate ("mickey"), and gamma hydroxy butyrate (GHB, or "liquid ecstasy").

Effects CNS depressants reduce anxiety and cause mood changes, impaired muscular coordination, slurring of speech, and drowsiness or sleep. Mental functioning is also affected, but the degree varies from person to person and also depends on the kind of task the person is trying to do. Most people become drowsy with small doses, although a few become more active.

Terms

V w

depressant, or sedative-hypnotic A drug that decreases nervous or muscular activity, causing drowsiness or sleep.

central nervous system (CNS) The brain and spinal cord.

sedation The induction of a calm, relaxed, often sleepy state.

tranquilizer A CNS depressant that reduces tension and anxiety.

anesthetic A drug that produces a loss of sensation with or without a loss of consciousness.

stimulant A drug that increases nervous or muscular activity.

Medical Uses Barbiturates, antianxiety agents, and other sedative-hypnotics are widely used to treat insomnia and anxiety disorders and to control seizures. Some CNS depressants are used for their calming properties in combination with **anesthetics** before operations and other medical or dental procedures.

From Use to Abuse People are usually introduced to CNS depressants either through a medical prescription or through drug-using peers. The use of Rohypnol and GHB is often associated with dance clubs and raves (see the box "Club Drugs"). The abuse of CNS depressants by a medical patient may begin with repeated use for insomnia and progress to dependence through increasingly larger doses at night, coupled with a few capsules at stressful times during the day.

Most CNS depressants, including alcohol, can lead to classical physical dependence. Tolerance, sometimes for up to 15 times the usual dose, can develop with repeated use. Tranquilizers have been shown to produce physical dependence even at ordinary prescribed doses. Withdrawal symptoms can be more severe than those accompanying opioid dependence and are similar to the DTs of alcoholism (see Chapter 10). They may begin as anxiety, shaking, and weakness but may turn into convulsions and possibly cardiovascular collapse and death.

While intoxicated, people on depressants cannot function very well. They are mentally confused and are frequently obstinate, irritable, and abusive. Even prescription use of benzodiazepines has been associated with an increased risk of automobile crashes. After long-term use, depressants like alcohol can lead to generally poor health and brain damage, with impaired ability to reason and make judgments.

Overdosing with CNS Depressants Too much depression of the central nervous system slows respiration and may stop it entirely. CNS depressants are particularly dangerous in combination with another depressant, such as alcohol. People who combine depressants with alcohol account for thousands of emergency room visits and hundreds of overdose deaths each year. Rohypnol is ten times more potent than Valium and can be fatal if combined with alcohol. GHB is often produced clandestinely, resulting in widely varying degrees of purity; it has been responsible for many poisonings and a number of deaths.

In recent surveys, about 3% of college students report having used a CNS depressant (other than alcohol) within the past month.

Central Nervous System Stimulants

CNS **stimulants** speed up the activity of the nervous or muscular system. Under their influence, the heart rate accelerates, blood pressure rises, blood vessels constrict, the

In the United States and elsewhere, euphoria-inducing drugs known as club drugs have gained popularity in recent years. Club drugs include a variety of very different drugs that are part of the popular dance culture of clubs and raves—all-night dance parties held in fields or abandoned buildings. Some people refer to club drugs as soft drugs because they see them as recreational—more for the casual, weekend user—rather than as addictive. But club drugs have many potential negative effects and are particularly potent and unpredictable when mixed with alcohol. Substitute drugs are often sold in place of club drugs, putting users at risk for taking dangerous combinations of unknown drugs.

MDMA *(ecstasy, E, X, XTC, Adam, hug drug, lover's speed):* Taken in pill form, MDMA (methylenedioxymethamphetamine) is a stimulant with mildly hallucinogenic and amphetamine-like effects. Users may experience euphoria, increased energy, and a heightened sense of belonging. In club settings, using MDMA can produce dangerously high body temperature and potentially fatal dehydration; some users experience confusion, depression, anxiety, paranoia, muscle tension, involuntary teeth clenching, blurred vision, nausea, and seizures. Even low doses can affect concentration, judgment, and driving ability. Tolerance can develop, leading users to take the drug more frequently (on a daily basis), to use higher doses, or to combine MDMA with other drugs, including Prozac, to enhance the drug's effects. In addition to MDMA, many ecstasy tablets include other drugs such as methamphetamine, ephedrine, or cocaine. At high doses or mixed with other drugs, MDMA is extremely dangerous; most deaths linked to MDMA have occurred as a result of multidrug toxicity or traumatic injuries.

MDMA increases the activity of three neurotransmitters: serotonin, dopamine, and norepinephrine. Increases in serotonin are likely the cause of the drug's mood-elevating effects, but use of MDMA can deplete the brain of serotonin and may cause an emotional let-down (sadness, irritability, etc.) in the days following use. Animal studies have found that moderate to high doses of MDMA are toxic to nerve cells producing serotonin and may cause long-lasting damage; human studies are ongoing. MDMA users perform worse than nonusers on complex cognitive tasks of memory, attention, and general intelligence. Long-term effects may include physical symptoms and psychological problems such as confusion or paranoia. Research suggests that pregnant women who use MDMA are at increased risk for having a baby with congenital malformations and long-term impairment in memory and other cognitive functions.

LSD *(acid, boomers, yellow sunshines, red dragon):* A popular and potent hallucinogen, LSD (lysergic acid diethylamide) is sold in tablets or capsules, in liquid form, or on small squares of paper called blotters. LSD increases heart rate and body temperature and may cause nausea, tremors, sweating, numbness, and weakness. (See p. 256 for more on LSD.)

Ketamine *(special K, vitamin K, K, cat valium, jet):* A veterinary anesthetic that can be taken in powdered or liquid form, ketamine may cause hallucinations and impaired attention and memory. At higher doses, ketamine can cause delirium, amnesia, high blood pressure, and potentially fatal respiratory problems. Tolerance to ketamine develops rapidly.

GHB *(Georgia home boy, G, grievous bodily harm, liquid ecstasy):* GHB (gamma hydroxybutyrate) can be produced in clear liquid, white powder, tablet, and capsule form; it is often made in basement chemistry labs, where toxic substances may unintentionally be added or produced. GHB is a CNS depressant that in large doses or when taken in combination with alcohol or other depressants can cause sedation, loss of consciousness, respiratory arrest, and death. Evidence suggests that GHB may cause prolonged and potentially life-threatening withdrawal symptoms. Some products sold as dietary supplements for bodybuilding, weight loss, or insomnia contain the chemically similar compounds GBL (gamma butyrolactone) or BD (butanediol); the FDA considers these products dangerous and is working to remove them from the market.

Rohypnol *(roofies, roche, forget-me pill):* Taken in tablet form, Rohypnol (flunitrazepam) is a sedative that is ten times more potent than Valium. Its effects, which are magnified by alcohol, include reduced blood pressure, dizziness, confusion, gastrointestinal disturbances, and loss of consciousness. Users of Rohypnol may develop physical and psychological dependence on the drug.

An additional problem associated with GHB, Rohypnol, and several other club drugs is their potential use as "date rape drugs." Because they can be added to beverages surreptitiously, these drugs may be unknowingly consumed by intended rape victims. In addition to depressant effects, some drugs also cause *anterograde amnesia,* the loss of memory of things occurring while under the influence of the drug. Because of concern about GHB, Rohypnol, and other similarly abused drugs, Congress passed the "Drug-Induced Rape Prevention and Punishment Act," which increased federal penalties for use of any controlled substance to aid in sexual assault (see Chapter 23).

pupils of the eyes and the bronchial tubes dilate, and gastric and adrenal secretions increase. There is greater muscular tension and sometimes an increase in motor activity. Small doses usually make people feel more awake and alert, less fatigued and bored. The most common CNS stimulants are cocaine, amphetamines, nicotine (discussed in Chapter 11), ephedrine, and caffeine.

Cocaine Usually derived from the leaves of coca shrubs that grow high in the Andes Mountains in South America, cocaine is a potent CNS stimulant. For centuries, natives of the Andes have chewed coca leaves both for pleasure and to increase their endurance. For a short time during the nineteenth century, some physicians were enthusiastic about the use of cocaine to cure alcoholism and addiction to the painkiller morphine. Enthusiasm waned after the adverse side effects became apparent.

Cocaine—also known as coke, or snow—quickly produces a feeling of euphoria, which makes it a popular recreational drug. Cocaine use surged in popularity during the early 1980s, when the drug's high price made it a status drug. The introduction of crack cocaine during the 1980s made the drug available in smaller quantities and at lower prices to more people. The typical recreational user shifted rapidly from the wealthy professional snorting powdered cocaine to poor inner-city smokers of crack cocaine. In the general population, cocaine use peaked in 1985 with an estimated 3% of adult Americans reporting use. In recent surveys, about 1% of all adults and 2% of college students surveyed reported using cocaine in the previous month.

METHODS OF USE   Cocaine is usually snorted and absorbed through the nasal mucosa or injected intravenously, providing rapid increases of the drug's concentration in the blood and therefore fast, intense effects. Another method of use involves processing cocaine with baking soda and water, yielding the ready-to-smoke form of cocaine known as crack. Crack is typically available as small beads or pellets smokable in glass pipes. The tiny but potent beads can be handled more easily than cocaine powder and marketed in smaller, less expensive doses.

EFFECTS   The effects of cocaine are usually intense but short-lived. The euphoria lasts from 5 to 20 minutes and ends abruptly, to be replaced by irritability, anxiety, or slight depression. When cocaine is absorbed via the lungs, by either smoking or inhalation, it reaches the brain in about 10 seconds, and the effects are particularly intense. This is part of the appeal of smoking crack. The effects from IV injections occur almost as quickly—in about 20 seconds. Since the mucous membranes in the nose briefly slow absorption, the onset of effects from snorting takes 2–3 minutes. Heavy users may inject cocaine intravenously every 10–20 minutes to maintain the effects.

The larger the cocaine dose and the more rapidly it is absorbed into the bloodstream, the greater the immediate—and sometimes lethal—effects. Sudden death from cocaine is most commonly the result of excessive CNS stimulation that causes convulsions and respiratory collapse, irregular heartbeat, extremely high blood pressure, blood clots, and possibly heart attack or stroke. Although rare, fatalities can occur in healthy young people; among people age 18–59, cocaine users are seven times more likely than nonusers to have a heart attack. Chronic cocaine use produces inflammation of the nasal mucosa, which can lead to persistent bleeding and ulceration of the septum between the nostrils. The use of cocaine may also cause paranoia and/or aggressiveness.

Although the use of cocaine decreased in the general U.S. population after 1985, cocaine is responsible for more deaths and emergency room visits than any other illicit drug. This presumably reflects the fact that smoking crack is more toxic than snorting powdered cocaine. Most deaths result from people using cocaine in combination with another substance, such as alcohol or heroin.

ABUSE AND DEPENDENCE   When steady cocaine users stop taking the drug, they experience a sudden "crash" characterized by depression, agitation, and fatigue, followed by a period of withdrawal. Their depression can be temporarily relieved by taking more cocaine, so its continued use is reinforced. A binge cocaine user may go for weeks or months without using any cocaine and then take large amounts repeatedly. Although not physically dependent, a binge cocaine user who misses work or school and risks serious health consequences is clearly abusing the drug.

COCAINE USE DURING PREGNANCY   Cocaine rapidly passes from the mother's bloodstream into the placenta and can have serious effects on the fetus. A woman who uses cocaine during pregnancy is at higher risk for miscarriage, premature labor, and stillbirth. She is more likely to deliver a low-birth-weight baby who has a small head circumference. Her infant may be at increased risk for defects of the genitourinary tract, cardiovascular system, central nervous system, and extremities. It is difficult to pinpoint the effects of cocaine because many women who use cocaine also use tobacco and/or alcohol.

Infants whose mothers use cocaine may also be born intoxicated. They are typically irritable and jittery and do not eat or sleep normally. These characteristics may affect their early social and emotional development because it may be more difficult for adults to interact with them. Cocaine also passes into breast milk and can intoxicate a breastfeeding infant.

Research on the long-term effects of prenatal exposure to cocaine has been inconclusive. Initial findings of devastating effects have not been borne out. Recent studies suggest that prenatal cocaine exposure may cause subtle changes in the brain that affect specific cognitive and motor skills; behavioral problems—disorganization, poor social skills, and hyperactivity—have also been reported. Although fetal cocaine exposure is an important issue, the type and magnitude of effects produced by nicotine are similar, and there are nearly 20 times more infants exposed to cigarettes than to cocaine.

Amphetamines   Amphetamines (uppers) are a group of synthetic chemicals that are potent CNS stimulants. Some common drugs in this family are amphetamine (Benzedrine), dextroamphetamine (Dexedrine), and methamphetamine (Methedrine). Popular names for these drugs include "speed," crank, chalk, crystal, and "meth." Crystal methamphetamine (ice), a smokable, high-potency form of methamphetamine, is popular in some cities. Easy to manufacture, ice is cheaper than crack and produces a similar but longer-lasting euphoria.

The use of ice can quickly lead to dependence. In a recent survey of high school students, about 2% reported having used ice in the past year.

EFFECTS Small doses of amphetamines usually make people feel more alert and wide-awake and less fatigued or bored. Amphetamines generally increase motor activity but do not measurably alter a normal, rested person's ability to perform tasks calling for challenging motor skills or complex thinking. When amphetamines do improve performance, it is primarily by counteracting fatigue and boredom. Amphetamines in small doses also increase heart rate and blood pressure and change sleep patterns.

Amphetamines are sometimes used to curb appetite, but after a few weeks the user develops tolerance and higher doses are necessary. When people stop taking the drug, their appetite usually returns, and they gain back the weight they lost unless they have made permanent changes in eating behavior.

FROM USE TO ABUSE Much amphetamine abuse begins as an attempt to cope with a temporary situation. A student cramming for an exam or an exhausted long-haul truck driver can go a little longer by taking amphetamines, but the results can be disastrous. The likelihood of making bad judgments significantly increases. The stimulating effects may also wear off suddenly, and the user may precipitously feel exhausted or fall asleep ("crash").

Another problem is **state dependence**, the phenomenon whereby information learned in a certain drug-induced state is difficult to recall when the person is not in that same physiological state. Test performance may deteriorate when students use drugs to study and then take tests in their normal, nondrug state. (Users of antihistamines may also experience state dependence.)

Methamphetamine intoxication leads to unsafe and uncharacteristic behavior. It has been linked to high-risk sexual activity and increased rates of STDs, including HIV infection (see Chapter 18 for more information).

DEPENDENCE Repeated use of amphetamines, even in moderate doses, often leads to tolerance and the need for increasingly larger doses. The result can be severe disturbances in behavior, including a temporary state of paranoid **psychosis**, with delusions of persecution and unprovoked violence. If injected in large doses, amphetamines produce a feeling of intense pleasure, followed by sensations of vigor and euphoria that last for several hours. As these feelings wear off, they are replaced by feelings of irritability and vague uneasiness. Long-term use of amphetamines at high doses can cause paranoia, hallucinations, delusions, and incoherence. Methamphetamine users have signs of brain damage similar to those seen in Parkinson's disease patients that appear to persist even after drug use ceases, causing impaired memory and motor coordination. Withdrawal symptoms may include

muscle aches and tremors, along with profound fatigue, deep depression, despair, and apathy. Chronic high-dose use is often associated with pronounced psychological cravings and obsessive drug-seeking behavior.

Women who use amphetamines during pregnancy risk premature birth, stillbirth, low birth weight, and early infant death. Babies born to amphetamine-using mothers have a higher incidence of cleft palate, cleft lip, and deformed limbs. They may also experience symptoms of withdrawal from amphetamines.

Ritalin A stimulant with amphetamine-like effects, Ritalin (methylphenidate) is used to treat attention-deficit/hyperactivity disorder. When taken orally at prescribed levels, it has little potential for abuse. When injected or snorted, however, dependence and tolerance can rapidly result. Ritalin abuse among high school and college students began to be reported in the 1990s; in a 2003 survey, 4.7% of college students reported having used Ritalin in the previous year.

Ephedrine Amphetamine was made in the 1920s by modifying the chemical ephedrine, which was originally isolated from a Chinese herbal tea. Although somewhat less potent than amphetamine, ephedrine does produce stimulant effects. Ephedrine has been linked to heart arrhythmia, stroke, psychotic reactions, seizures, and some deaths, and it may be particularly dangerous at high doses or when combined with another stimulant such as caffeine. Until 2004, ephedrine was a common ingredient in over-the-counter dietary supplements for weight loss. But following the publication of studies about its dangers, the FDA banned the sale of ephedrine; lawsuits to overturn the ban were filed in several states.

Caffeine Caffeine is probably the most popular psychoactive drug and also one of the most ancient. It is found in coffee, tea, cocoa, soft drinks, headache remedies, and OTC preparations like NōDōz. In ordinary doses, caffeine produces greater alertness and a sense of well-being. It also decreases feelings of fatigue or boredom; using caffeine may enable a person to keep at physically exhausting or repetitive tasks longer. Such use is usually followed, however, by a sudden letdown. Caffeine does not noticeably influence a person's ability to perform complex mental tasks unless fatigue, boredom, or other factors have already affected normal performance.

Terms

state dependence A situation in which information learned in a drug-induced state is difficult to recall when the effect of the drug wears off.

psychosis A severe mental disorder characterized by a distortion of reality; symptoms might include delusions or hallucinations.

Caffeine mildly stimulates the heart and respiratory system, increases muscular tremor, and enhances gastric secretion. Higher doses may cause nervousness, anxiety, irritability, headache, disturbed sleep, and gastric irritation or peptic ulcers. In people with high blood pressure, caffeine can cause blood pressure to rise even further above normal; in people with type 2 diabetes, caffeine may cause glucose and insulin levels to rise after meals. Some people, especially children, are quite vulnerable to the adverse effects of caffeine. They become wired: hyperactive and overly sensitive to any stimulation in their environment. In rare instances, the disturbance is so severe that there is misperception of their surroundings—a toxic psychosis.

Drinks containing caffeine are rarely harmful for most individuals, but some tolerance develops, and withdrawal symptoms of irritability, headaches, and even mild depression do occur. Thus, although we don't usually think of caffeine as a dependence-producing drug, for some people it is. People can usually avoid problems by simply decreasing their daily intake of caffeine (Figure 9-4); if intake is decreased gradually, withdrawal symptoms can be reduced or avoided. About 80–90% of American adults consume caffeine regularly; the average daily intake is about 280 mg.

Marijuana and Other Cannabis Products

Marijuana is the most widely used illegal drug in the United States (cocaine is second). More than 40% of Americans—more than 90 million—have tried marijuana at least once; among 21–25-year-olds, more than 50% have tried marijuana. In recent surveys, about 18% of college students report using marijuana within the past month.

Marijuana is a crude preparation of various parts of the Indian hemp plant *Cannabis sativa*, which grows in most parts of the world. THC (tetrahydrocannabinol) is the main active ingredient in marijuana. Based on THC content, the potency of marijuana preparations varies widely. Marijuana plants that grow wild often have less than 1% THC in their leaves, whereas when selected strains are cultivated by separation of male and female plants (*sinsemilla*), the bud leaves from the flowering tops may contain 7–8% THC. Hashish, a potent preparation made from the thick resin that exudes from the leaves, may contain up to 14% THC. These various preparations have all been known and used for centuries, so the frequently heard claim that today's marijuana is more potent than the marijuana of the 1970s is not strictly true. However, a greater proportion of the marijuana sold today is the higher-potency (and more expensive) sinsemilla; hence, the average potency of street marijuana has increased.

Marijuana is usually smoked, but it can also be ingested. The classification of marijuana is a matter of some debate. For this reason, it is treated separately here.

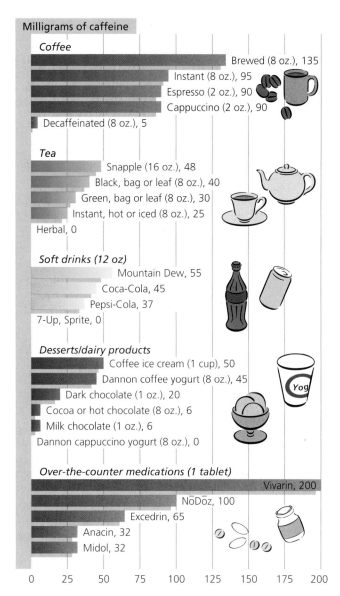

Figure 9-4 Common sources of caffeine. The caffeine content of products varies with the brand and preparation method; the values shown here are averages. SOURCES: Become a bean counter. 2000. *Prevention*, July; International Food Information Council. 1998. *Everything You Need to Know About Caffeine* (http://ific.org/publications/brochures/caffeinebroch.cfm; retrieved December 8, 2004); Caffeine content of foods and drugs. 1996. *Nutrition Action Healthletter*, December.

Short-Term Effects and Uses As is true with most psychoactive drugs, the effects of a low dose of marijuana are strongly influenced both by the user's expectations and by past experiences. At low doses, marijuana users typically experience euphoria, a heightening of subjective sensory experiences, a slowing down of the perception of passing time, and a relaxed, laid-back attitude. These pleasant effects are the reason this drug is so widely used. With moderate doses, these effects become stronger, and the user can also expect to have impaired memory function, disturbed thought patterns, lapses of attention, and feelings of **depersonalization,** in which the mind seems to be separated from the body.

The effects of marijuana in higher doses are determined mostly by the drug itself rather than by the user's expectations and setting. Very high doses produce feelings of depersonalization, as well as marked sensory distortion and changes in body image (such as a feeling that the body is very light). Inexperienced users sometimes think these sensations mean they are going crazy and become anxious or even panicky. Such reactions resemble a bad trip on LSD, but they happen much less often, are less severe, and do not last as long. However, unexpected reactions are the leading reason for emergency room visits by users of marijuana or hashish. And marijuana/hashish is now cited more frequently than heroin as a reason for emergency room visits.

Physiologically, marijuana increases heart rate and dilates certain blood vessels in the eyes, which creates the characteristic bloodshot eyes. The user may also feel less inclined toward physical exertion and may feel particularly hungry or thirsty (see the box "Medical Marijuana"). THC affects parts of the brain controlling balance, coordination, and reaction time, thus marijuana use reduces driving performance. The combination of alcohol and marijuana is even more dangerous: Even a low dose of marijuana, when combined with alcohol, significantly impairs driving performance and increases crash risk.

Long-Term Effects The most probable long-term effect of smoking marijuana is respiratory damage, including impaired lung function, chronic bronchial irritation, and precancerous changes in the lungs. People who smoke marijuana may be at increased risk for emphysema and cancer of the head and neck; among people with chronic conditions like cancer and AIDS, marijuana use is associated with increased risk of fatal lung infections. (These negative effects from smoking marijuana are key reasons why the Institute of Medicine report on medical marijuana recommended the development of alternative methods of delivering the potentially beneficial compounds in marijuana.) Heavy users who are frequently intoxicated experience subtle impairments of attention and memory that may or may not be reversible following long-term abstinence. Long-term use may also decrease testosterone levels and sperm counts and increase sperm abnormalities.

Heavy marijuana use during pregnancy may cause impaired fetal growth and development and low birth weight. Marijuana may act synergistically with alcohol to increase the damaging effects of alcohol on the fetus. THC rapidly enters breast milk and may impair an infant's early motor development.

When we consider the long-term effects of marijuana (and of any other drugs), we should keep in mind the time-lag factor. Tobacco, for example, was long thought to be a "harmless" drug. Widespread marijuana use has been com-

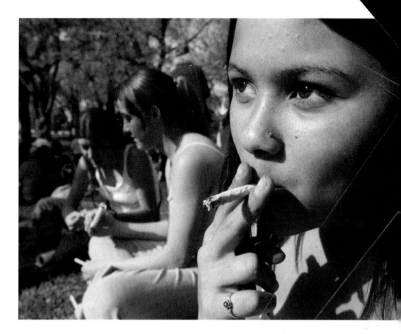

Marijuana is the most widely used illegal drug in the United States. At low doses, marijuana users typically experience euphoria and a relaxed attitude. Further research is needed to determine its precise physiological and psychological effects, particularly for chronic use.

mon for only about 30 years, and some effects may take longer than that to appear and be linked to marijuana.

Dependence Regular users of marijuana can develop tolerance; some develop dependence, and researchers estimate that 1.5% of Americans meet the APA criteria for marijuana dependence. Withdrawal symptoms may occur in the majority of dependent or heavy users; common symptoms include anger or aggression, irritability, nervousness or restlessness, sleep difficulties, and decreased appetite or weight loss. Withdrawal symptoms begin about 1–2 days after cessation of marijuana use and typically last 1–2 weeks, although some symptoms may last longer. As with all drugs that relieve "bad" feelings and produce "good" feelings, marijuana can become the focus of the user's life, to the exclusion of other activities. Drug uses appear to be related, and the chronic marijuana user is more likely to be a heavy user of tobacco, alcohol, and other dangerous drugs.

Hallucinogens

Hallucinogens are a group of drugs whose predominant pharmacological effect is to alter the user's perceptions,

Terms

depersonalization A state in which a person loses the sense of his or her reality or perceives his or her body as unreal.

hallucinogen Any of several drugs that alter perception, feelings, or thoughts; examples are LSD, mescaline, and PCP.

The question of whether marijuana has any medical uses has been hotly debated. Cannabis preparations were once medically prescribed for a variety of illnesses, but most such uses are no longer supported by research. A legal, prescription form of THC called dronabinol has been available in a capsule for some patients since 1985. However, many patients argue that oral THC is not as effective as smoked marijuana; the chemicals are absorbed more rapidly when marijuana is smoked, and it is possible that compounds in marijuana other than THC contribute to its effects. Part of the difficulty in making a case for or against medical marijuana based on current research is that most patient testimonials are based on smoked marijuana, whereas most published research utilized THC in pill form.

A 1999 government-commissioned report from the Institute of Medicine (IOM) concluded that substances in marijuana have potential therapeutic value for pain relief, for control of nausea and vomiting in chemotherapy patients, and for stimulating appetite in people with AIDS-related wasting. Although effective drugs already exist for these conditions, marijuana may be suitable for patients who do not respond to other therapies. The report said that short-term use of marijuana could be considered for patients with debilitating symptoms.

The IOM report recommended further studies and the development of alternative methods of drug delivery—inhalers, patches, or under-the-tongue sprays, for example—that would safely deliver set doses of specific compounds in marijuana. As described in the chapter, smoking marijuana can cause respiratory damage and impair lung function; it may also increase cancer risk. Some people already use vaporizers to heat marijuana rather than burning it. Beyond the risks from smoking, the IOM report found that the range of problems associated with marijuana is not out of line with problems associated with other medications available in the United States.

Researchers are currently studying how THC affects the brain and body and how to turn on similar, naturally occurring, brain chemicals. THC and related synthetic compounds are being tested for conditions such as chronic pain, multiple sclerosis, and Alzheimer's disease. It is hoped that further research will clarify potential risks, benefits, and uses of THC for medical purposes.

A number of states have passed laws legalizing marijuana for medical uses; these laws are intended to shield users from laws against possessing marijuana and to protect physicians who recommend its use. However, purchasing, prescribing, or possessing marijuana is a federal crime. Under federal drug laws, marijuana is classified as a schedule I drug, defined as being potentially addictive, having no medical uses, and being unsafe for use under medical supervision (heroin and LSD are also schedule I drugs; cocaine is a schedule II drug because it has accepted medical uses). Opponents of allowing medical use of marijuana fear that making the drug more available would expand nonmedical use among the general population.

Several cases relating to medical marijuana have been heard by the U.S. Supreme Court. In 2003, the Court upheld the right of physicians to discuss marijuana with patients for medical purposes; however, an earlier ruling found that a so-called cannabis cooperative that was distributing marijuana to patients was not exempt from federal drug laws. And in June 2005, the Court ruled that patients using homegrown marijuana on the advice of a physician for personal, noncommercial use are still subject to federal drug law and can be prosecuted—even if they live in a state that allows such use. The debate over medical marijuana is likely to continue.

SOURCES: Reefer Rx: Marijuana as medicine. 2004. *Harvard Health Letter,* September; U.S. Department of Justice. 2004. *Supreme Court Briefs: No. 03-1454: Ashcroft v. Raich* (http://www.usdoj.gov/osg/briefs/2004/3mer/2mer/toc3index.html; retrieved December 7, 2004); Institute of Medicine. 1999. *Marijuana and Medicine: Assessing the Science Base.* Washington, D.C.: National Academy Press.

feelings, and thoughts. Hallucinogens include LSD (lysergic acid diethylamide), mescaline, psilocybin, STP (4-methyl-2,5-dimethoxyamphetamine), DMT (dimethyltryptamine), MDMA (3,4-methylene-dioxymethamphetamine), ketamine, and PCP (phencyclidine). These drugs are most commonly ingested or smoked.

LSD LSD is one of the most powerful psychoactive drugs. Tiny doses will produce noticeable effects in most people, such as an altered sense of time, visual disturbances, an improved sense of hearing, mood changes, and distortions in how people perceive their bodies. Dilation of the pupils and slight dizziness, weakness, and nausea may also occur. With larger doses, users may experience a phenomenon known as **synesthesia**, feelings of depersonalization, and other alterations in the perceived relationship between the self and external reality.

Many hallucinogens induce tolerance so quickly that after only one or two doses their effects decrease substantially. The user must then stop taking the drug for several days before his or her system can be receptive to it again. These drugs cause little drug-seeking behavior and no physical dependence or withdrawal symptoms.

The immediate effects of low doses of hallucinogens are largely determined by expectations and setting. Many effects are hard to describe because they involve subjective and unusual dimensions of awareness—the **altered states of consciousness** for which these drugs are famous. For this reason, hallucinogens have acquired a certain aura not associated with other drugs. People have taken LSD in search of a religious or mystical experience or in the hope of exploring new worlds. During the 1960s, some psychiatrists gave LSD to their patients to help them talk about their repressed feelings.

A severe panic reaction, which can be terrifying in the extreme, can result from taking any dose of LSD. It is impossible to predict when a panic reaction will occur. Some LSD users report having had hundreds of pleasurable and ecstatic experiences before having a bad trip, or bummer. If the user is already in a serene mood and feels no anger or hostility and if he or she is in secure surroundings with trusted companions, a bad trip may be less likely, but a tranquil experience is not guaranteed.

Even after the drug's chemical effects have worn off, spontaneous flashbacks and other psychological disturbances can occur. **Flashbacks** are perceptual distortions and bizarre thoughts that occur after the drug has been entirely eliminated from the body. Although they are relatively rare phenomena, flashbacks can be extremely distressing. They are often triggered by specific psychological cues associated with the drug-taking experience, such as certain mood states or even types of music.

During the 1970s, researchers claimed that LSD damages chromosomes. But later evidence indicates that LSD in moderate doses, at least the pure LSD produced in the laboratory, does not damage chromosomes, cause detectable genetic damage, or produce birth defects.

Other Hallucinogens   Most other hallucinogens have the same general effects as LSD, but there are some variations. For example, a DMT or ketamine high does not last as long as an LSD high; an STP high lasts longer. MDMA has both hallucinogenic and amphetamine-like properties. Tolerance to MDMA develops quickly, and high doses can cause anxiety, delusions, and paranoia. (See the box "Club Drugs" on p. 251 for more on MDMA.)

PCP, also known as "angel dust," "hog," and "peace pill," reduces and distorts sensory input, especially **proprioception,** the sensation of body position and movement; it creates a state of sensory deprivation. PCP was initially used as an anesthetic but was unsatisfactory because it caused agitation, confusion, and delirium (loss of contact with reality). Because it can be easily made, PCP is often available illegally and is sometimes used as an inexpensive replacement for other psychoactive drugs. The effects of ketamine are similar to those of PCP—confusion, agitation, aggression, and lack of coordination—but they tend to be less predictable. Tolerance to either drug can develop rapidly.

Mescaline, derived from the peyote cactus, is the ceremonial drug of the Native American Church. It causes effects similar to LSD, including altered perception and feeling; increased body temperature, heart rate, and blood pressure; weakness and trembling; and sleeplessness. Obtaining mescaline is expensive, so most street mescaline is diluted LSD or a mixture of other drugs. Hallucinogenic effects can be obtained from certain mushrooms

Inhalant use is difficult to monitor and control because inhalants are found in many inexpensive and legal products. Low doses of inhalants may cause a user to feel slightly stimulated; higher concentrations can cause a loss of consciousness, heart failure, and death.

(*Psilocybe mexicana,* or "magic mushrooms"), certain morning glory seeds, nutmeg, jimsonweed, and other botanical products, but unpleasant side effects, such as dizziness, have limited the popularity of these products.

Inhalants

Inhaling certain chemicals can produce effects ranging from heightened pleasure to delirium and death. Inhalants fall into several major groups: (1) volatile solvents, which are found in products such as paint thinner, glue, and gasoline; (2) aerosols, which are sprays that contain propellants and solvents; (3) nitrites, such as butyl nitrite and amyl nitrite; and (4) anesthetics, which include nitrous oxide, or laughing gas. Inhalant use tends to be highest among younger adolescents and declines with age; in surveys, about 4% of eighth graders, 1.5% of twelfth graders, and 0.6% of college students report using inhalants in the past month.

Inhalant use is difficult to control because inhalants are easy to obtain. They are present in a variety of seemingly

Terms

synesthesia A condition in which a stimulus evokes not only the sensation appropriate to it but also another sensation of a different character, such as when a color evokes a specific smell.

altered states of consciousness Profound changes in mood, thinking, and perception.

flashback A perceptual distortion or bizarre thought that recurs after the chemical effects of a drug have worn off.

proprioception The sensation of body position and movement, from muscles, joints, and skin.

harmless products, from dessert-topping sprays to under-arm deodorants, that are both inexpensive and legal. Using the drugs also requires no illegal or suspicious paraphernalia. Inhalant users get high by sniffing, snorting, "bagging" (inhaling fumes from a plastic bag), or "huffing" (placing an inhalant-soaked rag in the mouth).

Although different in makeup, nearly all inhalants produce effects similar to those of anesthetics, which slow down body functions. Low doses may cause users to feel slightly stimulated; at higher doses, users may feel less inhibited and less in control. Sniffing high concentrations of the chemicals in solvents or aerosol sprays can cause a loss of consciousness, heart failure, and death. High concentrations of any inhalant can also cause death from suffocation by displacing the oxygen in the lungs and central nervous system. Deliberately inhaling from a bag or in a closed area greatly increases the chances of suffocation. Other possible effects of the excessive or long-term use of inhalants include damage to the nervous system (impaired perception, reasoning, memory, and muscular coordination); hearing loss; increased risk of cancer; and damage to the liver, kidneys, and bone marrow.

DRUG USE: THE DECADES AHEAD

Drug research will undoubtedly provide new information, new treatments, and new chemical combinations in the decades ahead. New psychoactive drugs may present unexpected possibilities for therapy, social use, and abuse. Making honest and unbiased information about drugs available to everyone, however, may cut down on their abuse. Misinformation about the dangers of drugs—using scare tactics—can lead some people to disbelieve any reports of drug dangers, no matter how soundly based and well documented they are.

Although the use of some drugs, both legal and illegal, has declined dramatically since the 1970s, the use of others has held steady or increased. Mounting public concern has led to great debate and a wide range of opinions about what should be done. Efforts to combat the problem include workplace drug testing, tougher law enforcement and prosecution, and treatment and education. With drugs entering the country on a massive scale from South America, Southeast Asia, and elsewhere and being distributed through tightly controlled drug-smuggling organizations and street gangs, it remains to be seen how effective any program will be.

Drugs, Society, and Families

The economic cost of drug use is staggering. Each year, Americans spend over $50 billion on illegal drugs, with an additional $100 billion going to cover enforcement, prevention, treatment, lost wages, and drug-related injuries and crime. But the costs are more than just financial; they are also paid in human pain and suffering.

The relationship between drugs and crime is complex. The criminal justice system is inundated with people accused of crimes related to drug possession, sale, or use. More than 2 million arrests are made each year for drug and alcohol violations, and over 100,000 people are in jail for violating drug laws. Many assaults and murders are committed when people try to acquire or protect drug territories, settle disputes about drugs, or steal from dealers. Violence and the use of guns are more common in neighborhoods where drug trafficking is prevalent. Addicts commit more robberies and burglaries than criminals not on drugs. People under the influence of drugs, especially alcohol, are more likely to commit violent crimes like rape and murder than people who do not use drugs. Although often associated with poor inner-city areas and ethnic minorities, drug-related problems affect all groups and every area of the country (see the box "Drug Use and Ethnicity: Risk and Protective Factors").

Drug use is also a health care issue for society. In the United States, illegal drug use leads to more than 500,000 emergency room admissions and nearly 20,000 deaths annually. Although it is in the best interest of society to treat addicts who want help, there is not nearly enough space in treatment facilities to help the estimated 5 million Americans in need of immediate treatment. Drug addicts who want to quit, especially those among the urban poor, often have to wait a year or more for acceptance into a residential care or other treatment program.

Drug abuse also takes a toll on individuals and families. Children born to women who use drugs such as alcohol, tobacco, or cocaine may have long-term health problems. Drug use in families can become a vicious cycle. Observing adults around them using drugs, children assume it is an acceptable way to deal with problems. Problems such as abuse, neglect, lack of opportunity, and unemployment become contributing factors to drug use and serve to perpetuate the cycle.

Legalizing Drugs

Pointing out that many of the social problems associated with drugs are related to prohibition rather than to the effects of the drugs themselves, some people have argued for various forms of drug legalization or decriminalization. Proposals range from making drugs such as marijuana and heroin available by prescription to allowing licensed dealers to sell some of these drugs to adults. Proponents argue that crimes by drug users are usually committed to buy drugs that cost relatively more than alcohol and tobacco because they are produced illegally and that making some currently illicit drugs legal—but putting controls on them similar to those used for alcohol, tobacco, and prescription drugs—could eliminate many of the problems related to drug use.

Opponents of drug legalization argue that allowing easier access to drugs would expose many more people to

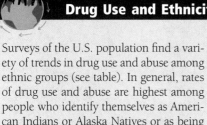

Dimensions of Diversity

Surveys of the U.S. population find a variety of trends in drug use and abuse among ethnic groups (see table). In general, rates of drug use and abuse are highest among people who identify themselves as American Indians or Alaska Natives or as being of two races; rates are lowest among Asian Americans. In addition to the general trends shown in the table, there are also trends relating to specific drugs; for example, hallucinogen use is relatively prevalent among whites and Latinos, inhalant use among Native Hawaiians and Pacific Islander Americans.

However, as is true for many areas of health, ethnic trends are influenced by a complex interplay of other factors:

- *Educational status:* Adults with four or more years of college are more likely to have *tried* illicit drugs than are people of the same age who never finished high school, but *current* drug use is lower among college graduates than among people with less education. Among teens, poor school performance is associated with increased risk for illicit drug use.

- *Employment status:* Most adult drug users are employed, but rates of current drug use are much higher among people who are unemployed or who work part-time compared with those who are employed full-time.

- *Parental education and socioeconomic status:* Students from poor families have higher rates of *early* drug use compared with students from

wealthier families, but by the twelfth grade, the differences disappear. Socioeconomic status and parental education are closely linked.

- *Geographic area:* Current drug use in the United States is highest in the West and Northeast; drug use is also somewhat higher in metropolitan and urban areas compared with more rural areas. People living in communities with high rates of poverty, crime, and unemployment have higher than average rates of drug use and abuse. Specific drugs may also be more available—and their abuse more prevalent—in certain regions or communities.

Strong cultural identity is associated with reduced risk of drug use and abuse among all groups. Researchers hope to learn more about other protective factors by studying groups that have relatively low rates of drug use and abuse, especially Asian Americans of all ages and African American adolescents. Some factors believed to contribute to lower rates of drug use among these groups include the following:

- *Parental and community disapproval of drug and alcohol use:* Parents of African American and Asian American children tend to have more restrictive drug and alcohol use norms than white parents, and black parents tend to monitor their children's activities and friendships more closely than white parents. Parental disapproval of

drug use is often tied to greater perceived risk of drug use—and lower rates of drug use—among teens.

- *Close family ties:* Asian American teens are the likeliest to come from intact homes. Black teens, although least likely to come from intact homes, often come from single-parent households with close extended family ties. Respect for authority and family loyalty are strongly valued among many Asian American populations. Teens from cohesive and stable families are less likely to use drugs.

- *Focus on schooling and education:* Teens from families who value education and where parents help with homework and limit weeknight time with friends have lower rates of drug use. Asian Americans have twice the rate of college graduation compared with other groups.

SOURCES: Office of Applied Studies, Substance Abuse and Mental Health Services Administration. 2004. *National Survey on Drug Use and Health* (http://oas.samhsa.gov/nhsda.htm; retrieved December 6, 2004); Johnston, L. D., et al. 2003. *Monitoring the Future: National Survey Results on Drug Use, 1975–2003: Volume I, Secondary School Students* (NIH Publication No. 04-5507). Bethesda, Md.: National Institute on Drug Abuse; National Center on Addiction and Substance Abuse at Columbia University. 2003. *The Formative Years: Pathways to Substance Abuse Among Girls and Young Women Ages 8–22.* New York: National Center on Addiction and Substance Abuse; National Asian Pacific American Families Against Substance Abuse. 2002. *Fact Sheet: Asian American and Pacific Islander Illicit Drug Use* (http://www.napafasa.org; retrieved December 7, 2004).

National Survey Results

	Lifetime Drug Use	Past Year Drug Use	Past Month Drug Use				Past Year Abuse or Dependence
			Age 12–17	Age 18–25	Age 26 and older	All ages	
Whites	49.2	14.9	11.8	22.5	5.8	8.3	2.8
African Americans	44.6	15.4	9.6	18.2	6.4	8.7	3.1
Latinos	37.0	14.7	11.0	15.6	5.2	8.0	3.4
Asian Americans	25.6	7.1	6.5	11.8	1.9	3.8	1.5
American Indians and Alaska Natives	62.4	18.9	19.3	31.0	6.8	12.1	4.8
Native Hawaiians and Pacific Islander Americans	51.0	18.5	n/a	n/a	n/a	11.1	5.6
Two or more races	60.1	20.1	15.1	29.2	7.9	12.0	5.0

possible abuse and dependence. Drugs would be cheaper and easier to obtain, and drug use would be more socially acceptable. Legalizing drugs could cause an increase in drug use among children and teenagers. Opponents point out that alcohol and tobacco are major causes of disease and death in our society and that they should not be used as models for other practices.

Drug Testing

One of the most controversial issues in American politics is drug testing in the workplace. It has been estimated that as many as 10% of workers use psychoactive drugs on the job. For some occupations, such as air traffic controllers, truck drivers, and train engineers, drug use can create significant hazards, sometimes involving hundreds of people. Some people believe that the dangers are so great that all workers should be tested and that anyone found with traces of drugs in the blood or urine should be either fired or treated. Others insist that this would violate people's right to privacy and to freedom from unreasonable search, guaranteed by the Fourth Amendment. Opponents point out that most jobs do not involve hazards, so employees who take drugs are not any more dangerous than employees who do not.

Despite the expense, many employers now test their employees, and the U.S. armed forces test military personnel regularly. People in jobs involving transportation—truck drivers, bus drivers, train engineers, airline pilots—are required by federal law to be tested regularly to ensure public safety. The primary criterion leading most companies to use drug testing is the company's liability if an employee under the influence of a drug makes a mistake that could potentially harm others.

Most drug testing involves a urine test; a test for alcohol involves a blood test or a breath test. The accuracy of these tests has improved in recent years, so there are fewer opportunities for people to cheat or for the tests to yield inaccurate results. If a person tests positive for drugs, the employer may provide drug counseling or treatment, suspend the employee until he or she tests negative, or fire the individual.

The FDA has approved several over-the-counter home drug testing kits designed to allow parents to check their children for drug use. Urine samples are collected at home; preliminary results may be available immediately, but final results require that the sample be sent to a laboratory for analysis. Many experts, including the American Academy of Pediatrics, advise against the use of home tests in cases of suspected drug use; instead, they recommend a comprehensive evaluation by a qualified health professional.

Treatment for Drug Dependence

A variety of programs is available to help people break their drug habits, but there is no single best method of

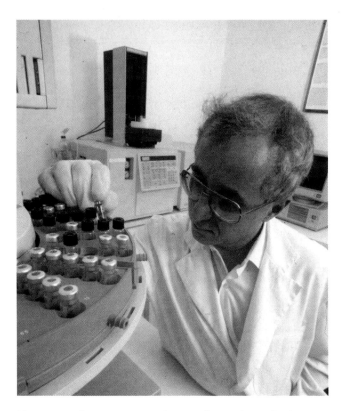

Many companies test current and prospective employees for drug use. Most drug testing involves a urine test that can detect recent use of marijuana, heroin, cocaine, amphetamines, codeine, and many other psychoactive drugs.

treatment. The relapse rate is high for all types of treatment but is similar to the rate of relapse seen in people being treated for diabetes, high blood pressure, and asthma. Numerous studies have shown that being treated is better than not being treated. To be successful, treatment must deal with the reasons behind people's drug abuse and help them develop behaviors, attitudes, and a social support system that will help them remain drug-free.

Medication-Assisted Treatment Medications are increasingly being used in addiction treatment—to reduce the craving for the abused drug or to block or oppose its effects. Perhaps the best-known medication for drug abuse is methadone, a synthetic drug used as a substitute for heroin. Use of methadone prevents withdrawal reactions and reduces the craving for heroin; it enables dependent people to function normally in social and vocational activities, although they remain dependent on methadone. The narcotic buprenorphine, approved in 2002 for treatment of opioid addiction, also reduces cravings; researchers are studying long-acting forms of this drug, which may be even more effective than use of a daily pill. Many other medications are under study; drugs used specifically in the treatment of nicotine and alcohol dependence are discussed in Chapters 10 and 11.

Medication therapy is relatively simple and inexpensive and is therefore popular among patients, health care providers, and insurance companies. However, the relapse rate is high. Combining drug therapy with psychological and social services improves success rates, underscoring the importance of psychological factors in drug dependence.

Treatment Centers   Treatment centers offer a variety of short-term and long-term services, including hospitalization, detoxification, counseling, and other mental health services. The therapeutic community is a specific type of center, a residential program run in a completely drug-free atmosphere. Administered by ex-addicts, these programs use confrontation, strict discipline, and unrelenting peer pressure to attempt to resocialize the addict with a different set of values. Halfway houses, transitional settings between a 24-hour-a-day program and independent living, are an important phase of treatment for some people. Strategies for evaluating programs are given in the box "Choosing a Drug-Treatment Program."

Self-Help Groups and Peer Counseling
Groups such as Alcoholics Anonymous (AA) and Narcotics Anonymous (NA) have helped many people. People treated in drug substitution programs or substance-abuse treatment centers are often urged or required to join a self-help group as part of their recovery. These groups follow a 12-step program. Group members' first step is to acknowledge that they have a problem over which they have no control. Peer support is a critical ingredient of these programs, and members usually meet at least once a week. Each member is paired with a sponsor to call on for advice and support if the temptation to relapse becomes overwhelming. With such support, thousands of substance-dependent people have been able to recover, remain abstinent, and reclaim their lives. Chapters of AA and NA meet on some college campuses; community-based chapters are listed in the phone book and in local newspapers. (Also see the For More Information section at the end of the chapter.)

Many colleges also have peer counseling programs, in which students are trained to help other students who have drug problems. A peer counselor's role may be as limited as referring a student to a professional with expertise in substance dependence for an evaluation or as involved as helping arrange a leave of absence from school for participation in a drug-treatment program. Most peer counseling programs are founded on principles of strict confidentiality. Peer counselors may also be able to help students who are concerned about a classmate or loved one with an apparent drug problem (see the box "If Someone You Know Has a Drug Problem . . ." on p. 263). Information about peer counseling programs is usually available from the student health center.

Harm Reduction Strategies   Recognizing that many attempts at treatment are at first unsuccessful and that a drug-free society may be an unobtainable goal, some experts advocate the use of harm reduction strategies. The goal of harm reduction is to minimize the negative effects of drug use and abuse; a common example is the use of designated drivers to reduce alcohol-related motor vehicle crashes. In terms of illicit drugs, drug substitution programs such as methadone maintenance are one form of harm reduction; although participants remain drug dependent, the negative individual and social consequences of their drug use is reduced. Syringe exchange programs, designed to reduce transmission of HIV and hepatitis C, are another harm reduction approach. Some experts have also suggested free testing of street drugs for purity and potency to help users avoid unintentional toxicity or overdose. Harm reduction strategies are controversial, in part because they measure success not in terms of overall levels of drug use and dependence but rather in terms of the harm caused by drug use in terms of illness, death, and crime.

Codependency   Many treatment programs also offer counseling for those who are close to drug abusers. Drug abuse takes a toll on friends and family members, and counseling can help people work through painful feelings of guilt and powerlessness. **Codependency,** in which a person close to the drug abuser is controlled by the abuser's behavior, sometimes develops. Codependent people may come to believe that love, approval, and security are contingent on their taking care of the abuser. People can become codependent naturally because they want to help when someone they love becomes dependent on a drug. They may assume that their good intentions will persuade the drug user to stop.

Codependent people often engage in behaviors that remove or soften the effects of the drug use on the user—so-called *enabling* behaviors. However, the habit of enabling can inhibit a drug-dependent person's recovery because the person never has to experience the consequences of his or her behavior. Often, the enabler is dependent, too—on the patterns of interaction in the relationship. People who need to take care of people often marry people who need to be taken care of. Children in these families often develop the same behavior pattern as one of their parents, by either becoming helpless or becoming a caregiver. For this reason, many treatment programs involve the whole family.

Term

codependency A relationship in which a non–substance-abusing partner or family member is controlled by the abuser's behavior; codependent people frequently engage in enabling behaviors.

When evaluating different facilities or programs for drug treatment, consider the following issues:

- *What type of treatment or facility is most appropriate?* Intensive outpatient treatment is available through many community mental health centers, as well as through specialized drug-treatment facilities. Such programs typically require several sessions per week, combining individual therapy, group counseling, and attendance at 12-step meetings. Residential, or inpatient, facilities may be associated with a medical facility such as a hospital, or they may be freestanding programs that focus solely on substance-abuse treatment. Some residential treatment programs last longer or cost more per week than many health insurance plans will cover.

- *How will treatment be paid for?* Many health insurance plans limit residential treatment to a maximum of 3 weeks or less. They may also require that you first attempt a less expensive form of treatment before they will approve coverage for a residential facility.

- *Is there likely to be a need for medical support?* Chronic alcoholics or abusers of other CNS depressants may experience life-threatening seizures or other withdrawal symptoms during the first few days of detoxification. Malnutrition is common among substance abusers, and injection drug users may suffer from local infections and bloodborne diseases such as hepatitis or HIV infection. Medical problems such as these are best handled in an inpatient program with good medical support.

- *What is the level of professional training of the staff?* Is there a medical doctor on-site or making frequent visits? Are there trained nurses? Licensed psychologists or social workers? Many successful programs are staffed primarily by recovering alcoholics or drug users. Do those staff members have training and certification as addiction specialists or some other license or certificate?

- *Does the program provide related services, such as family and job counseling and post-treatment follow-up?* These types of services are extremely important for the long-term success of drug-abuse treatment.

- *Can you visit the facility and speak with the staff and clients?* A prospective client and his or her family should be allowed to visit any treatment center or program.

Have you ever been an enabler in a relationship? You may have, if you've ever done any of the following:

- Given someone one more chance to stop abusing drugs, then another, and another . . .
- Made excuses or lied for someone to his or her friends, teachers, or employer
- Joined someone in drug use and blamed others for your behavior
- Loaned money to someone to continue drug use
- Stayed up late waiting for or gone out searching for someone who uses drugs
- Felt embarrassed or angry about the actions of someone who uses drugs
- Ignored the drug use because the person got defensive when you brought it up
- Not confronted a friend or relative who was obviously intoxicated or high on a drug

If you come from a codependent family or see yourself developing codependency relationships or engaging in enabling behaviors, consider acting now to make changes in your patterns of interaction. Remember, you cannot cause or cure drug dependence in another person.

Preventing Drug Abuse

Obviously, the best solution to drug abuse is prevention. Government attempts at controlling the drug problem tend to focus on stopping the production, importation, and distribution of illegal drugs. Creative effort also has to be put into stopping the demand for drugs. Developing persuasive antidrug educational programs offers the best hope for solving the drug problem in the future. Indirect approaches to prevention involve building young people's self-esteem, improving their academic skills, and increasing their recreational opportunities. Direct approaches involve giving information about the adverse effects of drugs and teaching tactics that help students resist peer pressure to use drugs in various situations. Developing strategies for resisting peer pressure is one of the more effective techniques.

Prevention efforts need to focus on the different motivations individuals have for using and abusing specific drugs at different ages. For example, grade-school children seem receptive to programs that involve their parents or well-known adults such as professional athletes. Adolescents in junior or senior high school are often more responsive to peer counselors. Many young adults tend to be influenced by efforts that focus on health education. For all ages, it is important to provide nondrug alternatives—such as recreational facilities, counseling, greater opportunities for leisure activities, and places to socialize—that speak to the individual's or group's specific reasons for using drugs. Reminding young people that most people, no matter what age, are *not* users of illegal drugs, do *not* smoke cigarettes, and do *not* get drunk frequently is a critical part of preventing substance abuse.

If you notice changes in behavior and mood in someone you know, they may signal a growing dependence on drugs. Signs that a person's life is beginning to focus on drugs include the following:

- Sudden withdrawal or emotional distance
- Rebellious or unusually irritable behavior
- A loss of interest in usual activities or hobbies
- A decline in school performance
- A sudden change in the chosen group of friends
- Changes in sleeping or eating habits
- Frequent borrowing of money or stealing
- Secretive behavior about personal possessions, such as a backpack or the contents of a drawer
- Deterioration of physical appearance

If you believe a family member or friend has a drug problem, obtain information about resources for drug treatment available on your campus or in your community. Communicate your concern, provide him or her with information about treatment options, and offer your support during treatment. If the person continues to deny having a problem, you may want to talk with an experienced counselor about setting up an intervention—a formal, structured confrontation designed to end denial by having family, friends, and other caring individuals present their concerns to the drug user. Participants in an intervention would indicate the ways in which the individual is hurting others as well as himself or herself. If your friend or family member agrees to treatment, encourage him or her to attend a support group such as Narcotics Anonymous or Alcoholics Anonymous. And finally, examine your relationship with the abuser for signs of codependency. If necessary, get help for yourself; friends and family of drug users can often benefit from counseling.

The Role of Drugs in Your Life

Where do you fit into this complex picture of drug use and abuse? Chances are that you've had experience with OTC and prescription drugs, and you may or may not have had experience with one or more of the drugs described in this chapter. You probably know someone who has used or abused a psychoactive drug. Whatever your experience has been up to now, it's likely that you will encounter drugs at some point in your life. To make sure you'll have the inner resources to resist peer pressure and make your own decision, cultivate a variety of activities you enjoy doing, realize that you are entitled to have your own opinion, and don't neglect your self-esteem.

Issues to Consider Before you try a psychoactive drug, consider the following questions:

- *What are the risks involved?* Many drugs carry an immediate risk of injury or death. Most involve the longer-term risk of abuse and dependence.
- *Is using the drug compatible with your goals?* Consider how drug use will affect your education and career objectives, your relationships, your future happiness, and the happiness of those who love you.
- *What are your ethical beliefs about drug use?* Consider whether using a drug would cause you to go against your personal ethics, religious beliefs, social values, or family responsibilities.
- *What are the financial costs?* Many drugs are expensive, especially if you become dependent on them.

- *Are you trying to solve a deeper problem?* Drugs will not make emotional pain go away; in the long run, they will only make it worse. If you are feeling depressed or anxious, seek help from a mental health professional instead of self-medicating with drugs.

Like all aspects of health-related behavior, making responsible decisions about drug use depends on information, knowledge, and insight into yourself. Many choices are possible; making the ones that are right for you is what counts.

What to Do Instead of Drugs If you have used or considered using drugs, think carefully about your reasons for doing so. Consider trying healthier strategies for dealing with difficult emotions and peer pressure. For ideas, look over the following list of reasons for drug use and suggested alternative activities:

- *Bored?* Go for a walk or a run; stimulate your senses at a museum or a movie; challenge your mind with a new game or book; introduce yourself to someone new.
- *Stressed?* Practice relaxation or visualization; try to slow down and open your senses to the natural world; get some exercise.
- *Shy or lonely?* Talk to a counselor; enroll in a shyness clinic; learn and practice communication techniques.
- *Feeling low on self-esteem?* Focus on the areas in which you are competent; give yourself credit for the things you do well. A program of regular exercise can also enhance self-esteem.

- *Depressed or anxious?* Talk to a friend, parent, or counselor.

- *Apathetic or lethargic?* Force yourself to get up and get some exercise to energize yourself; assume responsibility for someone or something outside yourself; volunteer.

- *Searching for meaning?* Try yoga or meditation; explore spiritual experiences through religious groups, church, prayer, or reading.

- *Afraid to say no?* Take a course in assertiveness training; get support from others who don't want to use drugs; remind yourself that you have the right and the responsibility to make your own decisions.

- *Still feeling peer pressure?* Begin to look for new friends or roommates. Take a class or join an organization that attracts other health-conscious people.

SUMMARY

- Addictive behaviors are reinforcing. Addicts experience a strong compulsion for the behavior and a loss of control over it; an escalating pattern of abuse with serious negative consequences may result.

- The sources or causes of addiction include heredity, personality, lifestyle, and environmental factors. People may use an addictive behavior as a means of alleviating stress or painful emotions.

- Many common behaviors are potentially addictive, including gambling, shopping, sexual activity, Internet use, eating, and working.

- Drug abuse is a maladaptive pattern of drug use that persists despite adverse social, psychological, or medical consequences.

- Drug dependence involves taking a drug compulsively, which includes neglecting constructive activities because of it and continuing to use it despite experiencing adverse effects resulting from its use. Tolerance and withdrawal symptoms are often present.

- Reasons for using drugs include the lure of the illicit; curiosity; rebellion; peer pressure; and the desire to alter one's mood or escape boredom, anxiety, depression, or other psychological problems.

- Psychoactive drugs affect the mind and body by altering brain chemistry. The effect of a drug depends on the properties of the drug and how it's used (drug factors), the physical and psychological characteristics of the user (user factors), and the physical and social environment surrounding the drug use (social factors).

- Opioids relieve pain, cause drowsiness, and induce euphoria; they reduce anxiety and produce lethargy, apathy, and an inability to concentrate.

- CNS depressants slow down the overall activity of the nerves; they reduce anxiety and cause mood changes, impaired muscular coordination, slurring of speech, and drowsiness or sleep.

- CNS stimulants speed up the activity of the nerves, causing acceleration of the heart rate, a rise in blood pressure, dilation of the pupils and bronchial tubes, and an increase in gastric and adrenal secretions.

- Marijuana usually causes euphoria and a relaxed attitude at low doses; very high doses produce feelings of depersonalization and sensory distortion. The long-term effects may include chronic bronchitis and cancer; use during pregnancy may impair fetal growth.

- Hallucinogens alter perception, feelings, and thought and may cause an altered sense of time, visual disturbances, and mood changes.

- Inhalants are present in a variety of harmless products; they can cause delirium. Their use can lead to loss of consciousness, heart failure, suffocation, and death.

- Economic and social costs of drug abuse include the financial costs of law enforcement, treatment, and health care and the social costs of crime, violence, and family problems. Drug testing and drug legalization have been proposed to address some of the problems related to drug abuse.

- Approaches to treatment include medication, treatment centers, self-help groups, and peer counseling; many programs also offer counseling to family members.

Changing Your Drug Habits

This behavior change strategy focuses on one of the most commonly used drugs—caffeine. If you are concerned about your use of a different drug or another type of addictive behavior, you can devise your own plan based on this one and on the steps outlined in Chapter 1.

Because caffeine supports certain behaviors that are characteristic of our culture, such as sedentary, stressful work, you may find yourself relying on coffee (or tea, chocolate, or cola) to get through a busy schedule. Such habits often begin in college. Fortunately, it's easier to break a habit before it becomes entrenched as a lifelong dependency.

When you are studying for exams, the forced physical inactivity and the need to concentrate even when fatigued may lead you to overuse caffeine. But caffeine doesn't help unless you are already sleepy. And it does not relieve any underlying condition (you are just more tired when it wears off). How can you change this pattern?

Self-Monitoring

Keep a log of how much caffeine you eat or drink. Use a measuring cup to measure coffee or tea. Using Figure 9-4, convert the amounts you eat or drink into an estimate expressed in milligrams of caffeine. Be sure to include all forms, such as chocolate bars and OTC medications, as well as caffeine candy, colas, cocoa or hot chocolate, chocolate cake, tea, and coffee.

Self-Assessment

At the end of the week, add up your daily totals and divide by 7 to get your daily average in milligrams. How much is too much? At more than 250 mg per day, you may well be experiencing some adverse symptoms. If you are experiencing at least five of the following symptoms, you may want to cut down.

- Restlessness
- Nervousness
- Excitement
- Insomnia
- Flushed face
- Excessive sweating
- Gastrointestinal problems
- Muscle twitching
- Rambling thoughts and speech
- Irregular heartbeat
- Periods of inexhaustibility
- Excessive pacing or movement

Set Limits

Can you restrict your caffeine intake to a daily total, and stick to this contract? If so, set a cutoff point, such as one cup of coffee. Pegging it to a specific time of day can be helpful, because then you won't confront a decision at any other point (and possibly fail). If you find you cannot stick to your limit, you may want to cut out caffeine altogether; abstinence can be easier than moderation for some people. If you experience caffeine withdrawal symptoms (headache, fatigue), you may want to cut your intake more gradually.

Find Other Ways to Keep Up Your Energy

If you are fatigued, it makes sense to get enough sleep or exercise more, rather than drowning the problem in coffee or tea. Different people need different amounts of sleep; you may also need more sleep at different times, such as during a personal crisis or an illness. Also, exercise raises your metabolic rate for hours afterward—a handy fact to exploit when you want to feel more awake and want to avoid an irritable caffeine jag. And if you've been compounding your fatigue by not eating properly, try filling up on complex carbohydrates such as whole-grain bread or crackers instead of candy bars.

Tips on Cutting Out Caffeine Here are some more ways to decrease your consumption of caffeine:

- Keep some noncaffeinated drinks on hand, such as decaffeinated coffee, herbal teas, mineral water, bouillon, or hot water.
- Alternate between hot and very cold liquids.
- Fill your coffee cup only halfway.
- Avoid the office or school lunchroom or cafeteria and the chocolate sections of the grocery store. (Often people drink coffee or tea and eat chocolate simply because they're available.)
- Read labels of over-the-counter medications to check for hidden sources of caffeine.

Take Action

1. **Research local addiction services:** Find out what types of services are available on your campus or in your community to handle drug dependence and other addictive behaviors. If there are none, what services are needed? Locate the school official and public health agency responsible for your campus and community, and ask why these needs aren't being met.

2. **Survey attitudes:** Survey three older adults and three young students about their attitudes toward legalizing marijuana. Are there any differences? If so, what accounts for these differences? What kinds of reasons do they give for their positions?

3. **Analyze media portrayals:** Look at a current movie or television program, paying special attention to how drug use is portrayed. What messages are being conveyed? If possible, compare a recent movie with one made 10–20 years ago. Has the presentation of drug use changed? If so, how?

4. **Be a mentor or role model:** Consider volunteering at your local YMCA or with Boys and Girls Clubs or Big Brothers Big Sisters. By providing positive role models and activities, such organizations help keep young people away from drugs and other unhealthy behaviors. You can also just take time out to talk with the young people in your life about making smart choices.

Books

Booth, M. 2004. *Cannabis: A History*. New York: Thomas Dunne Books. *Provides historical information and covers current issues about marijuana from a variety of perspectives.*

Ginther, C. 2004. *Drug Abuse Sourcebook: Basic Consumer Health Information About Illicit Substances of Abuse and the Misuse of Prescription and Over-the-Counter Medications*. Detroit, Mich.: Omnigraphics. *Provides basic information about a wide variety of drugs.*

Julien, R. M. 2004. *A Primer of Drug Action*, 10th ed. New York: Worth. *A guide to the actions, uses, and side effects of psychoactive drugs.*

Kuhn, C., S. Swartzwelder, and W. Wilson. 2003. *Buzzed: The Straight Facts About the Most Used and Abused Drugs from Alcohol to Ecstasy*, 2nd ed. New York: W. W. Norton. *Provides straightforward information about the effects of drugs.*

Ray, O. S., and C. Ksir. 2006. *Drugs, Society, and Human Behavior*, 11th ed. New York: McGraw-Hill. *Examines drugs and behavior from the behavioral, pharmacological, historical, social, legal, and clinical perspectives.*

Roleff, T. L., and H. Cothran. 2004. *Drug Abuse: Opposing Viewpoints*. San Diego: Greenhaven Press. *Explores key issues relating to drug use and abuse.*

Organizations, Hotlines, and Web Sites

Addiction: Close to Home. Created to accompany a PBS television series on addiction, this site provides information about prevention, treatment, and public policy; it also includes animated illustrations of how drugs affect the brain.

http://www.pbs.org/wnet/closetohome/home.html

Center for On-Line Addiction. Contains information about Internet and cybersex addiction.

http://netaddiction.com

ClubDrugs.Org. Provides information on drugs commonly classified as "club drugs."

http://www.clubdrugs.org

Do It Now Foundation. Provides youth-oriented information about drugs.

http://www.doitnow.org

Drug Enforcement Administration: Drugs of Abuse. Provides basic facts about major drugs of abuse, including penalties for drug trafficking.

http://www.dea.gov/concern/concern.htm

Frontline: Drug Wars. Includes information on key drugs, drug abusers, and the issues surrounding America's "war on drugs."

http://www.pbs.org/wgbh/pages/frontline/shows/drugs

Gamblers Anonymous. Includes questions to help diagnose gambling problems and resources for getting help.

http://www.gamblersanonymous.org

Habitsmart. Contains information about addictive behavior, including tips for effectively managing problematic habitual behaviors, a self-scoring alcohol check-up, and links.

http://www.habitsmart.com

Higher Eduction Center for Alcohol and Other Drug Prevention. Gives information about alcohol and drug abuse on campus and links to related sites.

http://www.edc.org/hec

Indiana Prevention Resource Center. A clearinghouse of information and links on substance-abuse topics, including specific psychoactive drugs and issues such as drug testing and drug legalization.

http://www.drugs.indiana.edu

Narcotics Anonymous (NA). Similar to Alcoholics Anonymous, NA sponsors 12-step meetings and provides other support services for drug abusers.

818-773-9999

http://www.na.org

There are also 12-step programs that focus on specific drugs:

Cocaine Anonymous

http://www.ca.org

Marijuana Anonymous

http://www.marijuana-anonymous.org

National Center on Addiction and Substance Abuse (CASA) at Columbia University. Provides information about the costs of substance abuse to individuals and society.

http://www.casacolumbia.org

National Clearinghouse for Alcohol and Drug Information. Provides statistics, information, and publications on substance abuse, including resources for people who want to help friends and family members overcome substance-abuse problems.

http://www.health.org

National Council on Problem Gambling. Provides information and help for people with gambling problems and their families, including a searchable directory of counselors.

800-522-4700

http://www.ncpgambling.org

National Drug Information, Treatment, and Referral Hotlines. Sponsored by the SAMHSA Center for Substance Abuse Treatment, these hotlines provide information on drug abuse and on HIV infection as it relates to substance abuse; referrals to support groups and treatment programs are available.

800-662-HELP

800-729-6686 (Spanish)

800-487-4889 (TDD for hearing impaired)

National Institute on Drug Abuse. Develops and supports research on drug-abuse prevention programs; fact sheets on drugs of abuse are available on the Web site or via recorded phone messages, fax, or mail.

http://www.drugabuse.gov

Office of National Drug Control Policy (ONDCP). Provides information on national and international drug-related topics, including U.S. policies related to prevention, education, treatment, and enforcement.

http://www.whitehousedrugpolicy.gov

Society for the Advancement of Sexual Health. Provides information, resources, and a self-quiz relating to sexual addiction.

http://www.ncsac.org

Substance Abuse and Mental Health Services Administration (SAMHSA). Provides statistics, information, and other resources related to substance-abuse prevention and treatment.

http://www.samhsa.gov

See also the listings for Chapters 10 and 11.

American Psychiatric Association. 2000. *Diagnostic and Statistical Manual of Mental Disorders,* Fourth Edition, Text Revision. *(DSM-IV).* Washington, D.C.: American Psychiatric Association.

Braine, N. 2004. Long-term effects of syringe exchange on risk behavior and HIV prevention. *AIDS Education and Prevention* 16(3): 264–275.

Budney, A. J., et al. 2004. Review of the validity and significance of cannabis withdrawal syndrome. *American Journal of Psychiatry* 161(11): 1967–1977.

Colfax, G., et al. 2005. Longitudinal patterns of methamphetamine, popper (amyl nitrite), and cocaine use and high-risk sexual behavior among a cohort of San Francisco men who have sex with men. *Journal of Urban Health,* epub February 28.

Compton, W. M., et al. 2004. Prevalence of marijuana use disorder in the United States. *Journal of the American Medical Association* 291(17): 2114–2121.

Delaney-Black, V., et al. 2004. Prenatal cocaine: Quantity of exposure and gender moderation. *Journal of Developmental and Behavioral Pediatrics* 25(4): 254–263.

Drugs approved for opiate dependence. 2003. *FDA Consumer,* January/February.

Dyer, J. E., B. Roth, and B. A. Hyma. 2001. Gamma-hydroxybutyrate withdrawal syndrome. *American College of Emergency Physicians* 37: 147–153.

Elkins, I. J., et al. 2004. The effect of parental alcohol and drug disorders on adolescent personality. *American Journal of Psychiatry* 161(4): 670–676.

Engwall, D., R. Hunter, and M. Steinberg. 2004. Gambling and other risk behaviors on university campuses. *Journal of American College Health* 52(6): 245–255.

Ernst, T., et al. 2000. Evidence for long-term neurotoxicity associated with methamphetamine abuse. *Neurology* 54(6): 1344–1349.

Fried, P., et al. 2002. Current and former marijuana use: Preliminary findings of a longitudinal study of effects on IQ in young adults. *Canadian Medical Association Journal* 166(7): 887–891.

Herning, R. I., et al. 2005. Cerebrovascular perfusion in marijuana users during a month of monitored abstinence. *Neurology* 64(3): 488–493.

Hurd, Y. L., et al. 2005. Marijuana impairs growth in mid-gestation fetuses. *Neurotoxicology and Teratology* 27(2): 221–229.

Johnston, L. D., et al. 2004. *Monitoring the Future: National Survey Results on Drug Use, 1975–2003. Volume I: Secondary School Students* (NIH Publication No. 04-5507). Bethesda, Md.: National Institute on Drug Abuse.

Johnston, L. D., et al. 2004. *Monitoring the Future: National Survey Results on Drug Use, 1975–2003. Volume II: College Students and Adults Ages 19–45* (NIH Publication No. 04-5508). Bethesda, Md.: National Institute on Drug Abuse.

Juliano, L. M., and R. R. Griffiths. 2004. A critical review of caffeine withdrawal: Empirical validation of symptoms and signs, incidence, severity, and associated features. *Psychopharmacology* 176(1): 1–29.

Kish, S. J., et al. 2000. Striatal serotonin is depleted in brain of a human MDMA (ecstasy) user. *Neurology* 55(2): 294–296.

Kloner, R. A., and S. H. Rezkalla. 2003. Cocaine and the heart. *New England Journal of Medicine* 348(6): 487–488.

Kubley, R., and M. Csikszentmihalyi. 2002. Television addiction is no mere metaphor. *Scientific American,* February.

LaBrie, R. A., et al. 2003. Correlates of college student gambling in the United States. *Journal of American College Health* 52(2): 53–62.

Lane, J. D., et al. 2004. Caffeine impairs glucose metabolism in type 2 diabetes. *Diabetes Care* 27(8): 2047–2048.

Lynch, W. J., P. K. Maciejewski, and M. N. Potenza. 2004. Psychiatric correlates of gambling in adolescents and young adults grouped by age at gambling onset. *Archives of General Psychiatry* 61(11): 1116–1122.

Lynskey, M. T., et al. 2003. Escalation of drug use in early-onset cannabis users vs. co-twin controls. *Journal of the American Medical Association* 289(4): 427–433.

Maglione, M., et al. 2005. Psychiatric effects of ephedra use: An analysis of Food and Drug Administration reports of adverse events. *American Journal of Psychiatry* 162(1): 189–191.

Mahowald, M. L., J. A. Singh, and P. Majeski. 2005. Opioid use by patients in an orthopedics spine clinic. *Arthritis and Rheumatology* 52(1): 312–321.

McBride, B. F., et al. 2004. Electrocardiographic and hemodynamic effects of a multicomponent dietary supplement containing ephedra and caffeine. *Journal of the American Medical Association* 291(4): 216–221.

National Clearinghouse for Alcohol and Drug Information. 2002. *Drugs of Abuse* (http://www.health.org/govpubs/rpo926; retrieved November 12, 2002).

National Institute on Drug Abuse. 2004. *Inhalant Abuse: What Are the Medical Consequences of Inhalant Abuse?* (http://www.drugabuse.gov/ResearchReports/Inhalants/Inhalants4.html; retrieved December 6, 2004).

Opioid abuse. 2004. *Journal of the American Medical Association* 291(11): 1394.

Parrott, A. C. 2005. Chronic tolerance to recreational MDMA (3,4-methylenedioxymethamphetamine) or ecstasy. *Journal of Psychopharmacology* 19(1): 71–83.

Qureshi, A. I., et al. 2001. Cocaine use and the likelihood of nonfatal myocardial infarction and stroke: Data from the Third National Health and Nutrition Examination Survey. *Circulation* 103: 502–506.

Ramaekers, J. G., et al. 2004. Dose-related risk of motor vehicle crashes after cannabis use. *Drug and Alcohol Dependence* 73(2): 109–119.

Savoca, M. R., et al. 2005. Association of ambulatory blood pressure and dietary caffeine in adolescents. *American Journal of Hypertension* 18(1): 116–120.

Singer, L. T., et al. 2004. Cognitive outcomes of preschool children with prenatal cocaine exposure. *Journal of the American Medical Association* 291(20): 2448–2456.

Solowij, N., et al. 2002. Cognitive functioning of long-term heavy cannabis users seeking treatment. *Journal of the American Medical Association* 287(9): 1123–1131.

Strote, J., J. E. Lee, and H. Wechsler. 2002. Increased MDMA use among college students: Results of a national survey. *Journal of Adolescent Health* 30: 64–72.

Substance Abuse and Mental Health Services Administration. 2005. Nonmedical oxycodone users: A comparison with heroin users. *The NSDUH Report,* January.

Substance Abuse and Mental Health Services Administration. 2002. *Drug Abuse Warning Network: Club Drugs, 2001 Update.* Rockville, Md.: Substance Abuse and Mental Health Services Administration.

Tuncel, M., et al. 2002. Mechanism of the blood pressure–raising effect of cocaine in humans. *Circulation* 105(9): 1054–1059.

U.S. Drug Enforcement Agency. 2002. *DEA Drug Briefs: OxyContin* (http://www.dea.gov/concern/oxycodone.html; retrieved November 12, 2002).

U.S. Food and Drug Administration. 2001. *OxyContin: Questions and Answers* (http://www.fda.gov/cder/drug/infopage/oxycontin/oxycontin-qa.htm; retrieved November 12, 2002).

U.S. Food and Drug Administration. 2002. *Subutex and Suboxone: Questions and Answers* (http://www.fda.gov/cder/drug/infopage/subutex_suboxone/subutex-qa.htm; retrieved November 12, 2002).

Wareing, M., et al. 2005. Visuo-spatial working memory deficits in current and former users of MDMA ('ecstasy'). *Human Psychopharmacology* 20(2): 115–23.

World Health Organization. 2004. *Facts and Figures: Management of Substance Abuse* (http://www.who.int/substance_abuse/facts/en; retrieved September 15, 2004).

Zakzanis, K. K., and D. A. Young. 2001. Memory impairment in abstinent MDMA ("ecstasy") users: A longitudinal investigation. *Neurology* 56: 966–969.

10

After reading this chapter, you should be able to

- Explain how alcohol is absorbed and metabolized by the body

- Describe the immediate and long-term effects of drinking alcohol

- Define alcohol abuse, binge drinking, and alcoholism and discuss their effects on the drinker and others

- Evaluate the role of alcohol in your life, and list strategies for using it responsibly

The Responsible Use of Alcohol

Knowledge

Test Your

1. "Moderate drinking" is having three or fewer drinks per day.
True or false?

2. How many adults in the United States do not drink any alcohol?
a. 1 in 10
b. 1 in 5
c. 1 in 3

3. If a man and a woman of the same weight drink the same amount of alcohol, the woman will become intoxicated more quickly than the man.
True or false?

4. Drinking too much alcohol in too short a time can cause death from alcohol poisoning.
True or false?

5. Drinking coffee will help you sober up.
True or false?

6. About 10,000 college students between the ages of 18 and 24 are victims of alcohol-related sexual assault or date rape each year.
True or false?

ANSWERS

1. FALSE. Moderate drinking is no more than one drink per day for women and no more than two drinks per day for men.

2. C. Most other adults drink lightly and occasionally; a small number of heavy drinkers, about 7% of adults, consume more than half of all the alcohol in the United States. Overall, college students drink more alcohol and are more likely to binge drink than young adults who are not in college, but nonstudents are more likely to be dependent on alcohol.

3. TRUE. Women usually have a higher percentage of body fat than men and a less active form of a stomach enzyme that breaks down alcohol. Both factors cause them to become intoxicated more quickly and to a greater degree.

4. TRUE. Consuming a number of drinks over a period of several hours is likely to cause intoxication, followed by a hangover; chugging the same amount in an hour or less can be lethal.

5. FALSE. Once alcohol has been absorbed by the body, nothing speeds its metabolism.

6. FALSE. The figure is more than 70,000 students; each year, a half million students report having unsafe sex while drunk or having sex when they are too intoxicated to know whether they have consented.

VW Visit the *Core Concepts in Health* Online Learning Center (www.mhhe.com/insel10e) for study aids and many additional resources.

269

Alcohol has been used in religious ceremonies, in feasts and celebrations, and as a medicine for thousands of years. Throughout history, alcohol has been more popular than any other drug in the Western world, despite numerous prohibitions against it. Alcohol has a somewhat contradictory role in human life. Most of us think of alcohol the way it is portrayed in advertisements, on television, and in movies—as part of good times at the beach, social occasions, and elegant gatherings. Used in moderation, alcohol can enhance social occasions by loosening inhibitions and creating a pleasant feeling of relaxation. But the use of alcohol can also be unhealthy. Like other drugs, alcohol has definite physiological effects on the body that can impair functioning in the short term and cause devastating damage in the long term. For some people, alcohol becomes an addiction, leading to a lifetime of recovery or, for a few, to debilitation and death. Many of our slang expressions for intoxication reflect its less positive aspects; we say we're "smashed," "bombed," or "wasted."

About 49% of American adults abstain from alcohol or drink fewer than 12 drinks per year. About 22% are light or occasional drinkers, and about 29% are risky drinkers, meaning they occasionally or regularly drink excessively. Among risky drinkers are the approximately 8% of U.S. adults who meet the diagnostic criteria for alcohol abuse or dependence. If the total amount of alcohol consumed in the United States in a year were evenly divided among drinkers, each would consume the equivalent of 4 gallons of whiskey, 20 gallons of wine, or 50 gallons of beer. But heavy drinkers, who constitute about 7% of the American drinking population, account for over half of all the alcohol consumed, as well as a disproportionate amount of the social, economic, and medical costs of alcohol abuse (estimated at over $180 billion per year). Alcohol is responsible for about 85,000 deaths per year among Americans, and it is the leading cause of death among people age 15 to 24. Worldwide, alcohol causes 1.8 million deaths per year.

The use of alcohol is a complex issue, one that demands conscious thought and informed decisions. In our society, some people choose to drink in moderation, some choose not to drink at all, and others realize too late that they've made an unwise choice—when they become dependent on alcohol, are involved in an alcohol-related car crash, or simply wake up to discover they've done something they regret. This chapter discusses the complexities of alcohol use and provides information that will help you make the choices that are right for you.

THE NATURE OF ALCOHOL

How does alcohol affect people? Does it affect some people differently than others? Can some people handle alcohol? Is it possible to drink a safe amount of alcohol?

Many of the misconceptions about the effects of alcohol can be cleared up by taking a closer look at the chemistry of alcohol and how it is absorbed and metabolized by the body.

The Chemistry of Alcohol

Ethyl alcohol is the psychoactive ingredient in all alcoholic beverages. Beer, a mild intoxicant brewed from a mixture of grains, usually contains 3–6% alcohol by volume. Ales and malt liquors are 6–8% alcohol by volume. Wines are made by *fermenting* the juices of grapes or other fruits. The concentration of alcohol in table wines is about 9–14%. *Fortified wines,* so named because alcohol has been added to them, contain about 20% alcohol; these include sherry, port, and Madeira. Stronger alcoholic beverages, called *hard liquors,* are made by *distilling* brewed or fermented grains or other products. These beverages, including gin, whiskey, brandy, rum, tequila, vodka, and liqueurs, usually contain 35–50% alcohol.

The concentration of alcohol in a beverage is indicated by the **proof value,** which is two times the percentage concentration. For example, if a beverage is 100 proof, it contains 50% alcohol. Two ounces of 100-proof whiskey contain 1 ounce of pure alcohol. The proof value of hard liquors can usually be found on the bottle labels. When alcohol consumption is discussed, "one drink" refers to a 12-ounce bottle of beer, a 5-ounce glass of table wine, or a cocktail with 1.5 ounces of 80-proof liquor. Each of these different drinks contains approximately the same amount of alcohol: 0.5–0.6 ounce.

Alcohol provides 7 calories per gram, and the alcohol in one drink (14–17 grams) supplies about 100–120 calories. Most alcoholic beverages also contain some carbohydrate, so, for example, one beer provides about 150 total calories. The "light" in light beer refers to calories; a light beer typically has close to the same alcohol content as a regular beer and about two-thirds the calories. People who choose to drink alcohol should remember to count the calories in alcoholic beverages toward their total daily calorie intake to avoid unintentional weight gain.

There are a number of different kinds of alcohol. In this book, the term **alcohol** refers to ethyl alcohol, which is the only kind of alcohol that can be consumed. Other kinds of alcohol such as methanol (wood alcohol) and isopropyl alcohol (rubbing alcohol) are highly toxic and can cause blindness and other serious problems when consumed even in low doses.

Absorption

When a person ingests alcohol, about 20% is rapidly absorbed from the stomach into the bloodstream. About 75% is absorbed through the upper part of the small intestine. Any remaining alcohol enters the bloodstream further along the gastrointestinal tract. Once in the bloodstream, alcohol

Ethyl alcohol is the common psychoactive drug found in all alcoholic beverages. One drink—a 12-ounce beer, a 1.5-ounce cocktail, or a 5-ounce glass of wine—contains about 0.5–0.6 ounce of ethyl alcohol.

Alcohol Intake and Blood Alcohol Concentration

Blood alcohol concentration (BAC), a measure of intoxication, is determined by the amount of alcohol consumed in a given amount of time and by individual factors:

- *Body weight:* In most cases, a smaller person develops a higher BAC than a larger person after drinking the same amount of alcohol. A smaller person has less overall body tissue into which alcohol can be distributed.

- *Percent body fat:* A person with a higher percentage of body fat will usually develop a higher BAC than a more muscular person of the same weight. Alcohol does not concentrate as much in fatty tissue as in muscle and most other tissues, in part because fat has fewer blood vessels.

- *Sex:* Women metabolize less alcohol in the stomach than men do because the stomach enzyme that breaks down alcohol before it enters the bloodstream is four times more active in men than in women. This means that more unmetabolized alcohol is released into the bloodstream in women. Because women are also generally smaller than men and have a higher percentage of body fat, women will have a higher BAC than men after consuming the same amount of alcohol. Hormonal fluctuations may also affect the rate of alcohol metabolism, making a woman more susceptible to high BACs at certain times during her menstrual cycle (usually just prior to the onset of menstruation).

BAC also depends on the balance between the rate of alcohol absorption and the rate of alcohol metabolism. A man who weighs 150 pounds and has normal liver function metabolizes about 0.3 ounce of alcohol per hour, the equivalent of about half a 12-ounce bottle of beer or a 5-ounce glass of wine.

The rate of alcohol metabolism varies among individuals and is largely determined by genetic factors and drinking behavior. (Chronic drinking activates enzymes that metabolize alcohol in the liver, so people who drink frequently metabolize alcohol at a more rapid rate than nondrinkers.)

produces feelings of intoxication. The rate of absorption is affected by a variety of factors. For example, the carbonation in a beverage like champagne increases the rate of alcohol absorption. Food in the stomach slows the rate of absorption, as does the drinking of highly concentrated alcoholic beverages such as hard liquor. But remember: *All* alcohol a person consumes is eventually absorbed.

Metabolism and Excretion

Alcohol is quickly transported throughout the body by the blood. Because alcohol easily moves through most biological membranes, it is rapidly distributed throughout most body tissues. The main site of alcohol **metabolism** is the liver, though a small amount of alcohol is metabolized in the stomach. (See the box "Metabolizing Alcohol: Our Bodies Work Differently" for more information.)

About 2–10% of ingested alcohol is not metabolized in the liver or other tissues but is excreted unchanged by the lungs, kidneys, and sweat glands. Excreted alcohol causes the telltale smell on a drinker's breath and is the basis of breath and urine analyses for alcohol levels. Although such analyses do not give precise measurements of alcohol concentrations in the blood, they do provide a reasonable approximation if done correctly.

Terms

proof value Two times the percentage of alcohol by volume; a beverage that is 50% alcohol by volume is 100 proof.

alcohol The intoxicating ingredient in fermented liquors; a colorless, pungent liquid.

metabolism The chemical transformation of food and other substances in the body into energy and wastes.

blood alcohol concentration (BAC) The amount of alcohol in the blood in terms of weight per unit volume; used as a measurement of intoxication.

Dimensions of Diversity

Do you notice that you react differently to alcohol than some of your friends do? If so, you may be noticing genetic differences in alcohol metabolism that are associated with ethnicity. Alcohol is metabolized mainly in the liver, where it is broken down by an enzyme called alcohol dehydrogenase, producing a by-product called acetaldehyde (see the figure). Acetaldehyde is responsible for many of the unpleasant effects of alcohol abuse. Another enzyme, acetaldehyde dehydrogenase, breaks this product down further.

Some people, including many of Asian descent or of certain Jewish population groups, have genes that cause them to produce somewhat different forms of the two enzymes that metabolize alcohol. The result is high concentrations of acetaldehyde in the brain and other tissues, producing a host of unpleasant symptoms. When

people with these enzymes drink alcohol, they experience a physiological reaction referred to as *flushing syndrome*. Their skin feels hot, their heart and respiration rates increase, and they may get a headache, vomit, or break out in hives. Drinking makes some people so uncomfortable that it's unlikely they could ever become addicted to alcohol.

The body's response to acetaldehyde is the basis for treating alcohol abuse with the drug disulfiram (Antabuse), which inhibits the action of acetaldehyde dehydrogenase. When a person taking disulfiram ingests alcohol, acetaldehyde levels increase rapidly, and he or she develops an intense flushing reaction along with weakness, nausea, vomiting, and other disagreeable symptoms.

How people behave in relation to alcohol is influenced in complex ways by

many factors, including social and cultural ones. But in this case at least, individual choices and behavior are strongly influenced by a specific genetic characteristic.

Contrary to popular myths, this metabolic rate *cannot* be influenced by exercise, breathing deeply, eating, drinking coffee, or taking other drugs. The rate of alcohol metabolism is the same whether a person is asleep or awake.

If a person absorbs slightly less alcohol each hour than he or she can metabolize in an hour, the BAC remains low. People can drink large amounts of alcohol this way over a long period of time without becoming noticeably intoxicated; however, they do run the risk of significant long-

term health hazards (described later in the chapter). If a person is absorbing alcohol more quickly than it can be metabolized, the BAC will steadily increase, and he or she will become more and more drunk (Table 10-1). How fast you drink makes a big difference in how high your BAC will be. Consuming several drinks over a period of 2 or 3 hours is likely to cause intoxication, followed on the next day by a hangover; chugging the same amount of alcohol in an hour or less could be lethal.

Table 10-1	The Effects of Alcohol	
BAC (%)	**Common Behavioral Effects**	**Hours Required to Metabolize Alcohol**
0.00–0.05	Slight change in feelings, usually relaxation and euphoria. Decreased alertness.	2–3
0.05–0.10	Emotional instability, with exaggerated feelings and behavior. Reduced social inhibitions. Impairment of reaction time and fine motor coordination. Increasingly impaired during driving. Legally drunk at 0.08%.	3–6
0.10–0.15	Unsteadiness in standing and walking. Loss of peripheral vision. Driving is extremely dangerous.	6–10
0.15–0.30	Staggering gait. Slurred speech. Pain and other sensory perceptions greatly impaired.	10–24
More than 0.30	Stupor or unconsciousness. Anesthesia. Death possible at 0.35% and above. Can result from rapid or binge drinking with few earlier effects.	More than 24

Alcoholic beverages like beer and wine are an integral part of social occasions for many people. A central nervous system depressant, alcohol loosens inhibitions; when used in moderation, it tends to make people feel more relaxed and sociable.

ALCOHOL AND HEALTH

The effects of alcohol consumption on health depend on the individual, the circumstances, and the amount of alcohol consumed.

The Immediate Effects of Alcohol

BAC is a primary factor determining the effects of alcohol (see Table 10-1). At low concentrations, alcohol tends to make people feel relaxed and jovial, but at higher concentrations people are more likely to feel angry, sedated, or sleepy. Alcohol is a CNS depressant, and its effects vary because body systems are affected to different degrees at different BACs. At any given BAC, the effects of alcohol are more pronounced when the BAC is rapidly increasing than when it is slowly increasing, steady, or decreasing. The effects of alcohol are more pronounced if a person drinks on an empty stomach, because alcohol is absorbed more quickly and the BAC rises more quickly.

Low Concentrations of Alcohol The effects of alcohol can first be felt at a BAC of about 0.03–0.05%. These effects may include light-headedness, relaxation, and a release of inhibitions. Most drinkers experience mild euphoria and become more sociable. When people drink in social settings, alcohol often seems to act as a stimulant, enhancing conviviality or assertiveness. This apparent stimulation occurs because alcohol depresses inhibitory centers in the brain.

Higher Concentrations of Alcohol At higher concentrations, the pleasant effects tend to be replaced by more negative ones: interference with motor coordination, verbal performance, and intellectual functions. The drinker often becomes irritable and may be easily angered or given to crying. When the BAC reaches 0.1%, most sensory and motor functioning is reduced, and many people become sleepy. Vision, smell, taste, and hearing become less acute. At 0.2%, most drinkers are completely unable to function, either physically or psychologically, because of the pronounced depression of the central nervous system, muscles, and other body systems. Coma usually occurs at a BAC of 0.35%, and any higher level can be fatal.

Shakespeare accurately described the effects of alcohol on sexual functioning. He said (in *Macbeth*) that "it stirs up desire, but it takes away the performance." Small doses may improve sexual functioning for individuals who are especially anxious or self-conscious, but higher doses usually have a negative effect. Excessive alcohol use can result in reduced erection response and reduced vaginal lubrication. Testicular atrophy (shrinking) may result from the long-term overuse of alcohol.

Alcohol causes blood vessels near the skin to dilate, so drinkers often feel warm; their skin flushes, and they may sweat more. Flushing and sweating contribute to heat loss, and so the internal body temperature falls. High doses of alcohol may impair the body's ability to regulate temperature, causing it to drop sharply, especially if the surrounding temperature is low. Drinking alcoholic beverages to keep warm in cold weather does not work and can even be dangerous.

Drinking alcohol, particularly in large amounts, disturbs normal sleep patterns. Alcohol may facilitate falling asleep more quickly, but the sleep is often light, punctuated with awakenings, and unrefreshing. Even after the habitual drinker stops drinking, his or her sleep may be altered for weeks or months.

Alcohol Hangover Despite all the jokes about hangovers, anyone who has experienced a severe hangover knows they are no laughing matter. The symptoms include headache, shakiness, nausea, diarrhea, fatigue, and impaired mental functioning. It is estimated that hangovers cost the U.S. economy about $148 billion each year because of absenteeism and poor job performance. Hangovers represent a substantial portion of the money lost to society as a result of alcohol use.

A hangover is probably caused by a combination of the toxic products of alcohol breakdown, dehydration, and hormonal effects. During a hangover, heart rate and blood

Take Charge

Remember: Being very drunk is potentially life-threatening. Helping a drunken friend could save a life.

- Be firm but calm. Don't engage the person in an argument or discuss her drinking behavior while she is intoxicated.

- Get the person out of harm's way—don't let her drive or wander outside. Don't let her drink any more alcohol.

- If the person is unconscious, don't assume she is just "sleeping it off." Place her on her side with her knees up. This position will help prevent choking if the person should vomit.

- Stay with the person—you need to be ready to help if she vomits or stops breathing.

- Don't try to give the person anything to eat or drink, including coffee or other drugs. Don't give cold showers or try to make her walk around. None of these things help anyone to sober up, and they can be dangerous.

Call 911 immediately in any of the following instances:

- You can't wake the person even with shouting or shaking.

- The person is taking fewer than 8 breaths per minute or her breathing seems shallow or irregular.

- You think the person took other drugs in addition to alcohol.

- The person has had an injury, especially a blow to the head.

- The person drank a large amount of alcohol within a short period of time and then became unconscious. Death caused by alcohol poisoning most often occurs when the blood alcohol level rises very quickly due to rapid ingestion of alcohol.

If you aren't sure what to do, call 911. You may save a life.

---

pressure increase, making some individuals more vulnerable to heart attacks. Electroencephalography (brain wave measurement) shows diffuse slowing of brain waves for up to 16 hours after BAC drops to zero. Studies of pilots, drivers, and skiers all indicate that coordination and cognition are impaired in a person with a hangover, increasing the risk of injury.

The best treatment for hangover is prevention. Nearly all men can expect a hangover if they drink more than 5 or 6 drinks; for women, the number is 3 or 4 drinks. Drinking less, drinking more slowly, and consuming plenty of nonalcoholic liquids decrease the risk of hangover. If you do get a hangover, remember that your ability to drive is definitely impaired, even after your BAC has returned to zero.

Alcohol Poisoning   Acute alcohol poisoning occurs much more frequently than most people realize, and all too often it can cause death. Drinking large amounts of alcohol over a short period of time can rapidly raise the BAC into the lethal range. Alcohol, either alone or in combination with other drugs, is responsible for more toxic overdose deaths than any other drug. A common scenario for alcohol poisoning is that inexperienced drinkers try to outdo each other by consuming glass after glass of alcohol as rapidly as possible. Coma and death can result before the participants in this game have any awareness of how dangerous it can be. Children are at especially high risk for alcohol poisoning. Even a partially empty glass of liquor carelessly left out after a party can result in serious poisoning, or even death, if consumed by a toddler or small child.

Death from alcohol poisoning may be caused either by central nervous system and respiratory depression or by inhaling fluid or vomit into the lungs. The amount of alcohol it takes to make a person unconscious is dangerously close to a fatal dose. Special care should be taken to ensure the safety of anyone who has been drinking heavily, especially if the person becomes unconscious (see the box "Dealing with an Alcohol Emergency").

Using Alcohol with Other Drugs   Alcohol-drug combinations are the number-one cause of drug-related deaths in this country. Using alcohol while taking any other drug that can cause CNS depression increases the effects of both drugs, potentially leading to coma, respiratory depression, and death. Examples of common drugs that can result in oversedation when combined with alcohol include barbiturates, Valium-like drugs, narcotics such as codeine, and OTC antihistamines such as Benadryl. For people who consume three or more drinks per day, use of OTC pain relievers like aspirin, ibuprofen, or acetaminophen increases the risk of stomach bleeding or liver damage. Some antibiotics and diabetes medications can also interact dangerously with alcohol.

Many illegal drugs are especially dangerous when combined with alcohol. Life-threatening overdoses occur at much lower doses when heroin and other narcotics are combined with alcohol. When cocaine and alcohol are used together, a toxic substance called cocaethylene is formed; this substance is responsible for more than half of all cocaine-related deaths.

The safest strategy is to avoid combining alcohol with any other drug—prescription, over-the-counter, or illegal. If in doubt, ask your pharmacist or physician before using any drug in combination with alcohol, or just don't do it.

Alcohol-Related Injuries and Violence

The combination of impaired judgment, weakened sensory perception, reduced inhibitions, impaired motor coordination, and, often, increased aggressiveness and hostility that characterizes alcohol intoxication can be dangerous or even deadly. Illness and injuries caused by alcohol use result in about 7.5 million emergency room visits per year in the United States. Through homicide, suicide, automobile crashes (discussed in the next section), and other incidents, alcohol kills over 75,000 Americans each year. Alcohol use contributes to over 50% of all murders, assaults, and rapes, and alcohol is frequently found in the bloodstream of both perpetrators and victims. Nearly 80% of people who attempt suicide have been drinking, and about half of all successful suicides are alcoholics. Alcohol use more than triples the chances of fatal injuries during leisure activities such as swimming and boating, and more than half of all fatal falls and serious burns happen to people who have been drinking. Being drunk is clearly hazardous to your health.

Alcohol and Sexual Decision Making

Alcohol seriously affects a person's ability to make wise decisions about sex. A recent survey of college students revealed that frequent binge drinkers were five times more likely to engage in unplanned sexual activity and five-and-a-half times more likely to have unprotected sex than non–binge drinkers. Heavy drinkers are also more likely to have multiple sex partners and to engage in other forms of high-risk sexual behavior. For all these reasons, rates of sexually transmitted diseases and unwanted pregnancy are higher among people who drink heavily than among people who drink moderately or not at all. A study comparing rates of gonorrhea (a sexually transmitted disease) in states with varying minimum drinking ages and beer taxes found that gonorrhea rates dropped significantly among young people when beer taxes were increased and the minimum drinking age was raised.

Women who binge-drink are at increased risk for rape and other forms of nonconsensual sex. The laws regarding sexual consent are clear: A person who is very drunk or passed out cannot consent to sex. If you have sex with a person who is drunk or unconscious, you are committing sexual assault. Claiming that you were drunk at the time won't absolve you of your legal and moral responsibility for this serious crime.

Drinking and Driving

Despite recent improvements, drunk driving continues to be one of the most serious public health and safety problems in the United States. Every year, more than 800,000 people are injured in alcohol-related automobile crashes—an average of *1 person every 40 seconds*

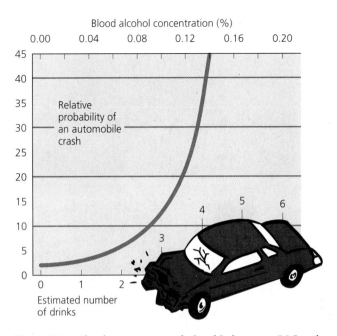

Figure 10-1 The dose-response relationship between BAC and automobile crashes.

(Figure 10-1). About 40% of the more than 44,000 crash fatalities in 2003 were alcohol-related, down from about 50% ten years ago. Increased public education about drunk driving and stiffer drunk driving laws are primarily responsible for this improvement. Still, in surveys, more than one in four of U.S. drivers admit to having used alcohol or another drug within 2 hours before driving a vehicle.

The *dose-response function* (see Chapter 9) is the relationship between the amount of alcohol or drug consumed and the type and intensity of the resulting effect. Higher doses of alcohol are associated with a much greater probability of automobile crashes. A person driving with a BAC of 0.14% is more than 40 times more likely to be involved in a crash than someone with no alcohol in his or her blood. For those with a BAC above 0.14%, the risk of a fatal crash is estimated to be 380 times higher. The risks for young drivers are even greater than indicated in Figure 10-1, especially at very low BACs. Younger drivers have less experience with both driving and alcohol, which results in significant impairment even with BACs as low as 0.02%.

In addition to an increased risk of injury and death, driving while intoxicated can have serious legal consequences. Drunk driving is against the law. In 2005, the legal limit for BAC was 0.08% in all states and the District of Columbia. Under current zero-tolerance laws in many states, drivers under age 21 who have consumed *any* alcohol may have their licenses suspended. There are stiff penalties for drunk driving, including fines, loss of license, confiscation of vehicle, and jail time. Many cities have checkpoints where drivers are stopped and checked for intoxication.

Alcohol interferes with judgment, perception, coordination, and other areas of mental and physical functioning, and it is a factor in a majority of all fatal automobile crashes. This driver is lucky that he was stopped by a suspicious police officer before a crash occurred. He is being given a breath test to determine his blood alcohol concentration.

drinks it takes the average person to reach various BACs is shown in Figure 10-2. However, some driving skills are affected at BACs of 0.02% and lower; at 0.05%, visual perception, reaction time, and certain steering tasks are all impaired. Any amount of alcohol impairs your ability to drive safely, and fatigue augments alcohol's effects.

If you are out of your home and drinking, find an alternative means of transportation or follow the practice of having a *designated driver,* an individual who refrains from drinking in order to provide safe transportation home for others in the group. The responsibility can be rotated for different occasions. Remember, you risk more than your own life when you drink and drive. Causing serious injury or death results in lifelong feelings of sadness and guilt for the driver and tremendous grief for the friends and families of victims.

It's more difficult to protect yourself against someone else who drinks and drives. Learn to be alert to the erratic driving that signals an impaired driver. Warning signs include wide, abrupt, and illegal turns; straddling the center line or lane marker; driving on the shoulder; weaving, swerving, or nearly striking an object or another vehicle; following too closely; erratic speed; driving with headlights off at night; and driving with the window down in very cold weather. If you see any of these signs, try the following strategies:

- If the driver is ahead of you, maintain a safe following distance. Don't try to pass.

- If the driver is behind you, turn right at the nearest intersection, and let the driver pass.

- If the driver is approaching your car, move to the shoulder and stop. Avoid a head-on collision by sounding your horn or flashing your lights.

- When approaching an intersection, slow down and stay alert for vehicles that don't appear to be slowing in preparation for stopping at a stop sign or red light.

Numerous studies have shown that alcohol-related highway deaths fall when states lower the legal BAC. Many developed countries have lower BAC limits than the United States. The most common BAC limit is 0.05%, a level used by Australia, Belgium, Denmark, France, Germany, Greece, Spain, and many other countries; Sweden and Russia have BAC limits of 0.02%.

People who drink and drive are unable to drive safely because their judgment is impaired, their reaction time is slower, and their coordination is reduced. The number of

Figure 10-2 Approximate blood alcohol concentration and body weight. This chart illustrates the BAC an average person of a given weight would reach after drinking the specified number of drinks in the time shown. The legal limit for BAC is 0.08%; for drivers under 21 years of age, many states have zero-tolerance laws that set BAC limits of 0.01% or 0.02%.

IMMEDIATE EFFECTS

Central nervous system: Impaired reaction time and motor coordination; impaired judgment and sedation; coma and death at high BACs

Senses: Less acute vision, smell, taste, and hearing

Stomach: Nausea, inflammation, and bleeding

Skin: Flushing; sweating; heat loss and hypothermia; formation of broken capillaries

Sexual functioning: In men, reduced erection response; in women, reduced vaginal lubrication

EFFECTS OF CHRONIC USE

Brain: Damaged/destroyed brain cells; impaired memory; loss of sensation in limbs; brain atrophy

Cardiovascular system: Weakened cardiac muscle; elevated blood pressure; irregular heartbeat; increased risk of stroke

Breast: Increased risk of breast cancer

Immune system: Lowered resistance to disease

Digestive system: Cirrhosis of the liver; inflammation of stomach and pancreas; increased risk of cancers of the lip, mouth, larynx, esophagus, liver, rectum, stomach, and pancreas

Kidney: Kidney failure associated with end-stage liver disease

Nutrition: Nutrient deficiencies; obesity

Reproductive system: In women, menstrual irregularities and increased risk of having children with fetal alcohol syndrome (FAS); in men, impotence and testicular atrophy

Bone: Increased risk of osteoporosis; increased risk of fractures from frequent falls

Figure 10-3   The immediate and long-term effects of alcohol use.

- Make sure your safety belt is fastened and children are in approved safety seats.
- Report suspected impaired drivers to the nearest police station by phone. Give a description of the vehicle, license number, location, and direction the vehicle is headed.

The Effects of Chronic Use

Because alcohol is distributed throughout most of the body, it can affect many different organs and tissues (Figure 10-3). Problems associated with chronic, or habitual, use of alcohol include diseases of the digestive and cardiovascular systems and some cancers. Drinking during pregnancy risks the health of both the woman and the developing fetus.

The Digestive System   Even in relatively small amounts, alcohol can alter the normal functioning of the liver. Within just a few days of heavy alcohol consumption, fat begins to accumulate in liver cells, resulting in

the development of "fatty liver." If drinking continues, inflammation of the liver can occur, resulting in alcoholic hepatitis, a frequent cause of hospitalization and death in alcoholics. Both fatty liver and alcoholic hepatitis are potentially reversible if the person stops drinking. With continued alcohol use, however, liver cells are progressively damaged and then permanently destroyed. The destroyed cells are replaced by fibrous scar tissue, a condition known as **cirrhosis.** As cirrhosis develops, a drinker may gradually lose his or her capacity to tolerate alcohol, because there are fewer and fewer healthy cells remaining in the liver to metabolize it. Alcohol-precipitated cirrhosis is the twelfth leading cause of death in the United States.

As with most health hazards, the risk of cirrhosis depends on an individual's susceptibility, largely genetically

Term

cirrhosis A disease in which the liver is severely damaged by alcohol, other toxins, or infection.

determined, and the amount of alcohol consumed over time. Some people show signs of cirrhosis after a few years of consuming three or four drinks per day. Women generally develop cirrhosis at lower levels of alcohol consumption than men. Alcoholics are especially susceptible to infection with hepatitis C virus (HCV); the combination of alcohol abuse and HCV infection greatly increases the risk for cirrhosis and liver cancer.

Signs of cirrhosis can include jaundice (a yellowing of the skin and white part of the eyes) and the accumulation of fluid in the abdomen and lower extremities. Some people with cirrhosis have no obvious outward signs of the disease. Treatment for cirrhosis includes a balanced diet and complete abstinence from alcohol. People with cirrhosis who continue to drink have only a 50% chance of surviving 5 or more years.

Alcohol can inflame the pancreas, causing nausea, vomiting, abnormal digestion, and severe pain. Acute alcoholic pancreatitis generally occurs in binge drinkers. Unlike cirrhosis, which usually occurs after years of fairly heavy alcohol use, pancreatitis can occur after just one or two severe binge-drinking episodes. Acute pancreatitis is often fatal and can also develop into a chronic condition.

Overuse of alcohol is a common cause of bleeding in the gastrointestinal tract. Vomiting after an alcohol binge can result in tearing of esophageal blood vessels. Chronic alcohol use with cirrhosis frequently results in the development of enlarged, fragile esophageal and rectal veins, which can easily burst with potentially fatal results. Even a relatively small amount of alcohol can cause painful irritation of the lining of the stomach.

The Cardiovascular System   The effects of alcohol on the cardiovascular system depend on the amount of alcohol consumed. Moderate doses of alcohol—less than one drink a day for women and two drinks a day for men—may reduce the risk of heart disease and heart attack in some people. (The possible health benefits of alcohol are discussed later in this chapter.) However, higher doses of alcohol have harmful effects on the cardiovascular system. In some people, more than two drinks a day will elevate blood pressure, making stroke and heart attack more likely. Some alcoholics show a weakening of the heart muscle, a condition known as **cardiac myopathy.** Binge drinking can cause "holiday heart," a syndrome characterized by serious abnormal heart rhythms, which usually appear within 24 hours of a binge episode.

Although the relationships between alcohol and cardiovascular disease are multiple and complex, it is clear that excessive drinking increases the risk of disease. These health risks progressively increase as the amount of excessive drinking increases.

Cancer   Alcoholics have a cancer rate about ten times higher than that of the general population. They are particularly vulnerable to cancers of the throat, larynx, esophagus, upper stomach, liver, and pancreas. Drinking three or more alcoholic beverages per day doubles a woman's risk of developing breast cancer. Some studies have linked even moderate drinking to increased risk for cancers of the breast, mouth, throat, and esophagus. In May 2000, the U.S. Department of Health and Human Services added alcoholic beverages to the list of known human carcinogens.

Brain Damage   Heavy social drinkers and alcoholics show evidence of brain damage. Men who have 100 or more drinks per month and women who have 80 or more drinks per month experience impairment of memory, processing speed, attention, and balance. Brain shrinkage has also been found among heavy drinkers; slight reduction in brain volume has been seen even in moderate drinkers, although it is unclear whether this indicates the death of nerve cells.

Mortality   As an ancient proverb states, "Those who worship Bacchus [the god of wine] die young." Excessive alcohol consumption is a factor in six of the ten leading causes of death for Americans. Average life expectancy among alcoholics is about 58 years; heavy drinkers may die in their 20s or 30s. About half the deaths caused by alcohol are due to chronic conditions such as cirrhosis and cancer; the other half are due to acute conditions or events such as car crashes, falls, and suicide. Because many deaths from acute conditions occur in youths and young adults, alcohol is responsible for 2.3 million years of potential life lost each year.

The Effects of Alcohol Use During Pregnancy

Alcohol ingested during pregnancy is harmful to the developing fetus. Alcohol and its metabolic product, acetaldehyde, readily cross the placenta. Damage to the fetus depends on the stage of pregnancy and the amount of alcohol consumed. Alcohol use in early pregnancy can cause a miscarriage. Moderate to heavy alcohol use can cause a collection of birth defects known as **fetal alcohol syndrome (FAS).** Children with FAS have a characteristic mixture of deformities that include a small head, abnormal facial structure, heart defects, and other physical abnormalities; most are mentally impaired, and their physical and mental growth is slower than normal.

FAS is a permanent, incurable condition that causes lifelong disability; it is by far the most common preventable cause of mental retardation in the Western world. Full-blown FAS occurs in 1 or 2 out of every 1000 live births in the United States. Many more babies are born with **alcohol-related neurodevelopmental disorder (ARND).** Children with ARND appear physically normal but often

A high level of alcohol consumption during pregnancy is associated with miscarriage, stillbirth, and a cluster of birth defects known as fetal alcohol syndrome. Total abstinence from alcohol during pregnancy is recommended.

have significant learning and behavioral disorders and are, as adults, more likely to develop substance-abuse problems and to have criminal records.

Heavy drinking early in pregnancy is responsible for most of the physical abnormalities associated with FAS. Binge drinking among women of childbearing age is thus of particular concern because women may drink heavily during the first few days and weeks of gestation before they become aware that they are pregnant. Fetal alcohol exposure later in pregnancy is more likely to cause brain damage without obvious external signs. Getting drunk just one time during the final 3 months of pregnancy, when brain cells are developing rapidly, can cause fetal brain damage.

No one is sure exactly how much alcohol use is required to cause FAS, but no amount of alcohol during pregnancy is considered safe. A 2002 study found that children born to mothers who drank as little as one-and-a-half drinks per week during their pregnancy weighed less and were shorter at age 14 than children of mothers who did not drink at all during pregnancy. This is one of the first studies to show a significant difference between the children of nondrinkers and those of light drinkers. The children in this study did not have FAS, but their smaller size may be a marker for subtle, persistent alcohol damage. The adverse effects of alcohol are especially pronounced when women drink early in pregnancy. For this reason, women who are trying to conceive or

who are sexually active without using effective contraception should abstain from alcohol in order to avoid inadvertently harming their fetus before they even know they are pregnant. Experts agree that the safest course of action is complete abstinence from alcohol during pregnancy. Despite this, about 10% of pregnant women do consume alcohol, and about 4% are binge drinkers. In 2005, the Surgeon General released an advisory to raise awareness about the dangers of drinking during pregnancy.

Any alcohol consumed by a nursing mother quickly enters the breast milk. What impact this has on the child or on the mother's milk production is a matter of controversy. Dosage may again be the key issue. However, many physicians advise nursing mothers to abstain from drinking alcohol because of the belief that any amount may have negative effects on the baby's brain development.

Possible Health Benefits of Alcohol

The relationship between alcohol use and health is complex and still under investigation. Numerous studies have shown that, on average, light to moderate drinkers live longer than either abstainers or heavy drinkers. Based on this and other research on the health benefits of alcohol, some have begun to think of alcohol—in particular, red wine—as the latest health drink. But although moderate alcohol consumption may provide some health benefits for a given individual, for many people the dangers of alcohol are much greater than the potential benefits.

A recent large-scale study found that the risks and benefits of drinking alcohol vary considerably with the age of the drinker. If you are 35 or younger, your odds of dying *increase* in direct proportion to the amount of alcohol you drink. Among people under age 35, even light drinkers have slightly higher mortality rates than nondrinkers. In other words, young adults who drink *any* amount of alcohol are more likely to die than nondrinkers of the same age. Alcohol consumption appears to confer health benefits primarily to older individuals, with the greatest benefits seen in people age 65 and older.

Moderate drinking may also benefit people who currently have or are at high risk for certain diseases such as

Terms

cardiac myopathy Weakening of the heart muscle through disease.

fetal alcohol syndrome (FAS) A characteristic group of birth defects caused by excessive alcohol consumption by the mother, including facial deformities, heart defects, and physical and mental impairments.

alcohol-related neurodevelopmental disorder (ARND) Cognitive and behavioral problems seen in people whose mothers drank alcohol during pregnancy.

coronary heart disease. Moderate drinking may improve heart health by raising blood levels of HDL (the beneficial form of cholesterol) and by reducing inflammation and the risk of dangerous blood clots, all of which can contribute to the risk of a heart attack. Individuals with heart disease or with strong risk factors should talk with their doctors about the possible health benefits of moderate drinking. Some evidence also suggests that moderate drinkers may be less likely to develop a variety of other conditions, including diabetes, strokes, arterial blockages in the legs, Alzheimer's disease, and benign prostate enlargement. Moderate wine consumption may also lower blood glucose levels, possibly reducing the risk of heart disease in some people.

Research is under way to determine whether the apparent health benefits of wine are due to the alcohol or to some other substance found in wine. Some experts believe that much of the apparent benefit of wine may merely reflect the fact that wine drinkers tend to be more affluent and to have healthier lifestyles than non–wine drinkers. (Much of the research on alcohol and health benefits has focused on wine, but moderate use of other forms of alcohol, such as beer, may have similar health benefits in some individuals.)

Moderate drinking is not without risk, however. It increases the risk of dying from unintentional injuries, violence, and certain types of cancer. In women, even moderate drinking may increase the risk of breast cancer; those who are at risk for breast cancer should discuss the potential risks and benefits of alcohol with their physician. There is also a risk that moderate drinking will not stay moderate. People who avoid alcohol because they or family members have had problems with dependence in the past should not start drinking for their health. People with conditions such as depression that are worsened by alcohol use should probably avoid even moderate drinking. Nor should drinkers use this information as an excuse to overindulge; any health benefits of alcohol are negated by heavy use. In addition, there are many situations in which consuming any amount of alcohol is unwise, including during pregnancy, while taking medication that may interact with alcohol, and when driving or engaging in another activity that requires attention, skill, or coordination. Sexually active women who are not consistently using effective contraception should also not drink.

The bottom line is that limited, regular consumption of alcohol may be beneficial for some adults, but there is a narrow window of benefit, and excessive drinking causes serious health problems. The *Dietary Guidelines for Americans* recommends that if you drink alcoholic beverages, you should do it in moderation, with meals, at times when consumption does not put you or others at risk. Moderate drinking means no more than one drink a day for women and two drinks a day for men.

ALCOHOL ABUSE AND DEPENDENCE

Abuse of and dependence on alcohol affect more than just the drinker. Friends, family members, coworkers, strangers that drinkers encounter on the road, and society as a whole pay the physical, emotional, and financial costs of the misuse of alcohol.

Alcohol Abuse

As explained in Chapter 9, the American Psychiatric Association's *Diagnostic and Statistical Manual of Mental Disorders* makes a distinction between substance abuse and substance dependence. **Alcohol abuse** is recurrent alcohol use that has negative consequences, such as drinking in dangerous situations (before driving, for instance), or drinking patterns that result in academic, professional, interpersonal, or legal difficulties. **Alcohol dependence,** or **alcoholism,** involves more extensive problems with alcohol use, usually involving physical tolerance and withdrawal. Alcoholism is discussed in greater detail later in the chapter.

Other authorities use different definitions to describe problems associated with drinking. The important point is that one does not have to be an alcoholic to have problems with alcohol. The person who drinks only once a month, perhaps after an exam, but then drives while intoxicated is an alcohol abuser.

How can you tell if you are beginning to abuse alcohol or if someone you know is doing so? Look for the following warning signs:

- Drinking alone or secretively
- Using alcohol deliberately and repeatedly to perform or get through difficult situations
- Feeling uncomfortable on certain occasions when alcohol is not available
- Escalating alcohol consumption beyond an already established drinking pattern
- Consuming alcohol heavily in risky situations, such as before driving
- Getting drunk regularly or more frequently than in the past
- Drinking in the morning or at other unusual times

Binge Drinking

A common form of alcohol abuse on college campuses is **binge drinking.** In surveys of students on over 100 college campuses, 44% reported binge drinking, defined as having five drinks in a row for men or four in a row for women on at least one occasion in the 2 weeks prior to the survey. Some 23% of all students were found to be frequent binge drinkers, defined as having at least three binges during the 2-week period. Students living at fraternity

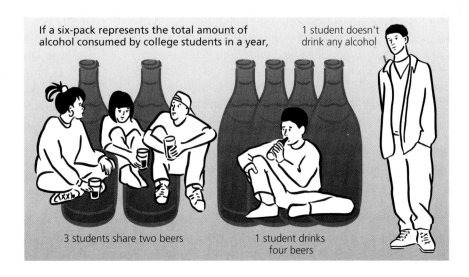

Figure 10-4 Alcohol consumption by college students. Alcohol consumption by students varies considerably, with some abstaining and some drinking large amounts. Only one in five college students is a frequent binge drinker, but this group accounts for nearly three-fourths of all the alcohol consumed by college students each year and causes or experiences the majority of alcohol-related problems. SOURCE: Wechsler, H., et al. 2000. *From Knowledge to Action: How Harvard's College Alcohol Study Can Help Your Campus Design a Campaign Against Student Alcohol Abuse* (http://www.hsph.harvard.edu/cas/test/articles/change2.html; retrieved July 17, 2000).

houses had the highest rate of binge drinking, up to 80%. Men were more likely to binge than women, and white students had higher rates of binge drinking than students of other ethnicities. Nineteen percent of students abstained from alcohol (Figure 10-4).

Binge drinking has a profound effect on students' lives. Frequent binge drinkers were found to be three to seven times more likely than non–binge drinkers to engage in unplanned or unprotected sex, to drive after drinking, and to get hurt or injured (Table 10-2). Binge drinkers were also more likely to miss classes, get behind in schoolwork,

and argue with friends. The more frequent the binges, the more problems the students encountered. Despite their experiences, fewer than 1% of the binge drinkers identified themselves as problem drinkers.

Binge drinking kills dozens of American college students each year. Some die from acute alcohol poisoning. The typical scenario involves a hazing ritual, a competition, or a bet that involves drinking a large amount of alcohol very quickly. This kind of fast, heavy drinking can result in unconsciousness and death very quickly, before anyone realizes that something is seriously wrong. Many other students die from alcohol-related injuries, including those from motor vehicle crashes.

Binge drinking also affects nonbingeing students. At schools with high rates of binge drinking, the nonbingers were up to twice as likely to report being bothered by the alcohol-related behaviors of others than were students at schools with lower rates of binge drinking. These problems included having sleep or studying disrupted; having to take care of a drunken student; being insulted or humiliated; experiencing unwanted sexual advances; and being pushed, hit, or assaulted.

The *Healthy People 2010* report sets the goal of reducing the rate of binge drinking to 20% among college students. Binge drinking is a difficult problem to address because many students arrive at college with drinking

VITAL STATISTICS

Table 10-2

The Effects of Binge Drinking on College Students

Alcohol-Related Problem	Percentage of Students Experiencing Problems	
	Non–Binge Drinkers	Frequent Binge Drinkers
Drove after drinking alcohol	18	58
Did something they regretted	17	62
Argued with friends	10	43
Engaged in unplanned sex	9	41
Missed a class	9	60
Got behind in schoolwork	9	42
Had unprotected sex	4	21
Got hurt or injured	4	28
Got into trouble with police	2	14
Had five or more of these problems since school year began	4	48

SOURCE: Wechsler, H., and B. Wuethrich. 2002. *Dying to Drink: Confronting Binge Drinking on College Campuses.* Emmaus, Pa.: Rodale.

Terms

alcohol abuse The use of alcohol to a degree that causes physical damage, impairs functioning, or results in behavior harmful to others.

alcohol dependence A pathological use of alcohol or impairment in functioning due to alcohol; characterized by tolerance and withdrawal symptoms; alcoholism.

alcoholism A chronic psychological disorder characterized by excessive and compulsive drinking.

binge drinking Periodically drinking alcohol to the point of severe intoxication.

patterns already established (binge drinking during high school is a strong predictor of binge drinking during college). The National Institutes of Health estimate that 3 million children between ages 14 and 17 are already problem drinkers. Many colleges have drinking cultures that perpetuate the pattern of binge drinking. On many campuses, drinking behavior that would be classified as abuse in another setting may be viewed as socially acceptable or even attractive, despite evidence that such behavior leads to automobile crashes, injuries, violence, suicide, and high-risk sexual behavior (see the box "College Binge Drinking").

Alcoholism

As mentioned earlier, alcoholism, or alcohol dependence, is usually characterized by tolerance to alcohol and withdrawal symptoms. Everyone who drinks—even nonalcoholics—develops tolerance after repeated alcohol use. As described in Chapter 9, *tolerance* means that a drinker needs more alcohol to achieve intoxication or the desired effect, that the effects of continued use of the same amount of alcohol are diminished, or that the drinker can function adequately at doses or a BAC that would produce significant impairment in a casual user. Heavy users of alcohol may need to consume about 50% more than they originally needed in order to experience the same degree of intoxication.

Withdrawal occurs when someone who has been using alcohol heavily for several days or more suddenly stops drinking or markedly reduces intake. Symptoms of withdrawal include trembling and nervousness and sometimes even **hallucinations** and seizures.

Patterns and Prevalence Alcoholism occurs among people of all ethnic groups and at all socioeconomic levels. The stereotype of the alcoholic skid-row bum actually accounts for fewer than 5% of all alcohol-dependent people and usually represents the final stage of a drinking career that began years earlier. There are different patterns of alcohol dependence, including these four common ones:

1. *Regular daily intake of large amounts.* This continuous pattern is the most common adult pattern of excessive consumption in most countries.

2. *Regular heavy drinking limited to weekends.* This pattern of binge drinking is often followed by teenagers and college students.

3. *Long periods of sobriety interspersed with binges of daily heavy drinking lasting for weeks or months.* This episodic, or bender, pattern is common in the United States but quite uncommon in France, although the per capita consumption of alcohol is higher in France.

4. *Heavy drinking limited to periods of stress.* This reactive pattern is associated with periods of anxiety or depression, such as at times of test anxiety or of other performance fears, interpersonal problems, or school or work pressures.

Once established, alcoholism often exhibits a pattern of exacerbations and remissions. The person may stop drinking and abstain from alcohol for days or months after a frightening problem develops. After a period of abstinence, an alcoholic often attempts controlled drinking, which almost inevitably leads to an escalation in drinking and more problems. Alcoholism is not hopeless, however; many alcoholics do achieve permanent abstinence.

According to the National Survey on Drug Use and Health, about 16.1 million Americans are heavy drinkers and 54 million are binge drinkers. Studies suggest that the lifetime risk of alcoholism in the United States is about 10% for men and about 3% for women. The risk for women has been increasing in recent years as women's roles in our society have expanded.

Health Effects Tolerance and withdrawal can have a serious impact on health. An alcoholic requires increasingly larger amounts to produce the desired effects, and these larger doses increase the chance of adverse physical effects. When alcoholics stop drinking or sharply decrease their intake, they experience withdrawal. Symptoms include trembling hands (shakes, or jitters), a rapid pulse and accelerated breathing rate, insomnia, nightmares, anxiety, and gastrointestinal upset. These symptoms usually begin 5–10 hours after alcohol intake is decreased and improve after 4–5 days. After a week, most people feel much better, but occasionally anxiety, insomnia, and other symptoms persist for 6 months or more.

More severe withdrawal symptoms occur in about 5% of alcoholics. These include seizures (sometimes called rum fits), confusion, and hallucinations. Still less common is **DTs (delirium tremens)**, a medical emergency characterized by severe disorientation, confusion, epileptic-like seizures, and vivid hallucinations, often of vermin and small animals. The mortality rate from DTs can be as high as 15%, especially in very debilitated people with preexisting medical illnesses.

Because alcohol is distributed throughout the body's organs and tissues, alcoholism takes a heavy physical and psychological toll. Alcoholics face all the physical health risks associated with intoxication and chronic drinking

Terms

V w

hallucination A false perception that does not correspond to external reality, such as seeing visions or hearing voices that are not there.

DTs (delirium tremens) A state of confusion brought on by the reduction of alcohol intake in an alcohol-dependent person; other symptoms are sweating, trembling, anxiety, hallucinations, and seizures.

In the News

College Binge Drinking

College binge drinking, a serious problem for more than 30 years, finally began receiving national attention in the past decade, due in part to alcohol-related tragedies. Highly publicized cases of deaths caused by alcohol overdose, alcohol-related injuries (including motor vehicle crashes) and violent crimes, student riots, and serious vandalism have all drawn attention to the epidemic of heavy drinking on college campuses.

An estimated 1700 college students age 18–24 die from alcohol-related injuries and alcohol overdoses each year. To many people, heavy drinking is considered a normal and integral part of college life. But research has shown that the pattern of excessive binge drinking common on many of today's college campuses has had a devastating impact on far too many students, as well as on their families and communities.

Much of the current data on college drinking comes from the ongoing Harvard School of Public Health College Alcohol Study, the first large-scale national study of college drinking habits. Since 1993, studies of college students across the United States have confirmed that nearly half (44%) of all college students binge-drink. The statistics have shocked many students, college administrators, and parents into demanding a change in our attitudes and policies regarding alcohol use on campus.

In response to this increased awareness of the college alcohol problem, the Task Force of the National Advisory Council on Alcohol Abuse and Alcoholism was formed. Its report documents the extent of the alcohol problem and is a call to action for colleges and their surrounding communities to reexamine their alcohol policies.

What are some of the facts about college drinking? A recent survey of 14,000 students at U.S. 4-year colleges found that 31% of college students meet the medical criteria for a diagnosis of alcohol abuse and 6% for a diagnosis of alcohol dependence. More students drink alcohol than use cigarettes, marijuana, or cocaine combined. Alcohol use and abuse are linked to many serious problems on campus; the annual toll includes the following:

- A total of 500,000 students between 18 and 24 are unintentionally injured in alcohol-related incidents (motor vehicle crashes, fights, falls, and so on).

- College students currently spend $5.5 billion a year on alcohol, more than they spend on textbooks, soft drinks, tea, milk, juice, and coffee combined.

- More than 600,000 students are assaulted by another student who has been drinking.

- More than 70,000 students are victims of alcohol-related sexual assault, including date rape. Nearly 75% of female rape victims were raped while intoxicated.

- Hundreds of thousands of students engage in unsafe sex while intoxicated, resulting in dramatically increased risk for STDs and unwanted pregnancy.

- As many as 2.1 million students drive while under the influence of alcohol.

- About 1.2–1.5% of college students attempt suicide because of drinking or drug use.

- Among students who live on campus and don't binge-drink, 61% say that drinkers have disrupted their study or sleep time, 50% say they have had to take care of a drunken student, and 29% say they have been insulted or humiliated by a drunken student.

Heavy alcohol use detracts from the college experience of drinkers and non-drinkers alike. The National Advisory Council Task Force calls for an overhaul of the campus drinking culture. Unfortunately, drinking to excess has been a college tradition for decades. Changing long-entrenched campus drinking habits will require effort on the part of students, college administrators, parents, and communities alike. According to the Task Force, changes must occur on three levels:

1. Ultimately, *individual students* must take responsibility for their own behavior. Motivating and encouraging students to develop a new, healthier relationship to alcohol is the focus of this part of the Task Force's recommendation. Students who enter college as nonbingers should be supported, and treatment should be readily available to problem drinkers. Groups at special risk for increasing or established problem drinking behavior include first-year students, Greek organization members and athletes.

2. The *student body as a whole* must work to discourage alcohol abuse. This effort might include promoting alcohol-free activities for students, reducing the availability of alcohol, and avoiding the social and commercial promotion of alcohol on campus. Fraternities and sororities must be involved in these changes, as the most serious binge drinking tends to occur among their members. Currently, 80% of fraternity members and 69% of sorority members are binge drinkers. The Greek system must substitute genuine camaraderie for alcohol-saturated events.

3. *Colleges and surrounding communities* must cooperate to discourage excessive drinking. College administrators, law enforcement, bar and liquor store owners, residents who live near the campus, and the court system all must work together to reduce the availability of cheap alcohol. Laws that prohibit excessive and underage drinking must be fairly enforced. Students who commit crimes while under the influence must receive appropriate punishment, including restitution to any victims. College administrators must find other funding sources to replace the financial support that currently flows in from the alcohol industry in exchange for advertising and promotion of their products on college campuses.

Excessive binge drinking undermines the quality of colleges. Solutions to the problem of alcohol overuse are complex, but change is possible. Individual students can find out about the alcohol problems on their campus and work together with their college administrators and the community to find solutions. Colleges can say no to the alcohol industry when it comes to alcohol promotion on campus, even if it means a loss of substantial revenue. Working together, students, faculty, administrators, parents, and the community can put an end to the destructive culture of heavy drinking on college campuses.

SOURCES: Harvard College Alcohol Study. 2005. *Binge Drinking on Campus Lower in States with Fewer Adult Binge Drinkers and Stronger Alcohol Control Laws* (http://www.hsph.harvard.edu/cas/Documents/state/state_pr.html; retrieved March 14, 2005). Hingson, R., et al. 2005. Magnitude of alcohol-related mortality and morbidity among U.S. college students ages 18–24. Annual Review of Public Health 26: 259–279. Mohler-Kuo, M., et al. 2004. Correlates of rape while intoxicated in a national sample of college women. *Journal of Studies on Alcohol* 65(1): 37–45; Wechsler, H., and B. Wuethrich. 2002. *Dying to Drink: Confronting Binge Drinking on College Campuses.* Emmaus, Pa.: Rodale; National Institute on Alcohol Abuse and Alcoholism. 2002. *A Call to Action: Changing the Culture of Drinking at U.S. Colleges* (http://www.collegedrinkingprevention.gov/Reports/TaskForce/TaskForce_TOC.aspx; retrieved October 10, 2002).

In Focus — Children of Alcoholics

About one out of eight Americans grows up in an alcoholic household. For these children, life is a struggle to deal with constant stress, anxiety, and embarrassment. They may be victims of violence, abuse, or neglect in the home. Family life centers on the drinking parent, and children's needs are often ignored.

Children in alcoholic households often cope by learning patterns of interaction that help them survive childhood but that don't support their own healthy development. Many adult children of alcoholics fear losing control, and they try to control their own feelings and behavior and those of people around them. They may fear emotions, even pleasant feelings such as happiness and joy. They avoid conflict and are easily upset by criticism from authority figures. Other common traits include an overdeveloped sense of responsibility and hypersensitivity to the needs of others. Children of alcoholics often feel guilty if they stand up for themselves and acknowledge their own needs. All these characteristics can be stumbling blocks to forming healthy relationships.

Children of alcoholics are more likely than other children to become alcoholic themselves and to marry alcoholics. An estimated 13–25% of children of alcoholics will become alcoholic at some point in their lives. They are more likely to abuse other drugs and develop an eating disorder. They are also particularly prone to stress-related medical illnesses.

If you are the child of an alcoholic, be aware, first, that you are not alone. Millions of people have been through the same problem and have dreamed of having a happy family life in which drinking is not an issue. Realize, too, that other people can understand what you have been through and can help. Find a person you can trust, and confide in her or him. It may seem safer to keep your feelings secret, but talking about the problem is the first step toward a healthy readjustment. Many adult children of alcoholics benefit greatly from therapy with a counselor who is experienced in treating people who have been affected by an alcoholic family. Individual or group therapy can be a critical step in recovery. (The For More Information section at the end of this chapter lists agencies that can provide help and referrals.)

Finally, acknowledge that your parent's alcoholism is not your fault. Many children of alcoholics carry a burden of guilt from early childhood, when they could not understand that they weren't the cause of their parent's behavior. This unexamined assumption is often part of the emotional pain experienced by children of alcoholics.

---

described earlier in the chapter. Some of the damage is compounded by nutritional deficiencies that often accompany alcoholism. A mental problem associated with alcohol use is profound memory gaps (commonly known as blackouts), which are sometimes filled by conscious or unconscious lying.

The specific health effects of alcoholism tend to vary from person to person. For example, one individual may suffer from problems with memory and CNS defects and have no liver or gastrointestinal problems. Another person with a similar drinking and nutritional history may have advanced liver disease but no memory gaps.

Social and Psychological Effects   Alcohol use causes more serious social and psychological problems than all other forms of drug abuse combined. For every person who is an alcoholic, another three or four people are directly affected (see the box "Children of Alcoholics"). In a 2004 Gallup poll, about a third of Americans reported that alcohol had been a source of trouble in their family.

Alcoholics frequently suffer from mental disorders in addition to their substance dependence. Alcoholics are much more likely than nonalcoholics to suffer from clinical depression, panic disorder, schizophrenia, and antisocial personality disorders. People with anxiety or panic attacks may try to use alcohol to lessen their anxiety, even though alcohol often makes these disorders worse. Alcoholics also often have other substance-abuse problems.

An estimated 3 million Americans age 14–17 show signs of potential alcohol dependence. These numbers are far greater than those associated with cocaine, heroin, or marijuana use. The social and psychological consequences of excessive drinking in young people are more difficult to measure than the risks to physical health. One consequence is that excessive drinking interferes with learning the interpersonal and job-related skills required for adult life. Excessive drinkers sometimes narrow their circle of friends to other heavy drinkers and thus limit the range of people they can learn from. Perhaps most important is that people who were excessive drinkers in college are more likely to have social, occupational, and health problems 20 years later. Despite media attention on cocaine and other drugs, alcohol abuse remains our society's number-one drug-abuse problem.

Causes of Alcoholism   The precise causes of alcoholism are unknown, but many factors are probably involved. Studies of twins and adopted children clearly demonstrate the importance of genetics. If one of a pair of fraternal twins is alcoholic, then the other has about twice the chance of becoming alcoholic. For the identical twin of an alcoholic, the risk of alcoholism is about four times that of the general population. These risks persist even when the twins have little contact with each other or their biological parents. Similarly, adoption studies show an increased risk among children of alcoholics, even if they were adopted at birth into nondrinking families. Alcoholism in adoptive parents, contrarily, doesn't make individuals more or less likely to become alcoholic. Some studies suggest that as much as 50–60% of a person's risk for alcoholism is determined by genetic factors. Many genes are thought to be involved in shaping the risk for alcoholism.

Not all children of alcoholics become alcoholic, however, and it is clear that other factors are involved. A person's risk of developing alcoholism may be increased by certain personality disorders, having grown up in a violent or otherwise troubled household, and imitating the alcohol abuse of peers and other role models. People who begin drinking excessively in their teens are especially prone to binge drinking and alcoholism later in life. Common psychological features of individuals who abuse alcohol are denial ("I don't have a problem") and rationalization ("I drink because I need to socialize with my customers"). Certain social factors have also been linked with alcoholism, including urbanization, disappearance of the extended family, a general loosening of kinship ties, increased mobility, and changing values.

Treatment   Some alcoholics recover without professional help. How often this occurs is unknown, but possibly as many as one third stop drinking on their own or reduce their drinking enough to eliminate problems. Often these spontaneous recoveries are linked to an alcohol-related crisis, such as a health problem or the threat of being fired. Not all alcoholics must hit bottom before they are motivated to stop. People vary markedly in what induces them to change their behavior. For some, the first blackout or alcohol-related automobile crash fosters abstinence.

Most alcoholics, however, require a treatment program of some kind in order to stop drinking. Many different kinds of programs exist. No single treatment works for everyone, so a person may have to try different programs before finding the right one. Over 1 million Americans enter treatment for alcoholism every year.

Although treatment is not successful for all alcoholics, considerable optimism has replaced the older view that nothing could be done. Many alcoholics have patterns of drinking that fluctuate widely over time. These fluctuations indicate that their alcohol abuse is a response to environmental factors, such as life stressors or social pressures, and therefore may be influenced by treatment.

One of the oldest and best-known recovery programs is Alcoholics Anonymous (AA). AA consists of self-help groups that meet several times each week in most communities and follow a 12-step program. Important steps for people in these programs include recognizing that they are "powerless over alcohol" and must seek help from a "higher power" in order to regain control of their lives. By verbalizing these steps, the alcoholic directly addresses the denial that is often prominent in alcoholism and other addictions. Many AA members have a sponsor of their choosing who is available by phone 24 hours a day for individual support and crisis intervention. AA convincingly shows the alcoholic that abstinence can be achieved and also provides a sober peer group of people who share the same identity—that of recovering alcoholics.

Alcoholics Anonymous is generally recognized as an effective mutual help program, but not everyone responds to its style and message, and other recovery approaches are available. Some, like Rational Recovery and Women for Sobriety, deliberately avoid any emphasis on higher spiritual powers. Even people who are helped by AA often find that it works best in combination with counseling and medical care. A more controversial approach to problem drinking is offered by the group Moderation Management, which encourages people to manage their drinking behavior by limiting intake or abstaining.

Al-Anon is a companion program to AA that consists of groups for families and friends of alcoholics. In Al-Anon, spouses and others explore how they enabled the alcoholic to drink by denying, rationalizing, or covering up his or her drinking and how they can change this codependent behavior.

Employee assistance programs and school-based programs represent another approach to alcoholism treatment that works for some people. One of the advantages of these programs is that they can deal directly with work and campus issues, often important sources of stress for the alcohol abuser. These programs sometimes encourage learning effective coping responses for internal and external sources of distress. Individuals might also benefit from learning new cognitive concepts, such as a self-identity that does not involve drinking.

Inpatient hospital rehabilitation is useful for some alcoholics, especially if they have serious medical or mental problems or if life stressors threaten to overwhelm them. When the person returns to the community, however, it is critical that there be some form of active, continuing, long-term treatment. Patients who return to a spouse or family often require ongoing treatment on issues involving those significant others, such as establishing new routines and planning shared recreational activities that do not involve drinking.

There are also some pharmacological treatments for alcoholism:

- *Disulfiram* (Antabuse) inhibits the metabolic breakdown of acetaldehyde and causes patients to flush and feel ill when they drink, thus theoretically inhibiting impulse drinking. However, it is potentially dangerous if the user does also drink, and it works best combined with ongoing therapy.

- *Naltrexone* reduces the craving for alcohol and decreases the pleasant, reinforcing effects of alcohol without making the user ill. It also works most effectively in combination with counseling and other forms of psychosocial treatment.

- *Acamprosate* (Campral), approved by the FDA in 2004, helps people maintain alcohol abstinence after they have stopped drinking. It is unclear precisely how it works, but it appears to act on the brain pathways related to alcohol abuse.

Research is currently under way on other medications, including baclofen and gabapentin.

In people who abuse alcohol and have significant depression or anxiety, the use of antidepressant or anti-anxiety medication can improve both mental health and drinking behavior. In addition, drugs such as diazepam (Valium) are sometimes prescribed to replace alcohol during initial stages of withdrawal. Such chemical substitutes are usually useful for only a week or so, because alcoholics are at particularly high risk for developing dependence on other drugs. Counseling and peer-group support are generally the most essential elements of alcoholism treatment.

Alcohol-treatment programs are successful in achieving an extended period of sobriety for about half of those who participate. Success rates of conventional treatment programs are about the same for men and women and for people from different ethnic groups. Women, minorities, and the poor often face major economic and social barriers to receiving treatment. Most inpatient treatment programs are financially out of reach for people of low income or those without insurance coverage. AA remains the mainstay of treatment for most people and is often a component of even the most expensive treatment programs. Special AA groups exist in many communities for young people, women, gay men and lesbians, non–English speakers, and a variety of interest groups. You can find out about AA meetings in your community by looking in the phone book or consulting the For More Information section at the end of the chapter.

Gender and Ethnic Differences

Alcohol abusers come from all socioeconomic levels and cultural groups, but there are notable differences in patterns of drinking between men and women and among different ethnic groups (Table 10-3).

Men Among white American men, excessive drinking often begins in the teens or twenties and progresses gradually through the thirties until the individual is clearly identifiable as an alcoholic by the time he is in his late thirties or early forties. Other men remain controlled

W**W** VITAL STATISTICS

Table 10-3 — Prevalence of Alcohol Abuse and Dependence

	Past Year Prevalence (Percentage)	
	Alcohol Abuse	Alcohol Dependence
Gender		
Men	6.9	5.4
Women	2.6	2.3
Ethnicity		
White	5.1	3.8
African American	3.3	3.6
American Indians and Alaska Natives	5.8	6.4
Asian Americans and Pacific Islander Americans	2.1	2.4
Latinos	4.0	4.0
Total population	**4.7**	**3.8**

SOURCE: Grant, B., et al. 2004. The 12-month prevalence and trends in DSM-IV alcohol abuse and dependence: United States, 1991–1992 and 2001–2002. *Drug and Alcohol Dependence* 74(3): 223–234.

drinkers until later in life, sometimes becoming alcoholic in association with retirement, the inevitable losses of aging, boredom, illness, or psychological disorders. (See the box "Gender and Alcohol Use and Abuse.")

Women The progression of alcoholism in women is usually different. Women tend to become alcoholic at a later age and with fewer years of heavy drinking. It is not unusual for women in their forties or fifties to become alcoholic after years of controlled drinking. Women alcoholics develop cirrhosis and other medical complications somewhat more often than men. Women alcoholics may have more medical problems because they are less likely to seek early treatment. In addition, there may be an inherently greater biological risk for women who drink.

African Americans Alcohol abuse is a serious problem for African Americans. Although as a group they use less alcohol than most other groups (including whites), they face disproportionately high levels of alcohol-related birth defects, cirrhosis, cancer, hypertension, and other medical problems. In addition, blacks are more likely than members of other ethnic groups to be victims of alcohol-related homicides, criminal assaults, and injuries. African American women are more likely to abstain from

Men are more likely than women to drink alcohol, to abuse alcohol, and to have alcohol dependency. Men account for the majority of alcohol-related deaths and injuries in the United States, the greater proportion occurring in men age 35 and younger. Most alcohol-related deaths and injuries among men result from acute conditions related to intoxication, such as motor vehicle crashes, falls, drowning, suicide, and homicide.

A variety of factors contributes to the higher rates of alcohol use and abuse among men. Traditional or stereotypic gender roles and ideas regarding masculinity and drinking behavior may promote excessive alcohol consumption among men. Young men in particular are also more likely to engage in all types of risky health behaviors. Men drive more miles, drive more dangerously, and are more likely to drive while intoxicated. They tend to have greater access to firearms, contributing to their increased rates of suicide and homicide. Men may also be more likely than

women to use alcohol to cope with stress and other life challenges.

Women are not immune to alcohol problems, however, and rates of alcohol abuse and dependence among women have increased in the past decade. Whether a woman is a "social drinker," a binge drinker, or a heavy daily user, the impact of alcohol on her will be different from and generally greater than the impact of comparable use on a man. And because of the social stigma attached to problem drinking, particularly among women, women are less likely to seek early treatment.

Women become intoxicated at lower doses of alcohol than men, and they tend to experience the adverse physical effects of chronic drinking sooner and at lower levels of alcohol consumption than men. Female alcoholics have higher death rates than male alcoholics, including death rates from cirrhosis. They develop alcohol liver disease and alcohol-related brain damage after a comparatively shorter period of heavy drinking and a lower level of drinking than

men. Some alcohol-related health problems are unique to women, including an increased risk of breast cancer, menstrual disorders, infertility, and, in pregnant women, giving birth to a child with FAS.

Women from all walks of life and all ethnic groups can develop alcohol problems, but those who have never married or are divorced are more likely to drink heavily than married or widowed women. Women who have multiple life roles, such as parent, worker, and spouse, are less vulnerable to alcohol problems than women who have fewer roles.

Both men and women are likely to be the perpetrator or victim of a crime when they have been drinking. Sexual assaults of all types, and date rape in particular, are more likely to occur when people are intoxicated. Alcohol use also makes men and women much less likely to practice safer sex, leaving them vulnerable to significant and lasting health problems as the result of sexually transmitted diseases and, for women, to unintended pregnancy.

alcohol use than white women, but among black women who drink there is a higher percentage of heavy drinkers. Urban black males commonly start drinking excessively and develop serious neurological illnesses at an earlier age than urban white males. They also have a higher rate of alcoholism-related suicide.

AA groups of predominantly African Americans have been shown to provide effective treatment, perhaps because essential elements of AA—sharing common experiences, mutual acceptance of one another as human beings, and trusting a higher power—are already a part of African American culture. Treatment efforts that use the extended family and include occupational training are also especially effective.

Latinos Drinking patterns among Latinos vary significantly, depending on their specific cultural background and how long they and their families have lived in the United States. Drunk driving and cirrhosis are the most common causes of alcohol-related death and injury among Hispanic men. Hispanic women are more likely to abstain from alcohol than white or black women, but those who do drink are at special risk for problems. Treating the entire family as a unit is an important part of treatment because family pride, solidarity, and support are important aspects of Latino culture. Some Hispanics do better during treatment

if treatment efforts are integrated with the techniques of *curanderos* (folk healers) and *espiritistas* (spiritists).

Asian Americans As a group, Asian Americans have lower-than-average rates of alcohol abuse. However, acculturation may somewhat weaken the generally strong Asian taboos and community sanctions against alcohol use. For many Asian Americans, though, the genetically based physiological aversion to alcohol remains a deterrent to abuse. For those needing treatment, ethnic agencies, health care professionals, and ministers seem to be the most effective sources.

American Indians and Alaska Natives Alcohol abuse is one of the most widespread and severe health problems among American Indians and Alaska Natives, especially for adolescents and young adults. Excessive drinking varies from tribe to tribe but is generally high in both men and women. The rate of alcoholism among American Indians is twice that of the general population, and the death rate from alcohol-related causes is about eight times higher. Treatment may be more effective if it reflects tribal values. Some healers have incorporated aspects of American Indian religions into the therapeutic process, using traditional sweat houses, prayers, and dances.

Helping Someone with an Alcohol Problem

Helping a friend or relative with an alcohol problem requires skill and tact. One of the first steps is making sure you are not an enabler or codependent, perhaps unknowingly allowing someone to continue excessively using alcohol. Enabling takes many forms. One of the most common is making excuses or covering up for the alcohol abuser—for example, saying "he has the flu" when it is really a hangover. Whenever you find yourself minimizing or lying about someone's drinking behavior, a warning bell should sound. Another important step is open, honest labeling—"I think you have a problem with alcohol." Such explicit statements usually elicit emotional rebuttals and may endanger a relationship. In the long run, however, you are not helping your friends by allowing them to deny their problems with alcohol or other drugs. Taking action shows that you care.

Even when problems are acknowledged, there is usually reluctance to get help. You can't cure a friend's drinking problem, but you can guide him or her to appropriate help. Your best role might be to obtain information about the available resources and persistently encourage their use. Consider making an appointment for your friend at the student health center and then go with him or her to the appointment. Most student health centers will be able to recommend local options for self-help groups and formal treatment; the counseling center is another excellent source for help. You can also check the phone book and the Internet for local chapters of AA and other groups (see For More Information at the end of the chapter). And don't underestimate the power of families to help. An honest phone call to your friend's parents could save a life if your friend is in serious trouble with alcohol.

DRINKING BEHAVIOR AND RESPONSIBILITY

The responsible use of alcohol means drinking in such a way that you keep your BAC low, so that your behavior is always under your control. In addition to controlling your own drinking, there are things you can do to promote responsible alcohol use in others.

Examine Your Attitudes About Alcohol Use

Think about how you really feel about drinking. Is it of little consequence to you or perhaps even an intrusion into your college experience? Or is alcohol the key ingredient for any and all fun activities? Can you imagine having a good time at a party or at the beach without alcoholic beverages? How do you perceive nondrinkers at a party where others are drinking? Do they seem mature or odd? What do your answers to these questions say about your attitude about alcohol and the role of alcohol in your life?

Attitudes toward drinking are usually based on a multitude of experiences, including your family background. Consider how alcohol was used in your family when you were growing up. Was it used for family celebrations? Was alcohol a big deal in your family, or was it treated as a relatively unimportant occasional addition to dinner? Was alcohol a source of problems, with a parent or relative becoming dependent on alcohol and/or abusive when drunk? Do you think that alcohol problems run in your family? Understanding the source of some of your beliefs and feelings about alcohol may give you insight into your current drinking habits as well as your feelings about other people's use of alcohol.

Also examine your ideas about alcohol use on your college campus. Does it seem to you as if everyone at your college drinks? Do you feel pressure to drink or use illegal drugs, even if you don't really feel like it? Who pressures you? Why do you think some people push others to engage in heavy drinking? A recent survey of college students found that over half felt pressured to use alcohol or illegal drugs and that this pressure hampered their schoolwork. Even though it may seem that everyone drinks, about one in five college students is a nondrinker, with a higher percentage of abstainers at many schools. Remember that the majority of American adults drink moderately or not at all. Frequent binge drinking is far outside the norm in the adult world.

Examine Your Drinking Behavior

When you want to drink responsibly, it's helpful to know, first of all, why you drink. The following are common reasons given by college students:

- "It lets me go along with my friends."
- "It makes me less self-conscious and more social."
- "It makes me less inhibited in thinking, saying, or doing certain things."
- "It relieves depression, anxiety, tension, or worries."
- "It enables me to experience a different state of consciousness."

If you drink alcohol, what are your reasons for doing so? Are you attempting to meet underlying needs that could best be addressed by other means?

After examining your reasons for drinking, take a closer look at your drinking behavior. Is it moderate and responsible? Or do you frequently overindulge and suffer negative consequences? The Behavior Change Strategy at the end of the chapter explains how to keep and analyze

Do You Have a Problem with Alcohol?

For each question, choose the answer that best describes your behavior. Then total your scores.

Questions	Points					Your Score
	0	1	2	3	4	
1. How often do you have a drink containing alcohol?	Never	Monthly or less	2–4 times a month	2–3 times a week	4 or more times a week	_____
2. How many drinks containing alcohol do you have on a typical day when you are drinking?	1 or 2	3 or 4	5 or 6	7–9	10 or more	
3. How often do you have 6 or more drinks on one occasion?	Never	Less than monthly	Monthly	Weekly	Daily or almost daily	_____
4. How often during the past year have you found that you were not able to stop drinking once you had started?	Never	Less than monthly	Monthly	Weekly	Daily or almost daily	_____
5. How often during the past year have you failed to do what was normally expected because of drinking?	Never	Less than monthly	Monthly	Weekly	Daily or almost daily	_____
6. How often during the past year have you needed a first drink in the morning to get yourself going after a heavy drinking session?	Never	Less than monthly	Monthly	Weekly	Daily or almost daily	_____
7. How often during the past year have you had a feeling of guilt or remorse after drinking?	Never	Less than monthly	Monthly	Weekly	Daily or almost daily	_____
8. How often during the past year have you been unable to remember what happened the night before because you had been drinking?	Never	Less than monthly	Monthly	Weekly	Daily or almost daily	_____
9. Have you or someone else been injured as a result of your drinking?	No	Yes, but not in the past year (2 points)		Yes, during the past year (4 points)		_____
10. Has a relative, friend, doctor, or other health worker been concerned about your drinking or suggested you cut down?	No	Yes, but not in the past year (2 points)		Yes, during the past year (4 points)		_____

Total _____

A total score of 8 or more indicates a strong likelihood of hazardous or harmful alcohol consumption. Even if you score below 8, if you are encountering drinking-related problems with your academic performance, job, relationships, health, or the law, you should consider seeking help. The effects of alcohol abuse can be extremely serious—even fatal—both to you and to others.

SOURCE: Sanders, J. B., et al. 1993. Development of the Alcohol Use Disorders Identification Test (AUDIT): WHO collaborative project on early detection of persons with harmful alcohol consumption—II. *Addiction* 88: 791–804. Reprinted with permission from Carfax Publishing, a division of Taylor & Francis Ltd. (http://www.tandf.co.uk).

a record of your drinking. The CAGE screening test can help you determine whether you, or someone close to you, may have a drinking problem. Answer yes or no to the following questions:

Have you ever felt you should
Cut down on your drinking?
Have people
Annoyed you by criticizing your drinking?
Have you ever felt bad or
Guilty about your drinking?

Have you ever had an
Eye-opener (a drink first thing in the morning to steady your nerves or get rid of a hangover)?

One "yes" response suggests a possible alcohol problem; if you answered yes to more than one question, it is highly likely that a problem exists. For a more detailed evaluation of your drinking habits, complete the questionnaire in the box "Do You Have a Problem with Alcohol?" If the results of either assessment test indicate a potential problem, get help right away.

People who choose to drink should do so responsibly—in moderation and when doing so does not put themselves or others in danger. By choosing a designated driver, these men help ensure a safe trip home.

Drink Moderately and Responsibly

Sometimes people lose control when they misjudge how much they can drink. At other times, they set out deliberately to get drunk. Following are some strategies for keeping your drinking and your behavior under control.

Drink Slowly Learn to sip your drinks rather than gulp them. Do not drink alcoholic beverages to quench your thirst. Avoid drinks made with carbonated mixers, especially if you're thirsty; you'll be more likely to gulp them down.

Space Your Drinks Learn to drink nonalcoholic drinks at parties, or alternate them with alcoholic drinks. Learn to refuse a round: "I've had enough for right now." Parties are easier for some people if they hold a glass of something nonalcoholic that has ice and a twist of lime floating in it so it looks like an alcoholic drink.

Eat Before and While Drinking Avoid drinking on an empty stomach. Food in your stomach will not prevent the alcohol from eventually being absorbed, but it will slow down the rate somewhat and thus often lower the peak BAC. In restaurants, order your food before you order a drink. Try to have something to eat before you go out to a party where alcohol will be served.

Know Your Limits and Your Drinks Learn how different BACs affect you. In a safe setting such as your home, with your roommate or a friend, see how a set amount—say, two drinks in an hour—affects you. A good test is walking heel to toe in a straight line with your eyes closed or standing with your feet crossed and trying to touch your finger to your nose with your eyes closed.

But be aware that in different settings your performance, and especially your ability to judge your behavior, may change. At a given BAC, you will perform less well when surrounded by activity and boisterous companions than you will in a quiet test setting with just one or two other people. This impairment results partially because alcohol reduces your ability to perform when your brain is bombarded by multiple stimuli. It is useful to discover the rate at which you can drink without increasing your BAC. Be able to calculate the approximate amount a given drink increases your BAC.

Promote Responsible Drinking in Others

Although you cannot completely control the drinking behavior of others, there are things you can do to help promote responsible drinking.

Encourage Responsible Attitudes Our society teaches us attitudes toward drinking that contribute to alcohol-related problems. Many of us have difficulty expressing disapproval about someone who has drunk too much, and we are amused by the antics of a funny drunk. We accept the alcohol industry's linkage of drinking with virility or sexuality (see the box "Alcohol Advertising"). And many people treat nondrinkers as nonconformists in social settings. Recognize that the choice to abstain is neither odd nor unusual. More than one-third of adults do not drink at all or drink very infrequently. Most adults are capable of enjoying their leisure time without alcohol or drugs. In hazardous situations,

Alcohol Advertising

To be a careful and informed health consumer, you need to consider the effects that advertisements have on you. Are alcohol ads, such as those featuring young musicians, talking frogs, or football games between beer bottles, harmless fun? Or can they have more serious effects? How do such ads affect you?

Alcohol manufacturers spend $6 billion every year on advertising and promotions. They claim that the purpose of their advertising is to persuade adults who already drink to choose a certain brand. But in reality, ads cleverly engage young people and children—never overtly suggesting that young people should drink, but clearly linking alcohol and good times.

Alcohol ads are common during televised sporting events and other shows popular with teenagers. By age 18, the average American teen will have seen 100,000 TV beer commercials, and teens are more likely than adults to see alcohol ads in their favorite magazines. Studies show that the more TV adolescents watch, the more likely they are to take up drinking in their teens. New alcoholic drinks geared to the tastes of young people are heavily promoted. "Hard lemonade" and other fruity or sweetened drinks ("alcopops" or "low-alcohol refreshers") have been described by teens as a way to get drunk without suffering the bitter taste of most alcoholic beverages. Though only recently introduced, these drinks have been tried by almost half of 14–18-year-olds.

Alcohol manufacturers also reach out to young people at youth-oriented activities like concerts and sporting events.

Product logos are heavily marketed through sales of T-shirts, hats, and other items. Many colleges allow alcohol manufacturers to advertise at campus events in exchange for sponsorship.

What is the message of all these advertisements? Think about the alcohol ads you've seen. Many give the impression that drinking alcohol is a normal part of everyday life and good times. This message seems to work well on the young, many of whom believe that heavy-duty drinking at parties is normal and fun. The use of famous musicians, athletes, or actors in commercials increases the appeal of alcohol by associating it with fame, wealth, sex, and popularity. The "Whassup?!" Bud ads feature the humorous use of guy talk to portray beer drinking as a supposedly critical aspect of men's relationships.

What ads don't show is the darker side of drinking. You never see hangovers, car crashes, slipping grades, or violence. Although some ads include a brief message such as "know when to say when," the impact of such cautions is small compared to that of the image of happy, attractive young people having fun while drinking.

The next time you see an advertisement for alcohol, take a critical look. What is the message of the ad? What audience is being targeted, and what is the ad implying about alcohol use? Be aware of its effect on you.

---

such as driving or operating machinery, abstinence is the only appropriate choice.

Be a Responsible Host   When you are the host, serve nonalcoholic beverages as well as alcohol. Popular nonalcoholic choices include soft drinks, sparkling water, fruit juice, and alcohol-free wine, beer, and mixers. Serve only enough alcohol for each guest to have a moderate number of drinks. Don't put out large kegs of beer, as these invite people to overindulge. For parties hosted by a dorm, fraternity, or other campus group, don't allow guests to have unlimited drinks for a single admission fee, as this also encourages binge drinking.

Always serve food along with alcohol, and stop serving alcohol an hour or more before people will leave. If possible, arrange carpools with designated nondrinking drivers in advance. Remind your guests who are under 21 about the new zero-tolerance laws in many states—even a single drink can result in an illegal BAC. Insist that guests who drink too much take a taxi, ride with someone else, or stay overnight rather than drive.

Plan social functions with no alcohol at all. Outdoor parties, hikes, and practically every other type of social occasion can be enjoyable without alcohol. If that doesn't seem possible to you, then examine your drink-

ing patterns and attitudes toward alcohol. If you can't have fun without drinking, you may have a problem with alcohol.

Hold the Drinker Responsible   The individual who consumes alcohol must take full responsibility for his or her behavior. Pardoning unacceptable behavior fosters the attitude that the behavior is caused by the drug. The drinker is thereby excused from responsibility and learns to expect minimal adverse consequences for his or her behavior. The opposite approach—holding the individual fully accountable for his or her behavior—is a more effective policy. For example, alcohol-impaired drivers who receive legal penalties have fewer subsequent rearrests than those who receive only mandatory treatment. Restrictions on public smoking gained momentum after nonsmokers learned about the dangers that environmental tobacco smoke posed to them. Other people's drunkenness can impinge on your living or study environment. Speak up against this behavior—and insist on your rights.

Learn About Prevention Programs   What alternatives are being developed on your campus or in your community to keg parties and other events where heavy drinking occurs? Does your campus have dormitories, fraternities, or sororities where members agree to abstain from alcohol or drug use? Are programs available for students who are at high risk for alcohol abuse, such as those whose parents abused alcohol? Are counseling or self-help programs like AA available?

Take Community Action Consider joining an action group such as Students Against Destructive Decisions (SADD). The goal of SADD is to address the issues of drinking, impaired driving, drug use, and other destructive decisions and killers of young people. Lesson plans, peer counseling, and the promotion of better communication between students and parents are all used to help protect students from the dangers of drinking, drug use, and impaired driving.

SUMMARY

- Although alcohol has been a part of human celebrations for a long time, it is a psychoactive drug capable of causing addiction.

- After being absorbed into the bloodstream in the stomach and small intestine, alcohol is transported throughout the body. The liver metabolizes alcohol as blood circulates through it.

- If people drink more alcohol each hour than the body can metabolize, blood alcohol concentration (BAC) increases. The rate of alcohol metabolism depends on a variety of individual factors.

- Alcohol is a CNS depressant. At low doses, it tends to make people feel relaxed.

- At higher doses, alcohol interferes with motor and mental functioning; at very high doses, alcohol poisoning, coma, and death can occur. Effects may be increased if alcohol is combined with other drugs.

- Alcohol use increases the risk of injury and violence; drinking before driving is particularly dangerous, even at low doses.

- Continued alcohol use has negative effects on the digestive and cardiovascular systems and increases cancer risk and overall mortality.

- Pregnant women who drink risk giving birth to children with a cluster of birth defects known as fetal alcohol syndrome (FAS). Even occasional drinking during pregnancy can cause brain injury in the fetus.

- Moderate drinking may decrease the risk of coronary heart disease in some people.

- Alcohol abuse involves drinking in dangerous situations or drinking to a degree that causes academic, professional, interpersonal, or legal difficulties.

- Alcohol dependence, or alcoholism, is characterized by more extensive problems with alcohol, usually involving tolerance and withdrawal.

- Binge drinking is a common form of alcohol abuse on college campuses that has negative effects on both drinking and nondrinking students.

- Physical consequences of alcoholism include the direct effects of tolerance and withdrawal, as well as all the problems associated with chronic drinking. Psychological problems include memory loss and additional mental disorders such as depression.

- Treatment approaches include mutual support groups like AA, job- and school-based programs, inpatient hospital programs, and pharmacological treatments.

- Helping someone who abuses alcohol means avoiding being an enabler and obtaining information about available resources and persistently encouraging their use.

- Strategies for keeping drinking under control include examining attitudes about drinking and drinking behavior, drinking slowly, spacing drinks, eating before and while drinking, and knowing one's limits.

- Strategies for promoting responsible drinking in others include encouraging responsible attitudes, being a responsible host, holding the drinker responsible for his or her actions, learning about prevention programs, and taking community action.

Developing Responsible Drinking Habits

How much do you drink? Is it the right amount for you? You may know the answer to this question already, or you may not have given it much thought. Many people learn through a single unpleasant experience how alcohol affects them. Others suffer ill effects but choose to ignore or deny them.

To make responsible and informed choices about using alcohol, consider, first, whether there is any history of alcohol abuse in your family. If someone in your family is dependent on alcohol, you have a higher-than-average likelihood of becoming dependent too. Second, consider whether you are dependent on other substances or behaviors. Do you smoke, drink strong coffee every day, or use other drugs regularly? Does some habit control your life? Some people have more of a tendency to become addicted than others, and a person with one addiction is often likely to have other addictions as well. If this is the case for you, again you may need to be more cautious with alcohol.

Keep a Record

Once you have answered these questions, find out more about your alcohol-related behavior by keeping track of your drinking for 2 weeks in your health journal. Keep a daily alcohol behavior record like the one illustrated in Chapter 1 for eating behavior. Include information on

- *The drinking situation,* including type of drink, time of day, how fast you drank it, where you were, and what else you were doing.

- *Your internal state,* including what made you want to drink and your feelings, thoughts, and concerns at the time. Note how others influenced you.

- *The consequences of drinking,* including any changes in your feelings or behavior while or after you were drinking, such as silliness, assertiveness, aggressiveness, or depression.

Analyze Your Record

Next, analyze your record to detect patterns of feelings and environmental cues. Do you always drink when you're at a certain place or with certain people? Do you sometimes drink just to be sociable, when you don't really want a drink and would be satisfied with a nonalcoholic beverage? Refer to the list of warning signs of alcohol abuse given in the text. Are any of them true for you? For example, do you feel uncomfortable in a social situation if alcohol is *not* available?

Set Goals

Now that you've analyzed your record, think about whether you want to change any of your behaviors. Would you do better academically if you drank less? Has drinking had a negative impact on any of your relationships? Have you risked infection and unplanned pregnancy by having unprotected sex while drunk? Do you depend on alcohol in order to have a good time? Have you been injured while drinking? If you drink and drive or if you feel you are becoming dependent on alcohol, it is time to change your drinking behavior. Decide on goals that will give you the best health and safety returns, such as a beer or a glass of wine with dinner, one drink per hour at a party, or no alcohol at all.

Devise a Plan

Refer to your health journal to see what kinds of patterns your drinking falls into and where you can intervene to break the behavior chain. If you have determined that your life would be improved if you changed your drinking habits, now is the time to make changes. For some people, simple changes in the environment such as stocking the refrigerator with alternative beverages like juices or sparkling water can be helpful. If you feel self-conscious about ordering a nonalcoholic drink when you're out with a group, try recruiting a friend to do the same. If it's too difficult to avoid drinking in some situations, such as at a bar or a beer party, you may decide to avoid those situations for a period of time.

Examine your friendships. If drinking is becoming a problem for you and some of your friends drink heavily, you may need to think about letting those relationships go. If you find support groups helpful, check with your college counseling center or health clinic; most schools sponsor peer group activities for those who are working to change their drinking habits. Local chapters of AA and other organizations may have groups geared toward college-age people.

Instead of drinking, you can try other activities that produce the same effect. For example, if you drink to relieve anxiety or tension, try adding 20–30 minutes of exercise to your schedule to help you manage stress. Or try doing a relaxation exercise or going for a brisk walk to help reduce anxiety before a party or date. If you drink to relieve depression or to stop worrying, consider finding a trustworthy person (perhaps a professional counselor) to talk to about the problem that's bothering you. If you drink to feel more comfortable sexually, consider ways to improve communication with your partner so you can deal with sexual issues more openly. When these activities are successful, they will reinforce your responsible drinking decisions and make it more likely that you'll make the same decisions again in the future.

For other ways to monitor and control your drinking behavior, see the suggestions in the section "Drinking Behavior and Responsibility."

Reward Yourself and Monitor Your Progress

If changing your drinking behavior turns out to be difficult, it may be a clue that drinking was becoming a problem for you—all the more reason to get it under control now. Be sure to reward yourself as you learn to drink responsibly (or not at all). You may lose weight, look better, feel better, and have higher self-esteem as a result of limiting your drinking. Keep track of your progress in your health journal, and use the strategies described in Chapter 1 for maintaining your program. Remember, when you establish sensible drinking habits, you're planning not just for this week or month—but for your whole life.

1. **Interview peers:** Interview some of your fellow students about their drinking habits. How much do they drink, and how often? Are they more likely to drink on certain days or in certain circumstances? Are there any habits that seem to be common to most students? How do your own drinking habits compare to those of people you interviewed?

2. **Visit a local AA or Al-Anon group:** Some AA groups encourage visitors. If your local chapter does so, attend a meeting to see how the organization functions. What behavioral techniques are used to help people stop drinking? How effective do these techniques seem to be? If there is a local codependent or Al-Anon group, attend one of the group's meetings. What themes are emphasized? Do any themes apply to your relationships?

3. **Plan an alcohol-free party:** What would you serve to eat and drink? What would you tell people about the party when you invite them?

4. **Identify alcohol ads and points of sale in your community:** Look around your neighborhood and note the types of alcohol advertisements you find. How many are there, and what groups are being targeted—for example, young people, college students, or people of a particular ethnic group? Also identify where alcohol is sold: in what types of stores, and in how many locations? Is there a cluster of bars in a particular location? If you notice patterns that suggest marketing or sales targeted at particular groups, consider bringing your findings to the attention of community leaders.

For More Information

Books

Kinney, J., and G. Leaton. 2006. *Loosening the Grip: A Handbook of Alcohol Information,* 8th ed. New York: McGraw-Hill. *A fascinating book about alcohol, including information on physical effects, abuse, alcoholism, and cultural aspects of alcohol use.*

Nuwer, H. 2002. *Wrongs of Passage: Fraternities, Sororities, Hazing and Binge Drinking.* Bloomington: Indiana University Press. *Describes how hazing and binge drinking destroy the college experience for many students; written by a hazing expert.*

Shaw, B. F. 2004. *Addiction and Recovery for Dummies.* Hoboken, N.J.: For Dummies. *Provides information on identifying abuse and dependence, a review of approaches to treatment, and advice for helping others.*

Wechsler, H., and B. Wuethrich. 2003. *Dying to Drink: Confronting Binge Drinking on College Campuses.* Emmaus, Pa.: Rodale. *An in-depth review of the problem of binge drinking that lays out solutions for students, schools, parents, and communities; written by the lead researcher of the College Alcohol Study.*

Zailckas, K. 2005. *Smashed: Story of a Drunken Girlhood.* New York: Viking. *A 24-year-old writes about her own experiences of drinking through high school and college; also includes information from surveys and research into the effects of alcohol use.*

Organizations, Hotlines, and Web Sites

Al-Anon Family Group Headquarters. Provides information and referrals to local Al-Anon and Alateen groups. The Web site includes a self-quiz to determine if you are affected by someone's drinking.
888-4AL-ANON
http://www.al-anon.alateen.org

Alcoholics Anonymous (AA) World Services. Provides general information on AA, literature on alcoholism, and information about AA meetings and related 12-step organizations.
212-870-3400
http://www.alcoholics-anonymous.org

AlcoholScreening.Org. Provides information about alcohol and health, referrals for treatment and support groups, and a drinking self-assessment.
http://www.alcoholscreening.org

Alcohol Treatment Referral Hotline. Provides referrals to local intervention and treatment providers.
800-ALCOHOL

Bacchus and Gamma Peer Education Network. An association of college- and university-based peer education programs that focus on prevention of alcohol abuse.
http://www.bacchusgamma.org

The College Alcohol Study. Harvard School of Public Health. Provides information about and results from the recent studies of binge drinking on college campuses.
http://www.hsph.harvard.edu/cas

College Drinking Prevention: Students. Includes information about alcohol, including myths about alcohol use and an interactive look at how alcohol affects the body.
http://www.collegedrinkingprevention.gov/students

Facts on Tap. Provides information about alcohol and college life, sex and alcohol, and children of alcoholics, as well as suggestions for students who have been negatively affected by other students' alcohol use.
http://www.factsontap.org

Habitsmart. Contains an online self-scoring alcohol-use assessment, tips for outsmarting cravings, and links to related sites.
http://www.habitsmart.com

HadEnough.Org. Provides information and a self-quiz on binge drinking among college students.
http://www.hadenough.org

Higher Education Center for Alcohol and Other Drug Prevention. Provides support for campus alcohol and illegal drug prevention efforts; a Web site gives information about alcohol and drug abuse on campus and links to related sites.
http://www.edc.org/hec

Intoximeters Drink Wheel Blood Alcohol Test. Calculate your approximate BAC based on body weight, gender, and amount of alcohol consumed.
http://www.intox.com/wheel/drinkwheel.asp

Moderation Management Network. Controversial self-help program designed to help early problem drinkers limit their drinking; not intended for serious alcohol abusers or alcoholics.
http://www.moderation.org

Mothers Against Drunk Driving (MADD). Supports efforts to develop solutions to the problems of drunk driving and underage drinking; provides news, information, and brochures about many topics, including a guide for giving a safe party.
http://www.madd.org

National Association for Children of Alcoholics (NACoA). Provides information and support for children of alcoholics.

888-554-COAS

http://www.nacoa.net

National Clearinghouse for Alcohol and Drug Information/Prevention Online. Provides statistics and information on alcohol abuse, including resources for people who want to help friends and family members overcome alcohol-abuse problems.

800-729-6686

http://www.health.org

National Council on Alcoholism and Drug Dependence (NCADD). Provides information and counseling referrals.

212-269-7797; 800-NCA-CALL (24-hour Hope Line)

http://www.ncadd.org

National Institute on Alcohol Abuse and Alcoholism (NIAAA). Provides booklets and other publications on a variety of alcohol-related topics, including fetal alcohol syndrome, alcoholism treatment, and alcohol use and minorities.

http://www.drugabuse.gov

Rational Recovery. A free self-help program that offers an alternative to 12-step programs; the emphasis is on learning the skill of abstinence.

http://www.rational.org

See also the listings for Chapter 9.

Selected Bibliography

Centers for Disease Control and Prevention. 2004. Alcohol-attributable deaths and years of potential life lost, United States, 2001. *Morbidity and Mortality Weekly Report* 53(37): 866–870.

Dawson, D. A., et al. 2005. Recovery from DSM-IV alcohol dependence: United States, 2001–2002. *Addiction* 100(3): 281–292.

Day, N., et al. 2002. Prenatal alcohol exposure predicts continued deficits in offspring size at 14 years of age. *Alcoholism: Clinical and Experimental Research* 26(10): 1584–1591.

Ding, J., et al. 2004. Alcohol intake and cerebral abnormalities on magnetic resonance imaging in a community-based population of middle-aged adults: The Atherosclerosis Risk in Communities (ARIC) study. *Stroke* 35(1): 16–21.

Food and Drug Administration. 2004. New drug to treat alcoholism. *FDA Consumer,* September/October.

Gallup Poll. 2004. *Americans and Alcohol: Drink, Drank, Drunk?* (http://www.gallup.com/content/print.aspx?ci=12790; retrieved September 7, 2004).

Grant, B., et al. 2004. The 12-month prevalence and trends in DSM-IV alcohol abuse and dependence: United States, 1991–1992 and 2001–2002. *Drug and Alcohol Dependence* 74(3): 223–234.

Hingson, R., et al. 2005. Magnitude of alcohol-related mortality and morbidity among U.S. college students ages 18–24. *Annual Review of Public Health* 26: 259–279.

Insurance Institute for Highway Safety. 2004. *DUI/DWI Laws as of July 2004* (http://www.hwysafety.org/safety_facts/state_laws/dui.htm; retrieved December 13, 2004).

Jacobson, S. W., et al. 2004. Maternal age, alcohol abuse history, and quality of parenting as moderators of the effects of prenatal alcohol exposure on 7.5-year intellectual function. *Alcoholism: Clinical and Experimental Research* 28(11): 1732–1745.

Jernigan, D. H., et al. 2004. Sex differences in adolescent exposure to alcohol advertising in magazines. *Archives of Pediatrics and Adolescent Medicine* 158(7): 629–634.

Kesmodel, U., et al. 2002. Moderate alcohol intake during pregnancy and the risk of stillbirth and death in the first year of life. *American Journal of Epidemiology* 155(4): 305–312.

Klatsky, A. L. 2003. Drink to your health? *Scientific American,* February.

McCarty, C. A., et al. 2004. Continuity of binge and harmful drinking from late adolescence to early adulthood. *Pediatrics* 114(3): 714–719.

Meyerhoff, D. J., et al. 2004. Effects of heavy drinking, binge drinking, and family history of alcoholism on regional brain metabolites. *Alcoholism: Clinical and Experimental Research* 28(4): 650–651.

Monti, P. M., et al. 2005. Adolescence: Booze, brains, and behavior. *Alcohol: Clinical and Experimental Research* 29(2): 207–220.

Moos, R. H., et al. 2004. High-risk alcohol consumption and late-life alcohol use problems. *American Journal of Public Health* 94(11): 1985–1991.

Mukamal, K. J., et al. 2005. Alcohol and risk for ischemic stroke in men: The role of drinking patterns and usual beverage. *Annals of Internal Medicine* 142(1): 11–19.

National Institute on Alcohol Abuse and Alcoholism. 2005. *2001–2002 Survey Finds That Many Recover from Alcoholism; Researchers Identify Factors Associated with Abstinent and Non-Abstinent Recovery* (http://www.niaaa.nih.gov/press/2005/Recovery.htm; retrieved March 14, 2005).

National Institute on Alcohol Abuse and Alcoholism. 2003. *The Genetics of Alcoholism.* Alcohol Alert No. 60. Bethesda, Md.: National Institute on Alcohol Abuse and Alcoholism.

National Institute on Alcohol Abuse and Alcoholism. 2003. *State of the Science Report on the Effects of Moderate Drinking* (http://www.niaaa.nih.gov/publications/ModerateDrinking-03.htm; retrieved September 15, 2004).

National Institute on Alcohol Abuse and Alcoholism. 2004. *Alcohol—An Important Women's Health Issue.* Alcohol Alert No. 62. Bethesda, Md.: National Institute on Alcohol Abuse and Alcoholism.

National Institute on Alcohol Abuse and Alcoholism. 2004. *Neuroscience Research and Therapeutic Targets.* Alcohol Alert No. 61. Bethesda, Md.: National Institute on Alcohol Abuse and Alcoholism.

Nelson, T. F., et al. 2005. The state sets the rate: The relationship of college binge drinking to state binge drinking rates and selected state alcohol control policies. *American Journal of Public Health* 95(3): 441–446.

Office of Applied Studies, Substance Abuse and Mental Health Services Administration. 2004. *National Survey on Drug Use and Health* (http://oas.samhsa.gov/nhsda.htm; retrieved December 6, 2004).

Pletcher, M. J., et al. 2005. Alcohol consumption, binge drinking, and early coronary calcification: Findings from the coronary artery risk development in young adults (CARDIA) study. *American Journal of Epidemiology* 161(5): 423–433.

Slutske, W. S. 2005. Alcohol use disorders among US college students and their non-college-attending peers. *Archives of General Psychiatry* 62(3): 321–327.

Smothers, B. A., H. T. Yahr, and C. E. Ruhl. 2004. Detection of alcohol use disorders in general hospital admissions in the United States. *Archives of Internal Medicine* 164(7): 749–756.

Spurling, M. C., and D. C. Vinson. 2005. Alcohol-related injuries: Evidence for the prevention paradox. *Annals of Family Medicine* 3(1): 47–52.

U.S. Surgeon General. 2005. *U.S. Surgeon General Releases Advisory on Alcohol Use in Pregnancy* (http://www.hhs.gov/surgeongeneral/pressreleases/sg02222005.html; retrieved March 13, 2005).

Weitzman, E. R. 2004. Poor mental health, depression, and associations with alcohol consumption, harm and abuse in a national sample of young adults in college. *Journal of Nervous and Mental Disease* 192(4): 269–277.

Wilson, G. S., M. E. Pritchard, and J. Schaffer. 2004. Athletic status and drinking behavior in college students. *Journal of American College Health* 52(6): 269–273.

World Health Organization. 2004. *Burden of Disease Attributable to Alcohol* (http://www.who.int/substance_abuse/facts/alcohol/en; retrieved September 15, 2004).

11

Emphysema Ultra Lights!

LOW TAR & NICOTINE

FILTER CIGARETTES

Got Emphysema?

Looking AHEAD

After reading this chapter, you should be able to

- List the reasons people start using tobacco and why they continue to use it

- Explain the short- and long-term health risks associated with tobacco use

- Discuss the effects of environmental tobacco smoke on nonsmokers

- Describe the social costs of tobacco, and list actions that have been taken to combat smoking in the public and private sectors

- Prepare plans to stop using tobacco and to avoid environmental tobacco smoke

Toward a Tobacco-Free Society

1. **People who smoke "light" or low-tar cigarettes reduce their risk of smoking-related diseases compared to people who smoke other cigarettes.**
   True or false?

2. **Which of the following substances is found in tobacco smoke?**
   a. acetone (nail polish remover)
   b. ammonia (cleaner)
   c. hexamine (lighter fluid)
   d. toluene (industrial solvent)

3. **The health care costs associated with smoking work out to about $0.84 per pack of cigarettes, the average tax collected by states to offset these costs.**
   True or false?

4. **Cigarette smoking increases the risk for which of the following conditions?**
   a. facial wrinkling
   b. miscarriage
   c. impotence
   d. automobile crashes

5. **A person who quits smoking now will reduce his or her risk of lung cancer within 10 years.**
   True or false?

6. **Every cigarette a person smokes reduces life expectancy by about 1 minute.**
   True or false?

ANSWERS

1. FALSE. Smokers who choose "light" or low-tar cigarettes do not reduce tar intake or smoking-related disease risks, nor is there any evidence that switching to "light" cigarettes helps smokers quit.

2. ALL FOUR. Tobacco contains thousands of chemical substances, including many that are poisonous or linked to the development of cancer.

3. FALSE. States collect about $0.84 per pack in taxes, but the total cost of smoking-related medical care and lost productivity is about $157 billion a year, or $7.18 per pack.

4. ALL FOUR. Cigarette smoking reduces the quality of life and is the greatest preventable cause of death in the United States.

5. TRUE. The lung cancer rate of a former smoker is 50% of that of a continuing smoker within 10 years of quitting.

6. FALSE. Every cigarette reduces life expectancy by about 11 minutes; one carton represents a day and a half of lost life.

WW Visit the *Core Concepts in Health* Online Learning Center (www.mhhe.com/insel10e) for study aids and many additional resources.

297

O nce considered a glamorous and sophisticated habit, smoking is now viewed with increasing disapproval. The recognition of the health risks of smoking is a primary cause of this change in public opinion, and it has led to significant changes in the behavior of many Americans. Over the past four decades, the proportion of cigarette smoking among adults in the United States has dropped 30%. Private businesses and all levels of government have jumped on the nonsmoking bandwagon: Almost every state now restricts smoking in public places, and several have introduced statewide smoking bans for indoor workplaces. The U.S. Surgeon General has proposed that America become completely smoke-free.

Despite such progress, tobacco use is still widespread. About one in four Americans age 12 and older smokes cigarettes. Smoking is the leading cause of preventable death in the United States and has negative health effects on people at all stages of life: It harms unborn babies, infants, children, adolescents, adults, and seniors. Each year 440,000 Americans die prematurely from tobacco-related causes (Figure 11-1). This accounts for nearly one in every five adult deaths each year—equivalent to one death every 80 seconds or three fully loaded airliners crashing each day. Male and female smokers lose an average of 13.2 and 14.5 years of life, respectively. Nonsmokers, particularly children whose parents smoke, also suffer. Exposure to environmental tobacco smoke (ETS) causes more than 60,000 deaths annually among nonsmokers. Smoking by pregnant women is responsible for about 10% of all infant deaths in this country. Children exposed to ETS suffer higher rates of asthma, bronchitis, and pneumonia. Spit (smokeless) tobacco and cigars are regaining popularity: The use of spit tobacco products has tripled since 1972, and cigar smoking has increased 50% since 1993.

Given the overwhelming evidence against tobacco, why would anyone today begin using it? How does it exercise its hold over users? What can smokers and nonsmokers do to help achieve a tobacco-free society? In this chapter, we explore answers to these and other questions about nicotine addiction.

WHY PEOPLE USE TOBACCO

Roughly 70 million Americans, including nearly 4 million adolescents, use tobacco. Each day more than 2000 teenagers become regular smokers, and at least one-third of them will die prematurely because of tobacco. Most smokers understand the risks of tobacco use: More than 80% of adult smokers believe tobacco will shorten their life and would like to quit. Each year roughly 40% of smokers quit for at least a day, but 9 out of 10 of them are smoking again within a year, most within 3 months.

Nicotine Addiction

The primary reason people continue to use **tobacco** despite the health risks is that they have become addicted to a powerful psychoactive drug: **nicotine.** Although the tobacco industry long maintained that there was insufficient evidence about the addictiveness of nicotine, scientific evidence overwhelmingly supports the conclusion that nicotine is highly addictive. In fact, many researchers consider nicotine to be the most physically addictive of all the psychoactive drugs.

Some neurological studies indicate that nicotine acts on the brain in much the same way as cocaine and heroin. Nicotine reaches the brain via the bloodstream seconds after it is inhaled or, in the case of spit tobacco, absorbed through membranes of the mouth or nose. It triggers the release of powerful chemical messengers in the brain, including epinephrine, norepinephrine, and dopamine. But unlike street drugs, most of which are used to achieve a high, nicotine's primary attraction seems to lie in its ability to modulate everyday emotions.

At low doses, nicotine acts as a stimulant: It increases heart rate and blood pressure and, in adults, can enhance

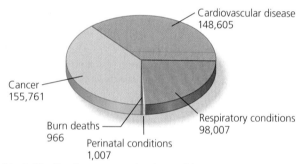

(a) Mortality: Deaths per year due to smoking

Cardiovascular disease 148,605
Cancer 155,761
Burn deaths 966
Perinatal conditions 1,007
Respiratory conditions 98,007

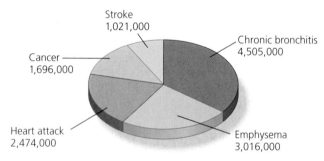

(b) Morbidity: Number of people with chronic illnesses due to smoking

Stroke 1,021,000
Chronic bronchitis 4,505,000
Cancer 1,696,000
Heart attack 2,474,000
Emphysema 3,016,000

VITAL STATISTICS

Figure 11-1 Annual mortality and morbidity among smokers attributable to smoking. SOURCE: Centers for Disease Control and Prevention. 2003. Cigarette smoking attributable morbidity—United States, 2000. *Morbidity and Mortality Weekly Report* 52(35): 842–844; Centers for Disease Control and Prevention. 2002. Annual smoking-attributable mortality, years of potential life lost, and economic costs. *Morbidity and Mortality Weekly Report* 51(14): 300–303.

Assess Yourself

Nicotine Dependence: Are You Hooked?

Answer each question in the list below, giving yourself the appropriate number of points.

_____ 1. How soon after you wake up do you have your first cigarette?
   a. within 5 minutes (3)
   b. 6–30 minutes (2)
   c. 31–60 minutes (1)
   d. after 60 minutes (0)

_____ 2. Do you find it difficult to refrain from smoking in places where it is forbidden, such as the library, a theater, or a doctor's office?
   a. yes (1)
   b. no (0)

_____ 3. Which cigarette would you most hate to give up?
   a. the first one in the morning (1)
   b. any other (0)

_____ 4. How many cigarettes a day do you smoke?
   a. 10 or less (0)
   b. 11–20 (1)
   c. 21–30 (2)
   d. 31 or more (3)

_____ 5. Do you smoke more frequently during the first hours after waking than during the rest of the day?
   a. yes (1)
   b. no (0)

_____ 6. Do you smoke if you are so ill that you are in bed most of the day?
   a. yes (1)
   b. no (0)

_____ TOTAL

A total score of 7 or more indicates that you are very dependent on nicotine and are likely to experience withdrawal symptoms when you stop smoking. A score of 6 or less indicates low to moderate dependence.

SOURCE: Heatherton, T. F., et al. 1991. The Fagerstrom Test for Nicotine Dependence: A revision of the Fagerstrom Tolerance Questionnaire. *British Journal of Addictions* 86(9): 1119–1127.

alertness, concentration, rapid information processing, memory, and learning. People type faster on nicotine, for instance. The opposite effect occurs in teens who smoke, however; they show impairment in memory and other cognitive functions.

In some circumstances, nicotine acts as a mild sedative. Most commonly, nicotine relieves symptoms such as anxiety, irritability, and mild depression in tobacco users who are experiencing withdrawal. Some studies have shown that high doses of nicotine and rapid smoking cause increases in levels of glucocorticoids and endorphins, chemicals that act in the brain to moderate moods and reduce stress. Tobacco users are able to fine-tune nicotine's effects and regulate their moods by increasing or decreasing their intake of the drug. Studies have shown that smokers experience milder mood variation than nonsmokers while performing long, boring tasks or while watching emotional movies, for example.

All tobacco products contain nicotine, and the use of any of them can lead to addiction (see the box "Nicotine Dependence: Are You Hooked?"). Nicotine addiction fulfills the criteria for substance dependence described in Chapter 9, including loss of control, tolerance, and withdrawal.

Loss of Control   Three out of four smokers want to quit but find they cannot. Although 60–80% of people who attend stop-smoking clinics are able to quit, three-quarters of them start smoking again within a year—a relapse rate similar to rates for alcoholics and heroin addicts. Quitting may be even harder for smokeless users: In one study, only 1 of 14 spit tobacco users who participated in a tobacco-cessation clinic was able to stop for more than 4 hours.

Regular tobacco users live according to a rigid cycle of need and gratification. On average, they can go no more than 40 minutes between doses of nicotine; otherwise, they begin feeling edgy and irritable and have trouble concentrating. If ignored, nicotine cravings build until getting a cigarette or some spit tobacco becomes a paramount concern, crowding out other thoughts. Tobacco users may plan their daily schedule around opportunities to satisfy their nicotine cravings; this loss of control and personal freedom can affect all the dimensions of wellness (see the box "Tobacco Use and Religion: Global Views" on p. 300).

Tobacco users become adept, therefore, at keeping a steady amount of nicotine circulating in the blood and going to the brain. In one experiment, smokers were given cigarettes that looked and tasted alike but varied in nicotine content. The subjects automatically adjusted their rate and depth of inhalation so that they absorbed

Terms

tobacco The leaves of cultivated tobacco plants prepared for smoking, chewing, or use as snuff.

nicotine A poisonous, addictive substance found in tobacco and responsible for many of the effects of tobacco.

Mind/Body/Spirit

What contributions can the world's religions make to efforts to limit tobacco use? This was the question behind a meeting attended by representatives of the major religions of the world at the headquarters of the World Health Organization (WHO).

Tobacco Use as a Violation of Religious Principles

A primary thread among all the religions is a condemnation of tobacco use for its damaging effects on the body. Most religions regard the human body as the dwelling place of the spirit; as such, it deserves care and respect.

The Baha'i faith, for example, strongly discourages smoking as unclean and unhealthy. Some Protestant churches consider tobacco use a violation of the body. For Hindus, smoking goes against one of the primary spiritual practices, the care of the body. The Roman Catholic Church endorses the age-old adage "a sound mind in a sound body." For Muslims, one of the five essential principles on which religious law is based is the protection of the integrity of the individual. In Judaism, people are urged to "choose life" and to choose whatever strengthens the capacity to live. Buddhists believe that the body doesn't belong to the person at all—even suicide is considered murder—and one must do nothing to harm it.

A second thread common to most religions is the notion that dependence and addiction run counter to ideas of freedom, choice, and human dignity. Buddhism teaches a path of freedom—a way of life without dependence on anything.

Hindus regard tobacco use as a *vyasana*, a dependence that is not necessary for the preservation of health. Protestant churches caution that any form of dependence is contrary to the notion of Christian freedom.

A third argument against tobacco use is the immorality of imposing secondhand smoke on nonsmokers, which is seen as inflicting harm on others. In Hinduism, harming others is sinful. In the Jewish tradition, those who force nonsmokers to breathe smoke jeopardize the lives of others, and to do so is to jeopardize the whole universe.

The Role of Individual Responsibility

Most religions focus on the role of individual responsibility in overcoming dependence on tobacco. In Buddhism, for example, people must assume responsibility for their habits; they practice introspection to understand the cause of problems within themselves and the effects of their actions on others. The principles of Islam are based on notions of responsibility and protection; a fundamental message is that you are responsible for your body and for your health.

Religion and Tobacco Control

Common threads again emerged in discussions of how the problem of tobacco use should be approached. The Islamic view is that the campaign to control tobacco use must be based on awareness, responsibility, and justice. Developing awareness means providing information

on the global problem. Fostering responsibility means helping people understand what they need to do to attain well-being. Emphasizing social and human justice means helping the farmers and societies that depend on tobacco cultivation to find alternative crops.

According to the representative from the Geneva Interreligious Platform (a project involving Hindus, Buddhists, Jews, Christians, Muslims, and Baha'is), the best approach is prevention. Here, the rights of nonsmokers clearly prevail over the freedom of smokers. In support of this position, the common religious exhortation not to do unto others what you would not have them do unto you can be invoked. Further, adequate information should be provided to counter the deceptive images projected by tobacco industry advertising, especially where minors are concerned. Protection of the weak and denunciation of dishonesty are underlying values of all religious traditions.

Religious traditions can best assist adult smokers by reminding them of two principles: one, the value of liberation from any form of slavery, and two, respect for life out of deference to the source of all life, which religions call by different names—God, ultimate reality, and so on—but which is the supreme value of any religious commitment.

SOURCE: World Health Organization Tobacco Free Initiative. 1999. *Meeting Report: Meeting on Tobacco and Religion* (3 May 1999). Geneva: World Health Organization.

their usual amount of nicotine. In other studies, heavy smokers were given nicotine without knowing it, and they cut down on their smoking without a conscious effort. Spit tobacco users maintain blood nicotine levels as high as those of cigarette smokers.

Tolerance and Withdrawal Using tobacco builds up tolerance. Where one cigarette may make a beginning smoker nauseated and dizzy, a long-term smoker may have to chain-smoke a pack or more to experience the same effects. For most regular tobacco users, sudden abstinence from nicotine produces predictable withdrawal

symptoms as well. These symptoms, which come on several hours after the last dose of nicotine, can include severe cravings, insomnia, confusion, tremors, difficulty concentrating, fatigue, muscle pains, headache, nausea, irritability, anger, and depression. Users undergo measurable changes in brain waves, heart rate, and blood pressure, and they perform poorly on tasks requiring sustained attention. Although most of these symptoms of physical dependence pass in 2 or 3 days, the craving associated with addiction persists. Many ex-smokers report intermittent, intense urges to smoke for years after quitting.

Many teenagers believe they will be able to stop smoking when they want. In fact, adolescents are more vulnerable to nicotine than are older tobacco users. Compared with older smokers, adolescents become heavy smokers and develop dependence after fewer cigarettes. Nicotine addiction can start within a few days of smoking and after just a few cigarettes. Over half of teenagers who try cigarettes progress to daily use, and about half of those who ever smoke daily progress to nicotine dependence. In polls, about 75% of smoking teens state they wish they had never started. Another survey revealed that only 5% of high school smokers predicted they would definitely be smoking in 5 years; in fact, close to 75% were smoking 7–9 years later.

Social and Psychological Factors

Why do tobacco users have such a hard time quitting even when they want to? Social and psychological forces combine with physiological addiction to maintain the tobacco habit. Many people, for example, have established habits of smoking while doing something else—while talking, working, drinking, and so on. The spit tobacco habit is also associated with certain situations—studying, drinking coffee, or playing sports. It is difficult for these people to break their habits because the activities they associate with tobacco use continue to trigger their urge. Such activities are called **secondary reinforcers**; they act together with the physiological addiction to keep the user dependent on tobacco.

Genetic Factors

Genetic makeup does not guarantee protection against nicotine dependence or make addiction inevitable. But inherited characteristics do play an important role in some aspects of tobacco use. Studies that look for differences in behavior among twins and other sibling pairs suggest that genetic factors are more important than social and environmental factors in smoking initiation and in the development of nicotine dependence when people do start to smoke.

Scientists have begun to identify specific genes associated with biological response to tobacco use. For example, a gene that influences the way in which nicotine is metabolized, or broken down in the body, helps regulate the activity of an enzyme called CYP2A6. When people with slow CYP2A6 metabolism use tobacco, the nicotine remains in their blood longer than in people who have the gene for a faster metabolizing form of the enzyme. The slow metabolizers are more likely to feel nausea or dizziness when they first use tobacco, are less likely to continue smoking if they try it, and find it easier to quit if they do become regular smokers. Further research will likely identify other genes involved in nicotine dependence.

The average age of new smokers is 13, and most adult smokers began as teenagers. In polls, about 75% of teen smokers state they wish they had never started.

Why Start in the First Place?

A junior high school girl takes up smoking in an attempt to appear older. A high school boy uses spit tobacco in the bullpen, emulating the major league ball players he admires. An overweight first-year college student turns to cigarettes, hoping they will curb her appetite. Smoking rates among American youth rose steadily through the 1990s but have begun to decline. Between 2000 and 2002, use of any tobacco product among high school students declined; cigarette use dropped from 28.5% to 22.9%, and use of cigars, bidis, and kreteks also dropped. Moreover, use of spit tobacco and pipes among high school students held steady, suggesting that high school students were not just switching from cigarettes to other tobacco products. There was no similar drop in tobacco use among middle school students, however.

It is not clear why middle school and high school students appear to respond differently to the current

Term

V\w

secondary reinforcers Stimuli that are not necessarily pleasurable in themselves but that are associated with other stimuli that are pleasurable.

Take Charge

A common misconception among smokers is that a few cigarettes a day aren't enough to cause harm. Perhaps this is why a recent survey showed that among college students who smoke, 75% smoke 10 or fewer cigarettes a day. These smokers are ignoring the very real health risks of even one cigarette. The U.S. Public Health Service suggests a "5 R's" strategy to enhance motivation to quit. If you are a smoker or are trying to help one, think about these areas of concern and see if they help develop a desire and readiness to make a real attempt at quitting.

Relevance: Think about the personal relevance of quitting tobacco use. What would the effects be on your family and friends? How would your daily life improve? What is the most important way that quitting would change your life?

Risks: There are immediate risks, such as shortness of breath, infertility, and impotence, and long-term risks, including cancer, heart disease, and respiratory problems. Remember, smoking is harmful both to you and to anyone exposed to your smoke.

Rewards: The list of the rewards of quitting is almost endless, including improving immediate and long-term health, saving money, and feeling better about yourself. You can also stop worrying about quitting and set a good example for others.

Roadblocks: What are the potential obstacles to quitting? Are you worried about withdrawal symptoms, weight gain, or lack of support? How can these barriers be overcome?

Repetition: Revisit your reasons for quitting and strengthen your resolve until you are ready to prepare a plan. Most people make several attempts to quit before they succeed. Relapsing once does not mean that you will never succeed.

SOURCES: Rigotti, N. A., J. E. Lee, and H. Wechsler. 2000. U.S. college students' use of tobacco products. *Journal of the American Medical Association* 284(6): 699–705; Fiore, M. C., et al. 2000. *Treating Tobacco Use and Dependence.* Clinical Practice Guidelines. Rockville, Md.: U.S. Department of Health and Human Services.

anti-smoking environment, which includes increases in cigarette prices; more widespread smoke-free laws and policies; restrictions on tobacco advertising; and local, state, and national anti-tobacco campaigns such as the truth® campaign. However, promotional spending by the tobacco industry has increased substantially, and industry-sponsored media efforts may be diluting the impact of public health campaigns.

Children and teenagers constitute 90% of all new smokers in this country: Every day, an estimated 2000 adolescents become regular cigarette smokers, while hundreds of others take up snuff or chewing tobacco. The average age for starting smokers is 13; for spit tobacco users, 10. Meanwhile, children—especially girls—are beginning to experiment with tobacco at ever-younger ages. The earlier people begin smoking, the more likely they are to become heavy smokers—and to die of tobacco-related disease.

Rationalizing the Dangers   Making the decision to smoke requires minimizing or denying both the health risks of tobacco use and the tremendous pain, disability, emotional trauma, family stress, and financial expense involved in tobacco-related diseases such as cancer and emphysema. A sense of invincibility, characteristic of many adolescents and young adults, also contributes to the decision to use tobacco. Young people may persuade themselves they are too intelligent, too lucky, or too healthy to be vulnerable to tobacco's dangers (see the box "Building Motivation to Quit Smoking"). "I'm not dumb enough to get hooked," they may argue. "I'll be able to quit before I do myself any real harm." Other typical rationalizations:

"My grandmother smoked and she lived to be 80" and "You can get killed just by crossing the street."

Listening to Advertising   Advertising is a powerful influence. The tobacco industry spends more than $12 billion each year on advertising that links tobacco products with desirable traits such as confidence, popularity, sexual attractiveness, and slenderness. Young people are a prime target of these ads. Once a teen begins smoking, nicotine addiction can lead to a lifetime of smoking. As one teenager said, "It may have been my decision to smoke my first cigarette, and maybe even my second. But now *needing* to smoke is no longer a choice."

The tobacco industry has perfected techniques that target young people, for it is young smokers who are the likeliest to purchase familiar brands. Thus, the most heavily advertised cigarettes—Marlboro, Camel, and Newport—are the choice of 90% of teen smokers. Only a third of adult smokers, who prefer less expensive generic cigarettes, choose these brands. R. J. Reynolds Tobacco Company's promotion of the Camel brand, the most notorious tobacco campaign ever aimed at young people, recruited millions of new smokers and quadrupled Camel's share of tobacco companies' most coveted demographic—the FUBYAS, or "first usual brand younger adult smoker." To tobacco companies, "younger adult" means 14 or older, and Joe Camel became as familiar to children as Mickey Mouse. In surveys, more than 90% of 6-year-olds recognized the character and associated it with cigarettes.

Young people are not the only group targeted. Certain brands are designed to appeal primarily to men, women, or particular ethnic groups. For example, Virginia Slims tries to appeal to women by associating the brand with confidence and sexual attractiveness. Magazines that are targeted at African American audiences receive proportionately more revenues from cigarette advertising than do other consumer magazines. Billboards advertising tobacco products are placed in black communities four or five times more often than in primarily white communities.

The government began regulating tobacco advertising in 1967. Under the Fairness Doctrine, the Federal Communications Commission (FCC) required broadcasters to air anti-smoking messages along with industry-sponsored cigarette advertisements on television and radio. Anti-smoking ads featuring unattractive older people smoking or cigarettes used as coffin nails effectively counteract the glamorous images that appear in tobacco ads. Between 1967 and 1971, when anti-smoking messages were first broadcast, per capita cigarette consumption declined by 7%—one of the largest declines ever. Cigarette advertising on television and radio was banned altogether in 1971. In 1996, the FDA issued strict advertising regulations designed to reduce minors' exposure and access to tobacco advertising and products; however, the Supreme Court ruled in March 2000 that the FDA does not have the authority to regulate tobacco. Debate continues over legislation that would give the FDA regulatory authority.

In November 1998, controls on advertising were enacted as part of the $206 billion deal to settle lawsuits brought against the tobacco industry by the attorneys general of 39 states (see pp. 315–317 for more information). This settlement limits or bans billboard and transit advertising of tobacco products; cartoon characters in advertisements and packaging; tobacco logos on T-shirts, hats, and other promotional items; brand-name sponsorship of sporting events; and payments for product placement in movies, television, and concerts.

The 1998 advertising limits changed the environment but not the intensity of tobacco marketing. For example, the industry spent nearly twice as much on advertising and other promotions in 2002—$12.47 billion, or more than $34 million each day—as in 1998, the year before the settlement restrictions took effect. About 63% ($7.87 billion) of the expenditure went for cost discounts that allowed retailers to keep cigarette prices low in the face of increasing taxes on tobacco products. Other point-of-sale expenditures ("buy two, get one free," give-away discount coupons, and payments for preferential placement of displays) accounted for an additional 21% ($2.9 billion) of the overall marketing budget. The concentration of the industry's promotional effort is most apparent in neighborhood convenience stores, where tobacco products and promotional displays are prominently placed—often at child's eye-level—at the store's most-visited location, the checkout counter. In this carefully engineered setting, tobacco products are presented as a colorful and commonplace part of the neighborhood retail environment—as acceptable as a candy bar or quart of milk.

Emulating Smoking Onscreen Tobacco companies agreed to end paid product placement in movies as part of the 1998 settlement; a voluntary ban had been in effect since 1990. This ban does not appear to be having the intended effect, however. Researchers have found that smoking in movies has actually increased significantly since 1990, to levels not seen since 1960. In the 2 years following the settlement, smoking in PG-13 movies increased by 50%. Half the tobacco shots in the top movies from 2002 to 2003 were in G, PG, and PG-13 movies.

The portrayal of smoking in films does not reflect U.S. patterns of tobacco use. The prevalence of smoking among lead characters is three to four times that among comparable Americans. Films typically show the smoker as white, male, well educated, successful, and attractive. In reality, smokers tend to be poor and to have less education. In the top-grossing films in 2002–2003, smoking was portrayed in more than 73% of the films, including 82% of PG-13 films; smoking was often shown positively as a means to relieve tension or as something to do while socializing. Negative consequences resulting from tobacco use were depicted for only 3% of the major characters who used tobacco. By showing smoking in an unrealistically positive light, films may be acting as advertisement.

Does smoking on-screen affect real-life smoking habits? Studies of adolescents have consistently found a strong association between seeing tobacco use in films and trying cigarettes. Adolescents who see more smoking in films or whose favorite movie stars frequently use tobacco on-screen have more positive attitudes about smoking and are as much as three times more likely to have tried smoking than teens with less exposure to films. Teens may be particularly sensitive to on-screen portrayals of smoking because they are in the process of developing adult identities; during this period, they may try out different personas, including those of their favorite movie stars.

Some groups equate seeing a favorite actor smoke on-screen with now-banned celebrity television advertisements for cigarettes. They suggest an automatic R rating for any film that shows tobacco use, equating smoking with violence, strong language, sexuality, and nudity in determining a film's rating. The debate over the prevalence and effects of smoking is likely to continue.

Who Uses Tobacco?

Not all young people are equally vulnerable to the lure of tobacco. Research suggests that the more of the following characteristics that apply to a child or adolescent, the more likely he or she is to use tobacco:

- A parent or sibling uses tobacco.
- Peers use tobacco.

Table 11-1   Who Smokes?

	Percentage of Smokers		
	Men	Women	Total
Ethnic group (age ≥ 18)			
White	26	22	24
Black	27	19	22
Asian	19	7	13
American Indian/ Alaska Native	40	41	41
Latino	23	11	17
Education (age ≥ 25)			
≤8 years	25	13	20
9–11 years	39	31	34
12 years (no diploma)	32	30	31
GED diploma	48	38	42
12 years (diploma)	30	22	26
Associate degree	24	20	22
Undergraduate degree	14	11	12
Graduate degree	8	6	7
Total	25	20	22

SOURCE: Centers for Disease Control and Prevention. 2004. Cigarette smoking among adults—United States, 2002. *Morbidity and Mortality Weekly Report* 53(20): 427–431.

- The child comes from a blue-collar family.
- The child comes from a low-income home.
- The family is headed by a single parent.
- The child performs poorly in school.
- The child drops out of school.
- The child has positive attitudes about tobacco use.

In 2002, about 25% of men and 20% of women smoked cigarettes (Table 11-1). Rates of smoking varied, based on gender, age, ethnicity, and education level (see the box "Smoking Among U.S. Ethnic Populations"). Adults with less than a twelfth-grade education were three times as likely to smoke cigarettes as those with a college degree. The reverse is true for cigars: Cigar smoking is most common among the affluent and those with high educational attainment.

Between 1996 and 2001 the percentage of smokers who said they smoked only occasionally rose in 38 states and the District of Columbia, and recent surveys indicate the trend is continuing. Most of those who describe themselves as occasional smokers (smoke on some days but not daily) are young adults age 18–25 who say they smoke only at parties or when they are with friends who smoke. Health officials warn that occasional smokers are as vulnerable as other smokers to developing dependence and addiction to nicotine. They are also less likely to try to quit.

Although all states ban the sale of tobacco to anyone under 18 years of age, at least 500 million packs of cigarettes and 26 million containers of chewing tobacco are consumed by minors each year. About 15% of middle school students use some form of tobacco. Among high school students, about 28% smoke cigarettes at least occasionally and 15% smoke cigars. An estimated 8%, including 11% of white male students, use spit tobacco. Male college athletes and professional baseball players report even higher rates of spit tobacco use.

Men and women with other drug-abuse problems frequently use tobacco. For example, studies show that roughly 80% of alcoholics and more than 90% of heroin addicts are heavy smokers. Smoking also is more prevalent among people with mental disorders than among the rest of the population: 40% of people with major depression, social phobias, and generalized anxiety disorder—and eight out of ten people with schizophrenia—are smokers. Such findings suggest that underlying psychological or physiological traits may predispose people to drug use, including tobacco.

HEALTH HAZARDS

Tobacco adversely affects nearly every part of the body, including the brain, stomach, mouth, and reproductive organs.

Tobacco Smoke: A Toxic Mix

Tobacco smoke contains hundreds of damaging chemical substances, including acetone (nail polish remover), ammonia, hexamine (lighter fluid), and toluene (industrial solvent). Smoke from a typical unfiltered cigarette contains about 5 billion particles per cubic millimeter—50,000 times as many as are found in an equal volume of smoggy urban air. These particles, when condensed, form the brown, sticky mass called **cigarette tar**.

Carcinogens and Poisons   At least 43 chemicals in tobacco smoke are linked to the development of cancer. Some, such as benzo(a)pyrene and urethane, are **carcinogens**; that is, they directly cause cancer. Other chemicals, such as formaldehyde, are **cocarcinogens**; they do not themselves cause cancer but combine with other chemicals to stimulate the growth of certain cancers, at least in laboratory animals. Other substances in

Terms

VW

cigarette tar A brown, sticky mass created when the chemical particles in tobacco smoke condense.

carcinogen Any substance that causes cancer.

cocarcinogen A substance that works with a carcinogen to cause cancer.

The overall rate of tobacco use among Americans age 12 and older was 30.4% in 2003. That means on average that any group of a dozen people is likely to include three or four who use tobacco. But averages include wide variations among populations, and ethnic differences appear in the earliest stages of tobacco use.

Among all eighth graders, roughly one in ten (10.2%) is a current smoker, but African American students (6.9%) are less likely than either whites (10.9%) or Latinos (11.9%) to smoke at that age. By senior year, these differences become more pronounced—whites (29.4%) are half again as likely as Latinos (19.0%) and three times as likely as blacks (10.0%) to be current smokers. Use of spit tobacco shows similar disparities: African Americans in eighth grade are less likely than whites to use spit tobacco, and their rate of use declines through twelfth grade. Among whites, usage increases from eighth through twelfth grades.

Wide ethnic variations also exist among older smokers. More than 40% of American Indian and Alaska Native adults are smokers; among Asian Americans, only 12% of adults smoke, less than half the rate for the general population. Within the broad ethnic categories even greater variation occurs: Among people grouped under the broad category Latinos, 30% of Puerto Ricans but only 19% of Cuban Americans are smokers. There are higher smoking rates among population groups who trace their origins to Southeast Asia (for example, Vietnam, Cambodia, or Laos) than among other population groups within the general Asian American grouping (for exam-

ple, people from the Philippines, China, or Japan). Time in the United States, English proficiency, and level of educational attainment also influence smoking rates.

In populations of Asian and Pacific Islander Americans, rates of smoking are much higher among men than among women, regardless of country of origin. Although smoking among women decreases with age in the general population, smoking rates among Asian and Pacific Islander women increase with age. Asian and Pacific Islander Americans, male and female, who do smoke tend to smoke fewer cigarettes per day (a half a pack daily or less) than whites who smoke.

The variations between and within ethnic populations reflect a complex interplay of social, environmental, and cultural factors. For example, in some Latino populations, strong parental disapproval of smoking, particularly for girls, holds down the rate of smoking initiation; for other groups, smoking may have a mature and masculine aura, thereby promoting smoking. In some populations, socioeconomic factors may limit access to stop-smoking programs; prevention programs may also not be available to non–English speaking groups.

Tobacco companies understand the value of marketing strategies based on ethnic, cultural, age, and other differences. In 2004, a New York Supreme Court justice ruled that Brown & Williamson Tobacco Company was illegally appealing to young people with its "Kool MIXX" marketing campaign, which focused on hip-hop music and culture. R. J. Reynolds Tobacco

Company (RJRT) is continuing an extensive marketing effort for "Exotic Blends"—fruit- and spice-flavored, premium-priced, and imaginatively packaged versions of Camel cigarettes—in minority communities and to women. To increase Camel cigarette sales in the gay and lesbian community, RJRT developed a marketing plan designated Project Sub Culture Urban Marketing, or "Project SCUM." The campaign identified gays, "rebellious generation X," and street people as markets where "opportunity exists for a cigarette manufacturer to dominate." (A memo describing Camel's SCUM strategy is available at http://www.projectscum.org.)

Examine your own attitudes toward smoking and smokers—where do your ideas come from? Also consider the tobacco advertising you encounter: What groups are being targeted and how are they being targeted? As a smoker, a parent, or a concerned member of your community, it is important to be aware of the amount and type of tobacco advertising that you encounter and how your own background may influence your smoking attitudes and behavior.

SOURCES: Office of Applied Studies, Substance Abuse and Mental Health Services Administration. 2004. *National Survey on Drug Use and Health* (http://oas.samhsa.gov/nhsda.htm; retrieved December 6, 2004); Centers for Disease Control and Prevention. 2004. Prevalence of cigarette use among 14 racial/ethnic populations—United States, 1990–2001. *Morbidity and Mortality Weekly Report* 53(3): 49–52; Centers for Disease Control and Prevention. 2003. Tobacco use among middle and high school students—United States, 2002. *Morbidity and Mortality Weekly Report* 52(45): 1096–1098.

tobacco cause health problems because they damage the lining of the respiratory tract or decrease the lungs' ability to fight off infection.

Tobacco also contains poisonous substances, including arsenic and hydrogen cyanide. In addition to being an addictive psychoactive drug, nicotine is also a poison and can be fatal in high doses. Many cases of nicotine poisoning occur each year in toddlers and infants who pick up and eat cigarette butts they find at home or on the playground.

Cigarette smoke contains carbon monoxide, the deadly gas in automobile exhaust, in concentrations

400 times greater than is considered safe in industrial workplaces. Not surprisingly, smokers often complain of breathlessness when they require a burst of energy to run across campus for their next class. Carbon monoxide displaces oxygen in red blood cells, depleting the body's supply of life-giving oxygen for extra work. Carbon monoxide also impairs visual acuity, especially at night.

Additives Tobacco manufacturers use additives to manipulate the taste and effect of cigarettes and other

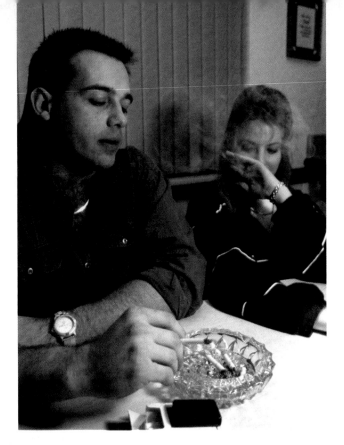

Cigarette smoke contains many toxic and carcinogenic chemicals that affect both the person smoking and the people breathing the environmental tobacco smoke. A growing body of evidence links ETS with lung cancer and respiratory and cardiovascular diseases.

tobacco products. Nearly 600 chemicals, approved as safe when used as food additives, are used in manufacturing cigarettes. In 1994, U.S. cigarette manufacturers submitted a list of tobacco additives to the Department of Health and Human Services, which made the list public and accompanied it with the notice that "although these ingredients are regarded as safe when ingested in foods, some may form carcinogens when heated or burned."

Additives account for roughly 10%, by weight, of a cigarette, and include sugars and other flavoring agents, humectants (compounds that keep tobacco from drying out), and chemicals that enhance the addicting properties of nicotine. The added sugars—including licorice, cocoa, and honey—have a dual role. As flavor enhancers, sugars mask the harsh, bitter taste of tobacco, making it possible for smokers, particularly first-time smokers, to inhale larger volumes of smoke and therefore absorb more nicotine. When sugars burn, they produce acetaldehyde, a chemical that enhances the addictive effect of nicotine and is a carcinogen. Other flavor components, such as the theobromine found in cocoa and the glycyrrhizin in licorice, share one of the properties of menthol—they act as bronchodilators, opening the lungs' airways and making it easier for nicotine to get

into the bloodstream. (Menthol cigarettes are discussed below.)

Ammonia plays a complex role in tobacco products, but its chief purpose is to boost the amount of addictive nicotine delivered by cigarettes. Ammonia reduces the acidity of tobacco smoke and releases nicotine in the form of a base (alkaline) rather than a salt (acid) bound to other acid components of smoke. As a free base, nicotine is more readily absorbed into the blood.

Ammonia and other additives are essential to the technology of reconstituted tobacco, which enables manufacturers to make cigarettes from leaf scraps and stems of tobacco plants (high in nicotine but harsh and bitter tasting). Flavor additives improve the taste, and ammonia delivers higher levels of nicotine. Cigarettes made from reconstituted tobacco treated with flavor enhancers and ammonia contain nearly twice as much available nicotine as cigarettes made from tobacco leaf. A study of free-base nicotine content in 11 brands of cigarettes available in the United States found that some contained 10–20 times higher percentages of free-base nicotine than experts had previously believed. Content ranged from less than 2% in some brands to as high as 36% for the specialty brand American Spirit. Marlboro brands contained up to 9.6% free-base nicotine.

Some additives are intended to make sidestream smoke (the uninhaled smoke from a burning cigarette) less obvious and objectionable. For example, potassium citrate, aluminum and other metal hydroxides, and clay are added to cigarette wrappers to convert particulate ash into an invisible gas with less irritating odor than would be given off by a conventional paper wrapper. These additives serve no purpose in making cigarettes more desirable and addicting to the smoker; instead, they are intended to reduce social pressures from nonsmokers.

Effects of Smoking Behavior All smokers absorb some gases, tar, and nicotine from cigarette smoke, but smokers who inhale bring most of these substances into their bodies and keep them there. In 1 year, a typical pack-a-day smoker takes in 50,000–70,000 puffs. Smoke from a cigarette, pipe, or cigar directly assaults the mouth, throat, and respiratory tract. The nose, which normally filters about 75% of foreign matter we breathe, is completely bypassed.

In a cigarette, the unburned tobacco itself acts as a filter. As a cigarette burns down, there is less and less filter. Thus, more chemicals are absorbed into the body during the last third of a cigarette than during the first. A smoker can cut down on the absorption of harmful chemicals by not smoking cigarettes down to short butts. Any gains, of course, will be offset by smoking more cigarettes, inhaling more deeply, or puffing more frequently.

"Light" and Low-Tar Cigarettes Some smokers switch to low-tar, low-nicotine, or filtered cigarettes because they believe them to be healthier alternatives. But there is no such thing as a safe cigarette, and smoking behavior is a more important factor in tar and nicotine intake than the type of cigarette smoked. Smokers who switch to a low-nicotine brand often compensate by smoking more cigarettes, inhaling more deeply, taking larger or more frequent puffs, or blocking ventilation holes with lips or fingers to offset the effects of filters. Studies have found that people who smoke "light" cigarettes inhale up to eight times as much tar and nicotine as printed on the label. Use of "light" and low-tar cigarettes does not reduce the risk of smoking-related illnesses, and the National Cancer Institute has concluded that they provide *no* benefit to smokers' health.

Menthol Cigarettes Concerns have also been raised about menthol cigarettes. About 70% of African American smokers smoke these cigarettes, as compared to 22% of whites. Studies have found that blacks absorb more nicotine than other groups and metabolize it more slowly; they also have lower rates of successful quitting. The anesthetizing effect of menthol, which may allow smokers to inhale more deeply and hold smoke in their lungs for a longer period, may be partly responsible for these differences. Further research is needed to determine if chemical effects of menthol and differences in smoking behavior can help explain the higher rates of smoking-related diseases seen among blacks.

The Immediate Effects of Smoking

The beginning smoker often has symptoms of mild nicotine poisoning: dizziness; faintness; rapid pulse; cold, clammy skin; and sometimes nausea, vomiting, and diarrhea. The seasoned smoker occasionally suffers these effects of nicotine poisoning, particularly after quitting and then returning to a previous level of consumption. The effects of nicotine on smokers vary, depending greatly on the size of the nicotine dose and how much tolerance previous smoking has built up. Nicotine can either excite or tranquilize the nervous system, depending on dosage.

Nicotine has many other immediate effects. It stimulates the part of the brain called the **cerebral cortex.** It also stimulates the adrenal glands to discharge adrenaline. And it inhibits the formation of urine; constricts the blood vessels, especially in the skin; accelerates the heart rate; and elevates blood pressure. Higher blood pressure, faster heart rate, and constricted blood vessels require the heart to pump more blood. In healthy people, the heart can usually meet this demand, but in people whose coronary arteries are damaged enough to interfere with the flow of blood, the heart muscle may be strained.

Smoking depresses hunger contractions and dulls the taste buds; smokers who quit often notice that food tastes much better. Smoking is not useful for weight loss, however. (Smoking for decades may lessen or prevent age-associated weight gain for some smokers, but for people under 30, smoking is not associated with weight loss.) Figure 11-2 summarizes these immediate effects.

The Long-Term Effects of Smoking

Smoking is linked to many deadly and disabling diseases. Research indicates that the total amount of tobacco smoke inhaled is a key factor contributing to disease. People who smoke more cigarettes per day, inhale deeply, puff frequently, smoke cigarettes down to the butts, or begin smoking at an early age run a greater risk of disease than do those who smoke more moderately or who do not smoke at all. Many diseases have already been linked to smoking, and as more research is done, even more diseases associated with smoking are being uncovered. The costliest ones—to society as well as to the individual—are cardiovascular diseases, respiratory diseases such as emphysema and lung cancer, and other cancers.

Cardiovascular Disease Although lung cancer tends to receive the most publicity, one form of cardiovascular disease, **coronary heart disease (CHD),** is actually the most widespread single cause of death for cigarette smokers. CHD often results from **atherosclerosis,** a condition in which fatty deposits called **plaques** form on the inner walls of heart arteries, causing them to narrow and stiffen. Smoking and exposure to environmental tobacco smoke (ETS) permanently accelerate the rate of plaque accumulation in the coronary arteries—50% for smokers, 25% for ex-smokers, and 20% for people regularly exposed to ETS. The crushing chest pain of **angina pectoris,** a primary symptom of CHD, results when the heart muscle, or *myocardium,* does not get enough oxygen. Sometimes a plaque forms at a narrow point in a main coronary artery. If the plaque completely blocks the flow of blood to a portion of the heart, that portion may die. This type of heart attack is called a **myocardial infarction.**

CHD can also interfere with the heart's electrical activity, resulting in disturbances of the normal heartbeat rhythm.

Terms

V w

cerebral cortex The outer layer of the brain, which controls complex behavior and mental activity.

coronary heart disease (CHD) Cardiovascular disease caused by hardening of the arteries that supply oxygen to the heart muscle; also called *coronary artery disease.*

atherosclerosis Cardiovascular disease caused by the deposit of fatty substances in the walls of the arteries.

plaque A deposit on the inner wall of blood vessels; blood can coagulate around plaque and form a clot.

angina pectoris Chest pain due to coronary heart disease.

myocardial infarction A heart attack caused by the complete blockage of a main coronary artery.

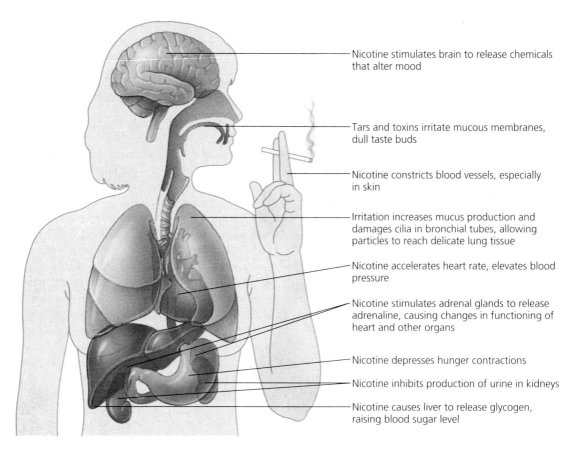

Figure 11-2 The short-term effects of smoking a cigarette.

Nicotine stimulates brain to release chemicals that alter mood

Tars and toxins irritate mucous membranes, dull taste buds

Nicotine constricts blood vessels, especially in skin

Irritation increases mucus production and damages cilia in bronchial tubes, allowing particles to reach delicate lung tissue

Nicotine accelerates heart rate, elevates blood pressure

Nicotine stimulates adrenal glands to release adrenaline, causing changes in functioning of heart and other organs

Nicotine depresses hunger contractions

Nicotine inhibits production of urine in kidneys

Nicotine causes liver to release glycogen, raising blood sugar level

Sudden and unexpected death is a common result of CHD, particularly among smokers. (See Chapter 15 for a more extensive discussion of cardiovascular disease.)

Smokers have a death rate from CHD that is 70% higher than that of nonsmokers. Deaths from CHD associated with cigarette smoking are most common in people age 40–50. (In contrast, deaths from lung cancer caused by smoking are most likely to occur in 60–70-year-olds.) Among people *under* age 40, smokers are five times more likely than nonsmokers to have a heart attack. Cigar and pipe smokers run a lower risk than cigarette smokers.

We do not completely understand how cigarette smoking increases the risk of CHD, but researchers are beginning to shed light on the process. Smoking reduces the amount of "good" cholesterol (high-density lipoprotein, or HDL) in the blood, thereby promoting plaque formation in artery walls. Smoking may also increase tension in heart muscle walls, speeding up the rate of muscular contraction and accelerating the heart rate. The workload of the heart thus increases, as does its need for oxygen and other nutrients. Carbon monoxide produced by cigarette smoking combines with hemoglobin in the red blood cells, displacing oxygen and thus providing less oxygen to the heart. One study showed that the additional blood supply available to the heart during stress was 21% less in smokers than in nonsmokers.

This reduced blood flow is an early indicator of future heart attacks or strokes.

The risks of CHD decrease rapidly when a person stops smoking; this is particularly true for younger smokers, whose coronary arteries have not yet been extensively damaged. Cigarette smoking has also been linked to other cardiovascular diseases, including the following:

- *Stroke*, a sudden interference with the circulation of blood in a part of the brain, resulting in the destruction of brain cells

- *Aortic aneurysm*, a bulge in the aorta caused by a weakening in its walls

- *Pulmonary heart disease*, a disorder of the right side of the heart, caused by changes in the blood vessels of the lungs

Lung Cancer and Other Cancers Cigarette smoking is the primary cause of lung cancer. A recent study identified the precise mechanism: Benzo(a)pyrene, a chemical found in tobacco smoke, causes genetic mutations in lung cells that are identical to those found in many patients with lung cancer. Those who smoke two or more packs of cigarettes a day have lung cancer death rates 12–25 times greater than those of nonsmokers. The dramatic rise in lung cancer rates among women in the past 40 years clearly parallels the increase of smoking in this group; lung cancer now exceeds breast cancer as the leading cause of cancer deaths among women. The risk of developing lung cancer increases with the number of cigarettes smoked each day, the number of years of smoking, and the age at which the person started smoking.

While cigar and pipe smokers have a higher risk of lung cancer than nonsmokers do, the risk is lower than that for cigarette smokers. Smoking filter-tipped cigarettes slightly reduces health hazards, unless the smoker compensates by smoking more, as is often the case.

Evidence suggests that after 1 year without smoking, the risk of lung cancer decreases substantially. After 10 years, the risk of lung cancer among ex-smokers is 50% of that of continuing smokers. The sooner one quits, the better: If smoking is stopped before cancer has started, lung tissue tends to repair itself, even if cellular changes that can lead to cancer are already present.

Research has also linked smoking to cancers of the trachea, mouth, pharynx, esophagus, larynx, pancreas, bladder, kidney, breast, cervix, stomach, liver, colon, and skin. For more information on cancer, see Chapter 16.

Chronic Obstructive Lung Disease The lungs of a smoker are constantly exposed to dangerous chemicals and irritants, and they must work harder to function adequately. The stresses placed on the lungs by smoking can permanently damage lung function and lead to *chronic obstructive lung disease (COLD)*, also known as chronic obstructive pulmonary disease. COLD is the fourth leading cause of death in the United States. This progressive and disabling disorder consists of several different but related diseases; emphysema and chronic bronchitis are two of the most common.

Cigarette smokers are up to 18 times more likely than nonsmokers to die from emphysema and chronic bronchitis. (Pipe and cigar smokers are more likely to die from COLD than are nonsmokers, but they have a smaller risk than cigarette smokers.) The risk of developing COLD rises with the number of cigarettes smoked and falls when smoking ceases. For most Americans, cigarette smoking is a more important cause of COLD than air pollution, but exposure to both is more dangerous than exposure to either by itself.

EMPHYSEMA Smoking is the primary cause of **emphysema,** a particularly disabling condition in which the walls of the air sacs in the lungs lose their elasticity and are gradually destroyed. The lungs' ability to obtain oxygen and remove carbon dioxide is impaired. A person with emphysema is breathless, is constantly gasping for air, and has the feeling of drowning. The heart must pump harder and may become enlarged. People with emphysema often die from a damaged heart. There is no known way to reverse this disease. In its advanced stage, the victim is bedridden and severely disabled.

CHRONIC BRONCHITIS Persistent, recurrent inflammation of the bronchial tubes characterizes **chronic bronchitis.** When the cell lining of the bronchial tubes is irritated, it secretes excess mucus. Bronchial congestion is followed by a chronic cough, which makes breathing more and more difficult. If smokers have chronic bronchitis, they face a greater risk of lung cancer, no matter how old they are or how many (or few) cigarettes they smoke. Chronic bronchitis seems to be a shortcut to lung cancer.

Other Respiratory Damage Even when the smoker shows no signs of lung impairment or disease, cigarette smoking damages the respiratory system. Normally the cells lining the bronchial tubes secrete mucus, a sticky fluid that collects particles of soot, dust, and other substances in inhaled air. Mucus is carried up to the mouth by the continuous motion of the cilia, hairlike structures that protrude from the inner surface of the bronchial tubes (Figure 11-3). If the cilia are destroyed or impaired, or if the pollution of inhaled air is more than the system can remove, the protection provided by cilia is lost.

Cigarette smoke first slows and then stops the action of the cilia. Eventually it destroys them, leaving delicate membranes exposed to injury from substances inhaled in cigarette smoke or from the polluted air in which the person lives or works. Special cells, *macrophages,* a type of white blood cell, also work to remove foreign particles from the respiratory tract by engulfing them. Smoking appears to make macrophages work less efficiently. This interference with the functioning of the respiratory system often leads rapidly to the conditions known as smoker's throat and smoker's cough, as well as to shortness of breath. Even smokers of high school age show impaired respiratory function, compared with nonsmokers of the same age. Other respiratory effects of smoking include a worsening of allergy and asthma symptoms and an increase in the smoker's susceptibility to colds.

Although cigarette smoking can cause many respiratory disorders and diseases, the damage is not always permanent. Once a person stops smoking, steady improvement in overall lung function usually takes place. Chronic coughing subsides, mucus production returns to normal, and breathing becomes easier. The likelihood of lung disease drops sharply. People of all ages, even those who have been smoking for decades, improve after they stop smoking. If given a chance, the human body has remarkable powers of restoring itself.

Terms

emphysema A disease characterized by a loss of lung tissue elasticity and breakup of the air sacs, impairing the lungs' ability to obtain oxygen and remove carbon dioxide.

chronic bronchitis Recurrent, persistent inflammation of the bronchial tubes.

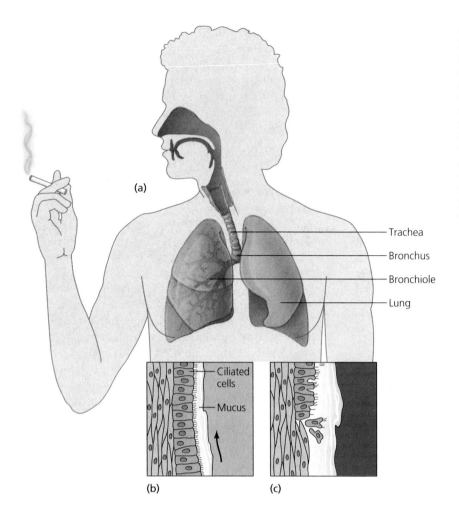

(a)

Trachea

Bronchus

Bronchiole

Lung

Ciliated cells

Mucus

(b)   (c)

Figure 11-3   Damage to the lungs caused by smoking.   (a) The respiratory system. (b) The inside of a bronchiole of a nonsmoker. Foreign particles are collected by a thin layer of sticky mucus and transported out of the lungs, up toward the mouth, by the action of cilia. (c) The inside of a bronchiole of a smoker. Smoking irritates the lung tissue and causes increased mucus production, which can overwhelm the action of the cilia. A smoker develops a chronic cough as the lungs try to rid themselves of foreign particles and excess mucus. Eventually the cilia are destroyed, leaving the delicate lung tissue exposed to injury from foreign substances.

Additional Health, Cosmetic, and Economic Concerns

- *Ulcers.* People who smoke are more likely to develop peptic ulcers and are more likely to die from them (especially stomach ulcers), because smoking impairs the body's healing ability. Smoking also increases the risk of gastroesophageal reflux, which causes heartburn and can, if severe, raise the risk of esophageal cancer.

- *Impotence.* Smoking affects blood flow in the veins and arteries of the penis, and it is an independent risk factor for impotence. In one recent study, smokers were twice as likely as nonsmokers to experience erectile dysfunction (impotence).

- *Reproductive health problems.* Smoking is linked to reduced fertility in both men and women. A study of 18-year-old smoking men found that they had a significantly higher proportion of abnormally shaped sperm and sperm with genetic defects than nonsmokers. In women, smoking can contribute to menstrual disorders, early menopause, and complications of pregnancy. See the box "Gender and Tobacco Use."

- *Dental diseases.* Smokers are at increased risk for tooth decay and gum and periodontal diseases, with symptoms appearing by the mid-20s.

- *Diminished physical senses.* Smoking dulls the senses of taste and smell. Over time, it increases the risk for hearing loss and cataracts (a serious eye condition that can result in partial or total blindness).

- *Injuries.* Smokers have higher rates of motor vehicle crashes, fire-related injuries, and back pain.

- *Cosmetic concerns.* Smoking can cause premature skin wrinkling, premature baldness, stained teeth, discolored fingers, and a persistent tobacco odor in clothes and hair.

- *Economic costs.* In 2003, the average per-pack price of cigarettes was $4.04. A pack-a-day habit costs nearly $1500 each year for cigarettes alone. Other costs include higher health and home insurance premiums; more frequent cleaning of clothes, teeth, home, office, and car; and repair of burnt clothing, upholstery, and carpeting—for a cost of $3000 per year. A study by researchers at Duke University estimated that the total cost for a 24-year-old—including cigarettes, lost earnings, insurance costs, and harm done by environmental tobacco smoke—is nearly $40 per pack.

American men are currently more likely than women to smoke, but women younger than age 23 are becoming smokers at a faster rate than any other population segment. As the rate of smoking among women approaches that of men, so do rates of tobacco-related illness and death. Lung cancer, emphysema, and cardiovascular diseases sicken and kill both men and women who smoke, and more American women now die each year from lung cancer than from breast cancer.

Although overall risks of tobacco-related illness are similar for women and men, sex appears to make a difference in some diseases. Women, for example, are more at risk for smoking-related blood clots and strokes than are men, and the risk is even greater for women using oral contraceptives. Among men and women with the same smoking history, the odds for developing three major types of cancer, including lung cancer, is 1.2–1.7 times higher in women than in men. One possible explanation for this difference is that women are more likely to use low-tar cigarettes and thus engage in compensatory behaviors such as deep inhalation, which is linked to increased respiratory damage. Women may also have a greater biological vulnerability to lung cancer.

For both men and women, tobacco use is associated with increased incidence of sex-specific health problems. Men who smoke increase their risk of erectile dysfunction and infertility due to reduced sperm density and motility. Women who smoke have higher rates of osteoporosis (a bone-thinning disease that can lead to fractures), thyroid-related diseases, and depression.

Women who smoke also have risks associated with reproduction and the reproductive organs. Smoking is associated with greater menstrual bleeding, greater duration of painful menstrual cramps, and more variability in menstrual cycle length. Smokers have a more difficult time becoming pregnant, and they reach menopause on average a year or two earlier than nonsmokers. When women smokers become pregnant, they face increased chances of miscarriage or placental disorders that lead to bleeding and premature delivery; rates of ectopic pregnancy, preeclampsia, and stillbirth are also higher among women who smoke. Smoking is a risk factor for cervical cancer.

When women decide to try to stop smoking, they are more likely than men to join a support group. Overall, though, women are less successful than men in quitting. Women report more severe withdrawal symptoms when they stop smoking and are more likely than men to report cravings in response to social and behavioral cues associated with smoking. For men, relapse to smoking is often associated with work or social pressure; women are more likely to relapse when sad or depressed or concerned about weight gain. Women and men also respond differently to medications: Nicotine replacement therapy appears to work better for men, whereas the non-nicotine medication bupropion appears to work better for women.

In addition, smoking contributes to osteoporosis, increases the risk of complications from diabetes, and accelerates the course of multiple sclerosis. Further research may link tobacco use to still other disorders.

Cumulative Effects The cumulative effects of tobacco use fall into two general categories. The first category is reduced life expectancy. A male who takes up smoking before age 15 and continues to smoke is only half as likely to live to age 75 as a male who never smokes. If he inhales deeply, he risks losing a minute of life for every minute of smoking. Females who have similar smoking habits also have a reduced life expectancy. Smoking reduces their life expectancy by more than 10 years.

The second category involves quality of life. A national health survey begun in 1964 shows that smokers spend one-third more time away from their jobs because of illness than nonsmokers. Female smokers spend 17% more days sick in bed than female nonsmokers. Lost work days due to smoking number in the millions.

Both men and women smokers show a greater rate of acute and chronic disease than people who have never smoked. Smokers become disabled at younger ages than nonsmokers and have more years of unhealthy life in addition to a shorter life span. The U.S. Public Health Service estimates that if all people had the same rate of disease as those who never smoked, there would be 1 million fewer cases of chronic bronchitis, 1.8 million fewer cases of **sinusitis**, and 1 million fewer cases of peptic ulcers in the country every year.

Other Forms of Tobacco Use

Many smokers have switched from cigarettes to other forms of tobacco, such as spit (smokeless) tobacco, cigars and pipes, and clove cigarettes and bidis. However, each of these alternatives is far from safe.

Spit (Smokeless) Tobacco More than 5 million adults and about 6% of all high school students are current spit tobacco users. Spit tobacco use has increased in recent years and is especially common among Native Americans, adolescent males (especially white males),

Term

sinusitis Inflammation of the sinus cavities; symptoms include headache, fever, and pain.

Cigars contain more tobacco than cigarettes and so produce more tar when smoked. Cigar smokers face an increased risk of cancer even if they don't inhale the smoke.

male college athletes, and professional baseball players. About 80% of users start by the ninth grade.

Spit tobacco comes in two major forms: snuff and chewing tobacco (chew). In snuff, the tobacco leaf is processed into a coarse, moist powder and mixed with flavorings. Snuff is usually sold in small tins. Users place a "pinch," "dip," or "quid" between the lower lip or cheek and gum and suck on it. In chewing tobacco, the tobacco leaf may be shredded ("leaf"), pressed into bricks or cakes ("plugs"), or dried and twisted into rope-like strands ("twists"). Chew is usually sold in pouches. Users place a wad of tobacco in their mouth and then chew or suck it to release the nicotine. All types of smokeless tobacco cause an increase in saliva production, and the resulting tobacco juice is spit out or swallowed.

The nicotine in spit tobacco—along with flavorings and additives—is absorbed through the gums and lining of the mouth. Holding an average-size dip in the mouth for 30 minutes delivers about the same amount of nicotine as two or three cigarettes. Because of its nicotine content, spit tobacco is highly addictive. Some users keep it in their mouth even while sleeping.

Although not as dangerous as smoking cigarettes, the use of spit tobacco carries many health risks. Changes can occur in the mouth after only a few weeks of use: Gums and lips become dried and irritated and may bleed. White or red patches may appear inside the mouth; this condition, known as *leukoplakia,* can lead to oral cancer (see below). A study of major league baseball players found dangerous mouth lesions in 83

out of the 141 spit tobacco–using players who were examined. Other studies have found even higher rates of oral sores. About 25% of regular spit tobacco users have *gingivitis* (inflammation) and recession of the gums and bone loss around the teeth, especially where the tobacco is usually placed. The senses of taste and smell are usually dulled. In addition, other people find the presence of wads of tobacco in the mouth, stained teeth, bad breath, and behaviors such as frequent spitting to be unpleasant.

One of the most serious effects of spit tobacco is an increased risk of oral cancer—cancers of the lip, tongue, cheek, throat, gums, roof and floor of the mouth, and larynx. Spit tobacco contains at least 28 chemicals known to cause cancer, and long-term snuff use may increase the risk of oral cancer by as much as 50 times. Surgery to treat oral cancer is often disfiguring and may involve removing parts of the face, tongue, cheek, or lip.

Data on the incidence of heart disease among spit tobacco users have not yet been collected. But it is known that dipping and chewing tobacco produce blood levels of nicotine similar to those in cigarette smokers. High blood levels of nicotine have dangerous effects on the cardiovascular system, including elevation of blood pressure, heart rate, and blood levels of certain fats. Other chemicals in spit tobacco are believed to pose risks to developing fetuses.

Cigars and Pipes   After more than two decades of decline, cigar smoking has increased by nearly 50% since 1993. The popularity of cigars is highest among white males age 18–44 with higher-than-average income and education, but women are also smoking cigars in record numbers. Cigar use is also growing among young people: In the latest government surveys, 12% of high school students reported having smoked at least one cigar in the previous month. An estimated 2% of Americans, mostly males who also smoke cigarettes, are pipe smokers.

Cigars are made from rolled whole tobacco leaves; pipe tobacco is made from shredded leaves and often flavored. Because cigar and pipe smoke are more alkaline than cigarette smoke, users of cigars and pipes do not need to inhale in order to ingest nicotine; instead, they absorb nicotine through the gums and lining of the mouth. Cigars contain more tobacco than cigarettes and so contain more nicotine and produce more tar when smoked. Large cigars may contain as much tobacco as a whole pack of cigarettes and take 1–2 hours to smoke.

The smoke from cigars contains many of the same toxins and carcinogens as the smoke from cigarettes, some in much higher quantities. The health risks of cigars depend on the number of cigars smoked and whether the smoker inhales. Because most cigar and pipe users do not inhale, they have a lower risk of cancer and cardiovascular and respiratory diseases than cigarette smokers. However, their risks are substantially higher than those of nonsmokers. For example, compared to nonsmokers, people who smoke one or two cigars per day without inhaling have six times the risk of cancer of the larynx. The risks are much higher for cigar smokers who do inhale: They have 27 times the risk of oral cancer and 53 times the risk of cancer of the larynx compared to nonsmokers, and their risk of heart and lung diseases approaches that of cigarette smokers. Smoking a cigar immediately impairs the ability of blood vessels to dilate, reducing the amount of oxygen delivered to tissues, including heart muscle, especially during times of stress. Pipe and cigar smoking are also risk factors for pancreatic cancer, which is almost always fatal.

Nicotine addiction is another concern. Most adults who smoke cigars do so only occasionally, and there is little evidence that use of cigars by adults leads to addiction. The recent rise in cigar use among teens has raised concerns, however, because nicotine addiction almost always develops in the teen or young adult years. More research is needed to determine if cigar use by teens will develop into nicotine addiction and frequent use of either cigarettes or spit tobacco. In June of 2000 the FTC announced an agreement to put warning labels on cigar packages, 34 years after warning labels first appeared on cigarette packages.

Clove Cigarettes and Bidis   Clove cigarettes, also called "kreteks" or "chicartas," are made of tobacco mixed with chopped cloves; they are imported primarily from Indonesia and Pakistan. Clove cigarettes contain almost twice as much tar, nicotine, and carbon monoxide as conventional cigarettes and so have all the same health hazards. Some chemical constituents of cloves may also be dangerous. For example, eugenol, an anesthetic compound found in cloves, may impair the respiratory system's ability to detect and defend against foreign particles. There have been a number of serious respiratory injuries and deaths from the use of clove cigarettes.

Bidis, or "beadies," are small cigarettes imported from India that contain species of tobacco different from those used by U.S. cigarette manufacturers. The tobacco in bidis is hand-rolled in Indian ebony leaves (tendu) and then often flavored; clove, mint, chocolate, and fruit varieties are available. Bidis contain up to four times more nicotine than and twice as much tar as U.S. cigarettes. Use of bidis has been growing among teens, possibly because of the flavorings they contain or because they look and smell somewhat like marijuana cigarettes (joints); they do not have the same effects as marijuana, however.

Currently, an estimated 3% of high school students use clove cigarettes or bidis (Figure 11-4). Neither is a safe or healthy alternative to conventional tobacco cigarettes.

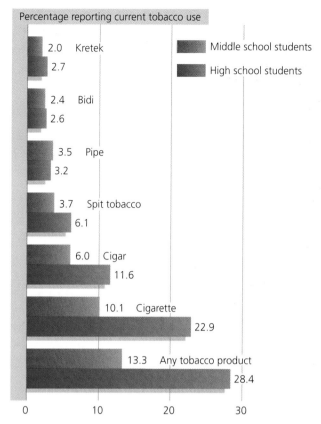

Percentage reporting current tobacco use

Middle school students
High school students

	Middle school	High school
Kretek	2.0	2.7
Bidi	2.4	2.6
Pipe	3.5	3.2
Spit tobacco	3.7	6.1
Cigar	6.0	11.6
Cigarette	10.1	22.9
Any tobacco product	13.3	28.4

VITAL STATISTICS

Figure 11-4   Tobacco use among middle school and high school students.   Although it is illegal for those under age 18 to purchase tobacco, 13.3% of middle school and 28.4% of high school students report having used some form of tobacco within the past month.
SOURCE: Centers for Disease Control and Prevention. 2003. Tobacco use among middle and high school students—United States, 2002. *Morbidity and Mortality Weekly Report* 52(45): 1096–1098.

THE EFFECTS OF SMOKING ON THE NONSMOKER

In a watershed decision in 1993, the U.S. Environmental Protection Agency (EPA) designated **environmental tobacco smoke (ETS)** a Class A carcinogen—an agent known to cause cancer in humans. In 2000, the Department of Health and Human Services' National Toxicology Program classified ETS as a "known human carcinogen." These designations put ETS in the same category as notorious cancer-causing agents like asbestos. Every year, ETS causes thousands of deaths from lung cancer and heart

Term

environmental tobacco smoke (ETS) Smoke that enters the atmosphere from the burning end of a cigarette, cigar, or pipe, as well as smoke that is exhaled by smokers; also called *secondhand smoke.*

disease and is responsible for hundreds of thousands of respiratory infections in young children. The health effects of ETS are the basis for efforts to limit or ban smoking in public and in the workplace.

Environmental Tobacco Smoke

Environmental tobacco smoke, or *secondhand smoke,* consists of mainstream smoke and sidestream smoke. Smoke exhaled by smokers is referred to as **mainstream smoke. Sidestream smoke** enters the atmosphere from the burning end of a cigarette, cigar, or pipe. Undiluted sidestream smoke, because it is not filtered through either a cigarette filter or a smoker's lungs, has significantly higher concentrations of the toxic and carcinogenic compounds found in mainstream smoke. For example, compared to mainstream smoke, sidestream smoke has (1) twice as much tar and nicotine; (2) three times as much benzo(a)pyrene, a carcinogen; (3) almost three times as much carbon monoxide, which displaces oxygen from red blood cells and forms *carboxyhemoglobin,* a dangerous compound that seriously limits the body's ability to use oxygen; and (4) three times as much ammonia.

Nearly 85% of the smoke in a room where someone is smoking comes from sidestream smoke. Of course, sidestream smoke is diffused through the air, so nonsmokers don't inhale the same concentrations of toxic chemicals that the smoker does. Still, the concentrations can be high. In rooms where people are smoking, levels of carbon monoxide, for instance, can exceed those permitted by Federal Air Quality Standards for outside air. In a typical home with the windows closed, it takes about 6 hours for 95% of the airborne cigarette smoke particles to clear.

The secondhand smoke from a cigar can be even more dangerous than that from cigarettes. The EPA has found that the output of carcinogenic particles from a cigar exceeds that of three cigarettes, and cigar smoke contains up to 30 times more carbon monoxide.

ETS Effects Studies show that up to 25% of nonsmokers subjected to ETS develop coughs, 30% develop headaches and nasal discomfort, and 70% suffer from eye irritation. Other symptoms range from breathlessness to sinus problems. People with allergies tend to suffer the most. The odor of tobacco smoke clings to skin and clothes—another unpleasant effect of ETS.

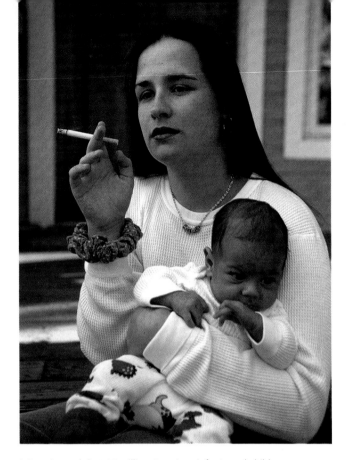

It is estimated that 19 million American infants and children are regularly exposed to environmental tobacco smoke. ETS can cause SIDS, trigger respiratory infections, cause or aggravate asthma, contribute to middle-ear infections, and impair development.

But ETS causes more than just annoyance and discomfort; it causes 3000 lung cancer deaths annually. People who live, work, or socialize among smokers face a 24–50% increase in lung cancer risk. ETS is also responsible for about 60,000 deaths from cardiovascular disease each year. As described earlier, exposure to ETS is associated with a 20% increase in the progression of atherosclerosis. ETS also aggravates asthma, an increasing cause of sudden death in otherwise healthy adults, and increases the risk for breast and cervical cancers. Scientists have been able to measure changes that contribute to lung tissue damage and potential tumor promotion in the bloodstreams of healthy young test subjects who spend just 3 hours in a smoke-filled room. After just 30 minutes of exposure to ETS, the endothelial function in the coronary arteries of healthy nonsmokers is reduced to the same level as that of smokers. And nonsmokers can still be affected by the harmful effects of ETS hours after they have left a smoky environment. Carbon monoxide, for example, lingers in the bloodstream 5 hours later.

Infants, Children, and ETS Recent studies have shown that infants exposed to smoke from more than 21 cigarettes a day are more than 23 times more likely to die of sudden infant death syndrome (SIDS) than babies not exposed to ETS. The National Cancer Institute recently estimated that ETS causes up to 18,600 cases of low birth

Terms

mainstream smoke Smoke that is inhaled by a smoker and then exhaled into the atmosphere.

sidestream smoke Smoke that comes from the burning end of a cigarette, cigar, or pipe.

weight each year. Children under 5 whose primary care-giver smokes 10 or more cigarettes per day have measurable blood levels of nicotine and tobacco carcinogens. Chemicals in tobacco smoke also show up in breast milk, and breastfeeding may pass more chemicals to the infant of a smoking mother than direct exposure to ETS.

ETS triggers 150,000–300,000 cases of bronchitis, pneumonia, and other respiratory infections in infants and toddlers up to age 18 months each year, resulting in 7,500–15,000 hospitalizations. Older children suffer, too. ETS is a risk factor for asthma in children who have not previously displayed symptoms of the disease, and it aggravates the symptoms of the 200,000 to 1 million children who already have asthma. ETS is also linked to reduced lung function and fluid buildup in the middle ear, a contributing factor in middle-ear infections, a leading reason for childhood surgery. Children and teens exposed to ETS score lower on tests of reading and reasoning. Later in life, people exposed to ETS as children are at increased risk for lung cancer, emphysema, and chronic bronchitis.

Why are infants and children so vulnerable? Because they breathe faster than adults, they inhale more air—and more of the pollutants in the air. Because they also weigh less, they inhale three times more pollutants per unit of body weight than adults do. And because their young lungs are still growing, this intake can impair optimal development. The problem is widespread: About 19 million American children are exposed to ETS.

Avoiding ETS Given the health risks of exposure to ETS, try these strategies to keep the air around you safe:

- *Speak up tactfully.* Smokers may not know the dangers they are causing or may not know it bothers you.
- *Display reminders.* Put up signs asking smokers to refrain in your home, work area, and car.
- *Don't allow smoking in your home or room.* Get rid of ashtrays and ask smokers to light up outside.
- *Open a window.* If you cannot avoid being in a room with a smoker, at least try to provide some ventilation.
- *Sit in the nonsmoking section in restaurants and other public areas.* Complain to the manager if none exists.
- *Fight for a smoke-free work environment.* Join with your coworkers to either eliminate all smoking indoors or confine it to certain areas.
- *Discuss quitting strategies.* Social pressure is a major factor in many former smokers' decisions to quit. Help the smokers in your life by sharing quitting strategies with them.

Smoking and Pregnancy

Smoking almost doubles a pregnant woman's chance of having a miscarriage, and it significantly increases her risk of ectopic pregnancy. Maternal smoking causes an estimated 4600 infant deaths in the United States each year, primarily due to premature delivery and smoking-related problems with the placenta. Maternal smoking is a major factor in low birth weight, which puts newborns at high risk for infections and other serious problems. If a nonsmoking mother is regularly exposed to ETS, her infant is also at greater risk for low birth weight. Recent studies have also shown that babies whose mothers smoked during pregnancy had higher rates of colic, clubfoot, cleft lip and palate, and impaired lung function; they may also have genetic damage.

Babies born to mothers who smoke more than two packs a day perform poorly on developmental tests in the first hours after birth, compared to babies of nonsmoking mothers. Later in life, obesity, hyperactivity, short attention span, and lower scores on spelling and reading tests all occur more frequently in children whose mothers smoked during pregnancy than in those born to nonsmoking mothers. Prenatal tobacco exposure has also been associated with behavioral problems in children, including immaturity, emotional instability, physical aggression, and hyperactivity. Other research shows that teenagers whose mothers smoked during pregnancy have lower scores on tests of general intelligence and poorer performance on tasks requiring auditory memory than do children who were not exposed to cigarette smoke before birth. Males born to smoking mothers have higher rates of adolescent and adult criminal activity, suggesting that maternal smoking may cause brain damage that increases the risk of criminal behavior. Nevertheless, about 11% of pregnant women smoke and only about 14% of female smokers quit while pregnant; *Healthy People 2010* sets a goal of increasing this to 30%.

The Cost of Tobacco Use to Society

The health care costs associated with smoking exceed $75 billion per year. If the cost of lost productivity from sickness, disability, and premature death is included, the total is closer to $157 billion. This works out to $7.18 per pack of cigarettes, far more than the average $0.84 per pack tax collected by states to offset tobacco-related medical costs.

In order to recoup public health care expenditures, 43 state attorneys general filed suit against tobacco companies. In March 1997, Liggett Group settled its part of the suit by agreeing to turn over internal documents and to pay a portion of its profits to cover tobacco-related medical expenses and anti-smoking campaigns. In November 1998, an agreement was reached that settled 39 state lawsuits and applied to seven states that never filed suit. (Four states—Florida, Minnesota, Mississippi, and Texas—settled their suits separately for a total of $40 billion.) The 1998 Master Settlement Agreement (MSA) requires the tobacco companies to pay states $206 billion over 25 years; it also limits or bans certain types of advertising, promotions, and lobbying. Many of the provisions of the deal are designed to limit youth exposure and access to tobacco. In exchange, the tobacco industry settled the state lawsuits and is protected

In the News

In the 1998 Master Settlement Agreement (MSA), the tobacco industry agreed to pay states more than $200 billion over 25 years as compensation for tobacco-related health care costs and as a penalty for deceptive marketing of their addictive and dangerous products. The legal, economic, and social impact of the MSA continues to influence tobacco use and control. Since the settlement, tobacco use has begun declining, acceptance of smoking—in public buildings and private workplaces—is decreasing, and quit-smoking programs are becoming more widely available.

Tobacco companies are fighting these trends. In 2004, industry lobbying contributed to the decision by Congress to abandon legislative efforts to permit the FDA to regulate tobacco—the only legal product that kills at least a third of those who use it regularly—in the same way that the agency now regulates products such as breakfast cereal or lip gloss. Industry expenditures on marketing have increased, emphasizing discounts, promotion of existing brands, and the introduction of new products—still addictive and dangerous but promoted as stylish or less harmful.

Not all of the new products are cigarettes and not all of them are new. The Smokeless Tobacco Company petitioned the FTC to allow spit tobacco, identified by the U.S. Surgeon General 20 years ago as a cause of oral cancer, to be advertised as less harmful than cigarettes. The smokeless tobacco industry is also attempting to improve its less than elegant image by going spitless. Revel is a tea bag–like product that is sucked and "discarded." A lozenge called Ariva, made of compressed tobacco, dissolves in the user's mouth.

Conventional cigarettes are also being promoted with a new look and new less harmful identity. Philip Morris introduced a product called Accord, which looks like a conventional cigarette but does not burn; instead it is heated in an electronic device the size of a pager. Brands called Eclipse and Advance were touted as less harmful but delivered increased carbon monoxide; in one test, smokers inhaled 25% more nicotine from Advance than from their standard brand.

Recent reductions in smoking rates are in part the result of actions by state governments. Legislatures passed increases in tobacco taxes, driving up the price of smoking. Research suggests that a 10% increase in the price of cigarettes reduces youth smoking by 7% and overall cigarette sales by 3–5%. States have also used settlement funds to pay for educational campaigns that reduce the number of new smokers and encourage quitting. This spending, too, pays dividends: Each dollar spent to control tobacco yields a savings of $3 in smoking-related health costs.

In recent years, however, states have shifted settlement money from tobacco control to other budget obligations. Overall, states cut tobacco control spending from the settlement fund by nearly a third—from $750 million to $538 million—in fiscal years 2002–2005. Most states spend less than half the recommended amount, and several spend no settlement money on tobacco control.

Tobacco use will soon become the leading cause of death worldwide. The World Health Organization (WHO) estimates that tobacco accounted for more than 3 million deaths in 1990 and 5 million in 2000. Deaths are projected to more than double by 2020, with 70% of these deaths taking place in developing countries. The tobacco industry—faced with increased regulation, growing awareness of the health risks of smoking, and declining sales in Europe and North America—has stepped up activities to establish and expand markets in the developing world. The poor will be increasingly victimized by tobacco and its burden of disease.

To help protect health worldwide, WHO developed the Framework Convention on Tobacco Control (FCTC), a global public health treaty designed to reduce tobacco-related deaths and disease. FCTC sets international standards on tobacco price and tax increases, tobacco advertising and sponsorship, health warnings and labeling, illicit trade, and secondhand smoke. FCTC attained the status of international law in 2004, when Peru became the 40th country to ratify the protocol; it entered into force in February 2005. The United States signed the treaty in 2004, but the treaty has not yet been ratified by the Senate and written into U.S. law.

SOURCES: Hatsukami, D. K., and M. Zeller. 2004. Tobacco harm reduction: The need for research to inform policy. *Psychological Science Agenda,* April (http://www.apa.org/science/psa/sb-hatsukami.html; retrieved December 6, 2004); Lee, E. M., et al. 2004. Quantitative comparisons between a nicotine delivery device (Eclipse) and conventional cigarette smoking. *Nicotine and Tobacco Research* 6(1): 95–102; Wahlberg, D. 2004. Smoking: Products claim to lower risks. Is less bad good? Health officials wary of claims that new products lower smoking dangers. *Atlanta Journal-Constitution,* October 3 (http://www.ajc.com/news/content/health/1004/04smoking.html; retrieved December 6, 2004); Breland, A. B., et al. 2002. Evaluating acute effects of potential reduced-exposure products for smokers: Clinical laboratory methodology. *Nicotine and Tobacco Research* 4(Suppl 2): 131–140.

from future suits by states, counties, towns, and other public entities. Tobacco companies passed the costs of the settlement on to smokers, increasing the average price of a pack of cigarettes by approximately 45 cents.

The governors involved in the MSA unanimously declared themselves "committed to spending a significant portion of the tobacco settlement funds on smoking cessation programs, health care, education, and programs benefiting children." A report prepared on the fifth anniversary of the settlement found that only four states—Maine, Delaware, Mississippi, and Arkansas—fund tobacco prevention and cessation programs at minimum levels recommended by the CDC. In a survey by the U.S. General Accounting Office, only nine states reported plans to spend more than 10% of their settlement money on tobacco control programs in 2004; nine planned to spend more than half on budget deficits (see the box "After the Master Settlement Agreement").

In March 2000 the Supreme Court ruled that the FDA lacks the authority to regulate tobacco products, stopping the FDA's efforts to prevent tobacco sales and marketing aimed at minors. Among the FDA's guidelines affected by the ruling is the requirement that retailers ask for identification from tobacco purchasers who appear to be under age 27.

In 2004, the U.S. Congress passed a major spending and corporate tax reform bill after dropping a provision that would have reestablished FDA authority over tobacco products. However, both House and Senate voted to retain in the bill a provision that pays tobacco farmers nearly $10 billion to give up a federal quota program that has propped up tobacco prices.

In July 2000, a Florida jury ordered tobacco companies to pay a $145 billion penalty in a class-action suit filed on behalf of sick Florida smokers, the largest penalty in U.S. history. A Florida appeals court ruled that the MSA did not allow punitive damages; that decision has been appealed. The Justice Department is arguing in a federal court that tobacco companies violated racketeering laws by conspiring to mislead the public about the dangers of smoking. For current information on political and legal activities, call or visit the Web site of one of the tobacco control advocacy groups listed in the For More Information section at the end of the chapter.

WHAT CAN BE DONE?

Every hour, 60 Americans die from preventable smoking-related diseases. Today there are more avenues than ever before for individual and group action against this major public health threat.

Action at the Local Level

Before the EPA issued its report declaring ETS to be a carcinogen, most efforts to limit smoking focused on enacting local laws and ordinances. Tobacco interests have been able to block actions at the national and state levels through lobbying and political contributions. However, during the 1980s and 1990s, tobacco restrictions were passed by local school boards, town councils, and county boards of supervisors, over which the tobacco industry has little or no influence.

There are now thousands of local ordinances across the nation that restrict or ban smoking in restaurants, stores, and workplaces. Since the EPA classification of environmental tobacco smoke as a carcinogen, local governments and businesses have become bolder about protecting nonsmokers. Even public outdoor areas are not exempt from regulations: Sharon, Massachusetts, has banned smoking at all beaches and playgrounds. Honolulu, Hawaii, has also banned smoking at the beach, but for a different reason—to protect sea turtles from being poisoned by eating cigarette butts.

As local no-smoking rules proliferate, evidence is mounting that such restrictions encourage smokers to quit. The smoking rate dropped from one in three adults in 1980 to one in four in 2004.

Action at the State and Federal Levels

The EPA report fundamentally changed the politics of tobacco by declaring that smokers not only shorten their own lives but also kill innocent bystanders. It became harder for politicians who are sympathetic to the tobacco industry—and who often accept sizable contributions from tobacco interests—to argue that anti-tobacco laws constitute unwarranted intrusions into voters' private lives.

State legislatures have passed many tough new anti-tobacco laws. California has one of the most aggressive—and successful—tobacco control programs, combining taxes on cigarettes, graphic advertisements, and bans on smoking in bars and restaurants. In the past decade, per-capita cigarette consumption fell by 50% in California, lung cancer cases dropped 14%, and heart disease deaths were reduced by more than 30,000. California now has the second lowest rate of smoking among U.S. states. Utah, with a smoking rate of 12%, is the first (and only) state to meet the *Healthy People 2010* target. Kentucky has the highest rate, 31%.

California, Delaware, New York, Connecticut, Maine, Massachusetts, and Rhode Island have smoke-free workplace laws that cover all workers. Florida, Idaho, and Utah have passed similar legislation, excluding stand-alone bars. Other states are considering similar protection for their citizens. An assessment made in 2004 found that 33% of Americans live in municipalities with smoke-free restaurants, 21% in locations with smoke-free workplaces and government buildings, and 11% in cities and towns with protection in all three areas.

The federal government is also acting to protect non-smokers from ETS. Smoking has been banned on virtually all domestic airplane flights, and the U.S. Defense Department has banned smoking at all military work sites. And the U.S. Occupational Safety and Health Administration considered nationwide rules that would, in effect, ban smoking on the job except in specially ventilated areas.

International Action

Many countries are following the United States' lead in restricting smoking. Smoking is now banned on many international air flights, as well as in many restaurants and hotels and on public transportation in some countries. The World Health Organization has taken the lead in international anti-tobacco efforts by sponsoring the Framework Convention on Tobacco Control, an international treaty designed to improve tobacco control efforts worldwide. Another international activity is the annual commemoration of World No Tobacco Day (May 31), on which smokers are encouraged to stop smoking for one day. (This is similar to the American Cancer Society's Great American Smokeout®, held each November.) The smoker who successfully takes the first step of quitting for a day may be

The U.S. Public Health Service recommends a "Five A's" approach for physicians to help patients quit tobacco use. If someone you care about uses tobacco, you can try the same strategies to help them quit.

1. **Ask** about tobacco use. How many cigarettes does your girlfriend smoke each day? How long has your roommate been dipping snuff?

2. **Advise** tobacco users to stop. Express your concern over the tobacco user's habit. "When we're close, the smell of smoke on your hair and breath bothers me. I've noticed you cough a lot and your voice is raspy. I'm worried about your health. You should stop."

3. **Assess** the tobacco user's willingness to quit. "Next week would be a good time to try to quit. Would you be willing to give it a try?"

4. **Assist** the tobacco user who is willing to stop. To coincide with your partner's quit date, take him away for a romantic weekend far from the places he associates with smoking. Offer to be an exercise partner. Call once a day to offer support and help. Bring gifts of low-calorie snacks or projects that occupy the hands. If the quitter lapses, be encouraging. A lapse doesn't have to become a relapse.

5. **Arrange** follow-up. Maintaining abstinence is an ongoing process. Celebrate milestones of 1 week, 1 month, 1 year without tobacco. Note how much better your friend's or partner's car, room, and person smell, how much healthier he or she is, and how much you appreciate not having to breathe tobacco smoke.

Keep in mind the special influence that a partner or loved one can have on someone who is trying to quit using tobacco. Recent research has shown that certain kinds of behavior by a partner are consistently related to successful quitting, whereas other behaviors are related to relapse. Behaviors linked to success include expressing pleasure at the smoker's efforts to quit, actively rewarding the smoker's efforts (for example, giving a small gift), helping to calm the smoker when he or she is feeling stressed or irritable, and actively sharing in an activity such as dancing, jogging, or hiking that serves as a distraction from smoking.

Sometimes a tobacco user's partner does things that are intended to be helpful but actually interfere with the user's efforts to quit. These behaviors include hiding ashtrays, keeping track of the amount of tobacco used, hiding or throwing out the smoker's cigarettes, frequently mentioning the health risks associated with tobacco, ignoring the smoker during efforts to quit, downplaying the difficulty of quitting, and complaining about the partner's irritability during attempts to quit.

If your partner is trying to quit and you are uncertain how to help, ask what would be most helpful. Recognize that tobacco use is your partner's problem, and although there may be things you can do to help, your partner is ultimately in control of his or her own body. If your partner asks you to back off, then do so within the limits you have established in your relationship. If your partner gets angry or irritable, recognize that this hypersensitivity is a normal but temporary side effect of nicotine withdrawal and remind yourself that it will pass. Listen to your partner, communicate your feelings as clearly as possible, and do what you can to reduce your partner's stress level, such as temporarily taking over a household chore. If you smoke, you can help your partner by not smoking in open view and by providing positive support. Even better, take inspiration from your partner's efforts and quit.

SOURCE: "Five A's" from Fiore, E. M. C., et al. 2000. *Treating Tobacco Use and Dependence.* Clinical Practice Guideline. Rockville, Md.: U.S. Department of Health and Human Services.

encouraged enough to follow through on the commitment and become a permanent nonsmoker. With more than 1 billion smokers worldwide, addressing the global impact of tobacco use will require a massive coordinated effort.

Action in the Private Sector

The EPA report also shook up the private sector, giving employers reason to fear worker's compensation claims based on exposure to workplace smoke. The year after the report was issued, businesses including McDonald's and Taco Bell banned smoking in thousands of their restaurants across the country. The number of smoke-free restaurants has increased dramatically in recent years, and the vast majority of the nation's shopping malls now prohibit smoking.

Such local, state, national, and international efforts represent progress, but health activists warn that tobacco industry influence remains strong. The tobacco industry contributes heavily to sympathetic legislative officeholders and candidates. Many states have relatively weak antismoking laws that are backed by the tobacco industry and include clauses that prevent the passage of stricter local ordinances. Since 1999, tobacco interests have spent more than $112 million on federal lobbying activities. During the 2003–2004 election cycle, the industry gave nearly $2.8 million to federal candidates, political parties, and political committees.

Individual Action

When a smoker violates a no-smoking designation, complain. If your favorite restaurant or shop doesn't have a nonsmoking policy, ask the manager to adopt one. If you see children buying tobacco, report this illegal activity to the facility manager or the police. Learn more about addiction and tobacco cessation so you can better support the tobacco users you know (see the box "Helping a Friend or Partner Stop Using Tobacco"). Vote for candidates who support anti-tobacco measures; contact local, state, and national representatives to express your views.

Cancel your subscriptions to magazines that carry tobacco advertising; send a letter to the publisher explaining your decision. Voice your opinion about other positive representations of tobacco use. (A recent study found that more than two-thirds of children's animated feature films have featured tobacco or alcohol use with no clear message that such practices were unhealthy.) Volunteer with the American Lung Association, the American Cancer Society, or the American Heart Association.

These are just some of the many ways in which individuals can help support tobacco prevention and stop-smoking efforts. Nonsmokers not only have the right to breathe clean air but also have the right to take action to help solve one of society's most serious public health threats.

Controlling the Tobacco Companies

With their immensely profitable industry shrinking, tobacco companies are concentrating on appealing to narrower and narrower market segments with an ever-increasing array of brands and styles—over 350 in all. As tobacco use has declined among better-educated, wealthier segments of the American population, tobacco companies have redirected their marketing efforts toward minorities, the poor, and young women, populations among whom smoking rates are still high. This practice of targeting specific segments of the market has become controversial, especially when the segment has an unusually high risk for fatal diseases caused by tobacco use.

With cigarette sales falling in the United States, tobacco companies have begun focusing on increasing the export of cigarettes, particularly to developing nations. As companies compete for customers in the years ahead, the need to exercise public pressure to keep the powerful tobacco companies in check will persist.

HOW A TOBACCO USER CAN QUIT

Since 1964, over 50% of all adults who have ever smoked have quit. Giving up tobacco is a long-term, intricate process. Heavy smokers who say they have just stopped cold turkey don't tell of the thinking and struggling and other mental processes that contributed to their final conquest over this powerful addiction. Olympic diver Greg Louganis, who began smoking at the age of 8, has said that he considers quitting, at the age of 23, the greatest accomplishment of his life.

Research shows that tobacco users move through predictable stages—from being uninterested in stopping, to thinking about change, to making a concerted effort to stop, to finally maintaining abstinence. But most attempt to quit several times before they finally succeed. Relapse is a normal part of the process.

The Benefits of Quitting

Giving up tobacco provides immediate health benefits to men and women of all ages (Table 11-2). People who quit smoking find that food tastes better. Their sense of smell is

Table 11-2	Benefits of Quitting Smoking

Within 20 minutes of your last cigarette: • You stop polluting the air • Blood pressure drops to normal • Pulse rate drops to normal • Temperature of hands and feet increases to normal **8 hours:** • Carbon monoxide level in blood drops to normal • Oxygen level in blood increases to normal **24 hours:** • Chance of heart attack decreases **48 hours:** • Nerve endings start regrowing • Ability to smell and taste is enhanced **2–3 months:** • Circulation improves • Walking becomes easier • Lung function increases up to 30%	**1–9 months:** • Coughing, sinus congestion, fatigue, and shortness of breath all decrease **1 year:** • Heart disease death rate is half that of a smoker **5 years:** • Stroke risk drops nearly to the risk for nonsmokers **10 years:** • Lung cancer death rate drops to 50% of that of continuing smokers • Incidence of other cancers (mouth, throat, larynx, esophagus, bladder, kidney, and pancreas) decreases • Risk of ulcer decreases **15 years:** • Risk of lung cancer is about 25% of that of continuing smokers • Risks of heart disease and death are close to those for nonsmokers

SOURCES: American Lung Association. 2002. *Benefits of Quitting* (http://www.lungusa.org/tobacco/quit_ben.html; retrieved November 25, 2002); American Cancer Society. 2000. *Quitting Smoking* (http://www.cancer.org/tobacco/quitting.html; retrieved July 10, 2000).

Quitting smoking improves the quality of life. In addition to reducing his long-term disease risks, this ex-smoker has more energy and an improved capacity for exercise.

sharper. Circulation improves, heart rate and blood pressure drop, and lung function and heart efficiency increase. Ex-smokers can breathe more easily, and their capacity for exercise improves. Many ex-smokers report feeling more energetic and alert. They experience fewer headaches. Even their complexion may improve. Quitting also has a positive effect on long-term disease risk. From the first day without tobacco, ex-smokers begin to decrease their risk of cancer of the lung, larynx, mouth, pancreas, bladder, cervix, and other sites. Risk of heart attack, stroke, and other cardiovascular diseases drops quickly, too.

The younger people are when they stop smoking, the more pronounced the health improvements. And these improvements gradually but invariably increase as the period of nonsmoking lengthens. It's never too late to quit, though. According to a U.S. Surgeon General's report, people who quit smoking, regardless of age, live longer than people who continue to smoke. Even smokers who have already developed chronic bronchitis or emphysema may show some improvement when they quit.

Options for Quitting

Most tobacco users—76% in a recent survey—want to quit, and half of those who want to quit will make an attempt this year. What are their options? No single method works for everyone, but each does work for some people some of the time. In June 2000, the U.S. Public Health Service issued new guidelines for medical professionals on how to help their patients quit smoking, emphasizing the benefits of both behavioral and pharmacological interventions.

Choosing to quit requires developing a strategy for success. Some people quit cold turkey, whereas others taper off slowly. There are over-the-counter and prescription products that help many people (see the box "Smoking Cessation Products" for more on these options). Behavioral factors that have been shown to increase the chances of a smoker's permanent smoking cessation are support from others and regular exercise. Support can come from friends and family and/or formal group programs sponsored by organizations such as the American Cancer Society, the American Lung Association, and the Seventh-Day Adventist Church or by your college health center or community hospital. Programs that combine group support with nicotine replacement therapy have rates of continued abstention as high as 35% after 1 year.

Free telephone quitlines are emerging as a popular and effective strategy to help stop smoking. Quitlines are staffed by trained counselors who help each caller plan a personal quitting strategy, usually including a combination of nicotine replacement therapy, changes in daily habits, and emotional support. Counselors provide printed materials that match the smoker's needs and schedule phone counseling sessions for key days after a smoker quits. Smokers can schedule sessions to fit their schedule, and some quitlines may provide stop-smoking medications at reduced prices. Almost all smokers make more than one attempt to stop before they succeed in quitting for good; and quitline

Smoking Cessation Products

V ̇w

Nicotine Replacement Therapy

As the name suggests, nicotine replacement therapy involves supplying the tobacco user with nicotine from a source other than standard tobacco products. This allows a user to overcome the psychological and behavioral aspects of a tobacco habit without simultaneously having to endure the physical symptoms of withdrawal. Although still harmful, nicotine replacement provides a cleaner form of nicotine. It avoids the thousands of poisons and tars that are found in burning tobacco and delivers a lower dose of nicotine than most smokers receive. After a few weeks or months of use, the reforming tobacco user begins to taper off use of the replacement, alleviating withdrawal symptoms.

There are several types of nicotine replacements, each with advantages and disadvantages. None of them are safe to use if the smoker plans to continue using tobacco; nicotine is a powerful stimulant, and an overdose can cause serious health complications. Studies have shown that combining nicotine replacement therapy with behavioral counseling can double the number of smokers who quit.

Nicotine patches can be purchased in varying strengths without a prescription. The patches release a controlled and steady supply of nicotine through the skin for 16 or 24 hours, depending on the type selected. Smokers often begin by using a full-strength patch and then switch to a weaker one to decrease the nicotine dosage. The most common side effects of the patch are skin irritation and redness, which can often be cleared up by switching to another brand.

Another nonprescription option is *nicotine gum*. When chewed, the gum releases nicotine that is absorbed through the mucous membranes of the mouth. Most users chew one or two pieces per hour. An advantage of the gum versus the patch is that it allows the user to control the nicotine doses, so that the smoker can chew more during a craving. Long-term dependence seems to be a problem for some gum users. Research has shown that 15–20% of gum users who successfully quit

smoking continued using the gum for a year or longer, despite the recommended 6-month limit on use.

A new over-the-counter nicotine replacement product, the *nicotine lozenge* Commit, was approved by the FDA in 2002. The lozenge comes in two strengths and is designed to be taken for 12 weeks. Side effects may include nausea and heartburn.

Nicotine nasal spray and *nicotine inhalers* are available only by prescription. The nasal spray immediately relieves withdrawal symptoms by delivering nicotine to the bloodstream through the nose. The most common side effects are nasal irritation and sinus problems. Inhalers are plastic rods with a nicotine plug. When the smoker puffs on the rod, the plug produces a nicotine vapor that goes to the mouth instead of the lungs. A benefit of the inhaler is that it mimics hand and mouth actions of smoking.

Non-Nicotine Medications

One of the most exciting developments in smoking cessation has been the use of bupropion (Zyban), a prescription antidepressant that affects neurotransmitters related to nicotine cravings. In one study of quitting success, 36% of nicotine patch users quit for at least the month, 49% of bupropion users quit, and 58% of users of both the patch and bupropion quit. Another study found that quitters who use bupropion tend to gain less weight than quitters who do not; an especially significant difference was seen among women. Bupropion has also been shown to be successful in helping even the most hardened smokers quit. If bupropion is not effective, there are two other drugs that may be prescribed, clonidine and nortriptyline; however, neither has been approved by the FDA specifically for nicotine dependence.

Each smoking cessation product may be successful for some people, but any attempt to quit must address both the psychological and the physical aspects of nicotine dependence. Plan carefully how you will quit, to maximize your chance of conquering this powerful addiction.

counselors can help smokers understand what leads to relapse, review their reasons for wanting to quit, and make a better plan for the next attempt. The goal is for smokers to find a support system and techniques that work for them. In 2004, the Department of Health and Human Services established a national toll-free number, 1-800-QUITNOW (1-800-784-8669), to serve as a single access point for smokers seeking information and assistance in quitting. Callers are routed to their state's smoking cessation quitline or, in states that have not established quitlines, to one maintained by the National Cancer Institute.

Most smokers in the process of quitting experience both physical and psychological effects of nicotine withdrawal, and exercise can help with both. For many smokers, their tobacco use is associated with certain times and places—following a meal, for example. Resolving to walk

after dinner instead of lighting up provides a distraction from cravings and eliminates the cues that trigger a desire to smoke. In addition, many people worry about weight gain associated with quitting. Although most ex-smokers do gain a few pounds, at least temporarily, incorporating exercise into a new tobacco-free routine lays the foundation for healthy weight management. The health risks of adding a few pounds are far outweighed by the risks of continued smoking; it's estimated that a smoker would have to gain 75–100 pounds to equal the health risks of smoking a pack a day.

As with any significant change in health-related behavior, giving up tobacco requires planning, sustained effort, and support. It is an ongoing process, not a one-time event. The Behavior Change Strategy describes the steps that successful quitters follow.

Kicking the Tobacco Habit

You can look forward to a longer and healthier life if you join the 47 million Americans who have quit using tobacco. The steps for quitting described below are discussed in terms of the most popular tobacco product in the United States—cigarettes—but they can be adapted for all forms of tobacco.

Gather Information

Collect personal smoking information in a detailed journal about your smoking behavior. Write down the time you smoke each cigarette of the day, the situation you are in, how you feel, where you smoke, and how strong your craving for the cigarette is, plus any other information that seems relevant. Part of the job is to identify patterns of smoking that are connected with routine situations (for example, the coffee break smoke, the after-dinner cigarette, the tension-reduction cigarette). Use this information to discover the behavior patterns involved in your smoking habit.

Make the Decision to Quit

Choose a date in the near future when you expect to be relatively stress-free and can give quitting the energy and attention it will require. Don't choose a date right before or during finals week, for instance. Consider making quitting a gift: Choose your birthday as your quit date, for example, or make quitting a Father's Day or Mother's Day present. You might also want to coordinate your quit date with a buddy—a fellow tobacco user who wants to quit or a nonsmoker who wants to give up another bad habit or begin an exercise program. Tell your friends and family when you plan to quit. Ask them to offer encouragement and help hold you to your goal.

Decide what approach to quitting will work best for you. Will you go cold turkey, or will you taper off? Will you use nicotine patches or gum? Will you join a support group or enlist the help of a buddy? Prepare a contract for quitting, as discussed in Chapter 1. Set firm dates and rewards, and sign the contract. Post it in a prominent place.

Prepare to Quit

One of the most important things you can do to prepare to quit is to develop and practice nonsmoking relaxation techniques. Many smokers find that they use cigarettes to help them unwind in tense situations or to relax at other times. If this is true for you, you'll need to find and develop effective substitutes. It takes time to become proficient at relaxation techniques, so begin practicing before your quit date. Refer to the detailed discussion of relaxation techniques in Chapter 2.

Other things you can do to help prepare for quitting include the following:

- Make an appointment to see your physician. Ask about OTC and prescription aids for tobacco cessation and whether one or more might be appropriate for you.

- Make a dentist's appointment to have your teeth cleaned the day after your target quit date.

- Start an easy exercise program, if you're not exercising regularly already.

- Buy some sugarless gum. Stock your kitchen with low-calorie snacks.

- Clean out your car, and air out your house. Send your clothes out for dry cleaning.

- Throw away all your cigarette-related paraphernalia (ashtrays, lighters, etc.).

- The night before your quit day, get rid of all your cigarettes. Have fun with this—get your friends or family to help you tear them up.

- Make your last few days of smoking inconvenient: Smoke only outdoors and when alone. Don't do anything else while you smoke.

Quitting

Your first few days without cigarettes will probably be the most difficult. It's hard to give up such a strongly ingrained habit, but remember that millions of Americans have done it—and you can, too. Plan and rehearse the steps you will take when you experience a powerful craving. Avoid or control situations that you know from your journal are powerfully associated with your smoking (see the table). If your hands feel empty without a cigarette, try holding or fiddling with a small object such as a paper clip or pencil.

Social support can also be a big help. Arrange with a buddy to help you with your weak moments, and call him or her whenever you feel overwhelmed by an urge to smoke. Tell people you've just quit. You may discover many inspiring former smokers who can encourage you and reassure you that it's possible to quit and lead a happier, healthier life. Find a formal support group to join if you think it will help.

Maintaining Nonsmoking

The lingering smoking urges that remain once you've quit should be carefully

Smoking is the leading preventable cause of death in the United States. Most smokers get hooked before they realize it, providing a market of millions to the tobacco industry. For most smokers, quitting is one of the hardest things they'll ever do. The best choice is never to start.

Right now you can

- If you smoke, put your cigarette out and go brush your teeth. Throw the pack and matches away.

- If you smoke, think about the next time you'll want a cigarette, such as while talking on the phone this afternoon or relaxing after dinner tonight. Visualize yourself enjoying this activity without a cigarette in your hand. Imagine yourself as a healthier, more robust person. See if you get pleasure or satisfaction from thinking of yourself as a nonsmoker, as an ex-smoker, or as someone liberated from dependence on cigarettes.

- If you use tobacco, go outside for a short walk or a stretch to limber up. Breathe deeply. Tell a friend you've just decided to quit.

- Resolve to talk to someone you know who uses tobacco, offering support and assistance if the person is interested in quitting.

tracked and controlled because they can cause relapses if left unattended. Keep track of these urges in your journal to help you deal with them. If certain situations still trigger the urge for a cigarette, change something about the situation to break past associations. If stress or boredom causes strong smoking urges, use a relaxation technique, take a brisk walk, have a stick of gum, or substitute some other activity for smoking.

Don't set yourself up for a relapse. If you allow yourself to get overwhelmed at school or work or to gain weight, it will be easier to convince yourself that now isn't the right time to quit. This is the right time. Continue to practice time-management and relaxation techniques. Exercise regularly, eat sensibly, and get enough sleep. These habits will not only ensure your success at remaining tobacco-free but also serve you well in stressful times throughout your life. In fact, former smokers who have quit for at least 3 months report reduced stress levels, probably because quitting smoking lowers overall arousal.

Watch out for patterns of thinking that can make nonsmoking more difficult. Focus on the positive aspects of not smoking, and give yourself lots of praise—you deserve it. Stick with the schedule of rewards you developed for your contract.

Keep track of the emerging benefits that come from having quit. Items that might appear on your list include improved stamina, an increased sense of pride at having kicked a strong addiction, a sharper sense of taste and smell, no more smoker's cough, and so on. Keep track of the money you're saving by not smoking, and spend it on things you really enjoy. And if you do lapse, be gentle with yourself. Lapses are a normal part of quitting. Forgive yourself, and pick up where you left off.

Strategies for Dealing with High-Risk Smoking Situations

Cues and High-Risk Situations	Suggested Strategies
Awakening in morning	Brush your teeth as soon as you wake up. Take a shower or bath.
Drinking coffee	Do something else with your hands. Drink tea or another beverage instead.
Eating meals	Sit in nonsmoking sections of restaurants. Get up from the table right after eating, and start another activity. Brush your teeth right after eating.
Driving a car	Have the car cleaned when you quit smoking. Chew sugarless gum or eat a low-calorie snack. Take public transportation or ride your bike. Turn on the radio and sing along.
Socializing with friends who smoke	Suggest nonsmoking events (movies, theater, shopping). Tell friends you've quit and ask them not to smoke around you, offer you cigarettes, or give you cigarettes if you ask for them.
Drinking at a bar, restaurant, or party	Try to take a nonsmoker with you, or associate with nonsmokers. Let friends know you've just quit. Moderate your intake of alcohol (it can weaken your resolve).
Encountering stressful situations	Practice relaxation techniques. Take some deep breaths. Get out of your room or house. Go somewhere that doesn't allow smoking. Take a shower, chew gum, call a friend, or exercise.

SOURCES: Strategies adapted with permission from *Postgraduate Medicine* 90(1), July 1991; Antonuccio, D. O. 1993. *Butt Out, The Smoker's Book: A Compassionate Guide to Helping Yourself Quit Smoking, With or Without a Partner.* Saratoga, Calif.: R & E.

SUMMARY

- Smoking is the largest preventable cause of ill health and death in the United States. Nevertheless, millions of Americans continue to use tobacco.

- Regular tobacco use causes physical dependence on nicotine, characterized by loss of control, tolerance, and withdrawal. Habits can become associated with tobacco use and trigger the urge for a cigarette.

- People who begin smoking are usually imitating others or responding to seductive advertising. Smoking is associated with low education level and the use of other drugs.

- Tobacco smoke is made up of hundreds of different chemicals, including some that are carcinogenic or poisonous or that damage the respiratory system.

- Nicotine acts on the nervous system as a stimulant or a depressant. It can cause blood pressure and heart rate to increase, straining the heart.

- Cardiovascular disease is the most widespread cause of death for cigarette smokers. Cigarette smoking is the primary cause of lung cancer and is linked to many other cancers and respiratory diseases.

- Cigarette smoking is linked to ulcers, impotence, reproductive health problems, dental diseases, and other conditions. Tobacco use leads to lower life expectancy and to a diminished quality of life.

- The use of spit tobacco leads to nicotine addiction and is linked to oral cancers.

- Cigars, pipes, clove cigarettes, and bidis are not safe alternatives to cigarettes.

- Environmental tobacco smoke (ETS) contains high concentrations of toxic chemicals and can cause headaches, eye and nasal irritation, and sinus problems. Long-term exposure to ETS can cause lung cancer and heart disease.

- Infants and young children take in more pollutants than adults do; children whose parents smoke are especially susceptible to respiratory diseases.

- Smoking during pregnancy increases the risk of miscarriage, stillbirth, congenital abnormalities, premature birth, and low birth weight. SIDS, behavior problems, and long-term impairments in development are also risks.

- The overall cost of tobacco use to society includes the cost of both medical care and lost worker productivity.

- There are many avenues individuals and groups can take to act against tobacco use. Nonsmokers can use social pressure and legislative channels to assert their rights to breathe clean air.

- Giving up smoking is a difficult and long-term process. Although most ex-smokers quit on their own, some smokers benefit from stop-smoking programs, OTC and prescription medications, and support groups.

Take Action

1. Interview successful quitters: Interview one or two former tobacco users about their experiences with tobacco and the methods they used to quit. Why did they start smoking or using tobacco, how old were they when they started, and how long did their habit continue? What made them decide to quit? How did they quit? What could a current tobacco user learn from their experience of quitting?

2. Identify community smoking restrictions: Make a tour of the public facilities in your community and on your campus, such as movie theaters, auditoriums, business and school offices, and classrooms. What kinds of restrictions on smoking do these places have? In your opinion, are they appropriate? If you feel more or different restrictions are in order, write a letter to the editor of your school or local newspaper, and state your case. Support it with convincing arguments and appropriate facts.

For More Information

Books

Gilman, S. L., ed. 2004. *Smoke: A Global History of Smoking.* London: Reaktion Books. *A look at smoking and its effects, including history and issues related to culture, art, and gender.*

Kessler, D. 2001. *A Question of Intent: A Great American Battle with a Deadly Industry.* New York: Public Affairs. *A description of the federal government's attempts to regulate tobacco, written by the former head of the FDA.*

Sloan, F. A., et al. 2004. *The Price of Smoking.* Cambridge, Mass.: MIT Press. *A careful examination of the economic and social consequences of smoking.*

Watson, R. R., and M. L. Witten, eds. 2001. *Environmental Tobacco Smoke.* Boca Raton, Fla.: CRC Press. *A scientific look at the health effects of environmental tobacco smoke.*

Self-help books designed to help smokers quit:

Carr, A. 2005. *The Easy Way to Stop Smoking.* New York: Sterling.

Kicking Butts: Quit Smoking and Take Charge of Your Health. 2002. Atlanta: American Cancer Society.

Kleinman, L. 2000. *The Complete Idiot's Guide to Quitting Smoking.* Indianapolis, Ind.: Macmillan.

ⓦ Organizations, Hotlines, and Web Sites

Action on Smoking and Health (ASH). An advocacy group that provides statistics, news briefs, and other information.
202-659-4310
http://ash.org

American Cancer Society (ACS). Sponsor of the annual Great American Smokeout; provides information on the dangers of tobacco, as well as tools for prevention and cessation for both smokers and users of spit tobacco.

800-ACS-2345
http://www.cancer.org

American Lung Association. Provides information on lung diseases, tobacco control, and environmental health.
800-LUNG-USA; 212-315-8700
http://www.lungusa.org

CDC's Tobacco Information and Prevention Source (TIPS). Provides research results, educational materials, and tips on how to quit smoking; Web site includes special sections for kids and teens.
800-CDC-1311
http://www.cdc.gov/tobacco

Environmental Protection Agency Indoor Air Quality/ETS. Provides information and links about secondhand smoke.
866-SMOKE-FREE
http://www.epa.gov/smokefree

Nicotine Anonymous. A 12-step program for tobacco users.
http://www.nicotine-anonymous.org

Quitnet. Provides interactive tools and questionnaires, support groups, a library, news on tobacco issues, and quitting programs for both smokers and spit tobacco users.
http://www.quitnet.com

Smokefree.Gov. Provides step-by-step strategies for quitting as well as expert support via telephone or instant messaging.
http://www.smokefree.gov
1-800-QUITNOW (1-800-784-8669)
http://www.cancer.gov (additional information)

Tobacco BBS. A resource center on tobacco and smoking issues that includes news and information, assistance for smokers who want to quit, and links to related sites.
http://www.tobacco.org

Tobacco Control Resource Center and Tobacco Products Liability Project (TPLP). Provides current information about tobacco-related court cases and legislation.
http://www.tobacco.neu.edu
World Health Organization Tobacco Free Initiative. Promotes the goal of a tobacco-free world.
http://www.who.int/tobacco/en

World No Tobacco Day (WNTD). Provides information on the annual worldwide event to encourage people to quit smoking; includes general information about tobacco use and testimonials of ex-smokers.
http://www.worldnotobaccoday.com

See also the listings for Chapters 9, 15, and 16.

Selected Bibliography

American Cancer Society. 2005. *Cancer Facts and Figures, 2005.* Atlanta, Ga.: American Cancer Society.

American Nonsmokers' Rights Foundation. 2004. *Overview List—How Many Local Smokefree Laws?* (http://www.no-smoke.org/pdf/mediaordlist.pdf; retrieved December 20, 2004).

Anthonisen, N. R., et al. 2005. The effects of a smoking cessation intervention on 14.5-year mortality: A randomized clinical trial. *Annals of Internal Medicine* 142(4): 233–239.

Campaign for Tobacco-Free Kids. 2004. *State Cigarette Excise Tax Rates and Rankings* (http://tobaccofreekids.org/research/factsheets/pdf/0097.pdf; retrieved December 19, 2004).

Centers for Disease Control and Prevention. 2004. Smoking during pregnancy—United States, 1990–2002. *Morbidity and Mortality Weekly Report* 53(39): 911–915.

Centers for Disease Control and Prevention. 2004. State-specific prevalence of current cigarette smoking among adults—United States, 2002. *Morbidity and Mortality Weekly Report* 52(53): 1277–1280.

Centers for Disease Control and Prevention. 2004. *Tobacco-Related Mortality Fact Sheet* (http://www.cdc.gov/tobacco/factsheets/Tobacco_Related_Mortality_factsheet.htm; retrieved December 20, 2004).

Collins, S. L., and S. Izenwasser. 2004. Chronic nicotine differentially alters cocaine-induced locomotor activity in adolescent vs. adult male and female rats. *Neuropharmacology* 46(3): 349–362.

de la Chica, R. A., et al. 2005. Chromosomal instability in amniocytes from fetuses of mothers who smoke. *Journal of the American Medical Association* 293(10): 1212–1222.

Distefan, J. M., J. P. Pierce, and E. A. Gilpin. 2004. Do favorite movie stars influence adolescent smoking initiation? *American Journal of Public Health* 94(7): 1239–1244.

Doll, R., et al. 2004. Mortality in relation to smoking: 50 years' observations on male British doctors. *British Medical Journal* 328(7455): 1519.

Etter, J. F., L. T. Kozlowski, and T. V. Perneger. 2003. What smokers believe about light and ultralight cigarettes. *Preventive Medicine* 36(1): 92–98.

Ezzati, M., and A. D. Lopez. 2004. Regional, disease specific patterns of smoking-attributable mortality in 2000. *Tobacco Control* 13(4): 388–395.

Farrelly, M. C., et al. 2005. Evidence of a dose-response relationship between "truth" antismoking ads and youth smoking prevalence. *American Journal of Public Health* 95(3): 425–431.

Federal Trade Commission. 2004. *2004 Report on Cigarette Sales, Advertising and Promotion* (http://www.ftc.gov/bcp/menu-tobac.htm; retrieved December 20, 2004).

Fiore, M. C., et al. 2000. *Treating Tobacco Use and Dependence.* Clinical Practice Guidelines. Rockville, Md.: U.S. Department of Health and Human Services.

Fried, P. A., B. Watkinson, and R. Gray. 2003. Differential effects on cognitive functioning in 13- to 16-year-olds prenatally exposed to cigarettes and marihuana. *Neurotoxicology and Teratology* 25(4): 427–436.

Gades, N. M., et al. 2005. Association between smoking and erectile dysfunction: A population-based study. *American Journal of Epidemiology* 161(4): 346–351.

Gidwani, P. P., et al. 2002. Television viewing and initiation of smoking among youth. *Pediatrics* 110(3): 505–508.

Giovino, G. A., et al. 2004. Epidemiology of menthol cigarette use. *Nicotine & Tobacco Research* 6(Suppl 1): 67–81.

Government Accountability Office. 2004. *Tobacco Settlement: States' Allocations of Fiscal Year 2003 and Expected Fiscal Year 2004 Payments.* GAO 04–518. Washington, D.C.: Government Accountability Office.

Hanaoka, T., et al. 2005. Active and passive smoking and breast cancer risk in middle-aged Japanese women. *International Journal of Cancer* 114(2): 317–322.

Henschke, C. I., and O. S. Miettinen. 2004. Women's susceptibility to tobacco carcinogens. *Lung Cancer* 43(1): 1–5.

Jacobsen, L. K., et al. 2005. Effects of smoking and smoking abstinence on cognition in adolescent tobacco smokers. *Biological Psychiatry* 57(1): 56–66.

Lerman, C., et al. 2004. Interacting effects of the serotonin transporter gene and neuroticism in smoking practices and nicotine dependence. *Molecular Psychiatry.* In press.

Mahonen, M. S., et al. 2004. Current smoking and the risk of non-fatal myocardial infarction in the WHO MONICA Project populations. *Tobacco Control* 13(3): 244–250.

McCabe, R. E., et al. 2004. Smoking behaviors across anxiety disorders. *Journal of Anxiety Disorders* 18(1): 7–18.

Moran, S., H. Wechsler, and N. A. Rigotti. 2004. Social smoking among U.S. college students. *Pediatrics* 114(4): 1028–1034.

National Cancer Institute. 2004. *The Truth About "Light" Cigarettes: Questions and Answers* (http://cis.nci.nih.gov/fact/3_74.htm; retrieved September 3, 2004).

National Center for Health Statistics. 2003. Cigarette smoking behavior of adults. *Advance Data from Vital and Health Statistics* No. 331.

Ng, C., and B. Dakake. 2002. *Tobacco Use in PG-13 Films.* Boston: MASSPIRG.

O'Loughlin, J., et al. 2004. Genetically decreased CYP2A6 and the risk of tobacco dependence: A prospective study of novice smokers. *Tobacco Control* 13(4): 422–428.

Prochazka, A. J., et al. 2004. A randomized trial of nortriptyline combined with transdermal nicotine for smoking cessation. *Archives of Internal Medicine* 164(20): 2229–2233.

Schroeder, S. A. 2004. Tobacco control in the wake of the 1998 Master Settlement Agreement. *New England Journal of Medicine* 350(3): 293–301.

Shiffman, S., M. E. Di Marino, and J. L. Pillitteri. 2005. The effectiveness of nicotine patch and nicotine lozenge in very heavy smokers. *Journal of Substance Abuse Treatment* 28(1): 49–55.

Sloan, F. A., et al. 2004. *The Price of Smoking.* Cambridge, Mass.: MIT Press.

Smoke Free Movies. 2004. *Now Showing* (http://smokefreemovies.ucsf.edu/problem/now_showing.html; retrieved December 20, 2004).

Trimble, C. L., et al. 2005. Active and passive cigarette smoking and the risk of cervical neoplasia. *Obstetrics and Gynecology* 105(1):174–81.

Vineis, P., et al. 2005. Environmental tobacco smoke and risk of respiratory cancer and chronic obstructive pulmonary disease in former smokers and never smokers in the EPIC prospective study. *British Medical Journal* 330(7486): 277.

World Health Organization. 2003. *Gender, Health, and Tobacco.* Geneva: World Health Organization.

Yolton, K., et al. 2005. Exposure to environmental tobacco smoke and cognitive abilities among U.S. children and adolescents. *Environmental Health Perspectives* 113(1): 98–103.

Zhang, X., et al. 2005. Association of passive smoking by husbands with prevalence of stroke among Chinese women nonsmokers. *American Journal of Epidemiology* 161(3): 213–218.

12

After reading this chapter, you should be able to

- List the essential nutrients, and describe the functions they perform in the body

- Describe the guidelines that have been developed to help people choose a healthy diet, avoid nutritional deficiencies, and reduce their risk of diet-related chronic diseases

- Discuss nutritional guidelines for vegetarians and for special population groups

- Explain how to use food labels and other consumer tools to make informed choices about foods

- Put together a personal nutrition plan based on affordable foods that you enjoy and that will promote wellness, today as well as in the future

Nutrition Basics

1. **It is recommended that all adults consume one to two servings each of fruits and vegetables every day.**
   True or false?

2. **How many french fries are considered to be one ½-cup serving?**
   a. 10
   b. 15
   c. 25

3. **Candy is the leading source of added sugars in the American diet.**
   True or false?

4. **Which of the following is not a whole grain?**
   a. brown rice
   b. wheat flour
   c. popcorn

5. **Nutritionists advise reduced intake of saturated and trans fats for which of the following reasons?**
   a. They increase levels of low-density lipoproteins (LDL), or "bad" cholesterol.
   b. They provide more calories than other types of fat.
   c. They increase the risk of heart disease.

ANSWERS

1. FALSE. For someone consuming 2000 calories, a minimum of nine servings per day—four of fruits and five of vegetables—is recommended, the equivalent of 4½ cups per day. The majority of Americans fail to meet this goal; half of all the vegetables we *do* eat are potatoes—and half of those are french fried.

2. A. Many people underestimate the size of the portions they eat, leading to overconsumption of calories and fat.

3. FALSE. Regular (nondiet) sodas are the leading source of sugar and of calories, with an average of 55 gallons consumed per person per year. Each 12-ounce soda supplies about 10 teaspoons of sugar, or nearly 10% of the calories in a 2000-calorie diet.

4. B. Unless labeled *whole* wheat, wheat flour is processed to remove the bran and the germ and is not a whole grain.

5. A AND C. High intake of saturated and trans fats raises LDL levels and the risk of heart disease. Saturated and trans fats provide the same number of calories as other types of fat—9 calories per gram (compared to 4 calories per gram for protein and carbohydrate).

WW Visit the *Core Concepts in Health* Online Learning Center (www.mhhe.com/insel10e) for study aids and many additional resources.

327

In your lifetime, you'll spend about 6 years eating—about 70,000 meals and 60 tons of food. What you choose to eat can have profound effects on your health and well-being. Of particular concern is the connection between lifetime nutritional habits and the risk of major chronic diseases, including heart disease, cancer, stroke, and diabetes. Choosing foods that provide adequate amounts of the nutrients you need while limiting the substances linked to disease should be an important part of your daily life. The food choices you make will significantly influence your health—both now and in the future.

Choosing a healthy diet that supports maximum wellness and protects against disease is a two-part process. First, you have to know which nutrients are necessary and in what amounts. Second, you have to translate those requirements into a diet consisting of foods you like to eat that are both available and affordable. Once you have an idea of what constitutes a healthy diet for you, you may want to make adjustments in your current diet to bring it into line with your goals.

This chapter provides the basic principles of **nutrition.** It introduces the six classes of essential nutrients, explaining their roles in the functioning of the body. It also provides different sets of guidelines that you can use to design a healthy diet plan. Finally, it offers practical tools and advice to help you apply the guidelines to your own life. Diet is an area of your life in which you have almost total control. Using your knowledge and understanding of nutrition to create a healthy diet plan is a significant step toward wellness.

NUTRITIONAL REQUIREMENTS: COMPONENTS OF A HEALTHY DIET

When you think about your diet, you probably do so in terms of the foods you like to eat—a turkey sandwich and a glass of milk or black beans and rice. What's important for your health, though, are the nutrients contained in those foods. Your body requires proteins, fats, carbohydrates, vitamins, minerals, and water—about 45 **essential nutrients.** The word *essential* in this context means that you must get these substances from food because your body is unable to manufacture them at all, or at least not fast enough to meet your physiological needs. Plants obtain all the chemicals they need from air, water, soil, and sunlight. Animals, including humans, must eat foods to obtain the nutrients necessary to keep their bodies growing and functioning properly. Your body obtains these nutrients through the process of **digestion,** in which the foods you eat are broken down into compounds your gastrointestinal tract can absorb and your body can use (Figure 12-1). A diet containing adequate amounts of all essential nutrients is vital because various nutrients provide energy, help build and

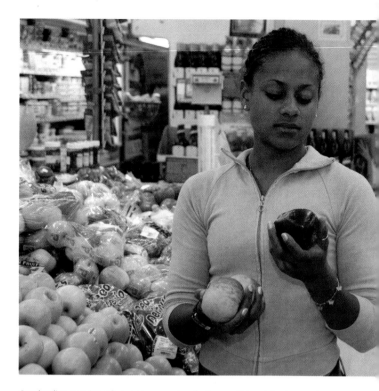

Our bodies require adequate amounts of all essential nutrients—water, proteins, carbohydrates, fats, vitamins, and minerals—in order to grow and function properly. Choosing foods to satisfy these nutritional requirements is an important part of a healthy lifestyle.

maintain body tissues, and help regulate body functions (see the box "Eating Habits and Total Wellness").

The energy in foods is expressed as **kilocalories.** One kilocalorie represents the amount of heat it takes to raise the temperature of 1 liter of water 1°C. A person needs about 2000 kilocalories per day to meet his or her energy needs. In common usage, people usually refer to kilocalories as *calories*, which is technically a much smaller energy unit: (1 kilocalorie contains 1000 calories). We use the familiar word *calorie* in this chapter to stand for the larger energy unit; you'll also find the word *calorie* used on food labels.

Of the six classes of essential nutrients, three supply energy:

- Fat = 9 calories per gram
- Protein = 4 calories per gram
- Carbohydrate = 4 calories per gram

(Alcohol, although it is not an essential nutrient, also supplies energy, providing 7 calories per gram.) The high caloric content of fat is one reason experts often advise against high fat consumption; most of us do not need the extra calories to meet energy needs. Regardless of their source, calories consumed in excess of energy needs are converted to fat and stored in the body.

But just meeting energy needs is not enough; our bodies require adequate amounts of all the essential nutrients to

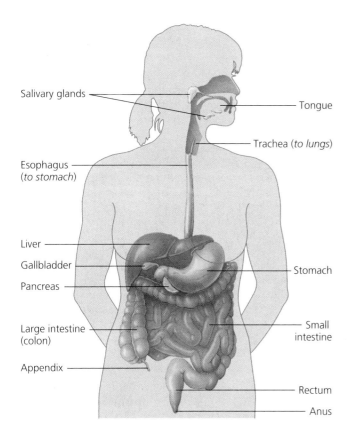

Salivary glands

Tongue

Trachea (*to lungs*)

Esophagus
(*to stomach*)

Liver

Gallbladder

Pancreas

Stomach

Large intestine
(colon)

Small
intestine

Appendix

Rectum

Anus

Figure 12-1 The digestive system. Food is partially broken down by being chewed and mixed with saliva in the mouth. After traveling to the stomach via the esophagus, food is broken down further by stomach acids. As food moves through the digestive tract, it is mixed by muscular contractions and broken down by chemicals. Most absorption of nutrients occurs in the small intestine, aided by secretions from the pancreas, gallbladder, and intestinal lining. The large intestine reabsorbs excess water; the remaining solid wastes are collected in the rectum and excreted through the anus.

grow and function properly. Practically all foods contain mixtures of nutrients, although foods are commonly classified according to the predominant nutrient; for example, spaghetti is thought of as a carbohydrate. Let's take a closer look at the function and sources of each class of nutrients.

Proteins—The Basis of Body Structure

Proteins form important parts of the body's main structural components: muscles and bones. Proteins also form important parts of blood, enzymes, some hormones, and cell membranes. As mentioned above, proteins can provide energy (4 calories per gram) for the body.

Amino Acids The building blocks of proteins are called **amino acids.** Twenty common amino acids are found in food; nine of these are essential: histidine, isoleucine, leucine, lysine, methionine, phenylalanine, threonine, tryptophan, and valine. The other eleven amino acids can be produced by the body, given the presence of the needed components supplied by foods.

Complete and Incomplete Proteins Individual protein sources are considered *complete* if they supply all the essential amino acids in adequate amounts and *incomplete* if they do not. Meat, fish, poultry, eggs, milk, cheese, and soy provide complete proteins. Incomplete proteins, which come from other plant sources such as **legumes** and nuts, are good sources of most essential amino acids but are usually low in one or two.

Certain combinations of vegetable proteins, such as wheat and peanuts in a peanut butter sandwich, allow each vegetable protein to make up for the amino acids missing in the other protein. The combination yields a complete protein. Many traditional food pairings, such as beans and rice or corn and beans, emerged as dietary staples because they are complementary proteins. It was once believed that vegetarians had to complement their proteins at each meal in order to receive the benefit of a complete protein. It is now known, however, that proteins consumed throughout the course of the day can complement each other to form a pool of amino acids the body can draw from to produce the necessary proteins. Vegetarians should include a variety of vegetable protein sources in their diets to make sure they get all the essential amino acids in adequate amounts. (Healthy vegetarian diets are discussed later in the chapter.) About two-thirds of the protein in the American diet comes from animal sources (red meat and milk); therefore, the American diet is rich in essential amino acids.

Recommended Protein Intake Adequate daily intake of protein for adults is 0.8 gram per kilogram (0.36 gram per pound) of body weight, corresponding to 50 grams of protein per day for someone who weighs 140 pounds and 65 grams of protein for someone who weighs 180 pounds. This amount of protein is easily obtained from popular foods: 3 ounces of lean

Terms

nutrition The science of food and how the body uses it in health and disease.

essential nutrients Substances the body must get from foods because it cannot manufacture them at all or fast enough to meet its needs. These nutrients include proteins, fats, carbohydrates, vitamins, minerals, and water.

digestion The process of breaking down foods in the gastrointestinal tract into compounds the body can absorb.

kilocalorie A measure of energy content in food; 1 kilocalorie represents the amount of heat needed to raise the temperature of 1 liter of water 1°C; commonly referred to as *calorie.*

protein An essential nutrient; a compound made of amino acids that contain carbon, hydrogen, oxygen, and nitrogen.

amino acids The building blocks of proteins.

legumes Vegetables such as peas and beans that are high in fiber and are also important sources of protein.

Healthy eating does more than nourish your body—it enhances your ability to enjoy life to the fullest by improving overall wellness, both physical and mental. A recent study examined a group of adults who followed a healthy eating plan for four years. At the end of this period, the study subjects were more confident with their food choices and more satisfied with their lives in general than their peers who did not make any dietary changes. The reverse is also true—when people overeat they often have feelings of guilt, anger, discouragement, and even self-loathing. Out-of-control eating can erode self-confidence and lead to depression. How we eat is a reflection of how we feel about ourselves. Enjoying food and eating well is a major part of a healthy and happy life.

Can individual foods affect the way we feel? Limited scientific evidence points to some correlation between certain foods and one's mood. Many people, especially women, seem to crave chocolate when they feel down. Studies show that chocolate, in small quantities, may indeed give you a lift. The fat found in chocolate acts to increase endorphins, brain chemicals that reduce pain and increase feelings of well-being. Chocolate also contains caffeine, theobromine, phenylethylamine,

and a variety of other less studied chemicals that may have a positive influence on mood. Sugary foods tend to temporarily raise serotonin levels in the brain, which can improve mood (serotonin is a neurotransmitter associated with a calm, relaxed state).

A commonly held belief about the connection between food and the mind is that eating sugary foods makes people (especially children) hyperactive. However, several carefully controlled studies showed no correlation between behavior and the consumption of sugary foods. Researchers speculate that high-sugar foods tend to be eaten at birthday parties and other exciting occasions when children tend to be highly stimulated regardless of what they eat.

Some recent research shows that eating certain carbohydrate-rich foods, such as a plain baked potato or a bagel with jelly, can have a temporary calming effect. Scientists postulate that this occurs because carbohydrates stimulate insulin release, which improves the transport of the amino acid tryptophan (the major building block for serotonin) into the brain. This effect is most pronounced when rapidly digestible carbohydrates are consumed alone, with no fats or protein in the meal. The practical implications of this research are uncertain.

If you are looking for a mental boost, some scientists think that eating a meal consisting primarily of protein-rich foods may be helpful. The theory is that proteins contain the amino acid tyrosine, which is used by the body to manufacture the neurotransmitters dopamine and norepinephrine. Some researchers postulate that eating protein-containing foods could increase the synthesis of these neurotransmitters, which can speed reaction time and increase alertness. Whether this really works, especially in well-nourished individuals who have not been lacking these nutrients to begin with, remains to be seen. In the meantime, it wouldn't hurt, and might even help, to include some protein in the meal you eat prior to your next big exam.

What we know about how food affects mood remains limited. But evidence points to the commonsense conclusion that enjoying reasonable portions of a variety of healthy and tasty foods is a great way to optimize your physical and mental health.

SOURCE: Fahey, T. D., P. M. Insel, and W. T. Roth. 2005. *Fit and Well,* 6th ed. New York: McGraw-Hill. Copyright © 2005 The McGraw-Hill Companies, Inc. Reprinted with permission from The McGraw-Hill Companies, Inc.

meat, poultry, or fish or ½ cup of tofu contains about 20–25 grams of protein; 1 cup of dry beans (legumes such as pinto and kidney beans), 15–20 grams; 1 cup of milk or yogurt or 1½ ounces of cheese, 8–12 grams; and cereals, grains, nuts, and vegetables, about 2–4 grams of protein per serving.

Most Americans meet or exceed the protein intake needed for adequate nutrition. Protein consumed beyond what the body needs is synthesized into fat for energy storage or burned for energy requirements. Consuming somewhat above daily needs is not harmful, but it can contribute fat to the diet because protein-rich foods are often fat-rich as well. A very high protein intake can also strain the kidneys. A fairly broad range of protein intakes is associated with good health, and the Food and Nutrition Board recommends that the amount of protein adults eat should fall within the range of 10–35% of total daily calorie intake. The average American diet includes about 15–16% of total daily calories as protein.

Fats—Essential in Small Amounts

Fats, also known as *lipids,* are the most concentrated source of energy, at 9 calories per gram. The fats stored in your body represent usable energy, they help insulate your body, and they support and cushion your organs. Fats in the diet help your body absorb fat-soluble vitamins, as well as add important flavor and texture to foods. Fats are the major fuel for the body during rest and light activity. Two fats, linoleic acid and alpha-linolenic acid, are essential components of the diet. They are used to make compounds that are key regulators of such body functions as the maintenance of blood pressure and the progress of a healthy pregnancy.

Types and Sources of Fats Most of the fats in food are in the form of triglycerides, which are composed of a glycerol molecule (an alcohol) plus three fatty acids. A fatty acid is made up of a chain of carbon atoms with oxygen attached at one end and hydrogen atoms attached

Figure 12-2 Chemical structures of saturated and unsaturated fatty acids. This example of a triglyceride consists of a molecule of glycerol with three fatty acids attached. Fatty acids can differ in the length of their carbon chains and their degree of saturation.

along the length of the chain. Fatty acids differ in the length of their carbon atom chains and in their degree of saturation (the number of hydrogens attached to the chain). If every available bond from each carbon atom in a fatty acid chain is attached to a hydrogen atom, the fatty acid is said to be **saturated** (Figure 12-2). If not all the available bonds are taken up by hydrogens, the carbon atoms in the chain will form double bonds with each other. Such fatty acids are called *unsaturated fats.* If there is only one double bond, the fatty acid is called **monounsaturated.** If there are two or more double bonds, the fatty acid is called **polyunsaturated.** The essential fatty acids, linoleic and alpha-linolenic acids, are both polyunsaturated. The different types of fatty acids have different characteristics and different effects on your health.

Food fats are usually composed of both saturated and unsaturated fatty acids; the dominant type of fatty acid determines the fat's characteristics. Food fats containing large amounts of saturated fatty acids are usually solid at room temperature; they are generally found naturally in animal products. The leading sources of saturated fat in the American diet are red meats (hamburger, steak, roasts), whole milk, cheese, hot dogs, and lunch meats. Food fats containing large amounts of monounsaturated and polyunsaturated fatty acids are usually from plant sources and are liquid at room temperature. Olive, canola, safflower, and peanut oils contain mostly monounsaturated fatty acids. Soybean, corn, and cottonseed oils contain mostly polyunsaturated fatty acids.

There are notable exceptions to these generalizations. When unsaturated vegetable oils undergo the process of

hydrogenation, a mixture of saturated and unsaturated fatty acids is produced. Hydrogenation turns many of the double bonds in unsaturated fatty acids into single bonds, increasing the degree of saturation and producing a more solid fat from a liquid oil. Hydrogenation also changes some unsaturated fatty acids to **trans fatty acids,** unsaturated fatty acids with an atypical shape that affects their behavior in the body. Food manufacturers use hydrogenation to increase the stability of an oil so it can be reused for deep frying, to improve the texture of certain foods (to make pastries and pie crusts flakier, for example), and to extend the shelf life of foods made with oil. Hydrogenation is also used to transform a liquid oil into margarine or vegetable shortening.

Many baked and fried foods are prepared with hydrogenated vegetable oils, so they can be relatively high in saturated and trans fatty acids. Leading sources of trans fats in the American diet are deep-fried fast foods such as french fries and fried chicken (typically fried in vegetable shortening rather than oil); baked and snack foods such as pot pies, cakes, cookies, pastries, doughnuts, and chips; and stick margarine. In general, the more solid a hydrogenated oil is, the more saturated and trans fats it contains; for example, stick margarines typically contain more saturated and trans fats than do tub or squeeze margarines. Small amounts of trans fatty acids are found naturally in meat and milk.

Hydrogenated vegetable oils are not the only plant fats that contain saturated fats. Palm and coconut oils, although derived from plants, are also highly saturated. However, fish oils, derived from an animal source, are rich in polyunsaturated fats.

Fats and Health Different types of fats have very different effects on health. Many studies have examined the effects of dietary fat intake on blood **cholesterol** levels and the risk of heart disease. Saturated and trans fatty acids

Terms

saturated fat A fat with no carbon-carbon double bonds; usually solid at room temperature.

monounsaturated fat A fat with one carbon-carbon double bond; liquid at room temperature.

polyunsaturated fat A fat containing two or more carbon-carbon double bonds; liquid at room temperature.

hydrogenation A process by which hydrogens are added to unsaturated fats, increasing the degree of saturation and turning liquid oils into solid fats. Hydrogenation produces a mixture of saturated fatty acids and standard and trans forms of unsaturated fatty acids.

trans fatty acid A type of unsaturated fatty acid produced during the process of hydrogenation; trans fats have an atypical shape that affects their chemical activity.

cholesterol A waxy substance found in the blood and cells and needed for synthesis of cell membranes, vitamin D, and hormones.

raise blood levels of **low-density lipoprotein (LDL)**, or "bad" cholesterol, thereby increasing a person's risk of heart disease. Unsaturated fatty acids lower LDL. Monounsaturated fatty acids, such as those found in olive and canola oils, may also increase levels of **high-density lipoproteins (HDL)**, or "good" cholesterol, providing even greater benefits for heart health. In large amounts, trans fatty acids may lower HDL. Thus, to reduce the risk of heart disease, it is important to choose unsaturated fats instead of saturated and trans fats. (See Chapter 15 for more on cholesterol and a heart-healthy diet.)

Most Americans consume more saturated fat than trans fat (12% versus 2–4% of total daily calories). However, health experts are particularly concerned about trans fats because of their double negative effect on heart health—they both raise LDL and lower HDL—and because there is less public awareness of trans fats. The saturated fat content of prepared foods has been listed on nutrition labels since 1994. By January 2006, food labels will also include trans fat content. Until that time consumers can check for the presence of trans fats by examining the ingredient list of a food: If a food contains partially hydrogenated oil or vegetable shortening, it contains trans fat.

For heart health, it's important to minimize your consumption of both saturated and trans fats. The best way to reduce saturated fat in your diet is to lower your intake of meat and full-fat dairy products (whole milk, cream, butter, cheese, yogurt, ice cream). To lower trans fats, decrease your intake of deep-fried foods and crackers, cookies, and other baked goods made with hydrogenated vegetable oils, use liquid oils rather than margarine or shortening for cooking, and favor tub or squeeze margarines or those labeled low-trans or trans-free over standard stick margarines. Remember, the softer or more liquid a fat is, the less saturated and trans fat it is likely to contain.

Although saturated and trans fats pose health hazards, other fats can be beneficial. When used in place of saturated fats, monounsaturated fatty acids, as found in avocados, most nuts, and olive, canola, peanut, and safflower oils, improve cholesterol levels and may help protect against some cancers. **Omega-3 fatty acids**, a form of polyunsaturated fat found primarily in fish, may be even

more healthful. An omega-3 fatty acid has its endmost double bond three carbons from the end of the fatty acid chain. (The polyunsaturated fatty acid shown in Figure 12-2 is an omega-3 form.) Omega-3s and the compounds the body makes from them have a number of heart-healthy effects: They reduce the tendency of blood to clot, inhibit inflammation and abnormal heart rhythms, and reduce blood pressure and risk of heart attack and stroke in some people. Because of these benefits, nutritionists recommend that Americans increase the proportion of omega-3s in their diet by eating fish two or more times a week. Salmon, tuna, trout, mackerel, herring, sardines, and anchovies are all good sources of omega-3s; lesser amounts are found in plant sources, including dark-green leafy vegetables; walnuts; flaxseeds; and canola, walnut, and flaxseed oils.

Another form of polyunsaturated fat, omega-6 fatty acid, has its endmost double bond at the sixth carbon atom. Most of the polyunsaturated fats currently consumed by Americans are omega-6s, primarily from corn oil and soybean oil. Foods rich in omega-6s are important because they contain the essential nutrient linoleic acid. However, some nutritionists recommend that people reduce the proportion of omega-6s they consume in favor of omega-3s. To make this adjustment, use canola oil rather than corn oil in cooking, and check for corn, soybean, or cottonseed oil in products such as mayonnaise, margarine, and salad dressing.

In addition to its effects on heart disease risk, dietary fat can affect health in other ways. Diets high in fatty red meat are associated with an increased risk of certain forms of cancer, especially colon cancer. A high-fat diet can also make weight management more difficult. Because fat is a concentrated source of calories (9 calories per gram versus 4 calories per gram for protein and carbohydrate), a high-fat diet is often a high-calorie diet that can lead to weight gain. In addition, there is some evidence that calories from fat are more easily converted to body fat than calories from protein or carbohydrate.

Although more research is needed on the precise effects of different types and amounts of fat on overall health, a great deal of evidence points to the fact that most people benefit from keeping their overall fat intake at recommended levels and choosing unsaturated fats instead of saturated and trans fats. The types of fatty acids and their effects on health are summarized in Figure 12-3.

Recommended Fat Intake To meet the body's demand for essential fats, adult men need about 17 grams per day of linoleic acid and 1.6 grams per day of alpha-linolenic acid; adult women need 12 grams of linoleic acid and 1.1 grams of alpha-linolenic acid. Only 3–4 teaspoons (15–20 grams) of vegetable oil per day incorporated into your diet will supply the essential fats. Most Americans consume sufficient amounts of the essential

Terms

V**i**w

low-density lipoprotein (LDL) Blood fat that transports cholesterol to organs and tissues; excess amounts result in the accumulation of deposits on artery walls.

high-density lipoprotein (HDL) Blood fat that helps transport cholesterol out of the arteries, thereby protecting against heart disease.

omega-3 fatty acids Polyunsaturated fatty acids commonly found in fish oils that are beneficial to cardiovascular health; the endmost double bond occurs three carbons from the end of the fatty acid chain.

Type of Fatty Acid	Found In[a]	Possible Effects on Health
Keep Intake Low		
SATURATED	Animal fats (especially fatty meats and poultry fat and skin) Butter, cheese, and other high-fat dairy products Palm and coconut oils	Raises total cholesterol and LDL cholesterol levels Increases risk of heart disease May increase risk of colon and prostate
TRANS	French fries and other deep-fried fast foods Stick margarines, shortening Packaged cookies and crackers Processed snacks and sweets	Raises total cholesterol and LDL cholesterol levels Lowers HDL cholesterol levels May increase risk of heart disease and breast cancer
Choose Moderate Amounts		
MONOUNSATURATED	Olive, canola, and safflower oils Avocados, olives Peanut butter (without added fat) Many nuts, including almonds, cashews, pecans, pistachios	Lowers total cholesterol and LDL cholesterol levels May reduce blood pressure and lower triglyceride levels (a risk factor for CVD) May reduce risk of heart disease, stroke, and some cancers
POLYUNSATURATED (two groups)[b]		
Omega-3 fatty acids	Fatty fish, including salmon, white albacore tuna, mackerel, anchovies, and sardines Lesser amounts in walnut, flaxseed, canola, and soybean oils; tofu; walnuts; flaxseeds; and dark green leafy vegetables	Reduces blood clotting and inflammation and inhibits abnormal heart rhythms Lowers triglyceride levels (a risk factor for CVD) May lower blood pressure in some people May reduce risk of fatal heart attack, stroke and some cancers
Omega-6 fatty acids	Corn, soybean, and cottonseed oils (often used in margarine, mayonnaise, and salad dressing)	Lowers total cholesterol and LDL cholesterol levels May lower HDL cholesterol levels May reduce risk of heart disease May slightly increase risk of cancer if omega-6 intake is high and omega-3 intake is low

[a] Food fats contain a combination of types of fatty acids in various proportions; for example, canola oil is composed mainly of monounsaturated fatty acids (62%) but also contains polyunsaturated (32%) and saturated (6%) fatty acids. Food fats are categorized here according to their predominant fatty acid.

[b] The essential fatty acids are polyunsaturated: Linoleic acid is an omega-6 fatty acid and alpha-linolenic acid is an omega-3 fatty acid.

Figure 12-3   Types of fatty acids and their possible effects on health.   The health effects of dietary fats are still being investigated. In general, nutritionists recommend that we consume a diet moderate in fat overall and that we choose unsaturated fats instead of saturated and trans fats. Monounsaturated fats and omega-3 polyunsaturated fats may be particularly good choices for promoting health. Eating lots of fat of any type can provide excess calories because all types of fats are rich sources of energy (9 calories per gram).

fats; limiting unhealthy fats is a much greater health concern.

Limits for total fat, saturated fat, and trans fat intake have been set by a number of government and research organizations. In 2002, the Food and Nutrition Board of the Institute of Medicine released recommendations for the balance of energy sources in a healthful diet. These new recommendations, called Acceptable Macronutrient Distribution Ranges (AMDRs), are based on ensuring adequate intake of essential nutrients while also reducing the risk of chronic diseases such as heart disease and cancer. As with protein, a range of levels of fat consumption is associated with good health; the AMDR for total fat is 20–35% of total calories. Although more difficult for consumers to monitor, AMDRs have also been set for omega-6 fatty acids (5–10%) and omega-3 fatty acids (0.6–1.2%) as part of total fat intake. Because any amount of saturated and trans fats increases the risk of heart disease, the Food and Nutrition Board recommends that saturated fat and trans fat intake be kept as low as possible; most fat in a healthy diet should be unsaturated. American adults currently consume about 33% of total calories as fat, including 11–12% of calories as saturated fat and 2–4% as trans fat.

For advice on setting individual intake goals, see the box "Setting Intake Goals for Protein, Fat, and Carbohydrate." To determine how close you are to meeting your personal intake goals for fat, keep a running total over the course of the day. For prepared foods, food labels list the number of grams of fat, protein, and carbohydrate; the breakdown for popular fast-food items can be found in Appendix A. Nutrition information is also available in many grocery stores, in inexpensive published nutrition guides, and online (see For More Information at the end of the chapter). By checking these resources, you can keep track of the total grams of fat, protein, and carbohydrate you eat and assess your current diet.

Take Charge

Goals have been established by the Food and Nutrition Board to help ensure adequate intake of the essential amino acids, fatty acids, and carbohydrate. The daily goals for adequate intake for adults are as follow:

	Men	Women
Protein	56 grams	46 grams
Fat: Linoleic acid	17 grams	12 grams
Alpha-linolenic acid	1.6 grams	1.1 grams
Carbohydrate	130 grams	130 grams

Protein intake goals can be calculated more specifically by multiplying your body weight in kilograms by 0.8 or your body weight in pounds by 0.36. (Refer to the Nutrition Resources section at the end of the chapter for information for specific age groups and life stages.)

To meet your daily energy needs, you need to consume more than the minimally adequate amounts of the energy-providing nutrients listed above, which alone supply only about 800–900 calories. The Food and Nutrition Board provides additional guidance in the form of Acceptable Macronutrient Distribution Ranges (AMDRs). The ranges can help you balance your intake of the energy-providing nutrients in ways that ensure adequate intake while reducing the risk of chronic disease. The AMDRs for protein, total fat, and carbohydrate are as follow:

Protein	10–35% of total daily calories
Total fat	20–35% of total daily calories
Carbohydrate	45–65% of total daily calories

To set individual goals, begin by estimating your total daily energy (calorie) needs; if your weight is stable, your current energy intake is the number of calories you need to maintain your weight at your current activity level. Next, select percentage goals for protein, fat, and carbohydrate. You can allocate your total daily calories among the three classes of macronutrients to suit your preferences; just make sure that the three percentages you select total 100% and that you meet the minimum intake goals listed. Two samples reflecting different total energy intake and nutrient intake goals are shown in the table below.

To translate your own percentage goals into daily intake goals expressed in calories and grams, multiply the appropriate percentages by total calorie intake and then divide the results by the corresponding calories per gram. For example, a fat limit of 35% applied to a 2200-calorie diet would be calculated as follows: 0.35 × 2200 = 770 calories of total fat; 770 ÷ 9 calories per gram = 86 grams of total fat. (Remember that, fat has 9 calories per gram and that protein and carbohydrate have 4 calories per gram.)

Two Sample Macronutrient Distributions

Nutrient	AMDR	Sample 1 Individual Goals	Sample 1 Amounts for a 1600-Calorie Diet	Sample 2 Individual Goals	Sample 2 Amounts for a 2800-Calorie Diet
Protein	10–35%	15%	240 calories = 60 grams	30%	840 calories = 210 grams
Fat	20–35%	30%	480 calories = 53 grams	25%	700 calories = 78 grams
Carbohydrate	45–65%	55%	880 calories = 220 grams	45%	1260 calories = 315 grams

SOURCE: Food and Nutrition Board, Institute of Medicine, National Academies. 2002. *Dietary Reference Intakes: Applications in Dietary Planning,* Washington, D.C.: National Academies Press. © 2003 by the National Academy of Sciences. Reprinted with permission from the National Academies Press, Washington, D.C.

For most Americans, meeting recommendations for fat intake means lowering intake of saturated and trans fats and maintaining total fat intake within the healthy range (see Figure 12-3). You can still eat high-fat foods, but it makes good sense to limit the size of your portions and to balance your intake with low-fat foods. For example, peanut butter is high in fat, with 8 grams (72 calories) of fat in each 90-calorie tablespoon. Two tablespoons of peanut butter eaten on whole-wheat bread and served with a banana, carrot sticks, and a glass of fat-free milk makes a nutritious lunch—high in protein and carbohydrate, and relatively low in fat (500 calories, 18 grams of total fat, 4 grams of saturated fat). Four tablespoons of peanut butter on high-fat crackers with potato chips, cookies, and whole milk is a less healthy combination (1000 calories, 62 grams of total fat, 15 grams of saturated fat). So although it's important to evaluate individual food items for their fat content, it is more important to look at them in the context of your overall diet.

Carbohydrates—An Ideal Source of Energy

Carbohydrates are needed in the diet primarily to supply energy for body cells. Some cells, such as those found in the brain and other parts of the nervous system and in blood, use only carbohydrates for fuel. During high-intensity exercise, muscles also use primarily carbohydrates for fuel. When we don't eat enough carbohydrates to satisfy the needs of the brain and red blood cells, our bodies synthesize carbohydrates from proteins. In situations of extreme deprivation, when the diet lacks a sufficient amount of both carbohydrates and proteins, the body turns to its own organs and tissues, breaking down proteins in muscles, the heart, kidneys, and other vital organs to supply carbohydrate needs. This rarely occurs, however, because consuming the equivalent of just three or four slices of bread supplies the body's daily minimum need for carbohydrates.

Simple and Complex Carbohydrates   Carbohydrates are classified into two groups: simple and complex. Simple carbohydrates contain only one or two sugar units in each molecule; they include sucrose (table sugar), fructose (fruit sugar, honey), maltose (malt sugar), and lactose (milk sugar). Simple carbohydrates provide much of the sweetness in foods and are found naturally in fruits and milk and are added to soft drinks, fruit drinks, candy, and sweet desserts. There is no evidence that any type of simple sugar is more nutritious than others.

Complex carbohydrates consist of chains of many sugar molecules; they include starches and most types of dietary fiber. Starches are found in a variety of plants, especially grains (wheat, rye, rice, oats, barley, millet), legumes (dry beans, peas, and lentils), and tubers (potatoes and yams). Most other vegetables contain a mixture of starches and simple carbohydrates. Fiber, discussed in the next section, is found in grains, fruits, and vegetables.

During digestion in the mouth and small intestine, your body breaks down starches and double sugars into single sugar molecules, such as **glucose,** for absorption. Once glucose is in the bloodstream, the pancreas releases the hormone insulin, which allows cells to take up glucose and use it for energy. The liver and muscles also take up glucose to provide carbohydrate storage in the form of **glycogen.** Some people have problems controlling blood glucose levels, a disorder called diabetes mellitus (see Chapter 14 for more on diabetes). Carbohydrates consumed in excess of the body's energy needs are changed into fat and stored. Whenever calorie intake exceeds calorie expenditure, fat storage can lead to weight gain. This is true whether the excess calories come from carbohydrates, proteins, fat, or alcohol.

Refined Carbohydrates Versus Whole Grains
Complex carbohydrates can be further divided between refined, or processed, carbohydrates and unrefined carbohydrates, or whole grains. Before they are processed, all grains are **whole grains**, consisting of an inner layer, germ; a middle layer, the endosperm; and an outer layer, bran. During processing, the germ and bran are often removed, leaving just the starchy endosperm. The refinement of whole grains transforms whole-wheat flour to white flour, brown rice to white rice, and so on.

Refined carbohydrates usually retain all the calories of their unrefined counterparts, but they tend to be much lower in fiber, vitamins, minerals, and other beneficial compounds. (Many refined grain products are enriched or fortified with vitamins and minerals, but often the nutrients lost in processing are not replaced.) Unrefined carbohydrates tend to take longer to chew and digest than refined ones; they also enter the bloodstream more slowly. This slower digestive pace tends to make people feel full sooner and for a longer period. Also, a slower rise in blood glucose levels following consumption of complex carbohydrates may help in the management of diabetes. Whole grains are also high in dietary fiber and so have all the benefits of fiber. Consumption of whole grains has been linked to a reduced risk of heart disease, diabetes, high blood pressure, stroke, and certain forms of cancer. For all these reasons, whole grains are recommended over those that have been refined. This does not mean that you should never eat refined carbohydrates such as white bread or white rice, simply that whole-wheat bread, brown rice, and other whole grains are healthier choices. See the box "Choosing More Whole-Grain Foods" for tips on increasing your intake of whole grains.

Glycemic Index and Glycemic Response   Insulin and glucose levels rise and fall following a meal or snack containing any type of carbohydrate. Some foods cause a quick and dramatic rise in glucose and insulin levels; others have a slower, more moderate effect. A food that has a strong effect on blood glucose levels is said to have a high **glycemic index.** Research findings have been mixed, but some studies have found that consuming a meal containing high glycemic index foods may increase appetite, and that over the long term, diets rich in these foods may increase risk of diabetes and heart disease for some people. High glycemic index foods do not, as some popular diets claim, directly cause weight gain beyond the calories they contain.

Attempting to base food choices on glycemic index can be a difficult task, however. Although unrefined complex

Terms

carbohydrate An essential nutrient; sugars, starches, and dietary fiber are all carbohydrates.

glucose A simple sugar that is the body's basic fuel.

glycogen An animal starch stored in the liver and muscles.

whole grain The entire edible portion of a grain such as wheat, rice, or oats, consisting of the germ, endosperm, and bran. During milling or processing, parts of the grain are removed, often leaving just the endosperm.

glycemic index A measure of how the ingestion of a particular food affects blood glucose levels.

Whole-grain foods are good weapons against heart disease, diabetes, high blood pressure, stroke, and certain cancers. They are also low in fat and so can be a good choice for managing weight. Federal dietary guidelines recommend 6 or more total servings of grain products every day, with at least half of these servings from whole grains. However, Americans currently average less than 1 serving of whole grains per day.

What Are Whole Grains?

The first step in increasing your intake of whole grains is to correctly identify them. The following are whole grains:

whole wheat	whole-grain corn
whole rye	popcorn
whole oats	brown rice
oatmeal	whole-grain barley

More unusual choices include bulgur (cracked wheat), millet, kasha (roasted buckwheat kernels), quinoa, wheat and rye berries, amaranth, wild rice, graham flour, whole-grain kamut, whole-grain spelt, and whole-grain triticale.

Wheat flour, unbleached flour, enriched flour, and degerminated corn meal are not whole grains. Wheat germ and wheat bran are also not whole grains, but they are the constituents of wheat typically left out when wheat is processed and so are healthier choices than regular wheat flour, which typically contains just the endosperm.

Reading Food Packages to Find Whole Grains

To find packaged foods rich in whole grains, read the list of ingredients and check for special health claims related to whole grains. The *first* item on the list of ingredients should be one of the whole grains listed above. In addition, the FDA allows manufacturers to include special health claims for foods that contain 51% or more whole-grain ingredients. Such products may contain a statement such as the following on their packaging: "Rich in whole grain," "Made with 100% whole grain," or "Diets rich in whole-grain foods may help reduce the risk of heart disease and certain cancers." However, many whole-grain products will not carry such claims. Product names and food color can be misleading. *When in doubt, always check the list of ingredients, looking for "whole" as the first word on the list.*

Incorporating Whole Grains into Your Daily Diet

- *Bread:* Look for sandwich breads, bagels, English muffins, buns, and pita breads with a whole grain listed as the first ingredient.

- *Breakfast cereals:* Check the ingredient list for whole grains. Whole-grain choices include oatmeal, muesli, shredded wheat, and some types of raisin bran, bran flakes, wheat flakes, toasted oats, and granola.

- *Rice:* Choose brown rice or rice blends that include brown rice.

- *Pasta:* Look for whole-wheat, whole-grain kamut, or whole-grain spelt pasta.

- *Tortillas:* Choose whole-wheat or whole-corn tortillas.

- *Crackers and snacks:* Some varieties of crackers are made from whole grains, including some flatbreads or crispbreads, woven wheat crackers, and rye crackers. Other whole-grain snack possibilities include popcorn, popcorn cakes, brown rice cakes, whole-corn tortilla chips, and whole-wheat fig cookies. Be sure to check food labels for fat content, as many popular snacks are high in fat.

- *Mixed-grain dishes:* Combine whole grains with other foods to create healthy mixed dishes. Possibilities include tabouli; soups made with hulled barley or wheat berries; and pilafs, casseroles, and salads made with brown rice, whole-wheat couscous, kasha, millet, wheat bulgur, or quinoa.

If your grocery store doesn't carry all of these items, try your local health food store.

---

carbohydrates and high-fiber foods generally tend to have a low glycemic index, patterns are less clear for other types of foods and do not follow a easy distinction such as that of simple versus complex carbohydrates. For example, some fruits with fairly high levels of simple carbohydrates have only a moderate effect on blood glucose levels, whereas white rice, potatoes, and white bread, which are rich in complex carbohydrates, have a high glycemic index. Watermelon has a glycemic index more than twice that of strawberries, and the glycemic index of a banana changes dramatically as it ripens. The body's response to carbohydrates also depends on many other factors, such as how foods are combined and prepared and the fitness status of the individual.

This complexity is one reason major health organizations have not issued specific guidelines for glycemic index. For people with particular health concerns, glycemic index may be an important consideration; however, it should not be the sole criterion for food choices. For example, ice cream has a lower glycemic index than brown rice or carrots—but that doesn't make it a healthier choice overall. Glycemic index is discussed further in Chapters 14 and 15. For now, remember that most unrefined grains, fruits, vegetables, and legumes are rich in nutrients, have a relatively low energy density, and have low-to-moderate glycemic index. Choose a variety of vegetables daily, and avoid heavy consumption of white potatoes. Limit foods that are high in added sugars but provide few other nutrients. Some studies have singled out regular soda, with its large dose of rapidly absorbable sugar, as specifically linked to increased diabetes risk.

Recommended Carbohydrate Intake On average, Americans consume 200–300 grams of carbohydrate per day, well above the 130 grams needed to meet the body's requirement for essential carbohydrate. A range of intakes is associated with good health, and experts recommend that adults consume 45–65% of total daily calories as carbohydrate, about 225–325 grams of carbohydrate for someone consuming 2000 calories per day. The focus should be on consuming a variety of foods rich in complex carbohydrates, especially whole grains.

Although the Food and Nutrition Board set an AMDR for added sugars of 25% or less of total daily calories, many health experts recommend an even lower intake. World Health Organization guidelines suggested a limit of 10% of total daily calories from added sugars; limits set by the USDA in 2005 are even lower, with a maximum of about 8 teaspoons (32 grams) suggested for someone consuming 2000 calories per day. Foods high in added sugar are generally high in calories and low in nutrients and fiber, thus providing empty calories. To reduce your intake of added sugars, limit soft drinks, candy, sweet desserts, and sweetened fruit drinks. The simple carbohydrates in your diet should come mainly from fruits, which are excellent sources of vitamins and minerals, and from low-fat or fat-free milk and other dairy products, which are high in protein and calcium.

Athletes in training can especially benefit from high-carbohydrate diets (60–70% of total daily calories), which enhance the amount of carbohydrates stored in their muscles (as glycogen) and therefore provide more carbohydrate fuel for use during endurance events or long workouts. In addition, carbohydrates consumed during prolonged athletic events can help fuel muscles and extend the availability of the glycogen stored in muscles. Caution is in order, however, because overconsumption of carbohydrates can lead to fatigue and underconsumption of other nutrients.

Fiber—A Closer Look

Fiber is the term given to nondigestible carbohydrates provided by plants. Instead of being digested, like starch, fiber passes through the intestinal tract and provides bulk for feces in the large intestine, which in turn facilitates elimination. In the large intestine, some types of fiber are broken down by bacteria into acids and gases, which explains why consuming too much fiber can lead to intestinal gas. Because humans cannot digest fiber, it is not a source of carbohydrate in the diet; however, the consumption of fiber is necessary for good health.

Types of Fiber The Food and Nutrition Board has defined two types of fiber: dietary fiber and functional fiber.

Dietary fiber refers to the nondigestible carbohydrates (and the noncarbohydrate substance lignin) that are present naturally in plants such as grains, legumes, and vegetables. **Functional fiber** refers to nondigestible carbohydrates that have been either isolated from natural sources or synthesized in a lab and then added to a food product or dietary supplement. **Total fiber** is the sum of dietary and functional fiber.

Fibers have different properties that lead to different physiological effects in the body. For example, viscous fibers such as those found in oat bran or legumes can delay stomach emptying, slow the movement of glucose into the blood after eating, and reduce absorption of cholesterol. Other types of fiber, such as those found in wheat bran or psyllium seed, increase fecal bulk and help prevent constipation, hemorrhoids, and **diverticulitis.** A diet high in fiber can help reduce the risk of type 2 diabetes and heart disease as well as improve gastrointestinal health. Some studies have linked high-fiber diets with reduced risk of colon and rectal cancer; other studies have suggested that other characteristics of diets rich in fruits, vegetables, and whole grains may be responsible for this reduction in risk (see Chapter 16 for more on cancer and diet).

Sources of Fiber All plant foods contain some dietary fiber. Fruits, legumes, oats (especially oat bran), and barley all contain the viscous types of fiber that help lower blood glucose and cholesterol levels. Wheat (especially wheat bran), other grains and cereals, and vegetables are good sources of cellulose and other fibers that help prevent constipation. Psyllium, which is often added to cereals or used in fiber supplements and laxatives, improves intestinal health and also helps control glucose and cholesterol levels. The processing of packaged foods can remove fiber, so it is important to rely on fresh fruits and vegetables and foods made from whole grains as your main sources of fiber.

Recommended Fiber Intake To reduce the risk of chronic disease and maintain intestinal health, the Food and Nutrition Board recommends a daily fiber intake of 38 grams for adult men and 25 grams for adult women. Americans currently consume about half this amount. Fiber should come from foods, not supplements, which should be used only under medical supervision. To

Terms

dietary fiber Nondigestible carbohydrates and lignin that are intact in plants.

functional fiber Nondigestible carbohydrates either isolated from natural sources or synthesized; these may be added to foods and dietary supplements.

total fiber The total amount of dietary fiber and functional fiber in the diet.

diverticulitis A digestive disorder in which abnormal pouches form in the walls of the intestine and become inflamed.

increase the amount of fiber in your daily diet to recommended levels, try the following strategies:

- Choose whole-grain foods instead of those made from processed grains. Select high-fiber breakfast cereals (those with 5 or more grams of fiber per serving).
- Eat whole, unpeeled fruits rather than drinking fruit juice. Top cereals, yogurt, and desserts with berries, unpeeled apple slices, or other fruit.
- Include legumes in soups and salads. Combine raw vegetables with pasta, rice, or beans in salads.
- Substitute bean dip for cheese-based or sour cream–based dips or spreads. Use raw vegetables rather than chips for dipping.

Vitamins—Organic Micronutrients

Vitamins are organic (carbon-containing) substances required in small amounts to regulate various processes within living cells (Table 12-1). Humans need 13 vitamins; 4 are fat-soluble (A, D, E, and K), and 9 are water-soluble (C, and the 8 B-complex vitamins: thiamin, riboflavin, niacin, vitamin B-6, folate, vitamin B-12, biotin, and pantothenic acid). Solubility affects how a vitamin is absorbed, transported, and stored in the body. The water-soluble vitamins are absorbed directly into the bloodstream, where they travel freely; excess water-soluble vitamins are detected and removed by the kidneys and excreted in urine. Fat-soluble vitamins require a more complex absorptive process; they are usually carried in the blood by special proteins and are stored in the body in the liver and in fat tissues rather than excreted.

Functions of Vitamins
Many vitamins help chemical reactions take place. They provide no energy to the body directly but help unleash the energy stored in carbohydrates, proteins, and fats. Vitamins are critical in the production of red blood cells and the maintenance of the nervous, skeletal, and immune systems. Some vitamins act as **antioxidants,** which help preserve healthy cells in the body. Key vitamin antioxidants include vitamin E, vitamin C, and the vitamin A precursor beta-carotene. (Antioxidants are described later in the chapter.)

Terms

V̇ẇ

vitamins Carbon-containing substances needed in small amounts to help promote and regulate chemical reactions and processes in the body.

antioxidant A substance that can lessen the breakdown of food or body constituents by free radicals; actions include binding oxygen, donating electrons to free radicals, and repairing damage to molecules.

scurvy A disease caused by a lack of vitamin C, characterized by bleeding gums, loosening teeth, and poor wound healing.

Sources of Vitamins
The human body does not manufacture most of the vitamins it requires and must obtain them from foods. Vitamins are abundant in fruits, vegetables, and grains. In addition, many processed foods, such as flour and breakfast cereals, contain added vitamins. A few vitamins are made in certain parts of the body: The skin makes vitamin D when it is exposed to sunlight, and intestinal bacteria make vitamin K. Nonetheless, you still need to obtain vitamin D and vitamin K from foods.

Vitamin Deficiencies and Excesses
If your diet lacks sufficient amounts of a particular vitamin, characteristic symptoms of deficiency develop (see Table 12-1.) For example, vitamin A deficiency can cause blindness, and vitamin B-6 deficiency can cause seizures. The best-known deficiency disease is probably **scurvy,** caused by vitamin C deficiency. In the eighteenth century, it killed many sailors on long ocean voyages, until people realized that eating citrus fruits could prevent it. Even today people develop scurvy; its presence suggests a very poor intake of fruits and vegetables, which are rich sources of vitamin C.

Vitamin deficiency diseases are most often seen in developing countries; they are relatively rare in the United States because vitamins are readily available from our food supply. People suffering from alcoholism and malabsorption disorders probably run the greatest risk of vitamin deficiencies. However, intakes below recommended levels can have adverse effects on health even if they are not low enough to cause a deficiency disease. For example, low intake of folate and vitamins B-6 and B-12 has been linked to increased heart disease risk. Many Americans consume less-than-recommended amounts of several vitamins, including vitamins A, C, and D; vitamin E intake is also low among some groups, especially African Americans. Table 12-1 lists good food sources of vitamins.

Extra vitamins in the diet can also be harmful, especially when taken as supplements. High doses of vitamin A are toxic and increase the risk of birth defects, for example. Vitamin B-6 can cause irreversible nerve damage when taken in large doses. Megadoses of fat-soluble vitamins are particularly dangerous because the excess will be stored in the body rather than excreted, increasing the risk of toxicity. Even when vitamins are not taken in excess, relying on supplements for an adequate intake of vitamins can be a problem. There are many substances in foods other than vitamins and minerals, and some of these compounds may have important health effects. Later in the chapter we discuss specific recommendations for vitamin intake and when a vitamin supplement is advisable. For now, keep in mind that it's best to obtain most of your vitamins from foods rather than supplements.

Table 12-1 | Facts About Vitamins

Vitamin	Important Dietary Sources	Major Functions	Signs of Prolonged Deficiency	Toxic Effects of Megadoses
Fat-Soluble				
Vitamin A	Liver, milk, butter, cheese, and fortified margarine; carrots, spinach, and other orange and deep-green vegetables and fruits	Maintenance of vision, skin, linings of the nose, mouth, digestive and urinary tracts, immune function	Night blindness; dry, scaling skin; increased susceptibility to infection; loss of appetite; anemia; kidney stones	Liver damage, miscarriage and birth defects, headache, vomiting and diarrhea, vertigo, double vision, bone abnormalities
Vitamin D	Fortified milk and margarine, fish oils, butter, egg yolks (sunlight on skin also produces vitamin D)	Development and maintenance of bones and teeth, promotion of calcium absorption	Rickets (bone deformities) in children; bone softening, loss, and fractures in adults	Kidney damage, calcium deposits in soft tissues, depression, death
Vitamin E	Vegetable oils, whole grains, nuts and seeds, green leafy vegetables, asparagus, peaches	Protection and maintenance of cellular membranes	Red blood cell breakage and anemia, weakness, neurological problems, muscle cramps	Relatively nontoxic, but may cause excess bleeding or formation of blood clots
Vitamin K	Green leafy vegetables; smaller amounts widespread in other foods	Production of factors essential for blood clotting and bone metabolism	Hemorrhaging	None reported
Water-Soluble				
Biotin	Cereals, yeast, egg yolks, soy flour, liver; widespread in foods	Synthesis of fat, glycogen, and amino acids	Rash, nausea, vomiting, weight loss, depression, fatigue, hair loss	None reported
Folate	Green leafy vegetables, yeast, oranges, whole grains, legumes, liver	Amino acid metabolism, synthesis of RNA and DNA, new cell synthesis	Anemia, weakness, fatigue, irritability, shortness of breath, swollen tongue	Masking of vitamin B-12 deficiency
Niacin	Eggs, poultry, fish, milk, whole grains, nuts, enriched breads and cereals, meats, legumes	Conversion of carbohydrates, fats, and protein into usable forms of energy	Pellagra (symptoms include diarrhea, dermatitis, inflammation of mucous membranes, dementia)	Flushing of the skin, nausea, vomiting, diarrhea, liver dysfunction, glucose intolerance
Pantothenic acid	Animal foods, whole grains, broccoli, potatoes; widespread in foods	Metabolism of fats, carbohydrates, and proteins	Fatigue, numbness and tingling of hands and feet, gastrointestinal disturbances	None reported
Riboflavin	Dairy products, enriched breads and cereals, lean meats, poultry, fish, green vegetables	Energy metabolism; maintenance of skin, mucous membranes, and nervous system structures	Cracks at corners of mouth, sore throat, skin rash, hypersensitivity to light, purple tongue	None reported
Thiamin	Whole-grain and enriched breads and cereals, organ meats, lean pork, nuts, legumes	Conversion of carbohydrates into usable forms of energy, maintenance of appetite and nervous system function	Beriberi (symptoms include muscle wasting, mental confusion, anorexia, enlarged heart, nerve changes)	None reported
Vitamin B-6	Eggs, poultry, fish, whole grains, nuts, soybeans, liver, kidney, pork	Metabolism of amino acids and glycogen	Anemia, convulsions, cracks at corners of mouth, dermatitis, nausea, confusion	Neurological abnormalities and damage
Vitamin B-12	Meat, fish, poultry, fortified cereals	Synthesis of blood cells; other metabolic reactions	Anemia, fatigue, nervous system damage, sore tongue	None reported
Vitamin C	Peppers, broccoli, spinach, brussels sprouts, citrus fruits, strawberries, tomatoes, potatoes, cabbage, other fruits and vegetables	Maintenance and repair of connective tissue, bones, teeth, and cartilage; promotion of healing; aid in iron absorption	Scurvy, anemia, reduced resistance to infection, loosened teeth, joint pain, poor wound healing, hair loss, poor iron absorption	Urinary stones in some people, acid stomach from ingesting supplements in pill form, nausea, diarrhea, headache, fatigue

SOURCES: Food and Nutrition Board, Institute of Medicine, National Academies. 2001. *Dietary Reference Intakes Tables* (http://www.iom.edu/file.asp?id=21372; retrieved December 21, 2004). The complete Dietary Reference Intake reports are available from the National Academy Press (http://www.nap.edu); Shils, M. E., et al., eds. 1998. *Modern Nutrition in Health and Disease*, 9th ed. Baltimore: Williams & Wilkins.

Keeping the Nutrient Value in Food Vitamins and minerals can be lost or destroyed during the storage and cooking of foods. To retain nutrients, consume or process vegetables as soon as possible after purchasing. Store fruits and vegetables in the refrigerator in covered containers or plastic bags to minimize moisture loss; freeze foods that won't be eaten within a few days. (Frozen and canned vegetables are usually as high in nutrients as fresh vegetables because nutrients are locked in when produce is frozen or canned.) To reduce nutrient losses during food preparation, minimize the amount of water used and the total cooking time. Develop a taste for a crunchier texture in cooked vegetables. Baking, steaming, broiling, and microwaving are all good methods of preparing vegetables.

Minerals—Inorganic Micronutrients

Minerals are inorganic (non–carbon-containing) elements you need in relatively small amounts to help regulate body functions, aid in the growth and maintenance of body tissues, and help release energy (Table 12-2). There are about 17 essential minerals. The major minerals, those that the body needs in amounts exceeding 100 milligrams per day, include calcium, phosphorus, magnesium, sodium, potassium, and chloride. The essential trace minerals, those that you need in minute amounts, include copper, fluoride, iodide, iron, selenium, and zinc.

Characteristic symptoms develop if an essential mineral is consumed in a quantity too small or too large for good health. The minerals commonly lacking in the American diet are iron, calcium, potassium, and magnesium. Focus on good food choices for these (see Table 12-2). Lean meats are rich in iron, whereas low-fat or fat-free dairy products are excellent choices for calcium. Potassium is found in green leafy vegetables, white and sweet potatoes, bananas, and other fruits and vegetables. Plant foods such as whole grains and leafy vegetables are good sources of magnesium. Iron-deficiency **anemia** is a problem in many age groups, and researchers fear poor calcium intakes are sowing the seeds for future

Terms

V̇ẇ

minerals Inorganic compounds needed in relatively small amounts for regulation, growth, and maintenance of body tissues and functions.

anemia A deficiency in the oxygen-carrying material in the red blood cells.

osteoporosis A condition in which the bones become extremely thin and brittle and break easily.

free radical An electron-seeking compound that can react with fats, proteins, and DNA, damaging cell membranes and mutating genes in its search for electrons; produced through chemical reactions in the body and by exposure to environmental factors such as sunlight and tobacco smoke.

osteoporosis, especially in women. See Chapter 19 for more information on osteoporosis; the box "Eating for Healthy Bones" has tips for building and maintaining bone density.

Water—Vital but Often Ignored

Water is the major component in both foods and the human body: You are composed of about 50–60% water. Your need for other nutrients, in terms of weight, is much less than your need for water. You can live up to 50 days without food, but only a few days without water.

Water is distributed all over the body, among lean and other tissues and in blood and other body fluids. Water is used in the digestion and absorption of food and is the medium in which most of the chemical reactions take place within the body. Some water-based fluids, like blood, transport substances around the body, whereas other fluids serve as lubricants or cushions. Water also helps regulate body temperature.

Water is contained in almost all foods, particularly in liquids, fruits, and vegetables. The foods and fluids you consume provide 80–90% of your daily water intake; the remainder is generated through metabolism. You lose water each day in urine, feces, and sweat and through evaporation from your lungs.

Most people can maintain a healthy water balance by consuming beverages at meals and drinking fluids in response to thirst. Water and other beverages typically make up about 80% of your fluid intake; the remainder comes from foods, especially fruits and vegetables. In 2004, the Food and Nutrition Board set levels of adequate water intake to maintain hydration; all fluids, including those containing caffeine, can count toward your total daily fluid intake. Under these guidelines, men need to consume about 3.7 total liters of water, with 3.0 liters (about 13 cups) coming from beverages; women need 2.7 total liters, with 2.2 liters (about 9 cups) coming from beverages. (See Table 1 in the Nutrition Resources section at the end of the chapter for information on specific age groups.) If you exercise vigorously or live in a hot climate, you need to consume additional fluids to maintain a balance between water consumed and water lost. Severe dehydration causes weakness and can lead to death.

Other Substances in Food

Many substances in food are not essential nutrients but may influence health.

Antioxidants When the body uses oxygen or breaks down certain fats or proteins as a normal part of metabolism, it gives rise to substances called **free radicals.** Environmental factors such as cigarette smoke, exhaust

Table 12-2 Facts About Selected Minerals

Mineral	Important Dietary Sources	Major Functions	Signs of Prolonged Deficiency	Toxic Effects of Megadoses
Calcium M	Milk and milk products, tofu, fortified orange juice and bread, green leafy vegetables, bones in fish	Formation of bones and teeth, control of nerve impulses, muscle contraction, blood clotting	Stunted growth in children, bone mineral loss in adults; urinary stones	Kidney stones, calcium deposits in soft tissues, inhibition of mineral absorption, constipation
Fluoride	Fluoridated water, tea, marine fish eaten with bones	Maintenance of tooth and bone structure	Higher frequency of tooth decay	Increased bone density, mottling of teeth, impaired kidney function
Iodine	Iodized salt, seafood, processed foods	Essential part of thyroid hormones, regulation of body metabolism	Goiter (enlarged thyroid), cretinism (birth defect)	Depression of thyroid activity, hyperthyroidism in susceptible people
Iron	Meat and poultry, fortified grain products, dark green vegetables, dried fruit	Component of hemoglobin, myoglobin, and enzymes	Iron-deficiency anemia, weakness, impaired immune function, gastrointestinal distress	Nausea, diarrhea, liver and kidney damage, joint pains, sterility, disruption of cardiac function, death
Magnesium M	Widespread in foods and water (except soft water); especially found in grains, legumes, nuts, seeds, green vegetables, milk	Transmission of nerve impulses, energy transfer, activation of many enzymes	Neurological disturbances, cardiovascular problems, kidney disorders, nausea, growth failure in children	Nausea, vomiting, diarrhea, central nervous system depression, coma; death in people with impaired kidney function
Phosphorus M	Present in nearly all foods, especially milk, cereal, peas, eggs, meat	Bone growth and maintenance, energy transfer in cells	Impaired growth, weakness, kidney disorders, cardiorespiratory and nervous system dysfunction	Drop in blood calcium levels, calcium deposits in soft tissues, bone loss
Potassium M	Meats, milk, fruits, vegetables, grains, legumes	Nerve function and body water balance	Muscular weakness, nausea, drowsiness, paralysis, confusion, disruption of cardiac rhythm	Cardiac arrest
Selenium	Seafood, meat, eggs, whole grains	Defense against oxidative stress, regulation of thyroid hormone action	Muscle pain and weakness, heart disorders	Hair and nail loss, nausea and vomiting, weakness, irritability
Sodium M	Salt, soy sauce, salted foods, tomato juice	Body water balance, acid-base balance, nerve function	Muscle weakness, loss of appetite, nausea, vomiting; deficiency is rarely seen	Edema, hypertension in sensitive people
Zinc	Whole grains, meat, eggs, liver, seafood (especially oysters)	Synthesis of proteins, RNA, and DNA; wound healing; immune response; ability to taste	Growth failure, loss of appetite, impaired taste acuity, skin rash, impaired immune function, poor wound healing	Vomiting, impaired immune function, decline in blood HDL levels, impaired copper absorption

Chloride M

SOURCES: Food and Nutrition Board, Institute of Medicine, National Academies. 2001. *Dietary Reference Intakes Tables* (http://www.iom.edu/file.asp?id=21372; retrieved December 21, 2004). The complete Dietary Reference Intake reports are available from the National Academy Press (http://www.nap.edu); Shils, M. E., et al., eds. 1998. *Modern Nutrition in Health and Disease*, 9th ed. Baltimore: Williams & Wilkins.

fumes, radiation, excessive sunlight, certain drugs, and stress can increase free radical production. A free radical is a chemically unstable molecule that is missing an electron; it will react with any molecule it encounters from which it can take an electron. In their search for electrons, free radicals react with fats, proteins, and DNA, damaging cell membranes and mutating genes. Because of this, free radicals have been implicated in aging, cancer, cardiovascular disease, and other degenerative diseases like arthritis.

Antioxidants found in foods can help protect the body from damage by free radicals in several ways. Some dietary antioxidants prevent or reduce the formation of free radicals; others remove free radicals from the body by reacting with them directly by donating electrons. Antioxidants can also repair some types of free radical damage after it occurs. Some antioxidants, such as vitamin C, vitamin E, and selenium, are also essential nutrients; others, such as carotenoids, found in yellow, orange, and deep-green vegetables, are not. Obtaining a regular

Take Charge

Osteoporosis is a condition in which bones become dangerously thin and fragile over time. An estimated 10 million Americans over age 50 have osteoporosis, and another 34 million are at risk. Most bone mass is built by age 18, and after bone density peaks between ages 25 and 35, bone mass is slowly lost over time. To prevent osteoporosis, the best strategy is to build as much bone as possible during your youth and then do everything you can to maintain it as you age. Up to 50% of bone loss is determined by controllable lifestyle factors, especially diet and exercise habits. Key nutrients include the following:

Calcium　Consuming an adequate amount of calcium is important throughout life to build and maintain bone mass. Americans average 600–800 mg of calcium per day, only about half of what is recommended. Milk, yogurt, and calcium-fortified orange juice, bread, and cereals are all good sources. Nutritionists suggest that you obtain calcium from foods first and then take supplements only if needed to make up the difference.

Vitamin D　Vitamin D is necessary for bones to absorb calcium; a daily intake of 5 μg is recommended for adults age 19–50. Vitamin D can be obtained from foods and is manufactured by the skin when it is exposed to sunlight. Candidates for vitamin D supplements include people who don't eat many foods rich in vitamin D; those who have dark skin or who don't expose their face, arms, and hands to the sun (without sunscreen) for 5–15 minutes a few times each week; and people who live north of an imaginary line roughly between Boston and the Oregon–California border (the sun is weaker in northern latitudes).

Vitamin K　Vitamin K promotes the synthesis of proteins that help keep bones strong. Broccoli and leafy green vegetables are rich in vitamin K.

Other Nutrients　Several other nutrients may play an important role in bone health.

- *Vitamin C* works with calcium and other minerals to build bone; it also helps produce the connective tissue collagen, which forms the scaffolding in bones.

- *Magnesium* aids in bone formation.

- *Potassium* helps bones retain calcium.

- *Manganese* may help lessen calcium losses.

- *Zinc* and *copper* help maintain collagen.

- *Boron* may increase calcium absorption.

Several dietary substances may have a *negative* effect on bone health. Alcohol reduces the body's ability to absorb calcium and may interfere with the bone-protecting effects of the hormone estrogen. High sodium intake increases calcium loss in the urine, and thus may lead to loss of calcium from the skeleton. Caffeine may also cause small losses of urinary calcium, and experts often recommend that heavy caffeine consumers take special care to include calcium-rich foods in their diet. Adding milk to coffee or tea may offset the effect of caffeine on calcium loss. Protein can help build bone if intake of calcium and vitamin D is adequate; however, if calcium and vitamin D intake is low, high protein intake may lead to calcium loss. Chronic excess intake of retinol, one form of vitamin A, is associated with decreased bone density; if you consume a vitamin supplement or vitamin A–fortified foods, try to limit your daily intake of retinol to no more than 100% of the RDA. (You may need to check labels to determine what form of vitamin A is present; beta-carotene, which the body can convert to vitamin A, is not associated with problems.) Drinking lots of soda, which often replaces milk in the diet and which is high in phosphorus (a mineral that may interfere with calcium absorption), has been shown to increase the risk of bone fracture in teenage girls. For healthy bones, then, it is important to be moderate in your consumption of alcohol, protein, sodium, caffeine, retinol, and sodas.

Finally, it is important to combine a healthy diet with regular exercise. Weight-bearing aerobic activities, if performed regularly, help build and maintain bone mass throughout life. Strength training improves bone density, muscle mass, strength, and balance, protecting against both bone loss and falls, a major cause of fractures. See Chapter 13 for tips on creating a complete, personalized exercise program.

intake of these nutrients is vital for the health of the body. Many fruits and vegetables are rich in antioxidants.

Phytochemicals　Antioxidants fall into the broader category of **phytochemicals**, substances found in plant foods that may help prevent chronic disease. Researchers have just begun to identify and study all the different compounds found in foods, and many preliminary findings are promising. For example, certain substances found in soy foods may help lower cholesterol levels. Sulforaphane, a compound isolated from broccoli and other **cruciferous vegetables**, may render some carcinogenic compounds harmless. Allyl sulfides, a group of chemicals found in garlic and onions, appear to boost the activity of cancer-fighting immune cells. Further research on phytochemicals may extend the role of nutrition to the prevention and treatment of many chronic diseases.

If you want to increase your intake of phytochemicals, it is best to obtain them by eating a variety of fruits, vegetables, and grains rather than relying on supplements. Like many vitamins and minerals, isolated phytochemicals may be harmful if taken in high doses. In addition, it is likely that their health benefits are the result of chemical substances working in combination. The role of phytochemicals in disease prevention is discussed further in Chapters 15 and 16.

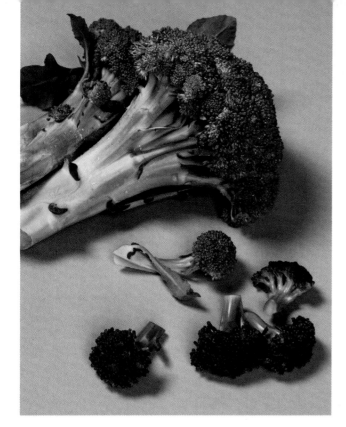

Cruciferous vegetables are rich in phytochemicals and essential vitamins and minerals. Most Americans can obtain adequate amounts of essential nutrients as well as other beneficial compounds by consuming a healthy, varied diet that favors nutrient-dense foods.

NUTRITIONAL GUIDELINES: PLANNING YOUR DIET

The second part of putting together a healthy food plan—after you've learned about necessary nutrients—is choosing foods that satisfy nutritional requirements and meet your personal criteria. Various tools have been created by scientific and government groups to help people design healthy diets. The **Dietary Reference Intakes (DRIs)** are standards for nutrient intake designed to prevent nutritional deficiencies and reduce the risk of chronic disease. **Dietary Guidelines for Americans** have been established to promote health and reduce the risk for major chronic diseases through diet and physical activity. Further guidance symbolized by **MyPyramid** provides daily food intake patterns that meet the DRIs and are consistent with the Dietary Guidelines for Americans.

Dietary Reference Intakes (DRIs)

How much vitamin C, iron, calcium, and other nutrients do you need to stay healthy? The Food and Nutrition Board establishes dietary standards, or recommended intake levels, for Americans of all ages. The current set of standards, called Dietary Reference Intakes (DRIs), is relatively new, having been introduced in 1997. An earlier set of stan-

dards, called the **Recommended Dietary Allowances (RDAs),** focused on preventing nutritional deficiency diseases such as anemia. The DRIs have a broader focus because of research that looked not just at the prevention of nutrient deficiencies but also at the role of nutrients in promoting optimal health and preventing chronic diseases such as cancer, osteoporosis, and heart disease.

The DRIs include standards for both recommended intakes and maximum safe intakes. The recommended intake of each nutrient is expressed as either a *Recommended Dietary Allowance (RDA)* or *Adequate Intake (AI)*. An AI is set when there is not enough information available to set an RDA value; regardless of the type of standard used, however, the DRI represents the best available estimate of intake for optimal health. The *Tolerable Upper Intake Level (UL)* sets the maximum daily intake that is unlikely to cause health problems in a healthy person. For example, the RDA for calcium for an 18-year-old female is 1300 mg per day; the UL is 2500 mg per day. Because of lack of data, ULs have not been set for all nutrients. This does not mean that people can tolerate chronic intakes of these vitamins and minerals above recommended levels. Like all chemical agents, nutrients can produce adverse effects if intakes are excessive. There is no established benefit from consuming nutrients at levels above the RDA or AI. The DRIs can be found in the Nutrition Resources section at the end of the chapter. (For more information, visit the Web site of the National Academies' Food and Nutrition Board; see For More Information at the end of the chapter.)

Should You Take Supplements? The aim of the DRIs is to guide you in meeting your nutritional needs primarily with food, rather than with vitamin and mineral supplements. Supplements lack potentially beneficial

Terms

phytochemical A naturally occurring substance found in plant foods that may help prevent and treat chronic diseases like cancer and heart disease; *phyto* means plant.

cruciferous vegetables Vegetables of the cabbage family, including cabbage, broccoli, brussels sprouts, kale, and cauliflower; the flower petals of these plants form the shape of a cross, hence the name.

Dietary Reference Intakes (DRIs) An umbrella term for four types of nutrient standards: Adequate Intake (AI), Estimated Average Requirement (EAR), and Recommended Dietary Allowance (RDA) set levels of intake considered adequate to prevent nutrient deficiencies and reduce the risk of chronic disease; Tolerable Upper Intake Level (UL) sets the maximum daily intake that is unlikely to cause health problems.

Dietary Guidelines for Americans General principles of good nutrition intended to help prevent certain diet-related diseases.

MyPyramid A food-group plan that provides practical advice to ensure a balanced intake of the essential nutrients.

Recommended Dietary Allowances (RDAs) Amounts of certain nutrients considered adequate to prevent deficiencies in most healthy people; will eventually be replaced by the broader Dietary Reference Intakes (DRIs).

phytochemicals and fibers that are found only in whole foods. Most Americans can obtain most of the vitamins and minerals they need to prevent deficiencies by consuming a varied, nutritionally balanced diet. The use of supplements to reduce heart disease or cancer risk remains controversial; intake levels above the UL should be avoided.

The question of whether to take supplements is a serious one. Some vitamins and minerals are dangerous when ingested in excess, as shown in Tables 12-1 and 12-2. Large doses of particular nutrients can also cause health problems by affecting the absorption of other vitamins and minerals. For these reasons, think carefully about whether to take supplements; consider consulting a physician or registered dietitian.

In setting the DRIs, the Food and Nutrition Board recommended supplements of particular nutrients for the following groups:

- Women who are capable of becoming pregnant should obtain 400 μg per day of folic acid (the synthetic form of the vitamin folate) from fortified foods and/or supplements in addition to folate from a varied diet. Research indicates that this level of folate intake will reduce the risk of neural tube defects. (This defect occurs early in pregnancy, before most women know they are pregnant; therefore, the recommendation for the folate intake applies to all women of reproductive age rather than only to pregnant women.) Since 1998, enriched breads, flours, cornmeals, rice, noodles, and other grain products have been fortified with small amounts of folic acid. Folate is found naturally in leafy green vegetables, legumes, oranges and orange juice, and strawberries.

- People over age 50 should consume foods fortified with vitamin B-12, B-12 supplements, or a combination of the two in order to meet the majority of the RDA of 2.4 μg of B-12 daily. Up to 30% of people over 50 may have problems absorbing protein-bound B-12 in foods. Vitamin B-12 in supplements and fortified foods is more readily absorbed and can help prevent a deficiency.

Because of the oxidative stress caused by smoking, the Food and Nutrition Board also recommends that smokers consume 35 mg *more* vitamin C per day than the RDA set for their age and sex (for adults, recommended daily vitamin C intakes for nonsmokers are 90 mg for men and 75 mg for women). However, supplements are not usually needed because this extra vitamin C can easily be obtained from foods. For example, one cup of orange juice has about 100 mg of vitamin C.

Supplements may also be recommended in other cases. Women with heavy menstrual flows may need extra iron to compensate for the monthly loss. The elderly, people with dark skin, and people exposed to little sunlight may need extra vitamin D from vitamin D–fortified foods and/or supplements that contain vitamin D. Some vegetarians may need supplemental calcium, iron, zinc, and vitamin B-12, depending on their food choices.

Newborns need a single dose of vitamin K, which must be administered under the direction of a physician. People who consume few calories, who have certain diseases, or who take certain medications may need specific vitamin and mineral supplements; such supplement decisions must be made by a physician because some vitamins and minerals counteract the actions of certain medications.

In deciding whether to take a vitamin and mineral supplement, consider whether you already regularly consume a fortified breakfast cereal. Many breakfast cereals contain almost as many nutrients as a multivitamin pill. If you do decide to take a supplement, choose a balanced formulation that contains 50–100% of the Daily Value (see below) for vitamins and minerals. Avoid supplements containing large doses of particular nutrients. See page 361 for more on choosing and using supplements.

Daily Values Because the DRIs are far too cumbersome to use as a basis for food labels, the U.S. Food and Drug Administration uses another set of dietary standards, the **Daily Values.** The Daily Values are based on several different sets of guidelines and include standards for fat, cholesterol, carbohydrate, dietary fiber, and selected vitamins and minerals. The Daily Values represent appropriate intake levels for a 2000-calorie diet. The percent Daily Value shown on a food label shows how well that food contributes to your recommended daily intake. Food labels are described in detail later in the chapter.

Dietary Guidelines for Americans

To provide general guidance for choosing a healthy diet, the U.S. Department of Agriculture (USDA) and the U.S. Department of Health and Human Services (DHHS) have jointly issued Dietary Guidelines for Americans, most recently in 2005. These guidelines are intended for healthy children age 2 and older and adults of all ages. Key recommendations include the following:

- Consume a variety of nutrient-dense foods within and among the basic food groups, while staying within energy needs.
- Control calorie intake to manage body weight.
- Be physically active every day.
- Increase daily intake of foods from certain groups: fruits and vegetables, whole grains, and fat-free or low-fat milk and milk products.
- Choose fats wisely for good health, limiting intake of saturated and trans fats.
- Choose carbohydrates wisely for good health, limiting intake of added sugars.
- Choose and prepare foods with little salt, and consume potassium-rich foods.
- If you drink alcoholic beverages, do so in moderation.
- Keep foods safe to eat.

Following these guidelines promotes health and reduces risk for chronic diseases, including heart disease, cancer, diabetes, stroke, osteoporosis, and obesity. Each of the recommendations in the 2005 Dietary Guidelines for Americans is supported by an extensive review of scientific and medical evidence. What follows is a brief summary of the guidelines.

Adequate Nutrients within Calorie Needs

Many people consume more calories than they need while failing to meet recommended intakes for all nutrients. Meeting the DRIs provides a foundation not only for current health but also for reducing chronic disease risk. Many adults don't eat enough calcium, potassium, fiber, magnesium, and vitamins A, C, and E; many children don't get enough calcium, potassium, fiber, magnesium, and vitamin E. Most people need to choose meals and snacks that are high in nutrients but low to moderate in calories.

Two eating plans that translate nutrient recommendations into food choices are the USDA's MyPyramid and the DASH eating plan. MyPyramid is described in detail in the next section (pp. 350–354); the DASH plan appears in the Nutrition Resources section at the end of the chapter. You can obtain all the nutrients and other substances you need by choosing the recommended number of daily servings from basic food groups and following the advice about selecting nutrient-dense foods within the groups. Following these plans would mean that many Americans would have to make some general dietary changes:

- Eat more dark green vegetables, orange vegetables, legumes, fruits, whole grains, and low-fat and fat-free milk and milk products.
- Eat less refined grains, saturated fat, trans fat, cholesterol, added sugars, and calories.

Your nutrients should come primarily from foods that contain not only the vitamins and minerals often found in supplements but also hundreds of naturally occurring substances that may benefit health, such as antioxidants. Situations in which a supplement might be recommended were described earlier in the chapter.

For maximum nutrition, it is important to consume foods from all the food groups daily and to consume a variety of nutrient-dense foods within the groups. Nutrient-dense foods are those that provide substantial amounts of vitamins and minerals and relatively few calories. Americans currently consume many foods and beverages that are low in nutrient density, making it difficult or impossible to meet nutrient needs without overconsuming calories. Selecting nutrient-dense foods—low-fat forms of foods in each group and those free of added sugars—allows you to meet your nutrient needs without overconsuming calories and unhealthy food components such as saturated and trans fats.

People's food choices can be affected by individual and cultural preferences, moral beliefs, the cost and availability of food, and food intolerances and allergies. But healthy eating is possible no matter how foods are prepared or combined (see the box "Ethnic Foods"). If you avoid most or all foods from any of the major food groups, be sure to get enough nutrients from the other groups. MyPyramid can be applied to vegetarian diets.

Weight Management

Overweight and obesity are a major public health problem in the United States. Calorie intake and physical activity (see next section) work together to influence body weight. Most Americans need to reduce the amount of calories they consume, increase their level of physical activity, and make wiser food choices. Many adults gain weight slowly over time, but even small changes in behavior can help avoid weight gain.

Evaluate your body weight in terms of body mass index (BMI), a measure of relative body weight that also takes height into account (see Chapter 14 for instructions on how to determine your BMI). If your current weight is healthy, aim to avoid weight gain. Do so by increasing physical activity and making small cuts in calorie intake. Choose nutrient-dense foods and sensible portion sizes. Avoiding weight gain is easier than losing weight: For example, for most adults, a reduction of 50 to 100 calories per day may prevent gradual weight gain, whereas a reduction of 500 calories or more per day may be needed initially for weight loss.

Monitoring weight regularly helps people know if they need to adjust their food intake or physical activity to maintain a healthy weight. Those who need to lose weight should aim for slow, steady weight loss by decreasing calorie intake, maintaining adequate nutrient intake, and increasing physical activity. In terms of macronutrient intake, use the AMDR ranges described earlier in the chapter for dietary planning; within these healthy ranges, total calorie intake is what counts for weight management rather than specific percentages of particular macronutrients.

Physical Activity

Regular physical activity improves fitness, helps manage weight, promotes psychological well-being, and reduces risk of heart disease, high blood pressure, cancer, and diabetes. Become active if you are inactive, and maintain or increase physical activity if you are already active. The amount of daily physical activity recommended for you depends on your current health status and goals.

- To reduce the risk of chronic disease, aim to accumulate at least 30 minutes (adults) or 60 minutes (children) of moderate physical activity—the equivalent of brisk walking at a pace of 3–4 miles per hour—beyond your usual activity at work, home, and school. Greater health benefits can be obtained by engaging in more vigorous activity or activity of longer duration.

Term

VW

Daily Values A simplified version of the RDAs used on food labels; also included are values for nutrients with no RDA per se.

Dimensions of Diversity

Ethnic Foods

There is no one ethnic diet that clearly surpasses all others in providing people with healthful foods. However, every diet has its advantages and disadvantages and, within each cuisine, some foods are better choices. The dietary guidelines described in this chapter can be applied to any ethnic cuisine. For additional guidance, refer to the table below.

Choose More Often

Chinese
- Dishes that are steamed, poached (jum), boiled (chu), roasted (kow), barbecued (shu), or lightly stir-fried
- Hoisin sauce, oyster sauce, wine sauce, plum sauce, velvet sauce, or hot mustard
- Fresh fish and seafood, skinless chicken, tofu
- Mixed vegetables, Chinese greens
- Steamed rice, steamed spring rolls, soft noodles

French
- Dishes prepared au vapeur (steamed), en brochette (skewered and broiled), or grillé (grilled)
- Fresh fish, shrimp, scallops, or mussels or skinless chicken, without sauces
- Clear soups

Greek
- Dishes that are stewed, broiled, or grilled, including shish kebabs (souvlaki)
- Dolmas (grape leaves) stuffed with rice
- Tzatziki (yogurt, cucumbers, and garlic)
- Tabouli (bulgur-based salad)
- Pita bread, especially whole wheat

Indian
- Dishes prepared masala (curry), tandoori (roasted in a clay oven), or tikke (pan roasted); kebabs
- Raita (yogurt and cucumber salad) and other yogurt-based dishes and sauces
- Dal (lentils), pullao or pilau (basmati rice)
- Chapati (baked bread)

Italian
- Pasta primavera or pasta, polenta, risotto, or gnocchi with marinara, red or white wine, white or red clam, or light mushroom sauce
- Dishes that are grilled or prepared cacciatore (tomato-based sauce), marsala (broth and wine sauce), or piccata (lemon sauce)
- Cioppino (seafood stew)
- Vegetable soup, minestrone or fagioli (beans)

Japanese
- Dishes prepared nabemono (boiled), shabu-shabu (in boiling broth), mushimono (steamed), nimono (simmered), yaki (broiled), or yakimono (grilled)
- Sushi or domburi (mixed rice dish)
- Steamed rice or soba (buckwheat), udon (wheat), or rice noodles

Mexican
- Soft corn or wheat tortillas
- Burritos, fajitas, enchiladas, soft tacos, and tamales filled with beans, vegetables, or lean meats
- Refried beans, nonfat or low-fat; rice and beans
- Ceviche (fish marinated in lime juice)
- Salsa, enchilada sauce, and picante sauce
- Gazpacho, menudo, or black bean soup
- Fruit or flan for dessert

Thai
- Dishes that are barbecued, sautéed, broiled, boiled, steamed, braised, or marinated
- Sâté (skewered and grilled meats)
- Fish sauce, basil sauce, chili or hot sauces
- Bean thread noodles, Thai salad

Choose Less Often

- Fried wontons or egg rolls
- Crab rangoon
- Crispy (Peking) duck or chicken
- Sweet-and-sour dishes made with breaded and deep-fried meat, poultry, or fish
- Fried rice
- Fried or crispy noodles
- Dishes prepared à la crème (in cream sauce), au gratin or gratinée (baked with cream and cheese), or en croûte (in pastry crust)
- Drawn butter, hollandaise sauce, and remoulade (mayonnaise-based sauce)
- Moussaka, saganaki (fried cheese)
- Vegetable pies such as spanakopita and tyropita
- Baba ghanoush (eggplant and olive oil)
- Deep-fried falafel (chickpea patties)
- Gyros stuffed with ground meat
- Baklava
- Ghee (clarified butter)
- Korma (meat in cream sauce)
- Samosas, pakoras (fried dishes)
- Molee and other coconut milk–based dishes
- Poori, bhatura, or paratha (fried breads)
- Antipasto (cheese, smoked meats)
- Dishes that are prepared alfredo, frito (fried), crema (creamed), alla panna (with cream), or carbonara
- Veal scaloppini
- Chicken, veal, or eggplant parmigiana
- Italian sausage, salami, and prosciutto
- Buttered garlic bread
- Cannoli
- Tempura (battered and fried)
- Agemono (deep fried)
- Katsu (fried pork cutlet)
- Sukiyaki
- Fried tofu
- Crispy, fried tortillas
- Dishes that are fried, such as chile relleños, chimichangas, flautas, and tostadas
- Nachos and cheese, chili con queso, and other dishes made with cheese or cheese sauce
- Guacamole, sour cream, and extra cheese
- Refried beans made with lard
- Fried ice cream
- Coconut milk soup
- Peanut sauce or dishes topped with nuts
- Mee-krob (crispy noodles)
- Red, green, and yellow curries, which typically contain coconut milk

SOURCES: National Heart, Lung, and Blood Institute. 1998. Tips for Healthy Multicultural Dining Out. In *Clinical Guidelines on the Identification, Evaluation, and Treatment of Overweight and Obesity in Adults*. Bethesda, Md.: National Institutes of Health; Duyff, R. L. 1998. *The American Dietetic Association's Complete Food and Nutrition Guide*. Minneapolis, Minn.: Chronimed; Kirby, J. 1998. *Dieting for Dummies*. Foster City, Calif.: IDG Books.

- To help manage body weight and prevent gradual, unhealthy weight gain, engage in 60 minutes of moderately to vigorously intense activity on most days of the week.
- To sustain weight loss in adulthood, engage daily in at least 60–90 minutes of moderate physical activity.

You can do the activity all at once or spread it out over several 10-minute or longer bouts during the day; choose activities you enjoy and can do regularly. You can boost fitness by engaging in exercises specifically designed for the health-related fitness components: cardiorespiratory endurance exercises, stretching exercises for flexibility, and resistance training for muscular strength and endurance. See Chapter 13 for advice on increasing daily physical activity and creating a complete fitness program.

Food Groups to Encourage   Many Americans do not consume the recommended amounts of fruits, vegetables, whole grains, and low-fat or fat-free milk products—all of which have health benefits.

FRUITS AND VEGETABLES   Fruits and vegetables are important sources of dietary fiber, vitamins, and minerals. For a 2000-calorie diet, about 4½ cups or the equivalent (9 servings) of fruits and vegetables each day is recommended. Eat a variety of fruits—fresh, frozen, canned, or dried—rather than fruit juice for most of your fruit choices. For vegetables, choose a variety of colors and kinds. Eat more of the following types of vegetables:

- Dark green vegetables, such as broccoli, kale, and other dark leafy greens
- Orange vegetables, such as carrots, sweet potatoes, pumpkin, and winter squash
- Legumes, such as pinto beans, kidney beans, black beans, garbanzo beans, split peas, and lentils

Other fruits and vegetables that are important sources of nutrients of concern include tomatoes and tomato products, red sweet peppers, cabbage and other cruciferous vegetables, bananas, citrus fruits, berries, and melons. See the discussion of MyPyramid for more advice on choosing fruits and vegetables.

WHOLE GRAINS   Whole grains provide more fiber and nutrients than refined grains, and intake of whole grains reduces the risk of chronic disease and helps with weight maintenance. For a 2000-calorie diet, 6 ounce-equivalents (6 servings) of grains each day are recommended; at least half of these servings should be whole grains. (One ounce is about 1 slice of bread, 1 cup of breakfast cereal flakes, or ½ cup of cooked pasta or rice.) The remaining grain servings should be from enriched or whole-grain products. Refer back to p. 336 for information on identifying whole-grain products.

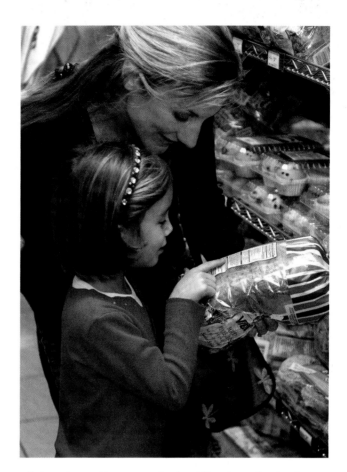

Whole grains provide more nutrients and fiber than refined grains, and they may help reduce the risk of chronic disease. Half of your daily grain servings should come from whole grains. To check if a food contains whole grains, read the ingredient list on a food label.

LOW-FAT AND FAT-FREE MILK AND MILK PRODUCTS   Milk and other dairy products are important sources of calcium and other nutrients. Regular consumption of milk and milk products can reduce the risk of low bone mass throughout life. Choosing low-fat and fat-free dairy products helps to control calorie intake and reduce intake of saturated fat and cholesterol. For adults, the equivalent of 3 daily cups of fat-free or low-fat milk or milk products is recommended; 1½ ounces of cheese is the equivalent of 1 cup of milk. Yogurt and lactose-free milk are options for people who are lactose intolerant, as is use of the enzyme lactase prior to the consumption of milk products. For individuals who avoid all milk products, nondairy calcium sources include fortified cereals and beverages, tofu prepared with calcium sulfate, green leafy vegetables, soybeans, and certain fish and seafood.

Fats   Fats and oils provide the essential fatty acids needed for a healthy diet, but, as described earlier in the chapter, the type and amount of fats consumed can make a difference for health. A diet low in saturated fat, trans fat, and cholesterol helps keep blood cholesterol low and reduces the risk for heart disease; a diet containing

Your overall goal is to limit total fat intake to no more than 35% of total calories. Within that limit, favor unsaturated fats from vegetable oils, nuts, and fish over saturated and trans fats from animal products and foods made with hydrogenated vegetable oils or shortening. Saturated and trans fat intake should be kept as low as possible within a nutritionally adequate diet.

- Be moderate in your consumption of foods high in fat, including fast food, commercially prepared baked goods and desserts, deep-fried foods, meat, poultry, nuts and seeds, and regular dairy products.

- When you do eat high-fat foods, limit your portion sizes, and balance your intake with foods low in fat.

- Choose lean cuts of meat, and trim any visible fat from meat before and after cooking. Remove skin from poultry before or after cooking.

- Drink fat-free or low-fat milk instead of whole milk, and use lower-fat varieties in puddings, soups, and baked products. Substitute plain low-fat yogurt, blender-whipped low-fat cottage cheese, or buttermilk for sour cream.

- Use vegetable oil instead of butter or margarine. Use tub or squeeze margarine instead of stick margarine. Look for margarines that are free of trans fats. Minimize intake of coconut or palm oil.

- Season vegetables, seafood, and meats with herbs and spices rather than with creamy sauces, butter, or margarine.

- Try lemon juice on salad, or use a yogurt-based salad dressing instead of mayonnaise or sour cream dressings.

- Steam, boil, bake, or microwave vegetables, or stir-fry them in a small amount of vegetable oil.

- Roast, bake, or broil meat, poultry, or fish so that fat drains away as the food cooks.

- Use a nonstick pan for cooking so that added fat will be unnecessary; use a vegetable spray for frying. Kitchen stores sell non-aerosol spray bottles to use with regular cooking oils.

- Chill broths from meat or poultry until the fat becomes solid. Spoon off the fat before using the broth.

- Substitute egg whites for whole eggs when baking; limit the number of egg yolks when scrambling eggs.

- Choose fruits as desserts most often.

- Eat a low-fat vegetarian main dish at least once a week.

---

omega-3 fats from fish also reduces the risk for heart disease. Goals for fat intake for most adults are as follows:

Total fat: 20–35% of total daily calories

Saturated fat: Less than 10% of total daily calories

Trans fat: As little as possible

Cholesterol: Less than 300 mg per day

Most fats in the diet should come from sources of unsaturated fats, such as fish, nuts, and vegetable oils. When selecting and preparing meat, poultry, dry beans, and milk or milk products, make choices that are lean, low-fat, or fat-free. To reduce trans fat intake, limit intake of foods made with hydrogenated vegetable oils. Refer to the box "Reducing the Saturated and Trans Fats in Your Diet" for additional specific suggestions.

Cholesterol is found only in animal foods. If you need to reduce your cholesterol intake, limit your intake of foods that are particularly high in cholesterol, including egg yolks, dairy fats, certain shellfish, and liver and other organ meats; watch your serving sizes of animal foods. Food labels list the fat and cholesterol content of foods.

Two servings per week of fish rich in heart-healthy omega-3 fatty acids are also recommended for people at high risk for heart disease. However, for certain groups, intake limits are set for varieties of fish that may contain mercury; see p. 364 for more information. Fish rich in omega-3 fatty acids include salmon, mackerel, and trout.

Carbohydrates Carbohydrates are an important energy source in a healthy diet. Foods rich in carbohydrates may also be rich in dietary fiber, which promotes healthy digestion and helps reduce the risk of type 2 diabetes and heart disease. Fruits, vegetables, whole grains, and fat-free or low-fat milk can provide the recommended amount of carbohydrate. Choose foods rich in fiber often—for example, choose whole fruits instead of juices and whole grains instead of refined grains. Legumes are another good source of fiber.

People who consume foods and beverages high in added sugars tend to consume more calories but smaller amounts of vitamins and minerals than those who limit their intake of added sugars. A food is likely high in sugar if one of the following appears first or second in the list of ingredients or if several are listed: sugar (any type, including beet, brown, invert, raw, and cane), corn syrup or sweetener, fruit juice concentrate, honey, malt syrup, molasses, syrup, cane juice, or dextrose, fructose, glucose, lactose, maltose, or sucrose.

To reduce added sugar consumption, cut back on soft drinks, candies, sweet desserts (cakes, cookies, pies), fruit drinks, and other foods high in added sugars. Drink water rather than sweetened drinks, and don't let sodas and other sweets crowd out more nutritious foods, such as low-fat milk. Regular soda is the leading source of both added sugars and calories in the American diet, but it provides little in the way of nutrients except sugar (Figure 12-4). The 10 teaspoons of sugar in a 12-ounce soda can exceed the

Nutrient	Recommended Daily Intake*	Orange Juice		Low-Fat (1%) Milk		Regular Cola		Bottled Iced Tea
Calories	2000 calories	168 calories		150 calories		152 calories		150 calories
Carbohydrate	300 g		40.5 g		18 g		38 g	37.5 g
Added sugars	32 g						38 g	34.5 g
Fat	65 g				3.9 g			
Protein	55 g				12 g			
Calcium	1000 mg		33 mg		450 mg		11 mg	
Potassium	4700 mg	15%	710 mg	12%	570 mg		4 mg	
Vitamin A	700 µg	4%	30 µg	31%	216 µg			
Vitamin C	75 mg		145.5 mg		3.6 mg			
Vitamin D	5 µg				3.7 µg			
Folate	400 µg		160 µg		20 µg			

*Recommended intakes and limits appropriate for a 20-year-old woman consuming 2000 calories per day.

Figure 12-4   Nutrient density of 12-ounce portions of selected beverages.   The four beverages shown have approximately the same number of calories in a 12-ounce serving. However, regular cola and iced tea provide few nutrients besides added sugars; both contain more than the total daily recommended limit of added sugars (about 8 teaspoons). Orange juice is rich in potassium, vitamin C, and folate; low-fat milk is an excellent source of protein, calcium, potassium, vitamin A, and vitamin D. (Color bars represent percentage of recommended daily intake or limit for each nutrient.)

recommended daily limit for added sugars for someone consuming 2000 calories per day; for more on added sugar limits, see the discussion of MyPyramid.

Keep your teeth and gums healthy by limiting consumption of sweet or starchy foods between meals and brushing and flossing regularly; drinking fluoridated water also reduces the risk of dental caries.

Sodium and Potassium   Many people can reduce their chance of developing high blood pressure or lower already elevated blood pressure by consuming less salt; reducing blood pressure lowers the risk for stroke, heart disease, and kidney disease. Salt is made up of the minerals sodium and chloride, and although both of these minerals are essential for normal body function, we need only small amounts (1500 mg per day for adults). Most Americans consume much more salt than they need. The goal is to reduce sodium intake to less than 2300 milligrams per day, the equivalent of about 1 teaspoon of salt. Certain groups, including people with hypertension, African Americans, and older adults, benefit from an even lower sodium intake (no more than 1500 mg per day).

Salt is found mainly in processed and prepared foods; smaller amounts may also be added during cooking or at the table. To lower your intake of salt, choose fresh or plain frozen meat, poultry, seafood, and vegetables most often; these are lower in salt than processed forms are. Check and compare the sodium content in processed foods, including frozen dinners, cheeses, soups, salad dressings, sauces, and canned mixed dishes. Add less salt during cooking and at the table, and limit your use of high-sodium condiments like soy sauce, ketchup, mustard, pickles, and olives. Use lemon juice, herbs, and spices instead of salt to enhance the flavor of foods.

Along with lowering salt intake, increasing potassium intake helps lower blood pressure. Fruits, vegetables, and most milk products are available in forms that contain no salt, and many of these are sources of potassium. Potassium-rich foods include leafy green vegetables, sweet and white potatoes, winter squash, soybeans, tomato sauce, bananas, peaches, apricots, cantaloupes, and orange juice.

Alcoholic Beverages   Alcoholic beverages supply calories but few nutrients. Drinking in moderation—that is, no more than one drink per day for women and no more than two drinks per day for men—is associated with mortality reduction among some groups, primarily males age 45 and older and women age 55 and older. Among younger people, alcohol use provides little if any health benefit, and heavy drinking is associated with motor vehicle injuries and deaths, liver disease, stroke, violence, and other health problems (see Chapter 10 for more on the health risks and potential benefits of alcohol use).

People who should not drink at all include individuals who cannot restrict their drinking to moderate levels; women who are pregnant or breastfeeding or who may become pregnant; children and adolescents; people with specific health conditions; individuals who plan to drive or

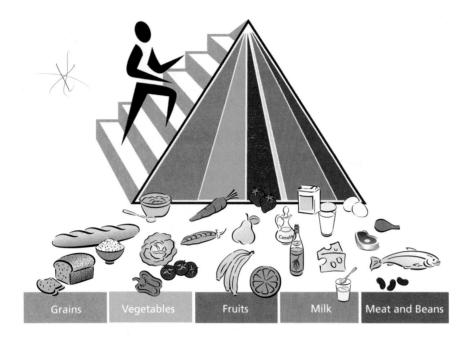

Figure 12-5 USDA's MyPyramid. The USDA food guidance system, called MyPyramid, can be personalized based on an individual's sex, age, and activity level; visit MyPyramid.gov to obtain a food plan appropriate for you. MyPyramid contains five main food groups plus oils (yellow band). Key consumer messages include the following:

- Grains: Make half your grains whole
- Vegetables: Vary your veggies
- Fruits: Focus on fruits
- Milk: Get your calcium-rich foods
- Meat and Beans: Go lean with protein

SOURCE: U.S. Department of Agriculture. 2005. *MyPyramid* (http://mypyramid.gov; retrieved April 20, 2005).

operate machinery or engage in any activity that requires attention, skill, or coordination; and individuals taking prescription or over-the-counter medications that can interact with alcohol. If you choose to drink alcoholic beverages, do so sensibly, moderately, and with meals. Never drink in situations where it may put you or others at risk.

Food Safety   Safe foods are those that pose little risk from harmful bacteria, viruses, parasites, toxins, or chemical or physical contaminants. Foodborne diseases affect about 76 million Americans each year. Actions by consumers can reduce the occurrence of foodborne illness significantly. It is especially important to be careful with perishable foods such as poultry, meats, eggs, shellfish, milk products, and fresh fruits and vegetables. Refer to the section "Protecting Yourself Against Foodborne Illness" (pp. 360–363) for specific food safety tips.

Some organizations, such as the American Cancer Society, have additional recommendations to reduce cancer risk, including not smoking and limiting intake of salt-cured, smoked, and nitrite-cured foods such as bacon or sausage. Curing and smoking of foods help prevent the growth of certain harmful bacteria. However, nitrites have been associated with an increased risk of colon and other gastrointestinal cancers in some people. The addition of vitamin C and other antioxidants to cured meats decreases the number of carcinogens, but salt-cured, smoked, and nitrite-cured foods should still be consumed in moderation because they are often high in saturated fat, cholesterol, and sodium.

Although the Dietary Guidelines apply to healthy Americans over age 2, not everyone has the same risk of developing high cholesterol, high blood pressure, obesity, cancer, and other health problems. You should consider your own health status and family history and apply these guidelines appropriately to address current or potential health problems. Chapters 15 and 16 have dietary advice relating to the prevention of heart disease and cancer.

USDA's MyPyramid

The first USDA daily food guide, published in 1916, emphasized the importance of fats and sugars in obtaining adequate calories to support daily activity. But nutrition needs have changed over time: Now the guidelines stress the importance of limiting additional fats and added sugars to keep calorie intake under control. Many Americans are familiar with the USDA Food Guide Pyramid, the food guidance system that was first released in 1992. Since the initial release of the Pyramid, scientists have updated both nutrient recommendations (the DRIs) and the Dietary Guidelines for Americans. So, as the 2005 Dietary Guidelines were prepared, the USDA reassessed its overall food guidance system and released MyPyramid in April 2005 (Figure 12-5).

A variety of experts have proposed other food-group plans. Some of these address perceived shortcomings in the USDA plans, and some adapt the basic 1992 Pyramid to special populations. Two alternative food plans appear in the Nutrition Resources section at the end of the chapter: The DASH eating plan and the Harvard Healthy Eating Pyramid. The USDA Center for Nutrition Policy and Promotion (www.usda.gov/cnpp) has more on alternative food plans for special populations such as young children, older adults, and people choosing particular ethnic diets.

Key Messages of MyPyramid   The new MyPyramid symbol (see Figure 12-5) has been developed to remind consumers to make healthy food choices and to be active every day. Consuming a balance of servings from each food group will not only meet nutrient needs but also help to reduce chronic disease risk. Key messages include the following:

- *Personalization* is represented by the person on the steps and the MyPyramid.gov site, which includes individualized recommendations, interactive assessments of food intake and physical activity, and tips for success.
- *Daily physical activity,* represented by the person climbing the steps, is important for maintaining a healthy weight and reducing the risk of chronic disease.
- *Moderation* of food intake is represented by the narrowing of each food group from bottom to top. The wider base stands for foods with little or no solid fats or added sugars, which should be selected more often; the narrower top represents food containing more solid fats and added sugars, which should be limited.
- *Proportionality* is represented by the different widths of the food group bands. The widths provide a general guide for how much food a person should choose from each group.
- *Variety* is represented by the six color bands representing the five food groups of MyPyramid and oils. Foods from all groups are needed daily for good health.
- *Gradual improvement* is a good strategy; people can benefit from taking small steps to improve their diet and activity habits each day.

The MyPyramid chart in Figure 12-6 (p. 352) shows the food intake patterns recommended for different levels of calorie intake; Table 12-3 (p. 353) provides guidance for determining an appropriate calorie intake for weight maintenance. Use the table to identify an energy intake that is about right for you; then refer to the appropriate column in Figure 12-6. A personalized version of MyPyramid recommendations can also be obtained by visiting MyPyramid. gov. Each food group is described briefly below. Past experiences have shown that many Americans have trouble identifying serving sizes, so recommended daily intakes from each group are now given in terms of cups and ounces; see the box "Judging Portion Sizes" for additional advice.

Grains   Foods from this group are usually low in fat and rich in complex carbohydrates, dietary fiber (if grains are unrefined), and many vitamins and minerals, including thiamin, riboflavin, iron, niacin, folic acid (if enriched or fortified), and zinc. Someone eating 2000 calories a day should include 6 ounce-equivalents each day, with half of those servings from whole grains such as whole-grain bread, whole-wheat pasta, high-fiber cereal, and brown rice. The following count as 1 ounce-equivalent:

- 1 slice of bread
- 1 small (2½-inch diameter) muffin
- 1 cup ready-to-eat cereal flakes

- ½ cup cooked cereal, rice, grains, or pasta
- 1 6-inch tortilla

Choose foods that are typically made with little fat or sugar (bread, rice, pasta) over those that are high in fat and sugar (croissants, chips, cookies, doughnuts).

Vegetables   Vegetables contain carbohydrates, dietary fiber, vitamin A, vitamin C, folate, potassium, and other nutrients. They are also naturally low in fat. In a 2000-calorie diet, 2½ cups (5 servings) of vegetables should be included daily. Each of the following counts as 1 serving (½ cup or equivalent) of vegetables:

- ½ cup raw or cooked vegetables
- 1 cup raw leafy salad greens
- ½ cup vegetable juice

Because vegetables vary in the nutrients they provide, it is important to consume a variety of types of vegetables to obtain maximum nutrition. Many Americans consume only a few types of vegetables, with white potatoes (baked or served as french fries) being the most popular. To help boost variety, MyPyramid recommends servings from five different subgroups within the vegetables group; try to consume vegetables from several subgroups each day. (For clarity, Figure 12-6 shows servings from the subgroups in terms of weekly consumption.)

- Dark green vegetables like spinach, chard, collards, bok choy, broccoli, kale, romaine, and turnip and mustard greens
- Orange and deep yellow vegetables like carrots, winter squash, sweet potatoes, and pumpkin
- Legumes like pinto beans, kidney beans, black beans, lentils, chickpeas, soybeans, split peas, and tofu; legumes can be counted as servings of vegetables *or* as alternatives to meat
- Starchy vegetables like corn, green peas, and white potatoes
- Other vegetables; tomatoes, bell peppers (red, orange, yellow, or green), green beans, and cruciferous vegetables like cauliflower are good choices

Fruits   Fruits are rich in carbohydrates, dietary fiber, and many vitamins, especially vitamin C. For someone eating a 2000-calorie diet, 2 cups (4 servings) of fruits are recommended daily. The following each count as 1 serving (½ cup or equivalent) of fruit:

- ½ cup fresh, canned, or frozen fruit
- ½ cup fruit juice (100% juice)
- 1 small whole fruit
- ¼ cup dried fruit

Good choices from this group are citrus fruits and juices, melons, pears, apples, bananas, and berries. Choose

Daily Amount of Food from Each Group

Food group amounts shown in cups (c) or ounce-equivalents (oz-eq), with number of daily servings (srv) shown in parentheses; vegetable subgroup amounts are per week

Calorie level	1600	1800	2000	2200	2400	2600	2800	3000
Grains	5 oz-eq	6 oz-eq	6 oz-eq	7 oz-eq	8 oz-eq	9 oz-eq	10 oz-eq	10 oz-eq
Whole grains	3 oz-eq	3 oz-eq	3 oz-eq	3.5 oz-eq	4 oz-eq	4.5 oz-eq	5 oz-eq	5 oz-eq
Other grains	2 oz-eq	3 oz-eq	3 oz-eq	3.5 oz-eq	4 oz-eq	4.5 oz-eq	5 oz-eq	5 oz-eq
Vegetables	2 c (4 srv)	2.5 c (5 srv)	2.5 c (5 srv)	3 c (6 srv)	3 c (6 srv)	3.5 c (7 srv)	3.5 c (7 srv)	4 c (8 srv)
Dark green	2 c/wk	3 c/wk	3 c/wk	3 c/wk	3 c/wk	3 c/wk	3 c/wk	3 c/wk
Orange	1.5 c/wk	2 c/wk	2 c/wk	2 c/wk	2 c/wk	2.5 c/wk	2.5 c/wk	2.5 c/wk
Legumes	2.5 c/wk	3 c/wk	3 c/wk	3 c/wk	3 c/wk	3.5 c/wk	3.5 c/wk	3.5 c/wk
Starchy	2.5 c/wk	3 c/wk	3 c/wk	6 c/wk	6 c/wk	7 c/wk	7 c/wk	9 c/wk
Other	5.5 c/wk	6.5 c/wk	6.5 c/wk	7 c/wk	7 c/wk	8.5 c/wk	8.5 c/wk	10 c/wk
Fruits	1.5 c (3 srv)	1.5 c (3 srv)	2 c (4 srv)	2 c (4 srv)	2 c (4 srv)	2 c (4 srv)	2.5 c (5 srv)	2.5 c (5 srv)
Milk	3 c	3 c	3 c	3 c	3 c	3 c	3 c	3 c
Lean meat and beans	5 oz-eq	5 oz-eq	5.5 oz-eq	6 oz-eq	6.5 oz-eq	6.5 oz-eq	7 oz-eq	7 oz-eq
Oils	5 tsp	5 tsp	6 tsp	6 tsp	7 tsp	8 tsp	8 tsp	10 tsp

The discretionary calorie allowances shown below are the calories remaining at each level after nutrient-dense foods in each food group are selected. Those trying to lose weight may choose not to use discretionary calories. For those wanting to maintain weight, discretionary calories may be used to increase the amount of food from each food group; to consume foods that are not in the lowest fat form or that contain added sugars; to add oil, fat, or sugars to foods; or to consume alcohol. The amounts below show how discretionary calories may be divided between solid fats and added sugars.

Discretionary calories	132	195	267	290	362	410	426	512
Solid fats	11 g	15 g	18 g	19 g	22 g	24 g	24 g	29 g
Added sugars	12 g (3 tsp)	20 g (5 tsp)	32 g (8 tsp)	38 g (9 tsp)	48 g (12 tsp)	56 g (14 tsp)	60 g (15 tsp)	72 g (18 tsp)

Figure 12-6   MyPyramid food intake patterns.   To determine an appropriate amount of food from each group, find the column with your approximate daily energy intake. That column lists the daily recommended intake from each food group. Visit MyPyramid.gov for a personalized intake plan and for intakes for other calorie levels.   SOURCE: U.S. Department of Health and Human Services and U.S. Department of Agriculture. *Dietary Guidelines for Americans,* 2005 (http://www.health.gov/dietaryguidelines; retrieved January 20, 2005).

whole fruits often—they are higher in fiber and often lower in calories than fruit juices. Fruit *juices* typically contain more nutrients and less added sugar than fruit *drinks.* For canned fruits, choose those packed in 100% fruit juice or water rather than in syrup.

Milk   This group includes all milk and milk products, such as yogurt, cheeses (except cream cheese), and dairy desserts, as well as lactose-free and lactose-reduced products. Foods from this group are high in protein, carbo-

hydrate, calcium, riboflavin, and vitamin D (if fortified). Those consuming 2000 calories per day should include 3 cups of milk or the equivalent daily. Each of the following counts as the equivalent of 1 cup:

- 1 cup milk or yogurt
- ½ cup ricotta cheese
- 1½ ounces natural cheese
- 2 ounces processed cheese

Studies have shown that most people underestimate the size of their food portions, in many cases by as much as 50%. If you need to retrain your eye, try using measuring cups and spoons and an inexpensive kitchen scale when you eat at home. With a little practice, you'll learn the difference between 3 and 8 ounces of chicken or meat, and what a half-cup of rice really looks like. For quick estimates, use the following equivalents:

- 1 teaspoon of margarine = the tip of your thumb

- 1 ounce of cheese = your thumb, four dice stacked together, or an ice cube

- 3 ounces of chicken or meat = a deck of cards or an audiocassette tape

- 1 cup of pasta = a small fist or a tennis ball

- $\frac{1}{2}$ cup of rice or cooked vegetables = an ice cream scoop or one-third of a can of soda

- 2 tablespoons of peanut butter = a ping-pong ball or large marshmallow

- 1 medium potato = a computer mouse

- 1–2-ounce muffin or roll = plum or large egg

- 2-ounce bagel = hockey puck or yo-yo

- 1 medium fruit (apple or orange) = baseball

- $\frac{1}{4}$ cup nuts = golf ball

- Small cookie or cracker = poker chip

Table 12-3 — MyPyramid Daily Calorie Intake Levels

Age (years)	Sedentary[a]	Moderately Active[b]	Active[c]
Child			
2–3	1000	1000–1400	1000–1400
Female			
4–8	1200–1400	1400–1600	1400–1800
9–13	1400–1600	1600–2000	1800–2200
14–18	1800	2000	2400
19–30	1800–2000	2000–2200	2400
31–50	1800	2000	2200
51+	1600	1800	2000–2200
Male			
4–8	1200–1400	1400–1600	1600–2000
9–13	1600–2000	1800–2200	2000–2600
14–18	2000–2400	2400–2800	2800–3200
19–30	2400–2600	2600–2800	3000
31–50	2200–2400	2400–2600	2800–3000
51+	2000–2200	2200–2400	2400–2800

[a]A lifestyle that includes only the light physical activity associated with typical day-to-day life.
[b]A lifestyle that includes physical activity equivalent to walking about 1.5 to 3 miles per day at 3 to 4 miles per hour (30–60 minutes a day of moderate physical activity), in addition to the light physical activity associated with typical day-to-day life.
[c]A lifestyle that includes physical activity equivalent to walking more than 3 miles per day at 3 to 4 miles per hour (60 or more minutes a day of moderate physical activity), in addition to the light physical activity associated with typical day-to-day life.

SOURCE: U.S. Department of Agriculture. 2005. *MyPyramid Food Intake Pattern Calorie Levels* (http://mypyramid.gov/professionals; retrieved April 20, 2005).

Cottage cheese is lower in calcium than most other cheeses; $\frac{1}{2}$ cup is equivalent to $\frac{1}{4}$ cup milk. Ice cream is also lower in calcium and higher in sugar and fat than many other dairy products; one scoop counts as $\frac{1}{3}$ cup milk. To limit calories and saturated fat in your diet, it is best to choose servings of low-fat and fat-free items from this group.

Meat and Beans   This group includes meat, poultry, fish, dry beans and peas, eggs, nuts, and seeds. These foods provide protein, niacin, iron, vitamin B-6, zinc, and thiamin; the animal foods in the group also provide vitamin B-12. For someone consuming a 2000-calorie diet, $5\frac{1}{2}$ ounce-equivalents is recommended. The following each count as equivalent to 1 ounce:

- 1 ounce cooked lean meat, poultry, or fish

- $\frac{1}{4}$ cup cooked dry beans (legumes) or tofu

- 1 egg

- 1 tablespoon peanut butter

- $\frac{1}{2}$ ounce nuts or seeds

One egg at breakfast, $\frac{1}{2}$ cup of pinto beans at lunch, and a 3-ounce (cooked weight) hamburger at dinner would add up to the equivalent of 6 ounces of lean meat for the day. To limit your intake of fat and saturated fat, choose lean cuts of meat and skinless poultry, and watch your serving sizes carefully. Choose at least one serving of plant proteins, such as black beans, lentils, or tofu, every day.

Oils   The Oils group represents the oils that are added to foods during processing, cooking, or at the table; oils and soft margarines include vegetables oils and soft vegetable oil table spreads that have no trans fats. These are major sources of vitamin E and unsaturated fatty acids, including the essential fatty acids. For a 2000-calorie diet, 6 tea-spoons of oils per day are recommended. One teaspoon is the equivalent of the following:

- 1 teaspoon vegetable oil or soft margarine
- 1 tablespoon salad dressing or light mayonnaise

Foods that are mostly oils include nuts, olives, avocados, and some fish. The following portions include about 1 teaspoon of oil: 8 large olives, 1/6 medium avocado, 1/2 tablespoon peanut butter, and 1/3 ounce roasted nuts. Food labels can help consumers identify the type and amount of fat in various foods.

Discretionary Calories, Solid Fats, and Added Sugars The suggested intakes from the basic food groups in MyPyramid assume that nutrient-dense forms are selected from each group; nutrient-dense forms are those that are fat-free or low-fat and that contain no added sugars. If this pattern is followed, then a small amount of additional calories can be consumed—the *discretionary calorie allowance*. Figure 12-6 shows the discretionary calorie allowance at each calorie level in MyPyramid.

People who are trying to lose weight may choose not to use discretionary calories. For those wanting to maintain weight, discretionary calories may be used to increase the amount of food from a food group; to consume foods that are not in the lowest fat form or that contain added sugars; to add oil, fat, or sugars to foods; or to consume alcohol. The amounts shown in Figure 12-6 show how discretionary calories may be divided between solid fats and added sugars. The values for additional fat target no more than 30% of total calories from fat and less than 10% of calories from saturated fat. Examples of discretionary solid fat calories include choosing higher-fat meats such as sausages, or chicken with skin, or whole milk instead of fat-free milk and topping foods with butter. For example, a cup of whole milk has 60 calories more than a cup of fat-free milk; these 60 calories would be counted as discretionary calories.

As described earlier in the chapter, added sugars are the sugars added to foods and beverages in processing or preparation, not the naturally occurring sugars in fruits or milk. The suggested amounts of added sugars may be helpful limits for including some sweetened foods or beverages in the daily diet without exceeding energy

needs or underconsuming other nutrients. For example, in a 2000-calorie diet, MyPyramid lists 32 grams (8 teaspoons) for discretionary intake of added sugars. In the American diet, added sugars are often found in sweetened beverages (regular soda, sweetened teas, fruit drinks), dairy products (ice cream, some yogurts), and grain products (bakery goods). For example, a 20-ounce regular soda has 260 calories from added sugars that would be counted as discretionary calories. The current American diet includes higher-than-recommended levels of sugar intake.

Remember, the amounts listed in Figure 12-6 for solid fats and added sugars assume that you selected foods in nutrient-dense forms from the major foods groups; don't just add fats and sugars to your diet. To control weight and obtain adequate amounts of essential nutrients, it is important to choose nutrient-dense forms of foods for most of your daily servings.

For an evaluation of your diet, complete the activity in the box "Your Diet Versus MyPyramid Recommendations."

The Vegetarian Alternative

Some people choose a diet with one essential difference from the diets we've already described—foods of animal origin (meat, poultry, fish, eggs, milk) are eliminated or restricted. Many do so for health reasons; vegetarian diets tend to be lower in saturated fat, cholesterol, and animal protein and higher in complex carbohydrates, dietary fiber, folate, vitamins C and E, carotenoids, and phyto-chemicals. Some people adopt a vegetarian diet out of concern for the environment, for financial considerations, or for reasons related to ethics or religion.

Types of Vegetarian Diets There are various veg-etarian styles; the wider the variety of the diet eaten, the easier it is to meet nutritional needs. **Vegans** eat only plant foods. **Lacto-vegetarians** eat plant foods and dairy prod-ucts. **Lacto-ovo-vegetarians** eat plant foods, dairy prod-ucts, and eggs. According to recent polls, over 5 million American adults never eat meat, poultry, or fish and fall into one of these three groups. Others can be categorized as **partial vegetarians, semivegetarians,** or **pescovege-tarians**; these individuals eat plant foods, dairy products, eggs, and usually a small selection of poultry, fish, and other seafood. Many other people choose vegetarian meals frequently but are not strictly vegetarian. Including some animal protein (such as dairy products) in a vegetarian diet makes planning easier, but it is not necessary.

A Food Plan for Vegetarians MyPyramid can be adapted for use by vegetarians with only a few key modi-fications. For the meat and beans group, vegetarians can focus on the nonmeat choices of dry beans (legumes), nuts, seeds, eggs, and soy foods like tofu (soybean curd) and tempeh (a cultured soy product). Vegans and other vegetarians who do not consume any dairy products must

Assess Yourself

1. **Keep a food record:** To evaluate your daily diet, begin by keeping a record of everything you eat on a typical day. To help with your analysis, break down each food item into its component parts and note your portion sizes; for example, a turkey sandwich might be listed as 2 slices sourdough bread, 3 ounces turkey, 1 tomato, 1 tablespoon mayonnaise, and so on.

2. **Compare your servings to the recommendations of MyPyramid:** Complete the chart below to compare your daily diet to MyPyramid. See Figure 12-6 for the recommended daily intake for your calorie level.

Food Group	Recommended Daily Amounts/Servings for Your Energy Intake	Your Actual Daily Intake (Amounts/Servings)	Serving Sizes and Equivalents
Grains (*total*)			1 oz equivalents = 1 slice of bread; 1 small muffin; 1 cup ready-to-eat cereal flakes; or ½ cup cooked cereal, rice, grains, or pasta
Whole grains			
Other grains			
Vegetables (*total*)			½ cup or equivalent (1 serving) = ½ cup raw or cooked vegetables; 1 cup raw leafy salad greens; or ½ cup vegetable juice
*Dark green**			
*Deep yellow**			
*Legumes**			
*Starchy**			
*Other**			
Fruits			½ cup or equivalent (1 serving) = ½ cup fresh, canned, or frozen fruit; ½ cup fruit juice; 1 small whole fruit; or ¼ cup dried fruit
Milk			1 cup or equivalent = 1 cup milk or yogurt; 1-½ oz natural cheese; or 2 oz processed cheese
Meat and Beans			1 oz equivalents = 1 oz lean meat, poultry, or fish; ¼ cup cooked dry beans or tofu; 1 egg; 1 tablespoon peanut butter; or ½ oz nuts or seeds
Oils			1 teaspoon or equivalent = 1 teaspoon vegetable oil or 1 tablespoon light mayonnaise or salad dressing
Solid Fats			
Added Sugars			

*Compare your daily intake with the approximate daily intake derived from the weekly pattern given in MyPyramid (Figure 12-6).

It may be difficult to track values for added sugars and, especially, oils and fats, but be as accurate as you can. Check food labels for information on fat and sugar. (NOTE: For a more complete and accurate analysis of your diet, keep food records for 3 days and then average the results.) MyPyramid.gov has additional guidelines for counting discretionary calories.

3. **Further evaluate your food choices within the groups:** Based on the data you collected and what you learned in the chapter, what were the especially healthy choices you made (for example, whole grains and citrus fruits) and what were your less healthy choices? Identify and list foods in the latter category, as these are areas where you can make changes to improve your diet. In particular, you may want to limit your intake of the following: processed, sweetened grains; high-fat meats and poultry skin; deep-fried fast foods; full-fat dairy products; regular sodas, sweetened teas, fruit drinks; alcoholic beverages; other foods that primarily provide sugar and fat and few other nutrients.

4. **Make healthy changes:** Bring your diet in line with MyPyramid by adding servings from food groups for which you fall short of the recommendations. To maintain a healthy weight, you may need to balance these additions by reductions in other areas—by eliminating some of the fats, oils, sweets, and alcohol you consume; by cutting extra servings from food groups for which your intake is more than adequate; or by making healthier choices within the food groups. Make a list of foods to add and a list of foods to eliminate; post your lists in a prominent location.

For a more detailed analysis of your current diet, including intakes of specific nutrients, use the online MyPyramid Tracker tool available at MyPyramid.gov.

When it comes to nutrition, men and women have a lot in common. Both sexes need the same essential nutrients, and the Dietary Guidelines for Americans apply equally to both. But beyond the basics, men and women need different amounts of essential nutrients and have different nutritional concerns.

Women tend to be smaller and weigh less than men, and thus have lower energy requirements and need to consume fewer calories than men to maintain a healthy weight. For most nutrients, women need the same or slightly lower amounts than men. But because women consume fewer calories, they may have more difficulty getting adequate amounts of all essential nutrients and need to focus on nutrient-dense foods.

Two nutrients of special concern to women are calcium and iron. Low calcium intake may be linked to the development of osteoporosis in later life. The *Healthy People 2010* report sets a goal of increasing from 40% to 75% the proportion of women age 20–49 who meet the dietary recommendation for calcium. Fat-free and low-fat dairy products and fortified cereal, bread, and orange juice are good choices for calcium-rich foods.

Menstruating women also have higher iron needs than other groups, and low iron intake can lead to iron-deficiency anemia. Lean red meat, green leafy vegetables, and fortified breakfast cereals are good sources of iron. As discussed earlier, all women capable of becoming pregnant should consume adequate folic acid from fortified foods and/or supplements.

Men are seldom thought of as having nutritional deficiencies because they generally have high-calorie diets. However, many men have a diet that does not follow recommended food intake patterns and includes more red meat and fewer fruits, vegetables, and whole grains than recommended. This dietary pattern is linked to heart disease and some types of cancer. A high intake of calories can lead to weight gain over time if a man's activity level decreases as he ages. To reduce chronic disease risk, men should focus on increasing their consumption of fruits, vegetables, and whole grains to obtain vitamins, minerals, fiber, and phytochemicals.

The "Eat 5 to 9 a Day for Better Health" program created by the National Cancer Institute and U.S. Department of Health and Human Services to promote increased intake of fruits and vegetables has been adapted to create the "Shoot for 9 for Better Health" message for men; for strategies and guidelines for consuming more fruits and vegetables, visit http://5aday.gov/9aday.

---

find other rich sources of calcium (see below). Fruits, vegetables, and whole grains are healthy choices for people following all types of vegetarian diets.

A healthy vegetarian diet emphasizes a wide variety of plant foods. Although plant proteins are generally of lower quality than animal proteins, choosing a variety of plant foods will supply all of the essential amino acids. Choosing minimally processed and unrefined foods will maximize nutrient value and provide ample dietary fiber. Daily consumption of a variety of plant foods in amounts that meet total energy needs can provide all needed nutrients, except vitamin B-12 and possibly vitamin D. Strategies for obtaining nutrients of concern include the following:

- *Vitamin B-12* is found naturally only in animal foods; if dairy products and eggs are limited or avoided, B-12 can be obtained from fortified foods such as ready-to-eat cereals, soy beverages, meat substitutes, and special yeast products or from supplements.

- *Vitamin D* can be obtained by spending 5–15 minutes a day in the sun, by consuming vitamin D–fortified products like ready-to-eat cereals and soy or rice milk, or by taking a supplement.

- *Calcium* is found in legumes, tofu processed with calcium, dark green leafy vegetables, nuts, tortillas made from lime-processed corn, and fortified orange juice, soy milk, bread, and other foods.

- *Iron* can be obtained from whole grains, fortified bread and breakfast cereals, dried fruits, green leafy vegetables, nuts and seeds, legumes, and soy foods. The iron in plant foods is more difficult for the body to absorb than is the iron from animal sources; consuming a good source of vitamin C with most meals is helpful because vitamin C improves iron absorption.

- *Zinc* is found in whole grains, nuts, legumes, and soy foods.

It takes a little planning and common sense to put together a good vegetarian diet. If you are a vegetarian or considering becoming one, devote some extra time and thought to your diet. It's especially important to eat as wide a variety of foods as possible to ensure that all your nutritional needs are satisfied. Consulting with a registered dietitian will make your planning even easier. Vegetarian diets for children, teens, and pregnant and lactating women warrant professional guidance.

Dietary Challenges for Special Population Groups

The Dietary Guidelines for Americans and MyPyramid provide a basis that everyone can use to create a healthy diet. However, some population groups face special dietary challenges (see the box "How Different Are the Nutritional Needs of Women and Men").

Children and Teenagers Young people often simply need to be encouraged to eat. Perhaps the best thing a parent can do for younger children is to provide them with a variety of foods. Add vegetables to casseroles and fruit to cereal; offer fruit and vegetable juices or homemade yogurt or fruit shakes instead of sugary drinks. Allowing children to help prepare meals is another good way to increase overall food consumption and variety. Many children and teenagers enjoy eating at fast-food restaurants; they should be encouraged to select the healthiest choices from fast-food menus (see Appendix A) and to complete the day's diet with low-fat, nutrient-rich foods.

College Students   Foods that are convenient for college students are not always the healthiest choices. It is easy for students who eat in buffet-style dining halls or food courts to overeat, and the foods offered are not necessarily high in essential nutrients and low in fat. The same is true of meals at fast-food restaurants, another convenient source of quick and inexpensive meals for busy students. Although no food is entirely bad, consuming a wide variety of foods is critical for a healthy diet. See the box "Eating Strategies for College Students" for tips on making healthy eating convenient and affordable.

Older Adults   Nutrient needs do not change much as people age; but because older adults tend to become less active, they require fewer calories to maintain body weight. At the same time, the absorption of nutrients tends to be lower in older adults because of age-related changes in the digestive tract. Thus, they must consume nutrient-dense foods in order to meet their nutritional requirements. As discussed earlier, foods fortified with vitamin B-12 and/or B-12 supplements are recommended for people over age 50. Because constipation is a common problem, consuming foods high in fiber and getting adequate fluids are important goals.

Athletes   Key dietary concerns for athletes are meeting their increased energy requirements and drinking enough fluids during practice and throughout the day to remain fully hydrated. Endurance athletes may also benefit from increasing the amount of carbohydrate in the diet to 60–70% of total daily calories; this increase should come in the form of complex, rather than simple, carbohydrates. Athletes for whom maintaining low body weight and body fat is important—such as skaters, gymnasts, and wrestlers—should consume adequate nutrients and avoid falling into unhealthy patterns of eating. Eating for exercise is discussed in more detail in Chapter 13; refer to Chapter 14 for information on eating disorders.

People with Special Health Concerns   Many Americans have special health concerns that affect their dietary needs. For example, women who are pregnant or breastfeeding require extra calories, vitamins, and minerals (see Chapter 8). People with diabetes benefit from a well-balanced diet that is low in simple sugars, high in

complex carbohydrates, and relatively rich in monounsaturated fats. People with high blood pressure need to control their weight and limit their sodium consumption. If you have a health problem or concern that may require a special diet, discuss your situation with a physician or registered dietitian.

A PERSONAL PLAN: MAKING INFORMED CHOICES ABOUT FOOD

Now that you understand the basis of good nutrition and a healthy diet, you can put together a diet that works for you. Focus on the likely causes of any health problems in your life, and make specific dietary changes to address them. You may also have some specific areas of concern, such as interpreting food labels and dietary supplement labels, avoiding foodborne illnesses and environmental contaminants, and understanding food additives. We turn to these and other topics next.

Reading Food Labels

Consumers can get help from food labels in applying the principles of the Dietary Guidelines for Americans. Since 1994, all processed foods regulated by either the FDA or the USDA have included standardized nutrition information on their labels. Every food label shows serving sizes and the amount of fat, saturated fat, cholesterol, sodium, total carbohydrate, dietary fiber, sugars, and protein in each serving. To make intelligent choices about food, learn to read and *understand* food labels (see the box "Using Food Labels").

Fresh meat, poultry, fish, fruits, and vegetables are not required to have food labels, and many of these products are not packaged. You can obtain information on the nutrient content of these items from basic nutrition books, registered dietitians, nutrient analysis computer software, the World Wide Web, and the companies that produce or distribute these foods. Also, supermarkets often have large posters or pamphlets listing the nutrient contents of these foods.

Reading Dietary Supplement Labels

Dietary supplements include vitamins, minerals, amino acids, herbs, glandular extracts, enzymes, and other compounds. They may come in the form of tablets, capsules, liquids, or powders. Surveys indicate that over half of American adults use dietary supplements at least occasionally, and sales have more than quadrupled since 1990, to over $15 billion per year. Although dietary supplements are often thought to be safe and "natural," they contain powerful, bioactive chemicals that have the potential for harm. About one-quarter of all pharmaceutical drugs are derived from botanical sources—morphine from poppies and digoxin from foxglove, for example.

General Guidelines

- Eat slowly, and enjoy your food. Set aside a separate time to eat, and don't eat while you study.

- Eat a colorful, varied diet. The more colorful your diet is, the more varied and rich in fruits and vegetables it will be. Many Americans eat few fruits and vegetables, despite the fact that these foods are typically inexpensive, delicious, rich in nutrients, and low in fat and calories.

- Eat breakfast. You'll have more energy in the morning and be less likely to grab an unhealthy snack later on.

- Choose healthy snacks—fruits, vegetables, grains, and cereals—as often as you can.

- Drink water more often than soft drinks or other sweetened beverages. Rent a mini-refrigerator for your dorm room and stock up on healthy beverages.

- Pay attention to portion sizes.

- Combine physical activity with healthy eating. You'll feel better and have a much lower risk of many chronic diseases. Even a little exercise is better than none.

Eating in the Dining Hall

- Choose a meal plan that includes breakfast, and don't skip it.

- Accept that dining hall food is not going to taste the same as home cooking. Find healthy dishes that you like.

- If menus are posted or distributed, decide what you want to eat before you get in line, and stick to your choices. Consider what you plan to do and eat for the rest of the day before making your choices.

- Ask for large servings of vegetables and small servings of meat and other high-fat main dishes. Build your meals around grains and vegetables.

- Try whole grains like brown rice, whole-wheat bread, and whole-grain cereals.

- Choose leaner poultry, fish, or bean dishes rather than high-fat meats and fried entrees.

- Ask that gravies and sauces be served on the side; limit your intake.

- Choose broth-based or vegetable soups rather than cream soups.

- At the salad bar, load up on leafy greens, beans, and fresh vegetables. Avoid mayonnaise-coated salads, bacon, croutons, and high-fat dressings. Put dressing on the side, and dip your fork into it rather than pouring it over the salad.

- Drink nonfat milk, water, mineral water, or 100% fruit juice rather than heavily sweetened fruit drinks, whole milk, or soft drinks.

- Choose fruit for dessert rather than pastries, cookies, or cakes.

- Do some research about the foods and preparation methods used in your dining hall or cafeteria. Discuss any suggestions you have with your food-service manager.

Eating in Fast-Food Restaurants

- Most fast-food chains can provide a brochure with a nutritional breakdown of the foods on the menu. Ask for it. (See also the information in Appendix A.)

- Order small single burgers with no cheese instead of double burgers with many toppings. If possible, ask for them broiled instead of fried.

- Ask for items to be prepared without mayonnaise, tartar sauce, sour cream, or other high-fat sauces. Ketchup, mustard, and fat-free mayonnaise or sour cream are better choices and are available at many fast-food restaurants.

- Choose whole-grain buns or bread for burgers and sandwiches.

- Choose chicken items made from chicken breast, not processed chicken.

- Order vegetable pizzas without extra cheese.

- If you order french fries or onion rings, get the smallest size, and/or share them with a friend.

Eating on the Run

Are you chronically short of time? The following healthy and filling items can be packed for a quick snack or meal: fresh or dried fruit, fruit juices, raw fresh vegetables like carrots, plain bagels, bread sticks, whole-wheat fig bars, low-fat cheese sticks or cubes, low-fat crackers or granola bars, nonfat or low-fat yogurt, snack-size cereal boxes, pretzels, rice or corn cakes, plain popcorn, soup (if you have access to a microwave), or water.

And, as described earlier, even essential vitamins and minerals can have toxic effects if consumed in excess.

In the United States, supplements are not legally considered drugs and are not regulated the way drugs are. Before they are approved by the FDA and put on the market, drugs undergo clinical studies to determine safety, effectiveness, side effects and risks, possible interactions with other substances, and appropriate dosages. The FDA does not authorize or test dietary supplements, and supplements are not required to demonstrate either safety or effectiveness prior to marketing. Although dosage guidelines exist for some of the compounds in dietary supplements, dosages for many are not well established.

Critical Consumer

Food labels are designed to help consumers make food choices based on the nutrients that are most important to good health. In addition to listing nutrient content by weight, the label puts the information in the context of a daily diet of 2000 calories that includes no more than 65 grams of fat (approximately 30% of total calories). For example, if a serving of a particular product has 13 grams of fat, the label will show that the serving represents 20% of the daily fat allowance. If your daily diet contains fewer or more than 2000 calories, you need to adjust these calculations accordingly.

Food labels contain uniform serving sizes. This means that if you look at different brands of salad dressing, for example, you can compare calories and fat content based on the serving amount. (Food label serving sizes may be larger or smaller than MyPyramid serving size equivalents, however.) Regulations also require that foods meet strict definitions if their packaging includes the terms *light, low-fat,* or *high-fiber* (see the sample label). Claims such as "good source of dietary fiber" or "low in saturated fat" on packages are signals that those products can wisely be included in your diet. Overall, the food label is an important tool to help you choose a diet that conforms to MyPyramid and the Dietary Guidelines.

Selected Nutrient Content Claims and What They Mean

Healthy A food that is low in fat, is low in saturated fat, has no more than 360–480 mg of sodium and 60 mg of cholesterol, *and* provides 10% or more of the Daily Value for vitamin A, vitamin C, protein, calcium, iron, or dietary fiber per serving.

Light or lite One-third fewer calories or 50% less fat than a similar product.

Reduced or fewer At least 25% less of a nutrient than a similar product; can be applied to fat ("reduced fat"), saturated fat, cholesterol, sodium, and calories.

Extra or added 10% or more of the Daily Value per serving when compared to what a similar product has.

Good source 10–19% of the Daily Value for a particular nutrient per serving.

High, rich in, or excellent source of 20% or more of the Daily Value for a particular nutrient per serving.

Low calorie 40 calories or less per serving.

High fiber 5 g or more of fiber per serving.

Good source of fiber 2.5–4.9 g of fiber per serving.

Fat-free Less than 0.5 g of fat per serving.

Low-fat 3 g of fat or less per serving.

Saturated fat-free Less than 0.5 g of saturated fat and 0.5 g of trans fatty acids per serving.

Low saturated fat 1 g or less of saturated fat per serving and no more than 15% of total calories.

Cholesterol-free Less than 2 mg of cholesterol and 2 g or less of saturated fat per serving.

Low cholesterol 20 mg or less of cholesterol and 2 g or less of saturated fat per serving.

Low sodium 140 mg or less of sodium per serving.

Very low sodium 35 mg or less of sodium per serving.

Lean Cooked seafood, meat, or poultry with less than 10 g of fat, 4.5 g or less of saturated fat, and less than 95 mg of cholesterol per serving.

Extra lean Cooked seafood, meat, or poultry with less than 5 g of fat, 2 g of saturated fat, and 95 mg of cholesterol per serving.

NOTE: As of April 2005, the FDA had not yet defined nutrient claims relating to carbohydrate, so foods labeled low- or reduced-carbohydrate do not conform to any approved standard.

1. Serving size: Determine how many servings there are in the food package and compare it to how much you actually eat. You may need to adjust the rest of the nutrient values based on your typical serving size.

2. Calories and calories from fat: Note whether a serving is high in calories and fat. The sample food shown here is low in fat, with only 30 of its 235 calories from fat.

3. Daily Values: Based on a 2000-calorie diet, Daily Value percentages tell you whether the nutrients in a serving of food contribute a lot or a little to your total daily diet.
    5% or less is low
    20% or more is high

4. Limit these nutrients: Look for foods low in fat, saturated fat, trans fat, cholesterol, and sodium. *(Trans fat content must be included on the label by January 2006 for any food with more than 0.5 g trans fat per serving.)*

5. Get enough of these nutrients: Look for foods high in dietary fiber, vitamin A, vitamin C, calcium, and iron.

Nutrition Facts

Serving Size 1 cup (265g)
Servings per Container 2

Amount per Serving

Calories 235   Calories from Fat 30

	% Daily Value*
Total Fat 3g	5%
Saturated Fat 1g	5%
Trans Fat 0.5g	
Cholesterol 30mg	10%
Sodium 775mg	32%
Total Carbohydrate 34g	11%
Dietary Fiber 9g	36%
Sugars 5g	
Protein 18g	

Vitamin A 25%	•	Vitamin C 0%
Calcium 12%	•	Iron 20%

*Percent Daily Values are based on a 2,000 calorie diet. Your daily values may be higher or lower depending on your calorie needs:

		Calories	2,000	2,500
Total Fat	Less than		65g	80
Sat Fat	Less than		20g	25g
Cholesterol	Less than		300mg	300mg
Sodium	Less than		2,400mg	2,400mg
Total Carbohydrate			300g	375g
Dietary Fiber			25g	30g

Calories per gram:
Fat 9 • Carbohydrate 4 • Protein 4

Note: This section shows recommended daily intake for two levels of calorie consumption and values for dietary calculations; it's the same on all labels.

Although many ingredients in dietary supplements have been used for centuries in Eastern or European herbal medicine, some have been found to be dangerous or to interact with prescription or over-the-counter drugs in dangerous ways. Garlic supplements, for example, can cause bleeding if taken with anticoagulant ("blood thinning") medications. Even products that are generally considered safe can have side effects—St. John's wort, for example, increases the skin's sensitivity to sunlight and may decrease the effectiveness of oral contraceptives, drugs used to treat HIV infection, and other medications.

There are also key differences in how drugs and supplements are manufactured. FDA-approved medications are standardized for potency, and quality control and proof of purity are required. Dietary supplement manufacture is not as closely regulated, and there is no guarantee that a product even contains a given ingredient, let alone in the appropriate amount. The potency of herbal supplements tends to vary widely due to differences in growing and harvesting conditions, preparation methods, and storage. Some manufacturers attempt to standardize their products by isolating the compounds believed to be responsible for an herb's action. However, potency is often still highly variable, and when several compounds are thought to be responsible for an herb's effect, often only one is standardized. In addition, herbs can be contaminated or misidentified at any stage from harvest to packaging. The FDA has recalled several products due to the presence of dangerous contaminants, including heavy metals and pharmaceutical drugs.

With increased consumer knowledge and demand, it is likely that both the research base and the manufacturing standards for supplements will improve. (The FDA proposed manufacturing standards in 2003.) To provide consumers with more reliable and consistent information about supplements, the FDA requires supplements to have labels similar to those found on foods (see the box "Using Dietary Supplement Labels" for more information). Label statements and claims about supplements are also regulated.

Finally, it is important to remember that dietary supplements are no substitute for a healthy diet. Supplements do not provide all the known—or yet-to-be-discovered—benefits of whole foods. Supplements should also not be used as a replacement for medical treatment for serious illnesses. (See Chapter 21 for more on herbal remedies.)

Protecting Yourself Against Foodborne Illness

Many people worry about additives or pesticide residues in their food. However, a greater threat to the safety of the food supply comes from microorganisms that cause foodborne illnesses. Raw or undercooked animal products, such as chicken, hamburger, and oysters, pose the greatest risk for causing illness. The CDC estimates that about 76 million illnesses, 325,000 hospitalizations, and 5000 deaths occur each year in the United States due to foodborne illness. Your last bout of "stomach flu" may very well have been a foodborne illness. The symptoms of both are often the same: diarrhea, vomiting, fever, and weakness. Although the effects of foodborne illnesses are usually not serious, some groups, such as children, pregnant women, and the elderly, are more at risk for severe complications such as rheumatic diseases, seizures, blood poisoning, other ailments, and death.

Causes of Foodborne Illnesses Most cases of foodborne illness are caused by **pathogens,** disease-causing microorganisms. Food can be contaminated with pathogens through improper handling; pathogens can grow if food is prepared or stored improperly. Causes of foodborne illness in the United States include the following pathogens:

• *Campylobacter jejuni* causes more cases of foodborne illness than any other bacteria. It is most commonly found in contaminated water, raw milk, and raw or undercooked poultry, meat, or shellfish; the majority of chickens sold in the United States test positive for the presence of *C. jejuni.* Symptoms of infection include diarrhea, fever, abdominal and muscle pain, and headache, which resolve in 7–10 days. However, in about 1 in 1000 cases, *Campylobacter* infection triggers Guillain-Barré syndrome, a neurological disease that can cause numbness, weakness, and (usually temporary) paralysis.

• *Salmonella* bacteria are most often found in raw or undercooked eggs, poultry, and meat; milk and dairy products; seafood; fruits and vegetables, including sprouts; and inadequately refrigerated and reheated leftovers. The recent identification of an antibiotic-resistant strain of *Salmonella* has raised concerns about a potential increase in serious illness from *Salmonella.*

• *Shigella* bacteria are found in the human intestinal tract and usually transmitted via fecal contamination of food and water. Outbreaks are typically traced to foods, especially salads, that have been handled by people using poor personal hygiene. Contaminated water, milk, and dairy products are other possible sources of infection.

• *Escherichia coli* bacteria, found in the intestinal tracts of humans and animals, most commonly contaminate water, raw milk, raw to rare ground beef, unpasteurized juices, and fruits and vegetables. A certain strain, known as *E. coli* O157:H7, is of particular concern because it produces a toxin that causes serious illness and up to 100 deaths annually. Children are particularly at risk for developing hemolytic uremic syndrome, which causes kidney failure.

Term

V **W**

pathogen A microorganism that causes disease.

Critical Consumer

Since 1999, specific types of information have been required on the labels of dietary supplements. In addition to basic information about the product, labels include a "Supplement Facts" panel, modeled after the "Nutrition Facts" panel used on food labels (see the label below). Under the Dietary Supplement Health and Education Act (DSHEA) and food labeling laws, supplement labels can make three types of health-related claims.

- *Nutrient-content claims,* such as "high in calcium," "excellent source of vitamin C," or "high potency." The claims "high in" and "excellent source of" mean the same as they do on food labels. A "high potency" single-ingredient supplement must contain 100% of its Daily Value; a "high potency" multi-ingredient product must contain 100% or more of the Daily Value of at least two-thirds of the nutrients present for which Daily Values have been established.

- *Health claims,* if they have been authorized by the FDA or another authoritative scientific body. The association between adequate calcium intake and lower risk of osteoporosis is an example of an approved health claim. Since 2003, the FDA has also allowed so-called *qualified* health claims for situations in which there is emerging but as yet inconclusive evidence for a particular claim. Such claims must include qualifying language such as "scientific evidence suggests but does not prove" the claim.

- *Structure-function claims,* such as "antioxidants maintain cellular integrity" or "this product enhances energy levels." Because these claims are not reviewed by the FDA, they must carry a disclaimer (see the sample label).

Tips for Choosing and Using Dietary Supplements

- Check with your physician before taking a supplement. Many are not meant for children, elderly people, women who are pregnant or breast-feeding, people with chronic illnesses, or people taking prescription or OTC medications.

- Choose brands made by nationally known food and drug manufacturers or house brands from large retail chains.

Due to their size and visibility, such sources are likely to have high manufacturing standards.

- Look for the USP-DSVP mark on the label, indicating that the product meets minimum safety and purity standards developed under the Dietary Supplement Verification Program (DSVP) by the United States Pharmacopeia (USP). The USP-DSVP mark means that the product (1) contains the ingredients stated on the label, (2) has the declared amount and strength of ingredients, (3) will dissolve effectively, (4) has been screened for harmful contaminants, and (5) has been manufactured using safe, sanitary, and well-controlled procedures. The National Nutritional Foods Association (NNFA) has a self-regulatory testing program for its members; other, smaller associations and labs, including ConsumerLab.Com, also test and rate dietary supplements.

- Follow the cautions, instructions for use, and dosage given on the label.

- If you experience side effects, discontinue use of the product and contact your physician. Report any serious reactions to the FDA's MedWatch monitoring program (800-FDA-1088; http://www.fda.gov/medwatch).

For More Information About Dietary Supplements

ConsumerLab.Com: http://www.consumerlab.com

Food and Drug Administration: http://vm.cfsan.fda.gov/~dms/supplmnt.html

National Institutes of Health, Office of Dietary Supplements: http://dietary-supplements.info.nih.gov

National Nutritional Foods Association: http://www.nnfa.org

U.S. Department of Agriculture: http://www.nal.usda.gov/fnic/etext/000015.html

U.S. Pharmacopeia: http://www.usp.org/dietarysupplements

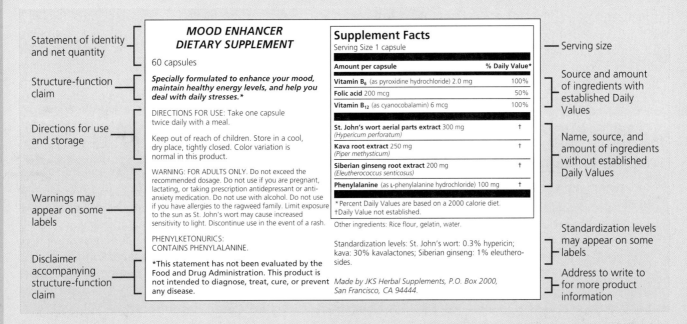

- *Listeria monocytogenes* sickens about 1200–1800 Americans a year, causing death in about 20% of cases. It is found in soft cheeses, raw milk, improperly processed ice cream, raw leafy vegetables, hot dogs and lunch meats, and other meat, poultry, and processed foods. *Listeria* is particularly dangerous for pregnant women and their fetuses, babies and children, older adults, and people with weakened immune systems.

- *Staphylococcus aureus* lives mainly in nasal passages and skin sores; it is transferred to food when people handle food or sneeze or cough over food. Foods contaminated with *S. aureus* may include cooked hams, egg and potato salads, cheese, seafood, whipped cream, and milk. *S. aureus* multiplies rapidly at room temperature to produce a toxin that causes illness.

- *Clostridium botulinum* is widely distributed in nature, but it grows only in environments with little or no oxygen; it produces a toxin that causes illness. Potential sources of *C. botulinum* include improperly canned foods, garlic in oil, sausages and other meat products, and vacuum-packed and tightly wrapped foods. Although rare, botulism is potentially fatal if untreated because the toxin affects the nervous system.

- Norovirus, the most common viral cause of foodborne illness, may be found in contaminated water, raw or insufficiently cooked shellfish, and salads contaminated by food handlers. Noroviruses typically cause vomiting, diarrhea, and abdominal pain, lasting 1–3 days.

Other causes of foodborne illness include the bacteria *Clostridium perfringens, Vibrio vulnificus,* and *Yersinia enterocolytica;* the hepatitis A virus; the parasites *Trichinella spiralis* (found in pork and wild game), *Anisakis* (found in raw fish), *Giardia lamblia, Cyclospora cayetanensis,* and tapeworms; and certain molds.

A potential new threat from food is bovine spongiform encephalopathy (BSE), or "mad cow disease," a fatal degenerative neurological disease caused by an abnormal protein that forms deposits in the brain. A variant form of the human version of this disease, known as Creutzfeldt-Jakob disease (CJD), is believed to be caused by eating beef contaminated with central nervous system tissue from BSE-infected cows. To date, there have been about 150 confirmed cases worldwide of this variant CJD among the hundreds of thousands of people who may have consumed BSE-contaminated products. In December 2003, the first BSE-infected cow in the United States was identified; no meat or organs from this animal had made it into the food supply. Although the USDA states

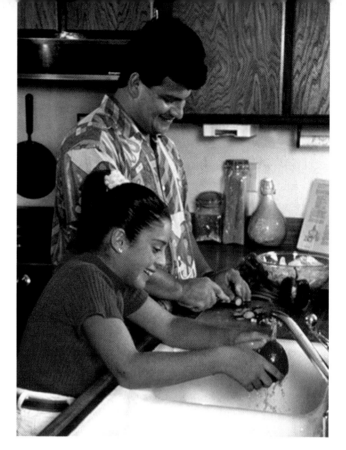

Careful food handling greatly reduces the risk of foodborne illness. Helpful strategies include washing hands and all fruits and vegetables, using separate cutting boards for meat and for foods that will be eaten raw, cooking meat thoroughly, and refrigerating leftovers promptly.

that the risk to human health from BSE is extremely low, additional steps are being taken to prevent the BSE protein from entering the food supply; visit the USDA Web site for more information (www.usda.gov/bse).

Preventing and Treating Foodborne Illnesses

Because every teaspoon of the soil that our food grows in contains about 2 billion bacteria (only some of them pathogenic), we are always exposed to the possibility of a foodborne illness. You can't tell by taste, smell, or sight whether a food is contaminated. Some studies have revealed high levels of contamination. In 2003, *Consumer Reports* tested 484 chickens purchased in grocery stores and found that half were contaminated with *Campylobacter* and/or *Salmonella;* many of the strains of bacteria found were resistant to antibiotics.

Although pathogens are usually destroyed during cooking, the U.S. government is taking steps to bring down levels of contamination. In addition to new microbiological testing methods for inspection of meat and poultry processing plants, raw meat and poultry products are now sold with safe handling and cooking instructions, and all packaged, unpasteurized fresh fruit and vegetable juices carry warnings about potential contamination. Foodborne illness outbreaks associated with food-processing plants

Term

V w

polychlorinated biphenyl (PCB) An industrial chemical used as an insulator in electrical transformers and linked to certain human cancers.

- Don't buy food in containers that leak, bulge, or are severely dented. Refrigerated foods should be cold, and frozen foods should be solid.

- Refrigerate perishable items as soon as possible after purchase. Use or freeze fresh meats within 3–5 days and fresh poultry, fish, and ground meat within 1–2 days.

- Store raw meat, poultry, fish, and shellfish in containers in the refrigerator so that the juices don't drip onto other foods. Keep these items away from other foods, surfaces, utensils, or serving dishes to prevent cross-contamination.

- Thaw frozen food in the refrigerator or in the microwave oven, not on the kitchen counter. Cook foods immediately after thawing.

- Thoroughly wash your hands with warm soapy water for 20 seconds before and after handling food, especially raw meat, fish, shellfish, poultry, or eggs.

- Make sure counters, cutting boards, dishes, utensils, and other equipment are thoroughly cleaned before and after use using hot soapy water. Wash dishcloths and kitchen towels frequently.

- If possible, use separate cutting boards for meat, poultry, and seafood and for foods that will be eaten raw, such as fruits and vegetables. Replace cutting boards once they become worn or develop hard-to-clean grooves.

- Thoroughly rinse and scrub fruits and vegetables with a brush, if possible, or peel off the skin.

- Cook foods thoroughly, especially beef, poultry, fish, pork, and eggs; cooking kills most microorganisms. Use a food thermometer to ensure that foods are cooked to a safe temperature. Hamburgers should be cooked to 160°F. Turn or stir microwaved food to make sure it is heated evenly throughout. When eating out, order hamburger cooked well-done and make sure foods are served piping hot.

- Cook stuffing separately from poultry; or wash poultry thoroughly, stuff immediately before cooking, and transfer the stuffing to a clean bowl immediately after cooking. The temperature of cooked stuffing should reach 165°F.

- Keep hot foods hot (140°F or above) and cold foods cold (40°F or below); harmful bacteria can grow rapidly between these two temperatures. Refrigerate foods within 2 hours of purchase or preparation, and within 1 hour if the air temperature is above 90°F. Refrigerate foods at or below 40°F and freeze at or below 0°F. Use refrigerated leftovers within 3–4 days.

- Don't eat raw animal products, including raw eggs in homemade hollandaise sauce or eggnog. Use only pasteurized milk and juice, and look for pasteurized eggs, which are now available in some states.

- Cook eggs until they're firm, and fully cook foods containing eggs. Store eggs in the coldest part of the refrigerator, not in the door, and use them within 3–5 weeks.

- Because of possible contamination with *E. coli* O157:H7 and *Salmonella,* avoid raw sprouts. Even sprouts grown under clean conditions in the home can be risky because bacteria may be present in the seeds. Cook sprouts before eating them.

- Read the food label and package information, and follow safety instructions such as "Keep Refrigerated" and the "Safe Handling Instructions."

- According to the USDA, "When in doubt, throw it out." Even if a food looks and smells fine, it may not be safe. If you aren't sure that a food has been prepared, served, and stored safely, don't eat it.

Additional precautions are recommended for people at particularly high risk for foodborne illness—pregnant women, young children, older persons, and people with weakened immune systems or certain chronic illnesses. If you are a member of one of these groups, don't eat or drink any of the following products: unpasteurized juices; raw sprouts; unpasteurized (raw) milk and products made from unpasteurized milk; raw or undercooked meat, poultry, eggs, fish, and shellfish; and soft cheeses such as feta, Brie, Camembert, or blue-veined cheeses. To protect against *Listeria,* it's also important to avoid ready-to-eat foods such as hot dogs, luncheon meats, and cold cuts unless they are reheated until they are steaming hot.

make headlines, but most cases of illness trace back to poor food handling in the home or in food-service establishments. To decrease your risk of foodborne illness, follow the guidelines in the box "Safe Food Handling."

If you think you may be having a bout of foodborne illness drink plenty of clear fluids to prevent dehydration and rest to speed recovery. To prevent further contamination, wash your hands often, and always before handling food. A fever higher than 102°F, blood in the stool, or dehydration deserves a physician's evaluation, especially if the symptoms persist for more than 2–3 days. In cases of suspected botulism—characterized by symptoms

such as double vision, paralysis, dizziness, and vomiting—consult a physician immediately to receive an antitoxin.

Environmental Contaminants and Organic Foods

Contaminants are also present in the food-growing environment, but few of them ever enter the food and water supply in amounts sufficient to cause health problems. Environmental contaminants include various minerals, antibiotics, hormones, pesticides, the industrial chemicals known as **PCBs (polychlorinated biphenyls)**, and naturally occurring substances such as cyanogenic glycosides (found in lima beans and the pits of some fruits) and certain molds. Their effects depend on many factors, including concentration, length of exposure, and the age and health status of the person involved. Safety regulations attempt to keep our exposure to contaminants at safe levels, but monitoring is difficult and many substances (such as pesticides) persist in the environment long after being banned from use.

Organic Foods Some people who are concerned about pesticides and other environmental contaminants choose to buy foods that are **organic.** In December 2000, the USDA enacted a new national standard for organic foods to replace the older system of local, state, and private standards. To be certified as organic, foods must meet strict production, processing, handling, and labeling criteria. Organic crops must meet limits on pesticide residues; for meat, milk, eggs, and other animal products to be certified organic, animals must be given organic feed and access to the outdoors and may not be given antibiotics or growth hormones. The use of genetic engineering, ionizing radiation, and sewage sludge is prohibited (see below for more on irradiated and genetically modified foods). Products can be labeled "100% organic" if they contain all organic ingredients and "organic" if they contain at least 95% organic ingredients; all such products may carry the USDA organic seal. A product with at least 70% organic ingredients can be labeled "made with organic ingredients" but cannot use the USDA seal.

Organic foods are not necessarily chemical-free, however. They may be contaminated with pesticides used on neighboring lands or on foods transported in the same train or truck. However, they do tend to have lower levels of pesticide residues than conventionally grown crops. There are strict pesticide limits for all foods—organic and conventional—and the debate about the potential health effects of long-term exposure to small amounts of pesticide residues is ongoing. The benefits of a diet rich in fruits and vegetables far outweigh any potential long-term risks of exposure to pesticide residues.

Supporters of organic foods also note that practices associated with organic farming help maintain biodiversity of crops and are less likely to degrade soil, contaminate water, or expose farm workers to dangerous chemicals. Organic foods tend to be more expensive than those grown conventionally, however, and there is no evidence that they consistently contain more nutrients or fewer foodborne pathogens. But some people choose to pay the higher prices for organic foods to support agricultural practices they believe promote a healthier environment.

Guidelines for Fish Consumption A specific area of concern has been possible mercury contamination in fish. Overall, fish and shellfish are healthy sources of protein, omega-3 fats, and other nutrients; and prudent choices can minimize the risk of any possible negative health effects. High mercury concentrations are most likely to be found in predator fish—large fish that eat smaller fish. Mercury can cause brain damage to fetuses and young children. In 2004, the FDA and Environmental Protection Agency (EPA) released an advisory with specific guidelines for certain groups. To reduce exposure to the harmful effects of mercury, women who are or who may become pregnant and nursing mothers should follow these guidelines:

- Do not eat shark, swordfish, king mackerel, or tilefish.
- Eat up to 12 ounces a week of a variety of fish and shellfish that is lower in mercury, such as shrimp, canned light tuna, salmon, pollock, and catfish. Limit consumption of albacore tuna to 6 ounces per week.
- Check advisories about the safety of recreationally caught fish from local lakes, rivers, and coastal areas; if no information is available, limit consumption to 6 ounces per week.

The same FDA/EPA guidelines apply to children, although they should consume smaller servings.

Some experts have also expressed concern about the presence of toxins such as PCBs in farmed fish, especially farmed salmon. Although no federal guidelines have been set, some researchers suggest that consumers limit themselves to 8 ounces of farmed salmon per month. Fish should be labeled with its country of origin and whether it is wild or farmed; most canned salmon is wild.

Additives in Food

Today, some 2800 substances are intentionally added to foods for one or more of the following reasons: (1) to maintain or improve nutritional quality, (2) to maintain freshness, (3) to help in processing or preparation, or (4) to alter taste or appearance. Additives make up less than 1% of our food. The most widely used are sugar, salt, and corn syrup; these three plus citric acid, baking soda,

Terms

V w

organic A designation applied to foods grown and produced according to strict guidelines limiting the use of pesticides, non-organic ingredients, hormones, antibiotics, irradiation, genetic engineering, and other practices.

food irradiation The treatment of foods with gamma rays, X rays, or high-voltage electrons to kill potentially harmful pathogens and increase shelf life.

genetically modified (GM) organism A plant, animal, or microorganism in which genes have been added, rearranged, or replaced through genetic engineering.

vegetable colors, mustard, and pepper account for 98% by weight of all food additives used in the United States.

Some additives may be of concern for certain people, either because they are consumed in large quantities or because they cause some type of reaction. Additives having potential health concerns include the following:

• *Nitrates and nitrites:* Used to protect meats from contamination with botulism. Their consumption is associated with the synthesis of cancer-causing agents in the stomach, but the cancer risk appears to be low, except for people with low stomach acid output (such as some elderly people).

• *BHA and BHT:* Used to help maintain the freshness of foods. Some studies indicate a potential link between BHT and an increased risk of certain cancers, but any risk from these agents is considered to be low. Some manufacturers have stopped using BHT and BHA.

• *Sulfites:* Used to keep vegetables from turning brown. They can cause severe reactions in some people. The FDA severely limits the use of sulfites and requires any foods containing sulfites to be clearly labeled.

• *Monosodium glutamate (MSG):* Typically used as a flavor enhancer. MSG may cause some people to experience episodes of increased blood pressure and sweating. If you are sensitive to MSG, check food labels when shopping, and ask to have it left out of dishes you order at restaurants.

Food additives pose no significant health hazard to most people because the levels used are well below any that could produce toxic effects. To avoid potential problems, eat a variety of foods in moderation. If you are sensitive to an additive, check food labels when you shop, and ask questions when you eat out.

Food Irradiation

Food irradiation is the treatment of foods with gamma rays, X rays, or high-voltage electrons to kill potentially harmful pathogens, including bacteria, parasites, insects, and fungi that cause foodborne illness. It also reduces spoilage and extends shelf life. For example, irradiated strawberries stay unspoiled in the refrigerator up to 3 weeks, versus only 3–5 days for untreated berries. Since 1963, the government has allowed the irradiation of certain foods; this growing list includes wheat and flour (1963); white potatoes (1964); pork, herbs and spices, and fruits and vegetables (1986); raw poultry (1992); and red meat (1999). The same irradiation process has also been used for decades on such items as plastic wrap, milk cartons, teething rings, contact lenses, and medical supplies.

Even though irradiation has been generally endorsed by agencies such as the World Health Organization, the Centers for Disease Control and Prevention, and the American Medical Association, few irradiated foods are

currently on the market due to consumer resistance and skepticism. Studies haven't conclusively identified any harmful effects of food irradiation, and the newer methods of irradiation involving electricity and X rays do not require the use of any radioactive materials. Some irradiated foods may taste slightly different, just as pasteurized milk tastes slightly different than unpasteurized milk.

Studies indicate that when consumers are given information about the process of irradiation and the benefits of irradiated foods, most want to purchase them. Without such information, many remain skeptical. All primary irradiated foods (meat, vegetables, and so on) are labeled with the flowerlike radura symbol and a brief information label; spices and foods that are merely ingredients do not have to be so labeled. It is important to remember that although irradiation kills most pathogens, it does not completely sterilize foods. Proper handling of irradiated foods is still critical for preventing foodborne illness.

Genetically Modified Foods

Genetic engineering involves altering the characteristics of a plant, animal, or microorganism by adding, rearranging, or replacing genes in its DNA; the result is a **genetically modified (GM) organism.** New DNA may come from related species or from entirely different types of organisms. Many GM crops are already grown in the United States: About 75% of the current U.S. soybean crop has been genetically modified to be resistant to an herbicide used to kill weeds, and about 34% of the U.S. corn crop carries genes for herbicide resistance or pest resistance. Products made with GM organisms include juice, soda, nuts, tuna, frozen pizza, spaghetti sauce, canola oil, chips, salad dressings, and soup.

The potential benefits of GM foods cited by supporters include improved yields overall and in difficult growing conditions, increased disease resistance, improved nutritional content, lower prices, and less pesticide use. Critics of biotechnology argue that unexpected effects may occur: Gene manipulation could elevate levels of naturally occurring toxins or allergens, permanently change the gene pool and reduce biodiversity, and produce pesticide-resistant insects through the transfer of genes. Experience has shown that GM products are difficult to keep separate from non-GM products; animal escapes, cross-pollination, and contamination during processing are just a few ways GM organisms could potentially appear unexpectedly in the food supply or the environment.

According to the National Academy of Sciences, there is currently no proof that the GM food already on the market is unsafe. However, experts have recommended regulatory changes and further study of key issues, particularly the environmental effects of the escape of GM animals. Labeling has been another major concern, with surveys indicating that most Americans want to know if their food contains GM ingredients. Under current rules, the FDA requires special labeling only when a food's composition is changed significantly or when a known allergen such as a peanut gene is introduced into a food. The only foods guaranteed not to contain GM ingredients are those certified as organic.

Food Allergies and Food Intolerances

For some people, consuming a particular food causes symptoms such as itchiness, swollen lips, or abdominal pain. Adverse reactions like these may be due to a food allergy or a food intolerance, and symptoms may range from annoying to life-threatening. If you've had an adverse reaction to a food, it's important to determine whether your symptoms are due to an allergy or an intolerance so that you can take appropriate action.

Food Allergies   A true **food allergy** is a reaction of the body's immune system to a food or food ingredient, usually a protein. The immune system perceives the reaction-provoking substance, or allergen, as foreign and acts to destroy it. This immune reaction can occur within minutes of ingesting the food, resulting in symptoms that affect the skin (hives), gastrointestinal tract (cramps or diarrhea), respiratory tract (asthma), or mouth (swelling of the lips or tongue). The most severe response is a systemic reaction called anaphylaxis, which involves a potentially life-threatening drop in blood pressure.

Food allergies affect only about 2% of the adult population and about 4–6% of infants; many infants outgrow food allergies. Although numerous food allergens have been identified, just a few foods account for more than 90% of the food allergies in the United States: cow's milk, eggs, peanuts, tree nuts (walnuts, cashews, and so on), soy, wheat, fish, and shellfish. Individuals with food allergies, especially those prone to anaphylaxis, must diligently avoid trigger foods. This involves carefully reading food labels and asking questions about ingredients when eating out. People at risk are usually advised to carry medications to treat anaphylaxis, such as injectable epinephrine. Refer to Chapter 17 for more on allergies.

Food Intolerances   Many people who believe they have food allergies may actually suffer from a much more common source of adverse food reactions, a **food intolerance**. In the case of a food intolerance, the problem usually lies with metabolism rather than with the immune system. Typically, the body cannot adequately digest a food or food component, often because of some type of chemical deficiency; in other cases, the body reacts to a particular compound in a food. Lactose intolerance, described in Chapter 8, is a fairly common food intolerance; it occurs in people who are deficient in the enzyme lactase, which is needed to digest milk sugar (lactose). A more serious condition is intolerance of gluten, a protein component of some grains; in affected individuals, consumption of gluten damages the lining of the small intestine. Sulfite, a common food additive, can produce severe asthmatic reactions in sensitive individuals. Food intolerances have also been attributed to tartrazine (a yellow food coloring), MSG, and the sweetener aspartame.

Food intolerance reactions often produce symptoms similar to food allergies, such as diarrhea or cramps, but reactions are typically localized and not life-threatening. Many people with food intolerances can consume small amounts of the food that affects them; exceptions are gluten and sulfite, which must be avoided by sensitive individuals. Through trial and error, most people with food intolerances can adjust their intake of the trigger food to an appropriate level.

If you suspect that you have a food allergy or intolerance, a good first step is to keep a food diary. Note everything you eat or drink, any symptoms you develop, and how long after eating the symptoms appear. Then make an appointment with your physician to go over your diary and determine if any additional tests are needed.

Staying Committed to a Healthy Diet

You've learned the basics of good nutrition, know how to interpret food and supplement labels, and have some guidelines for protecting yourself from food-related illness. With this foundation, you can now put together a diet that works for you. You can customize a food plan based on your age, sex, weight, activity level, medical risk factors—and, of course, personal tastes.

Sticking to a healthy diet is usually easiest when people choose and prepare their own food at home (see the box "America's Poor Eating Habits"). For meals prepared at home, advance planning is the key: Map out meals and shop appropriately, cook in advance when possible, and prepare enough food for leftovers later in the week. A tight budget need not make it more difficult to eat healthy meals. It makes good health sense and good budget sense to use only small amounts of meat and to have a few meatless meals each week.

Healthy eating becomes more challenging when you dine out. Portion sizes in restaurants are often far larger than the portion size used in MyPyramid. Try eating only

Terms

V w   **food allergy** An adverse reaction to a food or food ingredient in which the immune system perceives a particular substance (allergen) as foreign and acts to destroy it.

food intolerance An adverse reaction to a food or food ingredient that doesn't involve the immune system; intolerances are often due to a problem with metabolism.

The typical American diet has changed significantly in recent decades—and not for the better. The top ten sources of calories in the American diet, which together account for more than 30% total energy intake, do not reflect healthy eating habits (see table). Americans now consume too many calories, often in the form of added sugars and fats, but too few vitamins and minerals, in part because intake of fruits, vegetables, and milk products is relatively low.

Consumption of regular sodas and sweetened fruit drinks has nearly doubled since 1970, and Americans consume an average of 152 pounds of added sugars each year. Milk consumption has dropped 40% since 1970 as children and young adults have switched to sodas, which now account for nearly 10% of daily calories for 12–19-year-olds. Americans now eat out much more than in the past—more than 40% of Americans eat out at least once on a typical day—and foods eaten outside the home tend to be higher in calories and lower in nutrients than foods prepared at home.

Individual Choice

Individual choice is certainly a key component in recent dietary shifts. Low prices and convenience are valued by American consumers, and there has been a rapid increase in the availability of affordable, convenient, and tasty foods. Many foods with these characteristics do not have a healthy nutritional profile; they tend to be energy-dense and nutrient-poor. American consumers know they should make better choices—but they frequently fail to do so.

Environmental Influences

While acknowledging the role of personal responsibility, some experts also point to environmental factors. Convenience foods are now widely available for purchase, and in many urban neighborhoods in particular, it is easier to buy fast food than fruits and vegetables. In part because sugar is inexpensive, many foods high in added sugars are inexpensive. (Federal subsidies for corn make high-fructose corn syrup, which is found in a wide variety of processed foods, very inexpensive.)

The food industry spends over $30 billion a year on advertising, special promotions, and supermarket slotting fees, with $10 billion of this directed at children. McDonald's alone spends over $1 billion each year on ads, compared to just $1 million spent by the National Cancer Institute for its "5 to 9 a Day" fruits and vegetables campaign.

Many ads target children under age 10, who researchers have found cannot distinguish between advertising and informational programming. (A study of Australian children age 9–10 found that more than half believed that Ronald McDonald "knows best" when it comes to what children should eat.) Most ads during children's programming feature large portions of sweetened breakfast cereals, fruit-flavored drinks, and fast food. Teen programming features three times as many ads for soft drinks as for milk, a ratio that mirrors consumption patterns.

And young people can now consume fast food at school: About 30% of public high schools offer some type of brand-name fast food, and food ads are featured in television programming shown in schools. (Some school districts have raised money by accepting marketing deals with brand-name soda and fast-food companies.)

What Can Be Done?

Several different strategies have been proposed to promote personal responsibility and combat negative environmental forces:

• Change the price structure of food. Add small taxes on soft drinks, fast food, and other nutrient-poor foods to subsidize (and lower) the costs of healthy foods and to fund campaigns to promote healthy diet and activity habits.

• Prominently print or post basic nutrition information for meals ordered in restaurants and for convenience foods and fast foods. For example, the calorie, sugar, and fat content of sodas and popcorn could be printed on the cups in which they are served at schools, restaurants, and movie theaters.

• Restrict food advertising aimed at children, and ban commercials for unhealthy foods on school television programs.

Top Ten Sources of Calories in the American Diet

Food	Percent of Total Calories
Regular soft drinks	7.1
Cake, sweet rolls, doughnuts, pastries	3.6
Hamburgers, cheeseburgers, meatloaf	3.1
Pizza	3.1
Potato chips, corn chips, popcorn	2.9
Rice	2.7
Rolls, buns, English muffins, bagels	2.7
Cheese or cheese spread	2.6
Beer	2.6
French fries, fried potatoes	2.2

• Require that all meals sold on school grounds meet federal nutrition recommendations; ban paid marketing agreements between schools and fast-food and soft-drink companies.

• Increase public awareness of factors that promote unhealthy food choices, including low cost, accessibility, convenience, and taste (added sugars and fats).

If you're concerned about your own eating habits and those of people in your community, speak with your consumer dollars. Make it a priority to purchase healthy foods when they are offered. In addition, be aware of outside influences on your food choices. This chapter—and the resources listed at the end of the chapter—provide many suggestions for choosing delicious, convenient, and healthy foods.

SOURCES: Block, G. 2004. Foods contributing to energy intake in the US: Data from NHANES III and NHANES 1999–2000. *Journal of Food Composition and Analysis* 17(2004): 439–447; Brownell, K. D. 2004. *Food Fight.* New York: McGraw-Hill; Liebman, B. 2002. The changing American diet. *Nutrition Action HealthLetter,* December; Nestle, M., and M. F. Jacobson. 2000. Halting the obesity epidemic: A public health policy approach. *Public Health Reports* 115: 12–24.

part of your meal and take the rest home for a meal later in the week. Don't hesitate to ask questions about how menu selections are prepared and to ask for adjustments, such as salad dressings or sauces served on the side. To limit your fat and calorie intake, order dishes that have been broiled or grilled rather than fried, choose rice or a plain baked potato over french fries, and select a clear soup rather than a creamy one. Desserts that are irresistible can, at least, be shared.

Strategies like these can be helpful, but small changes cannot change a fundamentally high-fat, high-calorie meal into a moderate, healthful one. Often, the best advice is to bypass the sweet-and-sour pork with fried rice for an equally flavorful but low-fat entrée. Fast-food meals are often particularly high in calories, fat, sodium, and sugar and low in fiber and some vitamins and minerals. If you do eat at a fast-food restaurant, make sure the rest of your meals that day include healthier choices.

The information provided in this chapter should give you the tools you need to design and implement a diet that you enjoy and that promotes long-term health and well-being. If you need additional information or have questions about nutrition, be sure the source you consult is reliable.

Tips for Today

Eating is one of life's great pleasures. There are many ways to satisfy your nutrient needs, so you can create a healthy diet that takes into account your personal preferences and favorite foods. If your current eating habits are not as healthy as they could be, you can choose equally delicious foods that offer both short-term and long-term health benefits. Opportunities to improve your diet present themselves every day, and small changes add up.

Right now you can

- Substitute a healthy snack—an apple, a banana, or popcorn—for a bag of chips or cookies.

- Drink a glass of water, and put a bottle of water in your backpack for tomorrow.

- Plan to make healthy selections when you go to dinner, such as grilled or steamed vegetables instead of french fries or salmon instead of steak.

- Study the box on ethnic foods in this chapter and plan to order a healthy selection the next time you eat at your favorite ethnic restaurant. Do the same with the fast-food restaurants listed in Appendix A.

SUMMARY

- To function at its best, the human body requires about 45 essential nutrients in specific proportions. People get the nutrients needed to fuel their bodies and maintain tissues and organ systems from foods; the body cannot synthesize most of them.

- Proteins, made up of amino acids, form muscles and bones and help make up blood, enzymes, hormones, and cell membranes. Foods from animal sources provide complete proteins; plants provide incomplete proteins.

- Fats, a concentrated source of energy, also help insulate the body and cushion the organs; 1 tablespoon of vegetable oil per day supplies the essential fats. Dietary fat intake should be 20–35% of total daily calories. Unsaturated fats should be favored over saturated and trans fats.

- Carbohydrates supply energy to the brain and other parts of the nervous system as well as to red blood cells. The body needs about 130 grams of carbohydrates a day, but much more is recommended.

- Fiber includes nondigestible carbohydrates provided mainly by plants. Adequate intake of fiber (38 grams per day for men and 25 grams per day for women) can help people manage diabetes and high cholesterol levels and improve intestinal health.

- The 13 vitamins needed in the diet are organic substances that promote specific chemical and cell processes within living tissue. Deficiencies or excesses can cause serious illnesses and even death.

- The approximately 17 minerals needed in the diet are inorganic substances that regulate body functions, aid in the growth and maintenance of body tissues, and help in the release of energy from foods.

- Water is used to digest and absorb food, transport substances around the body, lubricate joints and organs, and regulate body temperature.

- Foods contain other substances such as phytochemicals, which may not be essential nutrients but which reduce chronic disease risk.

- Dietary Reference Intakes (DRIs) are recommended intakes for essential nutrients that meet the needs of healthy people.

- The Dietary Guidelines for Americans address the prevention of diet-related diseases such as CVD, cancer, and diabetes. The guidelines advise us to consume a variety of foods while staying within calorie needs; manage body weight through calorie control and regular physical activity; eat more fruits, vegetables, whole grains, and reduced-fat dairy products; choose fats and carbohydrates wisely; eat less salt and more potassium; be moderate with alcohol intake; and handle foods safely.

- Choosing foods from each group in MyPyramid every day helps ensure the appropriate amounts of necessary nutrients.

- A vegetarian diet can meet human nutritional needs.

- Almost all foods have labels that show how much fat, cholesterol, protein, fiber, and sodium they contain. Serving sizes are standardized, and health claims are carefully regulated. Dietary supplements also have uniform labels.

- Foodborne illnesses are a greater threat to health than additives and environmental contaminants. Other dietary issues of concern to some people include organic foods, food irradiation, genetic modification of foods, and food allergies and intolerances.

Improving Your Diet by Choosing Healthy Beverages

After reading this chapter and completing the dietary assessment on p. 355, you can probably identify several changes you could make to improve your diet. Here, we focus on choosing healthy beverages to increase intake of nutrients and decrease intake of empty calories from added sugars and fat. However, this model of dietary change can be applied to any modification you'd like to make to your diet. Additional specific plans for improving diet can be found in the Behavior Change Strategies in Chapter 15 (decreasing saturated and trans fat intake) and Chapter 16 (increasing intake of fruits and vegetables).

Gather Data and Establish a Baseline

Begin by tracking your beverage consumption in your health journal. Write down the types and amounts of beverages you drink, including water. Also note where you were at the time and whether you obtained the beverage there or brought it with you. At the same time, investigate your options. Find out what other beverages you can easily obtain over the course of your daily routine. For example, what drinks are available in the dining hall where you eat lunch or at the food court where you often grab snacks? How many drinking fountains do you walk by over the course of the day? This information will help you put together a successful plan for change.

Analyze Your Data and Set Goals

Evaluate your beverage consumption by dividing your typical daily consumption between healthy and less healthy choices. Use the following guide as a basis, and add other beverages to the lists as needed.

Choose less often:

- Regular soda
- Sweetened bottled iced tea
- Fruit beverages made with little fruit juice (usually labeled fruit drinks, punches, beverages, blends, or ades)
- Whole milk

Choose more often:

- Water—plain, mineral, and sparkling
- Low-fat or fat-free milk
- Fruit juice (100% juice)
- Unsweetened herbal tea

How many beverages do you consume daily from each category? What would be a healthy and realistic goal for change? For example, if your beverage consumption is currently evenly divided between the "choose more often" and "choose less often" categories (four from each list), you might set a final goal for your behavior change program of increasing your healthy choices by two (to six from the "more often" list and two from the "less often" list).

Develop a Plan for Change

Once you've set your goal, you need to develop strategies that will help you choose healthy beverages more often. Consider the following possibilities:

- Keep healthy beverages on hand; if you live in a student dorm, rent a small refrigerator or keep bottled water, juice, fat-free milk, and other healthy choices in the dorm kitchen's refrigerator.
- Plan ahead, and put a bottle of water or 100% juice in your backpack every day.

- Check food labels on beverages for serving sizes, calories, and nutrients; comparison shop to find the healthiest choices, and watch your serving sizes. Use this information to make your "choose more often" list longer and more specific.
- If you eat out frequently, examine all the beverages available at the places you typically eat your meals. You'll probably find that healthy choices are available; if not, bring along your own drink or find somewhere else to eat.
- For a snack, try water and a piece of fruit rather than a heavily sweetened beverage.
- Create healthy beverages that appeal to you; for example, try adding slices of citrus fruit to water or mixing 100% fruit juice with sparkling water.

You may also need to make some changes in your routine to decrease the likelihood that you'll make unhealthy choices. For example, you might discover from your health journal that you always buy a soda after class when you pass a particular vending machine. If this is the case, try another route that allows you to avoid the machine. And try to guard against impulse buying by carrying water or a healthy snack with you every day.

To complete your plan, try some of the other behavior change strategies described in Chapter 1: Develop and sign a contract, set up a system of rewards, involve other people in your program, and develop strategies for challenging situations. Once your plan is complete, take action. Keep track of your progress in your health journal by continuing to monitor and evaluate your beverage consumption.

Take Action

1. **Examine ingredients and nutrient content:** Read the list of ingredients on three or four canned or packaged foods that you enjoy eating. If any ingredients are unfamiliar to you, find out what they are and why they have been used. A nutrition textbook from the library may be a helpful resource. Also examine and compare nutrient content using the food label. Are you surprised by the energy or nutrient content of any of the foods you examine?

2. **Investigate nutritional and dietary guidelines:** What guidelines are used to prepare the food served in your school? Are they consistent with what you've learned in this chapter? If not, try to find out more about the guidelines that have been used and why they were chosen.

3. **Prepare a flavorful low-fat vegetarian and/or ethnic meal.** Use the suggestions in the chapter, and check your local

library for appropriate cookbooks. How do the foods included in the meal and the preparation methods differ from what you're used to?

4. **Keep a journal:** A nutrition journal is useful for evaluating and improving your diet. The very act of recording everything you eat may improve your dietary habits—you'll find yourself thinking before you eat and avoiding some unhealthy choices so that you don't have to record them in your journal. Keeping a journal boosts your awareness of your food choices and your portion sizes, and it reinforces your commitment to improving your diet.

5. **Volunteer in your community:** There are many opportunities for improving the nutritional status of members of your community. Consider volunteering at a food bank or a kitchen at a homeless shelter. Or find a community garden program for schoolchildren or low-income families—working in a vegetable garden increases your own connection to the food you eat and improves your community.

For More Information

Books

Duyff, R. L. 2002. *ADA Complete Food and Nutrition Guide,* 2nd ed. Chicago, Ill.: American Dietetic Association. *An excellent review of current nutrition information.*

Insel, P., R. E. Turner, and D. Ross. 2004. *Nutrition,* 2nd ed. Sudbury, Mass.: Jones & Bartlett. *An introductory nutrition textbook covering a variety of key topics.*

Katz, D., and M. Gonzalez. 2003. *The Way to Eat.* Chicago, Ill.: American Dietetic Association. *Guide to a lifetime of eating well and promoting good health, weight control, and enjoyment of food.*

Melina, V., and B. Davis. 2003. *The New Becoming Vegetarian: The Essential Guide to a Healthy Vegetarian Diet.* Summertown, Tn.: Healthy Living Publications. *Provides information on the health benefits of vegetarian diets and how to plan healthy meals.*

Selkowitz, A. 2000. *The College Student's Guide to Eating Well on Campus.* Bethesda, Md.: Tulip Hill Press. *Provides practical advice for students, including how to make healthy choices when eating in a dorm or restaurant and how to stock a first pantry.*

Wardlaw, G. M., and A. M. Smith. 2006. *Contemporary Nutrition.* New York: McGraw-Hill. *A review of major concepts in nutrition.*

Newsletters

Environmental Nutrition (800-829-5384; http://www. environmentalnutrition.com)

Nutrition Action Health Letter (202-332-9110; http://www. cspinet.org)

Tufts University Health & Nutrition Letter (800-274-7581; http:// www.healthletter.tufts.edu)

VW Organizations, Hotlines, and Web Sites

American Dietetic Association. Provides a wide variety of nutrition-related educational materials.
    800-877-1600
    http://www.eatright.org

American Heart Association: Delicious Decisions. Provides basic information about nutrition, tips for shopping and eating out, and heart-healthy recipes.
    http://www.deliciousdecisions.org

FDA Center for Food Safety and Applied Nutrition. Offers information about topics such as food labeling, food additives, dietary supplements, and foodborne illness.
    http://vm.cfsan.fda.gov

Food Safety Hotlines. Provide information on safe purchase, handling, cooking, and storage of food.
    888-SAFEFOOD (FDA)
    800-535-4555 (USDA)

Gateways to Government Nutrition Information. Provide access to government resources relating to food safety and nutrition.
    http://www.foodsafety.gov
    http://www.nutrition.gov

Harvard School of Public Health Nutrition Source. Provides recent key research findings, including advice on interpreting news on nutrition; an overview of the Healthy Eating Pyramid, an alternative to the basic USDA pyramid; and suggestions for building a healthy diet.
    http://www.hsph.harvard.edu/nutritionsource

International Food Information Council. Provides information on food safety and nutrition for consumers, journalists, and educators.
    http://ific.org

MyPyramid.Gov. Provides personalized dietary plans and interactive food and activity tracking tools.
    http://mypyramid.gov

National Academies' Food and Nutrition Board. Provides information about the Dietary Reference Intakes and related guidelines.
    http://www.iom.edu/board.asp?id=3788

National Cancer Institute: Eat 5 to 9 a Day for Better Health. Provides tips and recipes to help consumers increase their intake of fruits and vegetables.
    http://5aday.nci.nih.gov

Tufts University Nutrition Navigator. Provides descriptions and ratings for many nutrition-related Web pages.
    http://navigator.tufts.edu

USDA Center for Nutrition Policy and Promotion. Includes information on the Dietary Guidelines and MyPyramid.
    http://www.usda.gov/cnpp

USDA Food and Nutrition Information Center. Provides a variety of materials and extensive links relating to the Dietary Guidelines, food labels, MyPyramid, and many other topics.
    http://www.nal.usda.gov/fnic

Vegetarian Resource Group. Information and links for vegetarians and people interested in learning more about vegetarian diets.
    http://www.vrg.org

You can obtain nutrient breakdowns of individual food items from the following sites:

Nutrition Analysis Tool, University of Illinois, Urbana/Champaign
    http://nat.crgq.com

USDA Nutrient Data Laboratory
    http://www.nal.usda.gov/fnic/foodcomp

See also the resources listed in the dietary supplements box on p. 361 and in the For More Information sections in Chapters 13–16 and 19.

Selected Bibliography

Aldana, S. G., et al. 2005. Effects of an intensive diet and physical activity modification program on the health risks of adults. *Journal of the American Dietetic Association* 105(3): 371–381.

Block, G. 2004. Foods contributing to energy intake in the US: Data from NHANES III and NHANES 1999–2000. *Journal of Food Composition and Analysis* 17(2004): 439–447.

Clifton, P. M., J. B. Keogh, and M. Noakes. 2004. Trans fatty acids in adipose tissue and the food supply are associated with myocardial infarction. *Journal of Nutrition* 134: 874–879.

Cotton, P. A., et al. 2004. Dietary sources of nutrients among U.S. adults, 1994 to 1996. *Journal of the American Dietetic Association* 104: 921–930.

Ervin, R. B., et al. 2004. Dietary intake of selected minerals for the United States population: 1999–2000. *Advance Data from Vital and Health Statistics* No. 341.

Food and Drug Administration. 2004. *Backgrounder for the 2004 FDA/EPA Consumer Advisory: What You Need to Know About Mercury in Fish and Shellfish* (http://www.fda.gov/oc/opacom/hottopics/mercury/backgrounder.html; retrieved April 27, 2004).

Food and Drug Administration. 2004. *Commonly Asked Questions About BSE in Products Regulated by FDA's Center for Food Safety and Applied Nutrition* (http://www.cfsan.fda.gov/~comm/bsefaq.html; retrieved April 28, 2004).

Food and Drug Administration. 2004. *Fact Sheet: Carbohydrates* (http://www.fda.gov/oc/initiatives/obesity/factsheet.html; retrieved April 28, 2004).

Food and Nutrition Board, Institute of Medicine. 2002. *Dietary Reference Intakes for Energy, Carbohydrate, Fiber, Fat, Fatty Acids, Cholesterol, Protein, and Amino Acids.* Washington, D.C.: National Academy Press.

Food and Nutrition Board, Institute of Medicine. 2004. *Dietary Reference Intakes for Water, Potassium, Sodium, Chloride, and Sulfate.* Washington, D.C.: National Academy Press.

Foote, J. A., et al. 2004. Dietary variety increases the probability of nutrient adequacy among adults. *Journal of Nutrition* 134: 1779–1784.

Gilroy, C. M., et al. 2003. Echinacea and truth in labeling. *Archives of Internal Medicine* 163(6): 699–704.

Hanley, D. A., and K. S. Davison. 2005. Vitamin D insufficiency in North America. *Journal of Nutrition* 135(2): 332–337.

He, K., et al. 2004. Accumulated evidence on fish consumption and coronary heart disease mortality: A meta-analysis of cohort studies. *Circulation* 109: 2705–2711.

Hites, R. A., et al. 2004. Global assessment of organic contaminants in farmed salmon. *Science* 303(5655): 225–229.

Houston, D. K., et al. 2005. Dairy, fruit, and vegetable intakes and functional limitations and disability in a biracial cohort. *American Journal of Clinical Nutrition* 81(2): 515–522.

Joint WHO/FAO Expert Consultation. 2003. *Diet, Nutrition, and the Prevention of Chronic Diseases.* Geneva:World Health Organization.

Kranz, S., et al. 2005. Adverse effect of high added sugar consumption on dietary intake in American preschoolers. *Journal of Pediatrics* 46(1): 105–111.

Liu, S., et al. 2003. Is intake of breakfast cereals related to total and cause-specific mortality in men? *American Journal of Clinical Nutrition* 77(3): 594–599.

McKeown, N. M., et al. 2002. Whole-grain intake is favorably associated with metabolic risk factors for type 2 diabetes and cardiovascular disease in the Framingham Offspring Study. *American Journal of Clinical Nutrition* 76(2): 390–398.

Ma, Y., et al. 2005. Association between dietary carbohydrates and body weight. *American Journal of Epidemiology* 161(4): 359–367.

Michaelsson, K., et al. 2003. Serum retinol levels and the risk of fracture. *New England Journal of Medicine* 348(4): 287–294.

Nanney, M. S., et al. 2004. Rationale for a consistent "powerhouse" approach to vegetable and fruit messages. *Journal of the American Dietetic Association* 104(3): 352–356.

National Center for Health Statistics. 2003. Dietary intake of ten key nutrients for public health, United States: 1999–2000. *Advance Data from Vital and Health Statistics* No. 334.

Of birds and bacteria. 2003. *Consumer Reports,* January.

Opotowsky, A. R., et al. 2004. Serum vitamin A concentration and the risk of hip fracture among women 50 to 74 years old in the United States. *American Journal of Medicine* 117(3): 169–174.

Palmer, M. E., et al. 2003. Adverse events associated with dietary supplements: An observational study. *Lancet* 361(9352): 101–106.

Pereira, M. A., et al. 2004. Dietary fiber and risk of coronary heart disease: A pooled analysis of cohort studies. *Archives of Internal Medicine* 164(4): 370–376.

Tirodkar, M. A., and A. Jain. 2003. Food messages on African American television shows. *American Journal of Public Health* 93(3): 439–441.

U.S. Department of Agriculture, Center for Food Safety and Applied Nutrition. 2003. *Examples of Revised Nutrition Facts Panel Listing Trans Fat* (http://www.cfsan.fda.gov/~dms/labtr.html; retrieved January 5, 2004).

U.S. Department of Agriculture, Center for Nutrition Policy and Promotion. 2005. *MyPyramid* (http://www.mypyramid.gov; retrieved April 20, 2005).

U.S. Department of Agriculture, Center for Nutrition Policy and Promotion. 2004. *The Food Guide Pyramid Update* (http://www.cnpp.usda.gov/pyramid-update; retrieved January 5, 2005).

U.S. Department of Agriculture, Center for Nutrition Policy and Promotion. 2004. *2005 Dietary Guidelines Advisory Committee Report* (http://www.health.gov/dietaryguidelines/dga2005/report; retrieved January 5, 2005).

U.S. Department of Health and Human Services and U.S. Department of Agriculture. 2005. *Dietary Guidelines for Americans, 2005* (http://www.health.gov/dietary guidelines; retrieved January 20, 2005).

U.S. Department of Health and Human Services and U.S. Department of Agriculture. 2005. *Finding Your Way to a Healthier You: Based on the Dietary Guidelines for Americans.* Home and Garden Bulletin No. 232-CP.

Table 1 Dietary Reference Intakes (DRIs): Recommended Levels for Individual Intake

Life Stage	Group	Biotin (μg/day)	Choline (mg/day)[a]	Folate (μg/day)[b]	Niacin (mg/day)[c]	Pantothenic Acid (mg/day)	Riboflavin (mg/day)	Thiamin (mg/day)	Vitamin A (μg/day)[d]	Vitamin B-6 (mg/day)	Vitamin B-12 (μg/day)	Vitamin C (mg/day)[e]	Vitamin D (μg/day)[f]	Vitamin E (mg/day)[g]
Infants	0–6 months	5	125	65	2	1.7	0.3	0.2	400	0.1	0.4	40	5	4
	7–12 months	6	150	80	4	1.8	0.4	0.3	500	0.3	0.5	50	5	5
Children	1–3 years	8	200	150	6	2	0.5	0.5	300	0.5	0.9	15	5	6
	4–8 years	12	250	200	8	3	0.6	0.6	400	0.6	1.2	25	5	7
Males	9–13 years	20	375	300	12	4	0.9	0.9	600	1.0	1.8	45	5	11
	14–18 years	25	550	400	16	5	1.3	1.2	900	1.3	2.4	75	5	15
	19–30 years	30	550	400	16	5	1.3	1.2	900	1.3	2.4	90	5	15
	31–50 years	30	550	400	16	5	1.3	1.2	900	1.3	2.4	90	5	15
	51–70 years	30	550	400	16	5	1.3	1.2	900	1.7	2.4[h]	90	10	15
	>70 years	30	550	400	16	5	1.3	1.2	900	1.7	2.4[h]	90	15	15
Females	9–13 years	20	375	300	12	4	0.9	0.9	600	1.0	1.8	45	5	11
	14–18 years	25	400	400[i]	14	5	1.0	1.0	700	1.2	2.4	65	5	15
	19–30 years	30	425	400[i]	14	5	1.1	1.1	700	1.3	2.4	75	5	15
	31–50 years	30	425	400[i]	14	5	1.1	1.1	700	1.3	2.4	75	5	15
	51–70 years	30	425	400[i]	14	5	1.1	1.1	700	1.5	2.4[h]	75	10	15
	>70 years	30	425	400	14	5	1.1	1.1	700	1.5	2.4[h]	75	15	15
Pregnancy	≤18 years	30	450	600[j]	18	6	1.4	1.4	750	1.9	2.6	80	5	15
	19–30 years	30	450	600[j]	18	6	1.4	1.4	770	1.9	2.6	85	5	15
	31–50 years	30	450	600[j]	18	6	1.4	1.4	770	1.9	2.6	85	5	15
Lactation	≤18 years	35	550	500	17	7	1.6	1.4	1200	2.0	2.8	115	5	19
	19–30 years	35	550	500	17	7	1.6	1.4	1300	2.0	2.8	120	5	19
	31–50 years	35	550	500	17	7	1.6	1.4	1300	2.0	2.8	120	5	19
Tolerable Upper Intake Levels for Adults (19–70)			3500	1000[k]	35[k]				3000	100		2000	50	1000[k]

NOTE: The table includes values for the type of DRI standard—Adequate Intake (AI) or Recommended Dietary Allowance (RDA)—that has been established for that particular nutrient and life stage; RDAs are shown in **bold type**. The final row of the table shows the Tolerable Upper Intake Levels (ULs) for adults; refer to the full DRI report for information on other ages and life stages. A UL is the maximum level of daily nutrient intake that is likely to pose no risk of adverse effects. There is insufficient data to set ULs for all nutrients, but this does not mean that there is no potential for adverse effects; source of intake should be from food only to prevent high levels of intake of nutrients without established ULs. In healthy individuals, there is no established benefit from nutrient intakes above the RDA or AI.

[a] Although AIs have been set for choline, there are few data to assess whether a dietary supply of choline is needed at all stages of the life cycle, and it may be that the choline requirement can be met by endogenous synthesis at some of these stages.
[b] As dietary folate equivalents (DFE): 1 DFE = 1 μg food folate = 0.6 μg folate from fortified food or as a supplement consumed with food = 0.5 μg of a supplement taken on an empty stomach.
[c] As niacin equivalents (NE): 1 mg niacin = 60 mg tryptophan.

Table 1 Dietary Reference Intakes (DRIs): Recommended Levels for Individual Intake (Continued)

Life Stage	Group	Vitamin K (μg/day)	Calcium (mg/day)	Chromium (μg/day)	Copper (μg/day)	Fluoride (mg/day)	Iodine (μg/day)	Iron (mg/day)[l]	Magnesium (mg/day)	Manganese (mg/day)	Molybdenum (μg/day)	Phosphorus (mg/day)	Selenium (μg/day)	Zinc (mg/day)[m]
Infants	0–6 months	2.0	210	0.2	200	0.01	110	0.27	30	0.003	2	100	15	2
	7–12 months	2.5	270	5.5	220	0.5	130	11	75	0.6	3	275	20	3
Children	1–3 years	30	500	11	340	0.7	90	7	80	1.2	17	460	20	3
	4–8 years	55	800	15	440	1	90	10	130	1.5	22	500	30	5
Males	9–13 years	60	1300	25	700	2	120	8	240	1.9	34	1250	40	8
	14–18 years	75	1300	35	890	3	150	11	410	2.2	43	1250	55	11
	19–30 years	120	1000	35	900	4	150	8	400	2.3	45	700	55	11
	31–50 years	120	1000	35	900	4	150	8	420	2.3	45	700	55	11
	51–70 years	120	1200	30	900	4	150	8	420	2.3	45	700	55	11
	>70 years	120	1200	30	900	4	150	8	420	2.3	45	700	55	11
Females	9–13 years	60	1300	21	700	2	120	8	240	1.6	34	1250	40	8
	14–18 years	75	1300	24	890	3	150	15	360	1.6	43	1250	55	9
	19–30 years	90	1000	25	900	3	150	18	310	1.8	45	700	55	8
	31–50 years	90	1000	25	900	3	150	18	320	1.8	45	700	55	8
	51–70 years	90	1200	20	900	3	150	8	320	1.8	45	700	55	8
	>70 years	90	1200	20	900	3	150	8	320	1.8	45	700	55	8
Pregnancy	≤18 years	75	1300	29	1000	3	220	27	400	2.0	50	1250	60	13
	19–30 years	90	1000	30	1000	3	220	27	350	2.0	50	700	60	11
	31–50 years	90	1000	30	1000	3	220	27	360	2.0	50	700	60	11
Lactation	≤18 years	75	1300	44	1300	3	290	10	360	2.6	50	1250	70	14
	19–30 years	90	1000	45	1300	3	290	9	310	2.6	50	700	70	12
	31–50 years	90	1000	45	1300	3	290	9	320	2.6	50	700	70	12
Tolerable Upper Intake Levels for Adults (19–70)			2500		10,000	10	1100	45	350[k]	11	2000	4000	400	40

[d] As retinol activity equivalents (RAEs): 1 RAE = 1 μg retinol, 12 μg β-carotene, or 24 μg α-carotene or β-cryptoxanthin. Preformed vitamin A (retinol) is abundant in animal-derived foods; provitamin A carotenoids are abundant in some dark yellow, orange, red, and deep-green fruits and vegetables. For preformed vitamin A and for provitamin A carotenoids in supplements, 1RE = 1 RAE; for provitamin A carotenoids in foods, divide the REs by 2 to obtain RAEs. The UL applies only to preformed vitamin A.

[e] Individuals who smoke require an additional 35 mg/day of vitamin C over that needed by nonsmokers; nonsmokers regularly exposed to tobacco smoke should ensure they meet the RDA for vitamin C.

[f] As cholecalciferol: 1 μg cholecalciferol = 40 IU vitamin D. DRI values are based on the absence of adequate exposure to sunlight.

[g] As α-tocopherol. Includes naturally occurring RRR-α-tocopherol and the 2R-stereoisomeric forms from supplements; does not include the 2S-stereoisomeric forms from supplements.

[h] Because 10–30% of older people may malabsorb food-bound B-12, those over age 50 should meet their RDA mainly with supplements or foods fortified with B-12.

[i] In view of evidence linking folate intake with neural tube defects in the fetus. It is recommended that all women capable of becoming pregnant consume 400 μg from supplements or fortified foods in addition to consuming folate from a varied diet.

[j] It is assumed that women will continue consuming 400 μg from supplements or fortified food until their pregnancy is confirmed and they enter prenatal care, which ordinarily occurs after the end of the periconceptional period—the critical time for formation of the neural tube.

[k] The UL applies only to intake from supplements, fortified foods, and/or pharmacological agents and not to intake from foods.

[l] Because the absorption of iron from plant foods is low compared to that from animal foods, the RDA for strict vegetarians is approximately 1.8 times higher than the values established for omnivores (14 mg/day for adult male vegetarians; 33 mg/day for premenopausal female vegetarians). Oral contraceptives (OCs) reduce menstrual blood losses, so women taking them need less daily iron; the RDA for premenopausal women taking OCs is 10.9 mg/day. For more on iron requirements for other special situations, refer to *Dietary Reference Intakes for Vitamin A, Vitamin K, Arsenic, Boron, Chromium, Copper, Iodine, Iron, Manganese, Molybdenum, Nickel, Silicon, Vanadium, and Zinc* (visit http://www.nap.edu for the complete report).

[m] Zinc absorption is lower for those consuming vegetarian diets so the zinc requirement for vegetarians is approximately twofold greater than for those consuming a nonvegetarian diet.

Table 1 Dietary Reference Intakes (DRIs): Recommended Levels for Individual Intake (*continued*)

Life Stage	Group	Potassium (g/day)	Sodium (g/day)	Chloride (g/day)	Carbohydrate RDA/AI (g/day)	Carbohydrate AMDR[o] (%)	Total Fiber RDA/AI (g/day)	Total Fat AMDR[o] (%)	Linoleic Acid RDA/AI (g/day)	Linoleic Acid AMDR[o] (%)	Alpha-linolenic Acid RDA/AI (g/day)	Alpha-linolenic Acid AMDR[o] (%)	Protein[n] RDA/AI (g/day)	Protein[n] AMDR[o] (%)	Water[p] (L/day)
Infants	0–6 months	0.4	0.12	0.18	60	ND[q]	ND	r	4.4	ND[q]	0.5	ND[q]	9.1	ND[q]	0.7
	7–12 months	0.7	0.37	0.57	95	ND[q]	ND	r	4.6	ND[q]	0.5	ND[q]	13.5	ND[q]	0.8
Children	1–3 years	3.0	1.0	1.5	130	45–65	19	30–40	7	5–10	0.7	0.6–1.2	13	5–20	1.3
	4–8 years	3.8	1.2	1.9	130	45–65	25	25–35	10	5–10	0.9	0.6–1.2	19	10–30	1.7
Males	9–13 years	4.5	1.5	2.3	130	45–65	31	25–35	12	5–10	1.2	0.6–1.2	34	10–30	2.4
	14–18 years	4.7	1.5	2.3	130	45–65	38	25–35	16	5–10	1.6	0.6–1.2	52	10–30	3.3
	19–30 years	4.7	1.5	2.3	130	45–65	38	20–35	17	5–10	1.6	0.6–1.2	56	10–35	3.7
	31–50 years	4.7	1.5	2.3	130	45–65	38	20–35	17	5–10	1.6	0.6–1.2	56	10–35	3.7
	51–70 years	4.7	1.3	2.0	130	45–65	30	20–35	14	5–10	1.6	0.6–1.2	56	10–35	3.7
	>70 years	4.7	1.2	1.8	130	45–65	30	20–35	14	5–10	1.6	0.6–1.2	56	10–35	3.7
Females	9–13 years	4.5	1.5	2.3	130	45–65	26	25–35	10	5–10	1.0	0.6–1.2	34	10–30	2.1
	14–18 years	4.7	1.5	2.3	130	45–65	26	25–35	11	5–10	1.1	0.6–1.2	46	10–30	2.3
	19–30 years	4.7	1.5	2.3	130	45–65	25	20–35	12	5–10	1.1	0.6–1.2	46	10–35	2.7
	31–50 years	4.7	1.5	2.3	130	45–65	25	20–35	12	5–10	1.1	0.6–1.2	46	10–35	2.7
	51–70 years	4.7	1.3	2.0	130	45–65	21	20–35	11	5–10	1.1	0.6–1.2	46	10–35	2.7
	>70 years	4.7	1.2	1.8	130	45–65	21	20–35	11	5–10	1.1	0.6–1.2	46	10–35	2.7
Pregnancy	≤18 years	4.7	1.5	2.3	175	45–65	28	20–35	13	5–10	1.4	0.6–1.2	71	10–35	3.0
	19–30 years	4.7	1.5	2.3	175	45–65	28	20–35	13	5–10	1.4	0.6–1.2	71	10–35	3.0
	31–50 years	4.7	1.5	2.3	175	45–65	28	20–35	13	5–10	1.4	0.6–1.2	71	10–35	3.0
Lactation	≤18 years	5.1	1.5	2.3	210	45–65	29	20–35	13	5–10	1.3	0.6–1.2	71	10–35	3.8
	19–30 years	5.1	1.5	2.3	210	45–65	29	20–35	13	5–10	1.3	0.6–1.2	71	10–35	3.8
	31–50 years	5.1	1.5	2.3	210	45–65	29	20–35	13	5–10	1.3	0.6–1.2	71	10–35	3.8
Tolerable Upper Intake Level for Adults (19–70)			2.3	3.6											

[n]Daily protein recommendations are based on body weight for reference body weights. To calculate for a specific body weight, use the following values: 1.5 g/kg for infants, 1.1 g/kg for 1–3 years, 0.95 g/kg for 4–13 years, 0.85 g/kg for 14–18 years, 0.8 g/kg for adults, and 1.1 g/kg for pregnant (using prepregnancy weight) and lactating women.

[o]Acceptable Macronutrient Distribution Range (AMDR), expressed as a percent of total daily calories, is the range of intake for a particular energy source that is associated with reduced risk of chronic disease while providing adequate intakes of essential nutrients. If an individual consumes in excess of the AMDR, there is a potential for increasing the risk of chronic diseases and/or insufficient intakes of essential nutrients.

[p]Total water intake from fluids and food.

[q]Not determinable due to lack of data of adverse effects in this age group and concern with regard to lack of ability to handle excess amounts. Source of intake should be from food only to prevent high levels of intake.

[r]For infants, Adequate Intake of total fat is 31 grams/day (0–6 months) and 30 grams per day (7–12 months) from breast milk and, for infants 7–12 months, complementary food and beverages.

SOURCE: Food and Nutrition Board, Institute of Medicine, National Academies. 2004. *Dietary Reference Intakes Tables* (http://www.iom.edu/file.asp?id=21372; retrieved December 21, 2004). The complete Dietary Reference Intake reports are available from the National Academy Press (http://www.nap.edu).

Reprinted with permission from *Dietary Reference Intakes: Applications in Dietary Planning*, copyright © 2003 by the National Academy of Sciences. Reprinted with permission from the National Academies Press, Washington, D.C.

Number of servings per day (or per week, as noted)

Food groups	1600 calories	2000 calories	2600 calories	3100 calories	Serving sizes and notes
Grains	6	7–8	10–11	12–13	1 slice bread, 1 oz dry cereal, 1/2 cup cooked rice, pasta, or cereal; choose whole-grains
Vegetables	3–4	4–5	5–6	6	1 cup raw leafy vegetable, 1/2 cup cooked vegetable, 6 oz vegetable juice
Fruits	4	4–5	5–6	6	6 oz fruit juice, 1 medium fruit, 1/4 cup dried fruit, 1/2 cup fresh, frozen, or canned fruit
Low-fat or fat-free dairy foods	2–3	2–3	3	3–4	8 oz milk; 1 cup yogurt, 1-1/2 oz cheese; choose fat-free or low- fat types
Meat, poultry, fish	1–2	2 or less	2	2–3	3 oz cooked meats, poultry, or fish: select only lean; trim away visible fats; broil, roast, or boil instead of frying; remove skin from poultry
Nuts, seeds, legumes	3–4	4–5	1	1	1/3 cup or 1-1/2 oz nuts, 2 Tbsp or 1/2 oz seeds, 1/2 cup cooked dry beans/peas
Fats and oils	2 servings/ week	2–3	3	4	1 tsp soft margarine; 1 Tbsp low-fat mayonnaise, 2 Tbsp light salad dressing, 1 tsp vegetable oil; DASH has 27% of calories as fat (low in saturated fat)
Sweets	0	5 servings/ week	2	2	1 Tbsp sugar, 1 Tbsp jelly or jam, 1/2 oz jelly beans, 8 oz lemonade; sweets should be low in fat

Figure 1   The DASH Eating Plan.   SOURCE: U.S. Department of Health and Human Services and U.S. Department of Agriculture. 2005. *Dietary Guidelines for Americans, 2005* (http://www.health.gov/dietaryguidelines; retrieved January 20, 2005).

Figure 2   Healthy Eating Pyramid. The Healthy Eating Pyramid is an alternative food-group plan developed by researchers at the Harvard School of Public Health; this pyramid reflects many major research studies that have looked at the relationship between diet and long-term health. The Healthy Eating Pyramid differentiates between the various dietary sources of fat, protein, and carbohydrate, and it emphasizes whole grains, vegetable oils, fruits and vegetables, nuts, and dry peas and beans.   SOURCE: Reprinted by permission of Simon & Schuster Adult Publishing Group from *Eat, Drink, and Be Healthy: The Harvard Medical School Guide to Healthy Eating* by Walter C Willett, M.D. Copyright © 2001 by the President and Fellows of Harvard College.

After reading this chapter, you should be able to

- Define physical fitness, and list the health-related components of fitness

- Explain the wellness benefits of physical activity and exercise

- Describe how to develop each of the health-related components of fitness

- Discuss how to choose appropriate exercise equipment, how to eat and drink for exercise, how to assess fitness, and how to prevent and manage injuries

- Put together a personalized exercise program that you enjoy and that will enable you to achieve your fitness goals

Exercise for Health and Fitness

Knowledge

1. **Among American adults, about what percentage of trips of less than 1 mile in length are made by walking?**
   a. 15%
   b. 25%
   c. 50%

2. **Compared to sedentary people, those who engage in regular moderate exercise are likely to**
   a. have fewer colds.
   b. be less anxious and depressed.
   c. fall asleep more quickly and sleep better.
   d. be more alert and creative.

3. **For women, weight training typically results in which of the following?**
   a. bulky muscles
   b. significant increases in body weight
   c. improved body image

4. **If you want to lose fat around your middle to have a flat stomach, you should do sit-ups.**
   True or false?

5. **If all inactive American adults became physically active, the savings in direct costs for medical care would be about _____ per year.**
   a. $75 million
   b. $7.5 billion
   c. $75 billion

ANSWERS

1. A. The vast majority of short trips are made in automobiles. Most people have many opportunities to incorporate more physical activity into their daily routine.

2. ALL FOUR. Exercise has many immediate benefits that affect all the dimensions of wellness and improve overall quality of life.

3. C. Because women have lower levels of testosterone than men, they do not develop large muscles or gain significant amounts of weight in response to a moderate weight training program.

4. FALSE. The energy burned by sit-ups comes from fat stores throughout the body, not just from the abdomen, so sit-ups are no better at trimming fat from your stomach than any other calisthenic exercise.

5. C. People who engage in regular physical activity make fewer physician visits, use less medication, and have fewer hospital stays than physically inactive people.

Visit the Core Concepts in Health Online Learning Center (www.mhhe.com/insel10e) for study aids and many additional resources.

377

Your body is a wonderful moving machine. Your bones, joints, and ligaments provide a support system for movement; your muscles perform the motions of work and play; your heart and lungs nourish your cells as you move through your daily life. But your body is made to work best when it is physically active. It readily adapts to practically any level of activity and exercise: The more you ask of your body—your muscles, bones, heart, lungs—the stronger and more fit it becomes. The opposite is also true. Left unchallenged, bones lose their density, joints stiffen, muscles become weak, and cellular energy systems begin to degenerate. To be truly healthy, human beings must be active.

The benefits of physical activity are both physical and mental, immediate and far-reaching. Being physically fit makes it easier to do everyday tasks, such as lifting; it provides reserve strength for emergencies; and it helps people look and feel good. Over the long term, physically fit individuals are less likely to develop heart disease, cancer, high blood pressure, diabetes, and many other degenerative diseases. Their cardiorespiratory systems tend to resemble those of people 10 or more years younger than themselves. As they get older, they may be able to avoid weight gain, muscle and bone loss, fatigue, memory loss, and other problems associated with aging. With a healthy heart, strong muscles, a lean body, and a repertoire of physical skills they can call on for recreation and enjoyment, fit people can maintain their physical and mental well-being throughout their entire lives.

Unfortunately, modern life for most Americans provides few built-in occasions for vigorous activity. Technological advances have made our lives increasingly sedentary: We drive cars, ride escalators, watch television, and push papers around at school and work. According to *Healthy People 2010*, levels of physical activity remain low for all populations of Americans (Figure 13-1). In 1996, the U.S. Surgeon General published *Physical Activity and Health*, a report designed to reverse these trends and get Americans moving. The report's conclusions include the following:

- People of all ages, both male and female, benefit from regular physical activity.

- People can obtain significant health benefits by including a moderate amount of physical activity on most, if not all, days of the week. Through a modest increase in daily activity, most Americans can improve their health and quality of life.

- Additional health benefits can be gained through greater amounts of physical activity. People who can maintain a regular regimen of more vigorous or longer-duration activity are likely to obtain even greater benefits.

- Physical activity reduces the risk of premature mortality, improves psychological health, and is important for the health of muscle, bones, and joints.

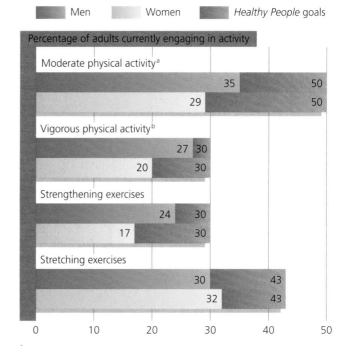

| | Men | Women | *Healthy People* goals |

Percentage of adults currently engaging in activity

Moderate physical activity[a] — 35 / 50; 29 / 50

Vigorous physical activity[b] — 27 / 30; 20 / 30

Strengthening exercises — 24 / 30; 17 / 30

Stretching exercises — 30 / 43; 32 / 43

[a]Moderate physical activity for 30 or more minutes on 5 or more days per week.
[b]Vigorous physical activity for 20 or more minutes on 3 or more days per week.

VITAL STATISTICS

Figure 13-1 Current levels of physical activity among American adults.   SOURCE: National Center for Health Statistics. 2004. *DATA2010: The Healthy People 2010 Database* (http://wonder.cdc.gov/data2010; retrieved January 1, 2005).

Are you one of the 55% of Americans who are not regularly active? Or one of the 25% who are not active at all? This chapter will give you the basic information you need to put together a physical fitness program that will work for you. If approached correctly, physical activity can contribute immeasurably to overall wellness, add fun and joy to life, and provide the foundation for a lifetime of fitness.

WHAT IS PHYSICAL FITNESS?

Physical fitness is a set of physical attributes that allows the body to respond or adapt to the demands and stress of physical effort—that is, to perform moderate-to-vigorous levels of physical activity without becoming overly tired. Physical fitness has many components, some related to general health and others related more specifically to particular sports or activities. The five components of fitness most important for health are cardiorespiratory endurance, muscular strength, muscular endurance, flexibility, and body composition (proportion of fat to fat-free mass).

Cardiorespiratory Endurance

Cardiorespiratory endurance is the ability to perform prolonged, large-muscle, dynamic exercise at moderate-

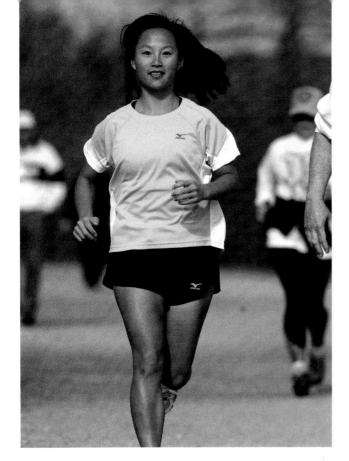

Cardiorespiratory endurance exercise conditions the heart, improves the function of the entire cardiorespiratory system, and has many other health benefits. An effective personal fitness program should be built around an activity like running, walking, biking, swimming, or group exercises such as aerobic dance or martial arts workouts.

the body's ability to use energy supplied by food and to do more exercise with less effort from the oxygen transport system.

Cardiorespiratory endurance is considered a critically important component of health-related fitness because the functioning of the heart and lungs is so essential to overall wellness. A person simply cannot live very long or very well without a healthy heart. Low levels of cardiorespiratory fitness are linked with heart disease, the leading cause of death in the United States. Cardiorespiratory endurance is developed by activities that involve continuous rhythmic movements of large-muscle groups like those in the legs—for example, walking, jogging, cycling, and aerobic dance.

Muscular Strength

Muscular strength is the amount of force a muscle can produce with a single maximum effort. Strong, powerful muscles are important for the smooth and easy performance of everyday activities, such as carrying groceries, lifting boxes, and climbing stairs, as well as for emergency situations. They help keep the skeleton in proper alignment, preventing back and leg pain and providing the support necessary for good posture. Muscular strength has obvious importance in recreational activities. Strong people can hit a tennis ball harder, kick a soccer ball farther, and ride a bicycle uphill more easily.

Muscle tissue is an important element of overall body composition. Greater muscle mass makes possible a higher rate of metabolism and faster energy use, which help to maintain a healthy body weight. Maintaining strength and muscle mass is vital for healthy aging. Older people tend to lose muscle cells (a condition called sarcopenia), and many of the remaining muscle cells become nonfunctional because they lose their attachment to the nervous system. Strength training helps maintain muscle mass, function, and balance in older people, which greatly enhances their quality of life and prevents life-threatening injuries. Strength training has also been shown to benefit cardiovascular health. Muscular strength can be developed by training with weights or by using the weight of the body for resistance during calisthenic exercises such as push-ups and sit-ups.

to-high levels of intensity. It depends on factors such as the ability of the lungs to deliver oxygen from the environment to the bloodstream, the heart's capacity to pump blood, the ability of the nervous system and blood vessels to regulate blood flow, the muscles' capacity to generate power, and the capability of the body's chemical systems to use oxygen and process fuels for exercise.

When levels of cardiorespiratory fitness are low, the heart has to work very hard during normal daily activities and may not be able to work hard enough to sustain high-intensity physical activity in an emergency. As cardiorespiratory fitness improves, the heart begins to function more efficiently. It doesn't have to work as hard at rest or during low levels of exercise. The heart pumps more blood per heartbeat, resting heart rate slows down, blood volume increases, blood supply to the tissues improves, the body is better able to cool itself, and resting blood pressure decreases. A healthy heart can better withstand the strains of everyday life, the stress of occasional emergencies, and the wear and tear of time. Endurance training also improves the functioning of biochemical systems, particularly in the muscles and liver, thereby enhancing

Terms

physical fitness A set of physical attributes that allows the body to respond or adapt to the demands and stress of physical effort.

cardiorespiratory endurance The ability of the body to perform prolonged, large-muscle, dynamic exercise at moderate-to-high levels of intensity.

muscular strength The amount of force a muscle can produce with a single maximum effort.

Muscular Endurance

Muscular endurance is the ability to resist fatigue and sustain a given level of muscle tension—that is, to hold a muscle contraction for a long period of time or to contract a muscle over and over again. Muscular endurance is important for good posture and for injury prevention. For example, if abdominal and back muscles are not strong enough or don't have the endurance to hold the spine correctly, the chances of low-back pain and back injury are increased. Muscular endurance helps people cope with the physical demands of everyday life and enhances performance in sports and work. It is also important for most leisure and fitness activities. Like muscular strength, muscular endurance is developed by stressing the muscles with a greater load (weight) than they are used to. The degree to which strength or endurance develops depends on the type and amount of stress that is applied.

Flexibility

Flexibility is the ability to move the joints through their full range of motion. Although range of motion is not a significant factor in everyday activities for most people, inactivity causes the joints to become stiffer with age. Stiffness often causes older people to assume unnatural body postures, and it can lead to back, shoulder, or neck pain. Stretching exercises can help ensure a normal range of motion and pain-free joints.

Body Composition

Body composition refers to the proportion of fat and fat-free mass (muscle, bone, and water) in the body. Healthy body composition involves a high proportion of fat-free mass and an acceptably low level of body fat. A person with excessive body fat is more likely to experience a variety of health problems, including heart disease, high blood pressure, stroke, joint problems, diabetes, gallbladder disease, cancer, and back pain. The best way to lose fat is through a lifestyle that includes a sensible diet and exercise. The best way to add muscle mass is through resistance training such as weight training. (Body composition is discussed in more detail in Chapter 14.)

Terms

V w

muscular endurance The ability of a muscle or group of muscles to remain contracted or to contract repeatedly for a long period of time.

flexibility The range of motion in a joint or group of joints; flexibility is related to muscle length.

body composition The proportion of fat and fat-free mass (muscle, bone, and water) in the body.

In addition to these five health-related components of physical fitness, physical fitness for a particular sport or activity might include any or all of the following: coordination, speed, reaction time, agility, balance, and skill. Sport-specific skills are best developed through practice. The skill and coordination needed to play basketball, for example, are developed by playing basketball.

THE BENEFITS OF EXERCISE

As mentioned above, the human body is very adaptable. The greater the demands made on it, the more it adjusts to meet the demands—it becomes fit. Over time, immediate, short-term adjustments translate into long-term changes and improvements (Figure 13-2). For example, when breathing and heart rate increase during exercise, the heart gradually develops the ability to pump more blood with each beat. Then, during exercise, it doesn't have to beat as fast to meet the body's demand for oxygen. The goal of regular physical activity is to bring about these kinds of long-term changes and improvements in the body's functioning.

Scientists have been actively studying these effects of exercise and their impact on health for over 40 years. They have found that exercise is one of the most important things you can do to improve your level of wellness. Regular exercise increases energy levels, improves emotional and psychological well-being, and boosts the immune system. It prevents heart disease, some types of cancer, stroke, high blood pressure, insulin resistance, type 2 diabetes, obesity, and osteoporosis. At any age, people who exercise are less likely to die from all causes than are their sedentary peers. Worldwide, it is estimated that physical inactivity causes 1.9 million deaths per year.

Improved Cardiorespiratory Functioning

Every time you take a breath, some of the oxygen in the air you take into your lungs is picked up by red blood cells and transported to your heart. From there, this oxygenated blood is pumped by the heart throughout the body to organs and tissues that use it. During exercise, the cardiorespiratory system (heart, lungs, and circulatory system) must work harder to meet the body's increased demand for oxygen. Regular endurance exercise improves the functioning of the heart and the ability of the cardiorespiratory system to carry oxygen to body tissues. It also reduces the risk of cardiovascular disease.

More Efficient Metabolism

Endurance exercise improves metabolism, the process by which food is converted to energy and tissue is built. This process involves oxygen, nutrients, hormones, and enzymes. A physically fit person is better able to generate

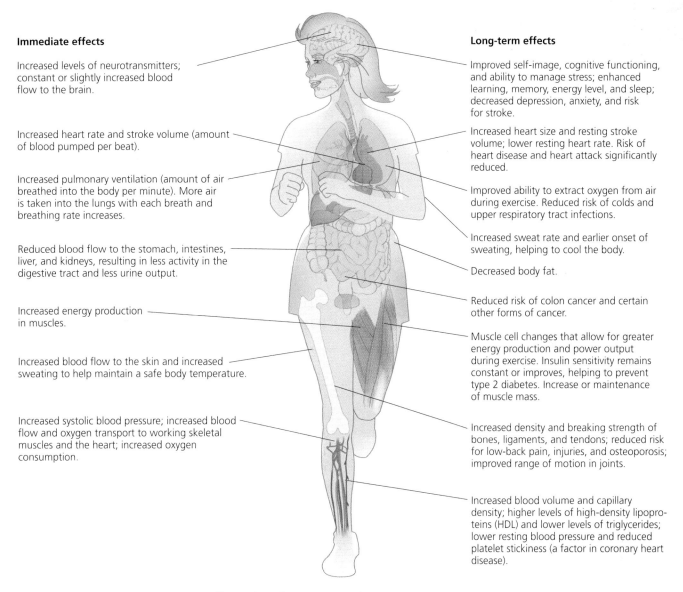

Immediate effects

Increased levels of neurotransmitters; constant or slightly increased blood flow to the brain.

Increased heart rate and stroke volume (amount of blood pumped per beat).

Increased pulmonary ventilation (amount of air breathed into the body per minute). More air is taken into the lungs with each breath and breathing rate increases.

Reduced blood flow to the stomach, intestines, liver, and kidneys, resulting in less activity in the digestive tract and less urine output.

Increased energy production in muscles.

Increased blood flow to the skin and increased sweating to help maintain a safe body temperature.

Increased systolic blood pressure; increased blood flow and oxygen transport to working skeletal muscles and the heart; increased oxygen consumption.

Long-term effects

Improved self-image, cognitive functioning, and ability to manage stress; enhanced learning, memory, energy level, and sleep; decreased depression, anxiety, and risk for stroke.

Increased heart size and resting stroke volume; lower resting heart rate. Risk of heart disease and heart attack significantly reduced.

Improved ability to extract oxygen from air during exercise. Reduced risk of colds and upper respiratory tract infections.

Increased sweat rate and earlier onset of sweating, helping to cool the body.

Decreased body fat.

Reduced risk of colon cancer and certain other forms of cancer.

Muscle cell changes that allow for greater energy production and power output during exercise. Insulin sensitivity remains constant or improves, helping to prevent type 2 diabetes. Increase or maintenance of muscle mass.

Increased density and breaking strength of bones, ligaments, and tendons; reduced risk for low-back pain, injuries, and osteoporosis; improved range of motion in joints.

Increased blood volume and capillary density; higher levels of high-density lipoproteins (HDL) and lower levels of triglycerides; lower resting blood pressure and reduced platelet stickiness (a factor in coronary heart disease).

Figure 13-2 Immediate and long-term effects of regular exercise.   When exercise is performed regularly, short-term changes in the body develop into more permanent adaptations; these long-term effects include improved ability to exercise, reduced risk of many chronic diseases, improved psychological and emotional well-being, and increased life expectancy.

energy, to use carbohydrates and fats for energy, and to regulate hormones. Physical training may also protect the body's cells from damage from free radicals, which are produced during normal metabolism (see Chapter 12), and from inflammation caused by high blood pressure or cholesterol, nicotine, and overeating. Training activates antioxidant enzymes that prevent free radical damage and maintain the health of the body's cells.

Improved Body Composition

Healthy body composition means that the body has a high proportion of fat-free mass (primarily composed of muscle) and a relatively small proportion of fat. Too much body fat is linked to a variety of health problems, includ-

ing heart disease, cancer, and diabetes. Healthy body composition can be difficult to achieve and maintain because a diet that contains all essential nutrients can be relatively high in calories, especially for someone who is sedentary. Excess calories are stored in the body as fat.

Exercise can improve body composition in several ways. Endurance exercise significantly increases daily calorie expenditure; it can also slightly raise *metabolic rate*, the rate at which the body burns calories, for several hours after an exercise session. Strength training increases muscle mass, thereby tipping the body composition ratio toward fat-free mass and away from fat. It can also help with losing fat because metabolic rate is directly proportional to fat-free mass: The more muscle mass, the higher the metabolic rate. (Metabolism, energy balance, and the

Relative risk of death

Amount of physical activity (hours per week)

Figure 13-3 Relationship among amount of physical activity, body weight, and risk of death. Physical activity reduces the risk of death for people at all levels of body fatness. SOURCE: Hu, F. B., et al. 2004. Adiposity compared with physical activity in predicting mortality among women. *New England Journal of Medicine* 351(26): 2694–2703.

role of exercise in improving body composition are discussed in detail in Chapter 14.)

It is important to note that physical activity reduces the risk of death regardless of its effect on body composition. That is, greater levels of activity are associated with lower death rates among people who are overweight or obese as well as people who are at a healthy weight (Figure 13-3). Physical activity does not eliminate the health risks associated with overweight, but it significantly reduces their effects.

Disease Prevention and Management

Regular physical activity lowers your risk of many chronic, disabling diseases. It can also help people with those diseases improve their health.

Cardiovascular Disease A sedentary lifestyle is one of the six major risk factors for **cardiovascular disease (CVD)**, including heart attack and stroke. The other major risk factors are smoking, unhealthy cholesterol levels, high blood pressure, diabetes, and obesity. People who are sedentary have CVD death rates significantly higher than those of fit individuals. Physical inactivity increases the risk of CVD by 50–240%. There is a dose-response relationship between exercise and CVD: The benefit of physical activity occurs at moderate levels of activity and increases with increasing levels of activity. Exercise positively affects the risk factors for CVD, including cholesterol levels and high blood pressure. Exercise also directly interferes with the disease process itself, directly lowering risk of heart disease and stroke. (See Chapter 15 for more information on CVD and associated risk factors.)

BLOOD FAT LEVELS Endurance exercise and strength training have a positive effect on the balance of lipids that circulate in the blood. High concentrations of lipids such as cholesterol and triglycerides are linked to heart disease because they contribute to the formation of fatty deposits on the linings of arteries. When such deposits block an artery, a heart attack or stroke can occur.

Cholesterol is carried in the blood by **lipoproteins**, which are classified according to size and density. Cholesterol carried by low-density lipoproteins (LDLs) tends to stick to the walls of coronary arteries. High-density lipoproteins (HDLs) tend to pick up excess cholesterol in the bloodstream and carry it back to the liver for excretion from the body. High LDL levels and low HDL levels are associated with a high risk of cardiovascular disease. High levels of HDL and low levels of LDL are associated with lower risk.

More information about cholesterol and heart disease is provided in Chapter 15. For our purposes in this chapter, it is important to know only that endurance exercise and strength training influence blood lipid, or fat, levels in a positive way, by increasing HDL and decreasing LDL and triglycerides—thereby helping to reduce the risk of CVD.

HIGH BLOOD PRESSURE Regular endurance exercise tends to reduce high blood pressure (hypertension) a contributing factor in diseases such as coronary heart disease, stroke, kidney failure, and blindness. People who exercise for a longer duration and at a higher intensity receive the greatest benefit, but even moderate exercise can produce significant improvements. Recent studies have found that strength training also reduces blood pressure.

CORONARY HEART DISEASE Coronary heart disease (CHD), also called coronary artery disease (CAD), involves blockage of one of the coronary arteries. These blood vessels supply the heart with oxygenated blood, and an obstruction in one of them can cause a heart attack. Exercise directly interferes with the disease process that causes coronary artery blockage. It also enhances the function of cells lining the arteries that help regulate blood flow. Finally, exercise minimizes other risk factors—such as obesity, high blood pressure, and blood fat levels—that contribute to CHD.

STROKE A stroke occurs when a blood vessel leading to the brain is blocked, often through the same disease process that leads to heart attacks. Regular exercise reduces the risk of stroke.

Cancer Some studies have shown a relationship between increased physical activity and a reduction in a person's risk of all types of cancer, but these findings are not conclusive. There is strong evidence that exercise reduces the risk of colon cancer and promising data that it reduces the risk of cancer of the breast and reproductive organs in women and cancer of the prostate in men. Exercise may decrease the risk of colon cancer by speeding the movement of food through the gastrointestinal tract (quickly eliminating potential carcinogens), enhancing immune function, and reducing blood fats. The protective mechanism in the case of reproductive system cancers is less clear, but physical activity during the high school and college years may be particularly important for preventing breast cancer later in life. Some studies have also found that regular physical activity reduces the risk of pancreatic cancer.

Osteoporosis   A special benefit of exercise, especially for women, is protection against osteoporosis, a disease that results in loss of bone density and poor bone strength. Weight-bearing exercise, which includes almost everything except swimming, helps build bone during the teens and twenties. Older people with denser bones can better endure the bone loss that occurs with aging. Strength training and impact exercises such as jumping rope can increase bone density throughout life. With stronger bones and muscles and better balance, fit people are less likely to experience debilitating falls and bone fractures. Along with exercise, a well-balanced diet containing adequate calcium and vitamin D and normal hormone function are also essential for strong bones. (One caution: Too much exercise can depress levels of estrogen, which helps maintain bone density, thereby leading to bone loss, even in young women.)

Type 2 Diabetes   People with diabetes are prone to heart disease, blindness, and severe problems of the nervous and circulatory systems. Recent studies have shown that exercise actually prevents the development of type 2 diabetes, the most common form. Exercise burns excess sugar and makes cells more sensitive to insulin. Exercise also helps keep body fat at healthy levels. (Obesity is a key risk factor for type 2 diabetes.) For people who have diabetes, physical activity is an important part of treatment. See Chapter 14 for more on diabetes.

Improved Psychological and Emotional Wellness

The joy of a well-hit cross-court backhand, the euphoria of a walk through the park, or the rush of a downhill schuss through deep powder snow provides pleasure that transcends health benefits alone. People who are physically active experience many social, psychological, and emotional benefits. For example,

• *Reduced stress.* In response to stressors, physically fit people experience milder physical responses and less emotional distress than sedentary individuals. Physical activity also provides protection against the effects of stress that have been linked to poor cardiorespiratory health. Psychological stress causes increased secretion of epinephrine and norepinephrine, compounds associated with the fight-or-flight reaction, which are thought to speed the development of atherosclerosis (hardening of the arteries). Excessive hostility is also associated with a risk of heart disease. Endurance exercise decreases the secretion of hormones and neurotransmitters triggered by emotional stress. It also can diffuse hostility and alleviate feelings of stress and anxiety by providing an emotional outlet and inducing feelings of relaxation. Regular exercise can also relieve sleeping problems.

• *Reduced anxiety and depression.* Sedentary adults have a much higher risk of feeling fatigue and depression than those who are physically active. Exercise is an effective treatment for people with depression and improves mood in nondepressed people who feel fine or who feel a little bit down.

• *Improved self-image.* Performing physical activities provides proof of skill and self-control, thus enhancing your self-concept. Sticking with an exercise program increases people's belief in their ability to be active, thereby boosting self-efficacy. Exercise also helps you look and feel better, boosting self-confidence and body image.

• *Learning and memory.* Exercise enhances the formation and survival of new nerve cells and the connections between nerves, which in turn improve memory and learning. Physical activity helps maintain mental functioning in older adults.

• *Enjoyment.* Exercise is fun. It offers an arena for harmonious interaction with other people, as well as opportunities to strive and excel. Physically fit people can perform everyday tasks—such as climbing stairs and carrying books or groceries—with ease. They have plenty of energy and can lead lives that are full and varied.

For more on the psychological benefits of physical activity, see the box "Exercise and the Mind on page 384."

Improved Immune Function

Exercise can have either positive or negative effects on the immune system, the physiological processes that protect us from disease. It appears that moderate endurance exercise boosts immune function, whereas excessive training depresses it. Physically fit people get fewer colds and upper respiratory tract infections than people who are not fit. The immune system—and ways to strengthen it—is discussed further in Chapter 17.

Prevention of Injuries and Low-Back Pain

Increased muscle strength provides protection against injury because it helps people maintain good posture and appropriate body mechanics when carrying out everyday

Terms

cardiovascular disease (CVD) A collective term for diseases of the heart and blood vessels.

lipoproteins Substances in blood, classified according to size, density, and chemical composition, that transport fats.

If you've ever gone for a long, brisk walk after a hard day's work, you know how refreshing exercise can be. Exercise can improve mood, stimulate creativity, clarify thinking, relieve anxiety, and provide an outlet for anger or aggression. But why does exercise make you feel good? Does it simply take your mind off your problems? Or does it cause a physical reaction that affects your mental state?

Current research indicates that exercise triggers many physical changes in the body that can alter mood. Scientists are now trying to explain how and why exercise affects the mind. One theory has to do with the physical structure of the brain. The area of the brain responsible for the movement of muscles is near the area responsible for thought and emotion. As muscles work vigorously, the resulting stimulation in the muscle center of the brain may also stimulate the thought and emotion center, producing improvements in mood and cognitive functions.

Other researchers suggest that exercise stimulates the release of brain chemicals that affect mood. Exercise increases levels of **endorphins,** brain chemicals that can suppress fatigue, decrease pain, and produce euphoria. Levels of a chemical called anandamide are increased in people who exercise at a moderate intensity for an extended period. Anandamide produces effects similar to those

of THC, the psychoactive chemical found in marijuana. The "runner's high" often experienced after running several miles may be due to the action of endorphins or anandamide.

Another area of research focuses on changes in brain activity during and after exercise. One change is an increase in alpha brain wave activity. Alpha waves indicate a highly relaxed state; meditation also induces alpha wave activity. Another change is an alteration in the levels of **neurotransmitters,** brain chemicals that increase alertness and reduce stress.

Higher levels of neurotransmitters such as serotonin may explain how exercise improves mild to moderate cases of depression. Researchers have found that exercise can be as effective as psychotherapy in treating depression, and even more effective when used in conjunction with other therapies. In addition to boosting neurotransmitter activity, exercise provides a distraction from stressful stimuli, enhances self-esteem, and may provide an opportunity for positive social interactions.

Another benefit of regular exercise is improved self-esteem and body image. According to a recent study, women who worked out on a regular basis rated their bodies as more attractive and healthier than did sedentary women. They actually weighed an average of 11–12 pounds

more than the less active women, suggesting that active women are more comfortable bucking cultural ideals of body shape. Other studies have found that athletes tend to have more positive images of their bodies than nonathletes, regardless of gender, sport, or level of expertise.

Although most people don't associate exercise with mental skills, physical activity has been shown to have positive effects on cognitive functioning in both the short term and the long term. Exercise improves alertness and memory and can help you perform cognitive tasks at your peak level. Exercise may also help boost creativity. In a study of college students, those who ran regularly or took aerobic dance classes scored significantly higher on standard psychological tests of creativity than sedentary students. Over the long term, exercise can slow and possibly even reverse certain age-related declines in cognitive performance, including slowed reaction time and loss of short-term memory and nonverbal reasoning skills.

The message from this research is that exercise is a critical factor in developing *all* the dimensions of wellness, not just physical health. Even moderate exercise like walking briskly a few times per week can significantly improve your well-being. A lifetime of physical activity can leave you with a healthier body and a sharper, happier, more creative mind.

---

activities such as walking, lifting, and carrying. Good muscle endurance in the abdomen, hips, lower back, and legs support the back in proper alignment and help prevent low-back pain, which afflicts over 85% of all Americans at some time in their lives.

Improved Wellness over the Life Span

Although people differ in the maximum levels of fitness they can achieve through exercise, the wellness benefits of exercise are available to everyone (see the box "Exercise

for People with Disabilities and Other Special Health Concerns"). Exercising regularly may be the single most important thing you can do now to improve the quality of your life in the future. All the benefits of exercise continue to accrue but gain new importance as the resilience of youth begins to wane. Simply stated, exercising can help you live a longer and healthier life.

DESIGNING YOUR EXERCISE PROGRAM

The best exercise program has two primary characteristics: It promotes your health, and it's fun for you to do. Exercise does not have to be a chore. On the contrary, it can provide some of the most pleasurable moments of your day, once you make it a habit. A little thought and planning will help you achieve these goals.

Terms

V.w

endorphins Brain chemicals that seem to be involved in modulating pain and producing euphoria.

neurotransmitters Brain chemicals that transmit nerve impulses.

Dimensions of Diversity

Regular, appropriate exercise is safe and beneficial for many people with chronic diseases, disabilities, or other special health conditions. For example, for people with asthma, regular exercise may reduce the risk of acute attacks during exertion. For people with diabetes, exercise can improve insulin sensitivity and body composition. For people who use wheelchairs, being active helps prevent secondary conditions that may result from prolonged inactivity, such as circulatory or muscular problems.

For everyone, activity provides an emotional boost that helps support a positive attitude as well as opportunities to make new friends, increase self-confidence, and gain a sense of accomplishment. For many people with special health concerns, the risks associated with *not* exercising are far greater than those associated with a moderate program of regular exercise.

If you have a special health concern and have hesitated becoming more active, one helpful strategy is to take a class or join an exercise group specifically designed for your condition. Many health centers and support groups sponsor specially tailored activity programs. For example, health clubs may have modified aerobics classes, special weight training machines, and classes involving mild exercise in warm water; popular sports and recreational activities include adapted golf, swimming, and skiing and wheelchair tennis, hockey, and basketball. Such a class or group activity can provide you with both expert advice and exercise partners who share your concerns and goals. If you prefer to exercise at home, exercise videos are available for people with a variety of conditions.

The fitness recommendations for the general population presented in this chapter can serve as general guidelines for any exercise program. However, for people with special health concerns, certain precautions and monitoring may be required. *Anyone with special health concerns should consult a physician before beginning an exercise program.* Guidelines and cautions for some common conditions are described below:

Asthma

• Carry medication during workouts and avoid exercising alone. Use your inhaler before exercise, if recommended by your physician.

• Exercise regularly, and warm up and cool down slowly to reduce the risk of acute attacks.

• When starting a fitness program, choose self-paced endurance activities, especially those involving interval training (short bouts of exercise followed by rest periods).

• When possible, avoid circumstances that may trigger an asthma attack, including cold, dry air or pollen or dust. Drink water to keep your airways moist, and in cold weather, cover your mouth with a mask or scarf to warm and humidify the air you breathe. Swimming is a good activity choice for people with asthma.

Diabetes

• Don't exercise alone; wear a bracelet identifying yourself as having diabetes.

• If you are taking insulin or another medication, you may need to adjust the timing and amount of each dose as you learn to balance your energy intake and output and your medication dosage.

• To prevent abnormally rapid absorption of injected insulin, inject it over a muscle that won't be exercised and wait at least an hour before exercising.

• Check blood sugar levels before, during, and after exercise, and adjust your diet or insulin dosage if needed. Avoid exercise if your blood sugar level is above 250 mg/dl, and ingest carbohydrates prior to exercise if your blood sugar level is below 100 mg/dl. Have high-carbohydrate foods available during a workout.

• Don't lift heavy weights. Check your skin regularly for blisters and abrasions, especially on your feet.

Obesity

• For maximum benefit and minimum risk, begin with low- to moderate-intensity activities and increase intensity slowly as your fitness improves.

• To lose weight or maintain lost weight, exercise moderately 60 minutes or more every day; you can exercise all at once or divide your total activity time into sessions of 10 or more minutes.

• Choose non- or low-weight-bearing activities like swimming, water exercises, cycling, or walking.

• Stay alert for symptoms of heat-related problems during exercise.

• Try to include as much lifestyle physical activity in your daily routine as possible.

• Include strength training in your program to build or maintain muscle mass.

Heart Disease and Hypertension

• Warm-up and cool-down sessions should be gradual and last at least 10 minutes.

• Exercise at a moderate rather than a high intensity; monitor your heart rate during exercise, and stop if you experience dizziness or chest pain.

• Increase exercise frequency, intensity, and time very gradually.

• Don't hold your breath when exercising as this can cause sudden, steep increases in blood pressure.

• Discuss the effects of your medication with your physician; for example, certain drugs for hypertension affect heart rate. If your physician has prescribed nitroglycerine, carry it with you during exercise.

Arthritis

• Begin an exercise program as early as possible in the course of the disease.

• Warm up thoroughly before each workout to loosen stiff muscles and lower the risk of injury.

• Avoid high-impact activities that may damage arthritic joints; consider swimming or water aerobics.

• In strength training, pay special attention to muscles that support and protect affected joints; add weight very gradually.

• Perform flexibility exercises regularly.

Osteoporosis

• If possible, choose low-impact, weight-bearing activities to help safely maintain bone density.

• To prevent fractures, avoid any activity or movement that stresses the back or carries a risk of falling.

• Weight train to improve strength and balance and reduce the risk of falls and fractures, but avoid lifting heavy weights.

No matter what your level of ability or disability, you can make physical activity an integral part of your life.

Physical Activity and Exercise for Health and Fitness

Physical activity can be defined as any body movement carried out by skeletal muscles and requiring energy. Different types of physical activity can be arranged on a continuum based on the amount of energy they require. Quick, easy movements such as standing up or walking down a hallway require little energy or effort; more intense, sustained activities such as cycling 5 miles or running in a race require considerably more.

The term *exercise* is commonly used to refer to a subset of physical activity—planned, structured, repetitive movement of the body designed specifically to improve or maintain physical fitness. As described earlier, levels of fitness depend on physiological factors such as the heart's ability to pump blood. To develop fitness, a person must perform a sufficient amount of physical activity to stress the body and cause long-term physiological changes. The precise type and amount of activity required to develop fitness is discussed in greater detail later in the chapter. For now, just remember that only some types of physical activity—those usually referred to as exercise—will develop fitness. This distinction is important for setting goals and developing a program.

Lifestyle Physical Activity for Health Promotion

The Surgeon General's report and joint guidelines from the CDC and the American College of Sports Medicine (ACSM) recommend that all Americans include a moderate amount of physical activity on most, preferably all, days of the week. The report suggests a goal of expending 150 calories per day, or about 1000 calories per week, in physical activity. Because energy expenditure is a function of both intensity and duration of activity, the same amount of benefit can be obtained in longer sessions of moderate-intensity activities as in shorter sessions of high-intensity activities. Thus, 15 minutes of running is equivalent to 30 minutes of brisk walking (Figure 13-4).

In this lifestyle approach to physical activity, the daily total of activity can be accumulated in multiple short bouts—for example, two 10-minute bicycle rides to and from class and a brisk 15-minute walk to the post office. Everyday tasks at school, work, and home can be structured to contribute to the daily activity total (see the box "Becoming More Active"). In addition to recommending moderate-intensity physical activity, the Surgeon General's report recommends that people perform resistance training (exercising against an opposing force such as a weight) at least twice a week to build and maintain strength.

By increasing lifestyle physical activity in accordance with the guidelines given in the Surgeon General's report, people can expect to significantly improve their health and well-being. Such a program may not, however, increase physical fitness. A program of 30 minutes of lifestyle activity

Washing and waxing a car for 45–60 minutes
Washing windows or floors for 45–60 minutes
Playing volleyball for 45 minutes
Playing touch football for 30–45 minutes
Gardening for 30–45 minutes
Wheeling self in wheelchair for 30–40 minutes
Walking 1¾ miles in 35 minutes (20 min/mile)
Basketball (shooting baskets) for 30 minutes
Bicycling 5 miles in 30 minutes
Dancing fast (social) for 30 minutes
Pushing a stroller 1½ miles in 30 minutes
Raking leaves for 30 minutes
Walking 2 miles in 30 minutes (15 min/mile)
Water aerobics for 30 minutes
Swimming laps for 20 minutes
Wheelchair basketball for 20 minutes
Basketball (playing a game) for 15–20 minutes
Bicycling 4 miles in 15 minutes
Jumping rope for 15 minutes
Running 1½ miles in 15 minutes (10 min/mile)
Shoveling snow for 15 minutes
Stairwalking for 15 minutes

Less Vigorous, More Time

More Vigorous, Less Time

Figure 13-4 Examples of moderate amounts of physical activity.   A moderate amount of physical activity is roughly equivalent to physical activity that uses approximately 150 calories of energy per day, or 1000 calories per week. Some activities can be performed at various intensities; the suggested durations correspond to expected intensity of effort.   SOURCE: U.S. Department of Health and Human Services. 1996. *Physical Activity and Health. A Report of the Surgeon General: At-a-Glance.* Washington, D.C.: U.S. Department of Health and Human Services.

per day may also not be enough activity for some people to achieve and maintain a healthy body weight.

Lifestyle Physical Activity for Health Promotion and Weight Management

Since the publication of the physical activity guidelines from the Surgeon General and the CDC/ACSM, other organizations have released physical activity recommendations that focus on specific health concerns. Because more than half of all U.S. adults are overweight, guidelines that focus on weight management are of particular interest. Guidelines from the Institute of Medicine, the 2005 Dietary Guidelines for Americans, and the World Health Organization/FAO Expert Report—all of which focus on weight control in addition to general health promotion—set higher daily goals for physical activity than the Surgeon General's report. These guidelines recognize that for people who need to prevent weight gain, to lose weight, or to maintain weight loss, 30 minutes per day of physical activity may not be enough—and so they recommend 60–90 or more minutes per day of physical activity. The different recommendations may seem confusing and contradictory, but all major health organizations have the same message: People can improve their health by becoming more active.

"Too little time" is a common excuse for not being physically active. Learning to manage your time successfully is crucial if you are to maintain a wellness lifestyle. You can begin by keeping a record of how you are currently spending your time; in your health journal, use a grid broken into blocks of 15, 20, or 30 minutes to track your daily activities. Then analyze your record: List each type of activity and the total time you engaged in it on a given day—for example, sleeping, 7 hours; eating, 1.5 hours; studying, 3 hours; and so on. Take a close look at your list of activities and prioritize them according to how important they are to you, from essential to somewhat important to not important at all.

Based on the priorities you set, make changes in your daily schedule by subtracting time from some activities in order to make time for physical activity. Look particularly carefully at your leisure time activities and your methods of transportation; these are areas where it is easy to build in physical activity. Make changes using a system of tradeoffs. For example, you may choose to reduce the total amount of time you spend playing computer games, listening to the radio, and chatting on the telephone in order to make time for an after-dinner bike ride or walk with a friend. You may decide to watch 10 fewer minutes of television in the morning in order to change your 5-minute drive to class into a 15-minute walk. In making these kinds of changes in your schedule, don't feel that you have to miss out on anything you enjoy. You can get more from less time by focusing on what you are doing and by combining activities. The following are just a few ways to become more active:

- Take the stairs instead of the elevator or escalator.
- Walk to the mailbox, post office, store, bank, or library whenever possible.
- Park your car a mile or even just a few blocks from your destination, and walk briskly.
- Do at least one chore every day that requires physical activity: wash the windows or your car, clean your room or house, mow the lawn, rake the leaves.
- Take study or work breaks to avoid sitting for more than 30 minutes at a time. Get up and walk around the library, your office, or your home or dorm; go up and down a flight of stairs.
- Stretch when you stand in line or watch TV.
- When you take public transportation, get off one stop down the line and walk to your destination.
- Go dancing instead of to a movie.
- Walk to visit a neighbor or friend rather than calling him or her on the phone. Go for a walk while you chat.
- Put your remote controls in storage; when you want to change TV channels or radio stations, get up and do it by hand.
- Take the dog for a walk (or an extra walk) every day.
- Play actively with your children or go for a walk pushing a stroller.
- If weather or neighborhood safety rule out walking outside, look for alternate locations—an indoor track, enclosed shopping mall, or even a long hallway. Look for locations near or on the way between your campus, workplace, or residence.
- Remember, being busy isn't the same thing as being active. Seize every opportunity to get up and walk around. Move more and sit less.

Exercise Programs to Develop Physical Fitness The Surgeon General's report also summarized the benefits of more formal exercise programs. It concluded that people can obtain even greater health benefits by increasing the duration and intensity of activity. Thus, a person who engages in a structured, formal exercise program designed to measurably improve physical fitness will obtain even greater improvements in quality of life and greater reductions in disease and mortality risk (Figure 13-5).

How Much Physical Activity Is Enough? Some experts believe that people get most of the health benefits of a formal exercise program simply by becoming more active over the course of the day. Others think that the lifestyle approach sets too low an activity goal; they argue that people should exercise long and intensely enough to improve the body's capacity for exercise—that is, to improve physical fitness. There is probably truth in both positions.

Most experts agree that some physical activity is better than none but that more—as long as it does not result in injury or become obsessive—is probably better than some. Regular physical activity, regardless of intensity, makes you healthier and can help protect you against many chronic diseases. However, exercising at low intensities does little to improve physical fitness. Although you get many of the health benefits of exercise by simply being more active, you obtain even more benefits when you are physically fit. In addition to long-term health benefits, fitness also significantly contributes to quality of life. Fit people have more energy and better body control. They can enjoy a more active lifestyle—cycling, hiking, skiing, and so on—than their more sedentary counterparts. Even if you don't like sports, you need physical energy and stamina in your daily life and for many nonsport leisure activities—visiting museums, playing with children, gardening, and so on.

A physical activity pyramid to guide you in meeting goals for physical activity is shown in Figure 13-6. If you are sedentary, start at the bottom of the pyramid and gradually increase the amount of moderate-intensity physical activity in your daily life. You don't have to exercise

Health and fitness benefits

Health

Fitness

Amount of physical activity/exercise

Figure 13-5 Relationship between amount of activity and health and fitness benefits. The health benefits of physical activity and exercise exist along a continuum. A fairly low level of physical activity (burning 1000 calories per week) can provide substantial health benefits, although it does little to increase fitness. Engaging in exercise that is more intense or of longer duration (burning 2000 calories per week) leads to greater health benefits and significant increases in fitness. Optimal fitness may require expending 3000 calories or more per week.   SOURCE: American College of Sports Medicine. 1998. *ACSM's Resource Manual for Guidelines for Exercise Testing and Prescription,* 3rd ed. Baltimore, Md.: Williams & Wilkins, p. 440.

vigorously, but you should experience a moderate increase in your heart and breathing rates; appropriate activities include walking, climbing stairs, doing yard work, and washing your car. As mentioned earlier, your activity time can be broken up into small blocks over the course of a day. Work up to meeting the goal set by the Surgeon General's report of using about 150 calories a day in physical activity. Choose to be active whenever you can. If weight management is a concern for you, begin by achieving the goal of 30 minutes per day and then gradually raise your activity level to 60 minutes per day or more.

For even greater benefits, move up to the next two levels of the pyramid, which illustrate parts of a formal exercise program. The American College of Sports Medicine has established guidelines for creating an exercise program that includes **cardiorespiratory endurance (aerobic) exercise,** strength training, and flexibility training (Table 13-1). Such a program will develop all the health-related components of physical fitness. The following sections of this chapter will show you how to develop a personalized exercise program that is fun and that will enable you to enjoy all the benefits of physical fitness.

For a summary of the health and fitness benefits of different levels of physical activity, refer to Figure 13-7.

First Steps

Are you thinking about starting a formal exercise program? A little planning can help make it a success.

Medical Clearance Previously inactive men over 40 and women over 50 should get a medical examination

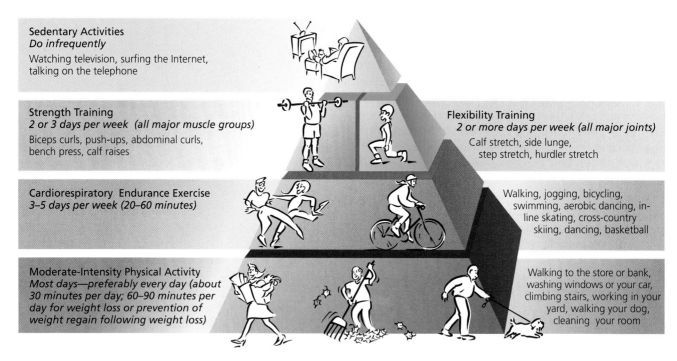

Sedentary Activities
Do infrequently
Watching television, surfing the Internet, talking on the telephone

Strength Training
2 or 3 days per week (all major muscle groups)
Biceps curls, push-ups, abdominal curls, bench press, calf raises

Flexibility Training
2 or more days per week (all major joints)
Calf stretch, side lunge, step stretch, hurdler stretch

Cardiorespiratory Endurance Exercise
3–5 days per week (20–60 minutes)

Walking, jogging, bicycling, swimming, aerobic dancing, in-line skating, cross-country skiing, dancing, basketball

Moderate-Intensity Physical Activity
Most days—preferably every day (about 30 minutes per day; 60–90 minutes per day for weight loss or prevention of weight regain following weight loss)

Walking to the store or bank, washing windows or your car, climbing stairs, working in your yard, walking your dog, cleaning your room

Figure 13-6 Physical activity pyramid. This physical activity pyramid is designed to help people become more active. If you are currently sedentary, begin at the bottom of the pyramid and gradually increase the amount of moderate-intensity physical activity in your life. If you are already moderately active, begin a formal exercise program that includes cardiorespiratory endurance exercise, flexibility training, and strength training to help you develop all the health-related components of fitness.

Table 13-1   Exercise Recommendations for Fitness Development in Healthy Adults

Exercise to Develop and Maintain Cardiorespiratory Endurance and Body Composition

Frequency of training	3–5 days per week.
Intensity of training	55/65–90% of maximum heart rate or 40/50–85% of maximum oxygen uptake reserve. Lower intensity values (55–64% of maximum heart rate and 40–49% of maximum oxygen uptake reserve) are most applicable to individuals who are quite unfit. For average individuals, intensities of 75–85% of maximum heart rate are appropriate; see p. 392 for instructions for determining target heart rate.
Time (duration) of training	20–60 total minutes of continuous or intermittent (in sessions lasting 10 or more minutes) aerobic activity. Duration is dependent on the intensity of activity; thus, lower-intensity activity should be conducted over a longer period of time (30 minutes or more). Lower- to moderate-intensity activity of longer duration is recommended for nonathletic adults.
Type (mode) of activity	Any activity that uses large-muscle groups, can be maintained continuously, and is rhythmical and aerobic in nature, such as walking-hiking, running-jogging, cycling-bicycling, cross-country skiing, aerobic dance and other forms of group exercise, rope skipping, rowing, stair climbing, swimming, skating, and endurance game activities.

Exercise to Develop and Maintain Muscular Strength and Endurance, Flexibility, and Body Composition

Resistance training	One set of 8–10 exercises that condition the major muscle groups should be performed 2 or 3 days per week. Most people should complete 8–12 repetitions of each exercise; for older or frailer people (approximately age 50–60 and above), 10–15 repetitions with a lighter weight may be more appropriate. Multiple-set regimens may provide greater benefits if time allows.
Flexibility training	Stretches for the major muscle groups should be performed a minimum of 2 or 3 days per week; at least four repetitions, held for 10–30 seconds, should be completed.

SOURCE: American College of Sports Medicine. 1998. ACSM position stand. The recommended quantity and quality of exercise for developing and maintaining cardiorespiratory and muscular fitness and flexibility in healthy adults. *Medicine and Science in Sports and Exercise* 30(6): 975–991.

---

before beginning an exercise program. Diabetes, asthma, heart disease, and extreme obesity are conditions that may call for a modified program. If you have an increased risk of heart disease because of smoking, high blood pressure, or obesity, have a physical checkup, including an **electrocardiogram (ECG or EKG)**, before beginning an exercise program. This checkup will help ensure that your program will be a benefit to your health, rather than a potential hazard. The Canadian Society for Exercise Physiology has developed questionnaires to help evaluate exercise safety; visit their Web site to complete an appropriate questionnaire (www.csep.ca/forms.asp).

Basic Principles of Physical Training Particular types and amounts of exercise are most effective in developing the various components of fitness. To put together an effective exercise program, a person should first understand the basic principles of physical training.

SPECIFICITY To develop a particular fitness component, you must perform exercises that are specifically designed for that component. This is the principle of *specificity*. Weight training, for example, develops muscular strength, but is less effective for developing flexibility. Specificity also applies to the skill-related fitness components—to improve at basketball, you must practice basketball—and to the differ-

ent parts of the body—to develop stronger arms, you must exercise your arms. A well-rounded exercise program includes exercises geared to each component of fitness, to different parts of the body, and to specific activities or sports.

PROGRESSIVE OVERLOAD Your body adapts to the demands of exercise by improving its functioning. When the amount of exercise, also called **overload**, is progressively increased, fitness continues to improve. The amount of overload is very important. Too little exercise will have no effect on fitness; too much may cause injury. The amount of exercise needed depends on your current level of fitness, your fitness goals, and the fitness components being developed. A novice, for example, might experience

Terms

cardiorespiratory endurance (aerobic) exercise Rhythmical, large-muscle exercise for a prolonged period of time; partially dependent on the ability of the cardiovascular system to deliver oxygen to tissues.

electrocardiogram (ECG or EKG) A recording of the changes in electrical activity of the heart.

overload The amount of stress placed on the body; a gradual increase in the amount of overload causes adaptations that improve fitness.

	Lifestyle physical activity	Moderate exercise program	Vigorous exercise program
Description	Moderate physical activity—an amount of activity that uses about 150 calories per day	Cardiorespiratory endurance exercise (20–60 minutes, 3–5 days per week); strength training and stretching exercises (2–3 days per week)	Cardiorespiratory endurance exercise (20–60 minutes, 3–5 days per week); interval training; strength training (3–4 days per week); and stretching exercises (3–5 days per week)
Sample activities or program	*One of the following:* • Walking to and from work, 15 minutes each way • Cycling to and from class, 10 minutes each way • Yardwork for 30 minutes • Dancing (fast) for 30 minutes • Playing basketball for 20 minutes	• Jogging for 30 minutes, 3 days per week • Weight training, 1 set of 8 exercises, 2 days per week • Stretching exercises, 3 days per week	• Running for 45 minutes, 3 days per week • Intervals: running 400 m at high effort 4 sets, 2 days per week • Weight training, 3 sets of 10 exercises, 3 days per week • Stretching exercises, 5 days per week
Health and fitness benefits	Better blood cholesterol levels, reduced body fat, better control of blood pressure, improved metabolic health, and enhanced glucose metabolism; improved quality of life; reduced risk of some chronic diseases Greater amounts of activity can help prevent weight gain and promote weight loss	All the benefits of lifestyle physical activity, plus improved physical fitness (increased cardiorespiratory endurance, muscular strength and endurance, and flexibility) and even-greater improvements in health and quality of life and reductions in chronic disease risk	All the benefits of lifestyle physical activity and a moderate exercise program, with greater increases in fitness and somewhat greater reductions in chronic disease risk Note: Participating in a vigorous exercise program may increase risk of injury and overtraining

Figure 13-7   Health and fitness benefits of different amounts of physical activity and exercise.

fitness benefits from jogging a mile in 10 minutes, but this level of exercise would cause no physical adaptations in a trained distance runner.

The amount of overload needed to maintain or improve a particular level of fitness is determined in four dimensions, represented by the acronym FITT:

Frequency

Intensity

Time

Type

• *Frequency, or how often.* Optimum exercise frequency, expressed in number of days per week, varies with the component being developed and your goals. A frequency of 3–5 days per week is recommended for cardiorespiratory endurance exercise, 2 or 3 days per week for strength training, and 2 or more days per week for stretching.

• *Intensity, or how hard.* Fitness benefits occur when you exercise harder than your normal level of activity. To develop cardiorespiratory endurance, you must raise your heart rate above normal; to develop muscular strength, you must lift a heavier weight than you normally

do; to develop flexibility, you must stretch your muscles beyond their normal length. A gradual increase in intensity is recommended to avoid injury.

• *Time (duration), or how long.* If fitness benefits are to occur, exercise sessions must last for an extended period of time. Depending on the component being developed and your intensity level, a duration of 20–60 minutes is usually recommended.

• *Type, or mode of activity.* The type of exercise in which you should engage varies with each fitness component and with your personal fitness goals. To develop cardiorespiratory endurance, you need to engage in continuous activities involving large-muscle groups—walking, cycling, or swimming, for example. Resistive exercises develop muscular strength and endurance; stretching exercises build flexibility. The frequency, intensity, and time of exercise will be different for each type of activity.

These dimensions of overload are described individually as they apply to the health-related components of fitness discussed in this chapter.

REVERSIBILITY   The body adjusts to lower levels of physical activity in the same way it adjusts to higher levels—

the principle of *reversibility*. When you stop exercising, you can lose up to 50% of fitness improvements within 2 months. Try to exercise consistently, and don't quit if you miss a few workouts. If a training schedule must be curtailed temporarily, fitness improvements are best maintained if exercise intensity is kept constant and frequency and/or time is reduced.

INDIVIDUAL DIFFERENCES Anyone watching the Olympics, a professional football game, or a tennis match can readily see that, from a physical standpoint, we are not all created equal. There are limits to the potential for improvement and large individual differences in our ability to improve fitness, achieve a desirable body composition, and perform and learn sports skills. Scientists have identified specific genes that influence body fat, strength, and endurance. In addition, men tend to have higher endurance capacity than women due to higher testosterone levels (which affect oxygen transport and cellular metabolism) and lower levels of body fat. However, men and women have the same capacity for improvement when gains are expressed as a percent of initial fitness. Although genetics and gender may place certain limits on your level of fitness and skill, physical training improves fitness and wellness regardless of heredity.

Selecting Activities
If you have been inactive, you should begin slowly by gradually increasing the amount of moderate physical activity in your life (the bottom of the activity pyramid). Once your body has adjusted to your new level of activity, you will be ready to choose additional activities for your exercise program.

Consider your choices carefully. First, be sure the activities you choose contribute to your overall wellness. Choose activities that make sense for you. Are you competitive? If so, try racquetball, basketball, or squash. Do you prefer to exercise alone? Then consider cross-country skiing or road running. Have you been sedentary? A walking program may be a good place to start.

If you think you may have trouble sticking with an exercise program, find a structured activity that you can do with a buddy or a group. If you don't have any favorite sports or activities, try something new. Take a physical education class, join a health club, or sign up for jazz dancing. You're sure to find an activity that's both enjoyable and good for you.

Be realistic about the constraints presented by some sports, such as accessibility, expense, and time. For example, if you have to travel for hours to get to a ski area, skiing may not be a good choice for your regular exercise program. If you don't have large blocks of time available, you may have trouble squeezing in 18 holes of golf. And if you've never played tennis, it will probably take you a fair amount of time to reach a reasonable skill level; you may be better off with a program of walking or jogging to get good workouts while you're improving your tennis game.

A general fitness program that supports an active lifestyle and promotes good health should contain the following components: cardiorespiratory endurance exercises, muscular strength and endurance exercises, flexibility exercises, and training in specific skills.

Cardiorespiratory Endurance Exercises

Exercises that condition your heart and lungs should have a central role in your fitness program. The best exercises for developing cardiorespiratory endurance stress a large portion of the body's muscle mass for a prolonged period of time. These include walking, jogging, running, swimming, bicycling, and aerobic dancing. Many popular sports and recreational activities, such as racquetball, tennis, basketball, and soccer, are also good if the skill level and intensity of the game are sufficient to provide a vigorous workout.

Frequency The optimal workout schedule for endurance training is 3–5 days per week. Beginners should start with 3 and work up to 5 days. Training more than 5 days a week often leads to injury for recreational athletes. Although you do get health benefits from exercising very vigorously only 1 or 2 days per week, you risk injury because your body never gets a chance to adapt fully to regular exercise training.

Intensity The most misunderstood aspect of conditioning, even among experienced athletes, is training intensity. Intensity is the crucial factor in attaining a significant training effect—that is, in increasing the body's cardiorespiratory capacity. A primary purpose of endurance training is to increase **maximal oxygen consumption (VO_{2max})**. VO_{2max} represents the maximum ability of the cells to use oxygen and is considered the best measure of cardiorespiratory capacity. Intensity of training is the crucial factor in improving VO_{2max}.

However, it's not true that the harder you work, the better it is for you. Working too hard can cause injury, just as not working hard enough provides less benefit. One of the easiest ways to determine exactly how intensely you should work involves measuring your heart rate. It is not necessary or desirable to exercise at your maximum heart rate—the fastest heart rate possible before exhaustion sets in—in order to improve your cardiorespiratory capacity. Beneficial effects occur at lower heart rates with a much lower risk of injury. **Target heart rate range** is the range of rates at which you should exercise to obtain cardiorespiratory

Terms

maximal oxygen consumption (VO_{2max}) The body's maximum ability to transport and use oxygen.

target heart rate range The range of heart rates at which exercise yields cardiorespiratory benefits.

Your target heart rate is the range of rates at which you should exercise to experience cardiorespiratory benefits. Your target heart rate range is based on your maximum heart rate, which can be estimated from your age. (If you are a serious athlete or face possible cardiovascular risks from exercise, you may want to have your maximum heart rate determined more accurately through a treadmill test in a physician's office, hospital, or sports medicine laboratory.) Your target heart rate is a range: The lower value corresponds to moderate-intensity exercise, and the higher value is associated with high-intensity exercise. Target heart rate ranges are shown in the table.

You can monitor the intensity of your workouts by measuring your pulse either at your wrist or at one of your carotid arteries, located on either side of your Adam's apple. Your pulse rate drops rapidly after exercise, so begin counting immediately after you have finished exercising. You will obtain the most accurate results by counting beats for 10 seconds and then multiplying by 6 to get your heart rate in beats per minute (bpm). The 10-second counts corresponding to each target heart rate range are also shown in the table.

Age (years)	Target Heart Rate Range (bpm)*	10-Second Count (beats)*
20–24	127–180	21–30
25–29	124–176	20–29
30–34	121–171	20–28
35–39	118–167	19–27
40–44	114–162	19–27
45–49	111–158	18–26
50–54	108–153	18–25
55–59	105–149	17–24
60–64	101–144	16–24
65+	97–140	16–23

*Target heart rates lower than those shown here are appropriate for individuals who are quite unfit. Ranges are based on the following formula: Target heart rate = 0.65 to 0.90 of maximum heart rate, assuming maximum heart rate = 220 − age.

benefits. To find out how you can determine the intensity at which you should exercise, refer to the box "Determining Your Target Heart Rate Range."

After you begin your fitness program, you may improve quickly because the body adapts readily to new exercises; the rate of improvement may slow after the first month or so. The more fit you become, the harder you will have to work to improve. By monitoring your heart rate, you will always know if you are working hard enough to improve, not hard enough, or too hard. For most people, a fitness program involves attaining an acceptable level of fitness and then maintaining that level. There is no need to keep working indefinitely to improve; doing so only increases the chance of injury. After you have reached the level you want, you can maintain fitness by exercising at the same intensity at least 3 nonconsecutive days per week.

Time (Duration) A total time of 20–60 minutes is recommended; exercise can take place in a single session or several sessions lasting 10 or more minutes. The total duration of exercise depends on its intensity. To improve cardiorespiratory endurance during a low- to moderate-intensity activity such as walking or slow swimming, you should exercise for 45–60 minutes. For high-intensity exercise performed at the top of your target heart rate zone, a duration of 20 minutes is sufficient. It is usually best to start off with less vigorous activities and only gradually increase intensity.

You can use these three dimensions of cardiorespiratory endurance training—frequency, intensity, and time—to

develop a fitness program that strengthens your heart and lungs and provides all the benefits described earlier in this chapter. Build your program around at least 20 minutes of endurance exercise at your target heart rate 3 to 5 days a week. Then add exercises that develop the other components of fitness.

The Warm-Up and Cool-Down It is always important to warm up before you exercise and to cool down afterward. Warming up enhances your performance and decreases your chances of injury. Your muscles work better when their temperature is elevated slightly above resting level. Warming up helps your body's physiology gradually progress from rest to exercise. Blood needs to be redirected to active muscles, and your heart needs time to adapt to the increased demands of exercise. A warm-up helps spread **synovial fluid** throughout the joints, which helps protect joint surfaces from wear and tear. (It's like warming up a car to spread oil through the engine parts before shifting into gear.)

A warm-up session should include low-intensity movements similar to those in the activity that will follow. Examples of low-intensity movements are hitting forehands and backhands before a tennis game and running a 12-minute mile before progressing to an 8-minute mile. Some people like to include stretching exercises in their warm-up. Experts recommend that you stretch *after* the active part of your warm-up, when your body temperature has been elevated. Studies have found that stretching prior to exercise can temporarily decrease muscle strength and power, so if a high-performance workout is

Gender Differences in Muscular Strength

Men are generally stronger than women because they typically have larger bodies overall and a larger proportion of their total body mass is made up of muscle. But when strength is expressed per unit of muscle tissue, men are only 1–2% stronger than women in the upper body and about equal to women in the lower body. Individual muscle cells are larger in men, but the functioning of the cells is the same in both sexes.

Two factors that help explain these disparities are testosterone levels and the speed of nervous control of muscle. Testosterone promotes the growth of muscle tissue in both males and females, but testosterone levels are about 6–10 times higher in men than in women, so men develop larger muscles. Also, because the male nervous system can activate muscles faster, men tend to have more power.

Some women are concerned that they will develop large muscles from strength training. Because of hormonal differences, most women do not develop large muscles unless they train intensely over many years or take steroids. Women do gain muscle and improve body composition through strength training, but they don't develop bulky muscles or gain significant amounts of weight. A study of average women who weight trained 2–3 days per week for 8 weeks found that the women gained about 1.75 pounds of muscle and lost about 3.5 pounds of fat.

Losing muscle over time is a much greater health concern for women than small gains in muscle weight in response to strength training, especially as any gains in muscle weight are typically more than balanced with loss of fat weight. Both men and women lose muscle mass and power as they age, but because men start out with more muscle when they are young and don't lose power as quickly as women, older women tend to have greater impairment of muscle function than older men. This may partially explain the higher incidence of life-threatening falls in older women.

The bottom line is that both men and women can increase strength through strength training. Women may not be able to lift as much weight as men, but pound for pound of muscle, they have nearly the same capacity to gain strength as men. The lifetime wellness benefits of strength training are available to everyone. Strength training is particularly beneficial for women because it helps prevent bone and muscle loss with aging and maintains fat-free weight during weight management programs.

SOURCES: Fahey, T. D. 2007. *Weight Training for Men and Women*, 6th ed. New York: McGraw-Hill; IDEA. 2001. *Fitness Tip—Why Women Need Weight Training* (http://www.ideafit.com/ftwomen.htm; retrieved October 22, 2002); Krivickas, L. S., et al. 2001. Age and gender-related differences in maximum shortening velocity of skeletal muscle fibers. *American Journal of Physical Medicine & Rehabilitation* 80: 447–455.

---

your goal, it is best to stretch after a workout. See pages 395–397 for more on stretching.

Cooling down after exercise is important to restore the body's circulation to its normal resting condition. When you are at rest, a relatively small percentage of your total blood volume is directed to muscles, but during exercise, as much as 85% of the heart's output is directed to them. During recovery from exercise, it is important to continue exercising at a low level to provide a smooth transition to the resting state. Cooling down helps regulate the return of blood to your heart.

Developing Muscular Strength and Endurance

Any program designed to promote health should include exercises that develop muscular strength and endurance. Your ability to maintain correct posture and move efficiently depends in part on adequate muscle fitness. Strengthening exercises also increase muscle tone, which improves the appearance of your body. A lean, healthy-looking body is certainly one of the goals and one of the benefits of an overall fitness program (see the box "Gender Differences in Muscular Strength").

Types of Strength Training Exercises Muscular strength and endurance can be developed in many ways, from weight training to calisthenics. Common exercises such as sit-ups, push-ups, pull-ups, and wall-sitting (leaning against a wall in a seated position and supporting yourself with your leg muscles) maintain the muscular strength of most people if they practice them several times a week. To condition and tone your whole body, choose exercises that work the major muscles of the shoulders, chest, back, arms, abdomen, and legs.

To increase muscular strength and endurance, you must do **resistance exercise**—exercises in which your muscles must exert force against a significant amount of resistance. Resistance can be provided by weights, exercise machines, or your own body weight. **Isometric (static) exercises** involve applying force without movement, such as when you contract your abdominal muscles. This static type of exercise is valuable for toning and strengthening muscles. Isometrics can be practiced anywhere and do not require

Terms

V|w

synovial fluid Fluid found within many joints that provides lubrication and nutrition to the cells of the joint surface.

resistance exercise Exercise that forces muscles to contract against increased resistance; also called *strength training*.

isometric (static) exercise The application of force without movement.

Gender Matters

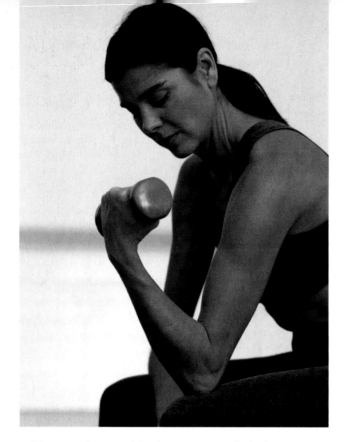

Building muscular strength is a key component of a fitness program. Weight training is just one way to increase strength, improve muscle tone, and enhance the overall appearance of the body.

any equipment. For maximum strength gains, hold an isometric contraction maximally for 6 seconds; do five to ten repetitions. Don't hold your breath—that can restrict blood flow to your heart and brain. Within a few weeks, you will notice the effect of this exercise. Isometrics are particularly useful when recovering from an injury.

Isotonic (dynamic) exercises involve applying force with movement, as, for example, in weight training exercises such as the bench press. These are the most popular type of exercises for increasing muscle strength and seem to be most valuable for developing strength that can be transferred to other forms of physical activity. They include exercises using barbells, dumbbells, weight machines, and body weight, as in push-ups or sit-ups.

Choosing Equipment Weight machines are preferred by many people because they are safe, convenient, and easy to use. You just set the resistance (usually by placing a pin in the weight stack), sit down at the machine, and start working. Machines make it easy to isolate and work specific muscles. Free weights require more

Term

Vi**w**

isotonic (dynamic) exercise The application of force with movement.

care, balance, and coordination to use, but they strengthen your body in ways that are more adaptable to real life. When using free weights, you need to use a spotter, someone who stands by to assist in case you lose control over a weight (see the box "Safe Weight Training").

Choosing Exercises A complete weight training program works all the major muscle groups: neck, upper back, shoulders, arms, chest, abdomen, lower back, thighs, buttocks, and calves. Different exercises work different muscles, so it usually takes about eight to ten exercises to get a complete workout for general fitness—for example, bench presses to develop the chest, shoulders, and upper arms; pull-ups to work the biceps and upper back; squats to develop the legs and buttocks; toe raises to work the calves; and so on. If you are also training for a particular sport, include exercises to strengthen the muscles important for optimal performance and those most likely to be injured.

Refer to the Online Learning Center for a sample recommended program for strength training using either free weights, weight machines, or no weight equipment. A sample workout card for monitoring your progress and video clips of selected exercises are also included.

Frequency For general fitness, the American College of Sports Medicine recommends a frequency of 2 or 3 days per week. Allow your muscles a day of rest between workouts to avoid soreness and injury. If you enjoy weight training and would like to train more often, try working different muscle groups on alternate days.

Intensity and Time The amount of weight (resistance) you lift in weight training exercises is equivalent to intensity in cardiorespiratory endurance training; the number of repetitions of each exercise is equivalent to time. In order to improve fitness, you must do enough repetitions of each exercise to temporarily fatigue your muscles. The number of repetitions needed to cause fatigue depends on the amount of resistance: the heavier the weight, the fewer repetitions to reach fatigue. In general, a heavy weight and a low number of repetitions (1–5) build strength, whereas a light weight and a high number of repetitions (20–25) build endurance. For a general fitness program to build both strength and endurance, try to do 8–12 repetitions of each exercise; a few exercises, such as abdominal crunches and calf raises, may require more. (For people who are 50–60 years of age and older, 10–15 repetitions of each exercise using a lighter weight is recommended.)

The first few sessions of weight training should be devoted to learning the exercises. To start, choose a weight that you can move easily through 8–12 repetitions. Add weight when you can do more than 12 repetitions of an exercise. If adding weight means you can do only 7 or 8 repetitions before your muscles fatigue, stay with that weight until you can again complete 12 repetitions. If you can do only 4–6 repetitions after adding weight, or if you can't maintain good form, you've added too much and should

Safe Weight Training

General Strategies

- Lift weights from a stabilized body position. Protect your back from dangerous positions. Don't twist your body while lifting.

- Don't lift beyond the limits of your strength.

- Be aware of what's going on around you so that you don't bump into someone or get too close to a moving weight stack.

- Don't use defective equipment; report any equipment problems immediately.

- Don't chew gum when exercising.

- *Don't hold your breath while doing weight training exercises.* Exhale when exerting the greatest force, and inhale when moving the weight into position. (Holding your breath raises blood pressure and causes a decrease in blood returning to the heart; it can make you become dizzy and faint.)

- Rest between lifts.

- Always warm up before training and cool down afterward.

Free Weights

- Use spotters to avoid injury. A spotter can help you if you cannot complete a lift or if the weight tilts.

- Secure weight plates to barbells with a collar to prevent them from sliding off.

- Keep weights as close to your body as possible. Do most of your lifting with your legs; keep your hips and buttocks tucked in.

- Lift weights smoothly and slowly; don't bounce or jerk them. Control the weight through the entire range of motion.

- When holding barbells and dumbbells, wrap your thumbs around the bar when gripping it.

Weight Machines

- Stay away from moving parts of the machine that could pinch your skin.

- Adjust each machine for your body so that you don't have to work in an awkward position.

- Beware of broken bolts, frayed cables, broken chains, or loose cushions that can give way and cause serious injury.

- Make sure the machines are clean. Carry a towel with you, and place it on the machine where you will sit or lie down.

take some off. As a general guideline, try increases of approximately ½ pound of additional weight for each 10 pounds you are currently lifting.

For developing strength and endurance for general fitness, a single set (group) of each exercise is sufficient, provided you use enough resistance (weight) to fatigue your muscles. Doing more than one set of each exercise may increase strength development, and most serious weight trainers do at least three sets of each exercise. If you do more than one set of an exercise, rest long enough between sets to allow your muscles to recover.

As with cardiorespiratory endurance exercise, you should warm up before every weight training session and cool down afterward. You can expect to improve rapidly during the first 6–10 weeks of training; gains will then come more slowly. Factors such as age, motivation, gender, and heredity will affect your program. Your ultimate goal depends on you. After you have achieved the level of strength and muscularity that you want, you can maintain your gains by training 2–3 days per week.

A Caution About Supplements No nutritional supplement or drug will change a weak, untrained person into a strong, fit person. Those changes require regular training that stresses the body and causes physiological adaptations. Supplements or drugs that promise quick, large gains in strength usually don't work and are often either dangerous, expensive, or both (see the box "Drugs and Supplements for Improved Athletic Performance"). The long-term effects of many supplements have not been studied, and over-the-counter supplements are not carefully regulated. The International Olympic Committee recently issued a warning after researchers tested hundreds of nutritional supplements and found that 15% contained unlabeled substances that would cause an athlete to fail a drug test. Use your critical thinking skills to evaluate claims made about supplements, and stay with the proven method of a steady, progressive fitness program to build strength.

Flexibility Exercises

Flexibility, or stretching, exercises are important for maintaining the normal range of motion in the major joints of the body. Some exercises, such as running, can actually decrease flexibility because they require only a partial range of motion. Like a good weight training program, a good stretching program includes exercises for all the major muscle groups and joints of the body: neck, shoulders, back, hips, thighs, hamstrings, and calves. Refer to the Online Learning Center for a sample recommended program for flexibility training.

Proper Stretching Technique Stretching should be performed statically. Ballistic stretching (known as

The 2004 Olympic Games in Athens made headlines not just for athletic achievements but also for the record number of athletes testing positive for performance-enhancing drugs. Some athletes were banned from competition before or during the games; others had medals taken away after they failed postcompetition drug tests. The Olympic Movement Anti-Doping Code calls for the elimination of the use of performance-enhancing drugs in sports in order to both ensure respect for sports ethics and protect the health of athletes. In the wake of the BALCO legal case, which focused attention on use of steroids and other compounds by Olympic and professional athletes, the U.S. Congress and additional sports organizations began to consider stricter regulations regarding performance-enhancing drugs.

Drugs intended to enhance athletic performance are used not only by elite Olympic and professional athletes but also by active individuals of all fitness levels. About 2–6% of high school and college students report having used anabolic steroids, and over-the-counter dietary supplements are much more popular. Many such substances are ineffective and expensive, and many are also dangerous. For example, supplements containing gamma butyrolactone or butanediol, CNS depressants related to the illegal drug gamma hydroxybutyrate (GHB), marketed to bodybuilders may cause vomiting, seizures, coma, and potentially fatal withdrawal reactions (see Chapter 9). A few of the most widely used compounds are described below.

Anabolic Steroids　　These synthetic derivatives of testosterone are taken to increase strength, power, speed, endurance, muscle size, and aggressiveness. **Anabolic steroids** have dangerous side effects, including disruption of the body's hormone system, liver disease, acne, breast development and testicular shrinkage in males, masculinization in women and children, and increased risk of heart disease and cancer.

Steroid users who inject the drugs face the same health risks as other injection drug users, including increased risk of HIV infection. Steroids have also been found to be a gateway to the use of other drugs. Steroid users who progress to heroin use typically obtain heroin from the same dealer who provided steroids; they also typically begin heroin use in an effort to blunt some of the side effects of steroid use and withdrawal, including irritability and depression.

Adrenal Androgens　　This group of drugs, which includes dehydroepiandrosterone (DHEA) and androstenedione, are typically taken to stimulate muscle growth and aid in weight control. The few studies of these agents done on humans show that they are of very little value in improving athletic performance, and they have side effects similar to those of anabolic steroids, especially when taken in high doses. In January 2005, androstenedione was reclassified and is no longer available without a prescription.

Ephedra and Other Stimulants　　These drugs may be taken to increase training intensity, to suppress hunger, to reduce fatigue, and to promote weight loss. They raise heart rate and blood pressure and, at high doses, may increase the risk of heart attack, stroke, and heat-related illness. Several stimulants, including ephedra and phenylpropanolamine, were recently banned by the FDA. See Chapters 9 and 14 for more information.

Erythropoietin (EPO)　　A naturally occurring hormone that boosts the concentration of red blood cells, EPO is typically used by endurance athletes to improve their performance. EPO can cause blood clots and death.

Creatine Monohydrate　　Use of creatine supplements may improve performance in short-term, high-intensity, repetitive exercise and decrease the risk of injury. These supplements may increase water retention in muscles, giving the feeling of increased muscularity without an actual increase in muscle size. The long-term effects of creatine use, especially among young people, are not well established.

Protein, Amino Acid, and Polypeptide Supplements　　Little research supports the use of such supplements, even in athletes on extemely heavy training regimens. The protein requirements of athletes are not much higher than those of sedentary individuals, and most people take in more than enough protein in their diets. By substituting supplements for food sources of protein, people may risk deficiencies in other key nutrients typically found in such foods, including iron and B vitamins.

Chromium Picolinate　　Sold over the counter, chromium picolinate is a more easily digested form of the trace mineral chromium. Although often marketed as a means to build muscle and reduce fat, most studies have found no positive effects. Long-term use of high dosages may have serious health consequences.

"bouncing") is dangerous and counterproductive. Stretching can be either active or passive. In active stretching, a muscle is stretched by a contraction of opposing muscles. In passive stretching, an outside force or resistance provided by yourself, a partner, gravity, or a weight helps your joints move through their range of motion. You can achieve a greater range of motion and a more intense stretch using passive stretching, but there is a greater risk of injury. The safest and most convenient technique may be active static stretching with a passive assist. For example, you might do a seated stretch of your calf muscles both by contracting the muscles on the top of your shin and by grabbing your feet and pulling them toward you.

Frequency　　Do stretching exercises a minimum of 2 or 3 days per week. You can set aside a special time for these exercises or do them after cardiorespiratory endurance exercise or strength training. You may develop

Term

anabolic steroids　Synthetic male hormones used to increase muscle size and strength.

When performed regularly, stretching exercises help maintain or improve the range of motion in joints. For each exercise, stretch to the point of tightness in the muscle and hold the position for 10–30 seconds.

more flexibility if you do them after exercise, during your cool-down, because your muscles are warmer then and can be stretched farther.

Intensity and Time   For each exercise, stretch to the point of tightness in the muscle, and hold the position for 10–30 seconds. Rest for 30–60 seconds, and then repeat, trying to stretch a bit farther. Relax and breathe easily as you stretch. You should feel a pleasant, mild stretch as you let the muscles relax; stretching should not be painful. Do at least four repetitions of each exercise. A complete flexibility workout usually takes about 20–30 minutes.

Increase your intensity gradually over time. Improved flexibility takes many months to develop. There are large individual differences in joint flexibility. Don't feel you have to compete with others during stretching workouts.

Training in Specific Skills

The final component in your fitness program is learning the skills required for the sports or activities in which you choose to participate. Taking the time and effort to acquire competence means that instead of feeling ridiculous, becoming frustrated, and giving up in despair, you achieve a sense of mastery and add a new physical activity to your repertoire.

The first step in learning a new skill is getting help. Sports like tennis, golf, sailing, and skiing require mastery of basic movements and techniques, so instruction from a qualified teacher can save you hours of frustration and increase your enjoyment of the sport. Skill is also important in conditioning activities such as jogging, swimming, and cycling. Even if you learned a sport as a child, additional instruction now can help you refine your technique, get over stumbling blocks, and relearn skills that you may have learned incorrectly.

Putting It All Together

Now that you know the basic components of a fitness program, you can put them all together in a program that works for you. Remember to include the following:

- *Cardiorespiratory endurance exercise:* Do at least 20 minutes of aerobic exercise at your target heart rate 3 to 5 days a week.

- *Muscular strength and endurance:* Work the major muscle groups (one or more sets of eight to ten exercises) 2 or 3 days a week.

- *Flexibility exercise:* Do stretches at least 2 or 3 days a week, preferably after exercise, when your muscles are warm.

- *Skill training:* Incorporate some or all of your aerobic or strengthening exercise into an enjoyable sport or physical activity.

Refer to Figure 13-8 for a summary of the FITT principle for the health-related fitness components; the fitness

	Cardiorespiratory Endurance Training	Strength Training	Flexibility Training
Frequency	3–5 days per week	2–3 days per week	2–3 days per week, or more
Intensity	55/65–90% of maximum heart rate	Sufficient resistance to fatigue muscles	Stretch to the point of tension
Time	20–60 minutes in sessions lasting 10 minutes or more	8–12 repetitions of each exercise, 1 or more sets	4 repetitions of each exercise, held for 10–30 seconds
Type	Continuous rhythmic activities using large-muscle groups	Resistance exercises for all major muscle groups	Stretching exercises for all major joints

Figure 13-8   A summary of the FITT principle for the health-related components of fitness

Table 13-2   A Summary of Sports and Fitness Activities

This table classifies sports and activities as high (H), moderate (M), or low (L) in terms of their ability to develop each of the five components of physical fitness: cardiorespiratory endurance (CRE), muscular strength (MS), muscular endurance (ME), flexibility (F), and body composition (BC). The skill level needed to obtain fitness benefits is noted: Low (L) means little or no skill is required to obtain fitness benefits, moderate (M) means average skill is needed to obtain fitness benefits, and high (H) means much skill is required to obtain fitness benefits. The fitness prerequisite, or conditioning needs of a beginner, is also noted: Low (L) means no fitness prerequisite is required, moderate (M) means some preconditioning is required, and high (H) means substantial fitness is required. The last two columns list the calorie cost of each activity when performed moderately and vigorously. To determine how many calories you burn, multiply the value in the appropriate column by your body weight and then by the number of minutes you exercise. Work up to using 300 or more calories per workout.

Sports and Activities	Components					Skill Level	Fitness Prerequisite	Approximate Calorie Cost (cal/lb/min)	
	CRE	MS*	ME*	F*	BC			Moderate	Vigorous
Aerobic dance	H	M	H	H	H	L	L	.046	.062
Backpacking	H	M	H	M	H	L	M	.032	.078
Badminton, skilled, singles	H	M	M	M	H	M	M	—	.071
Ballet (floor combinations)	M	M	H	H	M	M	L	—	.058
Ballroom dancing	M	L	M	L	M	M	L	.034	.049
Baseball (pitcher and catcher)	M	M	H	M	M	H	M	.039	—
Basketball, half court	H	M	H	M	H	M	M	.045	.071
Bicycling	H	M	H	M	H	M	L	.049	.071
Bowling	L	L	L	L	L	L	L	—	—
Calisthenic circuit training	H	M	H	M	H	L	L	—	.060
Canoeing and kayaking (flat water)	M	M	H	M	M	M	M	.045	—
Cheerleading	M	M	M	M	M	M	L	.033	.049
Fencing	M	M	H	H	M	M	L	.032	.078
Field hockey	H	M	H	M	H	M	M	.052	.078
Folk and square dancing	M	L	M	L	M	L	L	.039	.049
Football, touch	M	M	M	M	M	M	M	.049	.078
Frisbee, ultimate	H	M	H	M	H	M	M	.049	.078
Golf (riding cart)	L	L	L	M	L	L	L	—	—
Handball, skilled, singles	H	M	H	M	H	M	M	—	.078
Hiking	H	M	H	L	H	L	M	.051	.073
Hockey, ice and roller	H	M	H	M	H	M	M	.052	.078
Horseback riding	M	M	M	L	M	M	M	.052	.065
Interval circuit training	H	H	H	M	H	L	L	—	.062
Jogging and running	H	M	H	L	H	L	L	.060	.104
Judo	M	H	H	M	M	M	L	.049	.090

benefits of a variety of activities are provided in Table 13-2 to help you plan your program.

GETTING STARTED AND STAYING ON TRACK

Once you have a program that fulfills your basic fitness needs and suits your personal tastes, adhering to a few basic principles will help you improve at the fastest rate, have more fun, and minimize the risk of injury. These principles include buying appropriate equipment, eating and drinking properly, and managing your program so it becomes an integral part of your life.

Selecting Instructors, Equipment, and Facilities

Once you've chosen the activities for your program, you may need to obtain appropriate information, instruction, and equipment or find an appropriate facility.

Finding Help and Advice About Exercise
One of the best places to get help is an exercise class, where an expert instructor can help you learn the basics of training and answer your questions. A qualified personal trainer can also get you started on an exercise program or a new form of training. Make sure that your instructor or trainer has proper qualifications, such as a

| Sports and Activities | Components | | | | | Skill Level | Fitness Prerequisite | Approximate Calorie Cost (cal/lb/min) | |
	CRE	MS*	ME*	F*	BC			Moderate	Vigorous
Karate	H	M	H	H	H	L	M	.049	.090
Lacrosse	H	M	H	M	H	H	M	.052	.078
Modern dance (moving combinations)	M	M	H	H	M	L	L	—	.058
Orienteering	H	M	H	L	H	L	M	.049	.078
Outdoor fitness trails	H	M	H	M	H	L	L	—	.060
Popular dancing	M	L	M	M	M	M	L	—	.049
Racquetball, skilled, singles	H	M	M	M	H	M	M	.049	.078
Rock climbing	M	H	H	H	M	H	M	.033	.033
Rope skipping	H	M	H	L	H	M	M	.071	.095
Rowing	H	H	H	H	H	L	L	.032	.097
Rugby	H	M	H	M	H	M	M	.052	.097
Sailing	L	L	M	L	L	M	L	—	—
Skating, ice, roller, and in-line	M	M	H	M	M	H	M	.049	.095
Skiing, alpine	M	H	H	M	M	H	M	.039	.078
Skiing, cross-country	H	M	H	M	H	M	M	.049	.104
Soccer	H	M	H	M	H	M	M	.052	.097
Squash, skilled, singles	H	M	M	M	H	M	M	.049	.078
Stretching	L	L	L	H	L	L	L	—	—
Surfing (including swimming)	M	M	M	M	M	H	M	—	.078
Swimming	H	M	H	M	H	M	L	.032	.088
Synchronized swimming	M	M	H	H	M	H	M	.032	.052
Table tennis	M	L	M	M	M	M	L	—	.045
Tennis, skilled, singles	H	M	M	M	H	M	M	—	.071
Volleyball	M	L	M	M	M	M	M	—	.065
Walking	H	L	M	L	H	L	L	.029	.048
Water polo	H	M	H	M	H	H	M	—	.078
Water skiing	M	M	H	M	M	H	M	.039	.055
Weight training	L	H	H	H	M	L	L	—	—
Wrestling	H	H	H	H	H	H	H	.065	.094
Yoga	L	L	M	H	L	H	L	—	—

*Ratings are for the muscle groups involved.

SOURCE: Kusinitz, I., and M. Fine. 1995. *Your Guide to Getting Fit*, 3rd ed. Mountain View, Calif.: Mayfield. Copyright © 1995 by Consumers Union of U.S., Inc. Yonkers, NY 10703-1057, a nonprofit organization. Originally published in *Physical Fitness for Practically Everybody* by Kusinitz and Fine. Reprinted with permission for educational purposes only. No commercial use or reproduction permitted. www.ConsumerReports.org.

college degree in exercise physiology or physical education and certification by the American College of Sports Medicine (ACSM), National Strength and Conditioning Association (NSCA), or another professional organization. Don't seek out a person for advice simply because he or she looks fit. You can further your knowledge by reading articles by experts in fitness magazines.

Many Web sites provide fitness programs, including ongoing support and feedback via e-mail. Many of these sites charge a fee, so it is important to review the sites, decide which ones seem most appropriate, and if possible go through a free trial period before subscribing. Also remember to consider the reliability of the information at fitness Web sites, especially those that also advertise or sell products. A few popular sites are listed in For More Information at the end of the chapter.

Selecting Equipment Try to purchase the best equipment you can afford. Good equipment will enhance your enjoyment and decrease your risk of injury. Appropriate safety equipment, such as pads and helmets for in-line skating, is particularly important. If you shop around, you can often find bargains through mail-order companies and discount or used equipment stores.

Before you invest in a new piece of equipment, investigate it. Is it worth the money? Does it produce the results its proponents claim for it? Is it safe? Does it fit properly, and is it in good working order? Does it provide a genuine workout? Will you really use it? Before you buy an expensive piece of equipment, try it out at a local gym to make sure that you'll use it regularly. Also check whether you have space to use and store it at home. Ask the experts (coaches, physical educators, and sports instructors) for their opinion. Better yet, educate yourself. Every sport, from running to volleyball, has its own magazine. Expending a little effort to educate yourself will be well rewarded. Footwear is an important piece of equipment for almost any activity; see the box "Choosing Exercise Footwear" for shopping strategies.

Choosing a Fitness Center Are you thinking of becoming a member of a health club or fitness center? Be sure to choose one that has the right programs and equipment available at the times you will use them. You should feel comfortable with the classes and activities available; the age, fitness level, and dress of others in the club; and the types of music used in classes. The facility and equipment should be clean and well maintained, including the showers and lockers; the staff should be well trained and helpful. Ask for a free trial workout, a 1-day pass, or an inexpensive 1- to 2-week trial membership before committing to a long-term contract. Be wary of promotional gimmicks and high-pressure sales tactics. Also make sure the facility is certified; look for the displayed names American College of Sports Medicine (ACSM); National Strength and Conditioning Association (NSCA); American Council on Exercise (ACE); Aerobics and Fitness Association of America (AFAA); or International Health, Racquet, and Sportsclub Association (IHRSA). These trade associations have established standards to help protect consumer health, safety, and rights. Find a facility that you feel comfortable with and that meets your needs.

Eating and Drinking for Exercise

Most people do not need to change their eating habits when they begin a fitness program. Many athletes and other physically active people are lured into buying aggressively advertised vitamins, minerals, and protein supplements; but, in almost every case, a well-balanced diet contains all the energy and nutrients needed to sustain an exercise program (see Chapter 12).

A balanced diet is also the key to improving your body composition when you begin to exercise more. One of the promises of a fitness program is a decrease in body fat and an increase in muscular body mass. As mentioned earlier, the control of body fat is determined by the balance of energy in the body. If more calories are consumed than are expended through metabolism and exercise, then fat increases. If the reverse is true, fat is lost. The best way to control body fat is to follow a diet containing adequate but not excessive calories and to be physically active.

One of the most important principles to follow when exercising is to drink enough water. Your body depends on water to sustain many chemical reactions and to maintain correct body temperature. Sweating during exercise depletes the body's water supply and can lead to dehydration if fluids are not replaced. Serious dehydration can cause reduced blood volume, accelerated heart rate, elevated body temperature, muscle cramps, heat stroke, and other serious problems.

Drinking fluids before and during exercise is important to prevent dehydration and enhance performance. Thirst receptors in the brain make you want to drink fluids, but during heavy or prolonged exercise or exercise in hot weather, thirst alone isn't a good indication of how much fluid you need to drink. As a rule of thumb, drink at least 2 cups (16 ounces) of fluid 2 hours before exercise and then drink enough during exercise to match fluid loss in sweat—at least 1 cup of fluid every 20–30 minutes of exercise, more in hot weather or if you sweat heavily. To determine if you're drinking the right amount of fluid, weigh yourself before and after an exercise session: Any weight loss is due to fluid loss that needs to be replaced. Any weight gain is due to overconsumption of fluid.

Bring a bottle of water when you exercise so you can replace your fluids when they're depleted. For exercise sessions lasting less than 60–90 minutes, cool water is an excellent fluid replacement. For longer workouts, a sports drink that contains water and small amounts of electrolytes (sodium, potassium, and magnesium) and simple carbohydrates (sugar, usually in the form of sucrose or glucose) is recommended.

Managing Your Fitness Program

How can you tell when you're in shape? When do you stop improving and start maintaining? How can you stay motivated? If your program is going to become an integral part of your life, and if the principles behind it are going to serve you well in the future, these are key questions.

Consistency: The Key to Physical Improvement It is important to be able to recognize when you have achieved the level of fitness that is appropriate for you. This level will vary, of course, depending on your goals, the intensity of your program, and your natural ability. Your body gets into shape by adapting to increasing levels of physical stress. If you don't push yourself by increasing the intensity of your workout—by adding weight or running a little faster or a little longer—no change will occur in your body.

But if you subject your body to severe stress, it will break down and become distressed or injured. Overtraining (overdoing exercise) is just as bad as not exercising hard enough. No one can become fit overnight. Your body needs time to adapt to increasingly higher levels of stress. The process of improving fitness involves a countless number of stresses and adaptations. If you feel

Critical Consumer

Footwear is perhaps the most important item of equipment for most activities. Shoes protect and support your feet and improve your traction. When you jump or run, you place as much as six times more force on your feet than when you stand still. Shoes can help cushion against the stress that this additional force places on your lower legs, thereby preventing injuries. Some athletic shoes are also designed to help prevent ankle rollover, another common source of injury.

General Guidelines

When choosing athletic shoes, first consider the activity you've chosen for your exercise program. Shoes appropriate for different activities have very different characteristics. For example, running shoes typically have highly cushioned midsoles, rubber outsoles with elevated heels, and a great deal of flexibility in the forefoot. The heels of walking shoes tend to be lower, less padded, and more beveled than those designed for running. For aerobic dance, shoes must be flexible in the forefoot and have straight, nonflared heels to allow for safe and easy lateral movements. Court shoes also provide substantial support for lateral movements; they typically have outsoles made from white rubber that will not damage court surfaces.

Also consider the location and intensity of your workouts. If you plan to walk or run on trails, choose shoes with water-resistant, highly durable uppers and more outsole traction. If you work out intensely or have a relatively high body weight, you'll need thick, firm midsoles to avoid bottoming-out the cushioning system of your shoes.

Foot type is another important consideration. If your feet tend to roll inward excessively, you may need shoes with additional stability features on their inner side to counteract this movement. If your feet tend to roll outward excessively, you may need highly flexible and cushioned shoes that promote foot motion. For aerobic dancers with feet that tend to roll inward or outward, mid-cut to high-cut shoes may be more appropriate than low-cut aerobic shoes or cross-trainers (shoes designed to be worn for several different activities). Compared with men, women have narrower feet overall and narrower heels relative to the forefoot. Most women will get a better fit if they choose shoes that are specifically designed for women's feet rather than those that are downsized versions of men's shoes.

Successful Shopping

For successful shoe shopping, keep the following strategies in mind:

- Shop at an athletic shoe or specialty store that has personnel trained to fit athletic shoes and a large selection of styles and sizes.

- Shop late in the day or, ideally, following a workout. Your foot size increases over the course of the day and as a result of exercise.

- Wear socks like those you plan to wear during exercise. If you have an old pair of athletic shoes, bring them with you. The wear pattern on your old shoes can help you select a pair with extra support or cushioning in the places you need it the most.

- Ask for help. Trained salespeople know which shoes are designed for your foot type and your level of activity. They can also help fit your shoes properly.

- Don't insist on buying shoes in what you consider to be your typical shoe size. Sizes vary from shoe to shoe. In addition, foot sizes change over time, and many people have one foot that is larger or wider than the other. Try several sizes in several widths, if necessary. Don't buy shoes that are too small.

- Try on both shoes, and wear them for 10 or more minutes. Try walking on a noncarpeted surface. Approximate the movements of your activity: walk, jog, run, jump, and so on.

- Check the fit and style carefully:

   Is the toe box roomy enough? Your toes will spread out when your foot hits the ground or you push off. There should be at least one thumb's width of space from the longest toe to the end of the toe box.

   Do the shoes have enough cushioning? Do your feet feel supported when you bounce up and down? Try bouncing on your toes and on your heels.

   Do your heels fit snugly into the shoe? Do they stay put when you walk, or do they rise up?

   Are the arches of your feet right on top of the shoes' arch supports?

   Do the shoes feel stable when you twist and turn on the balls of your feet? Try twisting from side to side while standing on one foot.

   Do you feel any pressure points?

- If the shoes are not comfortable in the store, don't buy them. Don't expect athletic shoes to stretch over time in order to fit your feet properly.

- Replace athletic shoes about every 3 months or 300–500 miles of jogging or walking.

Collar
Upper
Toe box
Notched
Heel counter
Midsole
Outsole

Assess Yourself

The 1.5-Mile Run-Walk Test

You can obtain a general rating of your cardiorespiratory fitness by taking the 1.5-mile run-walk test. Don't attempt this test unless you have completed at least 6 weeks of some type of conditioning activity. Also, if you are over age 35 or have questions about your health, check with your physician before taking this test.

You'll need a stopwatch, clock, or watch with a second hand and a running track or course that is flat and provides measurements of up to 1.5 miles. You may want to practice pacing yourself prior to taking the test to avoid going too fast at the start and becoming fatigued before you finish. Allow yourself a day or two to recover from a practice run before taking the test.

Warm up before taking the test with some walking, easy jogging, and stretching exercises. The idea is to cover the distance as fast as possible, at a pace that is comfortable for you. You can run or walk the entire distance or use some combination of running and walking. If possible, monitor your own pace, or have someone call out your time at various intervals to help you determine whether your pace is correct. When you have completed the test, refer to the table for your cardiorespiratory fitness rating. Be sure to cool down by walking or jogging slowly for about 5 minutes.

Standards for the 1.5-Mile Run-Walk Test (minutes:seconds)

	Superior	Excellent	Good	Fair	Poor	Very Poor
Women						
Age: 18–29	11:00 or less	11:15–12:45	13:00–14:15	14:30–15:45	16:00–17:30	17:45 or more
30–39	11:45 or less	12:00–13:30	13:45–15:15	15:30–16:30	16:45–18:45	19:00 or more
40–49	12:45 or less	13:00–14:30	14:45–16:30	16:45–18:30	18:45–20:45	21:00 or more
50–59	14:15 or less	14:30–16:30	16:45–18:30	18:45–20:30	20:45–23:00	23:15 or more
60 and over	14:00 or less	14:15–17:15	17:30–20:15	20:30–22:45	23:00–24:45	25:00 or more
Men						
Age: 18–29	9:15 or less	9:30–10:30	10:45–11:45	12:00–12:45	13:00–14:00	14:15 or more
30–39	9:45 or less	10:00–11:00	11:15–12:15	12:30–13:30	13:45–14:45	15:00 or more
40–49	10:00 or less	10:15–11:45	12:00–13:00	13:15–14:15	14:30–16:00	16:15 or more
50–59	10:45 or less	11:00–12:45	13:00–14:15	14:30–15:45	16:00–17:45	18:00 or more
60 and over	11:15 or less	11:30–13:45	14:00–15:45	16:00–17:45	18:00–20:45	21:00 or more

SOURCES: Formula for maximal oxygen consumption taken from McArdle, W. D., F. I. Katch, and V. L. Katch. 1991. *Exercise Physiology: Energy, Nutrition, and Human Performance.* Philadelphia: Lea & Febiger, pp. 225–226. Ratings based on norms from The *Physical Fitness Specialist Certification Manual,* The Cooper Institute, Dallas, TX, revised 2005. Used with permission.

extremely sore and tired the day after exercising, then you have worked too hard. Injury will slow you down just as much as a missed workout.

Consistency is the key to getting into shape without injury. Steady fitness improvement comes when you overload your body consistently over a long period of time. The best way to ensure consistency is to keep a training journal in which you record the details of your workouts: how far you ran, how much weight you lifted, how many laps you swam, and so on. This record will help you evaluate your progress and plan your workout sessions intelligently. Don't increase your exercise volume by more than 5–10% per week.

Assessing Your Fitness When are you in shape? It depends. One person may be out of shape running a mile in 5 minutes; another may be in shape running a mile in 12 minutes. As mentioned earlier, your ultimate

level of fitness depends on your goals, your program, and your natural ability. The important thing is to set goals that make sense for you.

If you are interested in finding out exactly how fit you are before you begin a program, the best approach is to get an assessment from a sports medicine laboratory. Such laboratories can be found in university physical education departments and medical centers. Here you will receive an accurate profile of your capacity to exercise. Typically, your endurance will be measured on a treadmill or bicycle, your body fat will be estimated, and your strength and flexibility will be tested. This evaluation will reveal whether your physical condition is consistent with good health, and the staff members at the laboratory can suggest an exercise program that will be appropriate for your level of fitness. To assess your own approximate level of cardiorespiratory endurance, take the test in the box "The 1.5-Mile Run-Walk Test."

Table 13-3 Care of Common Exercise Injuries and Discomforts

Injury	Symptoms	Treatment
Blister	Accumulation of fluid in one spot under the skin	Don't pop or drain it unless it interferes too much with your daily activities. If it does pop, clean the area with antiseptic and cover with a bandage. Do not remove the skin covering the blister.
Bruise (contusion)	Pain, swelling, and discoloration	R-I-C-E: rest, ice, compression, elevation.
Joint sprain	Pain, tenderness, swelling, discoloration, and loss of function	R-I-C-E; apply heat when swelling has disappeared. Stretch and strengthen the affected area.
Muscle cramp	Painful, spasmodic muscle contractions	Gently stretch for 15–30 seconds at a time, and/or massage the cramped area. Drink fluids.
Muscle soreness or stiffness	Pain and tenderness in the affected muscle	Stretch the affected muscle gently; exercise at a low intensity; apply heat.
Muscle strain	Pain, tenderness, swelling, and loss of strength in the affected muscle	R-I-C-E; apply heat when swelling has disappeared. Stretch and strengthen the affected area.
Shin splints	Pain and tenderness on the front of the lower leg; sometimes also pain in the calf muscle	Rest; apply ice to the affected area several times a day and before exercise; wrap with tape for support. Stretch and strengthen muscles in the lower legs. Purchase good-quality footwear, and run on soft surfaces.
Side stitch	Pain on the side of the abdomen	Stretch the arm on the affected side as high as possible; if that doesn't help, try bending forward while tightening the abdominal muscles.

SOURCE: Fahey, T. D., P. M. Insel, and W. T. Roth. 2005. *Fit and Well: Core Concepts and Labs in Physical Fitness and Wellness*, 6th ed. New York: McGraw-Hill. Copyright © 2005 The McGraw-Hill Companies, Inc. Reprinted with permission.

Preventing and Managing Athletic Injuries

Although annoying, most injuries are neither serious nor permanent. However, an injury that is not cared for properly can escalate into a chronic problem. It is important to learn how to deal with injuries so they don't derail your fitness program (Table 13-3).

Some injuries require medical attention. Consult a physician for head and eye injuries, possible ligament injuries, broken bones, and internal disorders such as chest pain, fainting, and intolerance to heat. Also seek medical attention for apparently minor injuries that do not get better within a reasonable amount of time.

For minor cuts and scrapes, stop the bleeding and clean the wound with soap and water. Treat soft tissue injuries (muscles and joints) with the R-I-C-E principle:

Rest: Stop using the injured area as soon as you experience pain, protect it from further injury, and avoid any activity that causes pain.

Ice: Apply ice to the injured area to reduce swelling and alleviate pain. Apply ice immediately for 10–20 minutes, and repeat every few hours until the swelling disappears. Let the injured part return to normal temperature between icings, and do not apply ice to one area for more than 20 minutes (10 minutes if you are using a cold gel pack).

Compression: Wrap the injured area with an elastic or compression bandage between icings. If the area starts throbbing or begins to change color, the bandage may be wrapped too tightly. Do not sleep with the bandage on.

Elevation: Raise the injured area above heart level to decrease the blood supply and reduce swelling.

After about 36–48 hours, apply heat, if the swelling has completely disappeared, to help relieve pain, relax muscles, and reduce stiffness. Immerse the affected area in warm water or apply warm compresses, a hot water bottle, or a heating pad.

After a minor athletic injury, gradually reintroduce the stress of the activity until you are capable of returning to full intensity. Before returning to full exercise participation, you should have a full range of motion in your joints; normal strength and balance among your muscles;

no injury-compensation movements, such as limping; and little or no pain.

To prevent injuries in the future, follow a few basic guidelines:

1. Stay in condition; haphazard exercise programs invite injury.

2. Warm up thoroughly before exercise.

3. Use proper body mechanics when lifting objects or executing sports skills.

4. Don't exercise when you're ill or overtrained (experiencing extreme fatigue due to overexercising).

5. Use the proper equipment.

6. Don't return to your normal exercise program until athletic injuries have healed.

You can minimize the risk of injury by following safety guidelines, using proper technique and equipment, respecting signals from your body that something may be wrong, and treating any injuries that occur. Warm up, cool down, and drink plenty of fluids before, during, and after exercise. Use special caution in extreme heat or humidity (over 80°F and/or 60% humidity): Exercise slowly, rest frequently in the shade, wear clothing that "breathes," and drink plenty of fluids; slow down or stop if you begin to feel uncomfortable. During hot weather, it's best to exercise in the early morning or evening, when temperatures are lowest.

Staying with Your Program   Once you have attained your desired level of fitness, you can maintain it by exercising regularly at a consistent intensity, 3 to 5 days a week. You must work at the intensity that brought you to your desired fitness level. If you don't, your body will become less fit because less is expected of it. In general, if you exercise at the same intensity over a long period, your fitness will level out and can be maintained easily.

Adapt your program to changes in environment or schedule. Don't use wet weather or a new job as an excuse to give up your fitness program. If you walk in the summer, dress appropriately and walk in the winter as well. (Exercise is usually safe even in very cold temperatures as long as you dress warmly in layers and don't stay out too long.) If you can't go out because of darkness or an unsafe neighborhood, walk in a local shopping mall or on campus or join a gym and walk on a treadmill. Changes in your job or family situation can

It makes sense to choose activities that will add enjoyment to your life for years to come. In this group of older people, we can see the rewards of a lifetime of fitness and smart exercise habits.

also affect your exercise program. Remember that physical activity is important for your energy level, self-esteem, and well-being. You owe it to yourself to include physical activity in your day. Try to exercise before going to work or to do some physical activity during your lunch hour—even if it's only a short walk or a few trips up and down the stairs.

What if you run out of steam? Although good health is an important *reason* to exercise, it's a poor *motivator* for consistent adherence to an exercise program. A variety of specific suggestions for staying with your program are given in the box "Maintaining Your Exercise Program" and in the Behavior Change Strategy at the end of the chapter. It's a good idea to have a meaningful goal, anything from fitting into the same-size jeans you used to wear to successfully skiing down a new slope.

Varying your program is another key strategy. Some people alternate two or more activities—swimming and jogging, for example—to improve a particular component of fitness. The practice, called **cross-training**, can help prevent boredom and overuse injuries. Explore many exercise options. Consider competitive sports at the recreational level: swimming, running, racquetball, volleyball, golf, and so on. Find out how you can participate in an activity you've never done before: canoeing, hang gliding, windsurfing, backpacking. Try new activities, especially ones that you will be able to do for the rest of your life. Get maps of the recreational or wilderness areas near you, and go exploring. Fill a canteen, pack a good lunch, and take along a wildflower or bird book. Every step you take will bring you closer to your ultimate goal—fitness and wellness that last a lifetime.

Term

cross-training Participating in two or more activities to develop a particular component of fitness.

Take Charge

- *Set realistic goals.* Unrealistically high goals will only discourage you.

- *Sign a contract and keep a fitness journal.* A journal can help keep your program on track, identify sources of problems, and give you a continuing sense of accomplishment.

- *Start slowly, and increase your intensity and duration gradually.* Overzealous exercising can result in discouraging discomforts and injuries. Your program is meant to last a lifetime. The important first step is to break your established pattern of inactivity.

- *Make your program fun.* Participate in a variety of different activities that you enjoy. Vary the routes you take walking, running, or biking.

- *Exercise with a friend.* The social side of exercise is an important factor for many regular exercisers.

- *Focus on the positive.* Concentrate on the improvements you obtain from your program, how good you feel during and after exercise.

- *Revisit and revise.* If your program turns out to be unrealistic, revise it. Expect to make many adjustments in your program along the way.

- *Expect fluctuation.* On some days your progress will be excellent, whereas on others you'll barely be able to drag yourself through your scheduled activities.

- *Expect lapses.* Don't let lapses discourage you or make you feel guilty. Instead, feel a renewed commitment to your exercise program.

- *Plan ahead for difficult situations.* Think about what circumstances might make it tough to keep up with your fitness routine, and develop strategies for sticking with your program. For example, devise a plan for your program during vacation, travel, bad weather, and so on.

- *Reward yourself.* Give yourself frequent rewards for sticking with your program.

- *Renew your attitude.* If you notice you're slacking off, try to list the negative thoughts and behaviors that are causing noncompliance. Devise a strategy to decrease the frequency of negative thoughts and behaviors. Make changes in your program plan and reward system to help renew your enthusiasm and commitment.

- *Review your goals.* Visualize what it will be like to reach them, and keep these pictures in your mind as an incentive to stick to your program.

Tips for Today

Physical activity and exercise offer benefits in nearly every area of wellness, helping you generate energy, manage stress, control your weight, improve your mood, and, of course, become physically stronger and healthier. Building a program of regular exercise into your life is well worth the effort, even if it seems complicated or difficult at first. Even a low-to-moderate level of activity provides valuable health benefits. The important thing is to get moving: When in doubt, exercise!

Right now you can

- Get up and stretch.

- Go outside and take a brisk walk.

- Look at your calendar for the rest of the week and write in some physical activity—such as walking, running, biking, skating, swimming, hiking, or playing Frisbee—on as many days as you can; schedule the activity for a specific time, and stick to it.

- If you don't yet use the gym or fitness facility on your campus, go there now and begin planning how to use it.

- Call a friend and invite him or her to start a regular exercise program with you.

SUMMARY

- The five components of physical fitness most important to health are cardiorespiratory endurance, muscular strength, muscular endurance, flexibility, and body composition.

- Exercise improves the functioning of the heart and the ability of the cardiorespiratory system to carry oxygen to the body's tissues. It also increases the efficiency of the body's metabolism and improves body composition.

- Exercise lowers the risk of cardiovascular disease by improving blood fat levels, reducing high blood pressure, and interfering with the disease process that causes coronary artery blockage.

- Exercise reduces the risk of cancer, osteoporosis, and diabetes. It improves immune function and psychological health and helps prevent injuries and low-back pain.

- Everyone should accumulate at least 30–60 minutes per day of moderate endurance-type physical activity. Additional health and fitness benefits can be achieved through longer or more vigorous activity.

- Cardiorespiratory endurance exercises stress a large portion of the body's muscle mass. Endurance exercise should be performed 3–5 days per week for a total of 20–60 minutes per day. Intensity can be evaluated by measuring the heart rate.

Behavior Change Strategy

Although most people recognize the importance of incorporating exercise into their lives, many find it difficult to do. No single strategy will work for everyone, but the general steps outlined here should help you create an exercise program that fits your goals, preferences, and lifestyle. A carefully designed contract and program plan can help you convert your vague wishes into a detailed plan of action. And the strategies for program compliance outlined here and in Chapter 1 can help you enjoy and stick with your program for the rest of your life.

Step 1: Set Goals

Setting specific goals to accomplish by exercising is an important first step in a successful fitness program because it establishes the direction you want to take. Your goals might be specifically related to health, such as lowering your blood pressure and risk of heart disease, or they might relate to other aspects of your life, such as improving your tennis game or the fit of your clothes. If you can decide why you're starting to exercise, it can help you keep going.

Think carefully about your reasons for incorporating exercise into your life, and then fill in the goals portion of the Personal Fitness Contract.

Step 2: Select Activities

As discussed in the chapter, the success of your fitness program depends on the consistency of your involvement. Select activities that encourage your commitment: The right program will be its own incentive to continue; poor activity choices provide obstacles and can turn exercise into a chore.

When choosing activities for your fitness program, consider the following:

- Is this activity fun? Will it hold my interest over time?

- Will this activity help me reach the goals I have set?

- Will my current fitness and skill level enable me to participate fully in this activity?

- Can I easily fit this activity into my daily schedule? Are there any special requirements (facilities, partners, equipment, etc.) that I must plan for?

- Can I afford any special costs required for equipment or facilities?

- If you have special exercise needs due to a particular health problem: Does this activity conform to those exercise needs? Will it enhance my ability to cope with my specific health problem?

Refer to Table 13-2, which summarizes the fitness benefits and other characteristics of many activities. Using the guidelines listed above, select a number of sports and activities. Fill in the Program Plan portion of the Fitness Contract, using Table 13-2 to include the fitness components your choices will develop and the frequency, intensity, and time standard you intend to meet for each activity. Does your program meet the criteria of a complete fitness program discussed in the chapter?

Step 3: Make a Commitment

Complete your Fitness Contract and Program Plan by signing your contract and having it witnessed and signed by some-

one who can help make you accountable for your progress. By completing a written contract, you will make a firm commitment and will be more likely to follow through until you meet your goals.

Step 4: Begin and Maintain Your Program

Start out slowly to allow your body time to adjust. Be realistic and patient—meeting your goals will take time. The following guidelines may help you start and stick with your program:

- Set aside regular periods for exercise. Choose times that fit in best with your schedule, and stick to them. Allow an adequate amount of time for warm-up, cool-down, and a shower.

- Take advantage of any opportunity for exercise that presents itself (for example, walk to class, take the stairs instead of the elevator).

- Do what you can to avoid boredom. Do stretching exercises or jumping jacks to music, or watch the evening news while riding your stationary bicycle.

- Exercise with a group that shares your goals and general level of competence.

- Vary the program. Change your activities periodically. Alter your route or distance if biking or jogging. Change racquetball partners, or find a new volleyball court.

- Establish minigoals or a point system, and work rewards into your program. Until you reach your main goals, a series of small-rewards will help you stick with your program. Rewards should be things you enjoy that are easily obtainable.

- Warming up before exercising and cooling down afterward improve your performance and decrease your chances of injury.

- Exercises that develop muscular strength and endurance involve exerting force against a significant resistance. A strength training program for general fitness typically involves one set of 8–12 repetitions of 8–10 exercises, 2 or 3 days per week.

- A good stretching program includes exercises for all the major muscle groups and joints of the body. Do a series of active, static stretches (possibly with a passive assist) 2 or more days per week. Hold each stretch for 10–30 seconds; do at least four repetitions. Stretch when muscles are warm.

- Instructors, equipment, and facilities should be chosen carefully to enhance enjoyment and prevent injuries.

- A well-balanced diet contains all the energy and nutrients needed to sustain a fitness program. When exercising, remember to drink enough fluids.

- Rest, ice, compression, and elevation (R-I-C-E) are treatments for muscle and joint injuries.

- A desired level of fitness can be maintained by exercising 3 to 5 days a week at a consistent intensity.

- Strategies for maintaining an exercise program over the long term include having meaningful goals, varying the program, and trying new activities.

Personal Fitness Contract

I, _____, am contracting with myself to follow an exercise program to work at the following goals. I will begin my program on _____ .

Fitness Goals

1. _____   4. _____
2. _____   5. _____
3. _____   6. _____

Program Plan

Activities	Components (Check ✔)			Frequency (Check ✔)									Intensity	Time
	CRE	MS	ME	F	BC	M	Tu	W	Th	F	Sa	Su		
1. _____														
2. _____														
3. _____														
4. _____														
5. _____														

Note: You should conduct activities for achieving CRE goals at your target heart rate.

I agree to maintain a record of my activity, assess my progress periodically, and, if necessary, revise my goals.

Signed _____   Date _____

Witness _____

Step 5: Record and Assess Your Progress

Keeping a record that notes the daily results of your program will help remind you of your ongoing commitment to your program and give you a sense of accomplishment. Create daily and weekly program logs that you can use to track your progress. Record the activity frequency, intensity, time, and type. Keep your log handy, and fill it in immediately after each exercise session. Post it in a visible place to remind you of your activity schedule and to provide incentive for improvement.

SOURCE: Adapted from Kusinitz, I., and M. Fine. 1995. *Your Guide to Getting Fit*, 3rd ed. Mountain View, Calif.: Mayfield.

Take Action

1. **Investigate campus resources:** Go to your school's physical education office and ask for a comprehensive listing of all the exercise and fitness facilities available on your campus. Visit the facilities you haven't yet seen, and investigate the activities that take place there. If there are sports or activities you'd like to try, consider doing so.

2. **Investigate community resources:** Investigate the fitness clubs in your community. How do they compare with one another? How do they measure up in terms of the guidelines provided in this chapter?

3. **Count your steps:** One way to monitor physical activity is to purchase and wear a pedometer to count your daily steps. To begin, wear the pedometer for a week and determine your typical level of activity (average steps per day). Then record the number of steps you take during 10 minutes of brisk walking; three times that number would represent the Surgeon General's minimum of 30 minutes of brisk walking per day. With these numbers in mind, set a daily goal for physical activity, and continue to track and record your daily steps.

Books

Anderson, B., and J. Anderson. 2003. *Stretching,* 20th anniv. ed. Bolinas, Calif.: Shelter Publications. *Updated edition of a classic, with more than 200 stretches for 60 sports and activities.*

Bahrke, M., and C. Yesalis. 2002. *Performance-Enhancing Substances in Sport Exercise.* Champaign, Ill.: Human Kinetics. *Provides up-to-date coverage of the issues surrounding supplements as well as the current state of research on major types of supplements and their effects on athletic performance.*

Fahey, T. 2005. *Weight Training Basics.* New York: McGraw-Hill. *Weight training and plyometric exercises for fitness, weight control, and improved sports performance.*

Fahey, T., P. Insel, and W. Roth. 2005. *Fit and Well: Core Concepts and Labs in Physical Fitness and Wellness,* 6th ed. New York: McGraw-Hill. *A comprehensive guide to developing a complete fitness program.*

Nieman, D. C. 2007. *Exercise Testing and Prescription. A Health-Related Approach,* 6th ed. New York: McGraw-Hill. *A comprehensive discussion of the effects of exercise and exercise testing and prescription.*

U.S. Department of Health and Human Services. 1996. *Physical Activity and Health: A Report of the Surgeon General.* Atlanta, Ga.: Department of Health and Human Services. (Also available online: http://www.cdc.gov/nccdphp/sgr/sgr.htm.) *Provides a summary of the evidence for the benefits of physical activity as well as recommendations for activity and exercise.*

VW Organizations, Hotlines, and Web Sites

American Academy of Orthopaedic Surgeons. Provides fact sheets on many fitness and sports topics, including how to begin a program, how to choose equipment, and how to prevent and treat many types of injuries.
http://orthoinfo.aaos.org

American College of Sports Medicine. Provides brochures, publications, and audio- and videotapes on the positive effects of exercise.
317-637-9200
http://www.acsm.org

American Council on Exercise. Promotes exercise and fitness for all Americans; the Web site features fact sheets on many consumer topics, including choosing shoes, cross-training, steroids, and getting started on an exercise program.
800-529-8227
http://www.acefitness.org

American Heart Association: Just Move. Provides practical advice for people of all fitness levels plus an online fitness diary.
http://www.justmove.org

Canada's Physical Activity Guide. Offers many suggestions for incorporating physical activity into everyday life; also includes the Physical Activity Readiness Questionnaire (PAR-Q) to assess safety of exercise.
http://www.hc-sc.gc.ca/pau-uap/paguide

CDC Physical Activity Information. Provides information on the benefits of physical activity and suggestions for incorporating moderate physical activity into daily life.
http://www.cdc.gov/nccdphp/dnpa

Disabled Sports USA. Provides sport and recreation services to people with physical or mobility disorders.
http://www.dsusa.org

Exercise: A Guide from the National Institute on Aging and the National Aeronautics and Space Administration. Provides practical advice on fitness for seniors; includes animated instructions for specific weight training and flexibility exercises.
http://weboflife.ksc.nasa.gov/exerciseandaging/toc.html

Federal Trade Commission: Consumer Protection—Diet, Health, and Fitness. Provides several brochures with consumer advice about purchasing exercise equipment.
http://www.ftc.gov/bcp/menu-health.htm

Georgia State University: Exercise and Physical Fitness Page. Provides information about the benefits of exercise and how to get started on a fitness program.
http://www.gsu.edu/~wwwfit

Mayo Clinic Healthy Living Centers. Select the Fitness and Sports Medicine Health Living Center for more information on incorporating physical activity and exercise into your daily life.
http://www.MayoClinic.com/findinformation/
healthylivingcenter/index.cfm

MedlinePlus: Exercise and Physical Fitness. Provides links to news and reliable information about fitness and exercise from government agencies and professional associations.
http://www.nlm.nih.gov/medlineplus/exercisephysicalfitness.
html

National Institute on Drug Abuse: Anabolic Steroid Abuse. Provides information and links about the dangers of anabolic steroids.
http://www.steroidabuse.org

President's Council on Physical Fitness and Sports (PCPFS). Provides information on PCPFS programs and publications.
http://www.fitness.gov
http://www.presidentschallenge.org

SmallStep.Gov. Provides resources for increasing activity and improving diet through small changes in daily habits.
http://www.smallstep.gov

World Health Organization (WHO): Move for Health. Provides information about the WHO initiative to promote increased physical activity.
http://www.who.int/moveforhealth/en/

Commercial Web sites that feature fitness and nutrition programs include the following:

iShape
http://www.ishape.com
My Exercise Plan
http://www.myexerciseplan.com
Nutricise
http://www.nutricise.com

Web sites with links to information on a wide variety of activities and fitness issues include the following:

Fitness Partner Connection Jumpsite
http://www.primusweb.com/fitnesspartner
NetSweat: The Internet's Fitness Resource
http://www.netsweat.com
Yahoo! Recreation and Sports
http://dir.yahoo.com/Health/Fitness

See also the listings for Chapters 12, 14, and 15.

Akalan, C., L. Kravitz, and R. R. Roberts. 2004. VO$_{2max}$: Essentials of the most widely used test in exercise physiology. *ACSM's Health and Fitness Journal,* May/June.

American Cancer Society. 2005. *Cancer Prevention and Early Detection: Facts and Figures 2005.* Atlanta, Ga.: American Cancer Society.

American College of Sports Medicine. 2004. Position Stand: Physical activity and bone health. *Medicine and Science in Sports and Exercise* 36(11): 1985–1996.

American College of Sports Medicine. 2002. How much exercise is enough? Responding to the IOM report on dietary guidelines. *Sports Medicine Bulletin* 37(6): 5–6.

American Heart Association. 2005. *Heart Disease and Stroke Statistics—2005 Update.* Dallas: American Heart Association.

Brooks, G. A., et al. 2005. *Exercise Physiology: Human Bioenergetics and Its Applications,* 4th ed. New York: McGraw-Hill.

Brownson, R. C., T. K. Boehmer, and D. A. Luke. 2005. Declining rates of physical activity in the United States: What are the contributors? *Annual Review of Public Health* 26: 421–443.

Centers for Disease Control and Prevention. 2003. Prevalence of no leisure time physical activity. *Morbidity and Mortality Weekly Report* 53(4): 82–86.

Centers for Disease Control and Prevention. 2004. *Improving Nutrition and Increasing Physical Activity* (http://www.cdc.gov/nccdphp/bb_nutrition/index.htm; retrieved December 30, 2004).

Colbert, L. H., et al. 2004. Physical activity, exercise, and inflammatory markers in older adults: Findings from the health, aging and body composition study. *Journal of the American Geriatrics Society* 52: 1098–1104.

Cussler, E. C., et al. 2003. Weight lifted in strength training predicts bone change in postmenopausal women. *Medicine and Science in Sports and Exercise* 35(1): 10–17.

Dickey, C., and A. K. White. 2003. How many minutes a day? *ACSM's Health and Fitness Journal,* January/February.

Diet and fitness support, online. 2004. *Consumer Reports on Health,* October.

Dietrich A., and W. F. McDaniel. 2004. Endocannabinoids and exercise. *British Journal of Sports Medicine* 38: 536–541.

Dugan, S. 2005. Safe exercise for women. *ACSM Fit Society Page,* Winter.

Dunn, A. L., et al. 2005. Exercise treatment for depression: Efficacy and dose response. *American Journal of Preventive Medicine* 28(1): 1–8.

Evenson, K. R., et al. 2003. The effect of cardiorespiratory fitness and obesity on cancer mortality in women and men. *Medicine and Science in Sports and Exercise* 35(2): 270–277.

Fahey, T. D., P. M. Insel, and W. T. Roth. 2005. *Fit and Well: Core Concepts and Labs in Physical Fitness and Wellness,* 6th ed. New York: McGraw-Hill.

Fenicchia, L. M., et al. 2004. Influence of resistance exercise training on glucose control in women with type 2 diabetes. *Metabolism* 53(3): 284–289.

Food and Drug Administration. 2004. *Questions and Answers: Androstenedione* (http://cfsan.fda.gov/~androqa.html; retrieved April 8, 2004).

Food and Nutrition Board, Institute of Medicine, National Academies. 2002. *Dietary Reference Intakes for Energy, Carbohydrates, Fiber, Fat, Protein and Amino Acids (Macronutrients).* Washington, D.C.: National Academy Press.

Gleeson, M., D. C. Nieman, and B. K. Pedersen. 2004. Exercise, nutrition, and immune function. *Journal of Sports Science* 22(1): 115–125.

Green, J. S., et al. 2004. The effects of exercise training on abdominal visceral fat, body composition, and indicators of the metabolic syndrome in postmenopausal women with and without estrogen replacement therapy. *Metabolism* 53: 1192–1196.

Hulens, M., et al. 2002. Health-related quality of life in physically active and sedentary obese women. *American Journal of Human Biology* 14: 777–785.

Is easy-does-it exercise enough? 2004. *Consumer Reports on Health,* 2004.

John, E. M., P. L. Horn-Ross, and J. Koo. 2004. Lifetime physical activity and breast cancer risk in a multiethnic population. *Cancer Epidemiology, Biomarkers & Prevention* 12(11 Pt 1): 1143–1152.

Joint WHO/FAO Expert Consultation. 2003. *Diet, Nutrition, and the Prevention of Chronic Diseases.* Geneva: World Health Organization.

LaMonte, M. J., et al. 2002. Cardiorespiratory fitness and C-reactive protein among a tri-ethnic sample of women. *Circulation* 106(4): 403–406.

Laukkanen, J. A., S. Kurl, and J. T. Salonen. 2002. Cardiorespiratory fitness and physical activity as risk predictors of future atherosclerotic cardiovascular diseases. *Current Atherosclerosis Reports* 4: 468–476.

Lee, I. M., and R. S. Paffenbarger. 2000. Associations of light, moderate, and vigorous intensity physical activity with longevity. The Harvard Alumni Health Study. *American Journal of Epidemiology* 151(3): 293–299.

Le Masurier, G. C. 2004. Walk which way? *ACSM's Health and Fitness Journal,* January/February.

Pescatello, L. S., et al. 2004. American College of Sports Medicine Position Stand: Exercise and hypertension. *Medicine and Science in Sports and Exercise* 36(3): 533–553.

Rollo, I. 2004. Understanding the role of exercise in health promotion. *Nursing Times* 100: 36–38.

Salmon, P. 2001. Effects of physical exercise on anxiety, depression, and sensitivity to stress. *Clinical Psychology Review* 21(1): 33–61.

Sheel, A. W., et al. 2004. Sex differences in respiratory exercise physiology. *Sports Medicine* 34: 567–579.

Shekelle, P. G., et al. 2003. Efficacy and safety of ephedra and ephedrine for weight loss and athletic performance: A meta-analysis. *Journal of the American Medical Association* 289(12): 1537–1545.

Slattery, J. L. 2004. Physical activity and colorectal cancer. *Sports Medicine* 34(4): 239–252.

Stewart, K. J. 2004. Exercise training: Can it improve cardiovascular health in patients with type 2 diabetes? *British Journal of Sports Medicine* 38: 250–252.

Tanasescu, M., et al. 2002. Exercise type and intensity in relation to coronary heart disease in men. *Journal of the American Medical Association* 288(16): 1994–2000.

Thacker, S. B., et al. 2004. The impact of stretching on sports injury risk: A systematic review of the literature. *Medicine and Science in Sports and Exercise* 36(3): 371–378.

U.S. Department of Health and Human Services. 2005. *Dietary Guidelines for Americans, 2005* (http://www.healthierus.gov/dietaryguidelines; retrieved February 12, 2005).

Weuve, J., et al. 2004. Physical activity, including walking, and cognitive function in older women. *Journal of the American Medical Association* 292(12): 1454–461.

Wittink, H., et al. 2002. The association of pain with aerobic fitness in patients with chronic low back pain. *Archives of Physical Medicine and Rehabilitation* 83: 1467–1471.

Wong, S. L., et al. 2004. Cardiorespiratory fitness is associated with lower abdominal fat independent of body mass index. *Medicine and Science in Sports and Exercise* 36(2): 286–291.

World Health Organization. 2004. *Physical Activity* (http://www.who.int/dietphysicalactivity/publications/facts/pa/en; retrieved May 24, 2004).

14

After reading this chapter, you should be able to

- Discuss different methods for assessing body weight and body composition

- Explain the health risks associated with overweight and obesity

- Explain factors that may contribute to a weight problem, including genetic, physiological, lifestyle, and psychosocial factors

- Describe lifestyle factors that contribute to weight gain and loss, including the roles of diet, exercise, and emotional factors

- Identify and describe the symptoms of eating disorders and the health risks associated with them

- Design a personal plan for successfully managing body weight

Weight Management

1. **About what percentage of American adults are overweight?**
   a. 15%
   b. 35%
   c. 65%

2. **Genetic factors explain most cases of obesity.**
   True or false?

3. **The consumption of low-calorie sweeteners has helped Americans control their weight.**
   True or false?

4. **Approximately how many female high school and college students have either anorexia or bulimia?**
   a. 1 in 250
   b. 1 in 100
   c. 1 in 30

5. **Which of the following is the most significant risk factor for type 2 diabetes (the most common type of diabetes)?**
   a. smoking
   b. low-fiber diet
   c. overweight or obesity
   d. inactivity

6. **People who are overweight get less sleep than people who are at a healthy body weight.**
   True or false?

ANSWERS

1. C. About 65% of American adults are overweight, including more than 30% who are obese. The rate of obesity among adults has increased more than 75% since 1990.

2. FALSE. Genetic factors may increase an individual's tendency for weight gain; however, lifestyle is the key contributing factor.

3. FALSE. Since the introduction of low-calorie sweeteners, both total calorie intake and total sugar intake have increased, as has the proportion of Americans who are overweight.

4. C. About 2–4% of female students suffer from bulimia or anorexia, and many more occasionally engage in behaviors associated with anorexia or bulimia.

5. C. All four are risk factors for diabetes, but overweight or obesity is the most significant. It's estimated that 90% of cases of type 2 diabetes could be prevented if people adopted healthy lifestyle behaviors.

6. TRUE. It is unclear if there is a cause-and-effect relationship between lack of sleep and increased body weight, but insufficient sleep may affect hormones, metabolism, and appetite. Adequate sleep may also help prevent eating in response to feelings of stress and low energy.

VW Visit the *Core Concepts in Health* Online Learning Center (www.mhhe.com/insel10e) for study aids and many additional resources.

411

Achieving and maintaining a healthy body weight is a serious public health challenge in the United States and a source of distress for many Americans. Under standards developed by the National Institutes of Health, about 65% of American adults are overweight, including more than 30% who are obese (Figure 14-1). The number of severely obese people has nearly tripled in the past decade. At this rate, by 2030, it is estimated that the entire American adult population will be overweight or obese. Lifestyle changes may be at the root of this increase (see the box "The Growing American Waistline"). And while millions struggle to lose weight, others fall into dangerous eating patterns such as binge eating or self-starvation.

Although not completely understood, managing body weight is not a mysterious process. It's simply balancing calories consumed with calories expended in daily activities—in other words, eating a moderate diet and exercising regularly. Unfortunately, this is not as exciting as the latest fad diet or "scientific breakthrough" that promises slimness without effort. Many people fail in their efforts to manage their weight because they emphasize short-term weight loss rather than permanent changes in lifestyle. Successful weight management requires the long-term coordination of many aspects of a wellness lifestyle, including proper nutrition, adequate physical activity, and stress management.

This chapter explores the factors that contribute to the development of overweight and to eating disorders. It also takes a closer look at weight management through lifestyle behaviors and suggests specific strategies for reaching and maintaining a healthy weight. The information is designed to provide the tools necessary for integrating effective weight management into a wellness lifestyle.

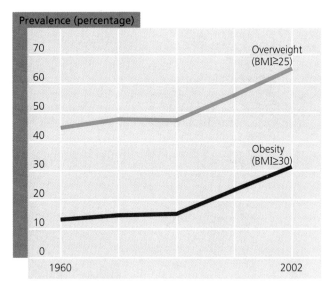

Figure 14-1 Prevalence of overweight and obesity among Americans. SOURCE: National Center for Health Statistics. 2004. *Health, United States, 2004.* Hyattsville, Md.: National Center for Health Statistics.

BASIC CONCEPTS OF WEIGHT MANAGEMENT

How many times have you or one of your friends said, "I'm too fat; I need to lose weight"? If you are like most people, you are concerned about what you weigh. But how do you decide if you are overweight? At what point does being overweight present a health risk? And how thin is too thin?

Body Composition

The human body can be divided into fat-free mass and body fat. Fat-free mass is composed of all the body's nonfat tissues: bone, water, muscle, connective tissue, organ tissues, and teeth. Body fat includes both essential and nonessential body fat. Remember that 1 pound of body fat is equal to 3500 calories. This means that having only an extra 10 calories a day will equal a 1-pound weight gain over a year; in just 10 years, this would amount to a 10-pound weight gain. **Essential fat** includes *lipids,* or fats, incorporated in the nerves, brain, heart, lungs, liver, and mammary glands. These fat deposits, crucial for normal body functioning, make up approximately 3–5% of total body weight in men and 8–12% in women. The larger percentage in women is due to fat deposits in the breasts, uterus, and other sites specific to females. Women naturally have more body fat than men because of their ability to bear children. Women tend to deposit fat in the lower body and thus develop a pear-shaped body. Men tend to deposit fat around their stomachs or abdomens, thus developing an apple-shaped body. As discussed later in the chapter, the accumulation of fat around the waist has an adverse effect on health.

Nonessential (storage) fat exists primarily within *adipose tissue,* or fat cells, often located just below the skin and around major organs. The amount of storage fat varies from person to person based on many factors, including gender, age, heredity, metabolism, diet, and activity level. When we talk about wanting to lose weight, most of us are referring to storage fat.

What is most important for health is not total weight but rather the proportion of the body's total weight that is fat—the **percent body fat.** For example, two women may both be 5 feet, 5 inches tall and weigh 130 pounds. But one woman, an endurance runner, may have only 15% of her body weight as fat, whereas the other, sedentary, woman may have 34% body fat. Although 130 pounds is not considered overweight for women of this height by most standards, the sedentary woman may be overfat. (Methods for measuring and evaluating percent body fat are presented later in this chapter.) Because most people use the word "overweight" to describe the condition of having too much body fat, we use it in this chapter, although "overfat" is actually a more accurate term.

By any measure, Americans are getting fatter. Since 1960, the average weight among adult men increased from 166 to 191 pounds; among women, from 140 to 164 pounds. The trend is also seen among young Americans: The number of overweight and obese children has more than tripled since 1960.

Along with rising rates of obesity come increased rates of obesity-related health problems, including a more than 60% rise in rates of type 2 diabetes since 1990. Inactivity and overweight may account for as many as 365,000 premature deaths annually in the United States, second only to tobacco-related deaths, and medical costs are more than $100 billion annually. Before long, rising rates of obesity may cut U.S. life expectancy.

At the same time that Americans have become fatter, more and more Americans report being unhappy with their bodies, obsessed with their weight, and on a diet. Despite widespread reports of dieting, however, the trend in body weight has been away from the *Healthy People 2010* goal of reducing the number of people who are obese to no more than 15% of adults and 5% of children and adolescents.

Contributing Factors

The basic facts of energy balance help explain the expanding American waistline: According to the CDC, average calorie intake among Americans has increased by about 250 calories per day since 1970, and levels of physical activity have declined. What are some of the factors underlying this change?

• *More meals eaten outside the home, especially fast-food meals:* Studies of adults have found that the more people eat out, the more calories they consume, especially when they choose a fast-food restaurant. One-third of American children eat fast food on any given day, and children who eat fast food consume almost 200 more calories per day than those who don't.

• *Underestimation of portion sizes and food consumption:* Many Americans underestimate the amount of food and calories they consume. When participants in one recent study were asked to report their food intake over the previous 24 hours, the majority underestimated their actual intake by about 600 calories.

• *Increased consumption of soft drinks and convenience snack foods:* Compared to 1970, Americans today consume significantly more carbohydrate, slightly more fat, and about the same amount of protein. The additional carbohydrate calories do not come from the fruits, vegetables, and whole grains recommended by health experts but rather from soft drinks, pizza, salty snacks, and desserts. Regular soft drinks are the leading source of calories in the American diet.

• *More time spent in sedentary activities:* Americans now spend far more time watching television and movies, sitting in cars, playing video games, and in other sedentary activities than they do in activities requiring more energy. We have greater numbers of labor-saving devices for household and work activities. For children, daily gym classes are no longer the norm.

Possible Solutions

Some possible strategies for improving America's food choices were outlined in Chapter 12; these include making healthy foods more attractive from a price perspective, placing consumer-friendly nutrition and serving-size information in prominent locations, restricting food advertising aimed at children, and improving food options sold on school grounds. Changes are needed at individual, family, school, community, and national levels.

Clear messages about physical activity and healthy food choices are needed from all sources, including public information campaigns, physicians, and school programs. Restaurants and food manufacturers should be encouraged to provide both more information and healthier choices and portion sizes. Support is also needed to get healthy food and activity options into communities that currently lack them. Residents of low-income and urban areas are less likely to have access to healthy foods and opportunities for safe physical activity.

As officials debate potential solutions, there are many actions you can take to manage your own weight and to promote healthy eating and activity habits among others. Refer to the suggestions in Chapters 12 and 13 as well as throughout this chapter.

SOURCES: Koplan, J. P., C. T. Liverman, and V. A. Kraak, eds. 2005. *Preventing Childhood Obesity: Health in the Balance.* Washington, D.C.: National Academy Press; Centers for Disease Control and Prevention. 2004. Mean body weight, height, and body mass index, United States 1960–2002. *Advance Data from Vital and Health Statistics* No. 347; Bowman, S. A., et al. 2004. Effects of fast-food consumption on energy intake and diet quality among children in a national household survey. *Pediatrics* 113(Pt 1): 112–118; Centers for Disease Control and Prevention. 2004. Trends in intake of energy and macronutrients—United States, 1971–2000. *Morbidity and Mortality Weekly Report* 53(4): 80–82.

Energy Balance

The key to keeping a healthy ratio of fat to fat-free mass is maintaining an energy balance (Figure 14-2). You take in energy (calories) from the food you eat. Your body uses energy (calories) to maintain vital body functions (resting metabolism), to digest food, and to fuel physical activity. When energy in equals energy out, you maintain your current weight. To change your

Terms

essential fat The fat in the body necessary for normal body functioning.

nonessential (storage) fat Extra fat or fat reserves stored in the body.

percent body fat The percentage of total body weight that is composed of fat.

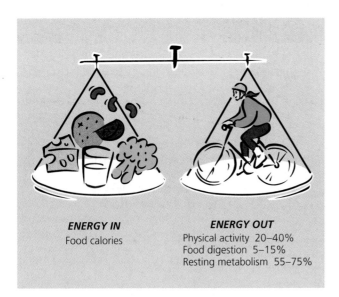

ENERGY IN
Food calories

ENERGY OUT
Physical activity 20–40%
Food digestion 5–15%
Resting metabolism 55–75%

Figure 14-2   The energy balance equation.   In order to maintain your current weight, you must burn as many calories as you take in as food each day.

weight and body composition, you must tip the energy balance equation in a particular direction. If you take in more calories daily than your body burns, the excess calories will be stored as fat, and you will gain weight over time. If you eat fewer calories than you burn each day, you will lose some of that storage fat and probably lose weight.

If we look at the energy balance equation today as expressed for the general American population, the equation is tipped heavily toward the energy-in side. Our environment is rich in large portion sizes; high-fat, high-calorie foods; and palatable, easily available, and inexpensive foods. Unfortunately, the energy-out side of the equation has not compensated for increased energy intake; instead, we've decreased work-related physical activity, decreased activity associated with daily living, and increased time spent in sedentary behaviors like TV watching and computer use.

The two parts of the energy balance equation over which you have the most control are the energy you take in as food and the energy you burn during physical activity. To create a negative energy balance and lose weight and body fat, you can increase the amount of energy you burn by increasing your level of physical activity and/or decrease the amount of energy you take in by consuming fewer calories. Specific strategies for altering energy balance are discussed later in the chapter.

Evaluating Body Weight and Body Composition

Overweight is usually defined as total body weight above the recommended range for good health (as determined by large-scale population surveys). **Obesity** is defined as

a more serious degree of overweight. Many methods are available for measuring and evaluating body weight and percent body fat; the cutoff points for defining overweight and obesity vary with the method chosen.

Height-Weight Charts   In the past, many people relied on height-weight charts to evaluate body weight. Based on insurance company statistics, these charts list a range of ideal or recommended body weights associated with the lowest mortality for people of a particular sex, age, and height. Although easy to use, height-weight charts can be highly inaccurate for some people, and they provide only an indirect measure of body fat.

Body Mass Index   Body mass index (BMI) is a measure of body weight that is useful for classifying the health risks of body weight if you don't have access to more sophisticated methods. Though more accurate than height-weight tables, BMI is also based on the concept that weight should be proportional to height. Easy to calculate and rate, BMI is a fairly accurate measure of the health risks of body weight for average people. Researchers frequently use BMI in studies that examine the health risks associated with body weight.

However, because BMI doesn't distinguish between fat weight and fat-free weight, it can be very inaccurate for some groups, including people of short stature, muscular athletes, and older adults with little muscle mass due to inactivity or an underlying disease. If you are in one of these groups, use one of the methods described in the next section for estimating percent body fat to assess whether your current weight and body composition are healthy. BMI is also not particularly useful for tracking changes in body composition—gains in muscle mass and losses of fat. Women are likely to have more body fat for a given BMI than men.

BMI is defined as body weight (in kilograms) divided by the square of height (in meters). You can determine your BMI by referring to Figure 14-3, or you can use the following short-cut formula to calculate it more precisely. The example below is for a person who is 5 feet, 6 inches tall (66 inches) and weighs 150 pounds:

1. Multiply weight (in pounds) by 704
    150 × 704 = 105,600

2. Multiply height (in inches) by height (in inches)
    66 × 66 = 4,356

3. Divide the answer in step 1 by the answer in step 2 to obtain a value for BMI.
    BMI = 105,600 ÷ 4,356 = 24.2

Under standards issued by the National Institutes of Health (NIH), a BMI between 18.5 and 24.9 is considered healthy; a person with a BMI of 25 or above is classified as overweight, and a person with a BMI of 30 or above is

	<18.5 Underweight		**18.5–24.9** Normal						**25–29.9** Overweight					**30–34.9** Obesity (Class I)					**35–39.9** Obesity (Class II)					**≥40** Extreme obesity
BMI	17	18	19	20	21	22	23	24	25	26	27	28	29	30	31	32	33	34	35	36	37	38	39	40
Height													Body Weight (pounds)											
4' 10"	81	86	91	96	101	105	110	115	120	124	129	134	139	144	148	153	158	163	168	172	177	182	187	192
4' 11"	84	89	94	99	104	109	114	119	124	129	134	139	144	149	154	159	163	168	173	178	183	188	193	198
5'	87	92	97	102	108	113	118	123	128	133	138	143	149	154	159	164	169	174	179	184	190	195	200	205
5' 1"	90	95	101	106	111	117	122	127	132	138	143	148	154	159	164	169	175	180	185	191	196	201	207	212
5' 2"	93	98	104	109	115	120	126	131	137	142	148	153	159	164	170	175	181	186	191	197	202	208	213	219
5' 3"	96	102	107	113	119	124	130	136	141	147	153	158	164	169	175	181	186	192	198	203	209	215	220	226
5' 4"	99	105	111	117	122	128	134	140	146	152	157	163	169	175	181	187	192	198	204	210	216	222	227	233
5' 5"	102	108	114	120	126	132	138	144	150	156	162	168	174	180	186	192	198	204	210	216	222	229	235	241
5' 6"	105	112	118	124	130	136	143	149	155	161	167	174	180	186	192	198	205	211	217	223	229	236	242	248
5' 7"	109	115	121	128	134	141	147	153	160	166	173	179	185	192	198	204	211	217	224	230	236	243	249	256
5' 8"	112	118	125	132	138	145	151	158	165	171	178	184	191	197	204	211	217	224	230	237	244	250	257	263
5' 9"	115	122	129	136	142	149	156	163	169	176	183	190	197	203	210	217	224	230	237	244	251	258	264	271
5' 10"	119	126	133	139	146	153	160	167	174	181	188	195	202	209	216	223	230	237	244	251	258	265	272	279
5' 11"	122	129	136	143	151	158	165	172	179	187	194	201	208	215	222	230	237	244	251	258	265	273	280	287
6'	125	133	140	148	155	162	170	177	184	192	199	207	214	221	229	236	243	251	258	266	273	280	288	295
6' 1"	129	137	144	152	159	167	174	182	190	197	205	212	220	228	235	243	250	258	265	273	281	288	296	303
6' 2"	132	140	148	156	164	171	179	187	195	203	210	218	226	234	242	249	257	265	273	281	288	296	304	312
6' 3"	136	144	152	160	168	176	184	192	200	208	216	224	232	240	248	256	264	272	280	288	296	304	312	320
6' 4"	140	148	156	164	173	181	189	197	206	214	222	230	238	247	255	263	271	280	288	296	304	312	321	329

Figure 14-3 Body mass index (BMI). To determine your BMI, find your height in the left column. Move across the appropriate row until you find the weight closest to your own. The number at the top of the column is the BMI at that height and weight. SOURCE: Ratings from National Heart, Lung, and Blood Institute. 1998. *Clinical Guidelines on the Identification, Evaluation, and Treatment of Overweight and Obesity in Adults: The Evidence Report.* Bethesda, Md.: National Institutes of Health.

classified as obese. A person with a BMI below 18.5 is classified as underweight, although low BMI values may be healthy in some cases if they are not the result of smoking, an eating disorder, or an underlying disease; a BMI of 17.5 or less is sometimes used as a diagnostic criterion for the eating disorder anorexia nervosa.

Body Composition Analysis
The most accurate and direct way to evaluate body composition is to determine percent body fat; a variety of methods are available. Refer to Table 14-1 for body composition ratings based on percent body fat; as with BMI, the percent body fat ratings indicate cutoff points for health risks associated with underweight and obesity.

HYDROSTATIC (UNDERWATER) WEIGHING One of the most accurate techniques is hydrostatic weighing. In this method, a person is submerged and weighed under water. Percent body fat can be calculated from body density. Muscle has a higher density and fat a lower density than water, so people with more fat tend to float and weigh less under water, while lean people tend to sink and weigh more under water.

SKINFOLD MEASUREMENTS The skinfold thickness technique measures the thickness of fat under the skin. A technician grasps a fold of skin at a predetermined location and measures it using a caliper. Measurements are taken at several sites and plugged into formulas that predict body fat percentages.

ELECTRICAL IMPEDANCE ANALYSIS In this method, electrodes are attached to the body and a harmless electrical current is transmitted from electrode to electrode. The electrical conduction through the body favors the path of the fat-free tissues over the fat tissues. A computer can calculate fat percentages from measurements of current.

SCANNING PROCEDURES High-tech scanning procedures are highly accurate means of assessing body composition, but they require expensive equipment. These procedures include computed tomography (CT), magnetic resonance imaging (MRI), dual-energy X-ray absorptiometry, and dual-photon absorptiometry.

Terms

overweight Body weight that falls above the range associated with minimum mortality.

obesity The condition of having an excess of nonessential body fat; having a body mass index of 30 or greater or having a percent body fat greater than about 24% for men and 38% for women.

body mass index (BMI) A measure of relative body weight that takes height into account and is highly correlated with more direct measures of body fat; calculated by dividing total body weight (in kilograms) by the square of height (in meters).

Table 14-1	Percent Body Fat Classification

	Percent Body Fat (%)		
	20–39 Years	40–59 Years	60–79 Years
Women			
Essential[a]	8–12	8–12	8–12
Low/athletic[b]	13–20	13–22	13–23
Recommended	21–32	23–33	24–35
Overfat[c]	33–38	34–39	36–41
Obese[c]	≥39	≥40	≥42
Men			
Essential[a]	3–5	3–5	3–5
Low/athletic[b]	6–7	6–10	6–12
Recommended	8–19	11–21	13–24
Overfat[c]	20–24	22–27	25–29
Obese[c]	≥25	≥28	≥30

The cutoffs for recommended, overfat, and obese ranges in this table are based on a study that linked body mass index classifications from the National Institutes of Health with predicted percent body fat (measured using dual energy X-ray absorptiometry).

[a]Essential body fat is necessary for the basic functioning of the body.
[b]Percent body fat in the low/athletic range may be appropriate for some people as long as it is not the result of illness or disordered eating habits.
[c]Health risks increase as percent body fat exceeds the recommended range.

SOURCES: Gallagher, D., et al. 2000. Healthy percentage body fat ranges: An approach for developing guidelines based on body mass index. *American Journal of Clinical Nutrition* 72: 694–701; American College of Sports Medicine. 2001. *ACSM's Resource Manual for Guidelines for Exercise Testing and Prescription*, 4th ed. Philadelphia: Lippincott, Williams & Wilkins.

Excess Body Fat and Wellness

The amount of fat in the body—and its location—can have profound effects on health.

The Health Risks of Excess Body Fat Obesity doubles mortality rates and can reduce life expectancy by 10–20 years. Obese individuals have a 50–100% increased risk of death from all causes, compared with normal weight persons. Obesity is associated with unhealthy cholesterol and triglyceride levels, impaired heart function, and death from cardiovascular disease. It is estimated that if all Americans had a healthy body composition, the incidence of coronary heart disease (CHD) would drop by more than 25%. Other health risks associated with obesity include hypertension, many kinds of cancer, impaired immune function, gallbladder and kidney diseases, skin problems, impotence, sleep and breathing disorders, back pain, arthritis, and other bone and joint disorders. Obesity is also associated with complications of pregnancy, menstrual irregularities, urine leakage (stress incontinence), psychological disorders, and increased surgical risk.

Of particular note is the strong association between excess body fat and diabetes mellitus, a disease that causes a disruption of normal metabolism. The pancreas, a long, thin organ located behind the stomach, normally secretes the hormone insulin, which stimulates cells to take up glucose to produce energy (Figure 14-4). In a person with diabetes, this process is disrupted, causing a buildup of glucose in the bloodstream. Over the long term, diabetes is associated with kidney failure; nerve damage; circulation problems and amputations; retinal damage and blindness; and increased rates of heart attack, stroke, and hypertension. Excess body fat is a major risk factor for type 2 diabetes (the most common form of diabetes). Obese people are more than three times as likely to develop diabetes, and the incidence of diabetes among Americans has increased dramatically as the rate of obesity has climbed. Diabetes is currently the sixth leading cause of death in the United States (see the box "Diabetes" for more information).

The risks from obesity increase with its severity, and they are much more likely to occur in people who are more than twice their desirable body weight. Controversy exists about the precise degree of risk at lower levels of overweight, particularly among overweight individuals who are physically active. The health risks associated with overweight depend in part on an individual's overall health and other risk factors, such as high blood pressure, unhealthy cholesterol levels, body fat distribution, and tobacco use. The NIH recommends weight loss for people whose BMI places them in the obese category and for those who are overweight *and* have two or more major risk factors for disease. If your BMI is 25 or above, consult a physician for help in determining a healthy BMI for you.

Many people who are overweight do have at least some of the risk factors associated with obesity. The Nurses' Health Study, in which Harvard researchers have followed more than 120,000 women since 1976, has found that even mildly to moderately overweight women have an 80% increased risk of developing CHD compared to leaner women. This study also confirmed that to reduce the risk of dying prematurely of any cause, maintaining a desirable body weight is important. But it is also important to realize that small weight losses—5% to 10% of total body weight—are associated with significant improvements in health.

Obesity can affect psychological as well as physical wellness. Being perceived as fat can be a source of ridicule, ostracism, and sometimes discrimination from others; it can contribute to psychological problems such as depression, anxiety, and low self-esteem (often caused by repeated failures at losing weight). For some, the stigma associated with obesity can give rise to a negative body image, body dissatisfaction, and eating disorders.

Symptoms of diabetes

• Frequent urination

• Extreme thirst and hunger

• Unexplained weight loss

• Extreme fatigue

• Blurred vision

• Frequent infections

• Slow wound healing

• Tingling or numbness in hands and feet

• Dry, itchy skin

Note: In the early stages, diabetes often has no symptoms

Esophagus

Stomach

Pancreas

Small intestine

Normal
Insulin binds to receptors on the surface of a cell and signals special transporters in the cell to transport glucose inside.

Glucose transporter

Cell

Insulin receptor

Glucose

Insulin

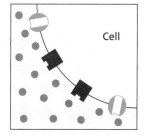

Type 1 diabetes
The pancreas produces little or no insulin. Thus, no signal is sent instructing the cell to transport glucose, and glucose builds up in the bloodstream.

Cell

Type 2 diabetes
The pancreas produces too little insulin and/or the body's cells are resistant to it. Some insulin binds to receptors on the cell's surface, but the signal to transport glucose is blocked. Glucose builds up in the bloodstream.

Cell

Figure 14-4   Diabetes mellitus.   During digestion, carbohydrates are broken down in the small intestine into glucose, a simple sugar that enters the bloodstream. The presence of glucose signals the pancreas to release insulin, a hormone that helps cells take up glucose; once inside a cell, glucose can be converted to energy. In diabetes, this process is disrupted, resulting in a buildup of glucose in the bloodstream.

Body Fat Distribution and Health   The distribution of body fat is also an important indicator of health. Men and postmenopausal women tend to store fat in the upper regions of their bodies, particularly in the abdominal area (the apple shape). Premenopausal women usually store fat in hips, buttocks, and thighs (the pear shape). Excess fat in the abdominal area increases risk of high blood pressure, diabetes, early-onset heart disease, stroke, certain types of cancer, and mortality. This risk is independent of a person's BMI. The reason for this increase in risk is not entirely clear, but it appears that abdominal fat is more easily mobilized and sent into the bloodstream, increasing disease-related blood fat levels.

The risks from body fat distribution are usually assessed by measuring waist circumference (the distance around the abdomen at the level of the hip bone, known as the iliac crest). Waist circumference can be used as a measure of abdominal obesity, an indicator of disease risk, and to monitor changes in body composition over time. More research is needed to determine the precise degree of risk associated with specific values for waist measurement. However, a total waist measurement of more than 40 inches for men and 35 inches for women is associated with a significantly increased risk of disease.

A person doesn't have to be technically overfat to have fat distribution be a risk factor, nor do all overfat people face this increased risk. The NIH BMI guidelines state that large waist circumference can be a marker for increased risk of diabetes, high blood pressure, and CVD even in people with a BMI in the normal range. And at any given level of overweight, people with a large waist circumference and/or additional disease risk factors are at greater risk for health problems. For example, a man with a BMI of 27, a waist circumference above 40 inches, and diabetes is at greater risk for health problems than another man who has a BMI of 27 but has a smaller waist and no other risk factors. Abdominal obesity and any two other risk factors associated with cardiovascular health put an individual at risk for metabolic syndrome. Abdominal obesity (as measured by waist circumference) is a primary component of metabolic syndrome and a forewarning of diabetes and heart disease.

Weight Cycling   It has been hypothesized that repeatedly losing and regaining weight, known as weight

Types of Diabetes

Approximately 18 million (1 in 14) Americans have one of two major forms of diabetes. About 5–10% of people with diabetes have the more serious form, known as type 1 diabetes. In this type of diabetes, the pancreas produces little or no insulin, so daily doses of insulin are required. (Without insulin, a person with type 1 can lapse into a coma.) Type 1 diabetes occurs when the body's immune system, triggered by a viral infection or some other environmental factor, mistakenly destroys the insulin-producing cells in the pancreas. It usually strikes before age 30.

The remaining 90–95% of Americans with diabetes have type 2 diabetes. This condition can develop slowly, and about a third of affected individuals are unaware of their condition. In type 2 diabetes, the pancreas doesn't produce enough insulin, cells are resistant to insulin, or both. This condition is usually diagnosed in people over age 40, although there has been a tenfold increase in type 2 diabetes in children in the past two decades. About one-third of people with type 2 diabetes must take insulin; others may take medications that increase insulin production or stimulate cells to take up glucose.

A third type of diabetes occurs in about 2–5% of women during pregnancy. *Gestational diabetes* usually disappears after pregnancy, but more than half of women who experience it eventually develop type 2 diabetes.

In 2002, the U.S. Department of Health and Human Services and the American Diabetes Association adopted the term *pre-diabetes* to describe blood glucose levels that are higher than normal but not high enough for a diagnosis of full-blown diabetes. About 41 million Americans have pre-diabetes, and most people with the condition will develop type 2 diabetes within 10 years unless they adopt preventive lifestyle measures. Pre-diabetes poses a risk to health beyond just the development of diabetes: Blood glucose levels in the pre-diabetes range increase the risk of heart attack or stroke by 50%. The insulin resistance and elevated glucose levels associated with pre-diabetes (and

diabetes) are one of the five defining risk factors of the condition known as metabolic syndrome, a collection of risk factors associated with heart disease; see Chapter 15 for more information on metabolic syndrome.

The major factors involved in the development of diabetes are age, obesity, physical inactivity, a family history of diabetes, and lifestyle. Excess body fat is a key risk factor because the cells of obese people are less responsive to insulin, and insulin resistance is almost always a precursor of type 2 diabetes. Ethnic background also plays a role. African Americans and Hispanics are 55% more likely than non-Hispanic whites to develop type 2 diabetes; over 20% of Hispanics over age 65 have diabetes. Native Americans also have a higher-than-average incidence of diabetes.

Prevention

It is estimated that 90% of cases of type 2 diabetes could be prevented if people adopted healthy lifestyle behaviors, including regular physical activity, a moderate diet, and modest weight loss. For people with pre-diabetes, lifestyle measures are more effective than medication for delaying or preventing the development of diabetes. Exercise (endurance and/or strength training) makes cells more sensitive to insulin and helps stabilize blood glucose levels; it also helps keep body fat at healthy levels.

A moderate diet to control body fat is perhaps the most important dietary recommendation for the prevention of diabetes. However, there is some evidence that the composition of the diet may also be important. Studies have linked diets low in fiber and high in sugar, refined carbohydrates, saturated fat, red meat, and high-fat dairy products to increased risk of diabetes; diets rich in whole grains, fruits, vegetables, legumes, fish, and poultry may be protective. The overall pattern of a person's diet is most important, but specific foods linked to higher risk of diabetes include regular (nondiet) soft drinks, white bread, white rice, french fries, processed meats (bacon, sausage, hot dogs), and sugary desserts. See Chapter 12 for information on different types of carbohydrates and

strategies for increasing fiber and whole-grain intake.

Treatment

There is no cure for diabetes, but it can be successfully managed. Treatment involves keeping blood sugar levels within safe limits through diet, exercise, and, if necessary, medication. Blood sugar levels can be monitored using a home test; close monitoring and control of glucose levels can significantly reduce the rate of serious complications among people with diabetes.

Nearly 90% of people with type 2 diabetes are overweight when diagnosed, including 55% who are obese. An important step in treatment is to lose weight; even a small amount of weight loss can be beneficial. People with diabetes should obtain carbohydrate from whole grains, fruits, vegetables, and low-fat dairy products; carbohydrate and monounsaturated fat together should provide 60–70% of total daily calories. Regular exercise and a healthy diet are often sufficient to control type 2 diabetes.

Warning Signs and Testing

A wellness lifestyle that includes a healthy diet and regular exercise is the best strategy for preventing diabetes. If you do develop diabetes, the best way to avoid complications is to recognize the symptoms and get early diagnosis and treatment. Be alert for the warning signs listed in Figure 14-4. Pre-diabetes and type 2 diabetes are often asymptomatic in the early stages, and routine screening is recommended for people over age 45 and anyone younger who is at high risk, including anyone who is obese.

The Web site for the American Diabetes Association, listed in the For More Information section at the end of the chapter, includes an interactive diabetes risk assessment. Screening involves a blood test to check glucose levels after either a period of fasting or the administration of a set dose of glucose. A fasting glucose level of 126 mg/dl or higher indicates diabetes; a level of 100–125 mg/dl indicates pre-diabetes. If you are concerned about your risk for diabetes, talk with your physician about being tested.

cycling or yo-yo dieting, might be harmful both to overall health and to efforts at weight loss. Weight cycling, it was thought, might make the body more efficient at extracting and storing calories from food; thus, with each successive diet, it would become more difficult to lose weight. Most studies, however, have not supported this idea or found weight cycling to be harmful to the health of an obese person. Most researchers believe that obese individuals should continue to try to control their weight. Losing even a few pounds brings substantial health benefits that appear to exceed any potential risks that might be incurred from weight loss or weight cycling.

Body Image   The collective picture of the body as seen through the mind's eye, **body image** consists of perceptions, images, thoughts, attitudes, and emotions. A negative body image is characterized by dissatisfaction with the body in general or some part of the body in particular. Recent surveys indicate that the majority of Americans, many of whom are not actually overweight, are unhappy with their body weight or with some aspect of their appearance.

Losing weight or getting cosmetic surgery does not necessarily improve body image. However, improvements in body image may occur in the absence of changes in weight or appearance. Many experts now believe that body image issues must be dealt with as part of treating obesity and eating disorders. See pp. 437–440 for more information on body image and eating disorders.

Problems Associated with Very Low Levels of Body Fat   Health experts have generally viewed very low levels of body fat—less than 8–12% for women and 3–5% for men—as a threat to wellness. Extreme leanness has been linked with reproductive, circulatory, and immune system disorders. Extremely lean people may experience muscle wasting and fatigue; they are also more likely to suffer from dangerous eating disorders.

In physically active women and girls, particularly those involved in sports where weight and appearance are important (ballet, gymnastics, skating, and distance running, for example), a condition called the **female athlete triad** may develop. The triad consists of three interrelated disorders: abnormal eating patterns (and excessive exercising), followed by **amenorrhea** (absence of menstruation), followed by decreased bone density (premature osteoporosis). Prolonged amenorrhea can cause bone density to erode to a point that a woman in her twenties will have the bone density of a woman in her sixties. Left untreated, the triad can lead to decreased physical performance, increased incidence of bone fractures, disturbances of heart rhythm and metabolism, and even death.

What Is the Right Weight for You?

For most of us, body weight and percentage of body fat fall somewhere below the levels associated with signifi-

cant health risks. For us, these assessment tests do not really answer the question How much should I weigh? BMI, percent body fat, and waist circumference measurement can best serve as general guides or estimates for body weight (Table 14-2, p. 420).

To answer the question of what you should weigh, let your lifestyle be your guide. Don't focus on a particular weight as your goal. Instead, focus on living a lifestyle that includes eating moderate amounts of healthful foods, getting plenty of exercise, thinking positively, and learning to cope with stress. Then let the pounds fall where they may. For most people, the result will be close to the recommended weight ranges discussed earlier. For some, their weight will be somewhat higher than societal standards—but right for them. By letting a healthy lifestyle determine your weight, you can avoid developing unhealthy patterns of eating and a negative body image.

FACTORS CONTRIBUTING TO EXCESS BODY FAT

Much research has been done in an effort to pinpoint the cause of overweight and obesity. It appears, however, that body weight and body composition are determined by multiple factors that may vary with each individual. These factors can be grouped into genetic, physiological, lifestyle, and psychosocial factors.

Genetic Factors

Estimates of the genetic contribution to obesity vary widely, from about 25% to 40% of an individual's body fat. More than 300 genes have been linked to obesity, but their actions are still under study. Genes influence body size and shape, body fat distribution, and metabolic rate. Genetic factors also affect the ease with which weight is gained as a result of overeating and where on the body extra weight is added. If both parents are overweight, their children are twice as likely to be overweight as are children who have only one overweight parent. In studies that compared adoptees and their biological parents, the

Terms   V̇w

body image   The mental representation a person holds about his or her body at any given moment in time, consisting of perceptions, images, thoughts, attitudes, and emotions about the body.

female athlete triad   A condition consisting of three interrelated disorders: abnormal eating patterns (and excessive exercising) followed by lack of menstrual periods (amenorrhea) and decreased bone density (premature osteoporosis).

amenorrhea   The absence of menstruation.

Table 14-2 Body Mass Index (BMI) Classification and Disease Risk

| Classification | BMI (kg/m²) | Obesity Class | Disease Risk Relative to Normal Weight and Waist Circumference[a] | |
			Men ≤ 40 in. (102 cm) Women ≤ 35 in. (88 cm)	> 40 in. (102 cm) > 35 in. (88 cm)
Underweight[b]	<18.5		—	—
Normal[c]	18.5–24.9		—	—
Overweight	25.0–29.9		Increased	High
Obesity	30.0–34.9	I	High	Very high
	35.0–39.9	II	Very high	Very high
Extreme obesity	≥ 40.0	III	Extremely high	Extremely high

[a]Disease risk for type 2 diabetes, hypertension, and cardiovascular disease. The waist circumference cutoff points for increased risk are 40 inches (102 cm) for men and 35 inches (88 cm) for women.

[b]Research suggests that a low BMI can be healthy in some cases, as long as it is not the result of smoking, an eating disorder, or an underlying disease process. A BMI of 17.5 or less is sometimes used as a diagnostic criterion for the eating disorder anorexia nervosa.

[c]Increased waist circumference can also be a marker for increased risk, even in persons of normal weight.

SOURCE: Adapted from National Heart, Lung, and Blood Institute. 1998. *Clinical Guidelines on the Identification, Evaluation, and Treatment of Overweight and Obesity in Adults: The Evidence Report.* Bethesda, Md.: National Institutes of Health.

weights of the adoptees were found to be more like those of the biological parents than the adoptive parents, again indicating a strong genetic link.

Research thus suggests a genetic component in the determination of body weight. However, hereditary influences must be balanced against the contribution of environmental factors. Not all children of obese parents become obese, and normal-weight parents may have overweight children. In a study comparing men born and raised in Ireland with their biological brothers who lived in the United States, the American men were found to weigh, on average, 6% more than their Irish brothers. Environmental factors like diet and exercise are probably responsible for this difference. Thus, the *tendency* to develop obesity may be inherited, but the expression of this tendency is affected by environmental influences.

The message you should take from this research is that genes are not destiny. It is true that some people have a harder time losing weight and maintaining weight loss than others. However, with increased exercise and attention to diet, even those with a genetic tendency toward obesity can maintain a healthy body weight. And regardless of genetic factors, lifestyle choices remain the cornerstone of successful weight management.

Term

V̇i̇ẇ

resting metabolic rate (RMR) The energy required to maintain vital body functions, including respiration, heart rate, body temperature, and blood pressure, while the body is at rest.

Physiological Factors

Metabolism is a key physiological factor in the regulation of body fat and body weight; hormones also play a role. Other factors that have been proposed as contributing to obesity include fat cells and carbohydrate craving.

Metabolism Metabolism is the sum of all the vital processes by which food energy and nutrients are made available to and used by the body. The largest component of metabolism, **resting metabolic rate (RMR)**, is the energy required to maintain vital body functions, including respiration, heart rate, body temperature, and blood pressure, while the body is at rest. As shown in Figure 14-2, RMR accounts for about 55–75% of daily energy expenditure. The energy required to digest food accounts for an additional 5–15% of daily energy expenditure. The remaining 20–40% is expended during physical activity.

Both heredity and behavior affect metabolic rate. Men, who have a higher proportion of muscle mass than women, have a higher RMR (muscle tissue is more metabolically active than fat). Also, some individuals inherit a higher or lower RMR than others. A higher RMR means that a person burns more calories while at rest and can therefore take in more calories without gaining weight.

Weight loss or gain also affects metabolic rate. When a person loses weight, both RMR and the energy required to perform physical tasks decrease. The reverse occurs when weight is gained. One of the reasons exercise is so important during a weight-loss program is that exercise, especially resistance training, helps maintain muscle mass and metabolic rate.

Exercise has a positive effect on metabolism. When people exercise, they slightly increase their RMR—the number of calories their bodies burn at rest. They also increase their muscle mass, which is associated with a higher metabolic rate. The exercise itself also burns calories, raising total energy expenditure. The higher the energy expenditure, the more the person can eat without gaining weight. (The role of exercise in weight management is discussed in greater detail later in the chapter.)

Hormones   Hormones clearly play a role in the accumulation of body fat, especially for females. Hormonal changes at puberty, during pregnancy, and at menopause contribute to the amount and location of fat accumulation. For example, during puberty, hormones cause the development of secondary sex characteristics, including larger breasts, wider hips, and a fat layer under the skin.

One hormone thought to be linked to obesity is leptin. Secreted by the body's fat cells, leptin is carried to the brain, where it appears to let the brain know how big or small the body's fat stores are. With this information, the brain can regulate appetite and metabolic rate accordingly. Other hormones that may be involved in the regulation of appetite are cholecystokinin (CCK), peptide YY, grelin, and gluconlike peptide-1 (GLP-1). Researchers hope to use these hormones to develop treatments for obesity based on appetite control; however, as most of us will admit, hunger is often *not* the primary reason we overeat. Cases of obesity based solely or primarily on hormone abnormalities do exist, but they are rare. Lifestyle choices still account for the largest proportion of the differences in body weight and body composition among individuals.

Fat Cells   The amount of fat the body can store is a function of the number and size of fat cells. These fat cells are like little compartments that can be inflated to hold body fat; when all or nearly all the fat cells are filled, the body makes more, thereby increasing its ability to store fat. Some people are born with an above-average number of fat cells and thus have the potential for storing more energy as body fat. Overeating at critical times, such as in childhood, can cause the body to expand the number of fat cells. It has been hypothesized that having more or larger fat cells creates biological pressure to keep eating to fill all the fat cells; however, this has not been substantiated by research. If a person loses weight, fat cell content is depleted, but it is unclear whether the number of fat cells can be decreased.

Carbohydrate Craving   It has been hypothesized that carbohydrate craving may cause overeating and thus lead to overweight and obesity. Animal studies have suggested that consuming carbohydrates increases brain levels of serotonin, a neurotransmitter that induces calmness. People with low levels of serotonin thus might crave and consume carbohydrates because they experience

The typical American lifestyle does not lead naturally to healthy weight management. Labor-saving devices such as escalators help reinforce our sedentary habits.

improved mood and reduced fatigue after eating foods such as bread, pasta, and candy. However, research in humans supporting this hypothesis remains incomplete.

A number of popular diets have been based on the idea that carbohydrates in general or foods with a high glycemic index cause weight gain (see Chapter 12 for a description of glycemic index). Carbohydrates do affect levels of glucose and insulin in the blood, but there is no real data that consumption of foods containing carbohydrates increases appetite and/or body weight beyond the effects of the calories contained in the foods. There are many other influences on appetite and caloric intake. In Asian nations such as China and Japan, people consume diets very high in carbohydrate and have low rates of obesity. Experts suggest that people follow the carbohydrate and calorie intake levels recommended by the Dietary Guidelines for Americans. It is most important to manage overall calorie intake and to choose healthy sources of carbohydrate.

Lifestyle Factors

Although genetic and physiological factors may increase risk for excess body fat, they are not sufficient to explain the increasingly high rate of obesity seen in the United States. The gene pool has not changed dramatically in the past 40 years, during which time the rate of obesity among Americans has more than doubled (see the box "Overweight and Obesity Among U.S. Ethnic Populations"). Clearly, other factors are at work—particularly lifestyle factors such as increased energy intake and decreased physical activity.

Eating   Americans have access to an abundance of highly palatable and calorie-dense foods, and many have eating habits that contribute to weight gain. Most overweight adults will admit to eating more than they should

Among all population groups in the United States, the prevalence of overweight and obesity is growing. However, rates and trends vary by ethnic group and by other population characteristics.

- Certain groups, including African Americans, Latinos, and American Indians and Alaska Natives, have higher-than-average rates of obesity. Asian Americans have a low rate of obesity.

- There is considerable variation within populations grouped into general ethnic categories. For example, Asian Americans, Vietnamese Americans, and Chinese Americans have very low rates of obesity, and Asian Indians have much higher rates of obesity.

- Within all groups, women have higher rates of overweight and obesity than men.

- Low socioeconomic status is associated with higher rates of overweight and obesity. Researchers theorize that people living in poor communities are more greatly affected by a toxic food and exercise environment—meaning there are fewer opportunities to purchase healthy foods and safely engage in regular physical activity. In addition, many foods low in price are high in calorie density (fast food, for example).

- Higher or increasing socioeconomic status is associated with lower rates of obesity among some groups and constant or increased rates of obesity

among other groups. Groups that are transitioning from poverty, food scarcity, and jobs that require significant energy expenditure may not have good family or community models of reducing energy intake and increasing leisure-time physical activity.

- Acculturation boosts body weight. The longer a foreign-born person lives in the United States, the more likely she or he is to become obese. BMI among immigrants begins to climb after about 10 years of U.S. residence, and after 15 years, it approaches the national average.

- Cultural factors that influence dietary and exercise behaviors appear to play a role in the development of obesity. There are also cultural differences in acceptance of larger body size and in body image perception. For example, one study found that African Americans were more likely to think they were thinner than they really were and whites were more likely to think they were fatter than they really were.

- Some studies have found that African Americans, on average, have lower resting metabolic rates than whites; in addition, weight loss may cause greater declines in RMR among African Americans. Further research is needed to determine the influence RMR differences may have on rates of obesity and successful weight loss among African Americans.

- The health consequences of obesity affect ethnic populations in different ways. At a given level of BMI, Latinos are significantly more likely to have type 2 diabetes. Obesity in African Americans is associated with increased risk of developing hypertension at a younger age and in a more severe form.

- For Asian Americans or persons of Asian descent, waist circumference is a better indicator of relative disease risk than BMI, and disease risk goes up at a lower level of BMI than for individuals of other groups. For Asian populations, WHO guidelines have a lower BMI cutoff for defining overweight and (BMI > 23).

SOURCES: Goel, M. S., et al. 2004. Obesity among U.S. immigrant subgroups by duration of residence. *Journal of the American Medical Association* 292(23): 2860–2867; Centers for Disease Control and Prevention. 2004. Prevalence of diabetes among Hispanics. *Morbidity and Mortality Weekly Report* 53(40): 941–944; Sanchez-Johnsen, L. A., et al. 2004. Ethnic differences in correlates of obesity between Latin-American and black women. *Obesity Research* 12(4): 652–660; Fitzgibbon, M. L., and M. R. Stolley. 2004. Environmental changes may be needed for prevention of overweight in minority children. *Pediatric Annals* 33(1): 45–49; American Obesity Association. 2004. *Obesity in Minority Populations* (http://www.obesity.org/subs/fastfacts/Obesity_Minority_Pop.shtml; September 29, 2004); Bhuiyan, A. R., et al. 2003. Differences in body shape representations among young adults from a biracial (black-white), semirural community. *American Journal of Epidemiology* 158(8): 792–797.

of high-fat, high-sugar, high-calorie foods. Americans eat out more frequently now than in the past, and we rely more heavily on fast food and packaged convenience foods. Restaurant and convenience food portion sizes tend to be large, and the foods themselves are likely to be high in fat, sugar, and calories and low in nutrients. Studies have consistently found that people underestimate portion sizes by as much as 25%.

The average calorie intake by Americans has increased by about 250 calories per day since 1970. Levels of physical activity declined during this period. The net result has been a substantial increase in the number of Americans who are overweight and obese. Healthy eating habits for successful weight management are described later in this chapter.

Physical Activity Research has shown that activity levels among Americans are declining, beginning in childhood and continuing throughout the life cycle. Many schools have cut back on physical education classes and recess. Most adults drive to work, sit all day, and then relax in front of the TV at night. During leisure time, both children and adults surf the Internet, play video games, or watch TV rather than bicycle, participate in sports, or just do yardwork or chores around the house. One study found that 60% of the incidence of overweight can be linked to excessive television viewing. On average, Americans exercise 15 minutes per day and watch 170 minutes of TV and movies. Modern conveniences such as remote controls, elevators, and power mowers have also reduced daily physical activity.

Psychosocial Factors

Many people have learned to use food as a means of coping with stress and negative emotions. Eating can provide a powerful distraction from difficult feelings—loneliness, anger, boredom, anxiety, shame, sadness, inadequacy. It can be used to combat low moods, low energy levels, and low self-esteem (see the box "What Triggers Your Eating?" on p. 424). When food and eating become the primary means of regulating emotions, binge eating or other disturbed eating patterns can develop.

Obesity is strongly associated with socioeconomic status. The prevalence of obesity goes down as income level goes up. More women than men are obese at lower income levels, but men are somewhat more obese at higher levels. These differences may reflect the greater sensitivity and concern for a slim physical appearance among upper-income women, as well as greater access to information about nutrition, to low-fat and low-calorie foods, and to opportunities for physical activity. It may also reflect the greater acceptance of obesity among certain ethnic groups, as well as different cultural values related to food choices.

In some families and cultures, food is used as a symbol of love and caring. It is an integral part of social gatherings and celebrations. In such cases, it may be difficult to change established eating patterns because they are linked to cultural and family values.

ADOPTING A HEALTHY LIFESTYLE FOR SUCCESSFUL WEIGHT MANAGEMENT

When all the research has been assessed, it is clear that most weight problems are lifestyle problems. Even though more and more young people are developing weight problems, most arrive at early adulthood with the advantage of having a normal body weight—neither too fat nor too thin. In fact, many young adults get away with terrible eating and exercise habits and don't develop a weight problem. But as the rapid growth of adolescence slows and family and career obligations increase, maintaining a healthy weight becomes a greater challenge. Slow weight gain is a major cause of overweight and obesity, so weight management is important for everyone, not just for people who are currently overweight. A good time to develop a lifestyle for successful weight management is during early adulthood, when healthy behavior patterns have a better chance of taking a firm hold.

Permanent weight loss is not something you start and stop. You need to adopt healthy behaviors that you can maintain throughout your life. Lifestyle factors that are critical for successful long-term weight management include eating habits, level of physical activity, an ability to think positively and manage your emotions effectively,

and the coping strategies you use to deal with the stresses and challenges in your life.

Diet and Eating Habits

In contrast to dieting, which involves some form of food restriction, diet refers to your daily food choices. Everyone has a diet, but not everyone is dieting. You need to develop a diet that you enjoy and that enables you to maintain a healthy body composition. Use MyPyramid or DASH as the basis for planning a healthy diet (see Chapter 12). For weight management, you may need to pay special attention to total calories, portion sizes, energy density, fat and carbohydrate intake, and eating habits.

Total Calories MyPyramid suggests approximate daily energy intakes based on gender, age, and activity level (see Table 12-3). However, energy balance may be a more important consideration for weight management than total calories consumed (see Figure 14-2). To maintain your current weight, the total number of calories you eat must equal the number you burn. To lose weight, you must decrease your calorie intake and/or increase the number of calories you burn; to gain weight, the reverse is true. (One pound of body fat represents 3500 calories.)

The best approach for weight loss is combining an increase in physical activity with moderate calorie restriction. Don't go on a crash diet. To maintain weight loss, you will probably have to maintain some degree of the calorie restriction you used to lose the weight. Therefore, you need to adopt a level of food intake that provides all the essential nutrients that you can live with over the long term. For most people, maintaining weight loss is more difficult than losing the weight in the first place.

Portion Sizes Overconsumption of total calories is closely tied to portion sizes. Many Americans are unaware that the portion sizes of packaged foods and of foods served at restaurants have increased in size, and most of us significantly underestimate the amount of food we eat. Limiting portion sizes is critical for maintaining good health. For many people, concentrating on portion sizes is also a much easier method of monitoring and managing total food intake than counting calories.

To counteract portion distortion, weigh and measure your food at home for a few days every now and then. In addition, check the serving sizes listed on packaged foods. With practice, you'll learn to judge portion sizes more accurately. When eating out, try to order the smallest-sized items on the menu. When a small isn't small enough, take half home or share it with a friend. It is especially important to limit serving sizes of foods that are high in calories and low in nutrients. Don't supersize your meals and snacks; although huge servings may seem like the best deal, it is more important to order just what you

What Triggers Your Eating?

Hunger isn't the only reason people eat. Efforts to maintain a healthy body weight can be sabotaged by eating related to other factors, including emotions, environment, and patterns of thinking. This quiz is designed to provide you with a score for five factors that describe many people's eating habits. This information will put you in a better position to manage your eating behavior and control your weight. Circle the number that indicates to what degree each situation is likely to make you start eating.

Social

		Very Unlikely							Very Likely	
1. Arguing or having a conflict with someone	1	2	3	4	5	6	7	8	9	10
2. Being with others when they are eating	1	2	3	4	5	6	7	8	9	10
3. Being urged to eat by someone else	1	2	3	4	5	6	7	8	9	10
4. Feeling inadequate around others	1	2	3	4	5	6	7	8	9	10

Emotional

5. Feeling bad, such as being anxious or depressed	1	2	3	4	5	6	7	8	9	10
6. Feeling good, happy, or relaxed	1	2	3	4	5	6	7	8	9	10
7. Feeling bored or having time on my hands	1	2	3	4	5	6	7	8	9	10
8. Feeling stressed or excited	1	2	3	4	5	6	7	8	9	10

Situational

9. Seeing an advertisement for food or eating	1	2	3	4	5	6	7	8	9	10
10. Passing by a bakery, cookie shop, or other enticement to eat	1	2	3	4	5	6	7	8	9	10
11. Being involved in a party, celebration, or special occasion	1	2	3	4	5	6	7	8	9	10
12. Eating out	1	2	3	4	5	6	7	8	9	10

Thinking

13. Making excuses to myself about why it's OK to eat	1	2	3	4	5	6	7	8	9	10
14. Berating myself for being fat or unable to control my eating	1	2	3	4	5	6	7	8	9	10
15. Worrying about others or about difficulties I'm having	1	2	3	4	5	6	7	8	9	10
16. Thinking about how things should or shouldn't be	1	2	3	4	5	6	7	8	9	10

Physiological

17. Experiencing pain or physical discomfort	1	2	3	4	5	6	7	8	9	10
18. Experiencing trembling, headache, or light-headedness associated with no eating or too much caffeine	1	2	3	4	5	6	7	8	9	10
19. Experiencing fatigue or feeling overtired	1	2	3	4	5	6	7	8	9	10
20. Experiencing hunger pangs or urges to eat, even though I've eaten recently	1	2	3	4	5	6	7	8	9	10

Scoring

Total your scores for each category, and enter them below. Then rank the scores by marking the highest score 1, next highest score 2, and so on. Focus on the highest-ranked categories first, but any score above 24 is high and indicates that you need to work on that category.

Category	Total Score	Rank Order
Social (Items 1–4)	_____	_____
Emotional (Items 5–8)	_____	_____
Situational (Items 9–12)	_____	_____
Thinking (Items 13–16)	_____	_____
Physiological (Items 17–20)	_____	_____

What Your Score Means

Social A high score here means you are very susceptible to the influence of others. Work on better ways to communicate more assertively, handle conflict, and manage anger. Challenge your beliefs about the need to be polite and the obligations you feel you must fulfill.

Emotional A high score here means you need to develop effective ways to cope with emotions. Work on developing skills in stress management, time management, and communication. Practicing positive but realistic self-talk can help you handle small daily upsets.

Situational A high score here means you are especially susceptible to external influences. Try to avoid external cues and respond differently to those you cannot avoid. Control your environment by changing the way you buy, store, cook, and serve food. Anticipate potential problems, and have a plan for handling them.

Thinking A high score here means that the way you think—how you talk to yourself, the beliefs you hold, your memories, and your expectations—have a powerful influence on your eating habits. Try to be less self-critical, less perfectionistic, and more flexible in your ideas about the way things ought to be. Recognize when you're making excuses or rationalizations that allow you to eat.

Physiological A high score here means that the way you eat, what you eat, or medications you are taking may be affecting your eating behavior. You may be eating to reduce physical arousal or deal with physical discomfort. Try eating three meals a day, supplemented with regular snacks if needed. Avoid too much caffeine. If any medication you're taking produces adverse physical reactions, switch to an alternative, if possible. If your medications may be affecting your hormone levels, discuss possible alternatives with your physician.

SOURCE: Adapted from Nash, J. D. 1997. *The New Maximize Your Body Potential.* Boulder, Colorado: Bull. Reprinted with permission from Bull Publishing Company.

Large portions can make it more difficult to consume a moderate diet and manage weight. Many people significantly underestimate the amount of food they eat.

need. Refer to Chapter 12 and the Online Learning Center for more information on choosing appropriate portion sizes.

Energy (Calorie) Density   Experts also recommend that you pay attention to energy density—the number of calories per ounce or gram of weight in a food. Studies suggest that it isn't consumption of a certain amount of fat or calories in food that reduces hunger and leads to feelings of fullness and satisfaction; rather, it is consumption of a certain weight of food. Foods that are low in energy density have more volume and bulk—that is, they are relatively heavy but have few calories. For example, for the same 100 calories, you could consume 21 baby carrots or 4 pretzel twists; you are more likely to feel full after eating the serving of carrots because it weighs 10 times that of the serving of pretzels (10 ounces versus 1 ounce).

To cut back on calories and still feel full, then, you should favor foods with a low energy density. Fresh fruits and vegetables, with their high water and fiber content, are low in energy density, as are whole-grain foods. Fresh fruits contain less calories and more fiber than fruit juices or drinks. Meat, ice cream, potato chips, croissants, crackers, and low-fat cakes and cookies are examples of foods high in energy density. Strategies for lowering the energy density of your diet include the following:

- Eat fruit with breakfast and for dessert.
- Add extra vegetables to sandwiches, casseroles, stir-fry dishes, pizza, pasta dishes, and fajitas.
- Start meals with a bowl of broth-based soup; include a green salad or fruit salad.
- Snack on fresh fruits and vegetables rather than crackers, chips, or other energy-dense snack foods.

- Limit serving sizes of energy-dense foods such as butter, mayonnaise, cheese, chocolate, fatty meats, croissants, and snack foods that are fried or high in added sugars (including reduced-fat products).

Fat Calories   Although some fat is needed in the diet to provide essential nutrients, you should avoid overeating fatty foods. There is some evidence that fat calories are more easily converted to body fat than calories from protein or carbohydrate. Limiting fat in the diet can also help you limit your total calories. As described in Chapter 12, fat should supply no more than 35% of your average total daily calories, which translates into no more than 78 grams of fat in a 2000-calorie diet each day. Most of the fat in your diet should be in the form of unsaturated fats from plant and fish sources. Saturated and trans fats should be limited for weight control and disease prevention; foods high in unhealthy fats include full-fat dairy products, fatty meats, stick margarine, deep-fried foods, and other processed and fast foods.

Some people are better fat burners than others; that is, they burn more of the fat they take in as calories and therefore have less fat to store. Low fat burners convert more dietary fat to stored body fat. This tendency to hoard fat calories may be an important part of the genetic tendency toward obesity. For low fat burners, restricting fat calories to a level below 35% may be helpful in weight management.

As Chapter 12 made clear, moving toward a diet strong in complex carbohydrates and fresh fruits and vegetables, and away from a reliance on meat and processed foods, is an effective approach to reducing fat consumption. Watch out for processed foods labeled "fat-free" or "reduced fat," as they may be high in calories (see the box "Evaluating Fat and Sugar Substitutes"). In addition, researchers have found that many Americans compensate for a lower-fat diet by consuming more calories overall. A low-fat diet that is high in calories will not lead to weight loss.

Carbohydrate   Most experts agree that people should consume about 45–65% of total daily calories as carbohydrate, with special emphasis on whole grains, vegetables, fruits, and other foods high in fiber. Americans currently consume most of their carbohydrate calories in the form of foods high in refined carbohydrates and added sugars—soft drinks and heavily sweetened fruit drinks, white rice, white potatoes, and breads, cereals, and snack foods made with refined grains. Such foods are typically high in calories and low in other essential nutrients; they also often cause dramatic swings in blood glucose and insulin levels and have been implicated in the development of type 2 diabetes and heart disease.

Foods high in whole grains and fiber are typically lower in calorie density, saturated fat, and added sugars and may promote feelings of satiety (fullness)—all characteristic features of a dietary pattern for successful weight management. They also help maintain normal

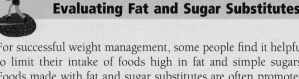

For successful weight management, some people find it helpful to limit their intake of foods high in fat and simple sugars. Foods made with fat and sugar substitutes are often promoted for weight loss. But just what are fat and sugar substitutes? And can they really contribute to weight management?

Fat Substitutes

A variety of substances are used to replace fats in processed foods and other products. Some contribute calories, protein, fiber, and/or other nutrients, whereas others do not. Fat replacers fall into three general categories:

• *Carbohydrate-based fat replacers* include starch, fibers, gums, cellulose, polydextrose, and fruit purees. They are the oldest and most widely used form of fat replacer and are found in dairy and meat products, baked goods, salad dressings, and many other prepared foods. Newer types such as Oatrim, Z-trim, and Nu-trim are made from types of dietary fiber that may actually lower cholesterol levels. Carbohydrate-based fat replacers contribute 0–4 calories per gram.

• *Protein-based fat replacers* are typically made from milk, egg whites, soy, or whey; trade names include Simplesse, Dairy-lo, and Supro. They are used in cheese, sour cream, mayonnaise, margarine spreads, frozen desserts, salad dressings, and baked goods. Protein-based fat replacers typically contribute 1–4 calories per gram.

• *Fat-based fat replacers* include glycerides, olestra, and other special types of fatty acids. Some of these compounds are not absorbed well by the body and so provide fewer calories per gram (5 calories compared with the standard 9 for fats); others are impossible for the body to digest and so contribute no calories at all. Olestra, marketed under the trade name Olean and used in fried snack foods, is an example of the latter type of compound. Concerns have been raised about the safety of olestra because it reduces the absorption of fat-soluble nutrients and certain antioxidants and because it causes gastrointestinal distress in some people.

Nonnutritive Sweeteners and Sugar Alcohols

Sugar substitutes are often referred to as nonnutritive sweeteners because they provide no calories or essential nutrients. By 2005, five types of nonnutritive sweeteners had been approved for use in the United States: acesulfame-K (Sunett, Sweet One), aspartame (NutraSweet, Equal, NatraTaste), saccharin (Sweet 'N Low), sucralose (Splenda), and neotame. They are used in beverages, desserts, baked goods, yogurt, chewing gum, and products such as toothpaste, mouthwash, and cough syrup. Another sweetener,

stevia, is an extract of a South American shrub; it is classified as a dietary supplement and so is not regulated by the FDA.

Sugar alcohols are made by altering the chemical form of sugars extracted from fruits and other plant sources; they include erythritol, isomalt, lactitol, maltitol, mannitol, sorbitol, and zylitol. Sugar alcohols provide 0.2–2.5 calories per gram, compared to 4 calories per gram in standard sugar. They have typically been used to sweeten sugar-free candies but are now being added to many sweet foods promoted as low-carbohydrate products, often combined with other sweeteners. Sugar alcohols are digested in a way that can create gas, cramps, and diarrhea if they are consumed in large amounts—more than about 10 grams in one meal. To avoid problems, check ingredient lists to determine if a food contains sugar alcohols.

Fat and Sugar Substitutes in Weight Management

Whether fat and sugar substitutes help you achieve and maintain a healthy weight depends on your lifestyle—your overall eating and activity habits. The increase in the availability of fat-free and sugar-free foods in the United States has *not* been associated with a drop in calorie consumption. When evaluating foods with fat and sugar substitutes, consider these issues:

• *Is the food lower in calories or just lower in fat?* Reduced-fat foods often contain extra sugar to improve the taste and texture lost when fat is removed, so such foods may be as high or even higher in total calories than their fattier counterparts. Limiting fat intake is an important goal for weight management, but so is controlling total calories.

• *Are you choosing foods with fat and/or sugar substitutes instead of foods you typically eat or in addition to foods you typically eat?* If you consume low-fat, no-sugar-added ice cream instead of regular ice cream, you may save calories. But if you add such ice cream to your daily diet simply because it is lower in fat and sugar, your overall calorie consumption—and your weight—may increase.

• *How many foods containing fat and sugar substitutes do you consume each day?* Although the FDA has given at least provisional approval to all the fat and sugar substitutes currently available, health concerns about some of these products linger. One way to limit any potential adverse effects is to read labels and monitor how much of each product you consume.

• *Is an even healthier choice available?* Many of the foods containing fat and sugar substitutes are low-nutrient snack foods. Although substituting a lower-fat or lower-sugar version of the same food may be beneficial, fruits, vegetables, and whole grains are healthier snack choices.

blood glucose and insulin levels and reduce the risk of heart disease. For weight management and overall health, choose a diet rich in complex carbohydrates from whole grains, vegetables, and fruits; avoid high-fat toppings, added sugars (especially sugary soft drinks, fruit drinks, and desserts), and refined carbohydrates.

Protein   The typical American consumes more than an adequate amount of protein. Special dietary supplements that provide extra protein are unnecessary for most people, and protein not needed by the body for growth and tissue repair will be stored as fat. Foods high in protein are often also high in fat. Stick to the recommended protein intake of

10–35% of total daily calories. High-protein diets promoted for weight loss are discussed later in the chapter.

Eating Habits   Equally important to weight management is eating small, frequent meals—three or more a day plus snacks—on a dependable, regular schedule. Skipping meals leads to excessive hunger, feelings of deprivation, and increased vulnerability to binge eating or snacking on high-calorie, high-fat, or sugary foods. A regular pattern of eating, along with some personal decision rules governing food choices, is a way of thinking about and then internalizing the many details that go into a healthy, low-fat diet. Decision rules for breakfast might be these, for example: Choose a sugar-free, high-fiber cereal with fat-free milk on most days; once in a while (no more than once a week), have a hard-boiled egg; save pancakes and waffles for special occasions.

Decreeing some foods off-limits generally sets up a rule to be broken. The better principle is "everything in moderation." If a particular food becomes troublesome, it might be placed off-limits temporarily until control over it is regained. The ultimate goal is to eat in moderation; no foods need to be entirely off-limits, though some should be eaten judiciously. Making the healthier choice more often than not is the essence of moderation.

Physical Activity and Exercise

Regular physical activity is another important lifestyle factor in weight management. Physical activity and exercise burn calories and keep the metabolism geared to using food for energy instead of storing it as fat. Making significant cuts in food intake in order to lose weight is a difficult strategy to maintain; increasing your physical activity is a much better approach. Regular physical activity also protects against weight gain and is essential for maintaining weight loss.

As described in Chapter 13, the first step in becoming more active is to incorporate more physical activity into your daily life. Accumulate 30 minutes or more of moderate-intensity physical activity—walking, gardening, housework, and so on—on most, or preferably all, days of the week. Moderate-intensity physical activities are equal, in effort, to walking briskly—1 mile in 15–20 minutes; other moderate-intensity activities include bicycling (10–12 mph), dancing, hiking, golfing (without a cart), raking leaves, vacuuming a carpet, playing volleyball, and washing a car. Take advantage of routine opportunities to be more active; in the long term, even a small increase in activity level can help maintain your current weight or help you lose a modest amount of weight. In fact, research suggests that fidgeting—stretching, squirming, standing up, and so on—may help prevent weight gain after overeating in some people. If you simply walked around during TV commercials while watching 2 hours of prime-time programming, you'd accumulate more than 30 minutes of physical activity. Short bouts of activity spread

throughout the day can produce many of the same health benefits as continuous physical activity.

If you are overweight or obese and want to lose weight and keep it off, a greater amount of physical activity is necessary. People who lose weight and don't regain it typically burn at least 2800 calories per week in physical activity—the equivalent of about 1 hour of brisk walking per day. The 2005 Dietary Guidelines for Americans recommend at least 60 minutes of daily physical activity to avoid slow weight gain in adulthood, and at least 60–90 minutes of activity to lose weight or to prevent weight regain after losing weight.

Once you become more active every day, consider beginning a formal exercise program that includes cardiorespiratory endurance exercise, resistance training, and stretching exercises. Moderate cardiorespiratory endurance exercise, sustained for 45 minutes to 1 hour, can help trim body fat permanently. Strength training helps increase fat-free mass, which results in more calorie burning even outside of exercise periods.

The message about exercise is that regular exercise, maintained throughout life, makes weight management easier and improves quality of life (see the box "Exercise, Body Image, and Self-Esteem" on p. 428). The sooner you establish good habits, the better. The key to success is making exercise an integral part of the lifestyle you can enjoy now and in the future. Chapter 13 contains many suggestions for becoming a more active, physically fit person.

Thinking and Emotions

What goes on in your head is another factor in a healthy lifestyle and successful weight management. The way you think about yourself and your world influences and is influenced by how you feel and how you act. Certain kinds of thinking produce negative emotions, which can undermine a healthy lifestyle.

Research on people who have a weight problem indicates that low self-esteem and the negative emotions that accompany it are significant problems. This often results in part from mentally comparing the actual self to an internally held picture of an ideal self. The greater the discrepancy, the larger the impact on self-esteem and the more likely the presence of negative emotions.

Often our internalized ideal self is the result of having adopted perfectionistic goals and beliefs about how we and others should be. Examples of such beliefs are "If I don't do things perfectly, I'm a failure" and "It's terrible if I'm not thin." These irrational beliefs may cause stress and emotional pain. The remedy is to challenge such beliefs and replace them with more realistic ones.

The beliefs and attitudes you hold give rise to self-talk, an internal dialogue about events that happen to and around you. Positive self-talk includes leading yourself through the steps of a job and then praising yourself when it's successfully completed. Negative self-talk takes

Exercise, Body Image, and Self-Esteem

Mind/Body/Spirit

If you gaze into the mirror and wish you could change the way your body looks, consider getting some exercise—not to re-shape your contours but to firm up your body image and enhance your self-esteem. In a recent study, 82 adults completed a 12-week aerobic exercise program and had 12 months of follow-up. Compared with the control group, these participants improved their fitness and also benefited psychologically in tests of mood, anxiety, and self-concept. These same physical and psychological benefits were still significant at the 1-year follow-up.

One reason for the findings may be that people who exercise regularly often gain a sense of mastery and competence that en-hances their self-esteem and body image. In addition, exercise contributes to a more toned look, which many adults prefer. Re-search suggests that physically active peo-ple are more comfortable with their body and their image than sedentary people are. In one workplace study, 60 employ-ees were asked to complete a 36-session stretching program whose main purpose was to prevent muscle strains at work. At the end of the program, besides the signif-icant increase by all participants in mea-surements of flexibility, their perceptions of their bodies improved and so did their overall sense of self-worth.

Similar results were obtained in a Norwegian study, in which 219 middle-aged people at risk for heart disease were randomly assigned to one of four groups: diet, diet plus exercise, exercise, and no intervention. The greater the participa-tion of individuals in the exercise compo-nent of the program, the higher were their scores in perceived competence/self-esteem and coping.

SOURCES: DiLorenzo, T. M., et al. 1999. Long-term effects of aerobic exercise on psychological outcomes. *Preventive Medicine* 28(1): 75–85; Sorensen, M., et al. 1999. The effect of exercise and diet on mental health and quality of life in middle-aged individuals with elevated risk factors for cardiovascular disease. *Journal of Sports Science* 17(5): 369–377; Moore, T. M. 1998. A workplace stretching program. *AAOHN Journal* 46(12): 563–568.

the form of self-deprecating remarks, self-blame, and an-gry and guilt-producing comments. Negative self-talk can undermine efforts at self-control and lead to feelings of anxiety and depression (see Chapter 3).

Your beliefs and attitude influence how you interpret what happens to you and what you can expect in the future, as well as how you feel and react. A healthy lifestyle is supported by having realistic beliefs and goals and by engaging in positive self-talk and problem-solving efforts.

Coping Strategies

Adequate and appropriate coping strategies for dealing with the stresses and challenges of life are another lifestyle factor in weight management. One strategy that some people adopt for coping is eating. (Others use drugs, al-cohol, smoking, spending, gambling, and so on, to cope.) When boredom occurs, eating can provide entertain-ment. Food may be used to alleviate loneliness or as a pickup for fatigue. Eating provides distraction from diffi-cult problems and is a means of punishing the self or oth-ers for real or imagined transgressions.

People with a healthy lifestyle have more effective ways to get their needs met. Having learned to communicate as-sertively and to manage interpersonal conflict effectively, they don't shrink from problems or overreact. The person with a healthy lifestyle knows how to create and maintain relationships with others and has a solid network of friends and loved ones. Food is used appropriately—to fuel life's ac-tivities and gain personal satisfaction, not to manage stress.

Obtaining adequate amounts of sleep is important for stress management and may be a key component of suc-cessful weight management. A recent study found a link between sleep and body mass index: People with a healthy BMI slept more than people who were overweight and obese. A cause-and-effect relationship is not yet es-tablished, but it is possible that insufficient sleep may affect hormones, metabolism, and appetite.

The healthy lifestyle that naturally and easily results in a reasonable body weight is one characterized by good nutrition, adequate exercise, positive thinking and emo-tions, and effective coping strategies and behavior pat-terns. You can make positive changes in your lifestyle to promote permanent weight control; see the box "Strate-gies for Successful Weight Management" for ideas.

APPROACHES TO OVERCOMING A WEIGHT PROBLEM

What should you do if you are overweight? Several op-tions are available to you.

Doing It Yourself

If you need to lose weight, focus on adopting the healthy lifestyle described throughout this book. The right weight for you will naturally evolve. Combine modest cuts in en-ergy intake with exercise, and avoid very-low-calorie diets. By producing a negative energy balance of 250–1000 calo-ries per day, you will produce the recommended weight loss of 0.5–2.0 pounds per week. Don't try to lose weight more rapidly. Realize that most low-calorie diets cause a rapid loss of body water at first. When this phase passes, weight loss declines. As a result, dieters are often misled into believing that their efforts are not working. They then give

Food Choices

- Follow the recommendations in the Food Guide Pyramid for eating a moderate, varied diet.

- Pay attention to the energy density and nutrient density of your food choices. Favor foods with a low energy density and a high nutrient density.

- Check food labels for serving sizes, calories, and nutrient levels.

- Watch for hidden calories. Reduced-fat foods often have as many calories as their full-fat versions. Fat-based condiments like butter, margarine, mayonnaise, and salad dressings provide about 100 calories per tablespoon; added sugars such as jams, jellies, and syrup are also packed with calories.

- Drink fewer calories. Many Americans consume high-calorie beverages such as soda, fruit drinks, sports drinks, alcohol, and specialty coffees and teas. (People who get extra calories from solid food tend to compensate by eating less later; those whose extra calories come in liquid form don't compensate and consume more calories overall.)

- For problem foods, try eating small amounts under controlled conditions. Go out for a scoop of ice cream, for example, rather than buying a half gallon for your freezer.

Planning and Serving

- Keep a log of what you eat. Before you begin your program, your log will provide a realistic picture of your current diet and what changes you can make. Once you start your program, a log will keep you focused on your food choices and portion sizes. Consider tracking the following:

      food eaten
      hunger level
      circumstances (location, other activities)
      outside influences (environment, other people)
      thoughts and emotions

- Eat three meals a day, *including breakfast.* In studies, people who eat breakfast consume fewer calories overall over the course of the day. Replace impulse snacking with planned, healthy snacks. Keep low-calorie snacks on hand to combat the munchies: baby carrots, popcorn, and fresh fruits and vegetables are good choices.

- When shopping, make a list and stick to it. Don't shop when you're hungry. Avoid aisles that contain problem foods.

- In a cafeteria, examine all the possible food choices before you begin making selections. This will help you avoid overloading your plate. Don't take dessert during your first trip through the line: What seems like an appropriate choice and portion size for dessert may look very different *after* you've eaten a meal.

- Pay special attention to portion sizes. Use measuring cups and spoons and a food scale to become more familiar with appropriate portion sizes.

- Serve meals on small plates and in small bowls to help you eat smaller portions without feeling deprived.

- Eat only in specifically designated spots. Remove food from other areas of your house or apartment.

- When you eat, just eat—don't do anything else, such as read or watch TV.

- Eat more slowly. It takes time for your brain to get the message that your stomach is full. Take small bites and chew food thoroughly. Pay attention to every bite, and enjoy your food. Between bites, try putting down your fork or spoon and taking sips of water or another beverage.

- When you're done eating, remove your plate. Cue yourself that the meal is over—drink a glass of water, suck on a mint, chew gum, or brush your teeth.

Special Occasions

- When you eat out, choose a restaurant where you can make healthy food choices. Ask the server not to put bread and butter on the table before the meal, and request that sauces and salad dressings be served on the side. If portion sizes are large, take half your food home for a meal later in the week.

- If you cook a large meal for friends, send leftovers home with your guests.

- If you're eating at a friend's, eat a little and leave the rest. Don't eat to be polite; if someone offers you food you don't want, thank the person and decline firmly: "No thank you, I've had enough" or "It's delicious, but I'm full."

- Take care during the winter holidays. Research indicates that people gain less than they think during the winter holidays (about a pound) but that the weight isn't lost during the rest of the year, leading to slow, steady weight gain.

Physical Activity and Stress Management

- Increase your level of daily physical activity. If you have been sedentary for a long time or are seriously overweight, increase your level of activity slowly. Start by walking 10 minutes at a time, and work toward 30–60 minutes or more of moderate physical activity per day.

- Begin a formal exercise program that includes cardiorespiratory endurance exercise, strength training, and stretching (see Chapter 13).

- Develop techniques for handling stress—go for a walk or use a relaxation technique. Practice positive self-talk. Get adequate sleep.

- Develop strategies for coping with non-hunger cues to eat, such as boredom, sleepiness, or anxiety. Try calling a friend, taking a shower, or reading a magazine.

- Tell family members and friends that you're making some changes in your eating and exercise habits. Ask them to be supportive.

For additional tips, visit the Department of Health and Human Services Small Steps Web site (www.smallstep.gov), which includes many specific suggestions to encourage individuals and families to take steps toward a healthier lifestyle.

up, not realizing that smaller, mostly fat, losses later in the diet are actually better than the initial larger, mostly fluid losses. Reasonable weight loss is 8–10% of body weight over 6 months. A registered dietitian or nutritionist can recommend an appropriate plan for you when you want to lose weight on your own. For more tips, refer to the Behavior Change Strategy at the end of the chapter.

For many Americans, maintaining weight loss is a bigger challenge than losing weight. Most weight lost during a period of dieting is regained. When planning a weight management program, it is extremely important to include strategies that you can maintain over the long term, both for food choices and for physical activity. Weight management is a lifelong project.

Diet Books

Many people who try to lose weight by themselves fall prey to one or more of the dozens of diet books on the market. Although some contain useful advice and tips for motivation, most make empty promises. Some guidelines for evaluating and choosing a diet book follow:

- Reject books that advocate an unbalanced way of eating. These include books advocating a high-carbohydrate-only diet or those advocating low-carbohydrate, high-protein diets. Also reject books promoting a single food, such as cabbage or grapefruit.
- Reject books that claim to be based on a "scientific breakthrough" or to have the "secret to success."
- Reject books that use gimmicks, such as matching eating to blood type, hyping insulin resistance as the single cause of obesity, combining foods in special ways to achieve weight loss, rotating levels of calories, or purporting that a weight problem is due to food allergies, food sensitivities, yeast infections, or hormone imbalances.
- Reject books that promise quick weight loss or that limit the selection of foods.
- Accept books that advocate a balanced approach to diet plus exercise and sound nutrition advice.

Many diets can cause weight loss if maintained; the real difficulty is finding a safe and healthy pattern of food choices and physical activity that results in long-term maintenance of a healthy body weight and reduced risk of chronic disease (see the box "Is Any Diet Best for Weight Loss?"). Check the Online Learning Center for worksheets that can help you evaluate diet books and commercial weight-loss programs.

Dietary Supplements and Diet Aids

The number of dietary supplements and other weight-loss aids on the market has also increased in recent years.

There are many plans and supplements promoted for weight loss, but few have any research supporting their effectiveness for long-term weight management. Developing lifelong healthy eating and exercise habits is the best approach for achieving and maintaining a healthy body composition.

Weight-loss supplements represent $1.8 billion in retail sales; in a recent survey of over-the-counter (OTC) weight-loss pill users, more than 25% were young obese women and 8% were normal-weight women. Promoted in advertisements, magazines, direct mail campaigns, infomercials, and Web sites, these products typically promise a quick and easy path to weight loss. Most of these products are marketed as dietary supplements and so are subject to fewer regulations than OTC medications. A 2002 report from the Federal Trade Commission stated that more than half of advertisements for weight-loss products made representations that are likely to be false. In addition, use of OTC products doesn't help in the adoption of lifestyle behaviors that can help people achieve and maintain a healthy weight over the long term.

The bottom line on nonprescription diet aids is caveat emptor—let the buyer beware. There is no quick and easy way to lose weight. The most effective approach is to develop healthy diet and exercise habits and make them a permanent part of your lifestyle. Some commonly marketed OTC products for weight loss are described below.

Formula Drinks and Food Bars Canned diet drinks, powders used to make shakes, and diet food bars and snacks are designed to achieve weight loss by substituting for some or all of a person's daily food intake. However, most people find it difficult to use these products for long periods, and muscle loss and other serious health problems may result if they are used as the sole source of nutrition for an extended period. Use of such products

Is Any Diet Best for Weight Loss?

Experts agree that reducing energy (calorie) intake promotes weight loss. However, many popular commercial and published weight-loss plans include a special hook and promote specific food choices and macronutrient (protein, fat, carbohydrate) combinations as best for weight loss. Research findings have been mixed, but two points are clear: Total calorie intake matters, and the best diet is probably the one that an individual can stick with.

Low-Carbohydrate Diets

Recent popular diet books have advocated a diet very low in carbohydrate—with fewer than 10% of total calories from carbohydrate, compared with the 45–65% recommended by the Food and Nutrition Board. Some suggest daily carbohydrate intake below the 130 grams needed to provide essential carbohydrate in the diet. Small studies have found that low-carbohydrate diets can help with weight loss and be safe for relatively short periods of time—although unpleasant effects such as bad breath, constipation, and headache are fairly common.

There are concerns about the long-term effects of low-carb diets, because they tend to be very high in saturated fat and protein and low in fiber, whole grains, vegetables, fruits, and some vitamins, minerals, and phytochemicals. Over the long term, this dietary pattern has been linked to increased risk of heart disease, high blood pressure, and cancer. Diets very high in protein can also stress the kidneys.

Low-Fat Diets

Many experts advocate diets that are relatively low in fat, high in carbohydrate, and moderate in protein. Critics of these diets blame them for rising rates of obesity and note that very-low-fat, very-high-carbohydrate diets can increase triglyceride levels and lower levels of good (HDL) cholesterol in some people. However, these negative effects can be counteracted with moderate-intensity exercise, and low-fat diets combined with physical activity can be safe and effective for many people.

Few experts take the position that low-fat, high-carbohydrate diets, apart from overall diet and activity patterns, are responsible for the increase in obesity among Americans. However, the debate has highlighted the importance of total calorie intake and the quality of carbohydrate choices. Most Americans consume large amounts of refined carbohydrates and added sugars from energy-dense, nutrient-poor foods; they do not consume the recommended whole grains, vegetables, and fruits. A low-fat diet is not a license to consume excess calories, even in the form of low-fat foods.

How Do Popular Diets Measure Up?

In one recent study, obese people on a very-low-carbohydrate, high-fat diet lost more weight over a 6-month period than people following a moderate-fat diet. However, after a year, the difference in weight loss between the two groups was no longer significant, and the dropout rate from both groups was high.

A 2005 study followed participants in four popular diets that emphasize different strategies—Weight Watchers (restricted portion sizes and calories), Atkins (low-carbohydrate, high-fat), Zone (relatively high protein, moderate fat and carbohydrate), and Ornish (very low fat). Each of these diets modestly reduced body weight and heart disease risk factors. There was no significant difference in weight loss at 1 year among the diets, and the more closely people adhered to each diet, the more weight they lost. The dropout rates were high—about 50% for Atkins and Ornish and about 35% for Weight Watchers and Zone. The message from this study? Finding a dietary approach that you can stick to is key to long-term success.

Energy Balance Counts: The National Weight Control Registry

Future research may determine that certain macronutrient patterns may be somewhat more helpful for disease reduction in people with particular risk profiles. However, in terms of weight loss, such differences among diets are likely overshadowed by the importance of total calorie intake and physical activity. Important lessons about energy balance can be drawn from the National Weight Control Registry, an ongoing study of people who have lost significant amounts of weight and kept it off. The average participant in the registry has lost 71 pounds and kept the weight off for more than 5 years. Nearly all participants use a combination of diet and exercise to manage their weight. Most consumed diets moderate in calories and relatively low in fat and fried foods; they monitor their body weight and their food intake frequently. Participants engage in an average of 60 minutes of moderate physical activity daily. The National Weight Control Registry study illustrates that to lose weight and keep it off, you must decrease daily calorie intake and/or increase daily physical activity—and continue to do so over your lifetime.

A Balanced Approach

For short-term weight loss, many types of diets can be safe and successful. However, long-term maintenance of healthy body weight and reduction of chronic disease risk requires permanent changes in lifestyle. Diets advocating strict limits on any nutrient or food groups may be impractical and difficult to maintain over the long term. The latest USDA guidelines provide a good model for healthy food and activity choices. Basic guidelines for weight loss and risk reduction advocated by many experts include the following:

- Set reasonable goals; even small amounts of weight loss benefit health.

- Reduce your intake of saturated and trans fats, refined carbohydrates, and added sugars. Favor unsaturated fats, lean protein sources, whole grains, vegetables, and fruits. Select nutrient-dense choices within each food group.

- Incorporate 60 or more minutes of physical activity into your daily routine; begin a formal exercise program for even greater health and fitness benefits.

- Choose a healthy dietary pattern that works for you over the long term.

SOURCES: Dansinger, M. L., et al. 2005. Comparison of the Atkins, Ornish, Weight Watchers, and Zone diets for weight loss and heart disease risk reduction. *Journal of the American Medical Association* 293(1): 43–53; Hays, N. P., et al. 2004. Effects of an ad libitum low-fat, high-carbohydrate diet on body weight, body composition, and fat distribution in older men and women. *Archives of Internal Medicine* 164(2): 210–217; Hill, J., and R. Wing. 2003. The National Weight Control Registry. *Permanente Journal* 7(3): 34–37; Bravata, D. M., et al. 2003. Efficacy and safety of low-carbohydrate diets. *Journal of the American Medical Association* 289: 1837–1850; Foster, G. D., et al. 2003. A randomized trial of low-carbohydrate diet for obesity. *New England Journal of Medicine* 348: 2082–2090; Samaha, F. F., et al. 2003. A low-carbohydrate as compared with a low-fat diet in severe obesity. *New England Journal of Medicine* 348: 2074–2081.

Critical Consumer

Table 14-3   Ingredients in Over-the-Counter Weight-Loss Aids

Common Name	Use/Claim	Safety Issues
Bitter orange extract	Stimulant chemically related to ephedrine; appetite suppressant	Concentrated extracts may increase blood pressure; contraindicated for people with cardiac problems
Chitosan (fiber derived from shellfish)	Interference with fat absorption	Can cause constipation or gas; contraindicated for people with shellfish allergies
Chromium picolinate	Increased muscle mass, decreased body fat	Short-term use of moderate doses generally considered safe; studies on effectiveness mixed
Conjugated linoleic acid (CLA)	Increased muscle mass, decreased body fat	Short-term use generally considered safe; no long-term studies support efficacy
Dieter's tea (made from aloe, buckthorn, senna, and other herbs)	Stimulant, diuretic, laxative	Acts as a stimulant laxative; in excess amounts can cause diarrhea, vomiting, nausea, fainting, laxative dependence, and electrolyte imbalances that can lead to heart rhythm problems
Garcinia cambogia	Interference with fat metabolism or appetite suppression	Generally considered safe, but common side effects include upper respiratory and gastrointestinal symptoms
HMB (beta-hydroxy-beta-methylbutyrate)	Increased muscle mass, decreased body fat	No reported side effects, but long-term effects unknown
Psyllium (fiber derived from seeds)	Appetite suppressant	Short-term use generally considered safe; hasn't been shown to be effective for weight loss
Pyruvate	Increased metabolism, decreased body fat	Generally considered safe
Yerba mate (tea); guarana; damiana	Stimulant, appetite suppression (active ingredient is caffeine)	Restlessness, anxiety, insomnia; symptoms of caffeine overdose in sensitive people

SOURCES: Fahey, T. D., P. M. Insel, and W. T. Roth. 2005. *Fit and Well*, 6th ed. New York: McGraw-Hill; Evaluating 10 ingredients in weight-loss pills: No clear winners. 2004. *Environmental Nutrition*, June; Sarubin, A. 2000. *The Health Professional's Guide to Popular Dietary Supplements*. Chicago: American Dietetic Association; Food and Drug Administration. 1998. *Supplements Associated with Illnesses and Injuries* (http://www.fda.gov/fdac/features/1998/dietchrt.html; retrieved January 15, 2004).

sometimes results in rapid short-term weight loss, but the weight is typically regained because users don't learn to change the eating and lifestyle behaviors that caused the weight problem in the first place.

Herbs and Herbal Products   As described in Chapter 12, herbs are marketed as dietary supplements, so there is little information about effectiveness, proper dosage, drug interactions, and side effects. In addition, labels may not accurately reflect the ingredients and dosages present, and safe manufacturing practices are not guaranteed. For example, the substitution of a toxic herb for another compound during the manufacture of a Chinese herbal weight-loss preparation caused more than 100 cases of kidney damage and cancer among users in Europe.

In 2004, the FDA banned the sale of ephedra (*ma huang*), stating that it presented a significant and unreasonable risk to human health. (Lawsuits to overturn the ban were subsequently filed in several states.) Ephedrine, the active ingredient in ephedra, is structurally similar to amphetamine and was widely used in weight-loss supplements. It may suppress appetite, but adverse effects have included elevated blood pressure, panic attacks, seizures, insomnia, and increased risk of heart attack or stroke, particularly when combined with another stimulant, such as caffeine. The synthetic stimulant phenylpropanolamine was banned in 2000 for similar reasons. Other herbal stimulants are still on the market (Table 14-3).

Other Supplements and Diet Aids   Fiber is another common ingredient in OTC diet aids, promoted for appetite control. However, dietary fiber acts as a bulking agent in the large intestine, not the stomach, so it doesn't have a pronounced effect on appetite. In addition, many diet aids contain only 3 or fewer grams of fiber, which does not contribute much toward the recommended daily intake of 25–38 grams. Other compounds marketed as diet aids include conjugated linoleic acid, carnitine, chromium, pyruvate, and a number of products labeled "fat absorbers," "fat blockers," and "starch blockers." Research has not found these products to be effective, and many have potentially adverse side effects.

Weight-Loss Programs

Weight-loss programs come in a variety of types, including noncommercial support organizations, commercial programs, Web sites, and medically supervised clinical programs.

Noncommercial Weight-Loss Programs Noncommercial programs such as TOPS (Take Off Pounds Sensibly) and Overeaters Anonymous (OA) mainly provide group support. They do not advocate any particular diet but do recommend seeking professional advice for creating an individualized plan. Like Alcoholics Anonymous, OA is a 12-step program with a spiritual orientation that promotes abstinence from compulsive overeating. These types of programs are generally free. Your physician or a registered dietitian can also provide information and support for weight loss.

Commercial Weight-Loss Programs Commercial programs such as Weight Watchers, Jenny Craig, Diet Workshop, and Richard Simmons Slimmons typically provide group support, nutrition education, physical activity recommendations, and behavior modification advice for changing habits. Some also make available packaged foods to assist in following dietary advice. Many programs voluntarily belong to the Partnership for Healthy Weight Management established by the Federal Trade Commission in 1999. By doing so, they agree to provide clients with information on staff training and education, the risks associated with overweight and obesity, the risks associated with each program or product, the costs of the program, and the expected outcomes of the program, including success rates.

Commercial programs can work, but only if you are motivated to decrease calorie intake and increase physical activity. A responsible and safe weight-loss program should have the following features:

1. The recommended diet should be safe and balanced, include all the food groups, and meet the DRIs for all nutrients. Physical activity and exercise should be strongly encouraged.

2. The program should promote slow, steady weight loss averaging 0.5–2.0 pounds per week. (There may be some greater weight loss initially due to fluid loss.)

3. If a participant plans to lose more than 20 pounds, has any health problems, or is taking medication on a regular basis, physician evaluation and monitoring should be recommended. The staff of the program should include qualified counselors and health professionals.

4. The program should include plans for weight maintenance after the weight-loss phase is over.

5. The program should provide information on all fees and costs, including those of supplements and prepackaged foods, as well as data on risks and expected outcomes of participating in the program.

In addition, you should consider whether a program fits your lifestyle and whether you are truly ready to make a commitment to it. A strong commitment and a plan for maintenance are especially important because only about 10–15% of program participants maintain their weight loss—the rest gain back all or more than they had lost. One study of participants found that regular exercise was the best predictor of maintaining weight loss, whereas frequent television viewing was the best predictor of weight gain. Successful weight management requires long-term lifestyle changes.

Online Weight-Loss Programs A recent addition to the weight-loss program scene is the Internet-based program. Most such Web sites include a cross between self-help and group support through chat rooms, bulletin boards, and e-newsletters. Many sites offer online self-assessment for diet and physical activity habits as well as a meal plan; some provide access to a staff professional for individualized help. Many are free, but some charge a small weekly or monthly fee. Preliminary research suggests that this type of program provides an alternative to in-person diet counseling and can lead to weight loss for some people. Studies found that people who logged on more frequently tended to lose more weight; weekly online contact in terms of behavior therapy proved most successful for weight loss. The criteria used to evaluate commercial programs can also be applied to Internet-based programs. In addition, check whether a program offers member-to-member support and access to staff professionals.

Clinical Weight-Loss Programs Medically supervised clinical programs are usually located in a hospital or other medical setting. Designed to help those who are severely obese, these programs typically involve a closely monitored very-low-calorie diet. The cost of a clinical program is usually high, but insurance will often cover part of the fee.

Prescription Drugs

For a medicine to cause weight loss, it must reduce energy consumption, increase energy expenditure, and/or interfere with energy absorption. The medications most often prescribed for weight loss are appetite suppressants that reduce feelings of hunger or increase feelings of fullness. Appetite suppressants usually work by increasing levels of catecholamine or serotonin, two brain chemicals that affect mood and appetite. All prescription weight-loss drugs have potential side effects. Those that affect catecholamine levels, including phentermine (Ionamin, Obenix, Fastin, and Adipex-P), diethylpropion (Tenuate), and mazindol (Sanorex), may cause sleeplessness, nervousness, and euphoria. Sibutramine (Meridia) acts on both the serotonin and catecholamine systems; it may trigger increases in blood pressure and heart rate. Headaches, constipation or diarrhea, dry mouth, and insomnia are other side effects.

Most appetite suppressants are approved by the FDA only for short-term use. Two drugs, however, are approved for longer-term use: sibutramine and orlistat (Xenical). Sibutramine's safety and efficacy record is good, but regular monitoring of blood pressure is required during therapy. Orlistat lowers calorie consumption by blocking fat absorption in the intestines; it prevents about 30% of the fat in food from being digested. Similar to the fat substitute olestra, orlistat reduces the absorption of fat-soluble vitamins and antioxidants. Therefore, taking a vitamin supplement is highly recommended if taking orlistat. Side effects include diarrhea, cramping, and other gastrointestinal problems if users do not follow a low-fat diet. If you have pizza and ice cream, for example, you will probably experience severe diarrhea. Using other weight-loss medications in combination or for long periods of time is considered off-label use; this means that although it is legal, the FDA has not approved such use. Certain antidepressants and other medications are also being evaluated as weight-loss drugs.

Medications for weight loss are prescribed to decrease the health risks associated with obesity. Both sibutramine and orlistat have proven to produce weight loss and weight maintenance and to decrease risk factors associated with obesity. It is important to remember that these medications work best in conjunction with behavior modification. Studies have generally found that appetite suppressants produce modest weight loss—about 5–22 pounds above the loss expected with nondrug obesity treatments. Individuals respond very differently, however, and some experience more weight loss than others. Unfortunately, weight loss tends to level off or reverse after 4–6 months on a medication, and many people regain the weight they've lost when they stop taking the drug.

Side effects and risks are other concerns. In 1997, the FDA removed from the market two prescription weight-loss drugs, fenfluramine (Pondimin) and dexfenfluramine (Redux), after their use was linked to potentially life-threatening heart valve problems. (Fenfluramine was used most often in combination with phentermine, an off-label combination referred to as "fen/phen.") It appears that people who took these drugs over a long period or at high dosages are at greatest risk for problems, but the FDA recommends that anyone who has taken either of these drugs be examined by a physician.

Prescription weight-loss drugs are not for people who want to lose a few pounds to wear a smaller size of jeans. The latest federal guidelines advise people to try lifestyle modification for at least 6 months before trying drug therapy. Prescription drugs are recommended—in conjunction with lifestyle changes—only in certain cases: for people who have been unable to lose weight with non-drug options and who have a BMI over 30 (or over 27 if two or more additional risk factors such as diabetes and high blood pressure are present). For severely obese people who have been unable to lose weight by other methods, prescription drugs may provide a good option. Even modest weight loss provides significant health benefits for obese individuals.

Surgery

About 3–5% of Americans are severely obese, meaning they have a BMI of 40 or higher or are 100 pounds or more over recommended weight. The number of severely obese people has nearly tripled in the past decade. For such people, obesity is a serious medical condition that is often complicated by other health problems such as diabetes, sleep disorders, heart disease, and arthritis. Surgical intervention may be necessary as a treatment of last resort for those who have not been successful in permanently reducing weight through other methods. According to a National Institutes of Health (NIH) Consensus Conference, gastric bypass surgery is recommended for patients with a BMI greater than 40, or greater than 35 with obesity-related illnesses.

In 2002, 65,000 people underwent gastric bypass surgery. Due to the increasing prevalence of severe obesity and the reduction of premature deaths, surgical treatment of obesity is growing worldwide. Obesity-related health conditions, as well as risk of premature death, generally improve after surgical weight loss. However, surgery is not without risks.

Gastric bypass surgery modifies the gastrointestinal tract by changing either the size of the stomach or how the intestine drains, thereby reducing food intake. The two most common surgeries are the Roux-en-Y gastric bypass and the vertical banded gastroplasty (VBG). The *Roux-en-Y gastric bypass* is named after the Swiss surgeon who developed the technique. In this procedure, the stomach is separated into two pouches, one large and one small. A "Y" segment of the small intestine is attached to the smaller pouch. The small stomach pouch restricts food intake, and the bypass of the lower stomach and part of the small intestine results in the absorption of fewer calories (and nutrients). Side effects include fat intolerance, nutritional deficiencies, and dumping syndrome; the latter is usually caused by foods like sugars and fats and results in nausea, cold sweats, cramps, and diarrhea.

In *vertical banded gastroplasty* (VBG), a small gastric pouch is created in the upper part of the stomach by applying a double row of staples that essentially elongates the esophagus. This small pouch empties into the remaining stomach through an outlet that is restricted with a band. The procedure controls the gastric emptying of food and the volume of foods eaten. Common complications associated with this kind of surgery are nausea, vomiting, band slippage, gastroesophageal reflux, and stenosis (constriction of the outlet). When compared with Roux-en-Y gastric bypass, VBG has a lower initial weight loss and a greater weight regain.

Weight loss from surgery generally ranges between 40% and 70% of total body weight over the course of a year. For both of these procedures the key to success is to have adequate follow-up and to stay motivated so that life behaviors and eating patterns are changed permanently.

Another procedure, *liposuction*, has become popular for removing localized fat deposits. This cosmetic procedure is for body contouring, not weight loss, and it doesn't improve health in the way that traditional weight loss does. In addition to being a medically serious operation, liposuction is associated with considerable pain and discomfort, bruising, swelling, discoloration, the risk of infection, and possible unexpected contour changes. Furthermore, it takes from 6 months to a year to see satisfactory results from a liposuction procedure, and the results are not always permanent. Unless patients adhere to healthy diet and activity habits, they gain weight.

Psychological Help

Many people can lose weight just by increasing their physical activity level and moderately restricting total calories. When concern about body weight and shape has developed into an eating disorder, the help of a professional is recommended. In choosing a therapist, be sure to ask about credentials and experience (see Chapter 3). The therapist should have experience working with weight management, body image issues, eating disorders, addictions, and abuse issues. Your physician may be able to provide a referral.

BODY IMAGE

As described earlier in the chapter, body image consists of perceptions, images, thoughts, attitudes, and emotions. Developing a positive body image is an important aspect of psychological wellness and an important component of successful weight management. See the box "Gender, Ethnicity, and Body Image" for suggestions on how to develope a healthy body image.

Severe Body Image Problems

Poor body image can cause significant psychological distress. A person can become preoccupied with a perceived defect in appearance, thereby damaging self-esteem and interfering with relationships. Adolescents and adults who have a negative body image are more likely to diet restrictively, eat compulsively, or develop some other form of disordered eating.

When dissatisfaction becomes extreme, the condition is called *body dysmorphic disorder (BDD)*. BDD affects

The image of the ideal body promoted by the fashion and fitness industries doesn't reflect the wide range of body shapes and sizes that are associated with good health. An overconcern with body image can contribute to low self-esteem and the development of eating disorders.

about 2% of Americans, males and females in equal numbers; BDD usually begins before age 18 but can begin in adulthood. Sufferers are overly concerned with physical appearance, often focusing on slight flaws of the face or head—things that are not obvious to others. Low self-esteem is common. Individuals with BDD may spend hours every day thinking about their flaws and looking at themselves in mirrors; they may desire and seek repeated cosmetic surgeries. BDD is related to obsessive-compulsive disorder and can lead to depression, social phobia, and suicide if left untreated. An individual with BDD needs to get professional evaluation and treatment; medication and therapy can help people with BDD.

In some cases, body image may bear little resemblance to fact. A person suffering from the eating disorder anorexia nervosa typically has a severely distorted body image—she believes herself to be fat even when she has become emaciated (see the next section for more on anorexia). Distorted body image is also a hallmark of *muscle dysmorphia*, a disorder experienced by some bodybuilders and other active people in which they see themselves as small and out of shape despite being very muscular. Those who suffer from muscle dysmorphia may let obsessive bodybuilding interfere with their work and relationships. They may also use steroids and other potentially dangerous muscle-building drugs.

Body Image and Gender

Women are much more likely than men to be dissatisfied with their bodies, often wanting to be thinner than they are. In one study, only 30% of eighth-grade girls reported being content with their bodies, while 70% of their male classmates expressed satisfaction with their looks. Girls and women are much more likely than boys and men to diet, develop eating disorders, and be obese.

One reason that girls and women are dissatisfied with their bodies is that they are influenced by the media—particularly advertisements and women's fashion magazines. Most teen girls report that the media influence their idea of the perfect body and their decision to diet. In a study of adult women, viewing pictures of thin models in magazines had an immediate negative effect on their mood. In another study, 68% of female college students felt worse about their own appearance after looking through women's magazines. Some 75% of normal-weight women think they are overweight, and 90% overestimate their body size. Clearly, media images affect women's self-image and self-esteem. For American women of all ages, success is still too often equated with how we look rather than who we are.

It is important to note that the image of the ideal woman presented in the media is often unrealistic and even unhealthy. In a review of BMI data for Miss America pageant winners since 1922, researchers noted a significant decline in BMI over time, with an increasing number of recent winners having BMIs in the underweight category. The average fashion model is 4–7 inches taller and more than 25 pounds lighter than the average American woman. Most fashion models are thinner than 98% of American women.

Our culture may be promoting an unattainable masculine ideal as well. Researchers surveying male undergraduates found that media consumption was positively associated with a desire for thinness and muscularity. Researchers studying male action figures such as GI Joe from the past 40 years noted that they have become increasingly muscular. A recent Batman action figure, if projected onto a man of average height, would result in someone with a 30-inch waist, 57-inch chest, and 27-inch biceps. Such media messages can be demoralizing, and, although not as commonly, boys and men do also suffer from body image problems.

Body Image and Ethnicity

The thin, toned look as a feminine ideal is just a fashion, one that is not shared by all cultures. Although some groups espouse thinness as an ideal body type, others do not. In many traditional African societies, for example, full-figured women's bodies are seen as symbols of health, prosperity, and fertility. African American teenage girls have a much more positive body image than do white girls; in one survey, two-thirds of them defined beauty as "the right attitude," whereas white girls were more preoccupied with weight and body shape.

A study of college students found that white and Latina students tend to have more body image problems than African American and Asian American students; black students had the most positive general body image among the groups of students in the study. Nevertheless, recent evidence indicates that African American women are as likely to engage in disordered eating behavior, especially binge eating and vomiting, as their Latina, American Indian, and white counterparts. These findings underscore the complex nature of eating disorders and body image.

Avoiding Body Image Problems

To minimize your risk of developing a body image problem, keep the following strategies in mind:

• Focus on healthy habits and good physical health. Eat a moderate, balanced diet, and choose physical activities you enjoy. Avoid chronic or repetitive dieting.

• Focus on good psychological health and put concerns about physical appearance in perspective. Your worth as a human being is not dependent on how you look.

• Practice body acceptance. You can influence your body size and type to some degree through lifestyle, but the basic fact is that some people are genetically designed to be bigger or heavier than others. Focus on healthy lifestyle behaviors and accept your body as it is.

• Find things to appreciate in yourself besides an idealized body image. Men and women whose self-esteem is based primarily on standards of physical attractiveness can find it difficult to age gracefully. Those who can learn to value other aspects of themselves are more accepting of the physical changes that occur naturally with age.

• View food choices as morally neutral—eating dessert isn't bad and doesn't make you a bad person. Healthy eating habits are an important part of a wellness lifestyle, but the things you really care about and do are more important in defining who you are.

• Don't judge yourself or others based on appearance. Watch your attitudes toward people of differing body sizes and shapes, and don't joke about someone's body type. Take people seriously for what they say and do, not for their appearance. Body size is just one external characteristic; millions of happy and successful people also just happen to have a weight problem.

• See the beauty and fitness industries for what they are. Realize that one of their goals is to prompt dissatisfaction with yourself so that you will buy their products.

Acceptance and Change

Most Americans, young and old, are unhappy with some aspect of their appearance, often their weight. The can-do attitude of Americans, together with the belief that there is a solution to this dissatisfaction, leads to more problems with body image, as well as to dieting, disordered eating, and the desire for cosmetic surgery to fix perceived defects.

In fact, there are limits to the changes that can be made to body weight and body shape, both of which are influenced by heredity. The changes that can and should be made are lifestyle changes—engaging in regular physical activity, obtaining adequate nutrition, and maintaining healthy eating habits. With these changes, the body weight and shape that develop will be natural and appropriate for an individual's particular genetic makeup.

Knowing when the limits to healthy change have been reached—and learning to accept those limits—is crucial for overall wellness. Women in particular tend to measure self-worth in terms of their appearance; when they don't measure up to an unrealistic cultural ideal, they see themselves as defective and their self-esteem falls. The result can be negative body image, disordered eating, or even a full-blown eating disorder.

Obesity is a serious health risk, but weight management needs to take place in a positive and realistic atmosphere. For an obese person, losing as few as 10 pounds can reduce blood pressure and improve mood. The hazards of excessive dieting and overconcern about body weight need to be countered by a change in attitude about what constitutes the perfect body and a reasonable body weight. A reasonable weight must take into account a person's weight history, social circumstances, metabolic profile, and psychological well-being.

EATING DISORDERS

Problems with body weight and weight control are not limited to excessive body fat. A growing number of people, especially adolescent girls and young women, experience **eating disorders,** characterized by severe disturbances in eating patterns and eating-related behaviors. The major eating disorders are anorexia nervosa, bulimia nervosa, and binge-eating disorder. More than 8 million Americans, most of them women, suffer from eating disorders. Many more people have abnormal eating habits and attitudes about food that, although not meeting the criteria for a major eating disorder, do disrupt their lives.

Anorexia nervosa is characterized by a refusal to maintain a minimally normal body weight. **Bulimia nervosa** is characterized by repeated episodes of binge eating followed by compensatory behaviors such as self-induced vomiting, the misuse of laxatives or diuretics, fasting, or excessive exercise. **Binge-eating disorder** is characterized by binge eating without regular use of compensatory behaviors. Eating disorders are associated with depression, anxiety, low self-esteem, and increased health risks, including, in some cases, increased risk of premature death.

Eating disorders are more prevalent in developed countries than in developing ones. At any given time, 0.5–2.0% of Americans suffer from anorexia and have bulimia. Research suggests that about 4% of college-aged women have bulimia. Binge-eating disorder may affect 2–5% of all adults and 8% of those who are obese. In the United States, anorexia and bulimia affect far more women than men: Of the 1 million Americans who develop anorexia or bulimia each year, 90% are female. Of those with binge-eating disorder, 60% are female. Eating disorders appear to be more prevalent among people of middle and upper-middle socioeconomic status. However, rates are increasing among males and females of all socioeconomic and cultural groups.

Factors in Developing an Eating Disorder

Many factors are probably involved in the development of an eating disorder. Although wildly different explanations have been proposed, they share one central feature: a dissatisfaction with body image and body weight. Such dissatisfaction is created by distorted thinking, including perfectionistic beliefs, unreasonable demands for self-control, and excessive self-criticism. Dissatisfaction with body weight leads to dysfunctional attitudes about eating, such as fear of fat and preoccupation with food, and problematic eating behaviors, including excessive dieting, constant calorie counting, and frequent weighing.

Heredity appears to play a role in the development of eating disorders, accounting for 30–50% of the risk. But as with other conditions, only the tendency to develop an eating disorder is explained by heredity; the expression of this tendency is affected by other factors. The home environment is one factor: Families in which there is hostility, abuse, or lack of cohesion provide fertile ground for the development of an eating disorder; a rigid or overprotective parent can also increase risk. Cultural messages, as well as family, friends, and peers, shape attitudes toward the self and others. Comparing oneself negatively with others can damage self-esteem and increase vulnerability. Young people who see themselves as lacking control over their lives are also at high risk for eating disorders. About 85% of eating disorders begin during adolescence.

Certain turning points in life, such as beginning to date, leaving home for college, or the breakup of an important relationship, often trigger the onset of an eating disorder. How a person reacts to and copes with such

Terms

Vw

eating disorder A serious disturbance in eating patterns or eating-related behavior, characterized by a negative body image and concerns about body weight or body fat.

anorexia nervosa An eating disorder characterized by a refusal to maintain body weight at a minimally healthy level and an intense fear of gaining weight or becoming fat; self-starvation.

bulimia nervosa An eating disorder characterized by recurrent episodes of binge eating and purging—overeating and then using compensatory behaviors such as vomiting, laxatives, and excessive exercise to prevent weight gain.

binge-eating disorder An eating disorder characterized by binge eating and a lack of control over eating behavior in general.

stresses can influence risk, particularly in individuals who have few stress-management skills. An eating disorder may become a means of coping: The abnormal eating behavior—starvation, **purging**, or binge eating—reduces anxiety by producing numbness and alleviating emotional pain. Restrictive dieting is another possible trigger for the development of eating disorders.

Anorexia Nervosa

A person with anorexia nervosa does not eat enough food to maintain a reasonable body weight. Anorexia affects 1–3 million Americans, 95% of them female. Although it can occur later, anorexia typically develops between the ages of 12 and 18.

Characteristics of Anorexia Nervosa People with anorexia have an intense fear of gaining weight or becoming fat. Their body image is so distorted that even when emaciated they think they are fat. People with anorexia may engage in compulsive behaviors or rituals that help keep them from eating, though some may also binge and purge. They often use vigorous and prolonged exercise to reduce body weight as well. Although they may express a great interest in food, even taking over the cooking responsibilities for the rest of the family, their own diet becomes more and more extreme. People with anorexia often hide or hoard food without eating it.

Anorexic people are typically introverted, emotionally reserved, and socially insecure. They are often model children who rarely complain and are anxious to please others and win their approval. Although school performance is typically above average, they are often critical of themselves and not satisfied with their accomplishments. For people with anorexia nervosa, their entire sense of self-esteem may be tied up in their evaluation of their body shape and weight.

Health Risks of Anorexia Nervosa Because of extreme weight loss, females with anorexia often stop menstruating, become intolerant of cold, and develop low blood pressure and heart rate. They develop dry skin that is often covered by fine body hair like that of an infant. Their hands and feet may swell and take on a blue tinge.

Anorexia nervosa has been linked to a variety of medical complications, including disorders of the cardiovascular, gastrointestinal, endocrine, and skeletal systems. When body fat is virtually gone and muscles are severely wasted, the body turns to its own organs in a desperate search for

Term

V_i_**W**

purging The use of vomiting, laxatives, excessive exercise, restrictive dieting, enemas, diuretics, or diet pills to compensate for food that has been eaten and that the person fears will produce weight gain.

protein. Death can occur from heart failure caused by electrolyte imbalances. About one in ten women with anorexia dies of starvation, cardiac arrest, or other medical complications—one of the highest death rates for any psychiatric disorder. Depression is also a serious risk, and about half the fatalities relating to anorexia are suicides.

Bulimia Nervosa

A person suffering from bulimia nervosa engages in recurrent episodes of binge eating followed by purging. Bulimia is often difficult to recognize because sufferers conceal their eating habits and usually maintain a normal weight, although they may experience weight fluctuations of 10–15 pounds. Although bulimia usually begins in adolescence or young adulthood, it has begun to emerge at increasingly younger (11–12 years) and older (40–60 years) ages.

Characteristics of Bulimia Nervosa During a binge, a bulimic person may rapidly consume anywhere from 1,000 to 60,000 calories. This is followed by an attempt to get rid of the food by purging, usually by vomiting or using laxatives or diuretics. During a binge, bulimics feel as though they have lost control and cannot stop or limit how much they eat. Some binge and purge only occasionally; others do so many times every day.

People with bulimia may appear to eat normally, but they are rarely comfortable around food. Binges usually occur in secret and can become nightmarish—ravaging the kitchen for food, going from one grocery store to another to buy food, or even stealing food. During the binge, food acts as an anesthetic, and all feelings are blocked out. Afterward, bulimics feel physically drained and emotionally spent. They usually feel deeply ashamed and disgusted with both themselves and their behavior and terrified that they will gain weight from the binge.

Major life changes such as leaving for college, getting married, having a baby, or losing a job can trigger a binge-purge cycle. At such times, stress is high and the person may have no good outlet for emotional conflict or tension. As with anorexia, bulimia sufferers are often insecure and depend on others for approval and self-esteem. They may hide difficult emotions such as anger and disappointment from themselves and others. Binge eating and purging become a way of dealing with feelings.

Health Risks of Bulimia Nervosa The binge-purge cycle of bulimia places a tremendous strain on the body and can have serious health effects. Contact with vomited stomach acids erodes tooth enamel. Bulimic people often develop tooth decay because they binge on foods that contain large amounts of simple sugars. Repeated vomiting or the use of laxatives, in combination with deficient calorie intake, can damage the liver and kidneys and cause cardiac arrhythmia. Chronic hoarseness and esophageal tearing with bleeding may also result from vomiting. More rarely, binge eating can lead to rupture of the stomach. Although many bulimic women maintain normal weight, even a small weight loss to lower-than-normal weight can cause menstrual problems. And although less often associated with suicide or premature death than anorexia, bulimia is associated with increased depression, excessive preoccupation with food and body image, and sometimes disturbances in cognitive functioning.

Binge-Eating Disorder

Binge-eating disorder is characterized by uncontrollable eating, usually followed by feelings of guilt and shame with weight gain. Common eating patterns are eating more rapidly than normal, eating until uncomfortably full, eating when not hungry, and preferring to eat alone. Binge eaters may eat large amounts of food throughout the day, with no planned mealtimes. Many people with binge-eating disorder mistakenly see rigid dieting as the only solution to their problem. However, rigid dieting usually causes feelings of deprivation and a return to overeating.

Compulsive overeaters rarely eat because of hunger. Instead, food is used as a means of coping with stress, conflict, and other difficult emotions or to provide solace and entertainment. People who do not have the resources to deal effectively with stress may be more vulnerable to binge-eating disorder. Inappropriate overeating often begins during childhood. In some families, eating may be used as an activity to fill otherwise empty time. Parents may reward children with food for good behavior or withhold food as a means of punishment, thereby creating distorted feelings about the use of food.

Binge eaters are almost always obese, so they face all the health risks associated with obesity. In addition, binge eaters may have higher rates of depression and anxiety. To overcome binge eating, a person must learn to put food and eating into proper perspective and develop other ways of coping with stress and painful emotions.

Borderline Disordered Eating

Eating habits and body image run a continuum from healthy to seriously disordered. Where each of us falls along that continuum can change depending on life stresses, illnesses, and many other factors. People with borderline disordered eating have some symptoms of eating disorders but do not meet the full diagnostic criteria for anorexia, bulimia, or binge-eating disorder. Behaviors such as excessive dieting, occasional bingeing or purging, or the inability to control eating turn food into the enemy and create havoc in the lives of millions of Americans.

How do you know if you have disordered eating habits? When thoughts about food and weight dominate your life, you have a problem. If you're convinced that your worth as a person hinges on how you look and how much you weigh, it's time to get help. Other danger signs include frequent feelings of guilt after a meal or snack, any use of vomiting or laxatives after meals, or overexercising or severely restricting your food intake to compensate for what you've already eaten.

If you suspect you have an eating problem, don't go it alone or delay getting help, as disordered eating habits can develop into a full-blown eating disorder. Check with your student health or counseling center—nearly all colleges have counselors and medical personnel who can help you or refer you to a specialist if needed. If you are concerned about eating habits of a family member or friend, refer to the suggestions in the box "If Someone You Know Has an Eating Disorder . . ."

Treating Eating Disorders

The treatment of eating disorders must address both problematic eating behaviors and the misuse of food to manage stress and emotions. Anorexia nervosa treatment first involves averting a medical crisis by restoring adequate body weight; then the psychological aspects of the disorder can be addressed. The treatment of bulimia nervosa or binge-eating disorder involves first stabilizing the eating patterns, then identifying and changing the patterns of thinking that led to disordered eating, and then improving coping skills. Concurrent problems, such as depression or anxiety, must also be addressed. In 1996, the antidepressant Prozac became the first medication approved by the FDA for the treatment of bulimia.

Treatment of eating disorders usually involves a combination of psychotherapy and medical management. The therapy may be carried out individually or in a group; sessions involving the entire family may be recommended. A support or self-help group can be a useful adjunct to such treatment. Medical professionals, including physicians, dentists, gynecologists, and registered dietitians, can evaluate and manage the physical damage caused by the disorder. If a patient is severely depressed or emaciated, hospitalization may be necessary. Depending on the severity of the disorder, treatment may last from a few months to several years.

Today's Challenge

Eating disorders can be seen as the logical extension of the concern with weight that pervades American society. Although most people don't succumb to irrational or distorted ideas about their bodies, many do become obsessed with dieting. The challenge facing Americans today is achieving a healthy body weight without excessive dieting—by adopting and maintaining sensible eating habits, an active lifestyle, realistic and positive attitudes and emotions, and creative ways of handling stress.

Take Charge

- Educate yourself about eating disorders and their risks and about treatment resources in your community. (See the For More Information section for suggestions.)

- Write down specific ways the person's eating problem is affecting you or others in the household. Call a house meeting to talk about how others are affected by the problem and how to take action.

- Consider consulting a professional about the best way to approach the situation. Research how and where your friend can get help. Attend a local support group.

- Arrange to speak privately with the person, along with other friends or family members. Let one person lead the group and do most of the talking. Discuss specific incidents and the consequences of disordered eating.

- If you are going to speak with your friend, write down ahead of time what your concerns are and what you would like to say. Expect that the person you are concerned about will deny there is a problem, minimize it, or become angry with you. Remain calm and nonjudgmental, and continue to express your concern.

- Avoid giving simplistic advice about eating habits. Gently encourage your friend to eat properly.

- Take time to listen to your friend, and express your support and understanding. Encourage honest communication. Emphasize your friend's good characteristics and compliment all her or his successes.

- Help maintain the person's sense of dignity by encouraging personal responsibility and decision making. Be patient and realistic; recovery is a long process. Continue to love and support your friend.

- If the situation is an emergency—if the person has fainted or attempted suicide, for example—take immediate action. Call 911 for help.

- If you feel very upset about the situation, seek professional help. Remember, you are not to blame for another person's eating disorder.

Tips for Today

Maintaining a healthy weight means balancing calories in with calories out. Many forces and factors in contemporary society work against a healthy balance, so it's imperative that individuals take active control of managing their weight. Many approaches work, but the simplest formula is moderate food intake coupled with regular exercise.

Right now you can

- Drink a glass of water instead of a soda.

- Throw away any high-calorie, low-nutrient snack foods in your kitchen and buy fruits and vegetables as snacks instead.

- Put a sign on your refrigerator reminding you of your weight-management goals.

- Go outside and walk or jog for 15 minutes or take a 15-minute bike ride.

- Review the information on portion sizes in Chapter 12 and consider whether the portions you usually take at meals are larger than they need to be.

SUMMARY

- Body composition is the relative amounts of fat-free mass and fat in the body. *Overweight* and *obesity* refer to body weight or the percentage of body fat that exceeds what is associated with good health.

- The key to weight management is maintaining a balance of calories in (food) and calories out (resting metabolism, food digestion, and physical activity).

- Standards for assessing body weight and body composition include body mass index (BMI) and percent body fat.

- Too much or too little body fat is linked to health problems; the distribution of body fat can also be a significant risk factor.

- An inaccurate or negative body image is common and can lead to psychological distress.

- Genetic factors help determine a person's weight, but the influence of heredity can be overcome with attention to lifestyle factors.

- Physiological factors involved in the regulation of body weight and body fat include metabolic rate, hormonal influences, and the size and number of fat cells.

- Nutritional guidelines for weight management include consuming a moderate number of calories; limiting portion sizes, energy density, and the intake of fat, simple sugars, refined carbohydrates, and protein to recommended levels; and developing an eating schedule and decision rules for food choices.

- Activity guidelines for weight management emphasize daily physical activity and regular sessions of cardiorespiratory endurance exercise and strength training.

- Weight management requires developing positive, realistic self-talk and self-esteem and a repertoire of appropriate techniques for handling stress and other emotional and physical challenges.

Behavior Change Strategy

The behavior management plan described in Chapter 1 provides an excellent framework for a weight-management program. Following are some suggestions about specific ways you can adapt that general plan to controlling your weight.

Motivation and Commitment

Make sure you are motivated and committed before you begin. Failure at weight loss is a frustrating experience that can make it more difficult to lose weight in the future. Think about why you want to lose weight. Self-focused reasons, such as to feel good about yourself or to have a greater sense of well-being, are often associated with success. Trying to lose weight for others or out of concern for how others view you is a poor foundation for a weight-loss program. Make a list of your reasons for wanting to lose weight, and post it in a prominent place.

Setting Goals

Choose a reasonable weight you think you would like to reach over the long term, and be willing to renegotiate it as you get further along. Break down your long-term weight and behavioral goals into a series of short-term goals. Develop a new way of behaving by designing small, manageable steps that will get you to where you want to go.

Creating a Negative Energy Balance

When your weight is constant, you are burning approximately the same number of calories as you are taking in. To tip the energy balance toward weight loss, you must either consume fewer calories, or burn more calories through physical activity, or both. One pound of body fat represents 3500 calories. To lose weight at the recommended rate of 0.5–2.0 pounds per week, you must create a negative energy balance of 1750–7000 calories per week or 250–1000 calories per day. To generate a negative energy balance, it's usually best to begin by increasing activity level rather than decreasing your calorie consumption.

Physical Activity

Consider how you can increase your energy output simply by increasing routine physical activity, such as walking or taking the stairs. (Figure 13-4 shows activities that use about 150 calories.) If you are not already involved in a regular exercise routine aimed at increasing endurance and building or maintaining muscle mass, seek help from someone who is competent to help you plan and start an appropriate exercise routine. If you are already doing regular physical exercise, evaluate your program according to the guidelines in Chapter 13.

Don't try to use exercise to spot reduce. Leg lifts, for example, contribute to fat loss only to the extent that they burn calories; they don't burn fat just from your legs. You can make parts of your body appear more fit by exercising them, but the only way you can reduce fat in any specific part of your body is to create an overall negative energy balance.

Diet and Eating Habits

If you can't generate a large enough negative energy balance solely by increasing physical activity, you may want to supplement exercise with modest cuts in your calorie intake. Don't think of this as going on a diet; your goal is to make small changes in your diet that you can maintain for a lifetime. Focus on cutting your intake of saturated and trans fats and added sugars and on eating a variety of nutritious foods in moderation. Don't skip meals, fast, or go on a very-low-calorie diet or a diet that is unbalanced.

Making changes in eating habits is another important strategy for weight management. If your program centers on a conscious restriction of certain food items, you're likely to spend all your time thinking about the forbidden foods. Focus on *how* to eat rather than *what* to eat. Refer to the box "Strategies for Successful Weight Management" for suggestions.

Self-Monitoring

Keep a record of your weight and behavior change progress. Try keeping a record of everything you eat. Write down what you plan to eat, in what quantity, *before* you eat. You'll find that just having to record something that is not OK to eat is likely to stop you from eating it. If you also note what seems to be triggering your urges to eat (for example, you feel bored, or someone offered you something), you'll become more aware of your weak spots and be better able to take corrective action. Also, keep track of your daily activities and your formal exercise program so you can monitor increases in physical activity.

Putting Your Plan into Action

• Examine the environmental cues that trigger poor eating and exercise habits, and devise strategies for dealing with them. For example, you may need to remove problem foods from your house temporarily or put a sign on the refrigerator reminding you to go for a walk instead of having a snack. Anticipate problem situations, and plan ways to handle them more effectively.

• Create new environmental cues that will support your new healthy behaviors. Put your walking shoes by the front door. Move fruits and vegetables to the front of the refrigerator.

• Get others to help. Talk to friends and family members about what they can do to support your efforts. Find a buddy to join you in your exercise program.

• Give yourself lots of praise and rewards. Think about your accomplishments and achievements and congratulate yourself. Plan special nonfood treats for yourself, such as a walk or a movie. Reward yourself often and for anything that counts toward success.

• If you do slip, tell yourself to get back on track immediately, and don't waste time on self-criticism. Think positively instead of getting into a cycle of guilt and self-blame. Don't demand too much of yourself.

• Don't get discouraged. Be aware that although weight loss is bound to slow down after the first loss of body fluid, the weight loss at this slower rate is more permanent than earlier, more dramatic, losses.

• Remember that weight management is a lifelong project. You need to adopt reasonable goals and strategies that you can maintain over the long term.

- People can be successful at long-term weight loss on their own, by combining diet and exercise.
- Diet books, OTC diet aids and supplements, and formal weight-loss programs should be assessed for safety and efficacy.
- Professional help is needed in cases of severe obesity; medical treatments include prescription drugs, surgery, and psychological therapy.

- Dissatisfaction with weight and shape are common to all eating disorders. Anorexia nervosa is characterized by self-starvation, distorted body image, and an intense fear of gaining weight. Bulimia nervosa is characterized by recurrent episodes of uncontrolled binge eating and frequent purging. Binge-eating disorder involves binge eating without regular use of compensatory purging.

Take Action

1. **Interview a successful dieter:** Identify some people who have successfully lost weight and kept it off, and interview them. What were their strategies and techniques? In what ways did they change their exercise and eating habits? Do you think their approach would work for others?

2. **Assess your body composition:** Find out what percentage of your body weight is fat by taking one of the tests described in this chapter at your campus health clinic, sports medicine clinic, or health club. If you have too high or too low a proportion of body fat, consider taking steps to change it.

3. **Critique advertisements:** Leaf through a few fashion and fitness magazines, and evaluate the "ideal" body types presented for women and men. Are they realistic? Are they healthy? How does looking at them affect you? Consider writing letters to advertisers; voice your opinion (positive or negative) about the body types and images they present.

For More Information

Books

Beck, C. 2003. *Anorexia and Bulimia for Dummies.* Hoboken, N.J.: John Wiley & Sons. *An easy-to-understand guide to eating disorders.*

Brownell, K. D. 2003. *Food Fight: The Inside Story of the Food Industry, America's Obesity Crisis, and What We Can Do About It.* New York: McGraw-Hill/Contemporary. *An in-depth look at environmental factors supporting the American lifestyle that contribute to obesity.*

Critser, G. 2004. *Fat Land: How Americans Became the Fattest People in the World.* Boston: Mariner Books. *A look at the many factors in American life that have contributed to the rapid increase in obesity rates.*

Ferguson, J. M., and C. Ferguson. 2003. *Habits Not Diets,* 4th ed. Boulder, Colo.: Bull. *A behavior-change approach to changing diet and activity habits that includes many helpful practical tips, assessment worksheets, and tracking forms.*

Hensrud, D. D. 2005. *Mayo Clinic Healthy Weight for Everyone.* Rochester, Minn.: Mayo Clinic. *Provides guidelines for successful weight management.*

Milchovich, S. K., and B. Dunn-Long. 2003. *Diabetes Mellitus: A Practical Handbook,* 8th. ed. Boulder, Colo.: Bull. *A user-friendly guide to diabetes.*

Nash, J. D. 2003. *Maximize Your Body Potential: Lifetime Skills for Successful Weight Management.* Boulder, Colo.: Bull. *A do-it-yourself guide that provides self-assessment tools and guidelines for setting realistic goals and developing an individualized weight management plan.*

Pope, H. G., K. A. Phillips, and R. Olivardia. 2000. *Adonis Complex: The Secret Crisis of Male Body Obsession.* New York: Free Press. *Provides a historical review of the changing fashions in male body type and information about body image problems.*

Organizations, Hotlines, and Web Sites

American Diabetes Association. Provides information, a free newsletter, and referrals to local support groups; the Web site includes an online diabetes risk assessment.

800-342-2383
http://www.diabetes.org

Calorie Control Council. Site includes a variety of interactive calculators, including an Exercise Calculator that estimates the calories burned from various forms of physical activity.
http://www.caloriecontrol.org

Cyberdiet. Provides a variety of assessment and planning tools as well as practical tips for adopting a healthy lifestyle.
http://www.cyberdiet.com

FDA Center for Food Safety and Applied Nutrition: Dietary Supplements. Provides background facts and information on the current regulatory status of dietary supplements, including compounds marketed for weight loss.
http://www.cfsan.fda.gov/~dms/supplmnt.html

Federal Trade Commission (FTC): Project Waistline. Provides advice for evaluating advertising about weight-loss products.
http://www.ftc.gov/bcp/consumer/edcams/waistline

National Heart, Lung, and Blood Institute (NHLBI): Aim for a Healthy Weight. Provides information and tips on diet and physical activity, as well as a BMI calculator.
http://www.nhlbi.nih.gov/health/public/heart/obesity/lose_wt

National Institute of Diabetes and Digestive and Kidney Diseases (NIDDK). Provides information and referrals for problems related to obesity, weight control, and nutritional disorders.
877-946-4627
http://win.niddk.nih.gov/

Partnership for Healthy Weight Management. Provides information on evaluating weight-loss programs and advertising claims.
http://www.consumer.gov/weightloss

SmallStep.Gov. Provides resources for increasing activity and improving diet through small changes in daily habits.
http://www.smallstep.gov

U.S. Consumer Gateway: Health—Dieting and Weight Control. Provides links to government sites with advice on evaluating claims about weight-loss products and programs.
http://www.consumer.gov/health.htm

USDA Food and Nutrition Information Center: Reports and Studies on Obesity. Provides links to recent reports and studies on the issue of obesity among Americans.
http://www.nal.usda.gov/fnic/reports/obesity.html

Resources for people concerned about eating disorders:

Eating Disorder Referral and Information Center
http://www.edreferral.com
Eating Disorders Shared Awareness
http://www.something-fishy.org

MedlinePlus: Eating Disorders
http://www.nlm.nih.gov/medlineplus/eatingdisorders.html
National Association of Anorexia Nervosa and Associated Disorders
847-831-3438 (referral line)
http://www.anad.org
National Eating Disorders Association
206-382-3587
http://www.nationaleatingdisorders.org

See also the listings in Chapters 12 and 13.

Selected Bibliography

American Diabetes Association. 2004. How to Tell if You Have Pre-Diabetes (http://www.diabetes.org/pre-diabetes/pre-diabetes-symptoms.jsp; retrieved March 27, 2005).

Bowman, S. A., et al. 2004. Effects of fast-food consumption on energy intake and diet quality among children in a national household survey. Pediatrics 113(1 Pt 1): 112–118.

Buchwald, H., et al. 2004. Bariatric surgery: A systematic review and meta-analysis. Journal of the American Medical Association 292(14): 1724–1737.

Calle, E. E., et al. 2003. Overweight, obesity, and mortality from cancer in a prospectively studied cohort of US adults. New England Journal of Medicine 348: 1625–1638.

Centers for Disease Control and Prevention. 2004. Overweight and Obesity: Economic Consequences (http://www.cdc.gov/nccdphp/dnpa/obesity/economic_consequences.htm; retrieved January 3, 2005).

Centers for Disease Control and Prevention. 2004. Prevalence of diabetes among Hispanics—selected areas, 1998–2002. Morbidity and Mortality Weekly Report 53(40): 941–944.

Dong, L., G. Block, and S. Mandel. 2004. Activities contributing to total energy expenditure in the United States: Results from the NHAPS Study. International Journal of Behavioral Nutrition and Physical Activity 1(4).

Farshchi, H. R., M. A. Taylor, and I. A. Macdonald. 2005. Deleterious effects of omitting breakfast on insulin sensitivity and fasting lipid profiles in healthy lean women. American Journal of Clinical Nutrition 81(2): 388–396.

Federal Trade Commission. 2002. Weight Loss Advertising: An Analysis of Current Trends. Washington, D.C.: Federal Trade Commission.

Fenicchia, L. M., et al. 2004. Influence of resistance exercise training on glucose control in women with type 2 diabetes. Metabolism 53(3): 284–289.

Fontaine, K. R., et al. 2003. Years of life lost due to obesity. Journal of the American Medical Association 289(2): 187–193.

Fung, T. T., et al. 2004. Dietary patterns, meat intake, and the risk of type 2 diabetes in women. Archives of Internal Medicine 164(20): 2235–2240.

Graves, B. S., and R. L. Welsh. 2004. Recognizing the signs of body dysmorphic disorder and muscle dysmorphia. ACSM's Health and Fitness Journal, January/February.

Hu, F. B., et al. 2003. Television watching and other sedentary behaviors in relation to risk of obesity and type 2 diabetes mellitus in women. Journal of the American Medical Association 289(14): 1785–1791.

Hu, F. B., et al. 2004. Adiposity as compared with physical activity in predicting mortality among women. New England Journal of Medicine 351(26): 2694–2703.

Irwin, M. L., et al. 2003. Effect of exercise on total and intra-abdominal body fat in postmenopausal women. Journal of the American Medical Association 289(3): 323–330.

Kaiser Family Foundation. 2004. The role of media in childhood obesity. Issue Brief, February.

Leit, R. A., J. J. Gray, and H. G. Pope, Jr. 2002. The media's representation of the ideal male body: A cause for muscle dysmorphia? International Journal of Eating Disorders 31(3): 334–338.

Ma, Y., et al. 2005. Association between dietary carbohydrates and body weight. American Journal of Epidemiology 161(4): 359–367.

Martinez-Gonzalez, M. A., et al. 2003. Parental factors, mass media influences, and the onset of eating disorders in a prospective population-based cohort. Pediatrics 111(2): 315–320.

McBride, B. F., et al. 2004. Electrocardiographic and hemodynamic effects of a multicomponent dietary supplement containing ephedra and caffeine. Journal of the American Medical Association 291(4): 216–221.

Mokdad, A. H., et al. 2003. Prevalence of obesity, diabetes, and obesity-related health risk factors, 2001. Journal of the American Medical Association 289: 76–79.

Mokdad, A. H., et al. 2005. Correction: Actual causes of death in the United States, 2000. Journal of the American Medical Association 293(3): 293–294.

Nestle, M. 2003. The ironic politics of obesity. Science 299: 781.

Nicklas, B. J., et al. 2004. Association of visceral adipose tissue with incident myocardial infarction in older men and women: The Health, Aging and Body Composition Study. American Journal of Epidemiology 160(8): 741–749.

Nielsen, S. J., and B. M. Popkin. 2003. Patterns and trends in food portion sizes, 1977–1996. Journal of the American Medical Association 289(4): 450–453.

Olshansky, S. J., et al. 2005. A potential decline in life expectancy in the United States in the 21st century. New England Journal of Medicine 352(11): 1138–1145.

Rubinstein, S., and B. Caballero. 2000. Is Miss America an undernourished role model? Journal of the American Medical Association 283(12): 1569.

Schulze, M. B., et al. 2004. Sugar-sweetened beverages, weight gain, and incidence of type 2 diabetes in young and middle-aged women. Journal of the American Medical Association 292(8): 927–934.

Sweeteners can sour your health. 2005. Consumer Reports on Health, January.

Tate, D. F., R. R. Wing, and R. A. Winett. 2001. Using Internet technology to deliver a behavioral weight loss program. Journal of the American Medical Association 285(9): 1172–1177.

Taylor, E. N., et al. 2005. Obesity, weight gain, and risk of kidney stones. Journal of the American Medical Association 293(4): 455–462.

Tsai, A. G., and T. A. Wadden. 2005. Systematic review: An evaluation of major commercial weight loss programs in the United States. Annals of Internal Medicine 142(1): 56–66.

U.S. Department of Health and Human Services. 2005. Dietary Guidelines for Americans (http://www.healthierus.gov/dietaryguidelines; retrieved January 15, 2005).

Vorona, R. D., et al. 2005. Overweight and obese patients in a primary care population report less sleep than patients with a normal body mass index. Archives of Internal Medicine 165: 25–30.

Walters, P. H., et al. 2003. Childhood obesity: Causes and treatment. ACSM's Health and Fitness Journal, January/February.

Weinstein, A. R., et al. 2004. Relationship of physical activity vs. body mass index with type 2 diabetes in women. Journal of the American Medical Association 292(10): 1188–1194.

Wong, S. L., et al. 2004. Cardiorespiratory fitness is associated with lower abdominal fat independent of body mass index. Medicine and Science in Sports and Exercise 36(2): 286–291.

Young, L. R., and M. Nestle. 2003. Expanding portion sizes in the U.S. marketplace: Implications for nutrition counseling. Journal of the American Dietetic Association 103(2): 231–234.

15

Looking

AHEAD

After reading this chapter, you should be able to

- List the major components of the cardiovascular system and describe how blood is pumped and circulated throughout the body

- Describe the controllable and uncontrollable risk factors associated with cardiovascular disease

- Discuss the major forms of cardiovascular disease and how they develop

- List the steps you can take to lower your personal risk of developing cardiovascular disease

Cardiovascular Health

1. **Reducing the amount of cholesterol you eat is the most important dietary change you can make to improve your blood cholesterol levels.**
   True or false?

2. **Women are about as likely to die of cardiovascular disease as they are to die of breast cancer.**
   True or false?

3. **How much earlier, on average, do people who do *not* exercise regularly develop heart disease compared with people who do exercise?**
   a. 6 months
   b. 2 years
   c. 6 years

4. **Healthy teenagers have no signs of cardiovascular disease.**
   True or false?

5. **Which of the following foods would be a good choice for promoting heart health?**
   a. tofu
   b. salmon
   c. bananas

ANSWERS

1. FALSE. Limiting your intake of saturated and trans fats, which promote the production of cholesterol by the liver, is the key dietary change for improving blood cholesterol levels; dietary cholesterol has much less of an effect on blood cholesterol.

2. FALSE. Cardiovascular disease kills far more. Among American women, about 1 in 2 deaths is due to cardiovascular disease and about 1 in 30 is due to breast cancer.

3. C. Both aerobic exercise and strength training significantly improve cardiovascular health.

4. FALSE. Autopsy studies of young trauma victims show that narrowing of the arteries that supply the heart with blood begins in adolescence in many people.

5. ALL THREE. Soy protein (tofu), foods with omega-3 fatty acids (salmon), and foods high in potassium and low in sodium (bananas) all improve cardiovascular health.

Visit the *Core Concepts in Health* Online Learning Center (www.mhhe.com/insel10e) for study aids and many additional resources.

445

ardiovascular disease (CVD) is the leading cause of death in the United States, claiming one life every 34 seconds. Nearly half of all Americans alive today will die from CVD. Heart attacks and strokes are the most common life-threatening manifestations of CVD. Though we typically think of CVD as primarily affecting men and older adults, heart attack is the number-one killer of American women, and nearly a third of heart attacks occur in people under age 65.

Much of the incidence of CVD is due to the American way of life. Too many Americans eat an unhealthy diet, are overweight and sedentary, smoke, manage stress ineffectively, have uncontrolled high blood pressure or high cholesterol levels, and don't know the signs of CVD. Not all the risk factors for CVD are controllable—for example, the older you are, the greater your risk for CVD. But many key risk factors can be changed, treated, or modified, and you have the power to significantly reduce your risk for CVD.

Exactly what is CVD, and how does it do its damage? More important, what steps can you take now to keep your heart healthy throughout your life? This chapter will provide some answers to these questions.

THE CARDIOVASCULAR SYSTEM

The cardiovascular system consists of the heart and blood vessels (veins, arteries, and capillaries); together, they

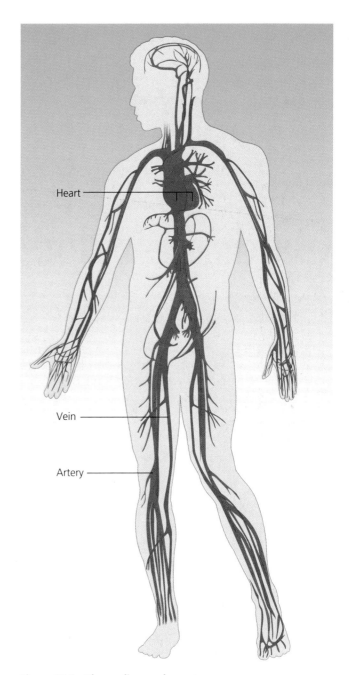

Figure 15-1   The cardiovascular system.

pump and circulate blood throughout the body. A person weighing 150 pounds has about 5 quarts of blood, which circulates about once every minute.

The heart is a four-chambered, fist-size muscle located just beneath the ribs under the left breast (Figure 15-1). Its role is to pump deoxygenated (oxygen-poor) blood to the lungs and oxygenated (oxygen-rich) blood to the rest of the body. Blood actually travels through two separate circulatory systems: The right side of the heart pumps blood to and from the lungs in what is called the **pulmonary circulation,** and the left side pumps blood through the rest of the body in the **systemic circulation.**

1 Waste-carrying, oxygen-poor blood enters the right atrium from the superior and inferior venae cavae.

Pulmonary artery

Aorta

Left lung

3 In the lungs, blood picks up oxygen and discards carbon dioxide; it then flows through the pulmonary veins into the left atrium.

Superior vena cava

Right lung

Pulmonary vein

Left atrium

Right atrium

4 Oxygen-rich blood flows from the left atrium into the left ventricle; from there it is pumped through the aorta into the rest of the body's blood vessels.

2 Blood flows from the right atrium into the right ventricle; from there, it is pumped through the pulmonary arteries into the lungs.

Left ventricle

Right ventricle

Inferior vena cava

Figure 15-2   Circulation in the heart.

Used, oxygen-poor blood enters the right upper chamber, or **atrium,** of the heart through the **vena cava,** the largest vein in the body (Figure 15-2). Valves prevent the blood from flowing the wrong way. As the right atrium fills, it contracts and pumps blood into the right lower chamber, or **ventricle,** which, when it contracts, pumps blood through the pulmonary artery into the lungs. There, blood picks up oxygen and discards carbon dioxide. Cleaned, oxygenated blood then flows through the pulmonary veins into the left atrium. As this chamber fills, it contracts and pumps blood into the powerful left ventricle, which pumps it through the **aorta,** the body's largest artery, to be fed into the rest of the body's blood vessels. The period of the heart's contraction is the **systole;** the period of relaxation is the **diastole.**

The heartbeat—the split-second sequence of contractions of the heart's four chambers—is controlled by electrical impulses. These signals originate in a bundle of specialized cells in the right atrium called the **sinus node.** Unless the pace is speeded up or slowed down by the brain in response to stimuli such as danger or exhaustion, the heart produces electrical impulses at a steady rate.

Blood vessels are classified by size and function. **Veins** carry blood to the heart; **arteries** carry blood away from the heart. Veins have thin walls; arteries have thick elastic walls that enable them to expand or contract with the volume of the blood being pumped through them. After leaving the heart, the aorta branches into smaller and smaller vessels. Two vital arteries, the left and right **coronary arteries,** branch off the aorta to carry blood back to the heart muscle itself (Figure 15-3).

The smallest arteries branch still further into **capillaries,** tiny vessels only one cell thick. The capillaries deliver oxygen and nutrient-rich blood to the tissues and receive oxygen-poor, waste-carrying blood. From the capillaries, this blood empties into small veins and then into larger veins that return it to the heart. From there the cycle is repeated.

RISK FACTORS FOR CARDIOVASCULAR DISEASE

Researchers have identified a variety of factors associated with an increased risk of developing cardiovascular disease. They are grouped into two categories: major risk factors and contributing risk factors. Some risk factors, such as diet, exercise habits, and use of tobacco, are linked to controllable aspects of lifestyle and can therefore be changed. Others, such as age, sex, and heredity, are beyond an individual's control.

Figure 15-3 Blood supply to the heart.

The labels in the figure are:
- Aorta
- Superior vena cava
- Pulmonary artery
- Left atrium
- Left coronary artery
- Right atrium
- Left ventricle
- Right coronary artery
- Right ventricle
- Inferior vena cava

Major Risk Factors That Can Be Changed

The American Heart Association (AHA) has identified six major risk factors for CVD that can be changed: tobacco use, high blood pressure, unhealthy blood cholesterol levels, physical inactivity, obesity, and diabetes.

Tobacco Use   About one in five deaths from CVD is attributable to smoking. Despite a 40% decline in smoking since 1965, it remains the number-one preventable cause of CVD in the United States. People who smoke a pack of cigarettes a day have twice the risk of heart attack that nonsmokers have; smoking two or more packs a day triples the risk. And when smokers do have heart attacks, they are 2 to 4 times more likely than nonsmokers to die from them. Women who smoke heavily and use oral contraceptives are up to 32 times more likely to have a heart attack and up to 20 times more likely to have a stroke than women who don't smoke and take the pill.

Smoking harms the cardiovascular system and raises the risk for CVD in several ways. Nicotine, a central nervous system stimulant, increases blood pressure and heart rate; the carbon monoxide in cigarette smoke displaces oxygen in the blood, reducing the amount of oxygen available to the heart and other parts of the body. Smoking damages the linings of arteries, and it contributes to unhealthy blood fat levels by reducing levels of high-density lipoproteins (HDL), good cholesterol, and raising levels of triglycerides and low-density lipoproteins (LDL), bad cholesterol. It causes the **platelets** in blood to become sticky and cluster, promoting clotting. Smoking also permanently accelerates the rate at which fatty deposits are laid down in arteries.

You don't have to smoke to be affected. The risk of death from coronary heart disease increases up to 30% among those exposed to environmental tobacco smoke (ETS) at home or at work. Researchers estimate that as many as 62,000 nonsmokers die from CVD each year as a result of exposure to ETS.

High Blood Pressure   High blood pressure, or **hypertension,** is a risk factor for many forms of cardiovascular disease, including heart attacks and strokes, and is itself considered a form of CVD. Hypertension can also cause kidney failure and damage to nearly every organ in the body. Blood pressure, the force exerted by the blood on the vessel walls, is created by the pumping action of the heart. When the heart contracts (systole), blood pressure increases. When the heart relaxes (diastole), pressure decreases. High blood pressure occurs when too much force is exerted against the walls of the arteries. Many

Table 15-1	Blood Pressure Classification for Healthy Adults			
Category[a]	Systolic (mm Hg)		Diastolic (mm Hg)	
Normal[b]	below 120	and	below 80	
Prehypertension	120–139	or	80–89	
Hypertension[c]				
Stage 1	140–159	or	90–99	
Stage 2	160 and above	or	100 and above	

[a]When systolic and diastolic pressure fall into different categories, the higher category should be used to classify blood pressure status.

[b]The risk of death from heart attack and stroke begins to rise when blood pressure is above 115/75.

[c]Based on the average of two or more readings taken at different physician visits. In persons older than 50 years, systolic blood pressure greater than 140 is a much more significant CVD risk factor than diastolic blood pressure.

SOURCE: *The Seventh Report of the Joint National Committee on Prevention, Detection, Evaluation, and Treatment of High Blood Pressure.* 2003. Bethesda, Md.: National Heart, Lung, and Blood Institute. National Institutes of Health (NIH Publication No. 03-5233).

factors affect blood pressure; for example, excitement or exercise causes the heart to pump more blood into the arteries, resulting in a rise in blood pressure. Short periods of high blood pressure are normal, but blood pressure that is continually at an abnormally high level constitutes hypertension.

Blood pressure is measured with a stethoscope and an instrument called a sphygmomanometer. It is expressed as two numbers—for example, 120 over 80—and measured in millimeters of mercury. The first and larger number is the systolic blood pressure; the second is the diastolic blood pressure. A normal blood pressure reading for a healthy adult is 115 systolic over 75 diastolic; CVD risk increases when blood pressure rises above this level. High blood pressure in adults is defined as equal to or greater than 140 over 90 (Table 15-1).

High blood pressure results from either an increased output of blood by the heart or, most often, increased resistance to blood flow in the arteries. The latter condition can be caused by **atherosclerosis,** discussed later in the chapter, or by constriction of smooth muscle surrounding the arteries. When a person has high blood pressure, the heart must work harder than normal to force blood through the narrowed arteries, thereby straining both the heart and arteries. Over time, a strained heart weakens and tends to enlarge, which weakens it more. Increased blood pressure also scars and hardens arteries, making them less elastic and further increasing blood pressure.

High blood pressure is often called a silent killer, because it usually has no symptoms. A person may have high blood pressure for years without realizing it. But during that time, it damages vital organs and increases the risk of heart attack, congestive heart failure, stroke, kidney failure, and blindness. In about 90% of people with high blood pressure, the cause is unknown. This type of high blood pressure is called primary (or essential) hypertension and is probably due to a mixture of genetic and environmental factors, including obesity, stress, excessive alcohol intake, inactivity, and a high-fat, high-salt diet. In the remaining 10% of people, the condition is caused by an underlying illness and is referred to as secondary hypertension.

Hypertension is common, occurring in nearly one in three adults. Its incidence rises dramatically with increasing age; however, it can occur among children and young adults, and women sometimes develop hypertension during pregnancy (blood pressure usually returns to normal following the pregnancy). High blood pressure is two to three times more common in women taking oral contraceptives, especially in obese and older women; this risk increases with the duration of use. The risk of developing hypertension is highest in African Americans, in whom, compared with other groups, the disorder is often more severe, more resistant to treatment, and more likely to be fatal at an early age. Among people age 20–39, African Americans also have higher rates of prehypertension. Overall, about 30% of adults have hypertension, 30% have prehypertension, and 40% have normal blood pressure.

Primary hypertension cannot be cured, but it can be controlled. Because hypertension has no early warning signs, it's crucial to have your blood pressure tested at least once every 2 years (more often if you have other CVD risk factors). Follow your physician's advice about lifestyle changes and medication. Unfortunately, only about 34% of Americans with hypertension have it under control.

Lifestyle changes are recommended for everyone with prehypertension and hypertension (see Table 15-1). These lifestyle changes include weight reduction, regular physical activity, a healthy diet, and moderation of alcohol consumption. The DASH diet, described in Chapter 12, is recommended; it emphasizes fruits, vegetables, and whole grains, foods that are rich in potassium and fiber, both of which may reduce blood pressure. Sodium restriction is also helpful. Many people are salt-sensitive, meaning that their blood pressure will decrease significantly when salt intake is restricted. Salt restriction has

Terms

platelets Microscopic disk-shaped cell fragments in the blood that disintegrate on contact with foreign objects and release chemicals that are necessary for the formation of blood clots.

hypertension Sustained abnormally high blood pressure.

atherosclerosis A form of CVD in which the inner layers of artery walls are made thick and irregular by plaque deposits; arteries become narrow, and blood supply is reduced.

less impact on those who are not salt-sensitive, but it may still be beneficial. The 2005 Dietary Guidelines for Americans recommend restricting consumption to less than 2300 mg of sodium (about 1 teaspoon of salt) per day. People with hypertension, African Americans, and middle-aged and older adults should aim to consume no more than 1500 mg of sodium per day. Adequate potassium intake is also important. For people whose blood pressure isn't adequately controlled with lifestyle changes, medication is prescribed. Many different types of antihypertensive drugs are available, and taking the right one can usually lower blood pressure effectively with a minimum of side effects.

Recent research has shed new light on the importance of lowering blood pressure to improve cardiovascular health. Death rates from CVD begin to rise when blood pressure is above 115 over 75, well below the traditional 140 over 90 cutoff for hypertension. People with blood pressures in the prehypertension range are at increased risk of heart attack and stroke as well as at significant risk of developing full-blown hypertension; preventive lifestyle measures are strongly recommended for people with prehypertension. The bottom line is that lowering your blood pressure through healthy lifestyle changes is beneficial, even if your current blood pressure is already below 140 over 90.

High Levels of Cholesterol
Cholesterol is a fatty, waxlike substance that circulates through the bloodstream and is an important component of cell membranes, sex hormones, vitamin D, the fluid that coats the lungs, and the protective sheaths around nerves. Adequate cholesterol is essential for the proper functioning of the body. However, excess cholesterol can clog arteries and increase the risk of cardiovascular disease. Our bodies obtain cholesterol in two ways: from the liver, which manufactures it, and from the foods we eat. Cholesterol levels vary depending on diet, age, sex, heredity, and other factors.

GOOD VERSUS BAD CHOLESTEROL Cholesterol is carried in the blood in protein-lipid packages called lipoproteins. Lipoproteins can be thought of as shuttles that transport cholesterol to and from the liver through the circulatory system (Figure 15-4). **Low-density lipoproteins (LDLs)** shuttle cholesterol from the liver to the organs and tissues

that require it. LDL is known as bad cholesterol because if there is more than the body can use, the excess is deposited in the blood vessels. LDL that accumulates and becomes trapped in artery walls may be oxidized by free radicals, speeding inflammation and damage to artery walls and increasing the likelihood of a blockage. If coronary arteries are blocked, the result may be a heart attack; if an artery carrying blood to the brain is blocked, a stroke may occur. **High-density lipoproteins (HDLs),** or good cholesterol, shuttle unused cholesterol back to the liver for recycling. By removing cholesterol from blood vessels, HDL helps protect against atherosclerosis.

RECOMMENDED BLOOD CHOLESTEROL LEVELS The risk for cardiovascular disease increases with increasing blood cholesterol levels, especially LDL (Table 15-2). The National Cholesterol Education Program (NCEP) recommends lipoprotein testing at least once every 5 years for all adults, beginning at age 20. The recommended test is

Table 15-2	Cholesterol Guidelines
LDL cholesterol (mg/dl)*	
Less than 100	Optimal
100–129	Near optimal/above optimal
130–159	Borderline high
160–189	High
190 or more	Very high
Total cholesterol (mg/dl)	
Less than 200	Desirable
200–239	Borderline high
240 or more	High
HDL cholesterol (mg/dl)	
Less than 40	Low (undesirable)
60 or more	High (desirable)
Triglycerides (mg/dl)	
Less than 150	Normal
150–199	Borderline high
200–499	High
500 or more	Very high

*These are general goals for LDL; specific LDL goals depend on a person's other risk factors (see pp. 472–473 for more information); for people at very high risk, an LDL goal of less than 70 mg/dl may be appropriate.

SOURCES: Grundy, S. M., et al. 2004. Implications of recent clinical trials for the National Cholesterol Education Program Adult Treatment Panel III Guidelines. *Circulation* 110: 227–239; Expert Panel on Detection, Evaluation, and Treatment of High Blood Cholesterol in Adults. 2001. Executive Summary of the Third Report of the National Cholesterol Education Program (NCEP) Expert Panel on Detection, Evaluation, and Treatment of High Blood Cholesterol in Adults (Adult Treatment Panel III). *Journal of the American Medical Association* 285(19).

Terms

ViW

low-density lipoproteins (LDL) Blood fat that transports cholesterol from the liver to organs and tissues; excess is deposited on artery walls, where it can eventually block the flow of blood to the heart and brain; "bad" cholesterol.

high-density lipoproteins (HDL) Blood fat that helps transport cholesterol out of the arteries and thus protects against heart diseases; "good" cholesterol.

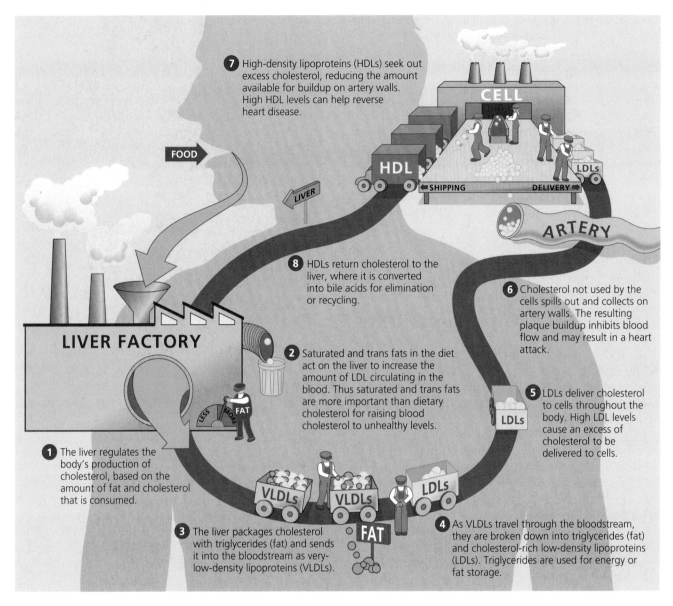

7 High-density lipoproteins (HDLs) seek out excess cholesterol, reducing the amount available for buildup on artery walls. High HDL levels can help reverse heart disease.

8 HDLs return cholesterol to the liver, where it is converted into bile acids for elimination or recycling.

2 Saturated and trans fats in the diet act on the liver to increase the amount of LDL circulating in the blood. Thus saturated and trans fats are more important than dietary cholesterol for raising blood cholesterol to unhealthy levels.

6 Cholesterol not used by the cells spills out and collects on artery walls. The resulting plaque buildup inhibits blood flow and may result in a heart attack.

5 LDLs deliver cholesterol to cells throughout the body. High LDL levels cause an excess of cholesterol to be delivered to cells.

1 The liver regulates the body's production of cholesterol, based on the amount of fat and cholesterol that is consumed.

3 The liver packages cholesterol with triglycerides (fat) and sends it into the bloodstream as very-low-density lipoproteins (VLDLs).

4 As VLDLs travel through the bloodstream, they are broken down into triglycerides (fat) and cholesterol-rich low-density lipoproteins (LDLs). Triglycerides are used for energy or fat storage.

Figure 15-4   Travels with cholesterol.

a fasting lipoprotein profile that measures total cholesterol, LDL cholesterol, HDL cholesterol, and triglycerides (another blood fat). General cholesterol and triglyceride guidelines are shown in Table 15-2. In general, high LDL levels and low HDL levels are associated with a high risk for CVD; low levels of LDL and high levels of HDL are associated with lower risk. HDL is important because a high HDL level seems to offer protection from CVD even in cases where total cholesterol is high. This seems to be especially true for women.

As shown in Table 15-2, LDL levels below 100 mg/dl (milligrams per deciliter) and total cholesterol levels below 200 mg/dl are desirable. An estimated 107 million American adults—over half the population—have total cholesterol levels of 200 mg/dl or higher. The CVD risk associated with elevated cholesterol levels also depends on other factors.

For example, an above-optimal level of LDL would be of more concern for an individual who also smokes and has high blood pressure than for an individual without these additional CVD risk factors, and it is especially a concern for diabetics. Specific NCEP guidelines for cholesterol based on risk factors are presented later in the chapter.

BENEFITS OF CONTROLLING CHOLESTEROL People can cut their heart attack risk by about 2% for every 1% that they reduce their total blood cholesterol levels. People who lower their total cholesterol from 250 to 200 mg/dl, for example, reduce their risk of heart attack by 40%. In addition, studies indicate that improving LDL and HDL levels not only reduces the likelihood that arteries will become clogged but can also reverse deposits on artery walls, thereby actually helping clean out diseased arteries.

How can you improve your cholesterol levels? Your primary goal should be to reduce LDL to healthy levels. Important dietary changes for reducing LDL levels include substituting unsaturated for saturated and trans fats and increasing fiber intake. Decreasing your intake of saturated and trans fats is particularly important because they promote the production of cholesterol by the liver. Exercising regularly and eating more fruits, vegetables, and whole grains also help. You can raise your HDL levels by exercising regularly, losing weight if you are overweight, quitting smoking, and altering the amount and type of fat you consume. These and other lifestyle changes promoting heart health are discussed in greater detail later in this chapter.

Physical Inactivity A sedentary lifestyle is a known major risk factor for CVD, but despite an increasing awareness of the risks of inactivity, only about 20% of American adults are active enough to derive health benefits from their physical activity. People, especially females, become less active as they age, and rates of activity are particularly low among certain ethnic populations and people with little education, low incomes, and living in the north-central and southern states.

Regular physical activity has direct and indirect benefits on the heart. Directly, it lowers heart rate and blood pressure, while improving the strength with which the heart pumps blood to the body and the ability of the tissues to extract oxygen from that blood. Indirectly, physical activity positively affects almost every risk factor for CVD. Exercise is thought to be the closest thing we have to a magic bullet against heart disease. It lowers CVD risk by helping decrease blood pressure, increase HDL levels, maintain desirable weight, and prevent or control diabetes; exercise also improves the functioning of the endothelial cells that line coronary arteries and decreases platelet aggregation, which can lead to clot formation in the coronary arteries.

In general, the more physical activity you engage in, the more cardiovascular benefit you derive. A minimum of 30–60 minutes per day of moderate physical activity is recommended. One recent study found that women who accumulated at least 3 hours of brisk walking each week cut their risk of heart attack and stroke by more than half. More intense or longer-duration exercise has even greater health benefits. Refer to Chapter 13 for more on the benefits of physical activity and guidelines for creating an exercise program.

A diet high in fiber and low in saturated and trans fats can help lower levels of total cholesterol and LDL. This young woman is eating a vegetable sandwich on whole-grain bread with fresh fruit for lunch.

Obesity As your weight increases, your risk of CVD increases. The risk of death from CVD is two to three times more likely in obese people (BMI $\geq$ 30) than it is in lean people (BMI 18.5–24.9), and for every 5-unit increment of BMI, a person's risk of death from coronary heart disease increases by 30%. BMI at age 18 predicts mortality due to CVD—the higher your BMI at age 18, the more likely you are to eventually die from CVD. Maintaining a healthy weight is also important. Researchers found that middle-aged women who had gained 22 pounds or more since age 18 had a significantly higher risk of subsequent death from CVD than those who were able to maintain their weight over time.

The increased risk of CVD associated with overweight is present even if a person has no other risk factors, but, unfortunately, overweight people usually do have other CVD risk factors. Excess body fat is strongly associated with hypertension, high cholesterol levels, insulin resistance, diabetes, physical inactivity, and increasing age. It is also associated with endothelial cell dysfunction and increased inflammatory markers, such as CRP (discussed later in this chapter). **Endothelial cells** line the inside of arteries, including the coronary arteries, and they help regulate blood flow to the heart and keep platelets and other cells from sticking to artery walls. When the endothelial cells are healthy, the coronary arteries dilate (widen) when the heart needs more blood, but when the cells are dysfunctional, the coronary arteries instead constrict, limiting blood flow to the heart. With excess weight, there is also more blood to pump and the heart has to work harder. This causes

Terms

V w

endothelial cells Cells lining the inside of arteries; they help regulate blood flow and prevent platelets from sticking.

hypertrophy Abnormal enlargement of an organ secondary to an increase in cell size.

chronically elevated pressures within the heart chambers that can lead to ventricular **hypertrophy,** and eventually the heart muscle can start to fail.

As discussed in Chapter 14, the distribution of body fat is significant: Fat that collects in the torso is more dangerous than fat that collects around the hips. Obesity in general, and abdominal obesity in particular, is significantly associated with narrowing of the coronary arteries, even in young adults in their twenties. Abdominal obesity can increase your risk even if your weight is normal.

A sensible diet and regular exercise are the best ways to achieve and maintain a healthy body weight. Physical activity and physical fitness also appear to have a strong positive influence on cardiovascular health in those who are overweight and obese. People who are obese but have at least moderate cardiorespiratory fitness may have lower rates of cardiovascular disease than their normal-weight but unfit peers. For someone who is overweight, even modest weight reduction—5–10% of body weight—can reduce CVD risk by lowering blood pressure, improving cholesterol levels, and reducing diabetes risk.

Diabetes As described in Chapter 14, diabetes is a disorder characterized by elevated blood glucose levels due to insufficient supply or action of insulin. Having diabetes doubles the risk of CVD for men and triples the risk for women. The most common cause of death in adults with diabetes is CVD, and they usually die at younger ages than people without diabetes. There is an estimated loss of 10–20 years of life in those with diabetes. The reason for the increased CVD risk among people with diabetes is complex. Diabetics have higher rates of other CVD risk factors, including hypertension, obesity, and unhealthy blood lipid levels (typically, high triglyceride levels and low HDL levels). The elevated blood glucose and insulin levels that occur in diabetes can damage the endothelial cells that line the arteries, making them more vulnerable to atherosclerosis; diabetics also often have platelet and blood coagulation abnormalities that increase the risk of heart attacks and strokes. People with pre-diabetes also face a significantly increased risk of CVD.

As described in Chapter 14, the number of people with diabetes and pre-diabetes continues to climb and is closely linked to obesity. It is estimated that for every kilogram increase in weight, the risk of diabetes increases by approximately 9%. The largest increase in prevalence of type 2 diabetes over the past decade has been among people age 30–39, and there has also been an alarming increase among children and adolescents. Children who are diagnosed with diabetes typically develop complications in their twenties or thirties. Complications of diabetes mainly affect the arteries. When small arteries are affected, the result can be problems with vision (retinopathy that can lead to blindness), kidney function (nephropathy that can require dialysis), and the nervous system (neuropathy that can lead to amputation). When the larger arteries are affected, all forms of CVD result, including heart attacks, strokes, and peripheral vascular disease. Having diabetes is considered to be a heart disease risk equivalent, meaning that your CVD morbidity and mortality risk is the same as if you already had coronary artery disease. And diabetics who do have CAD fare even worse; they have accelerated atherosclerosis and derive less benefit from common forms of treatment than non-diabetics.

Routine screening for diabetes is not currently recommended unless a person presents with symptoms of diabetes or has other CVD risk factors. For people diagnosed with diabetes, a healthy diet, exercise, and careful control of glucose levels is recommended to decrease chances of developing the complications listed above. But even people whose diabetes is under control face a high risk of CVD. For that reason, careful control of other CVD risk factors is critical for people with diabetes.

Contributing Risk Factors That Can Be Changed

Various other factors that can be changed have been identified as contributing to CVD risk, including triglyceride levels and psychological and social factors.

High Triglyceride Levels Like cholesterol, triglycerides are blood fats that are obtained from food and manufactured by the body. High triglyceride levels are a reliable predictor of heart disease, especially if associated with other risk factors, such as low HDL levels, obesity, and diabetes. Factors contributing to elevated triglyceride levels include excess body fat, physical inactivity, cigarette smoking, type 2 diabetes, excess alcohol intake, very high carbohydrate diets, and certain diseases and medications.

Much of the picture regarding triglycerides remains unclear, however. Studies have yet to show whether lowering triglyceride levels will actually decrease heart disease. Elevated triglyceride levels are most often seen in people with other lipid abnormalities; and the lifestyle modifications that help lower cholesterol also help decrease triglycerides, making it difficult to identify any potential independent benefit of lowering triglyceride levels.

A full lipid profile should include testing and evaluation of triglyceride levels (see Table 15-2). For people with borderline high triglyceride levels, increased physical activity, reduced intake of added sugars and starches, and weight reduction can help bring levels down into the healthy range; for people with high triglyceride levels, drug therapy may be recommended. Being moderate in the use of alcohol and quitting smoking are also important.

Psychological and Social Factors Many of the psychological and social factors that influence other areas of wellness are also important risk factors for CVD. The idea that the mind and the body are connected certainly seems to be true when it comes to the heart. When you become excited or stressed or angry, you can probably feel your heart pounding harder and faster. The cardiovascular system is affected by both sudden, acute episodes of mental stress and the more chronic, underlying emotions of anger, anxiety, and depression.

STRESS Excessive stress can strain the heart and blood vessels over time and contribute to CVD. With stress, the brain tells the adrenal glands to secrete cortisol and **catecholamines,** which in turn activate the sympathetic nervous system. As described in Chapter 2, the sympathetic nervous system causes the fight-or-flight response; this response increases heart rate and blood pressure so that more blood is distributed to the heart and other muscles in anticipation of physical activity. Blood glucose concentrations and cholesterol also increase to provide a source of energy, and the platelets become activated so that they will be more likely to clot in case of injury. Such a response can be adaptive if you're being chased by a hungry lion but may be more detrimental than useful if you're sitting at a desk taking an exam or feeling frustrated by a task given to you by your work supervisor.

If you are healthy, you can tolerate the cardiovascular responses that take place during stress, but if you already have CVD, stress can lead to adverse outcomes such as abnormal heart rhythms (arrhythmias), heart attacks, and sudden cardiac death. It has long been known that an increase in heart rhythm problems and deaths is associated with acute mental stress. For example, the rate of potentially life-threatening arrhythmias in patients who already had underlying heart disease doubled during the month after the September 11 terrorist attacks; interestingly, this increase was not limited to people in close proximity to Manhattan.

Because avoiding all stress is impossible, having healthy mechanisms to cope with it is your best defense. Instead of adopting unhealthy habits such as smoking or overeating to deal with stress, refer to Chapter 2 for more healthy coping strategies such as exercising, getting enough sleep, and talking to others.

CHRONIC HOSTILITY AND ANGER Certain traits in the hard-driving Type A personality—hostility, cynicism, and anger—are associated with increased risk of heart disease. Men prone to anger have two to three times the heart attack risk of calmer men and are much more likely to develop CVD at young ages. In a 10-year study of young adults age 18–30 years, those with high hostility levels were more than twice as likely to develop coronary artery calcification (a marker of early atherosclerosis) as those

---

Term

Víw

catecholamines A group of chemically similar hormones and neurotransmitters that are active during the fight-or-flight response; includes epinephrine and norepinephrine.

---

with low hostility levels. See the box "Anger, Hostility, and Heart Disease" for more information.

SUPPRESSING PSYCHOLOGICAL DISTRESS Consistently suppressing anger and other negative emotions may also be hazardous to a healthy heart. People who hide psychological distress appear to have higher rates of heart disease than people who experience similar distress but share it with others. People with Type D personalities tend to be pessimistic, negative, and unhappy and to suppress these feelings. Researchers are not yet certain why the Type D trait is dangerous. It may have physical effects, or it may lead to social isolation and poor communication with physicians.

DEPRESSION In both men and women, depression appears to increase the risk of CVD in healthy individuals, and it definitely increases the risk of adverse cardiac events in those who already have heart disease. You do not need to have a major depressive disorder to be affected: For each depressive symptom you have, the risk seems to increase in a linear fashion (see Chapter 3 for symptoms of depression).

Depression is common in people with coronary heart disease (CHD), and patients who are depressed tend to have worse outcomes than those who are not. Up to a third of patients experience major depression within 1 year of having a heart attack, and those who are depressed after having a heart attack are more likely to have another heart attack or die of a cardiac cause. Even in those with CHD who have not had a recent cardiac event, up to 20% have depression, and this number may be even higher in women. Major depressive disorder at the time of treatment for coronary artery disease is associated with both short- and long-term complications, including subsequent heart attack and death.

The relationship between depression and CHD is complex and not fully understood. Those who are depressed may engage in unhealthy behaviors such as smoking and inactivity that lead to heart disease. They may not consistently take prescribed medications, and they may not cope well with having an illness or undergoing a medical procedure. Depression also causes physiologic changes; for example, it elevates basal levels of catecholamines and cortisol, which, as described earlier, increases blood pressure, blood glucose levels, cholesterol levels, and platelet aggregation.

ANXIETY Chronic anxiety and anxiety disorders (such as phobias and panic disorder) are associated with up to a threefold increased risk of coronary heart disease, heart attack, and sudden cardiac death. There is some evidence that, similar to people with depression, people with anxiety are more likely to have a subsequent adverse cardiac event after having a heart attack. At the same time, people with anxiety and depression often have medically unexplained chest pain, meaning that no evidence of coronary artery disease can be found. This can create difficulties in diagnosis and disease management, but it is important to

Anger, Hostility, and Heart Disease

Mind/Body/Spirit

Current research suggests that people with a quick temper, a persistently hostile outlook, and a cynical, mistrusting attitude toward life are more likely to develop heart disease than those with a calmer, more trusting attitude. People who are angry frequently, intensely, and for long periods experience the stress response—and its accompanying boosts in heart rate, blood pressure, and stress hormone levels—much more often than more relaxed individuals. Over the long term, these effects may damage arteries and promote CVD.

Are You Too Hostile?

To help answer that question, Duke University researcher Redford Williams, M.D., has devised a short self-test. It's not a scientific evaluation, but it does offer a rough measure of hostility. Are the following statements true or false for you?

1. I often get annoyed at checkout cashiers or the people in front of me when I'm waiting in line.
2. I usually keep an eye on the people I work or live with to make sure they do what they should.
3. I often wonder how homeless people can have so little respect for themselves.
4. I believe that most people will take advantage of you if you let them.

5. The habits of friends or family members often annoy me.
6. When I'm stuck in traffic, I often start breathing faster and my heart pounds.
7. When I'm annoyed with people, I really want to let them know it.
8. If someone does me wrong, I want to get even.
9. I'd like to have the last word in any argument.
10. At least once a week, I have the urge to yell at or even hit someone.

According to Williams, five or more "true" statements suggest that you're excessively hostile and should consider taking steps to mellow out.

Managing Your Anger

Begin by monitoring your angry responses and looking for triggers—people or situations that typically make you angry. Familiarize yourself with the patterns of thinking that lead to angry or hostile feelings, and then try to head them off before they develop into full-blown anger. If you feel your anger starting to build, try reasoning with yourself by asking the following questions:

1. *Is this really important enough to get angry about?* For example, is having

to wait an extra 5 minutes for a late bus so important that you should stew about it for the entire 15-minute ride?
2. *Am I really justified in getting angry?* Is the person in front of you really driving slowly, or are you trying to speed?
3. *Is getting angry going to make a real and positive difference in this situation?* Will yelling and slamming the door really help your friend find the concert tickets he misplaced?

If you answer yes to all three questions, then calm but assertive communication may be an appropriate response. If your anger isn't reasonable, try distracting yourself or removing yourself from the situation. Exercise, humor, social support, and other stress-management techniques can also help (see Chapter 3 for additional anger-management tips). Your heart—and the people around you—will benefit from your calmer, more positive outlook.

SOURCES: Take it to heart: "Chill out." 2000. *Mind/Body Health Newsletter* 9(2): 1–2; Anger and heart-disease risk. 2000. *Harvard Heart Letter*, July. QUIZ SOURCE: Williams, Virginia, and Redford Williams. *Life Skills*. New York: Times Books. Reprinted by permission of the authors.

---

always seek medical attention if you are unsure about the cause of your chest pain.

SOCIAL ISOLATION Social isolation and low social support (living alone, having few friends or family members, and not belonging to organizations, clubs, or churches) are associated with an increased incidence of CHD and poorer outcomes after the first diagnosis of CHD. Elderly men and women who report less emotional support from others before they have a heart attack are almost three times more likely to die in the first 6 months after the attack. This is particularly true for men. A strong social support network is a major antidote to stress. Friends and family members can also promote and support a healthy lifestyle.

LOW SOCIOECONOMIC STATUS Low socioeconomic status and low educational attainment also increase risk for CVD. These associations are probably due to a variety of factors, including lifestyle and access to health care.

Alcohol and Drugs Although moderate drinking may have health benefits for some people, drinking too much alcohol raises blood pressure and can increase the risk of stroke and heart failure. Stimulant drugs, particularly cocaine, can also cause serious cardiac problems, including heart attack, stroke, and sudden cardiac death. Cocaine stimulates the nervous system, promotes platelet aggregation, and can cause spasm in the coronary arteries. The effect of cocaine on heart attack risk is unrelated to the amount ingested, the route of administration, and the frequency of use; the risk increases if cocaine use is combined with use of tobacco or another drug. Injection drug use can cause infection of the heart and stroke.

Major Risk Factors That Can't Be Changed

A number of major risk factors for CVD cannot be changed: heredity, aging, being male, and ethnicity.

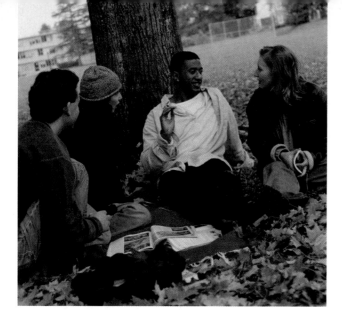

Stress and social isolation can increase the risk of cardiovascular disease. A strong social support network improves both heart health and overall wellness.

Heredity CVD is considered a genetically complex disease because there is no one gene that causes it. Instead, multiple genes contribute to the development of CVD and its associated risk factors, such as high cholesterol, hypertension, diabetes, and obesity. Having a favorable set of genes decreases your risk of developing CVD; having an unfavorable set of genes increases your risk. Risk, however, is modifiable by lifestyle factors such as whether you smoke, exercise, or eat a healthy diet.

Because of the genetic complexity of CVD, genetic screening is usually recommended for only a few specific conditions (for example, certain cholesterol disorders), but you can learn more about your personal risk just by assessing your family history. If you have a first-degree relative (parent, sibling, child) with CAD, you have a two-fold increased risk of someday developing CAD yourself. Genetics seem to play an especially strong role in early CAD, which occurs before age 60. Having a family member diagnosed with early CAD increases the risk of experiencing early CAD by as much as sevenfold; the risk is even higher if the affected relative is female, and the earlier the onset of the CAD, the higher the risk.

Don't forget the role of lifestyle factors, however. Coronary artery disease is usually the result of the interaction of several unfavorable genetic and lifestyle factors, and people with the greatest number of genetic and lifestyle risk factors will face the highest risks. People with favorable genes may not develop CAD despite having an unhealthy lifestyle, and people with many healthy habits may still develop CAD because they have an unfavorable genetic makeup. But it's important to remember that people who inherit a tendency for CVD are not destined to develop it. They may, however, have to work harder than other people to prevent CVD.

Aging The risk of heart attack increases dramatically after age 65. About 70% of all heart attack victims are age 65 or older, and more than four out of five who suffer fatal heart attacks are over 65. For people over 55, the incidence of stroke more than doubles in each successive decade. However, many people in their thirties and forties, especially men, have heart attacks.

Being Male Although CVD is the leading killer of both men and women in the United States, men face a greater risk of heart attack than women, especially earlier in life. Until age 55, men also have a greater risk of hypertension than women. Estrogen production, which is highest during the childbearing years, may offer premenopausal women some protection against CVD (see the box "Women and CVD"). By age 75, the gender gap nearly disappears.

Ethnicity Death rates from heart disease vary among ethnic groups in the United States, with African Americans having much higher rates of hypertension, heart disease, and stroke than other groups (see the box "Ethnicity and CVD" on p. 458). Puerto Rican Americans, Cuban Americans, and Mexican Americans are also more likely to suffer from high blood pressure and angina (a warning sign of heart disease) than non-Hispanic white Americans. These differences may be due in part to differences in education, income, and other socioeconomic factors. Asian Americans historically have had far lower rates of CVD than white Americans. However, cholesterol levels among Asian Americans appear to be rising, presumably because of the adoption of a high-fat American diet.

Possible Risk Factors Currently Being Studied

In recent years, a number of other possible risk factors for cardiovascular disease have been identified. These include homocysteine, specific types of cholesterol, infectious agents, inflammation, and others.

Inflammation and C-Reactive Protein Inflammation plays a key role in the development of CVD. When an artery is injured by smoking, cholesterol, infectious agents, or other factors, the body's response produces inflammation. A substance called C-reactive protein (CRP) is released into the bloodstream during the inflammatory response, and studies suggest that high levels of CRP indicate a substantially elevated risk of heart attack and stroke.

In 2003, the CDC and the American Heart Association jointly recommended testing of CRP levels for people at intermediate risk for CVD because people in this risk category who are found to also have high CRP levels may benefit from additional CVD testing or treatment. (This guideline assumes that people at high risk for CVD are already receiving treatment.) Lifestyle changes and

CVD has traditionally been thought of as a man's disease, and until recently, this has been the justification for carrying out almost all CVD research on men. It is true that men have a higher incidence of cardiovascular problems than women, especially before age 50. On average, women live 10–15 more years free of coronary heart disease than men do. But heart disease is the leading cause of death among women, and it has killed more women than men every year since 1984.

Polls indicate that women vastly underestimate their risk of dying of a heart attack and, in turn, overestimate their risk of dying of breast cancer. In reality, nearly 1 in 2 women dies of CVD, whereas 1 in 30 dies of breast cancer. Minority women face the highest risk of developing CVD, but their awareness of heart disease as a killer of women is lower than that of white women. To help raise awareness of CVD in women, the American Heart Association launched the "Go Red for Women" campaign in 2004; visit their Web site for more information (www.americanheart.org).

Risk factors for CVD are similar for men and women and include age, family history, smoking, hypertension, high cholesterol, and diabetes. There are some gender differences, however. HDL appears to be an even more powerful predictor of CAD risk in women than it is in men. Also, women with diabetes have a greater risk of having CVD events like heart attack and stroke than men with diabetes, so much so that diabetes appears to eliminate the 10- to 15-year advantage women traditionally have had over men for CVD.

Estrogen: A Heart Protector?

The hormone estrogen, produced naturally by a woman's ovaries until menopause,

improves blood lipid concentrations and other CVD risk factors. For the past several decades, many U.S. physicians encouraged menopausal women to take hormone replacement therapy (HRT) to relieve menopause symptoms and presumably reduce the risk of CVD. However, recent studies have found that HRT may actually *increase* a woman's risk for heart disease and certain other health problems, and the U.S. Preventive Services Task Force currently recommends against the use of HRT for the prevention of chronic diseases such as CVD (see Chapter 19 for more on HRT).

For younger women, the most common form of hormonal medication is oral contraceptives (OCs). Typical OCs contain estrogen and progestin in relatively low doses and are generally considered safe for most nonsmoking women. But women who smoke and use OCs are up to 32 times more likely to have a heart attack than nonsmoking OC users.

Postmenopausal Women: At Risk

When women do have heart attacks, they are more likely than men to die within a year. One reason is that because women develop heart disease at older ages, they are more likely to have other health problems that complicate treatment. Women have smaller hearts and arteries than men, possibly making diagnosis and treatment more difficult. There may also be unknown biological or psychosocial risk factors contributing to increased mortality among women.

Also, medical personnel appear to evaluate and treat women less aggressively than men. Women with positive stress tests and those with a recent MI are less likely to be referred to catheterization than are men

with similar findings, and coronary angiography is performed more often in men than in women.

Studies of heart attack patients have found that women usually have to wait longer than men to receive clot-dissolving drugs in an emergency room. Women are more likely than men to have a heart attack *without* chest pain. In one study, many women reported severe fatigue and disturbed sleep in the month leading up to the attack, and fatigue, weakness, and shortness of breath during the attack. Women are also more likely than men to report nausea and pain in the abdomen, back, neck, and/or jaw. A woman who experiences these symptoms should be persistent in seeking accurate diagnosis and appropriate treatment.

Careful diagnosis of cardiac symptoms is also key in cases of stress cardiomyopathy ("broken heart syndrome"), which occurs much more commonly in women. In this condition, exposure to hormones and neurotransmitters associated with a severe stress response stun the heart and produce heart-attack-like symptoms without any corresponding damage to the heart muscle. Typically, the condition can be reversed quickly, and correct diagnosis is important to avoid unnecessary invasive procedures.

Researchers are now focusing more attention on the health problems of women, and more accurate diagnostic techniques may soon be in use. Of course, positive lifestyle choices such as physical activity, quitting smoking, and management of risk factors like blood pressure and cholesterol levels are recommended for women of all ages.

---

certain drugs can reduce CRP levels. Statin drugs, widely prescribed to lower cholesterol, also decrease inflammation and reduce CRP levels; this may be one reason why statin drugs seem to lower CVD risk even in people with normal blood lipid levels. Studies published in 2005 found that patients who received intensive statin treatment, which lowered both LDL cholesterol and CRP levels, fared better than patients who received less aggressive treatment that primarily targeted LDL levels. The reduction in risk from decreased CRP levels was independent

of changes in LDL. Further research may help clarify who can benefit most from testing and treatment for CRP levels.

Insulin Resistance and Metabolic Syndrome

As described in Chapter 12, when you consume carbohydrate, your blood glucose level increases. This stimulates the pancreas to secrete insulin, which allows body cells to pick up glucose to use for energy (see Figure 14-4). The function of insulin is to maintain proper glucose levels in

Although cardiovascular disease is the leading cause of death for all Americans, there is a higher prevalence of CVD and its associated risk factors in adult African Americans and Mexican Americans than in whites and Asian Americans. The reasons for these disparities likely include both genetic and environmental factors.

African Americans are at substantially higher risk for death from CVD than other groups. The rate of hypertension among African Americans is among the highest of any group in the world. Blacks tend to develop hypertension at an earlier age than whites, and their average blood pressures are much higher. African Americans have a higher risk of stroke, have strokes at younger ages, and, if they survive, have more significant stroke-related disabilities. Some experts recommend that blacks be treated with antihypertensive drugs at an earlier stage—when blood pressure reaches 130/80 rather than the typical 140/90 cutoff for hypertension.

A number of genetic and biological factors may contribute to CVD in African Americans. They may be more sensitive to dietary sodium, leading to greater blood pressure elevation in response to a given amount of sodium. African Americans may also experience less dilation of blood vessels in response to stress, an attribute that also raises blood pressure.

Heredity also plays a large role in the tendency to develop diabetes, another important CVD risk factor that is more common in blacks than whites. However, Latinos are even more likely to develop diabetes and insulin resistance, and at a younger age, than African Americans.

There is variation within the Latino population, however, with a higher prevalence of diabetes occurring among Mexican Americans and Puerto Ricans and a relatively lower prevalence among Cuban Americans.

Another factor that likely contributes to the high incidence of CVD among ethnic minority groups is low income. Economic deprivation usually means reduced access to adequate health care and health insurance. Also associated with low income is low educational attainment, which often mean less information about preventive health measures, such as diet and stress management. And people with low incomes tend to smoke more, use more salt, and exercise less than those with higher incomes.

Discrimination may also play a role in CVD. Physicians and hospitals may treat the medical problems of ethnic minorities differently than those of whites. Discrimination, along with low income and other forms of deprivation, may also increase stress, which is linked with hypertension and CVD. In terms of access to care, factors such as insurance coverage and availability of high-tech cardiac equipment in hospitals used most often by minorities may also play a role.

CVD risk in ethnic groups is further affected by immigration and one's place of birth. Upon immigration to the United States, an Asian's risk for CVD tends to increase and reflect that of a typical American more than a typical Asian, perhaps in part because Asian immigrants often abandon their traditional (and healthier) diets.

However, birthplace (and its associated lifestyle factors) also seems to be a strong determinant of risk. One study found that among New Yorkers born in the Northeast, blacks and whites have nearly identical risk of CVD. But black New Yorkers who were born in the South have a sharply higher risk, and black New Yorkers born in the Caribbean have a significantly lower risk. Researchers speculate that instead of abandoning their traditional diets and lifestyles, blacks from the South instead bring these traditions with them. Some risk factors for CVD, including smoking and a high-fat diet, are more common in the South. When combined with urban stress, these factors create a lifestyle that is far from heart-healthy.

All Americans are advised to have their blood pressure checked regularly, exercise, eat a healthy diet, manage stress, and avoid smoking. These general preventive strategies may be particularly helpful for ethnic minorities. Tailoring your lifestyle to your particular ethnic risk may also be helpful in some cases. For example, studies have found that diets high in potassium and calcium may be particularly helpful in improving blood pressure in African Americans; fruits, vegetables, grains, and nuts are rich in potassium, and dairy products are high in calcium. Latinos, who are at greater risk for insulin resistance, may benefit from lifestyle strategies targeting metabolic syndrome. Discuss your particular risk profile with your physician to help identify lifestyle changes most appropriate for you.

---

the body, which it does by affecting the uptake of glucose from the blood by muscle and fat tissue and by limiting the liver's production of glucose. As people gain weight and engage in less physical activity, their muscles, fat, and liver become less sensitive to the effect of insulin—a condition known as insulin resistance (or pre-diabetes). As the body becomes increasingly insulin resistant, the pancreas must secrete more and more insulin (hyperinsulinemia) to keep glucose levels within a normal range. Eventually, however, even high levels of insulin may become insufficient, and blood glucose levels will also start to rise (hyperglycemia), resulting in type 2 diabetes.

Those who have insulin resistance tend to have several other related risk factors; as a group, this cluster of abnormalities is called metabolic syndrome, insulin resistance syndrome, or syndrome X (Table 15-3). Having metabolic syndrome significantly increases the risk of CVD—up to three times in men and six times in women. It is estimated that nearly 25% of the U.S. population has metabolic syndrome. Rates are highest among Mexican Americans, especially women. Among whites, the prevalence is similar in men and women, but among African Americans, the prevalence among women is 57% higher than in men. Some people are genetically predisposed, and among this

Table 15-3	Defining Characteristics of Metabolic Syndrome*	
Abdominal obesity (waist circumference)		
Men	>40 in (>102 cm)	
Women	>35 in (>88 cm)	
Triglycerides	≥150 mg/dl	
HDL cholesterol		
Men	<40 mg/dl	
Women	<50 mg/dl	
Blood pressure	≥130/≥85 mm Hg	
Fasting glucose	≥110 mg/dl	

*A person is diagnosed with metabolic syndrome if she or he has three or more of the risk factors listed here.

SOURCE: National Cholesterol Education Program. 2001. *ATP III Guidelines At-A-Glance Quick Desk Reference.* Bethesda, Md.: National Heart, Lung, and Blood Institute. NIH Publication No. 01-3305.

group, factors such as excess body fat and inactivity can elicit insulin resistance. However, metabolic syndrome is not limited to obese people.

To reduce your risk for metabolic syndrome, choose a healthy diet and get plenty of exercise. Regular physical activity increases your body's sensitivity to insulin in addition to improving cholesterol levels and decreasing blood pressure. Reducing calorie intake to prevent weight gain or losing weight if needed will also reduce insulin resistance. The amount and type of carbohydrate intake is also important: Diets high in carbohydrates, especially high-glycemic-index foods, can raise levels of glucose and triglycerides and lower HDL, thus contributing to the development or worsening of metabolic syndrome and CVD, particularly in people who are already sedentary and overweight. For people prone to insulin resistance, eating more unsaturated fats, protein, vegetables, and fiber while limiting added sugars and starches may be beneficial.

Homocysteine   Elevated levels of homocysteine, an amino acid circulating in the blood, are associated with an increased risk of CVD. Homocysteine appears to damage the lining of blood vessels, resulting in inflammation and the development of fatty deposits in artery walls. These changes can lead to the formation of clots and blockages in arteries, which in turn can cause heart attacks and strokes.

Men generally have higher homocysteine levels than women, as do individuals with diets low in folic acid, vitamin B-12, and vitamin B-6. Many genes may cause elevated homocysteine levels, and some genes associated with small-to-moderate elevations are quite common in the general population. Most people can lower homocysteine levels easily by adopting a healthy diet rich in fruits, vegetables, and grains and by taking supplements if needed. Studies are under way to determine if decreasing homocysteine

levels will actually reduce CVD risk. In the meantime, you can hedge your bet by eating plenty of the healthy foods known to be high in folate and B-vitamins. At this point, testing for elevated homocysteine is usually recommended only for people with heart disease who have few of the traditional risk factors.

Infectious Agents   Several infectious agents have been identified as possible culprits in the development of CVD. *Chlamydia pneumoniae*, a common cause of flulike respiratory infections, has been found in sections of clogged, damaged arteries but not in sections of healthy arteries. In one study, evidence of infection with *C. pneumoniae* was found in 90% of patients who had recently had a heart attack but in only 25% of healthy control subjects. It does not appear that antibiotic treatment for *C. pneumoniae* reduces risk, although further research is needed. Other infectious agents may also play a role in CVD, including *Cytomegalovirus*, *Helicobacter pylori*, and the bacteria that cause gingivitis (gum disease).

Lipoprotein(a)   A high level of a specific type of LDL called lipoprotein(a), or Lp(a), has been identified as a possible risk factor for coronary heart disease (CHD), especially when associated with high LDL or low HDL levels. Lp(a) is thought to contribute to CVD by promoting clots and by delivering cholesterol to a site of vascular injury. Lp(a) levels have a strong genetic component and are difficult to treat. Research suggests that a diet rich in omega-3 fatty acids and treatment for lowering elevated LDL levels may help reduce the associated risk.

LDL Particle Size   Research has shown that LDL particles differ in size and density and that the concentrations of different particles vary among individuals. LDL cholesterol profiles can be divided into three general types: People with pattern A have mostly large, buoyant LDL particles; people with pattern B have mostly small, dense LDL particles; and people with pattern C have a mixture of particle types. Small, dense LDL particles pose a greater CVD risk than large particles; thus, people with LDL pattern B are at greater risk for CVD. At this time, testing to identify LDL particle size is expensive and not widely available, and further research is needed before routine screening and treatment for LDL pattern B can be recommended. Exercise, a low-fat diet, and certain lipid-lowering drugs may help lower CVD risk in people with LDL pattern B. In a recent study of men who walked or jogged 12–20 miles per week, total cholesterol and LDL levels were often unchanged, but the LDL particles became larger and less dense. This may be one of the many ways exercise helps prevent CVD.

Fibrinogen   Fibrinogen is a protein that is essential for the formation of blood clots. High levels of fibrinogen are linked to increased risk of coronary heart disease and stroke. Elevated fibrinogen levels may be one way traditional risk factors such as smoking, obesity, diabetes, and elevated blood lipids cause CVD. Improvement in these risk factors, especially quitting smoking, tends to decrease fibrinogen levels. Fibrates and niacin can also lower fibrinogen levels.

Blood Viscosity and Iron High blood viscosity (thickness) may increase the risk of CVD; excess iron stores have also been linked to higher risk, especially for men and postmenopausal women (iron stores are usually lower in younger women because of menstrual blood loss). Regular blood donation, which reduces iron stores and blood viscosity, is associated with lower CVD risk in men. Drinking five or more glasses of water a day may also reduce risk by reducing blood viscosity. On the flip side, high consumption of heme iron—found in meat, fish, and poultry—is associated with an increased risk of heart attack. Men and postmenopausal women should consult a physician before taking iron supplements.

Uric Acid Recent research suggests a link between high blood levels of uric acid and CVD mortality, particularly among postmenopausal women and African Americans. Uric acid may raise CVD risk by increasing inflammation and platelet aggregation or by influencing the development of hypertension; high uric acid levels also cause gout (a type of arthritis), kidney stones, and certain forms of kidney disease. Medications to lower uric acid levels are available, but it is not yet known if they will be useful in preventing CVD.

Time of Day and Time of Year More heart attacks and sudden cardiac deaths occur in the morning hours between 6:00 A.M. and noon than during other times of the day. This trend may be explained by the natural increase in adrenaline and cortisol levels that occurs in the morning and by an increase in the sympathetic nervous system activity as people hurry around at the beginning of their day. Blood pressure is often lowest during sleep and highest in the morning, and endothelial function may be impaired in the early morning.

There is also a seasonal pattern of heart attacks, with up to 50% more occurring in winter months than in summer months. Heart attacks that occur in winter also tend to be more often fatal than those that occur during summer. Possible explanations include low temperature, which can constrict blood vessels; bursts of exertion, such as snow shoveling; increased rates of smoking; increased stress and depression, including seasonal affective disorder (see Chapter 3); holiday-related episodes of high-fat eating and binge drinking; and physiological factors, including levels of cholesterol and C-reactive protein, which appear to rise in winter. People who have symptoms of heart trouble may also be more reluctant to seek help during the holidays.

Additional studies may help to further explain these patterns and provide guidelines to reduce the effects of the underlying causes.

MAJOR FORMS OF CARDIOVASCULAR DISEASE

Collectively, the various forms of CVD kill more Americans than the next four leading causes of death combined (Figure 15-5). The financial burden of CVD, including the costs of medical treatments and lost productivity, is nearly $400 billion annually.

The main forms of CVD are atherosclerosis, heart disease and heart attack, stroke, peripheral arterial disease (PAD), congestive heart failure, congenital heart disease, rheumatic heart disease, and heart valve problems. Many forms are interrelated and have elements in common; we treat them separately here for the sake of clarity. Hypertension, which is both a major risk factor and a form of CVD, was described earlier in the chapter.

Atherosclerosis

Atherosclerosis is a form of arteriosclerosis, or thickening and hardening of the arteries. In atherosclerosis, arteries become narrowed by deposits of fat, cholesterol, and other substances. The process begins when the endothelial cells (cells that line the arteries) become damaged, most likely through a combination of factors such as smoking, high blood pressure, high insulin or glucose levels, deposits of oxidized LDL particles, and high homocysteine levels. The body's response to this damage results in inflammation and changes in the artery lining that create a sort of magnet for LDL, platelets, and other cells; these cells build up and cause a bulge in the wall of the artery. As these deposits, called **plaques,** accumulate on artery walls, the arteries lose their elasticity and their ability to expand and contract, restricting blood flow. Once narrowed by a plaque, an artery is vulnerable to blockage by blood clots (Figure 15-6, p. 462). The risk of life-threatening clots and heart attacks increases if the fibrous cap covering a plaque ruptures.

If the heart, brain, and/or other organs are deprived of blood, and thus the vital oxygen it carries, the effects of atherosclerosis can be deadly. Coronary arteries, which supply the heart with blood, are particularly susceptible to plaque buildup, a condition called **coronary heart disease (CHD),** or *coronary artery disease (CAD).* The blockage of a coronary artery causes a heart attack. If a cerebral artery (leading to the brain) is blocked, the result is a stroke. If an artery in a limb becomes narrowed or blocked, it causes *peripheral arterial disease,* a condition that causes pain and sometimes loss of the affected limb.

The main risk factors for atherosclerosis are cigarette smoking, physical inactivity, high levels of blood

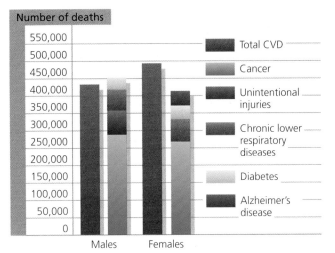

(a) Leading causes of death

Number of deaths

Legend:
- Total CVD
- Cancer
- Unintentional injuries
- Chronic lower respiratory diseases
- Diabetes
- Alzheimer's disease

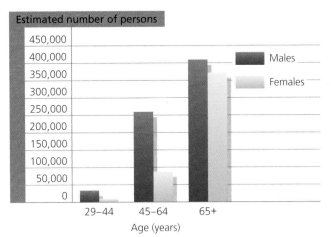

(b) Annual incidence of heart attack

Estimated number of persons

Age (years): 29–44, 45–64, 65+

Legend: Males, Females

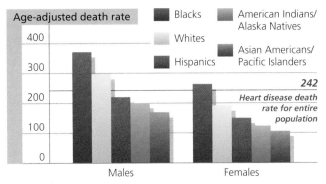

(c) Heart disease death rates

Age-adjusted death rate

Legend:
- Blacks
- Whites
- Hispanics
- American Indians/Alaska Natives
- Asian Americans/Pacific Islanders

242 Heart disease death rate for entire population

Males | Females

Vw VITAL STATISTICS

Figure 15-5 A statistical look at cardiovascular disease in the United States. (a) The leading causes of death. CVD causes more deaths than the next four causes combined. (b) Estimated numbers of Americans who have a heart attack each year. Among heart attack victims under age 65, men significantly outnumber women; after age 65, women start to catch up. (c) Heart disease death rates by gender and ethnicity. SOURCES: American Heart Association. 2005. *2005 Heart and Stroke Facts Statistical Update.* Dallas, Tex.: American Heart Association; National Center for Health Statistics. 2004. *Health, United States, 2004.* Hyattsville, Md.: U.S. Public Health Service.

cholesterol, high blood pressure, and diabetes. Atherosclerosis often begins in childhood.

Heart Disease and Heart Attack

Every year, about 1.2 million Americans have a heart attack (see Figure 15-5). Although a **heart attack,** or *myocardial infarction (MI),* may come without warning, it is usually the end result of a long-term disease process. The most common form of heart disease is coronary artery disease caused by atherosclerosis. When one of the coronary arteries, the arteries that branch off the aorta and supply blood directly to the heart muscle, becomes blocked, a heart attack results. A heart attack caused by a clot is called a **coronary thrombosis.** During a heart attack, part of the myocardium (heart muscle) may die from lack of oxygen. If an MI is not fatal, the heart muscle may sometimes partially repair itself.

Symptoms of MI may include chest pain or pressure; arm, neck, or jaw pain; difficulty breathing; excessive sweating; nausea and vomiting; and loss of consciousness. Although chest pain occurs in the majority of MI victims, a recent study of over 750,000 MI patients revealed that about one-third of people having a heart attack do not experience chest pain. Women, ethnic minorities, older adults, and people with diabetes were the most likely groups to experience heart attack without chest pain or to have several other accompanying symptoms.

Angina Arteries narrowed by disease may still be open enough to deliver blood to the heart. At times, however—primarily during emotional excitement, stress, or physical exertion—the heart requires more oxygen than narrowed arteries can accommodate. When the need for oxygen exceeds the supply, chest pain, called **angina pectoris,** may occur. Angina pain is felt as an extreme tightness in the chest and heavy pressure behind the breastbone or in the shoulder, neck, arm, hand, or back. This pain, although not actually a heart attack, is a warning that the load on the heart must be reduced. The symptoms of

Terms
Vw

plaque A deposit of fatty (and other) substances on the inner wall of the arteries.

coronary heart disease (CHD) Heart disease caused by atherosclerosis in the arteries that supply oxygen to the heart muscle; also called *coronary artery disease.*

heart attack Damage to, or death of, heart muscle, sometimes resulting in a failure of the heart to deliver enough blood to the body; also known as *myocardial infarction (MI).*

coronary thrombosis A clot in a coronary artery, often causing sudden death.

angina pectoris Pain in the chest, and often in the left arm and shoulder, caused by the heart muscle not receiving enough blood.

Plaque buildup begins when endothelial cells lining the arteries are damaged by smoking, high blood pressure, oxidized LDL, and other causes; excess cholesterol particles collect beneath these cells.

In response to the damage, platelets and other types of cells collect at the site; a fibrous cap forms, isolating the plaque within the artery wall. An early-stage plaque is called a fatty streak.

Chemicals released by cells in and around the plaque cause further inflammation and buildup; an advanced plaque contains LDL, white blood cells, connective tissue, smooth muscle cells, platelets, and other compounds.

The narrowed artery is vulnerable to blockage by clots. The risk of blockage and heart attack rises if the fibrous cap cracks (probably due to destructive enzymes released by white blood cells within the plaque).

Figure 15-6 Stages of plaque development.

angina are often very difficult to distinguish from a heart attack. Any severe chest pain that lasts more than a few minutes should be considered life-threatening, and emergency medical help should be obtained immediately. Angina may be controlled in a number of ways (with drugs and surgical or nonsurgical procedures), but its course is unpredictable. Over a period ranging from hours to years, the narrowing may go on to full blockage and a heart attack.

Arrhythmias and Sudden Cardiac Death   The pumping of the heart is controlled by electrical impulses from the sinus node that maintain a regular heartbeat of 60–100 beats per minute. If this electrical conduction system is disrupted, the heart may beat too quickly, too slowly, or in an irregular fashion, a condition known as **arrhythmia.** Arrhythmia can cause symptoms ranging from imperceptible to severe and even fatal.

Sudden cardiac death, also called cardiac arrest, is most often caused by an arrhythmia called ventricular fibrillation, a kind of quivering of the ventricle that makes it ineffective in pumping blood. If ventricular fibrillation continues for more than a few minutes, it is fatal. Cardiac defibrillation, in which an electrical shock is delivered to the heart, can be effective in jolting the heart into a more

efficient rhythm. Emergency personnel typically carry defibrillators, and automated external defibrillators (AEDs) are becoming increasingly available in public places for use by the general public. AEDs monitor the heart's rhythm and, if appropriate, deliver an electrical shock. (Training in the use of AEDs is available from organizations such as the American Red Cross and the American Heart Association.) Sudden cardiac death most often occurs in people with coronary heart disease. Serious arrhythmias frequently develop during or after a heart attack and are often the actual cause of death in cases of a fatal MI.

Other potential causes of arrhythmia include congenital heart abnormalities, infections, drug use, chest trauma, and congestive heart failure. Some arrhythmias cause no problems and resolve without treatment; more serious arrhythmias are usually treated with medication or a surgically implanted pacemaker or defibrillator that delivers electrical stimulation to the heart to create a more normal rhythm.

Helping a Heart Attack Victim   Most people who die from a heart attack do so within 2 hours from the time they experience the first symptoms. Unfortunately, half of all heart attack victims wait more than 2 hours before getting help. If you or someone you are with has any of the warning signs of heart attack listed in the box "What to Do in Case of a Heart Attack, Cardiac Arrest, or Stroke," take immediate action. Get help even if the person denies there is something wrong. One additional step recommended by many experts is for the affected individual to chew and swallow one adult aspirin tablet (325 mg); aspirin has an immediate anticlotting effect.

If the person loses consciousness, emergency **cardiopulmonary resuscitation (CPR)** should be initiated by a qualified person. Damage to the heart muscle increases with time. If the person receives emergency care quickly enough, a clot-dissolving agent can be injected to break up a clot in the coronary artery. These clot-busting

Heart Attack Warning Signs

Some heart attacks are sudden and intense—the "movie heart attack," where no one doubts what's happening. But most heart attacks start slowly, with mild pain or discomfort. Often people affected aren't sure what's wrong and wait too long before getting help. Here are signs that can mean a heart attack is happening:

- **Chest discomfort.** Most heart attacks involve discomfort in the center of the chest that lasts more than a few minutes, or that goes away and comes back. It can feel like uncomfortable pressure, squeezing, fullness, or pain.

- **Discomfort in other areas of the upper body.** Symptoms can include pain or discomfort in one or both arms, the back, neck, jaw or stomach.

- **Shortness of breath.** May occur with or without chest discomfort.

- **Other signs:** These may include breaking out in a cold sweat, nausea, or lightheadedness.

If you or someone you're with has chest discomfort, especially with one or more of the other signs, don't wait longer than a few minutes (no more than 5) before calling for help. Call 9-1-1 . . . Get to a hospital right away.

Calling 9-1-1 is almost always the fastest way to get lifesaving treatment. Emergency medical services staff can begin treatment when they arrive—up to an hour sooner than if someone gets to the hospital by car. The staff are also trained to revive someone whose heart has stopped. Patients with chest pain who arrive by ambulance usually receive faster treatment at the hospital, too.

If you can't access the emergency medical services (EMS), have someone drive you to the hospital right away. If you're the one having symptoms, don't drive yourself, unless you have absolutely no other option.

Stroke Warning Signs

The American Stroke Association says these are the warning signs of stroke:

- Sudden numbness or weakness of the face, arm, or leg, especially on one side of the body
- Sudden confusion, trouble speaking or understanding
- Sudden trouble seeing in one or both eyes
- Sudden trouble walking, dizziness, or loss of balance or coordination
- Sudden, severe headache with no known cause

If you or someone with you has one or more of these signs, don't delay! Immediately call 9-1-1 or the emergency medical services (EMS) number so an ambulance (ideally with advanced life support) can be sent for you. Also, check the time so you'll know when the first symptoms appeared. It's very important to take immediate action. If given within three hours of the start of symptoms, a clot-busting drug can reduce long-term disability for the most common type of stroke.

Cardiac arrest strikes immediately and without warning.

Here are the signs:

- Sudden loss of responsiveness. No response to gentle shaking.
- No normal breathing. The victim does not take a normal breath when you check for several seconds.
- No signs of circulation. No movement or coughing.

If cardiac arrest occurs, call 9-1-1 and begin CPR immediately. If an automated external defibrillator (AED) is available and someone trained to use it is nearby, involve her or him.

drugs, such as streptokinase, urokinase, and tissue plasminogen activator (TPA), are being used successfully to treat not only heart attacks but also some types of stroke. The sooner these drugs are used, the more effective they are. The other effective treatment used in larger hospitals is coronary angioplasty and stenting (discussed in more detail later).

Detecting and Treating Heart Disease Physicians have an expanding array of tools to evaluate the condition of the heart and arteries. Currently, the most common initial screening tool is the stress, or exercise, test, in which a patient runs or walks on a treadmill or pedals a stationary cycle while being monitored for abnormalities with an **electrocardiogram (ECG** or **EKG).**

Certain characteristic changes in the heart's electrical activity while under stress can reveal particular heart problems, such as restricted blood flow. Exercise testing can also be performed in conjunction with techniques such as nuclear medicine that provide further information about the heart and arteries.

Other non-invasive tests for evaluating CVD are becoming more widely used:

- Electron-beam computed tomography (EBCT) uses a sweeping electron beam to produce computerized cross-sectional images; it can detect calcium in the arteries, a marker for atherosclerosis.
- Echocardiographic equipment utilizes sound waves to examine the heart.

- **Magnetic resonance imaging** uses powerful magnets to look inside the body and generate pictures of the heart and blood vessels.

If symptoms or non-invasive tests suggest coronary artery disease, the next step is usually a coronary **angiogram.** In this test, a catheter (small plastic tube) is threaded into an artery, usually in the groin, and advanced through the aorta to the coronary arteries. The catheter is then placed into the opening of the coronary artery and a special dye is injected. The dye can be seen moving through the arteries under moving X ray, and any narrowings or blockages can be identified.

Treatments ranging from changes in diet to major surgery are available if a problem is detected. Along with a low-fat diet, regular exercise, and smoking cessation, one frequent nonsurgical recommendation for people at high risk for CVD is to take an aspirin tablet every day. Aspirin has an anticlotting effect, discouraging platelets in the blood from sticking to arterial plaques and forming clots; it also reduces inflammation. (Low-dose aspirin therapy appears to help prevent first heart attacks in men, second heart attacks in men and women, and strokes in women over age 65.) Prescription drugs can help control heart rate, dilate arteries, lower blood pressure, and reduce the strain on the heart—raising both quality and quantity of life in heart patients. In patients with coronary artery disease, a class of cholesterol-lowering drugs called statins is effective in preventing heart attacks; statins also have beneficial anti-inflammatory effects.

A common procedure for treating heart disease is **balloon angioplasty,** which is performed in a cardiac catheterization laboratory by specially trained cardiologists. This technique involves threading a catheter with a deflated balloon on it through the artery until it reaches the area of blockage. The balloon is then inflated, flattening the fatty plaque and widening the arterial opening. This is generally followed by placement of a stent, a small metal tube that helps keep the artery open. Repeat clogging of the artery, known as restenosis, can occur, but the introduction of stents coated in medication, which is slowly released over a few months, significantly decreases the chance of restenosis.

Every year, **coronary bypass surgery** is performed on over 300,000 people, about half of whom are under age 65. Cardiothoracic surgeons remove a healthy blood vessel, usually a vein from one of the patient's legs, and graft it from the aorta to one or more coronary arteries to bypass a blockage. A heart-lung machine maintains circulation during the surgery.

Whatever treatment is used, the person with heart disease is also advised to make behavior and lifestyle changes, such as changing the diet to improve blood cholesterol levels and quitting smoking. Otherwise, the arteries simply become clogged again, and the same problems recur a few years later.

Stroke

For brain cells to function as they should, they must have a continuous and ample supply of oxygen-rich blood. If brain cells are deprived of blood for more than a few minutes, they die. A **stroke,** also called a *cerebrovascular accident (CVA),* occurs when the blood supply to the brain is cut off. Many experts now refer to strokes as brain attacks to emphasize their similarity to heart attacks and the importance of early treatment. In the past, not much could be done for stroke victims; today, however, prompt treatment of stroke can greatly decrease the risk of permanent disability. Everyone should know the warning signs for a stroke and seek immediate medical help, just as they would at the first sign of a heart attack.

Types of Strokes There are two major types of strokes: **ischemic strokes,** which are caused by blockages in blood vessels, and **hemorrhagic strokes,** which are caused by rupture of blood vessels, leading to bleeding into the brain (Figure 15-7). One type of ischemic stroke, the *thrombotic stroke,* is caused by a **thrombus,** a blood clot that forms in a cerebral artery that has been narrowed or damaged by atherosclerosis. The other type of ischemic stroke, called an *embolic stroke,* is caused by an **embolus,** a

Terms

Vw

magnetic resonance imaging (MRI) A computerized imaging technique that uses a strong magnetic field and radio frequency signals to examine a thin cross section of the body; also known as *nuclear magnetic resonance imaging (NMR).*

angiogram A picture of the arterial system taken after injecting a dye that is opaque to X rays; also called *arteriogram.*

balloon angioplasty A technique in which a catheter with a deflated balloon on the tip is inserted into an artery; the balloon is then inflated at the point of obstruction in the artery, pressing the plaque against the artery wall to improve blood supply; also known as *percutaneous transluminal coronary angioplasty (PTCA).*

coronary bypass surgery Surgery in which a vein is grafted from a point above to a point below an obstruction in a coronary artery, improving the blood supply to the heart.

stroke An impeded blood supply to some part of the brain resulting in the destruction of brain cells; also called *cerebrovascular accident.*

ischemic stroke Impeded blood supply to the brain caused by the obstruction of a blood vessel by a clot.

hemorrhagic stroke Impeded blood supply to the brain caused by the rupture of a blood vessel.

thrombus A blood clot in a blood vessel that usually remains at the point of its formation.

embolus A blood clot that breaks off from its place of origin in a blood vessel and travels through the bloodstream.

aneurysm A sac formed by a distention or dilation of the artery wall.

transient ischemic attack (TIA) A small stroke; usually a temporary interruption of blood supply to the brain, causing numbness or difficulty with speech.

HEMORRHAGIC STROKE

- 20% of strokes
- Caused by ruptured blood vessels followed by blood leaking into tissue
- Usually more serious than ischemic stroke

Subarachnoid hemorrhage
- A bleed into the space between the brain and the skull
- Develops most often from an *aneurysm,* a weakened, ballooned area in the wall of an artery

Intracerebral hemorrhage
- A bleed from a blood vessel inside the brain
- Often caused by high blood pressure and the damage it does to arteries

ISCHEMIC STROKE

- 80% of strokes
- Caused by blockages in brain blood vessels; potentially treatable with clot-busting drugs
- Brain tissue dies when blood flow is blocked

Embolic stroke
- Caused by *emboli,* blood clots that travel from elsewhere in the body to the brain blood vessels
- 25% of embolic strokes are related to atrial fibrillation

Thrombotic stroke
- Caused by *thrombi,* blood clots that form where an artery has been narrowed by atherosclerosis
- Most often develops when part of a thrombus breaks away and causes a blockage in a downstream artery

Figure 15-7   Types of stroke.   SOURCE: Excerpted from the *Harvard Health Letter,* April 2000. Copyright © 2000, Harriet Greenfield, www.health.harvard.edu.

wandering blood clot that is carried in the bloodstream and may become wedged in one of the cerebral arteries. Many embolic strokes are linked to a type of abnormal heart rhythm called atrial fibrillation; when this arrhythmia occurs, blood may pool in the atria and form clots. Ischemic strokes, which account for 80% of all strokes, are potentially treatable with clot-busting drugs, so obtaining immediate medical help is critical to improving chances for recovery.

The other type of stroke, less common but more severe, is the hemorrhagic stroke. It occurs when a blood vessel in the brain bursts, spilling blood into the surrounding tissue. Cells normally nourished by the artery are deprived of blood and cannot function. In addition, accumulated blood from the burst vessel may put pressure on surrounding brain tissue, causing damage and even death. In a *subarachnoid hemorrhage,* a blood vessel on the brain's surface ruptures and bleeds into the space between the brain and the skull; a ruptured vessel within the brain causes an *intracerebral hemorrhage.* Hemorrhages can be caused by head injuries or the bursting of a malformed blood vessel or an **aneurysm,** a blood-filled pocket that bulges out from a weak spot in an artery wall. Aneurysms in the brain may remain stable and never break. But when they do, the result is a stroke. Aneurysms may be caused or worsened by high blood pressure.

The Effects of a Stroke   The interruption of the blood supply to any area of the brain prevents the nerve cells there from functioning—in some cases causing death. Of the 700,000 Americans who have strokes each year, nearly one-third die within a year. Those who survive usually have some lasting disability. Which parts of the body are affected depends on the area of the brain that has been damaged. Nerve cells control sensation and most of our body movements, and a stroke may cause paralysis, walking disability, speech impairment, memory loss, and changes in behavior. The severity of the stroke and its long-term effects depend on which brain cells have been injured, how widespread the damage is, how effectively the body can restore the blood supply, and how rapidly other areas of the brain can take over. Early treatment can significantly reduce the severity of disability resulting from a stroke.

Detecting and Treating Stroke   Death rates from stroke have declined significantly over the past decades. In 1950, nearly 90% of victims died; today, about two-thirds of stroke victims survive. Effective treatment requires the prompt recognition of symptoms and correct diagnosis of the type of stroke that has occurred. Signs of a stroke are listed in the box on p. 463.

Some stroke victims have a **transient ischemic attack (TIA),** or ministroke, days, weeks, or months before they have a full-blown stroke. A TIA produces temporary strokelike symptoms, such as weakness or numbness in an arm or a leg, speech difficulty, or dizziness; but these symptoms are brief, often lasting just a few minutes, and do not cause permanent damage. However, TIAs should be taken as warning signs of a stroke, and anyone with a suspected TIA should get immediate medical help.

Strokes should be treated with the same urgency as heart attacks. A person with stroke symptoms should be rushed to the hospital. A **computed tomography (CT)** scan, which uses a computer to construct an image of the brain from X rays, can assess brain damage and determine the type of stroke. Newer techniques using MRI and ultrasound are becoming increasingly available and should improve the speed and accuracy of stroke diagnosis.

If tests reveal that a stroke is caused by a blood clot—and if help is sought within a few hours of the onset of symptoms—the person can be treated with the same kind of clot-dissolving drugs that are used to treat coronary artery blockages. If the clot is dissolved quickly enough, brain damage is minimized and symptoms may disappear. (The longer the brain goes without oxygen, the greater the risk of permanent damage.) Drugs that help protect healthy brain cells from the effects of stroke are currently being tested. People who have had TIAs or who are at high risk for stroke due to narrowing of the carotid arteries may undergo a surgical procedure called *carotid endarterectomy,* in which plaque is removed. There is also a nonsurgical procedure, similar to coronary angioplasty and stenting, that can be done in the carotid arteries.

If tests reveal that a stroke was caused by a cerebral hemorrhage, drugs may be prescribed to lower the blood pressure, which will usually be high. Careful diagnosis is crucial, because administering clot-dissolving drugs to a person suffering a hemorrhagic stroke would cause more bleeding and potentially more brain damage.

If detection and treatment of stroke come too late, rehabilitation is the only treatment. Although damaged or destroyed brain tissue does not normally regenerate, nerve

Rehabilitation after a stroke can be a long and arduous process. Complete recovery eludes many stroke victims.

cells in the brain can make new pathways, and some functions can be taken over by other parts of the brain. Some spontaneous recovery starts immediately after a stroke and continues for a few months.

Rehabilitation consists of various types of therapy: physical therapy, which helps strengthen muscles and improve balance and coordination; speech and language therapy, which helps those whose speech has been damaged; and occupational therapy, which helps improve hand-eye coordination and everyday living skills. Progress varies from person to person and can be unpredictable. Some people recover completely in a matter of days or weeks, but most stroke victims who survive must adapt to some lifelong disability.

Peripheral Arterial Disease

Peripheral arterial disease (PAD) refers to atherosclerosis in the leg (or arm) arteries, which can eventually limit or completely obstruct blood flow. The same process that occurs in the heart arteries can occur in any artery of the body. In fact, patients with PAD frequently also have coronary artery disease and cerebrovascular disease, and they have an increased risk of death from CVD. Approximately 10 million people in the United States have PAD.

The risk factors associated with coronary atherosclerosis, such as smoking, diabetes, hypertension, and high cholesterol, also contribute to atherosclerosis in the peripheral

Terms

computed tomography (CT) The use of computerized X ray images to create a cross-sectional depiction (scan) of tissue density.

peripheral arterial disease (PAD) Atherosclerosis in arteries in the legs (or, less commonly, arms) that can impede blood flow and lead to pain, infection, and loss of the affected limb.

pulmonary edema The accumulation of fluid in the lungs.

congestive heart failure A condition resulting from the heart's inability to pump out all the blood that returns to it; blood backs up in the veins leading to the heart, causing an accumulation of fluid in various parts of the body.

congenital heart disease A defect or malformation of the heart or its major blood vessels, present at birth.

hypertrophic cardiomyopathy (HCM) An inherited condition in which there is an enlargement of the heart muscle, especially between the two ventricles.

rheumatic fever A disease, mainly of children, characterized by fever, inflammation, and pain in the joints; often damages the heart muscle, a condition called rheumatic heart disease.

circulation. The risk of PAD is significantly increased in people with diabetes and people who smoke. The likelihood of needing an amputation is increased in those who continue to smoke, and PAD in people with diabetes tends to be extensive and severe.

Symptoms of PAD include claudication and rest pain. *Claudication* is aching or fatigue in the affected leg with exertion, particularly walking, which resolves with rest. Claudication occurs when leg muscles do not get adequate blood and oxygen supply. *Rest pain* occurs when the limb artery is unable to supply adequate blood and oxygen even when the body is not physically active. This occurs when the artery is significantly narrowed or completely blocked. If blood flow is not restored quickly, cells and tissues may become infected and die; in severe cases, amputation may be needed. PAD is the leading cause of amputation in people over age 50.

Congestive Heart Failure

A number of conditions—high blood pressure, heart attack, atherosclerosis, alcoholism, viral infections, rheumatic fever, birth defects—can damage the heart's pumping mechanism. When the heart cannot maintain its regular pumping rate and force, fluids begin to back up. When extra fluid seeps through capillary walls, edema (swelling) results, usually in the legs and ankles, but sometimes in other parts of the body as well. Fluid can collect in the lungs and interfere with breathing, particularly when a person is lying down. This condition is called **pulmonary edema,** and the entire process is known as **congestive heart failure.**

Congestive heart failure can be controlled. Treatment includes reducing the workload on the heart, modifying salt intake, and using drugs that help the body eliminate excess fluid. Drugs used to treat congestive heart failure improve the pumping action of the heart, lower the blood pressure so the heart doesn't have to work as hard, and help the body eliminate excess salt and water. When medical therapy is ineffective, heart transplant is a solution for some patients with severe heart failure, but the need greatly exceeds the number of hearts available. There are about 2200 heart transplants performed each year.

The risk of heart failure increases with age, and being overweight is a significant independent risk factor. Experts fear that the incidence of heart failure will increase dramatically over the next few decades as our population ages and becomes increasingly obese.

Other Forms of Heart Disease

Other, less common, forms of heart disease include congenital heart disease, rheumatic heart disease, and heart valve disorders.

Congenital Heart Disease   About 40,000 children born each year in the United States have a defect or malformation of the heart or major blood vessels. These conditions are collectively referred to as **congenital heart disease,** and they cause about 4300 deaths a year. The most common congenital defects are holes in the wall that divides the chambers of the heart. With these defects the heart produces a distinctive sound, making diagnosis relatively simple. Another defect is *coarctation of the aorta,* a narrowing, or constriction, of the aorta. Heart failure may result unless the constricted area is repaired by surgery.

Most of the common congenital defects can now be accurately diagnosed and treated with medication or surgery. Early recognition that a newborn who has a bluish appearance or respiratory difficulty or who fails to thrive may be suffering from congenital heart disease is important in saving lives.

Hypertrophic cardiomyopathy (HCM) occurs in 1 out of every 500 people and is the most common cause of sudden death among athletes younger than age 35 (see the box "Sudden Death in Young Athletes"). It is an inherited condition that causes the heart muscle to become hypertrophic (enlarged), primarily in the septum, which is the area between the two ventricles. Young children with this disorder usually have no obvious symptoms; the hypertrophy generally develops gradually between ages 5 and 15. People with hypertrophic cardiomyopathy are at high risk for sudden death, mainly due to serious arrhythmias. A new test for hypertrophic cardiomyopathy using echocardiography may help health care providers diagnose the problem earlier, before serious problems arise.

Possible treatments include medication and surgery to implant a pacemaker or internal defibrillator. If the hypertrophy is mainly in the septum, some of the septum can be surgically removed or a nonsurgical procedure can be done to kill off the extra muscle. In either case, symptoms are significantly reduced, but the risk of arrhythmia and sudden death remains. The mortality rate is approximately 3% per year in adults and up to 6% per year in children. Individuals with hypertrophic cardiomyopathy should usually not participate in competitive sports because of the high risk of sudden death. In addition, if one person in a family is diagnosed with HCM, it is generally advised that all immediate family members get an echocardiogram.

Rheumatic Heart Disease   **Rheumatic fever,** a consequence of certain types of untreated streptococcal throat infections (group A beta-hemolytic), is a leading cause of heart trouble worldwide. Rheumatic fever can permanently damage the heart muscle and heart valves, a condition called rheumatic heart disease (RHD). Many of the approximately 100,000 operations on heart valves performed annually are related to RHD, and about 4000 Americans die each year from RHD. Fortunately, the incidence of rheumatic fever has declined significantly in the United States since the introduction of antibiotics; rates are highest among African Americans, Latinos, and American Indians.

Sudden, nontraumatic death in a young athlete is an unexpected and confusing tragedy. How could someone apparently so physically healthy and capable suddenly die? If it could happen to them, could it happen to anyone?

Although the sudden death of a young athlete (under age 35) tends to attract a lot of attention, it is fortunately an uncommon event, occurring in about 1 out of 200,000 athletes per year. The majority of these deaths are due to congenital cardiovascular conditions that are usually without prior symptoms and are therefore unlikely to be diagnosed during life without specific screening. Even with screening tests, they may be difficult or impossible to identify. These conditions also occur in the general population but may become more lethal during intense physical activity. Indeed, most young athletes who die suddenly do so during or immediately after athletic training or competition.

The most common cardiovascular cause of sudden death in young athletes is hypertrophic cardiomyopathy, accounting for about one-third of cases. In this condition, the heart muscle becomes very thick, which can impede the outflow of blood and cause fatal arrhythmias, especially during physical activity. Some people have a mild form that is hard to distinguish during screening tests from a normal athletic heart, which like any other muscle becomes bigger from physical activity.

The second most common cardiovascular cause of sudden death in athletes is congenital coronary artery anomalies, which account for about 20% of cases. In this condition, a coronary artery is malformed or doesn't arise from its normal position on the aorta; for example, if the left coronary artery originates from the right side of the aorta, near the right coronary artery, it may then have an unusual bend or shape. During physical activity, the anomalous artery may be unable to provide adequate blood flow to the heart muscle, leading to damage to the heart cells or to fatal arrhythmia.

Congenital malformations, including problems with the heart valves and the electrical conduction system, account for most other sudden deaths among athletes. Coronary artery disease is a more common cause in older athletes but rarely occurs in younger athletes. In about 2% of deaths, no cause can be identified. Some of these deaths may be due to noncardiac factors, including substance abuse (for example, cocaine) or use of the supplement ephedra. Use of anabolic steroids is associated with an increase in LDL cholesterol and early coronary artery disease, as well as risk of sudden cardiac death.

The majority (90%) of young athletes who have sudden cardiac death are male. Possible explanations are that men are more likely than women to participate in organized sports, to be exposed to more intensive training demands, and to participate in the sports most associated with sudden deaths (basketball, football). Men also have higher rates of certain cardiovascular problems, including hypertrophic cardiomyopathy. Ethnicity may also play a role, with the majority of reported sudden deaths in competitive athletes occuring in whites (52%) and African Americans (44%).

In most cases, underlying cardiovascular disease was completely unsuspected in affected individuals: Fewer than 20% report cardiovascular symptoms in the 36 months preceding their deaths. These symptoms include exertional chest pain, exertional shortness of breath, and exertional syncope (loss of consciousness) or dizziness.

There has been an effort to reduce the number of sudden deaths in young athletes by implementing preparticipation screening programs, although such programs are not foolproof. The American Heart Association has developed guidelines for screening high school and collegiate athletes. Those with a history of cardiovascular symptoms, a family history of sudden death, a murmur, or other worrisome physical findings should be referred to a cardiovascular specialist for further evaluation. If a cardiovascular condition that could lead to sudden cardiac death is identified, recommendations will be outlined for determining eligibility for continued participation in competitive sports.

Symptoms of strep throat include the sudden onset of a sore throat, painful swallowing, fever, swollen glands, headache, nausea, and vomiting. Careful laboratory diagnosis is important because strep throat is treated with antibiotics, which are not useful in the treatment of far more common viral sore throats. Symptoms of rheumatic fever generally occur about 3 weeks after the infection. They tend to be vague but in children can include weight loss or a failure to gain weight, fever, poor appetite, repeated nosebleeds, jerky body movements, fatigue, weakness, and pain in the arms, legs, or abdomen. Rheumatic fever can be prevented by treating strep throat, when it occurs, with antibiotics.

Heart Valve Disorders Congenital defects and certain types of infections can cause abnormalities in the valves between the chambers of the heart. Heart valve problems generally fall into two categories—the valve fails to open fully, or it fails to close completely. In either case, blood flow through the heart is impaired. Treatment for heart valve disorders depends on their location and severity; serious problems may be treated with surgery to repair or replace a valve. People with certain types of heart valve defects are advised to take antibiotics prior to some types of dental and surgical procedures in order to prevent

Term

mitral valve prolapse (MVP) A condition in which the mitral valve billows out during ventricular contraction, possibly allowing leakage of blood from the left ventricle into the left atrium; often asymptomatic and usually requiring treatment only in cases of significant leakage.

Figure 15-8   Strategies for reducing your risk of cardiovascular disease.

bacteria, which may be dislodged into the bloodstream during the procedure, from infecting the defective valve.

The most common heart valve disorder is **mitral valve prolapse (MVP),** which occurs in about 4% of the population. MVP is characterized by a billowing of the mitral valve, which separates the left ventricle and left atrium, during ventricular contraction; in some cases, blood leaks from the ventricle into the atrium. Most people with MVP have no symptoms; they have the same ability to exercise and live as long as people without MVP. The condition is often diagnosed during a routine medical exam when an extra heart sound (a click) or murmur is heard; the diagnosis can be confirmed with echocardiography. Treatment is usually unnecessary, although surgery may be needed in the rare cases where leakage through the faulty valve is severe. Experts disagree over whether patients with MVP should take antibiotics prior to dental procedures; most often, only those patients with significant leakage of blood from the valve are advised to take antibiotics.

PROTECTING YOURSELF AGAINST CARDIOVASCULAR DISEASE

There are several important steps you can take now to lower your risk of developing CVD in the future (Figure 15-8). If you are a young adult, you may be wondering how CVD prevention advice applies to you, as most cases of CVD show up in people who are decades older. Evidence is mounting that the development of CVD begins very early in life. For example, fatty streaks (very early atherosclerosis) can be seen on the aorta in children younger than age 10. Also, young adults with relatively low choles-terol levels go on to live substantially longer than those with higher levels. Reducing CVD risk factors when you are young can pay off with many extra years of life and health (see the box "Are You at Risk for CVD?").

Eat Heart-Healthy

For most Americans, eating a heart-healthy diet involves many of the changes suggested in the 2005 Dietary Guidelines for Americans: cutting total fat intake, substituting unsaturated fats for saturated and trans fats, and increasing intake of whole grains and fiber. Such changes can lower blood levels of total cholesterol, LDL cholesterol, and triglycerides. Reducing salt intake and obtaining adequate potassium can help lower blood pressure. A moderate amount of alcohol may also be beneficial for some people.

Decreased Fat and Cholesterol Intake   The National Cholesterol Education Program (NCEP) recommends that all Americans over age 2 adopt a diet in which total fat consumption is no more than 30% of total daily calories, with no more than one-third of total fat calories (10% of total daily calories) coming from saturated fat. For people with heart disease or high LDL levels, the NCEP recommends a total fat intake of 25–35% of total daily calories and a saturated fat intake of less than 7% of total calories. (As described earlier, the higher total fat allowance is for people with metabolic syndrome for whom high triglyceride and low HDL levels may also be a problem.)

Saturated fats are found in animal products; palm and coconut oil; and hydrogenated vegetable oils, which are also high in trans fats. Saturated and trans fats influence the production and excretion of cholesterol by the liver,

Assess Yourself

Are You at Risk for CVD?

Your chances of suffering an early heart attack or stroke depend on a variety of factors, many of which are under your control. The best time to identify your risk factors and change your behavior to lower your risk is when you are young. You can significantly affect your future health and quality of life if you adopt healthy behaviors. To help identify your risk factors, circle the response for each risk category that best describes you:

1. Gender and Age
   - 0 Female age 55 or younger; male age 45 or younger
   - 2 Female age 55 or older or male age 45 or older

2. Heredity
   - 0 Neither parent suffered a heart attack or stroke before age 60.
   - 3 One parent suffered a heart attack or stroke before age 60.
   - 7 Both parents suffered a heart attack or stroke before age 60.

3. Smoking
   - 0 Never smoked
   - 3 Quit more than 2 years ago and lifetime smoking is less than 5 pack-years*
   - 6 Quit less than 2 years ago and/or lifetime smoking is greater than 5 pack-years*
   - 8 Smoke less than ½ pack per day
   - 13 Smoke more than ½ pack per day
   - 15 Smoke more than 1 pack per day

4. Environmental Tobacco Smoke
   - 0 Do not live or work with smokers
   - 2 Exposed to ETS at work
   - 3 Live with a smoker
   - 4 Both live and work with smokers

5. Blood Pressure
   If available, average your last three readings:
   - 0 120/80 or below
   - 1 121/81–130/85
   - 3 Don't know
   - 5 131/86–150/90
   - 9 151/91–170/100
   - 13 Above 170/100

6. Total Cholesterol (mg/dl)
   - 0 Lower than 190
   - 1 190–210
   - 2 Don't know
   - 3 211–240
   - 4 241–270
   - 5 271–300
   - 6 Over 300

7. HDL Cholesterol (mg/dl)
   - 0 Over 60
   - 1 55–60
   - 2 Don't know
   - 3 45–54
   - 5 35–44
   - 7 25–34
   - 12 Lower than 25

8. Exercise
   - 0 Exercise three times a week
   - 1 Exercise once or twice a week
   - 2 Occasional exercise less than once a week
   - 7 Rarely exercise

9. Diabetes
   - 0 No personal or family history
   - 2 One parent with diabetes
   - 6 Two parents with diabetes
   - 9 Non–insulin-dependent diabetes
   - 13 Insulin-dependent diabetes

10. Body Mass Index (kg/m^2)
    - 0 <23.0
    - 1 23.0–24.9
    - 2 25.0–28.9
    - 3 29.0–34.9
    - 5 35.0–39.9
    - 7 ≥40

11. Stress
    - 0 Relaxed most of the time
    - 1 Occasional stress and anger
    - 2 Frequently stressed and angry
    - 3 Usually stressed and angry

Scoring

Total your risk factor points. Refer to the list below to get an approximate rating of your risk of suffering an early heart attack or stroke.

Score	Estimated Risk
Less than 20	Low risk
20–29	Moderate risk
30–45	High risk
Over 45	Extremely high risk

*Pack-years can be calculated by multiplying the number of packs you smoked per day by the number of years you smoked. For example, if you smoked a pack and a half a day for 5 years, you would have smoked the equivalent of 1.5 × 5 = 7.5 pack-years.

so decreasing saturated and trans fat intake is the most important dietary change you can make to achieve and maintain healthy cholesterol levels (see the Behavior Change Strategy at the end of the chapter). Choose unsaturated fats, especially monounsaturated fats, and omega-3 polyunsaturated fats, over saturated and trans fats.

Animal products contain cholesterol as well as saturated fat; vegetable products do not contain cholesterol. The NCEP recommends that most Americans limit dietary cholesterol intake to no more than 300 mg per day; for people with heart disease or high LDL levels, the suggested daily limit is 200 mg. The cholesterol content of packaged foods is provided on food labels, along with their total, saturated, and (beginning in 2006) trans fat content.

Increased Fiber Intake

Fiber traps the bile acids the liver needs to manufacture cholesterol and carries them to the large intestine, where they are excreted. It slows the production of proteins that promote blood clotting. Fiber may also interfere with the absorption of dietary fat and may help you cut total food intake because foods rich in fiber tend to be filling. Studies have shown that a high-fiber diet is associated with a 40–50% reduction in the risk of heart attack and stroke. To obtain the recommended 25–38 grams of dietary fiber per day, choose a diet rich in whole grains, fruits, and vegetables. Good sources of fiber include oatmeal, some breakfast cereals, barley, legumes, and most fruits and vegetables.

Decreased Sodium Intake and Increased Potassium Intake

Reducing sodium intake to recommended levels, while also increasing potassium intake, can help reduce blood pressure for many people. The recommended limit for sodium intake is 2300 mg per day; for population groups at special risk, including those with hypertension, middle-aged and older adults, and African Americans, the recommended limit is 1500 mg per day. About 10% of the sodium in the American diet occurs naturally in food, and another 10% is added during cooking or at the table; the remainder is added during processing. To limit sodium intake, read food labels carefully, and avoid foods particularly high in sodium; foods that are fresh, less processed, and less sodium-dense are good choices.

Adequate potassium intake is also important in control of blood pressure, and many Americans consume less than recommended amounts of the mineral. Good food sources include leafy green vegetables like spinach and beet greens, root vegetables like white and sweet potatoes, vine fruits like cantaloupe and honeydew melon, winter squash, bananas, many dried fruits, and tomato sauce.

Moderate Alcohol Consumption (For Some)

The Dietary Guidelines for Americans state that moderate alcohol consumption may lower the risk of CHD among middle-aged and older adults. (Moderate means no more than one drink per day for women and two drinks per day for men.) Moderate alcohol use may increase HDL cholesterol; it may also reduce stroke risk, possibly by dampening the inflammatory response or by affecting blood clotting. For most people under age 45, however, the risks of alcohol use probably outweigh any health benefit. Excessive alcohol consumption increases the risk of a variety of serious health problems, including hypertension, stroke, some cancers, liver disease, alcohol dependence, and injuries (see Chapter 10). If you do drink, do so moderately, with food, and at times when drinking will not put you or others at risk.

Other Dietary Factors

Researchers have identified other dietary factors that may affect CVD risk:

- *Omega-3 fatty acids.* Found in fish, shellfish, and some plant foods (nuts and canola, soybean, and flaxseed oils), omega-3 fatty acids may reduce clotting, abnormal heart rhythms, and inflammation and have other heart-healthy effects. The American Heart Association recommends eating fish two or more times a week; fish oil capsules may be appropriate for some people who won't eat fish or who have certain CVD risk factors, but they add fat and calories to the diet and may raise LDL levels. Plant sources of omega-3 fatty acids are also a good choice.

- *Plant stanols and sterols.* Plant stanols and sterols, found in some types of trans fat–free margarines and other products, reduce the absorption of cholesterol in the body and help lower LDL levels. For people with high LDL levels that do not respond to changes in fat intake, the NCEP suggests an intake of 2 grams per day of plant stanols or sterols.

- *Folic acid, vitamin B-6, and vitamin B-12.* These vitamins affect CVD risk by lowering homocysteine levels. In addition, folic acid has been found to reduce the risk of hypertension, possibly through its beneficial effects on endothelial function. See Chapter 12 for a list of foods rich in these vitamins and information on supplements.

- *Calcium.* Diets rich in calcium may help prevent hypertension and possibly stroke by reducing insulin resistance and platelet aggregation. The best way to ensure adequate intake of calcium is to consume the recommended number of servings of low-fat or fat-free dairy products and other calcium-rich foods (see Chapter 12).

- *Soy protein.* Replacing some animal proteins with soy protein may lower LDL cholesterol. Soy-based foods include tofu and tempeh.

- *Healthy carbohydrates.* Most of the carbohydrates in the current American diet come from added sugars, refined grains, and starchy foods, including soft drinks, sweets, white potatoes (including french fries and chips), white bread, and refined ready-to-eat cereals; these foods are often relatively low in nutrients and have a high glycemic index. Healthier carbohydrates choices, including whole grains, fruits, and nonstarchy vegetables, typically provide more nutrients and have a lower glycemic index. Choosing healthy carbohydrates may be of particular importance for people with insulin resistance.

- *Total calories.* Some studies have found that reducing energy intake can improve cholesterol and triglyceride levels as much as reducing fat intake does. Reduced calorie intake also helps control body weight, an extremely important risk factor for CVD.

DASH A diet plan that reflects many of the recommendations described above was released as part of a study called Dietary Approaches to Stop Hypertension, or DASH (see Chapter 12). The DASH study found that a diet low in fat and high in fruits, vegetables, and low-fat dairy products reduces blood pressure. (It also follows the recommendations for lowering the risk of heart disease, cancer, and osteoporosis.) The DASH diet plan is as follows:

- 7–8 servings per day of grains and grain products
- 4–5 servings per day of vegetables
- 4–5 servings per day of fruits
- 2–3 servings per day of low-fat or fat-free dairy products
- 2 or fewer servings per day of meats, poultry, and fish
- 4–5 servings per *week* of nuts, seeds, and legumes
- 2–3 servings per day of added fats, oils, and salad dressings
- 5 servings per *week* of snacks and sweets

Before you act on new dietary advice, remember not to seize on one particular food as a cure-all for CVD. The fight against CVD will not be won by any single dietary change; success depends on the collective effects of your entire diet. Eat a varied, moderate diet rich in fruits, vegetables, and whole grains, and use your common sense. For example, substituting olive oil or canola oil for butter is a helpful change because it lowers saturated fat intake. But adding a new oil to your diet—without subtracting fat elsewhere—will add calories and fat and not be nearly as beneficial.

Exercise Regularly

You can significantly reduce your risk of CVD with a moderate amount of physical activity. Follow the guidelines for physical activity and exercise described in Chapter 13. Begin by accumulating at least 30 minutes of moderate-intensity physical activity each day. Activities like brisk walking, gardening, and stair climbing are appropriate. Increasing the duration or intensity of exercise can provide even greater health benefits. The next step, then, is to begin a formal exercise program that develops cardiorespiratory endurance and other components of fitness. The American Heart Association recently recommended strength training in addition to aerobic exercise for building and maintaining

cardiovascular health. Strength training helps lower blood pressure, reduce body fat, and improve lipid levels and glucose metabolism.

Avoid Tobacco

Remember: The number-one risk factor for CVD that you can control is smoking. If you smoke, quit. If you don't, don't start. The majority of people who start don't believe they will become hooked, but most do. If you live or work with people who smoke, encourage them to quit— for their sake and yours. Regular exposure to ETS in social settings, at home, or at work raises your risk of CVD. If you find yourself breathing in smoke, take steps to prevent or stop the exposure.

Until recently, many experts believed that 5 or more years after quitting smoking, a former smoker's CVD risk would drop to about that of a person who had never smoked. However, research now indicates that the rate of plaque formation in arteries is significantly greater in former smokers than in those who have never smoked. What seems to matter most for CVD risk is the total amount of smoking over a lifetime rather than whether a person is currently smoking. The same study also showed that people exposed to environmental tobacco smoke have a significantly higher rate of plaque formation than nonsmokers who are not exposed to ETS.

The bottom line? Not smoking is highly beneficial. If you stop smoking, your risk of CVD will decrease, regardless of the age at which you quit. But abstaining from cigarette smoking and avoiding ETS throughout your entire life is even better.

Know and Manage Your Blood Pressure

Currently, only about 34% of Americans with hypertension have their blood pressure under control; the *Healthy People 2010* report sets the goal of increasing this number to 50%. If you have no CVD risk factors, have your blood pressure measured by a trained professional at least once every 2 years; yearly tests are recommended if you have other risk factors. If your blood pressure is high, follow your physician's advice on how to lower it. For those with hypertension that is not readily controlled with lifestyle changes, an array of antihypertension medications are available.

Know and Manage Your Cholesterol Levels

All people age 20 and over should have their cholesterol checked at least once every 5 years. The NCEP recommends a lipoprotein profile that measures total cholesterol, HDL, LDL, and triglyceride levels. Once you know your baseline numbers, you and your physician can develop an appropriate LDL goal and lifestyle plan. Your LDL

Religion and Wellness

In the past decade, numerous observational studies have shown a link between religious or spiritual factors and health. Regardless of why or how this relationship happens, the evidence clearly connects religion and wellness along several dimensions.

- *Reduced risk of disease and faster recovery.* Researchers have found that people who attend religious services regularly have especially low rates of heart disease, lung disease, cirrhosis of the liver, and some kinds of cancer. Older adults who attend religious services have healthier immune systems and recover from surgery more quickly.

- *Improved emotional health.* Religion also seems to aid in recovery from depression. Participating in religious activities, listening to religious programs on the radio, and watching religious programs on television are all associated with fewer symptoms of depression.

- *Longer life expectancy.* One study found that people who attend religious services one or more times a week live about 8 years longer than people who never attend services. How involved people are in their faith may be more important than was previously believed.

Although researchers are not sure why religion or spirituality seems to improve health, several explanations have been offered:

- *Social support.* Attending religious services helps people feel they are part of a community with similar values. It promotes social support and caring.

- *Healthy habits.* Religion may encourage healthy habits—such as eating less meat, drinking less alcohol, or eating a vegetarian diet—and also may discourage behavior that is harmful to health, such as smoking and indiscriminate sex.

- *Positive attitude.* Having a sense of meaning and purpose in life results in a positive attitude. This outlook may help patients participate more in their own care.

- *Moments of relaxation.* Deep relaxation during prayer may invoke benefits by eliciting the relaxation response.

SOURCES: Strawbridge, W. J., et al. 2001. Religious attendance increases survival by improving and maintaining good health behaviors, mental health, and social relationships. *Annals of Behavioral Medicine* 23(1): 68–74; Hummer, R. A., et al. 1999. Religious involvement and U.S. adult mortality. *Demography* 36: 273–285; Can spirituality uplift your health? 1998. *Consumer Reports on Health*, June, 7–8; Hafen, B., et al. 1996. *Mind/Body Health: The Effects of Attitudes, Emotions, and Relationships.* Needham Heights, Mass.: Allyn & Bacon.

---

goal depends in part on how many of the following major risk factors you have:

- Cigarette smoking
- High blood pressure
- Low HDL cholesterol (less than 40 mg/dl)
- A family history of heart disease
- Age (≥45 for men, ≥55 years for women)

An HDL level of 60 mg/dl or higher is protective and counts as a negative risk factor, meaning it removes one risk factor from your total count of risk factors. Depending on your LDL level and other risk factors, your physician may recommend changes in lifestyle alone or lifestyle changes in combination with drug therapy. The lifestyle modifications recommended by the 2001 NCEP guidelines, known collectively as "Therapeutic Lifestyle Changes" (TLC), include the TLC diet, weight management, and increased physical activity. The TLC diet includes total fat intake of 25–35% of total daily calories, saturated fat intake of less than 7% of total calories, and, for some people, 10–25 grams per day of viscous (soluble) fiber and 2 grams per day of plant stanols and sterols.

• If you have one or no risk factors, the NCEP sets an LDL goal of less than 160 mg/dl. If your LDL is below that level, maintain a healthy lifestyle by eating a heart-healthy diet, getting regular exercise, maintaining a healthy body weight, and not smoking. If your LDL is 160 mg/dl or higher, you should begin TLC; you may also need medication to bring your LDL into the healthy range.

• If you have two or more risk factors for heart disease, the NCEP sets an LDL goal of less than 130 mg/dl. If your LDL level is 130 or above, begin TLC; if your LDL level remains above the goal and your risk for CVD is fairly high, your physician may recommend medication.

• If you have heart disease or a condition such as diabetes that the NCEP considers the risk equivalent of heart disease, your goal for LDL is less than 100 mg/dl. For very-high-risk patients, the goal has been changed to less than 70 mg/dl. TLC is recommended for all people in this risk category. In addition, a variety of medications are available to lower LDL and improve other blood fat levels.

Develop Effective Ways to Handle Stress and Anger

To reduce the psychological and social risk factors for CVD, develop effective strategies for handling the stress in your life. Shore up your social support network, and try some of the techniques described in Chapter 2 for managing stress (see also the box "Religion and Wellness").

Manage Other Risk Factors and Medical Conditions

Know your CVD risk factors and follow your physician's advice for testing, lifestyle modification, and any drug treatments.

If you are at high risk for CVD, consult a physician about taking small doses of aspirin. Remember, aspirin reduces inflammation and the blood's tendency to clot, thereby reducing the risk of CVD for some people. Low doses of aspirin (50–325 mg) are recommended for men and women to treat TIA, stroke, angina, heart attack, and certain other cardiovascular problems. Because of possible side effects, including gastrointestinal bleeding and increased risk of certain types of strokes, the FDA cautions people to consult with their physician before taking aspirin regularly.

Tips for Today

Risk factors for cardiovascular disease fall into two categories—those you can do something about, such as physical activity and levels of stress, and those you can't, such as age and ethnicity. Because cardiovascular disease is a long-term process that can begin when you're young, it's important to develop heart-healthy habits early in life.

Right now you can

- Plan to have fish for dinner two times this week.
- Practice time management by prioritizing your day's activities; work on accomplishing the most important tasks first.
- Resolve to address any nagging interpersonal issue that's been causing you stress.
- Go to the gym or fitness facility on your campus and get started on an aerobic exercise program.

SUMMARY

- The cardiovascular system pumps and circulates blood throughout the body. The heart pumps blood to the lungs via the pulmonary artery and to the body via the aorta.
- The exchange of nutrients and waste products takes place between the capillaries and the tissues.

- The six major risk factors for CVD that can be changed are smoking, high blood pressure, unhealthy cholesterol levels, inactivity, obesity, and diabetes.
- Effects of smoking include lower HDL levels, increased blood pressure and heart rate, accelerated plaque formation, and increased risk of blood clots.
- Hypertension occurs when blood pressure exceeds normal limits most of the time. It weakens the heart, scars and hardens arteries, and can damage the eyes and kidneys.
- High LDL and low HDL cholesterol levels contribute to clogged arteries and increase the risk of CVD.
- Physical inactivity, obesity, and diabetes are interrelated and are associated with high blood pressure and unhealthy cholesterol levels.
- Contributing risk factors that can be changed include high triglyceride levels and psychological and social factors.
- Risk factors for CVD that can't be changed include being over 65, being male, being African American, and having a family history of CVD.
- Atherosclerosis is a progressive hardening and narrowing of arteries that can lead to restricted blood flow and even complete blockage.
- Heart attacks are usually the result of a long-term disease process. Warning signs of a heart attack include chest discomfort, light-headedness, nausea, and sweating.
- A stroke occurs when the blood supply to the brain is cut off by a blood clot or hemorrhage. A transient ischemic attack (TIA) is a warning sign of stroke.
- Congestive heart failure occurs when the heart's pumping action becomes less efficient and fluid collects in the lungs or in other parts of the body.
- Dietary changes that can protect against CVD include decreasing your intake of fat, especially saturated and trans fats, and cholesterol, and increasing your intake of fiber by eating more fruits, vegetables, and whole grains.
- CVD risk can also be reduced by engaging in regular exercise, avoiding tobacco and environmental tobacco smoke, knowing and managing your blood pressure and cholesterol levels, developing effective ways of handling stress and anger, and managing other risk factors and medical conditions.

Take Action

1. **Learn CPR:** The CPR courses given by the American Red Cross and other groups provide invaluable training that may help you save a life some day. Anyone can take these courses and become qualified to perform CPR and possibly use AED equipment. Investigate CPR courses in your community, and sign up to take one.

2. **Investigate your family's CVD history:** Do some research into your family medical history. Is there CVD in your family, as indicated by premature deaths from heart attack, stroke, or heart failure? Is there a family history of diabetes? Keep your family health history in mind as you consider whether you need to make lifestyle changes to avoid CVD.

Reducing the Saturated and Trans Fats in Your Diet

The American Heart Association recommends that no more than 10% of the calories in your diet come from cholesterol-raising saturated and trans fats. Foods high in saturated fat include meat, poultry skin, full-fat dairy products, coconut and palm oils, and hydrogenated vegetable oils. Hydrogenated fats and products such as snack foods that are made with them and deep-fried fast food are high in trans fats.

Monitor Your Current Diet

To see how your diet measures up, keep track of everything you eat for 3 days in your health journal. Information about the calorie and saturated fat content of foods is available on many food labels, in books, and on the Internet (see Chapter 12). Especially before 2006, trans fat content may be more difficult to determine; the list below gives a few average values for foods that are rich sources of trans fats in the American diet.

	Grams of trans fat/serving
Pot pie	6
French fries (large)	5
Pound cake	5
Fish sticks	5
Doughnut	4
Biscuit	4
Fried, breaded chicken	3
Danish pastry	3
Vegetable shortening	3
Margarine (stick)	2
Microwave popcorn	2
Sandwich cookies	2
Snack crackers	2
Margarine (tub)	1

At the end of the monitoring period, write in the calories and grams of saturated and trans fat for as many as possible of the foods you've eaten. Determine the percentage of daily calories as fat that you consumed for each day: multiply grams of saturated and trans fats by 9 (fat has 9 calories per gram) and then divide by total calories. For example, if you consumed 30 grams of saturated and trans fats and 2100 calories on a particular day, then your saturated and trans fat consumption as a percentage of total calories would be $30 \times 9 = 270$ calories of fat $\div$ 2100 total calories $= 0.13$, or 13%. If you have trouble obtaining all the data you need to do the calculations, you can still estimate whether your diet is high in saturated and trans fats by seeing how many servings of foods high in unhealthy fats you typically consume on a daily basis (see the list).

Making Heart-Healthy Changes

To reduce your intake of unhealthy fats, you may want to set a limit on the number of servings of foods high in saturated and trans fats that you consume each day. Or you may want to set a more precise goal and then continue to monitor your daily consumption. The 10% limit set by the American Heart Association corresponds to 18 grams of saturated and trans fats in a 1600-calorie diet, 24 grams in a 2200-calorie diet, and 31 grams in a 2800-calorie diet. (If you have high cholesterol, you may want to follow the 7% limit set by the NCEP, which corresponds to 12 grams of saturated and trans fats in a 1600-calorie diet, 17 grams in a 2200-calorie diet, and 22 grams in a 2800-calorie diet.)

To plan healthy changes, take a close look at your food record. Do you choose many foods high in saturated and trans fats? Do you limit your portion sizes to those recommended by MyPyramid? Try making healthy substitutions. Do you have a salami and cheese sandwich for lunch? Try turkey for a change. Do you always order french fries when you eat out? Try half a plain baked potato or a different vegetable next time. Do you snack on pastries, cookies, doughnuts, chips, or fatty crackers? Try fresh fruits and vegetables instead. If you frequently eat in fast-food restaurants or other places where the majority of the menu is heavy in saturated and trans fats, trying finding an appealing alternative—and recruit some friends to join you.

When you do choose foods that are rich in saturated and trans fats, *watch your portion sizes carefully*. Choose cuts of meat that have the least amount of visible fat, and trim off what you see. And try to balance your choices throughout the day: For example, if your lunch includes a hamburger and fries, choose broiled fish or poultry or a vegetarian pasta dish for dinner. There are plenty of delicious choices that are low in saturated and trans fats. Plan your diet around a variety of whole grains, vegetables, legumes, and fruits, which are nearly always low in fats and high in nutrients.

(continued)

For More Information

Books

Cohen, B. 2002. *Coronary Heart Disease: A Guide to Diagnosis and Treatment*. Omaha, Nebr.: Addicus Books. *Provides information about heart disease treatment and recovery for patients and their families.*

Freeman, M. W., and C. E. Junge. 2005. *Harvard Medical School Guide to Lowering Your Cholesterol*. New York: McGraw-Hill. *Information about cholesterol, including lifestyle changes and medication for improving cholesterol levels.*

Moore, T., et al. 2003. *The DASH Diet for Hypertension*. New York: Pocket Books. *Provides background information and guidelines for adopting the DASH diet; also includes recipes.*

Nelson, M. E., and A. Lichtenstein. 2005. *Strong Women, Strong Hearts*. New York: Putnam Adult. *Lifestyle advice for women to prevent heart disease.*

Reaven, G. M., et al. 2001. *Syndrome X, the Silent Killer: The New Heart Disease Risk*. St. Louis, Mo.: Fireside. *Provides information about metabolic syndrome and insulin resistance, including lifestyle strategies for affected individuals.*

Romaine, D. S., and O. S. Randall. 2005. *The Encyclopedia of Heart and Heart Disease*. New York: Facts on File. *Includes entries on the functioning of the cardiovascular system, types and causes of heart disease, and prevention and treatment.*

Instead of . . .	Try . . .
Butter, stick margarine, vegetable shortening, coconut and palm oils	Vegetable oils, trans fat–free tub or squeeze margarines
Whole or 2% milk; regular cheese, mayonnaise, and sour cream	Fat-free or 1% milk, low-fat cheese, fat-free or low-fat sour cream, yogurt, or mayonnaise
Chips, cheese puffs, crackers, buttered popcorn	Fruits, vegetables, rice cakes, plain popcorn, pretzels, fat-free chips, baked crackers
Cakes, cookies, pastries, doughnuts, cinnamon rolls, pie, regular ice cream	Fruit or a *small* serving of a low-fat sweet (angel food cake; fat-free ice cream, frozen yogurt, sherbet, or sorbet)
Biscuits, croissants, fried tortillas, regular granola, muffins, coffee cake	Whole-grain breads and rolls, baked tortillas, low-fat granola or cold cereal, English muffin, or bagel
Creamy or cheesy sauces and soups	Tomato- and other vegetable-based sauces, clam sauce, clear soups
Ground beef, hamburger patty, meatloaf, ribs, T-bone or flank steak, prime grades of beef	Ground turkey, veggie burger, extra lean ground beef, round steak, sirloin, choice or select grades of beef
Pork chops, roast, or ribs; bone-in ham; lamb chops or ribs	Pork sirloin or tenderloin, boneless ham, veal chops and cutlets, leg of lamb
Bacon, sausage, lunch meats, hot dogs	Canadian bacon; turkey ham or pastrami, other low-fat lunch meats
Poultry with skin; fried chicken or fish	Skinless poultry, especially breast or drumstick; baked, broiled, grilled, or roasted poultry or fish; ground turkey
French fries, onion rings	Baked potato or other nonfried vegetable, rice
Pizza, pot pie, macaroni and cheese, and other high-fat convenience foods	Vegetarian or turkey chili, pasta with vegetables, grilled poultry and fish dishes

SOURCES: American Heart Association. 2000. *An Eating Plan for Healthy Americans: The New 2000 Food Guidelines.* Dallas, Tex.: American Heart Association; U.S. Department of Agriculture and U.S. Department of Health and Human Services. 2000. *Nutrition and Your Health: Dietary Guidelines for Americans,* 5th ed. Home and Garden Bulletin No. 232; Food and Drug Administration. 1999. *Questions and Answers on Trans Fat Proposed Rule* (http://vm.cfsan.fda.gov/~dms/qatrans.html); Center for Science in the Public Interest. 1997. The sat fat switch. *Nutrition Action Healthletter,* January/February.

VIW Organizations, Hotlines, and Web Sites

American Heart Association. Provides information on hundreds of topics relating to the prevention and control of cardiovascular disease; sponsors a general Web site as well as several sites focusing on specific topics.

    800-AHA-USA1 (800-242-8721; general information)
    http://www.americanheart.org (general information)
    http://www.deliciousdecisions.org (dietary advice)
    http://www.justmove.org (fitness advice)

Dietary Approaches to Stop Hypertension (DASH). Provides information about the design, diets, and results of the DASH study, including tips on how to follow the DASH diet at home.

    http://www.nhlbi.nih.gov/health/public/heart/hbp/dash

Franklin Institute Science Museum/The Heart: An On-Line Exploration. An online museum exhibit containing information on the structure and function of the heart, how to monitor your heart's health, and how to maintain a healthy heart.

    http://www.fi.edu/biosci/heart.html

HeartInfo—Heart Information Network. Provides information for heart patients and others interested in learning how to identify and reduce their risk factors for heart disease; includes links to many related sites.

    http://www.heartinfo.org

MedlinePlus: Heart and Circulation Topics. Provides links to reliable sources of information on many topics relating to cardiovascular health.

    http://www.nlm.nih.gov/medlineplus/
      heartandcirculation.html

National Heart, Lung, and Blood Institute. Provides information on and interactive applications for a variety of topics relating to cardiovascular health and disease, including cholesterol, smoking, obesity, hypertension, and the DASH diet.

    800-575-WELL
    http://www.nhlbi.nih.gov
    http://rover.nhlbi.nih.gov/chd

National Stroke Association. Provides information and referrals for stroke victims and their families; the Web site has a stroke risk assessment.

    800-STROKES
    http://www.stroke.org

See also the listings for Chapters 2, 3, and 12–14.

Selected Bibliography

Ajani, U. A., et al. 2004. Body mass index and mortality among US male physicians. *Annals of Epidemiology* 14(10): 731–739.

American Heart Association. 2005. *Heart and Stroke Statistical Update, 2005.* Dallas, Tex.: American Heart Association.

Barrett-Connor, E., et al. 2004. Women and heart disease: The role of diabetes and hyperglycemia. *Archives of Internal Medicine* 164: 934–942.

Bradley, E. H., et al. 2004. Racial and ethnic differences in time to acute reperfusion therapy for patients hospitalized with myocardial infarction. *Journal of the American Medical Association* 292(13): 1563–1572.

Campia, U., et al. 2002. Reduced endothelium-dependent and -independent dilation of conductance arteries in African Americans. *Journal of the American College of Cardiology* 40(4): 754–760.

Cardiopulmonary resuscitation (CPR). 2005. *Journal of the American Medication Association* 293(3): 388.

Centers for Disease Control and Prevention. 2005. Differences in disability among black and white stroke survivors—United States, 2000–2001. *Morbidity and Mortality Weekly Report* 54(1): 3–9.

Centers for Disease Control and Prevention. 2005. Health disparities experienced by black or African Americans—United States. *Morbidity and Mortality Weekly Report* 54(1): 1–3.

Cooper, R. S., et al. 2005. An international comparative study of blood pressure in populations of European vs. African descent. *BMC Medicine* 3(1): 2.

Critchley, J. A., and S. Capewell. 2003. Mortality risk reduction associated with smoking cessation in patients with coronary heart disease. A systematic review. *Journal of the American Medical Association* 290: 86–97.

Daviglus, M. L., et al. 2004. Favorable cardiovascular risk profile in young women and long-term risk of cardiovascular and all-cause mortality. *Journal of the American Medical Association* 292(13): 1588–1592.

Douglas, J. G., et al. 2003. Management of high blood pressure in African Americans: Consensus statement of the Hypertension in African Americans Working Group of the International Society on Hypertension in Blacks. *Archives of Internal Medicine* 163(5): 525–541.

Eaker, E., et al. 2004. Anger and hostility predict the development of atrial fibrillation in men in the Framingham Offspring Study. *Circulation* 109: 1267–1271.

Forman, J. P., et al. 2005. Folate intake and risk of incident hypertension among U.S. women. *Journal of the American Medical Association* 293(3): 320–329.

Geerts, S. O., et al. 2004. Further evidence of the association between periodontal conditions and coronary artery disease. *Journal of Periodontology* 75(9): 1274–1280.

Hackman, D. G., and S. S. Anand. 2003. Emerging risk factors for atherosclerotic vascular disease. A critical review of the evidence. *Journal of the American Medical Association* 290: 932–940.

Jensen, M. K., et al. 2004. Intakes of whole grains, bran, and germ and the risk of coronary heart disease in men. *American Journal of Clinical Nutrition* 80(6): 1492–1499.

Kaiser Family Foundation and American College of Cardiology Foundation. 2002. *Racial/Ethnic Differences in Cardiac Care: The Weight of the Evidence.* Menlo Park, Calif.: Kaiser Family Foundation.

Kastrati, A., et al. 2005. Sirolimus-eluting stent or paclitaxel-eluting stent vs. balloon angioplasty for prevention of recurrences in patients with coronary in-stent restenosis. *Journal of the American Medical Association* 293(2): 165–171.

Koton, S., et al. 2004. Triggering risk factors for ischemic stroke. *Neurology* 63(11): 2006–2010.

Lloyd-Jones, D. M., et al. 2004. Parental cardiovascular disease as a risk factor for cardiovascular disease in middle-aged adults. *Journal of the American Medical Association* 291(18): 2204–2211.

Maron, B. J. 2003. Sudden death in young athletes. *New England Journal of Medicine* 349: 1064–1075.

McSweeney, J. C., et al. 2003. Women's early warning symptoms of acute myocardial infarction. *Circulation* 108: 2619–2623.

Kelemen, L. E., et al. 2005. Associations of dietary protein with disease and mortality in a prospective study of postmenopausal women. *American Journal of Epidemiology* 161(3): 239–249.

Meadows, M. 2005. Brain attack: A look at stroke prevention and treatment. *FDA Consumer,* March/April.

Mosca, L., et al. 2004. Evidence-based guidelines for cardiovascular disease prevention in women. *Circulation* 109: 672–693.

Mozaffarian, D., et al. 2005. Interplay between different polyunsaturated fatty acids and risk of coronary heart disease in men. *Circulation,* 111(2): 157–164.

Mukamal, K. J., et al. 2005. Alcohol and risk of ischemic stroke in men: The role of drinking patterns and usual beverage. *Annals of Internal Medicine* 142(1): 11–19.

Nissen, S. E., et al. 2005. Statin therapy, LDL cholesterol, C-reactive protein, and coronary artery disease. *New England Journal of Medicine* 352(1): 29–38.

O'Meara, J. G., et al. 2004. Ethnic and sex differences in the prevalence, treatment, and control of dyslipidemia among hypertensive adults in the GENOA study. *Archives of Internal Medicine* 164: 1313–1318.

Pearson, T. A., et al. 2003. AHA/CDC Scientific Statement: Markers of inflammation and cardiovascular disease: Application to clinical and public health practice. *Circulation* 107(3): 499–511.

Pereira, M. A., et al. 2004. Effects of a low-glycemic load diet on resting energy expenditure and heart disease risk factors during weight loss. *Journal of the American Medical Association* 292(20): 2482–2490.

Phillips, D. P., et al. 2004. Cardiac mortality is higher around Christmas and New Year's than at any other time. *Circulation* 110(25): 3781–3788.

Reaven, G. M. 2003. Insulin resistance/compensatory hyperinsulinemia, essential hypertension, and cardiovascular disease. *Journal of Clinical Endocrinology and Metabolism* 88(6): 2399–2403.

Ridker, P. M., et al. 2005. C-reactive protein levels and outcomes after statin therapy. *New England Journal of Medicine* 352(1): 20–28.

Ridker, P. M., et al. 2005. A randomized trial of low-dose aspirin in the primary prevention of cardiovascular disease in women. *New England Journal of Medicine,* epub, March 7.

Rothwell, P. M., and C. P. Warlow. 2005. Timing of TIAs preceding stroke: time window for prevention is very short. *Neurology* 64(5): 817–820.

Rozanski, A. S., et al. 2005. The epidemiology, pathophysiology, and management of psychosocial risk factors in cardiac practice: The emerging field of behavioral cardiology. *Journal of the American College of Cardiology* 45(5): 637–651.

Shai, I., et al. 2004. Homocysteine as a risk factor for coronary heart diseases and its association with inflammatory biomarkers, lipids and dietary factors. *Atherosclerosis* 177(2): 375–381.

Shai, I., et al. 2004. Multivariate assessment of lipid parameters as predictors of coronary heart disease among postmenopausal women. *Circulation* 110(18): 2824–2830.

Steffen, P. R., et al. 2003. Effects of perceived racism and anger inhibition on ambulatory blood pressure in African Americans. *Psychosomatic Medicine* 65(5): 746–750.

St.-Onge, M. P., I. Janssen, and S. B. Heymsfield. 2004. Metabolic syndrome in normal-weight Americans: New definition of the metabolically obese, normal-weight individual. *Diabetes Care* 27(9): 2222–2228.

Timing is everything: Fluctuations in cardiac risk. 2004. *Harvard Men's Health Watch,* December.

Turhan, H., et al. 2005. High prevalence of metabolic syndrome among young women with premature coronary artery disease. *Coronary Artery Disease* 16(1): 37–40.

Willingham, S. A., and E. S. Kilpatrick. 2005. Evidence of gender bias when applying the new diagnostic criteria for myocardial infarction. *Heart* 91(2): 237–238.

Wittstein, I. S., et al. 2005. Neurohumoral features of myocardial stunning due to sudden emotional stress. *New England Journal of Medicine* 352(6): 539–548.

Zhu, S., et al. 2004. Lifestyle behaviors associated with lower risk of having the metabolic syndrome. *Metabolism* 53(11): 1503–1511.

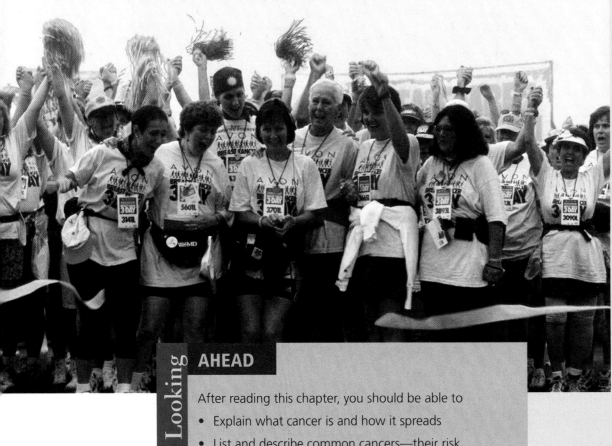

Looking AHEAD

After reading this chapter, you should be able to

- Explain what cancer is and how it spreads

- List and describe common cancers—their risk factors, signs and symptoms, treatments, and approaches to prevention

- Discuss some of the causes of cancer and how they can be avoided or minimized

- Describe how cancer can be detected, diagnosed, and treated

- List specific actions you can take to lower your risk of cancer

Cancer

1. Which type of cancer kills the most women each year?
a. breast cancer
b. lung cancer
c. ovarian cancer

2. Which type of cancer kills the most men each year?
a. prostate cancer
b. lung cancer
c. colon cancer

3. Testicular cancer is the most common cancer in men under age 30.
True or false?

4. The use of condoms during sexual intercourse can prevent cervical cancer in women.
True or false?

5. Because most college students now know that the use of tanning lamps can lead to premature aging of the skin and skin cancer, the rate of tanning lamp use among college students has declined significantly.
True or false?

6. Eating which of these foods may help prevent cancer?
a. chili peppers
b. broccoli
c. oranges

ANSWERS

1. B. There are more cases of breast cancer each year, but lung cancer kills more women. Smoking is the primary risk factor for lung cancer.

2. B. There are more cases of prostate cancer, but lung cancer kills about three times as many men as prostate cancer does each year.

3. TRUE. Although rare, testicular cancer is the most common cancer in men under age 30. Regular self-exams may aid in its detection.

4. TRUE. The primary cause of cervical cancer is infection with human papillomavirus (HPV), a sexually transmitted pathogen. The use of condoms helps prevent HPV infection.

5. FALSE. Nearly half of all college students report having used tanning lamps within the past year, and more than 90% of the tanning lamp users were aware of the dangers.

6. ALL THREE. These and many other fruits and vegetables are rich in phytochemicals, naturally occurring substances that may have anti-cancer effects.

Visit the *Core Concepts in Health* Online Learning Center (www.mhhe.com/insel10e) for study aids and many additional resources.

479

Cancer is derived from the Greek word for crab, *karkinos*. The early Greek physicians who first described cancerous tumors had no notion of their cause or true nature, but they were struck by the resemblance of some invasive tumors to crabs: a hard mass with clawlike extensions and an aggressive nature. Today, though we know a great deal about cancer, the old metaphor still has power; cancer has maintained its reputation as an alien presence in the body, capable of causing pain, great harm, even death. Cancer causes about 570,000 deaths in the United States each year and is the leading cause of death among people under age 85. Overall, cancer is the second most common cause of death, after heart disease.

While medical science struggles to find cures for the various cancers that plague us, evidence indicates that more than half of all cancers could be prevented by simple changes in lifestyle like those described in earlier chapters. Tobacco use is responsible for about one-third of all cancer deaths (Figure 16-1). Poor diet and exercise habits, including their effect on obesity, account for another large proportion of cancer deaths. Although cancer is primarily a disease of older adults, your behavior now will determine your cancer risk in the future. Experts estimate that through changes in lifestyle, most Americans can cut their lifetime cancer risk in half.

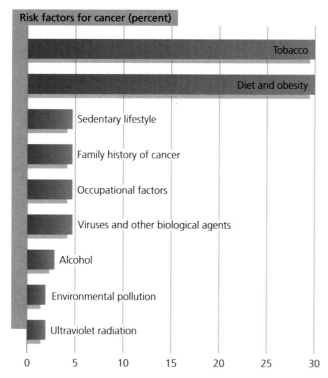

Risk factors for cancer (percent)

Tobacco
Diet and obesity
Sedentary lifestyle
Family history of cancer
Occupational factors
Viruses and other biological agents
Alcohol
Environmental pollution
Ultraviolet radiation

0   5   10   15   20   25   30

VITAL STATISTICS

Figure 16-1   Percentage of all cancer deaths linked to risk factors.   SOURCE: Harvard Center for Cancer Prevention. 1996. Harvard Report on Cancer Prevention. Vol. 1: Causes of Human Cancer. *Cancer Causes and Control* 7(Suppl).

WHAT IS CANCER?

Cancer is the abnormal, uncontrolled growth of cells, which, if left untreated, can ultimately cause death.

Benign Versus Malignant Tumors

Most cancers take the form of tumors, although not all tumors are cancerous. A tumor is simply a mass of tissue that serves no physiological purpose. It can be benign, like a wart, or malignant, like most lung cancers.

Benign tumors are made up of cells similar to the surrounding normal cells and are enclosed in a membrane that prevents them from penetrating neighboring tissues. They are dangerous only if their physical presence interferes with body functions. A benign brain tumor, for example, can cause death if it blocks the blood supply to the brain.

The term **malignant tumor** (or *neoplasm*) is synonymous with cancer. A malignant tumor is capable of invading surrounding structures, including blood vessels, the **lymphatic system,** and nerves. It can also spread to distant sites via the blood and lymphatic circulation, thereby producing invasive tumors in almost any part of the body. A few cancers, like leukemia, or cancer of the blood, do not produce a mass and therefore are not properly called tumors. But because leukemia cells do have the fundamental property of rapid, uncontrolled growth, they are still malignant and therefore cancers.

Every case of cancer begins as a change in a cell that allows it to grow and divide when it should not. Normally (in adults), cells divide and grow at a rate just sufficient to replace dying cells. When you cut your finger, for example, the cells around the wound divide more rapidly to heal the wound. When the wound is healed, the rate of cell growth and division returns to normal. In contrast, a malignant cell divides without regard for normal control mechanisms and gradually produces a mass of abnormal cells, or a tumor. It takes about a billion cells to make a mass the size of a pea, so a single tumor cell must go through many divisions, often taking years, before the tumor grows to a noticeable size (Figure 16-2).

Eventually a tumor produces a sign or symptom that is determined by its location in the body. In the breast, for example, a tumor may be felt as a lump and diagnosed as cancer by an X ray or **biopsy.** In less accessible locations, like the lung, ovary, or intestine, a tumor may be noticed only after considerable growth has taken place and may then be detected only by an indirect symptom—for instance, a persistent cough or unexplained bleeding or pain. In the case of leukemia, there is no lump, but the changes in the blood will eventually be noticed as increasing fatigue, infection, or abnormal bleeding.

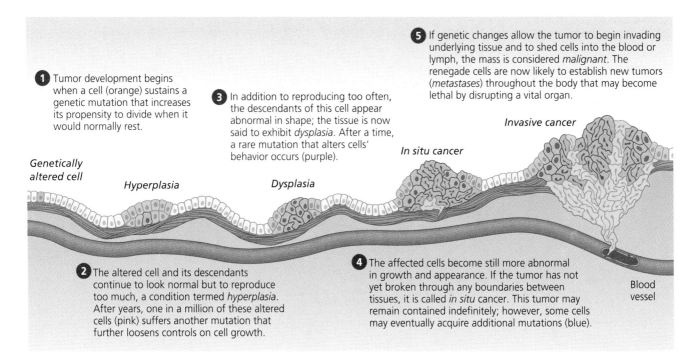

1 Tumor development begins when a cell (orange) sustains a genetic mutation that increases its propensity to divide when it would normally rest.

3 In addition to reproducing too often, the descendants of this cell appear abnormal in shape; the tissue is now said to exhibit *dysplasia*. After a time, a rare mutation that alters cells' behavior occurs (purple).

5 If genetic changes allow the tumor to begin invading underlying tissue and to shed cells into the blood or lymph, the mass is considered *malignant*. The renegade cells are now likely to establish new tumors (*metastases*) throughout the body that may become lethal by disrupting a vital organ.

Genetically altered cell

Hyperplasia

Dysplasia

In situ cancer

Invasive cancer

2 The altered cell and its descendants continue to look normal but to reproduce too much, a condition termed *hyperplasia*. After years, one in a million of these altered cells (pink) suffers another mutation that further loosens controls on cell growth.

4 The affected cells become still more abnormal in growth and appearance. If the tumor has not yet broken through any boundaries between tissues, it is called *in situ* cancer. This tumor may remain contained indefinitely; however, some cells may eventually acquire additional mutations (blue).

Blood vessel

Figure 16-2   Tumor development occurs in stages.   SOURCE: Weinberg, R. A. 1996. How cancer arises. *Scientific American,* September. Copyright © 1996 by Dana Burns-Pizer. Reprinted with permission.

How Cancer Spreads: Metastasis

Metastasis, the spreading of cancer cells, occurs because cancer cells do not stick to each other as strongly as normal cells do and therefore may not remain at the site of the *primary tumor,* the original location. They break away and can pass through the lining of lymph or blood vessels to invade nearby tissue. They can also drift to distant parts of the body, where they establish new colonies of cancer cells. This traveling and seeding process is called metastasizing, and the new tumors are called *secondary tumors,* or *metastases.*

Traveling cancer cells can follow two courses. They can produce secondary tumors in the lymph nodes and be carried through the lymph system to form secondary sites elsewhere, or they can invade blood vessels and circulate through the vessels to colonize other organs. This ability of cancer cells to metastasize makes early cancer detection critical. To control the cancer and prevent death, every cancerous cell must be removed. Once cancer cells enter either the lymphatic system or the bloodstream, it is extremely difficult to stop their spread to other organs of the body. In fact, counting the number of lymph nodes that contain cancer cells is one of the principal methods of predicting the outcome of the disease; the probability of a cure is much greater when the lymph nodes do not contain cancer cells.

Types of Cancer

The behavior of tumors arising in different body organs is characteristic of the tissue of origin. (Figure 16-3 shows the major cancer sites and the incidence of each type.) Because each cancer begins as a single (altered) cell with a specific function in the body, the cancer will retain some of the properties of the normal cell for a time. For instance, cancer of the thyroid gland may produce too much thyroid hormone and cause hyperthyroidism as well as cancer. Usually, however, cancer cells lose their resemblance to normal tissue as they continue to divide, becoming groups of rogue cells with increasingly unpredictable behavior.

Malignant tumors are classified according to the types of cells that give rise to them:

• **Carcinomas** arise from **epithelia,** tissues that cover external body surfaces, line internal tubes and

Terms

cancer Abnormal, uncontrolled cellular growth.

malignant tumor A tumor that is cancerous and capable of spreading.

benign tumor A tumor that is not cancerous.

lymphatic system A system of vessels that returns proteins, lipids, and other substances from fluid in the tissues to the circulatory system.

biopsy The removal and examination of a small piece of body tissue; a needle biopsy uses a needle to remove a small sample; some biopsies require surgery.

metastasis The spread of cancer cells from one part of the body to another.

carcinoma Cancer that originates in epithelial tissue (skin, glands, and lining of internal organs).

epithelial layer A layer of tissue that covers a surface or lines a tube or cavity of the body, enclosing and protecting other parts of the body.

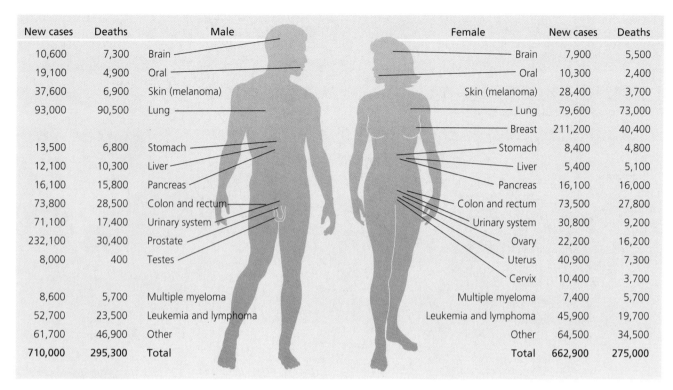

New cases	Deaths	Male	Female	New cases	Deaths
10,600	7,300	Brain	Brain	7,900	5,500
19,100	4,900	Oral	Oral	10,300	2,400
37,600	6,900	Skin (melanoma)	Skin (melanoma)	28,400	3,700
93,000	90,500	Lung	Lung	79,600	73,000
			Breast	211,200	40,400
13,500	6,800	Stomach	Stomach	8,400	4,800
12,100	10,300	Liver	Liver	5,400	5,100
16,100	15,800	Pancreas	Pancreas	16,100	16,000
73,800	28,500	Colon and rectum	Colon and rectum	73,500	27,800
71,100	17,400	Urinary system	Urinary system	30,800	9,200
232,100	30,400	Prostate	Ovary	22,200	16,200
8,000	400	Testes	Uterus	40,900	7,300
			Cervix	10,400	3,700
8,600	5,700	Multiple myeloma	Multiple myeloma	7,400	5,700
52,700	23,500	Leukemia and lymphoma	Leukemia and lymphoma	45,900	19,700
61,700	46,900	Other	Other	64,500	34,500
710,000	295,300	Total	Total	662,900	275,000

VITAL STATISTICS

Figure 16-3 Cancer cases and deaths by site and sex. The New cases column indicates the number of cancers that occurred in each site; the Deaths column indicates the number of cancer deaths that were attributed to each type. SOURCE: American Cancer Society. 2005. *Cancer Facts and Figures, 2005.* Atlanta: American Cancer Society.

cavities, and form the secreting portion of glands. They are the most common type of cancers; major sites include the skin, breast, uterus, prostate, lungs, and gastrointestinal tract.

- **Sarcomas** arise from connective and fibrous tissues such as muscle, bone, cartilage, and the membranes covering muscles and fat.

- **Lymphomas** are cancers of the lymph nodes, part of the body's infection-fighting system.

- **Leukemias** are cancers of the blood-forming cells, which reside chiefly in the **bone marrow.**

There is a great deal of variation in how easily different cancers can be detected and how well they respond to treatment. For example, certain types of skin cancer are easily detected, grow slowly, and are very easy to remove; virtually all of the 1 million cases that occur each year in the United States are cured. Cancer of the pancreas, on the other hand, is very difficult to detect or treat, and very few patients survive the disease. In general, it is very difficult for an **oncologist** to predict how a specific tumor will behave, because every tumor arises from a unique set of changes in a single cell.

The Incidence of Cancer

Each year, about 1.4 million people in the United States are diagnosed with cancer. Most will be cured, but about 36% will die as a result of their cancer within 5 years of diagnosis. These grim statistics exclude more than 1 million cases of the curable types of skin cancer. At current U.S. rates, nearly 1 in 2 men and more than 1 in 3 women will develop cancer at some point in their lives (see the box "Gender and Cancer").

Are cancer deaths increasing in the United States? Until 1991, the answer was yes, largely due to a wave of lethal lung cancers among men caused by smoking. In 1991, the death rate stopped increasing and began to fall slowly; it has dropped more than 10% since 1990. This is a very promising trend, as it suggests that efforts at prevention, early detection, and improved therapy are

Terms

sarcoma Cancer arising from bone, cartilage, or striated muscle.

lymphoma A tumor originating from lymphatic tissue.

leukemia Cancer of the blood or the blood-forming cells.

bone marrow Soft vascular tissue in the interior cavities of bones that produces blood cells.

oncologist A specialist in the study of tumors.

Gender Matters

Gender and Cancer

Men and women share most major risk factors for cancer, but they do have a different experience because more than a third of all cancers occur in sex organs (prostate, testes, breast, ovary, uterus, cervix). For women, this means that in addition to lifestyle factors such as smoking, diet, and exercise, hormonal factors relating to their menstrual and childbearing history are also important risk considerations. Women may also have a greater biological vulnerability to certain carcinogens, such as those in cigarettes.

Overall, however, men are more likely than women to have cancer and to die of cancer. For some cancers, the differences are especially significant. For example, men are much more likely than women to die from oral cancer, skin cancer, lung cancer, liver cancer, and urinary cancer. Here are some of the factors underlying the higher death rates among men:

• *Higher rates of tobacco use:* Particularly in the past, men had significantly higher rates of smoking than women, leading to much higher rates of the many cancers linked to smoking. Men also have much higher rates of spit tobacco and cigar use.

The graphs clearly show the powerful effects of smoking on cancer death rates since 1930. Lung cancer rates among men increased dramatically following significantly increased smoking rates beginning in the early 1900s (inexpensive machine-produced cigarettes were developed in the late 1800s). The lung cancer rate leveled off and (for men) started to decline after smoking rates began dropping. The smoking-related increase in lung cancer among women occurred about 20–30 years after that seen in men, as smoking among women became more socially acceptable and widespread beginning in the 1930s and 1940s.

• *Higher rates of alcohol use and abuse:* Alcohol abuse is more common in men and is a risk factor for several cancers, including oral and liver cancers.

• *Greater occupational exposure to carcinogens:* Men are more likely to work in jobs where they are exposed to chemicals—including asbestos, arsenic, coal tar, pitch, and dyes—or radiation, and such exposure is a risk factor for cancers of the bladder, lung, and skin. Men are also more likely to have outdoor jobs involving frequent sun exposure.

• *Less use of preventive measures and less contact with health care providers:* Traditional gender roles may make men more likely to minimize symptoms and less likely to seek help or to discuss cancer-related worries with a health care provider. Men may place a low status on preventive care or screenings, such as using sunscreen and wearing hats to protect the skin from the sun or performing self-exams.

Many of the factors underlying men's greater risk for cancer are controllable. It is important for both men and women to remember that there are many concrete steps they can take to significantly reduce their risk of cancer.

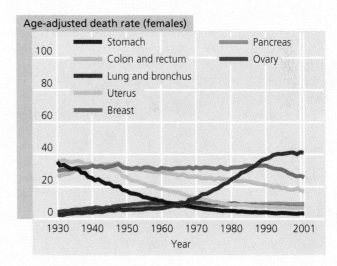

Change in cancer death rates since 1930   SOURCE: American Cancer Society's *Cancer Facts and Figures 2005,* © 2005 American Cancer Society, Inc. www.cancer.org. Reprinted with permission.

all bearing fruit. However, death rates from cancer are not declining as fast as those from heart disease, in large part because of the differing effects that quitting smoking has on disease risk: Heart-related damage of smoking reverses more quickly and more significantly than the cancer-related damage from smoking; smoking-related gene mutations cannot be reversed, although other mechanisms can sometimes control cellular changes. (Heart disease also has other risk factors like high cholesterol and blood pressure that can be tested for and controlled.) If heart disease death rates continue to decline faster than cancer death rates, cancer may overtake heart disease as the leading cause of death among Americans; cancer currently ranks number one for people under age 85.

Could more people be saved from cancer? The American Cancer Society (ACS) estimates that 90% of skin cancer could be prevented by protecting the skin from the rays of the sun and 87% of lung cancer could be prevented by avoiding exposure to tobacco smoke. Thousands of cases of colon, breast, and uterine cancer could be prevented by improving the diet and controlling body weight. Regular screenings and self-examinations have the potential to save an additional 100,000 lives per year. Although cancer may seem like a mysterious disease, there are many concrete strategies you can adopt to reduce your risk.

COMMON CANCERS

A discussion of all types of cancer is beyond the scope of this book. In this section we look at some of the most common cancers and their causes, prevention, and treatment.

Lung Cancer

Lung cancer is the most common cause of cancer death in the United States; it is responsible for about 163,000 deaths each year. For over 40 years, breast cancer was the major cause of cancer death in women, but since 1987 lung cancer has surpassed breast cancer as a killer of women.

Risk Factors The chief risk factor for lung cancer is tobacco smoke, which accounts for 87% of cancers. (Other negative effects of tobacco smoke on the lungs were discussed in Chapter 11.) When smoking is combined with exposure to other **carcinogens**, such as asbestos particles or certain pollutants, the risk of cancer can be multiplied by a factor of 10 or more.

The smoker is not the only one at risk. In 1993, the U.S. Environmental Protection Agency (EPA) classified environmental tobacco smoke (ETS) as a human carcinogen. Long-term exposure to ETS increases the risk of lung cancer. Secondhand smoke, the smoke from the burning end of the cigarette, has significantly higher concentrations of the toxic and carcinogenic compounds found in mainstream smoke. It is estimated that ETS causes about 3000 lung cancer deaths each year.

Detection and Treatment Lung cancer is difficult to detect at an early stage and hard to cure even when detected early. Symptoms of lung cancer do not usually appear until the disease has advanced to the invasive stage. Signals such as a persistent cough, chest pain, or

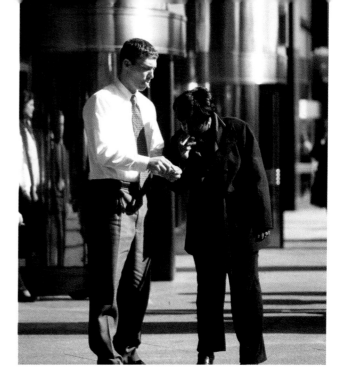

Smoking is responsible for about 30% of all cancer deaths. The benefits of quitting are substantial: Lung cancer risk decreases significantly after 1 smoke-free year and drops to half that of continuing smokers after 10 smoke-free years.

recurring bronchitis may be the first indication of a tumor's presence. Studies suggest that spiral CT (computed tomography) scans, a computer-assisted body imaging technique, can detect lung cancer significantly earlier than chest X rays. This screening method is expensive and often not covered by insurance, but further evaluation may determine that it is beneficial for high-risk individuals, such as chronic smokers. In cases where CT scanning is not available, a diagnosis can usually be made by chest X ray or by studying the cells in sputum. Because almost all lung cancers arise from the cells that line the bronchi, tumors can sometimes be visualized by fiber-optic bronchoscopy, a test in which a flexible lighted tube is inserted into the windpipe and the surfaces of the lung passages are directly inspected.

Treatment for lung cancer depends on the type and stage of the cancer. If caught early, localized cancers can be treated with surgery. But because only about 16% of lung cancers are detected before they spread, radiation and **chemotherapy** are often used in addition to surgery. For cases detected early, 49% of patients are alive 5 years after diagnosis; but overall, the survival rate is only 15%. Phototherapy, gene therapy, and immunotherapy (a vaccine) are being studied in the hope of improving these statistics. In addition, one form of lung cancer, known as small-cell lung cancer and accounting for about 20% of cases, can be treated fairly successfully with chemotherapy—alone or in combination with radiation. A large percentage of cases go into **remission,** which in some cases lasts for years.

Colon and Rectal Cancer

Another common cancer in the United States is colon and rectal cancer (also called colorectal cancer). It is the second leading cause of cancer death.

Risk Factors Age is a key risk factor for colon and rectal cancer, with more than 90% of cases diagnosed in people age 50 and older. Heredity also plays a role: Many cancers arise from preexisting **polyps,** small growths on the wall of the colon that may gradually develop into malignancies. The tendency to form colon polyps appears to be determined by specific genes, and 15–30% of colon cancers may be due to inherited gene mutations. Chronic inflammation of the colon as a result of disorders such as ulcerative colitis also increases the risk of colon cancer.

Lifestyle is also a risk factor for colon and rectal cancer. Regular physical activity appears to reduce a person's risk, whereas obesity increases risk. A diet rich in red and processed meats increases risk, although it is unclear whether fat or some other component of meat is the culprit. A diet rich in fruits, vegetables, and whole grains is associated with lower risk. However, research findings on whether dietary fiber prevents colon cancer have been mixed. Further investigation of different types and sources of fiber and other properties of plant-based diets may help clarify the relationship between diet and colon cancer. Studies have suggested a protective role for folic acid, magnesium, vitamin D, and calcium; in contrast, high intake of refined carbohydrates, simple sugars, and smoked meats and fish may increase risk. A plant-based, high-fiber diet is still recommended because it is associated with a lower risk of cancer overall and also helps prevent heart disease, hypertension, and diabetes.

Other lifestyle factors that may increase the risk of colon and rectal cancer include excessive alcohol consumption and smoking. Use of oral contraceptives or hormone replacement therapy may reduce risk in women. In addition, research indicates that regular use of nonsteroidal anti-inflammatory drugs such as aspirin and ibuprofen decreases the risk of developing colon cancer and other cancers of the digestive tract.

Detection and Treatment If identified early, precancerous polyps and early-stage cancers can be removed before they become malignant or spread. Because polyps may bleed as they progress, the standard warning signs of colon cancer are bleeding from the rectum and a change in bowel habits. Regular screening tests are recommended beginning at age 50 (earlier for people with a family history of the disease). A yearly stool blood test can detect small amounts of blood in the stool long before obvious bleeding would be noticed. More involved screening tests are recommended at 5- or 10-year intervals. In sigmoidoscopy or colonoscopy, a flexible fiber-optic device is inserted through the rectum; part or all of the colon can be examined, and polyps can be biopsied or even removed without major surgery. Although screening is effective, fewer than half of adults age 50 and over have undergone any of these tests in the past 5 years.

Surgery is the primary treatment for colon and rectal cancer. Radiation and chemotherapy may be used before surgery to shrink a tumor or after surgery to destroy any remaining cancerous cells. The survival rate is 90% for colon and rectal cancers detected early and 63% overall.

Breast Cancer

Breast cancer is the most common cancer in women and causes almost as many deaths in women as lung cancer. In men, breast cancer occurs only rarely. In the United States, about 1 woman in 7 will develop breast cancer during her lifetime, and 1 woman in 30 will die from the disease. About 210,000 American women are diagnosed with breast cancer each year. Although mortality rates declined during the early 1990s, about 40,000 women die from breast cancer each year.

Less then 1% of breast cancer cases occur in women under age 30, but a woman's risk doubles every 5 years between ages 30 and 45 and then increases more slowly, by 10–15% every 5 years after age 45. More than 75% of breast cancers are diagnosed in women over 50.

Risk Factors There is a strong genetic factor in breast cancer. A woman who has two close relatives with breast cancer is four to six times more likely to develop the disease than a woman who has no close relatives with it. However, even though genetic factors are important, only about 15% of cancers occur in women with a family history of breast cancer. (Genetic factors in breast cancer are discussed later in the chapter.)

Other risk factors include early onset of menstruation, late onset of menopause, having no children or having a first child after age 30, current use of hormone replacement therapy, obesity, and alcohol use. The unifying factor for many of these risk factors may be the female sex hormone estrogen, which circulates in a woman's body in high concentrations between puberty and menopause. Fat cells also produce estrogen, and estrogen levels are higher in obese women. Alcohol can interfere with estrogen metabolism in the liver and increase estrogen levels in the blood. Estrogen

---

Terms Vw

carcinogen Any substance that causes cancer.

chemotherapy The treatment of cancer with chemicals that selectively destroy cancerous cells.

remission A period during the course of cancer in which there are no symptoms or other evidence of disease.

polyp A small, usually harmless, mass of tissue that projects from the inner surface of the colon or rectum.

promotes the growth of cells in responsive sites, including the breast and the uterus, so any factor that increases estrogen exposure may raise breast cancer risk. Pregnancy and breastfeeding trigger changes in breast cells that make them less susceptible to cancerous changes.

Breast cancer has been called a "disease of civilization" because incidence is high in industrialized Western countries but remains low in developing non-Western countries. Differences in diet and exercise habits have been proposed to explain this pattern, but the connections are still being investigated. Monounsaturated fats have been linked with reduced risk, and certain types of polyunsaturated fat may increase risk. A diet rich in vegetables may also have a protective effect. Regular exercise is extremely important: A study of more than 25,000 women found that those who exercised regularly had a 37% lower risk of breast cancer than those who did not exercise. Vigorous exercise may reduce estrogen levels in the blood, and physical activity of all intensities helps control body weight. Both obesity and significant weight gain during adulthood are linked to increased risk of breast cancer.

A recent study found an interesting association between antibiotic use and increased breast cancer risk; however, this association may not be causal and could be related to other factors such as the patient's reasons for antibiotic use and her overall immune function. Antibiotics should be used only when prescribed and exactly as directed. Some research has also found that long-term use of aspirin and other nonsteroidal anti-inflammatory drugs reduces risk, possibly by affecting estrogen synthesis.

Although some of the risk factors for breast cancer—such as heredity and some hormonal factors—cannot be changed, important lifestyle risk factors are under the control of the individual. Eating a low-fat, vegetable-rich diet, exercising regularly, limiting alcohol intake, and maintaining a healthy body weight can minimize the chance of developing breast cancer, even for women at risk from family history or other factors.

Early Detection   A cure is most likely if breast cancer is detected early, so regular screening is a good investment, even for younger women. The ACS advises a three-part personal program for the early detection of breast cancer:

• *Mammography:* The ACS recommends a **mammogram** (low-dose breast X ray) every year for women over 40. Mammography is especially valuable as an early detection tool because it can identify breast abnormalities that may be cancer at an early stage, before physical symptoms develop. (Some physicians consider individual risk factors in determining a recommended frequency of mammograms.)

• *Clinical breast exam:* Women between ages 20 and 39 should have a clinical breast exam every 3 years, and women age 40 and older should have a breast exam by a health professional every year before their scheduled mammogram.

• *Breast self-exams:* Breast self-exam (BSE) allows a woman to become familiar with her breasts, so she can alert her health care provider to any changes. Starting at age 20, women should consider BSE an option for early detection (see the box "Breast Self-Examination").

Breast pain or tenderness is usually associated with benign conditions such as menstruation rather than breast cancer. The first physical signs of breast cancer are more likely to be a lump, swelling, or thickening; skin irritation or dimpling; or nipple pain, scaliness, or retraction. Although most breast lumps are benign, any breast lump should be taken seriously and brought to the attention of a health care provider.

Treatment   If a lump is detected, it may be scanned by **ultrasonography** and biopsied to see if it is cancerous. The biopsy may be done either by needle in the physician's office or surgically. In 90% of cases, the lump is found to be a cyst or other harmless growth, and no further treatment is needed. If the lump does contain cancer cells, a variety of surgeries may be called for, ranging from a lumpectomy (removal of the lump and surrounding tissue) to a mastectomy (removal of the breast). For small tumors, lumpectomy is as effective as mastectomy. To determine whether the cancer has spread, lymph nodes from the armpit may be removed and examined. If cancer cells are found, tumor cells remaining in the body can often be slowed or killed by additional therapy, such as radiation, chemotherapy, or both.

The chance of survival in cases of breast cancer varies, depending both on the nature of the tumor and whether it has metastasized. If the tumor is discovered early, before it has spread to the adjacent lymph nodes, the patient has about a 98% chance of surviving more than 5 years. The survival rate for all stages is 88% at 5 years and 77% at 10 years.

New Strategies for Treatment and Prevention   A number of new drugs have been developed for the treatment or prevention of breast cancer. A family of drugs called selective estrogen-receptor modulators, or SERMs, act like estrogen in some tissues of the body but block estrogen's effects in others. One SERM, tamoxifen, has long been used in breast cancer treatment because it blocks the action of estrogen in breast tissue. In 1998, the

Take Charge

The best time for a woman to examine her breasts is when the breasts are not tender or swollen. Women who are pregnant or breastfeeding or have breast implants can also choose to examine their breasts regularly. Women who examine their breasts should have their technique reviewed during their periodic health examinations by their health care professional. It is acceptable for women to choose not to do BSE or to do BSE occasionally. If you choose not to do BSE, you should still be familiar with your breasts and report any changes without delay to your doctor.

How to Examine Your Breasts

• Lie down and place your right arm behind your head. The exam is done while lying down, not standing up, because the breast tissue then spreads evenly over the chest wall and is as thin as possible, making it much easier to feel all the breast tissue.

• Use the finger pads of the three middle fingers on your left hand to feel for lumps in the right breast. Use overlapping dime-size circular motions of the finger pads to feel the breast tissue.

• Use three different levels of pressure to feel all the breast tissue. Light pressure is needed to feel the tissue closest to the skin; medium pressure to feel a little deeper; and firm pressure to feel the tissue closest to the chest and ribs. A firm ridge in the lower curve of each breast is normal. If you're not sure how hard to press, talk with your doctor or nurse. Use each pressure level to feel the breast tissue before moving on to the next spot.

• Move around the breast in an up-and-down pattern starting at an imaginary line drawn straight down your side from the underarm and moving across the breast to the middle of the chest bone (the sternum, or breastbone). Be sure to check the entire breast area, going down until you feel only ribs and going up to the neck or collar bone (clavicle).

• Repeat the exam on your left breast, using the finger pads of the right hand. Some evidence suggests that the up-and-down pattern (sometimes called the vertical pattern) is the most effective pattern for covering the entire breast, without missing any breast tissue.

• While standing in front of a mirror with your hands pressing firmly down on your hips, look at your breasts for any changes of size, shape, contour, or dimpling. (Pressing down on the hips contracts the chest wall muscles and enhances any breast changes.)

• Examine each underarm while sitting up or standing and with your arm only slightly raised so you can easily feel in this area. Raising your arm straight up tightens the tissue in this area and makes it difficult to examine.

SOURCE: American Cancer Society's Web site www.cancer.org, 2005. Copyright © 2005 American Cancer Society, Inc. Reprinted with permission.

FDA approved the use of tamoxifen to reduce the risk of breast cancer in healthy women who are at high risk for the disease. However, the drug has serious potential side effects, including increased risk of blood clots and uterine cancer, and its long-term effects are unknown. Another SERM currently being tested as a potential preventive agent is raloxifene, a drug, used to treat osteoporosis, that has fewer side effects than tamoxifen. Although still controversial, the use of SERMs in the prevention of breast cancer is a major breakthrough.

Women may take tamoxifen or other drugs or undergo chemotherapy to help reduce the risk of recurrence. A genetic test can help predict the risk of breast cancer recurrence and help identify women who will benefit most from chemotherapy; information from this test can help women make more informed treatment decisions. For advanced cancer, treatment with trastuzumab (Herceptin), a monoclonal antibody, is an option for some women.

Antibodies, discussed in Chapter 17, are proteins produced by the immune system that recognize and bind to foreign substances such as bacteria; monoclonal antibodies are a special type of antibody that is produced in the laboratory and designed to bind to a specific cancer-related target. About 30% of metastatic breast cancer tumors produce excess amounts of a growth-promoting protein called HER2. Herceptin binds to the excess HER2, thus blocking its action and slowing tumor growth. Herceptin is typically used alone or in combination with paclitaxel (Taxol), a drug that interferes with cell division.

Prostate Cancer

The prostate gland is situated at the base of the bladder in men. It produces seminal fluid; if enlarged, it can block the flow of urine. Prostate cancer is the most common cancer in men and, after lung cancer, the cause of the most deaths. More than 230,000 new cases are diagnosed each year, and about 30,000 American men die from the disease each year.

Risk Factors   Age is the strongest predictor of the risk, with about 75% of cases of prostate cancer diagnosed in men over age 65. Inherited genetic predisposition may be responsible for 5–10% of cases, and men with a family history of the disease should be particularly vigilant about screening. African American men have the highest rate of prostate cancer of any group in the world; both genetic and lifestyle factors may be involved. Diets high in calories, dairy products, and animal fats and low in plant foods have also been implicated as possible culprits, as have obesity, inactivity, and a history of sexually transmitted diseases. Compounds in soy foods, tomatoes, and cruciferous vegetables such as broccoli and cabbage are being investigated for their possible protective effects.

Detection   Early prostate cancer usually has no symptoms. Warning signs of prostate cancer can include changes in urinary frequency, weak or interrupted urine flow, painful urination, and blood in the urine. Screening tests for early detection are recommended annually for men age 50 and over—earlier for African Americans and those with a strong family history of the disease. Techniques for early detection include a digital rectal examination and the **prostate-specific antigen (PSA) blood test.** The American Cancer Society recommends that men be provided information about the benefits and limitations of the tests and that both the exam and the PSA test be offered annually, beginning at age 50 for men at average risk and age 45 for men at high risk, including African Americans and those with a family history of the disease.

During a digital rectal exam, a physician feels the prostate gland through the rectum to determine if the gland is enlarged or if lumps are present. The PSA blood test may detect an elevated level or a rapid increase in PSA: The PSA test can help catch early prostate cancer, but it also can register benign conditions (more than half of men over 50 have benign prostate disease) and very slow-growing cancers that are unlikely to kill affected individuals. Further, it is not rare for men with normal PSA levels to have prostate cancer.

Researchers are looking for ways to make the PSA test more sensitive. One strategy is to repeat the test over time to chart a rate of change. A newer approach involves measuring the percentage of PSA that is free-floating in the blood. PSA made by cancer cells is more likely to circulate bound to other proteins, whereas PSA from healthy prostate cells is more likely to be unbound. Thus, a low proportion of unbound, or free PSA indicates greater risk, while a high proportion of free PSA is associated with lower risk.

Ultrasound is used increasingly as a follow-up, to detect lumps too small to be felt and to determine their size, shape, and properties. A needle biopsy of suspicious lumps can be performed relatively painlessly, and whether the biopsied cells are malignant or benign can be determined by examining them under a microscope.

Treatment   Treatments vary based on the stage of the cancer and the age of the patient. A small, slow-growing tumor in an older man may be treated with watchful waiting because he is more likely to die from another cause before his cancer becomes life threatening. More aggressive treatment would be indicated for younger men or those with more advanced cancers. Treatment usually involves radical prostatectomy, in which the prostate is removed surgically. Although radical surgery has an excellent cure rate, it is major surgery and often results in **incontinence** and/or **impotence.**

A less-invasive alternative involves surgical implantation of radioactive seeds. Radiation from the seeds destroys the tumor and much of the normal prostate tissue but leaves surrounding tissue relatively untouched. Although there is less risk of incontinence or impotence, this procedure is relatively new, and its effectiveness for different stages of cancer is still being evaluated.

Alternative or additional treatments include external radiation, hormones that shrink tumors, cryotherapy, and anti-cancer drugs. Survival rates for all stages of this cancer have improved steadily since 1940; the 5-year survival rate is currently about 99%.

Cancers of the Female Reproductive Tract

Because the uterus, cervix, and ovaries are subject to similar hormonal influences, the cancers of these organs can be discussed as a group.

Cervical Cancer   Cervical cancer is at least in part a sexually transmitted disease. Probably more than 80% of cervical cancer stems from infection by the human papillomavirus (HPV), a large group of related viruses that cause both common warts and genital warts. When certain types of HPV are introduced into the cervix, usually by an infected sex partner, the virus infects cervical cells,

---

V·w
Terms

prostate-specific antigen (PSA) blood test   A diagnostic test for prostate cancer that measures blood levels of prostate-specific antigen (PSA).

incontinence   The inability to control the flow of urine.

impotence   The inability to have an erection or ejaculate; an inability to perform sexual intercourse.

Pap test   A scraping of cells from the cervix for examination under a microscope to detect cancer.

endometrium   The layers of tissue lining the uterus.

causing the cells to divide and grow. If unchecked, this growth can develop into cervical cancer. Cervical cancer is associated with multiple sex partners and is extremely rare in women who have not had heterosexual intercourse. The regular use of condoms can reduce the risk of transmitting HPV. Studies also suggest that women whose sexual partners are circumcised may be at reduced risk because circumcised men are less likely to be infected with HPV and to pass it to their partners.

Because only a very small percentage of HPV-infected women ever get cervical cancer, other factors must be involved. Two of the most important seem to be smoking and infection with genital herpes (discussed in Chapter 18 with other STDs). Both smoking and herpes infection can cause cancerous changes in cells in the laboratory and can speed and intensify the cancerous changes begun by HPV. Exposure to environmental tobacco smoke also appears to increase risk. Research suggests that women with high levels of HPV 16, a specific form of HPV, are at particularly high risk for the infection to develop into cancer. Some studies show that past exposure to the bacterium that causes the STD chlamydia may be a risk factor for cervical cancer that operates independently of HPV.

Screening for the changes in cervical cells that precede cancer is done chiefly by means of the **Pap test.** During a pelvic exam, loose cells are scraped from the cervix, spread on a slide, stained for easier viewing, and examined under a microscope to see whether they are normal in size and shape. If cells are abnormal, a condition commonly referred to as *cervical dysplasia,* the Pap test is repeated at intervals. Sometimes cervical cells spontaneously return to normal, but in about one-third of cases, the cellular changes progress toward malignancy. If this happens, the abnormal cells must be removed, either surgically or by destroying them with a cryoscopic (ultracold) probe or localized laser treatment. When the abnormal cells are in a precancerous state, the small patch of dangerous cells can be completely removed.

Without timely surgery, the malignant patch of cells goes on to invade the wall of the cervix and spreads to adjacent lymph nodes and to the uterus. At this stage, chemotherapy may be used with radiation to kill the fast-growing cancer cells, but chances for a complete cure are lower. Even when a cure can be achieved, it often means surgical removal of the uterus.

Because the Pap test is highly effective, all sexually active women and women between ages 18 and 65 should be tested. The recommended schedule for testing depends on risk factors, the type of Pap test performed, and whether the Pap test is combined with HPV testing. Unlike most cancers, which occur most often after the age of 60, cancer of the cervix occurs frequently in women in their thirties or even twenties. Although screening can clearly save lives, *Healthy People 2010* reports lower-than-average rates of Pap testing for certain groups, including women of low socioeconomic status and women with less than a high school education. Mortality rates for cervical cancer are twice as high for black women as for white women. Worldwide, cervical cancer kills about 230,000 women each year.

Encouraging results have been seen in studies of a vaccine designed to protect women from infection with HPV. A vaccine may be available in the United States by 2006; if effective, it could dramatically reduce rates of cervical cancer by preventing HPV infection.

Uterine, or Endometrial, Cancer Cancer of the lining of the uterus, or **endometrium,** most often occurs after the age of 55. The risk factors are similar to those for breast cancer: prolonged exposure to estrogen, early onset of menstruation, late menopause, never having been pregnant, and obesity; type 2 diabetes is also associated with increased risk. The use of oral contraceptives, which combine estrogen and progestin, appears to provide protection.

Endometrial cancer is usually detectable by pelvic examination. It is treated surgically, commonly by hysterectomy, or removal of the uterus; radiation treatment, hormones, and chemotherapy may be used in addition to surgery. When the tumor is detected at an early stage, about 96% of patients are alive and disease-free 5 years later. When the disease has spread beyond the uterus, the 5-year survival rate is less than 67%.

Ovarian Cancer Although ovarian cancer is rare compared with cervical or uterine cancer, it causes more deaths than the other two combined. It cannot be detected by Pap tests or any other simple screening method and is often diagnosed only late in its development, when surgery and other therapies are unlikely to be successful. The risk factors are similar to those for breast and endometrial cancer: increasing age (most ovarian cancer occurs after age 60), never having been pregnant, a family history of breast or ovarian cancer, obesity, and specific genetic mutations. A high number of ovulations appears to increase the chance that a cancer-causing genetic mutation will occur, so anything that lowers the number of lifetime ovulation cycles—pregnancy, breastfeeding, or use of oral contraceptives—reduces a woman's risk of ovarian cancer. A diet rich in fruits and vegetables may be associated with reduced risk.

There are often no warning signs of developing ovarian cancer. Early clues may include increased abdominal size and bloating, urinary urgency, and pelvic pain. Women with symptoms or who are at high risk because of family history or because they harbor a mutant gene should have thorough pelvic exams at regular intervals, as recommended by their physician. Pelvic exams may include the use of ultrasound to view the ovaries. Blood tests for a tumor marker called CA-125 and for a group of protein markers are being investigated as possible screening tests.

Ovarian cancer is treated by surgical removal of both ovaries, the fallopian tubes, and the uterus. Radiation and chemotherapy are sometimes used in addition to surgery. When the tumor is localized to the ovary, the survival rate after 5 years is 94%. But for all stages, the survival rate is only 44%, reflecting the difficulty of early detection.

Other Female Reproductive Tract Cancers

From 1938 to 1971, millions of women were given a synthetic hormone called DES (diethylstilbestrol), which was thought to help prevent miscarriage. It was later discovered that DES daughters (daughters born to these women) have an increased risk, about 1 in 1000, of a vaginal or cervical cancer called clear cell cancer. This cancer is extremely rare in unexposed women. DES daughters may also have an anatomically abnormal reproductive tract and have problems with fertility or miscarriage. Though this is primarily a health threat for daughters, there is also some risk to DES sons, who may have an increased risk of abnormalities of the reproductive tract, including undescended testicles, a risk factor for testicular cancer.

If you suspect you may be a DES daughter or son, you should ask your mother if she took any medications while pregnant and, if possible, review her medical records for that time. A DES daughter should find a physician who is familiar with the problems of DES exposure; more frequent and more thorough pelvic exams are recommended. A recent animal study suggested the possibility of an increased third-generation cancer risk from DES, but further research is needed to determine if the finding applies to DES granddaughters.

Skin Cancer

Skin cancer is the most common cancer of all when cases of the highly curable forms are included in the count. (Usually these forms are not included, precisely because they are easily treated.) Of the more than 1 million cases of skin cancer diagnosed each year, 54,000 are of the most serious type, **melanoma.** Treatments are usually simple and successful when the cancers are caught early.

Risk Factors Almost all cases of skin cancer can be traced to excessive exposure to **ultraviolet (UV) radiation**

The UVA radiation emitted by most tanning-salon beds doesn't usually cause an immediate sunburn, but it does cause premature wrinkling and aging of the skin and skin cancer.

from the sun, including longer-wavelength ultraviolet A (UVA) and shorter-wavelength ultraviolet B (UVB) radiation. UVB radiation causes sunburns and can damage the eyes and the immune system. UVA is less likely to cause an immediate sunburn, but by damaging connective tissue it leads to premature aging of the skin, giving it a wrinkled, leathery appearance. (Tanning lamps and tanning-salon beds emit mostly UVA radiation.) Both UVA and UVB radiation have been linked to the development of skin cancer, and the National Toxicology Program has declared both solar and artificial sources of UV radiation to be known human carcinogens.

Both severe, acute sun reactions (sunburns) and chronic low-level sun reactions (suntans) can lead to skin cancer. People with fair skin have less natural protection against skin damage from the sun and a higher risk of developing skin cancer; people with naturally dark skin have a considerable degree of protection (see the box "What's Your UV Risk?"). Caucasians are about 20 times more likely than African Americans to develop melanoma, but African Americans and Latinos are still at risk. Severe sunburns in childhood have been linked to a greatly increased risk of skin cancer in later life, so children in particular should be protected. Because of damage to the ozone layer of the atmosphere (discussed in Chapter 24), there is a chance that we may all be exposed to increasing amounts of UV radiation in the future. Take time now to understand the risks of excessive sun exposure, because the precautions suggested here will become increasingly critical if the ozone shield continues to thin.

Other risk factors for skin cancer include having many moles, particularly large ones; spending time at high altitudes; and a family history of the disease. Skin cancer may also be caused by exposure to coal tar, pitch, creosote, arsenic, and radioactive materials; but compared to sunlight, these agents account for only a small proportion of cases.

Types of Skin Cancer   There are three main types of skin cancer, named for the types of skin cells from which they develop. **Basal cell** and **squamous cell carcinomas** together account for about 95% of the skin cancers diagnosed each year. They are usually found in chronically sun-exposed areas, such as the face, neck, hands, and arms. They usually appear as pale, waxlike, pearly nodules or red, scaly, sharply outlined patches. These cancers are often painless, although they may bleed, crust, and form an open sore on the skin.

Melanoma is by far the most dangerous skin cancer because it spreads so rapidly. Since 1973, the incidence of melanoma has increased by about 4% per year. It is the most common cancer among women age 25–29. It can occur anywhere on the body, but the most common sites are the back, chest, abdomen, and lower legs. A melanoma usually appears at the site of a preexisting mole. The mole may begin to enlarge, become mottled or varied in color (colors can include blue, pink, and white), or develop an irregular surface or irregular borders. Tissue invaded by melanoma may also itch, burn, or bleed easily.

Prevention   One of the major steps you can take to protect yourself against all forms of skin cancer is to avoid lifelong overexposure to sunlight. Blistering, peeling sunburns from unprotected sun exposure are particularly

dangerous, but suntans—whether from sunlight or tanning lamps—also increase your risk of developing skin cancer later in life. People of every age, especially babies and children, need to be protected from the sun with **sunscreens** and protective clothing. For a closer look at sunlight and skin cancer, see the box "Choosing and Using Sunscreens and Sun-Protective Clothing" on page 492.

Detection and Treatment   The only sure way to avoid a serious outcome from skin cancer is to make sure it is recognized and diagnosed early. More than half of all melanomas are brought to a physician's attention by patients themselves. Make it a habit to examine your skin regularly. Most of the spots, freckles, moles, and blemishes on your body are normal; you were born with some of them, and others appear and disappear throughout your life. But if you notice an unusual growth, discoloration, sore that does not heal, or mole that undergoes a sudden or progressive change, see your physician or a dermatologist immediately.

The characteristics that may signal that a skin lesion is a melanoma—asymmetry, border irregularity, color change, and a diameter greater than ¼ inch—are illustrated in Figure 16-4. A mole that changes in size, shape, or color is also of concern. In addition, if someone in your family has had numerous skin cancers or melanomas, you may want to consult a dermatologist for a complete skin examination and discussion of your particular risk.

If you do have an unusual skin lesion, your physician will examine it and possibly perform a biopsy. If the lesion is cancerous, it is usually removed surgically, a

Critical Consumer

With consistent use of the proper clothing, sunscreens, and common sense, you can lead an active outdoor life *and* protect your skin against most sun-induced damage. Clothing should be your first and best line of defense. Sun-protective clothing can effectively block nearly all UVA and UVB rays. Sunscreens do provide protection, but many allow considerable UVA radiation to pass through to your skin. And even the best sunscreens are effective only when applied properly and reapplied frequently—something most people fail to do.

Clothing

• Wear long-sleeved shirts and long pants. Dark-colored, tightly woven fabrics provide reasonable protection from the sun. Another good choice is clothing made from special sun-protective fabrics; these garments have an Ultraviolet Protection Factor (UPF) rating, similar to the SPF for sunscreens. For example, a fabric with a UPF rating of 20 allows only one-twentieth of the sun's UV radiation to pass through. There are three categories of UPF protection: A UPF of 15–24 provides "good" UV protection, a UPF of 25–39 provides "very good" protection, and a UPF of 40–50 provides "excellent" protection. By comparison, typical shirts provide a UPF of only 5–9, a value that drops when clothing is wet.

• Consider washing some extra sun protection into your current wardrobe. A new laundry additive adds UV protection to ordinary fabrics and is recommended by the Skin Cancer Foundation.

• Put on a hat. Your face, ears, neck, and scalp are especially vulnerable to the sun's harmful effects, making hats an essential weapon in the battle against sun damage. Baseball caps are popular, but they don't protect the ears, the back of the neck and the lower face. A better choice is a broad-brimmed hat or a legionnaire-style cap that covers the ears and neck. You still need to wear sunscreen on your face even if you are wearing a hat, because sand, water, rocks, concrete, and snow all reflect the sun's rays onto your face.

Sunscreen

• Use a sunscreen and lip balm with a sun protection factor (SPF) of 15 or higher. (An SPF rating refers to the amount of time you can stay out in the sun before you burn, compared with not using sunscreen; for example, a product with an SPF of 15 would allow you to remain in the sun without burning 15 times longer, on average, than if you didn't apply sunscreen.) If you're fair-skinned, have a family history of skin cancer, are at high altitude, or will be outdoors for many hours, use a sunscreen with a high SPF (30+).

• Choose a broad-spectrum sunscreen that protects against both UVA and UVB radiation. The SPF rating of a sunscreen currently applies only to UVB, but a number of ingredients, especially titanium dioxide and zinc oxide, are effective at blocking most UVA radiation. Use a water-resistant sunscreen if you swim or sweat quite a bit. If you have sensitive skin, you may need to try several brands before finding one that doesn't irritate your skin. If you have acne, look for a sunscreen that is labeled "noncomedogenic," which means that it will not cause pimples.

• Shake sunscreen before applying. Apply it 30 minutes before exposure to allow it time to penetrate the skin. Reapply sunscreen frequently and generously to all sun-exposed areas (many people overlook their temples, ears, and sides and backs of their necks). Most people use less than half as much as they would need to attain the full SPF rating. One ounce of sunscreen—one-fourth of a 4-ounce container—is about enough to provide one application for an average-size adult in a swimsuit. Reapply sunscreen 15–30 minutes after sun exposure begins and then every few hours after that and/or following activities such as swimming or toweling that could remove sunscreen.

• If you're taking medications, ask your physician or pharmacist about possible reactions to sunlight or interactions with sunscreens. Medications for acne, allergies, and diabetes are just a few of the products that can trigger reactions. If you're using sunscreen and an insect repellent containing DEET, use extra sunscreen (DEET may decrease sunscreen effectiveness).

• Don't let sunscreens give you a false sense of security. Most of the sunscreens currently on the market allow considerable UVA radiation to penetrate the skin, with the potential for causing skin cancers (especially melanoma) as well as wrinkles and other forms of skin damage. Experts worry that our use of sunscreens may sometimes backfire by allowing us to spend many more hours in the sun than we would if we had to worry about getting a sunburn.

Time of Day and Location

• Avoid sun exposure between 10 A.M. and 4 P.M., when the sun's rays are most intense. Clouds allow as much as 80% of UV rays to reach your skin. Stay in the shade when you can.

• Consult the day's UV Index, which predicts UV levels on a 0–10+ scale, to get a sense of the amount of sun protection you'll need; take special care on days with a rating of 5 or above. UV Index ratings are available in local newspapers, from the weather bureau, or from certain Web sites. Also take special care in locations near the equator or at high altitudes, where the sun is more intense; use a stronger sunscreen and apply it more frequently.

• UV rays can penetrate at least 3 feet in water, so swimmers should wear water-resistant sunscreens. Snow reflects the sun's rays, so don't forget to apply sunscreen before skiing and other snow activities. Sand and water also reflect the sun's rays, so you still need to apply a sunscreen if you are under a beach umbrella. Concrete and white-painted surfaces are also highly reflective.

Tanning Salons

• Stay away from tanning salons! Despite advertising claims to the contrary, the lights used in tanning parlors are damaging to your skin. Tanning beds and lamps emit mostly UVA radiation, increasing your risk of premature skin aging (such as wrinkles) and skin cancer. If you *must* have a tan, consider using sunless self-tanning lotions. These can provide that bronzed look without the risks of UV radiation.

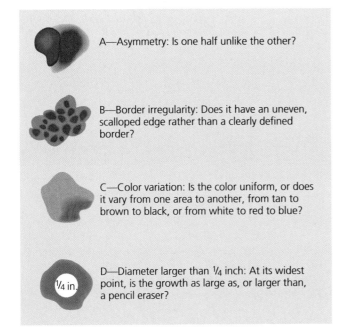

A—Asymmetry: Is one half unlike the other?

B—Border irregularity: Does it have an uneven, scalloped edge rather than a clearly defined border?

C—Color variation: Is the color uniform, or does it vary from one area to another, from tan to brown to black, or from white to red to blue?

D—Diameter larger than ¼ inch: At its widest point, is the growth as large as, or larger than, a pencil eraser?

Figure 16-4   The ABCD test for melanoma.   To see a variety of photos of melanoma and benign moles, visit the National Cancer Institute's Visuals Online site (http://visualsonline.cancer.gov).

procedure that can almost always be performed in the physician's office using a local anesthetic. Occasionally, other forms of treatment may be used. Even for melanoma, the outlook after removal in the early stages is good, with a 5-year survival rate of 98% if the tumor is localized but only 60% if the cancer has spread to adjacent lymph nodes. Since prevention requires a minimum of time and attention, it pays to be alert.

Oral Cancer

Oral cancer—cancers of the lip, tongue, mouth, and throat—can be traced principally to cigarette, cigar, or pipe smoking, the use of spit tobacco, and the excessive consumption of alcohol. These risk factors work together to multiply a person's risk of oral cancer. The incidence of oral cancer is twice as great in men as in women and most frequent in men over 40. Some prominent sufferers of oral cancer have included Sigmund Freud and Fidel Castro, both notorious cigar smokers. Sports figures who have cultivated a taste for spit tobacco are now also increasingly being diagnosed with oral cancer. Among long-term snuff users, the excess risk of cancers of the cheek, tongue, and gum is nearly 50-fold (see Chapter 11 for more on cigars and spit tobacco).

Oral cancers do have the virtue of being fairly easy to detect, but they are often hard to cure. Furthermore, among those who survive, a significant number will develop another primary cancer of the head and neck. The primary methods of treatment are surgery and radiation. The overall survival rate is about 59%.

Testicular Cancer

Testicular cancer is relatively rare, accounting for only 1% of cancer in men (about 7600 cases per year), but it is the most common cancer in men age 20–35. It is much more common among white Americans than Latinos, Asian Americans, or African Americans and among men whose fathers had testicular cancer. Men with undescended testicles are at increased risk for testicular cancer, and for this reason the condition should be corrected in early childhood. Men whose mothers took DES during pregnancy have an increased risk of undescended testicles and other genital anomalies. Thus, they may have a higher risk of testicular cancer.

Self-examination may help in the early detection of testicular cancer (see the box "Testicle Self-Examination" on p. 494). Tumors are treated by surgical removal of the testicle and, if the tumor has spread, by chemotherapy. The 5-year survival rate for testicular cancer is 95%.

Other Cancers

Several other cancers affect a significant number of people each year. Some have identifiable risk factors, particularly smoking and obesity, that are controllable; causes of others are still under investigation.

Pancreatic Cancer   The pancreas, a gland found deep within the abdomen behind the stomach, produces both digestive enzymes and insulin. Because of the gland's hidden location, pancreatic cancer is usually well advanced before symptoms become noticeable. No effective cure is available, and it is the fifth leading cause of cancer death in the United States: Each year there are about 32,000 new cases and about 32,000 deaths. About 3 out of 10 cases are linked to smoking. Other risk factors include being male, African American, obese, sedentary, or over age 60; having a family history of pancreatic cancer; having diabetes; and eating a diet high in fat and meat and low in vegetables.

Stomach Cancer   In many parts of the world, stomach cancer is the most common form of cancer. It is relatively unusual in the United States, with about 22,400 new cases and 12,100 deaths each year. It tends to occur after the age of 50 and is almost twice as common in men as in women. Risk factors include infection with the bacterium *Helicobacter pylori,* which has also been linked to the development of ulcers, and a diet high in smoked, salted, or pickled fish or meat. Bacteria, including *H. pylori,* can convert the nitrites in preserved foods into carcinogenic amines, and salt can break down the normal protective stomach coating, allowing these carcinogenic compounds access to the cells of the stomach wall. However, the great majority of people with *H. pylori* infection do not develop stomach cancer, particularly if they

Testicle Self-Examination

The best time to perform a testicular self-exam is after a warm shower or bath, when the scrotum is relaxed. First, stand in front of a mirror and look for any swelling of the scrotum. Then examine each testicle with both hands. Place the index and middle fingers under the testicle and the thumbs on top; roll the testicle gently between the fingers and thumbs. Don't worry if one testicle seems slightly larger than the other—that's common. Also, expect to feel the epididymis, the soft, sperm-carrying tube at the rear of the testicle.

Perform the self-exam each month. If you find a lump, swelling, or nodule, consult a physician right away. The abnormality may not be cancer, but only a physician can make a diagnosis. Other possible signs of testicular cancer include a change in the way a testicle feels, a sudden collection of fluid in the scrotum, a dull ache in the lower abdomen or groin, a feeling of heaviness in the scrotum, or pain in a testicle or the scrotum.

SOURCES: Testicular Cancer Resource Center. 2001. *How to Do a Testicular Self Examination* (http://www.acor.org/TCRC/tcexam.html; retrieved February 14, 2001); National Cancer Institute. 2000. *Questions and Answers About Testicular Cancer* (http://cis.nci.nih.gov/fact/6_34.htm; retrieved February 14, 2001).

maintain a low-salt diet with adequate amounts of fruits, vegetables, and whole grains. There is no screening test for stomach cancer; it is usually recognized only after it has spread, and the 5-year survival rate is only 23% for all stages.

Bladder Cancer   This cancer is almost three times as common in men as in women, and smoking is the key risk factor. People living in urban areas and workers exposed to chemicals used in the dye, rubber, and leather industries are also at increased risk. There is no screening test for it; the first symptoms are likely to be blood in the urine and/or increased frequency of urination. These symptoms can also signal a urinary infection but should trigger a visit to a physician, who can evaluate the possibility of cancer. With early detection, more than 90% of cases are curable. There are about 63,200 new cases and about 13,200 deaths each year.

Kidney Cancer   Although this cancer usually occurs in people over 50, anyone can develop it, and there are few controllable risk factors. Smoking and obesity are mild risk factors, as is a family history of the disease. Symptoms may include fatigue, pain in the side, and blood in the urine. Kidney cancer has been difficult to treat, with a 5-year survival rate of only 64% for all stages. Recently, immune cell therapies have shown some promise in the disease's advanced stage. There are about 36,200 new cases each year and about 12,700 deaths.

Brain Cancer   Tumors can arise from most of the many types of cells that are found in the brain. The vast majority of brain cancers develop for no apparent reason;

one of the few established risk factors is ionizing radiation, such as X rays. Before the risks were recognized, children with ringworm of the scalp (a fungal infection) often received low-dose radiation therapy, which substantially increased their risk of brain tumors later in life. Symptoms are often nonspecific and include headaches, fatigue, behavioral changes, and sometimes seizures. There has been a slight increase in the incidence of tumors over the past 20 years, but this may be due to improved methods of diagnosis. Some brain tumors are curable by surgery or by radiation and chemotherapy, but most are not. Survival time varies, depending on the type of the tumor, from 1 to 8 years. In the United States each year there are about 18,500 new cases and 13,000 deaths.

Leukemia   Leukemia, cancer of the white blood cells, can affect both children and adults. It starts in the bone marrow but can then spread to the lymph nodes, spleen, liver, other organs, and central nervous system. Like brain cancer, it is a complex disease with many different types and subtypes. Most people with leukemia have no known risk factors. About 20% of cases of adult leukemia are related to smoking; other possible risk factors include radiation and certain chemicals and infections. Most symptoms occur because leukemia cells crowd out the production of normal blood cells; the result can be fatigue, anemia, weight loss, and increased risk of infection. Treatment and survival rates vary, depending on the exact type and other factors. There are about 34,800 new cases and 22,600 deaths each year.

Lymphoma   Arising from the lymph cells, lymphoma begins in the lymph nodes and then may spread to almost

Take Charge

any part of the body. There are two types—Hodgkin's disease and non-Hodgkin's lymphoma (NHL). NHL is the more common and more deadly form of the disease. It is the sixth most common cancer in the United States, with about 56,000 people diagnosed annually; about half of all patients will eventually die from the disease. Risk factors for NHL are not well understood, but people with compromised immune systems are at much greater risk, especially when exposed to radiation or certain infections and chemicals. A new therapy based on the use of antibodies has shown promise in treating patients. Rates of Hodgkin's disease have fallen by more than 50% since the early 1970s, and there are now about 7300 cases and 1400 deaths each year.

Multiple Myeloma   Normal plasma cells play an important role in the immune system, producing antibodies. Malignant plasma cells may produce tumors in several sites, particularly in the bone marrow; when they grow in multiple sites, they are referred to as multiple myeloma (MM). By crowding out normal bone marrow cells, MM can lead to anemia, excessive bleeding, and decreased resistance to infection. Age is the most significant risk factor: Only 2% of cases are diagnosed in people under 40, and the average age at diagnosis is about 70. Other risk factors are not well understood, although MM is about twice as common among African Americans as among whites. Although treated with chemotherapy and slow in its progression, the disease is usually fatal. Researchers are working to develop new therapies. There are about 16,000 new cases each year and 11,000 deaths.

THE CAUSES OF CANCER

Although scientists do not know everything about what causes cancer, they have identified genetic, environmental, and lifestyle factors. (For information on possible factors involved in cancer incidence, see the box "Ethnicity, Poverty, and Cancer" on p. 496). There are usually several steps in the transformation of a normal cell into a cancer cell, and in many cases several factors may work together in the development of cancer.

The Role of DNA

Heredity and genetics are becoming increasingly important factors in assessing a person's risk of cancer. The inheritance of certain genes may predispose some people to develop cancers at a younger age, and various DNA techniques are used to identify specific genetic mutations associated with such cancers.

DNA Basics   The nucleus of each cell in your body contains 23 pairs of **chromosomes**, which are made up of tightly packed coils of **DNA** (deoxyribonucleic acid).

DNA consists of two long strands wound around each other in a spiral structure, like a twisted ladder; scientists refer to this spiral as a double helix. The rungs of the ladder are made from four different nucleotide bases: adenine, thymine, cytosine, and guanine, or A, T, C, and G. The arrangement of nucleotide bases along the double helix constitutes the genetic code. You can think of this code as a set of instructions for building, operating, and repairing your body.

A **gene** is a smaller unit of DNA made up of a specific sequence of nucleotide bases. Each chromosome contains hundreds, and in some cases thousands, of genes; you have about 25,000 genes in all. Each of your genes controls the production of a particular protein. The makeup of each protein—which amino acids it contains and in what sequence—is determined by its precise sequence of A, T, C, and G. Proteins build cells and make them work: They serve both as the structural material for your body and as the regulators of all chemical reactions and metabolic processes. By making different proteins at different times, genes can act as switches to alter the ways a cell works.

Except for sperm and egg cells, every cell in your body contains two copies of each gene, one on each of a pair of chromosomes. You inherit one copy of each gene from your mother and one from your father. Every cell contains a copy of the complete DNA sequence with all the genes. What makes the cells in your body different from one another in both structure and function—one a nerve cell and one a muscle cell, for example—is not which genes they contain, but which genes are expressed. Some genes are active and produce proteins all the time; others are expressed rarely.

Cells reproduce by dividing in two, and your body makes billions of new cells every day. When a cell divides, the DNA replicates itself so that each new cell has a complete set of chromosomes. Through the proteins for which they code, some genes are responsible for controlling the rate of cell division, and some types of cells divide much more rapidly than others. Genes that control the rate of cell division often play a critical role in the development of cancer.

DNA Mutations and Cancer   A mutation is any change in the normal sequence of nucleotide bases in a

Terms

chromosomes The threadlike bodies in a cell nucleus that contain molecules of DNA; most human cells contain 23 pairs of chromosomes.

DNA Deoxyribonucleic acid, a chemical substance that carries genetic information.

gene A section of a chromosome that contains the nucleotide base sequence for making a particular protein; the basic unit of heredity.

Rates of cancer have declined among all U.S. ethnic groups in recent years, but significant disparities still exist.

- Among U.S. ethnic groups, African Americans have the highest incidence of and death rates from cancer.

- White women have a higher incidence of breast cancer, but African American women have the highest death rate. Black women are less likely to receive regular mammograms and more likely to experience delays in follow-up.

- African American men have a higher rate of prostate cancer than any other U.S. group and more than twice the death rate of other groups. However, black men are less likely than white men to undergo PSA testing for prostate cancer.

- Latinas have the highest incidence of cervical cancer, but African American women have the highest death rate. Language barriers and problems accessing screening services are thought to particularly affect Latinas, who have relatively low rates of Pap testing.

- Asian Americans and Pacific Islander Americans have the highest rates of liver and stomach cancers. Recent immigration helps explain these higher rates, as these cancers are usually caused by infections that are more prevalent in the recent immigrant's country of origin.

- Significant disparities also exist within broad ethnic categories; for example, Vietnamese American women have a rate of cervical cancer four times higher than the overall rate among Asian American and Pacific Islander women.

Some of the disparities in cancer risks and rates may be influenced by genetic or cultural factors. For example, certain genetic/molecular features of aggressive breast cancer are more common among African American women with the disease; they are more likely to be diagnosed at a later stage and with more aggressive tumors. Genetic factors may also help explain the high rate of prostate cancer among black men. Women from cultures where early marriage and motherhood is common are likely to have a lower risk of breast cancer. People who don't smoke or who are vegetarians for religious or cultural reasons may have lower rates of many cancers.

Most of the differences in cancer rates and deaths, however, are thought to be the result of socioeconomic inequities, which influence the prevalence of many underlying cancer risk factors as well as access to early detection and quality treatment. People of low socioeconomic status are more likely to smoke, abuse alcohol, eat unhealthy foods, and be sedentary and overweight—all of which are associated with cancer. High levels of stress associated with poverty may impair the immune system, the body's first line of defense against cancer.

People with low incomes are more likely to live in unhealthy environments. For example, Latinos and Asian and Pacific Islander Americans are more likely than other groups to live in areas that do not meet federal air quality standards. Low-income people may also have jobs in which they come into daily contact with carcinogenic chemicals. They may face similar risks in their homes and schools, where they may be exposed to asbestos or other carcinogens.

People with low incomes also have less exposure to information about cancer, are less aware of the early warning signs of cancer, and are less likely to seek medical care when they have such symptoms. Lack of health insurance is a key factor explaining higher death rates among people with low incomes. A study comparing low-income Americans and Canadians found that the Canadians were more likely to survive cancer, possibly due to Canada's system of universal health care, which ensures access to treatment regardless of income. Discrimination and language and cultural barriers can also affect patients' use of the health care system.

Public education campaigns that encourage healthy lifestyle habits, routine cancer screening, and participation in clinical trials may be one helpful strategy to reduce cancer disparities. But the effects of poverty are more difficult to overcome. Some medical scientists look to policymakers for solutions and maintain that living and working conditions in the inner cities must be improved and that access to quality health care must be assured for all Americans. Then, even without new miracle drugs or medical breakthroughs, the United States could see a real decrease in cancer rates in low-income populations.

SOURCES: American Cancer Society. 2005. *Cancer Facts and Figures 2005*. Atlanta: American Cancer Society; Chlebowski, R. T., et al. 2005. Ethnicity and breast cancer: Factors influencing differences in incidence and outcome. *Journal of the National Cancer Institute* 97(6): 439–448; CDC National Center for Chronic Disease Prevention and Health Promotion. 2005. *Health Disparities: Minority Cancer Awareness* (http://www.cdc.gov/cancer/minorityawareness/index.htm; retrieved January 26, 2005); CDC Office of Minority Health. 2004. *Eliminate Disparities in Cancer Screening and Management* (http://www.cdc.gov/omh/AMH/factsheets/cancer.htm; retrieved January 26, 2005); National Cancer Institute. 2003. *Cancer Health Disparities: Fact Sheet* (http://www.cancer.gov/newscenter/healthdisparities; retrieved January 26, 2005).

gene. Like a typographical error, it may involve a deletion or a substitution of a certain base—for example, CAA may become CA or CTA. Some mutations are inherited: If the egg or sperm cell that produces a child contains a mutation, so will every one of the child's 30 trillion cells. Environmental agents can also produce mutational damage; these **mutagens** include radiation, certain viruses, and chemical substances in the air we breathe. (When a mutagen also causes cancer, it is called a carcinogen.) Some mutations are the result of copying errors that occur when DNA replicates itself as part of cell division.

A mutated gene no longer contains the proper code for producing its protein. Because a cell has two copies of each gene, it can sometimes get by with only one functioning version. In this case, the mutation may have no effect on health. However, if both copies of a gene are damaged or if the cell needs two normal copies to function properly, then the cell will cease to behave normally.

It requires several mutational changes over a period of years before a normal cell takes on the properties of a cancer cell. Genes in which mutations are associated with the conversion of a normal cell into a cancer cell are known as **oncogenes.** In their undamaged form, many oncogenes play a role in controlling or restricting cell growth; these are **tumor suppressor genes.** Mutational damage to these genes releases the brake on growth and leads to rapid and uncontrolled cell division—a precondition for the development of cancer.

A good example of how a series of mutational changes can produce cancer is provided by the p53 gene, located on chromosome 17. In its normal form, the protein that is coded for by this gene actually helps prevent cancer: If a cell's DNA is damaged, the p53 protein can either kill the cell outright or stop it from replicating until the damaged DNA is repaired. For example, if a skin cell's DNA is mutated by exposure to sunlight, the p53 protein activates the cell's "suicide" machinery. (The scientific term for this programmed cell death is **apoptosis.**) By thus preventing the replication of damaged DNA, the p53 protein keeps cells from progressing toward cancer. However, if the p53 gene itself undergoes a mutation, these controls are lost, and the cell can become cancerous. In fact, the damaged version of p53 can actually promote cell division and the spread of cancer.

A damaged p53 gene can be inherited, but carcinogenic damage or DNA copying errors are more common causes of p53 mutations. The carcinogen benzo(a)pyrene, found in tobacco smoke, causes a particular mutation in p53 that is linked to many cases of lung cancer. Other agents contribute to cancer by interfering with the p53 protein after it is produced. For example, human papillomavirus, the infectious agent linked to cervical cancer, neutralizes the p53 protein. Researchers believe that damage to the p53 gene and protein may be involved, directly and indirectly, in as many as 50–60% of all cancers.

Hereditary Cancer Risks

As we've described, one way to obtain a mutated oncogene is to inherit it. For example, a form of inherited colon cancer is believed to account for one in six colon cancer cases; children who inherit the altered gene are thought to face a 70–80% chance of developing the disease. Using information from the Human Genome Project, scientists have been able to identify the genes responsible for the condition. Another example is BRCA1 (breast cancer gene 1): Women who inherit a damaged copy of this suppressor gene face a significantly increased risk of breast and ovarian cancer.

It is important to remember, however, that most cancers are not linked to heredity; mutational damage usually occurs after birth. For example, only about 5–10% of breast cancer cases can be traced to inherited copies of a damaged BRCA1 gene. Lifestyle decisions are still important even for those who have inherited a damaged suppressor gene: Eating plenty of fruits and vegetables, exercising regularly, and maintaining a healthy body weight may protect against breast cancer.

Testing and identification of hereditary cancer risks can be helpful for some people, especially if it leads to increased attention to controllable risk factors and better medical screening. For more on hereditary cancer risks and the issues involved in genetic testing, see the box "Genetic Testing for Breast Cancer."

Cancer Promoters

Substances known as cancer promoters make up another important piece of the cancer puzzle. Carcinogenic agents such as UV radiation that cause mutational changes in the DNA of oncogenes are known as cancer *initiators.* Cancer *promoters,* on the other hand, don't directly produce DNA mutations. Instead, they accelerate the growth of cells without damaging or permanently altering their DNA. However, a faster growth rate means less time for a cell to repair DNA damage caused by initiators, so errors are more likely to be passed on. Estrogen, which stimulates cellular growth in the female reproductive organs, is an example of a cancer promoter. Cigarette smoke is a complete carcinogen because it acts as both an initiator and a promoter.

Colon cancer provides a good example of how the combination of initiators and promoters contributes to the development of cancer. Colon cells may divide more rapidly if the diet is high in red meat. Under these circumstances of growth promotion, a cell with a preexisting mutation in an oncogene has an increased chance of progressing toward cancer. Increasing intake of fruits, vegetables, and calcium may reverse this effect and slow the growth of cells that line the colon, thereby decreasing the possibility of cancer developing.

Although much still needs to be learned about the role of genetics in cancer, it's clear that minimizing mutation damage to our DNA will lower our risk of many cancers. Unfortunately, a great many substances produce cancer-causing mutations, and we can't escape them all. By

Terms

mutagen Any environmental factor that can cause mutation, such as radiation and atmospheric chemicals.

oncogene A gene involved in the transformation of a normal cell into a cancer cell.

tumor suppressor gene A type of oncogene that normally functions to restrain cellular growth.

apoptosis Genetically programmed cell death, in which the cell undergoes shrinkage, condensation of the nucleus, and fragmentation. Many cancer cells lose their ability to respond to the normal apoptosis triggers, such as DNA damage.

Linda's mother, sister, and grandmother all developed breast cancer at around age 40. Now Linda is wondering if she should be tested for mutations in the breast cancer genes, BRCA1 and BRCA2. She is not alone. Recent discoveries of disease-related genes are opening up a host of issues related to genetic testing and associated legal, financial, and ethical concerns. Tests for hereditary mutations in breast cancer genes are now commercially available, but who should be tested?

Researchers identified BRCA1 in 1994 and BRCA2 in 1995. About 1 or 2 in 1000 women in the general population carry a mutant copy of BRCA1 or BRCA2, but in certain groups, most notably women of Ashkenazi (Eastern European) Jewish descent, as many as 3 in 100 may carry an altered gene. Defects in these genes cause breast cancer in as many as 50–80% of affected women; they also increase the risk of ovarian cancer and, in men, prostate cancer. Women with an altered BRCA gene tend to develop breast cancer at younger ages than other women, and the cancers that develop are more malignant. The situation is complex, however, because hundreds of different mutations of BRCA1 and

BRCA2 have been identified, and not all of them carry the same risks. Additional genes influencing risk have been identified—TSG101 in 1997, BRAF35 in 2001, BASE in 2003—and others will no doubt be found in the future.

Genetic analysis of DNA from a blood sample can identify mutant copies of BRCA1 and BRCA2. The tests can be expensive, however, ranging from $350 to more than $2000. (Searching for a mutation on a large gene is a bit like looking for a single typo in a novel.) Good news from a genetic test is reassuring, but it doesn't guarantee freedom from disease. Only 5–10% of all cases of breast cancer occur among women who inherit an altered version of BRCA1 or BRCA2. And a woman with a family history of breast cancer must still be monitored closely, even if she carries normal versions of BRCA1 and BRCA2; the cancer-causing genetic defect in her family could be located on another gene.

What about women who test positive for an altered copy of the gene? Options include close monitoring, drug treatment with a SERM such as tamoxifen, and surgical removal of currently healthy breasts

or ovaries. None of these strategies completely eliminates risk, and they may expose a woman to a dangerous or drastic treatment that is actually unnecessary. And those who test positive can face problems in addition to an uncertain medical future. Some health insurers may use the results of a genetic test to justify canceling coverage. Although currently rare, such genetic discrimination could become a major problem as more and more disease-related genes are identified. Recent legislation has attempted to protect people from losing coverage due to the results of genetic tests.

In one study, 48% of women at risk for the BRCA1 mutation decided to take the test when it was offered. Women under the age of 50 and those with children were more likely to be tested. There is no simple answer to the question of who should undergo genetic testing for disease-related genes. If you think you are at high risk for a genetic abnormality because of your family or ethnic background, consider genetic counseling. A counselor can help you consider all the issues related to testing and can guide you in making the decision that is right for you.

---

identifying the important carcinogens and understanding how they produce their effects, we can help keep our DNA intact and avoid activating sleeping oncogenes. The careful study of oncogenes should also lead to more precise methods of assessing cancer risk and to new methods of diagnosis and treatment.

Dietary Factors

Diet is one of the most important factors in cancer prevention, but it is also one of the most complex and controversial. Diets high in meat, fast food, refined carbohydrates, and simple sugars and low in fruits and vegetables are associated with a higher risk of cancer than are plant-based diets rich in whole grains, fruits, and vegetables. The picture becomes less clear, however, when researchers attempt to identify the particular constituents of foods that affect cancer risk. The foods you eat contain many biologically active compounds, and your food choices affect your cancer risk by both exposing you to potentially dangerous compounds and depriving you of potentially protective ones. For example, snacking on a doughnut instead of an apple means that you consume

more fat and simple sugars *and* less fiber and fewer vitamins. Research into particular food components can help guide you in making dietary choices, but keep in mind that the overall quality of your diet is most important.

Let's take a look at some of the dietary factors that may affect cancer risk.

Dietary Fat and Meat   In general, diets high in fat and meat have been associated with higher rates of certain cancers, including those of the colon, esophagus, stomach, and prostate. Dietary fat may promote colon cancer by stimulating the production of bile acids, which are necessary to break down and digest material in the colon. Once produced, these bile acids remove layers of cells from the intestinal epithelium, which in turn are replaced by new cells. Newly formed and rapidly growing cells are particularly susceptible to carcinogens. Diets high in animal fats and low in plant fats may also increase the risk of aggressive forms of prostate cancer, possibly by affecting hormone levels.

As is the case for heart disease, certain types of fats may be riskier than others. Some studies suggest that diets favoring omega-6 polyunsaturated fats over the omega-3 forms commonly found in fish may be associated with a higher risk of certain cancers, and that monounsaturated fats may have a protective effect. Omega-3 fatty acids appear to slow the growth of colon cancer cells and may have protective factors against breast, prostate, and pancreatic cancers (see Chapter 12 for more on different types of fatty acids). The association between meat and cancer may be linked to the particular mix of fatty acids found in meat and how those fats are digested; in addition, high consumption of the iron in meat may promote the formation of free radicals. Curing, smoking, and grilling and other cooking methods utilizing a direct flame or high temperatures may also produce carcinogenic compounds such as polycyclic aromatic hydrocarbons. (Grilling vegetables does not produce these compounds.)

Alcohol   Alcohol is associated with an increased incidence of several cancers. An average alcohol intake of three drinks per day is associated with a doubling in the risk of breast cancer. Alcohol and tobacco interact as risk factors for oral cancer, and heavy users of both alcohol and tobacco have a risk of oral cancer up to 15 times greater than that of people who don't drink or smoke. Alcohol also increases the risk of colon cancer.

Fried Foods   In 2002, scientists in Sweden reported finding high levels of the chemical acrylamide in starch-based foods that had been fried or baked at high temperatures. Other labs have confirmed this finding and found substantial amounts of acrylamide in a variety of foods, especially french fries and certain types of snack chips and crackers. At high doses, acrylamide is toxic to humans and can induce mutations and cancer in lab animals; it is classified as a probable human carcinogen.

Studies are ongoing, but in 2005, WHO urged food companies to work to lower the acrylamide content of foods to reduce any risk to public health. Acrylamide levels vary widely in foods, and there are currently no warnings against eating specific foods. The wisest course may be to consume a variety of foods and avoid overindulging in any single class of foods, particularly foods like french fries and potato chips, which may contain other unhealthy substances such as saturated and trans fats. You can also limit your exposure to acrylamide by not smoking—you would likely get much more of the chemical from smoking than from food.

Fiber   Determining the effects of fiber intake on cancer risk is complicated by the fact that fiber is found in foods that also contain many other potential anti-cancer agents—fruits, vegetables, and whole grains. Various potential cancer-fighting actions have been proposed for fiber, but none of these actions has been firmly established. Further study is needed to clarify the relationship between fiber intake and cancer risk, and experts still recommend a high-fiber diet for its overall positive effect on health.

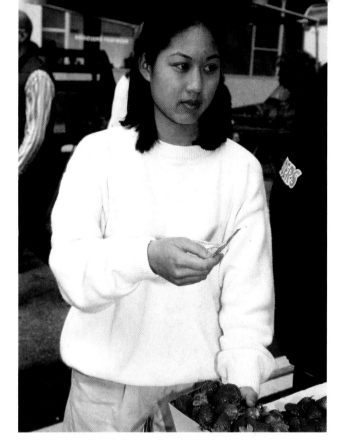

Your food choices significantly affect your risk of cancer. By consuming the recommended number of servings of fruits and vegetables per day, this young woman ensures that her diet is high in fiber and rich in cancer-fighting phytochemicals.

Fruits and Vegetables   Exactly which constituents of fruits and vegetables are responsible for reducing cancer risk is not clear, but researchers have identified many mechanisms by which food components may act against cancer: Some may prevent carcinogens from forming in the first place or block them from reaching or acting on target cells. Others boost enzymes that detoxify carcinogens and render them harmless. Still other anti-cancer agents act on cells that have already been exposed to carcinogens, slowing the development of cancer or starving cancer cells of oxygen and nutrients by cutting off their blood supply.

Some essential nutrients act as **anticarcinogens**. For example, vitamin C, vitamin E, selenium, and the **carotenoids** (vitamin A precursors) may help block the

Terms

anticarcinogen An agent that destroys or otherwise blocks the action of carcinogens.

carotenoid Any of a group of yellow-to-red plant pigments that can be converted to vitamin A by the liver; many act as antioxidants or have other anti-cancer effects. The carotenoids include beta-carotene, lutein, lycopene, and zeaxanthin.

Table 16-1	Choosing Foods with Phytochemicals

Food	Phytochemical and Its Potential Anti-Cancer Effects
Chili peppers (Note: Hotter peppers contain more capsaicin.)	Capsaicin: Neutralizes the effect of nitrosamines; may block carcinogens in cigarette smoke from acting on cells
Citrus fruits (oranges, lemons, limes), onions, apples, berries, eggplant	Flavonoids: Act as antioxidants; block access of carcinogens to cells; suppress malignant changes in cells; prevent cancer cells from multiplying
Citrus fruits, cherries	Monoterpenes: Help detoxify carcinogens; inhibit spread of cancer cells
Cruciferous vegetables (broccoli, cabbage, bok choy, cauliflower, kale, brussels sprouts, collards)	Isothiocyanates: Boost production of cancer-fighting enzymes; suppress tumor growth; block effects of estrogen on cell growth
Garlic, onions, leeks, shallots, chives	Allyl sulfides: Increase levels of enzymes that break down potential carcinogens; boost activity of cancer-fighting immune cells
Grapes, red wine, peanuts	Resveratrol: Acts as an antioxidant; suppresses tumor growth
Green, oolong, and black teas (Note: Drinking tea that is burning hot may *increase* cancer risk.)	Polyphenols: Increase antioxidant activity; prevent cancer cells from multiplying; help speed excretion of carcinogens from the body
Orange or deep yellow, red or pink, and dark green vegetables and some fruits	Carotenoids: Act as anitoxidants; reduce levels of cancer-promoting enzymes; inhibit spread of cancer cells
Soy foods, whole grains, flax seeds, nuts	Phytoestrogens: Block effects of estrogen on cell growth; lower blood levels of estrogen; inhibit angiogenesis
Whole grains, legumes	Phytic acid: Binds iron, which may prevent it from creating cell-damaging free radicals

initiation of cancer by acting as **antioxidants.** As described in Chapter 12, antioxidants prevent **free radicals** from damaging DNA. Vitamin C may also block the conversion of nitrites (food preservatives) into cancer-causing agents. Folic acid may inhibit the transformation of normal cells into malignant cells and strengthen immune function. Calcium inhibits the growth of cells in the colon and may slow the spread of potentially cancerous cells.

Many other anti-cancer agents in the diet fall under the broader heading of **phytochemicals,** substances in plants that help protect against chronic diseases. One of the first to be identified was **sulforaphane,** a potent anticarcinogen found in broccoli. Sulforaphane induces the cells of the liver and kidney to produce higher levels of protective enzymes, which then neutralize dietary carcinogens. Most fruits and vegetables contain beneficial phytochemicals, and researchers are just beginning to identify them. Some of the most promising are listed in Table 16-1.

To increase your intake of these potential cancer fighters, eat a wide variety of fruits, vegetables, legumes, and grains. Don't try to rely on supplements. Many of these compounds are not yet available in supplement form, and optimal intakes have not been determined. Like many vitamins and minerals, isolated phytochemicals may be harmful if taken in high doses. Beta-carotene pills, for example, may increase smokers' risk of lung cancer. In addition, it is likely that the anti-cancer effects of many foods are the result of many chemical substances working in combination. Some practical suggestions for maximizing your intake of anti-cancer agents are included in the Behavior Change Strategy at the end of the chapter.

Inactivity and Obesity

Several common types of cancer are associated with an inactive lifestyle, and research has shown a relationship between increased physical activity and a reduction in cancer risk. There is good evidence that exercise reduces the risk of colon cancer, perhaps by speeding the movement of food through the digestive tract, strengthening immune function, and decreasing blood fat levels. When young girls get adequate exercise, they tend to gain weight more slowly, menstruation begins later, and their risk of breast and ovarian cancers is reduced.

In addition, exercise is important because it helps prevent obesity, an independent risk factor for cancer (Figure 16-5). A high percentage of body fat appears to increase the risk of cancers of the prostate, breast, female reproductive tract, and kidney and possibly the colon and gallbladder. Obesity may affect hormone levels in the blood, slow the transit time of food through the colon, change the way the body metabolizes fat, and generally promote cell growth. All of these actions have the potential to increase cancer risk. Obesity is also associated with pre-diabetes and diabetes, and high blood sugar levels have also been linked to increased risk of cancer.

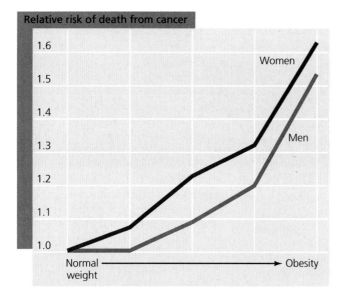

Figure 16-5 Body weight and cancer mortality. For both men and women, overweight and obesity are associated with significantly higher rates of death from cancer. From Thomas D. Fahey, Paul M. Insel, Walton T. Roth, *Fit & Well*, 6th ed., Fig. 6.3, p. 170. McGraw-Hill, 2004. Copyright © 2004 The McGraw-Hill Companies, Inc. Reprinted with permission. SOURCE: Calle, E. E., et al. 2003. Overweight, obesity, and mortality from cancer in a prospectively studied cohort of U.S. adults. *New England Journal of Medicine* 348(17): 1625–1638.

In the United States, about 170,000 cancer deaths per year appear to be due to a combination of dietary habits and a sedentary lifestyle. One expert estimates that if we were all to exercise for 20 minutes each day and make the dietary changes discussed in this chapter, about 40,000 cancer deaths could be prevented each year.

Microbes

It is estimated that about 15% of the world's cancers are caused by microbes, including viruses, bacteria, and parasites, although the percentage is much lower in developed countries like the United States. As discussed earlier, certain types of human papillomavirus cause many cases of cervical cancer, and the *Helicobacter pylori* bacterium has been definitely linked to stomach cancer.

Viruses seem to be the main cancer causers. The Epstein-Barr virus, best known for causing mononucleosis, is also suspected of contributing to Hodgkin's disease, cancer of the pharynx, and some stomach cancers. Human herpesvirus 8 has been linked to Kaposi's sarcoma and certain types of lymphoma. Hepatitis viruses B and C together cause as many as 80% of the world's liver cancers. Hepatitis B is spread mainly through sexual intercourse, though it can be passed through contact with any body fluid or with contaminated needles. A vaccine for hepatitis B is available. Hepatitis C is most commonly acquired through blood transfusions or injection drug use, but it, too, can be spread sexually. Although most people who develop hepatitis recover, up to 10% of people with

hepatitis B and 85% of people with hepatitis C become chronic carriers of the virus and are at high risk for liver cancer. The best way to avoid contracting these viruses is to limit the number of sex partners you have, practice safer sex, and avoid sharing needles. (See Chapters 17 and 18 for more information on hepatitis.)

Carcinogens in the Environment

Some carcinogens occur naturally in the environment, like the sun's UV rays. Others are manufactured or synthetic substances that show up occasionally in the general environment but more often in the work environments of specific industries.

Ingested Chemicals The food industry uses preservatives and other additives to prevent food from becoming spoiled or stale (see Chapter 12). Some of these compounds are antioxidants and may actually decrease any cancer-causing properties the food might have. Other compounds, like the nitrates and nitrites found in processed meat, are potentially more dangerous.

Nitrates and nitrites are added to foods like beer and ale, ham, bacon, hot dogs, and lunch meats. The nitrites inhibit the growth of bacteria, which could otherwise cause food poisoning. They also preserve the pink color of the meat, which has no bearing on taste but looks more appetizing to many people. While nitrates and nitrites are not themselves carcinogenic, they can combine with dietary substances in the stomach and be converted to **nitrosamines,** which are highly potent carcinogens. Foods cured with nitrites, as well as those cured by salt or smoke, have been linked to esophageal and stomach cancer, and they should be eaten only in modest amounts.

Environmental and Industrial Pollution Pollutants in urban air have long been suspected of contributing to the incidence of lung cancer. Fossil fuels and

Terms

antioxidant A substance that can lessen the breakdown of food or body constituents; actions include binding oxygen and donating electrons to free radicals.

free radicals Electron-seeking compounds that can react with fats, proteins, and DNA, damaging cell membranes and mutating genes in their search for electrons; produced through chemical reactions in the body and by exposure to environmental factors such as sunlight and tobacco smoke.

phytochemical A naturally occurring substance found in plant foods that may help prevent chronic diseases such as cancer and heart disease; *phyto* means "plant."

sulforaphane A compound found in cruciferous vegetables that can activate the body's detoxifying enzyme system.

nitrosamine A carcinogen made in the stomach from nitrates and nitrites.

In surveys, about one in four Americans agrees with the statement that there is nothing a person can do to keep from getting cancer. Many more focus most of their worry and attention on risk factors that account for relatively few cases of cancer—inherited gene mutations and chemicals in food, for example.

As in the case of heart disease—the other major killer of Americans—it is true that some cancer risk factors, such as age, are out of your control. However, you can significantly reduce your risk of cancer by making certain lifestyle changes.

Cancer—A Complex Disease

One reason people may feel powerless to protect themselves from cancer is that cancer is such a complex group of diseases, caused by the long-term interplay of genetic, environmental, and lifestyle factors. Some people engage in many unhealthy habits and never develop cancer; yet others seem to have near-ideal lifestyles but do develop cancer, possibly because they are more sensitive than others to cancer-causing agents.

In a relatively small proportion of cases, an inherited gene mutation may increase cancer risk; a family health history can help identify these situations and, in some cases, lead to increased screening and/or preventive therapies such as tamoxifen. In most cases, however, cancer develops from a series of gene mutations that occur after birth. Until researchers can pinpoint and test for elevated risk in the general population, the best cancer prevention strategy for most people is to follow the general advice for lifestyle changes and screening from major health organizations.

Cancer in the News

With new risk factors reported by the media nearly every week, it is difficult to know what to take seriously and act on and what to ignore. It also seems like the findings are constantly changing—one week, a specific dietary component is touted as a cancer protector, and a month later, a different study finds that it has no benefit. Some of the apparent flip-flops reflect the nature of science, because it often takes many studies to pinpoint the effects of a particular risk factor.

Often, too, the media may oversimplify the results of a study or exaggerate what it means for the average person. It is important to use your critical thinking skills when evaluating cancer news. In particular, consider whether a news story is a finding from a single research study or new health advice from a reputable source. Health behavior guidelines offered by government agencies or national research foundations are typically based on many long-term research studies and thus offer the best available advice.

Putting Risks into Perspective— and Taking Action

It is estimated that more than half of all cancer deaths could be prevented through individual action. On the positive side, surveys show that most Americans identify tobacco use and sun exposure as causes of cancer and that declines in smoking rates are now being mirrored by declines in lung cancer deaths. Pap tests to detect early cervical cancer are widely performed and have significantly reduced deaths from cervical cancer.

However, the same surveys indicate that more than half of Americans overlook other lifestyle factors that have been linked to more than a third of all cancer deaths: dietary choices, inactivity, obesity, and excessive consumption of alcohol. Instead, they focus attention on environmental carcinogens like food additives and pollutants that scientists believe are responsible for less than 5% of all cancers. In addition, many Americans do not keep up with recommended screening tests like colonoscopy and mammography that can detect cancer in its early, most treatable, stage.

Don't let cancer's complexity make you feel powerless and unmotivated to act. Perhaps the best advice is to focus your energy on the most significant risk factors and the known ways of reducing cancer risk: Don't use tobacco; be physically active; eat a diet rich in fruits, vegetables, and whole grains; and obtain recommended screening tests. These strategies may not seem as simple and sexy as the latest supplement or fad diet you see in a magazine, but they are based on the best available information and have the added benefit of improving quality of life and reducing the risk of many other chronic diseases.

SOURCES: American Cancer Society. 2005. *Cancer Facts and Figures 2005.* Atlanta: American Cancer Society; National Cancer Institute. 2002. *Possible Causes and Prevention of Cancer* (http://www.cancer.gov/cancertopics/wyntk/overview/page3; retrieved January 27, 2005); American Institute for Cancer Research. 2001. *New Survey of Americans Uncovers Widespread Fear of Cancer, But Little Knowledge About Reducing Risk* (http://www.aicr.org/press/pubsearchdetail.lasso?index=1318; retrieved January 27, 2005).

their combustion products, such as complex hydrocarbons, have been of special concern, and most gas stations are now required to provide special nozzles to reduce the amount of gasoline vapor released when you fill your tank. The effect of air pollutants has been difficult to study because of the overwhelmingly greater influence of smoking on lung cancer rates. Urban air pollution appears to have a measurable but limited role in causing lung cancer. (Chapter 24 has more information on air pollution.)

The best available data indicate that less than 2% of cancer deaths are caused by general environmental pollution, such as substances in our air and water (see the box "Putting Cancer Risks in Perspective"). Exposure to carcinogenic materials in the workplace is a more serious problem. Occupational exposure to specific carcinogens may account for up to 5% of cancer deaths. For example, diesel exhaust may contribute to lung cancer in truck operators and railroad workers, soot may cause skin cancer in firefighters and bricklayers, and hair dyes have been linked to bladder cancer in hairdressers and barbers. With increasing industry and government regulation, we can anticipate that the industrial sources of cancer risk will continue to diminish, at least in the United States. In contrast, in the former Soviet Union and Eastern European countries, where environmental concerns were sacrificed to industrial productivity for decades, cancer rates from industrial pollution continue to climb.

Radiation   All sources of radiation are potentially carcinogenic, including medical X rays, radioactive substances (radioisotopes), and UV rays from the sun. Striking examples of the effects of radiation can be seen in the survivors of the atomic bombings of Hiroshima and Nagasaki in 1945 and in residents of the area surrounding the Chernobyl nuclear reactor that blew up in 1986. In Japan, new cancers, especially leukemias, are still occurring over 50 years after the bombings. In Belarus, Russia, and Ukraine, the areas most affected by the radioactive debris from Chernobyl, rates of thyroid cancer in children are as much as 30 times higher than before the explosion. People living near Chernobyl suffered genetic damage that is being passed on to their children.

The continuing cancer cases in survivors of Hiroshima, Nagasaki, and Chernobyl are a warning to us that any unnecessary exposure to ionizing radiation should be avoided. Most physicians and dentists are quite aware of the risk of radiation, and successful efforts have been made to reduce the amount of radiation needed for mammograms, dental X rays, and other necessary medical X rays. Full-body CT scans are sometimes advertised for routine screening in otherwise well individuals in order to look for tumors. Such screening is not recommended; it is typically expensive and may have false-positive findings that lead to unnecessary and invasive additional tests. Also, the radiation in these full-body X rays may itself raise the risk of cancer; the radiation dose of one full-body CT scan is nearly 100 times that of a typical mammogram.

Another source of environmental radiation is radon gas. Radon is a radioactive decomposition product of radium, which is found in small quantities in some rocks and soils. Radon is inhaled with the air we breathe, so it comes into intimate contact with the cells of the lungs, where its radiation can produce mutations. Radon and smoking together create a more-than-additive risk of lung cancer. In most of our homes and classrooms, radon is rapidly dissipated into the atmosphere, and very low levels of radon do not appear to increase cancer risk. But in certain kinds of enclosed spaces, such as mines, some basements, and airtight houses built of brick or stone, it can rise to dangerous levels (see Chapter 24).

Sunlight is a very important source of radiation, but because its rays penetrate only a millimeter or so into the skin, it could be considered a surface carcinogen. Most cases of skin cancer are the relatively benign and highly curable basal cell carcinomas, but a substantial minority are the potentially deadly malignant melanomas. As discussed earlier, all types of skin cancer are increased by early and excessive exposure to the sun, and severe sunburn early in childhood appears to carry with it an added risk of melanoma later in life.

Cell phones generate low levels of non-ionizing radiation, a different type of radiation from that used for medical X rays (see Chapter 24). Studies of the effects of exposure to non-ionizing radiation from cell phones have had mixed results, and researchers have found no conclusive link between cell phone use and brain cancer. Research is ongoing, however, and until the effects of such radiation exposure have been determined, some health professionals suggest discouraging children from using mobile phones excessively because their brains are more susceptible to radiation than are those of adults.

DETECTING, DIAGNOSING, AND TREATING CANCER

Early cancer detection often depends on our willingness to be aware of changes in our own body and to make sure we keep up with recommended diagnostic tests. Although treatment success varies with individual cancers, cure rates have increased—sometimes dramatically—in this century.

Detecting Cancer

Unlike those of some other diseases, early signs of cancer are usually not apparent to anyone but the person who has them. Even pain is not a reliable guide to early detection, because the initial stages of cancer may be painless. Self-monitoring is the first line of defense, and the American Cancer Society recommends that you watch for the seven major warning signs shown in Figure 16-6. Remember them by the acronym CAUTION.

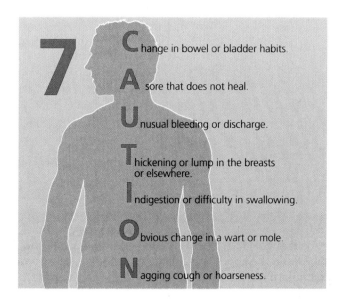

Figure 16-6   The seven major warning signs of cancer.

Table 16-2 Screening Guidelines for the Early Detection of Cancer in Asymptomatic People

Site	Recommendation
Breast	• Yearly mammograms are recommended starting at age 40. The age at which screening should be stopped should be individualized by considering the potential risks and benefits of screening in the context of overall health status and longevity. • Clinical breast exam should be part of a periodic health exam, about every 3 years for women age 20–39, and every year for women age 40 and older. • Women should know how their breasts normally feel and report any breast change promptly to their health care providers. Breast self-exam is an option for women starting at age 20. • Women at increased risk (e.g., family history, genetic tendency, past breast cancer) should talk with their doctors about the benefits and limitations of starting mammography screening earlier, having additional tests (i.e., breast ultrasound and MRI), or having more frequent exams.
Colon and rectum	Beginning at age 50, men and women should begin screening with one of the examination schedules below. • A fecal occult blood test (FOBT) or fecal immunochemical test (FIT) every year • A flexible sigmoidoscopy (FSIG) every 5 years • Annual FOBT or FIT and flexible sigmoidoscopy every 5 years* • A double-contrast barium enema every 5 years • A colonoscopy every 10 years *Combined testing is preferred over either annual FOBT or FIT, or FSIG every 5 years, alone. People who are at moderate or high risk for colorectal cancer should talk with a doctor about a different testing schedule.*
Prostate	The PSA test and the digital rectal examination should be offered annually, beginning at age 50, to men who have a life expectancy of at least 10 years. Men at high risk (African American men and men with a strong family history of one or more first-degree relatives diagnosed with prostate cancer at an early age) should begin testing at age 45. For men at both average risk and high risk, information should be provided about what is known and what is uncertain about the benefits and limitations of early detection and treatment of prostate cancer so that they can make an informed decision about testing.
Uterus	**Cervix:** Screening should begin approximately 3 years after a woman begins having vaginal intercourse, but no later than age 21. Screening should be done every year with regular Pap tests or every 2 years using liquid-based tests. At or after age 30, women who have had three normal test results in a row may get screened every 2 to 3 years. Alternatively, cervical cancer screening with HPV DNA testing and conventional or liquid-based cytology could be performed every 3 years. However, doctors may suggest a woman get screened more often if she has certain risk factors, such as HIV infection or a weak immune system. Women 70 years and older who have had three or more consecutive normal Pap tests in the past 10 years may choose to stop cervical cancer screening. Screening after total hysterectomy (with removal of the cervix) is not necessary unless the surgery was done as a treatment for cervical cancer. **Endometrium:** The American Cancer Society recommends that at the time of menopause all women should be informed about the risks and symptoms of endometrial cancer, and strongly encouraged to report any unexpected bleeding or spotting to their physicians. Annual screening for endometrial cancer with endometrial biopsy beginning at age 35 should be offered to women with or at risk for hereditary nonpolyposis colon cancer (HNPCC).
Cancer-related checkup	For individuals undergoing periodic health examinations, a cancer-related checkup should include health counseling and, depending on a person's age and gender, might include examinations for cancers of the thyroid, oral cavity, skin, lymph nodes, testes, and ovaries, as well as for some nonmalignant diseases.

SOURCE: American Cancer Society's *Cancer Facts and Figures 2005.* Copyright © 2005 American Cancer Society, Inc. www.cancer.org. Reprinted with permission.

Although none of the warning signs is a sure indication of cancer, the appearance of any one should send you to see your physician. By being aware yourself of the risk factors in your own life, including the cancer history of your immediate family and your own past history, you can often bring a problem to the attention of a physician long before it would have been detected at a routine physical.

In addition to self-monitoring, the ACS recommends routine cancer checkups, as well as specific screening tests for certain cancers (Table 16-2).

Diagnosing Cancer

Detection of a cancer by physical examination is only the beginning. Methods for determining the exact location, type, and degree of malignancy of a cancer continue to improve. Knowledge of the exact location and size of a tumor is necessary for precise and effective surgery or radiation therapy. This is especially true in cases where the tumor may be hard to reach, as in the brain.

Imaging studies or exploratory surgery may be performed to identify a cancer's *stage*—a designation based on a tumor's size, location, and spread that helps determine appropriate treatment. A biopsy may be performed to confirm the type of tumor. Several diagnostic imaging techniques have replaced exploratory surgery for some patients. In **magnetic resonance imaging (MRI),** a huge electromagnet is used to detect hidden tumors by mapping, on a computer screen, the vibrations of different atoms in the body. **Computed tomography (CT)** scanning uses X rays to examine the brain and other parts of the body. The process allows the construction of cross sections, which show a tumor's shape and location more accurately than is possible with conventional X rays. For patients undergoing radiation therapy, CT scanning enables the therapist to pinpoint the tumor more precisely, thereby providing more accurate radiation dosage while sparing normal tissue.

Ultrasonography has also been used increasingly in the past few years to view tumors. It has several advantages: It can be used in the physician's office, it is less expensive than other imaging methods, and it is completely safe. Prostate ultrasound (a rectal probe using ultrasonic waves to produce an image of the prostate gland) is being investigated for its ability to detect small, hidden tumors that would be missed by a digital rectal exam.

Treating Cancer

The ideal cancer therapy would kill or remove all cancerous cells while leaving normal tissue untouched. Sometimes this is almost possible, as when a surgeon removes a small superficial tumor of the skin. Usually the tumor is less accessible, and some combination of surgery, radiation therapy, and chemotherapy must be applied instead. Some patients choose to combine conventional therapies with alternative treatments (see the box "Avoiding Cancer Quackery" on p. 506).

Surgery   For most cancers, surgery is the most useful treatment. In many cases, the organ containing the tumor is not essential for life and can be partially or completely removed. This is true especially for localized breast, prostate, or testicular cancer, where the surgical removal of one breast, the prostate gland, or one testicle may give a long-lasting cure. Surgery is less effective when the tumor involves cells of the immune system, which are

widely distributed throughout the body, or when the cancer has already metastasized. In such cases, surgery must be combined with other techniques.

Chemotherapy   Chemotherapy, or the use of cell-killing drugs to destroy rapidly growing cancer cells, has been in use since the 1940s. Many of these drugs work by interfering with DNA synthesis and replication in rapidly dividing cells. Normal cells, which usually grow slowly, are not destroyed by these drugs. However, some normal tissues such as intestinal, hair, and blood-forming cells are always growing, and damage to these tissues produces the unpleasant side effects of chemotherapy, including nausea, vomiting, diarrhea, and hair loss.

Chemotherapy drugs are often used in combinations or with surgery. Recently, in a procedure called **induction chemotherapy,** physicians have begun to use chemotherapy before surgery, both to shrink the tumor and to kill any existing small metastases as soon as possible.

Radiation   In cancer radiation therapy, a beam of X rays or gamma rays is directed at the tumor, and the tumor cells are killed. Occasionally, when an organ is small enough, radioactive seeds are surgically placed inside the cancerous organ to destroy the tumor and then removed later if necessary. Radiation destroys both normal and cancerous cells, but because it can be precisely directed at the tumor it is usually less toxic for the patient than either surgery or chemotherapy, and it can often be performed on an outpatient basis. Radiation may be used as an exclusive treatment or in combination with surgery and/or chemotherapy.

New and Experimental Techniques   Many new and exciting possibilities for cancer therapy promise alternatives to the options of surgery, radiation, and chemotherapy. Although it is impossible to predict which of these new approaches will be most successful, researchers hope that cancer therapy overall will become increasingly safer and more effective.

- *Gene therapy.* Completion of the sequencing of the human genome in 2000 opened a treasure chest of new insights into cancer. Scientists have already

Terms

Vw

magnetic resonance imaging (MRI) A computerized imaging technique that uses a strong magnetic field and radio frequency signals to examine a thin cross section of the body; also known as *nuclear magnetic resonance imaging (NMR).*

computed tomography (CT) The use of computerized X ray images to create a cross-sectional depiction of tissue density.

induction chemotherapy The use of chemotherapy prior to surgery to shrink a cancerous tumor and prevent metastasis; sometimes eliminates the need for radical surgery.

Sometimes conventional treatments for cancer are simply not enough. A patient may be told that there is little conventional therapy can do, other than providing medication to ease pain. When therapy is available, it may be painful and even intolerable to some people. Not surprisingly, many cancer patients look for complementary and alternative therapies. As many as 80% of cancer patients report combining conventional treatments with some type of mind-body technique. A much smaller number of patients look for alternatives to the more conventional therapies. These may be therapies within the bounds of legitimate medical practice that have not yet proven themselves in clinical trials. Or, at the extreme, alternative therapies may be scientifically unsound and dangerous, as well as expensive.

Complementary therapies such as yoga, massage, meditation, music therapy, t'ai chi, and prayer can have positive physical and psychological benefits for patients and help them improve their quality of life as they deal with illness and the often difficult treatments for cancer. Mind-body practices can reduce pain and anxiety, improve sleep, and give people a sense of control and participation in their treatment; such practices may also enhance the immune system. (See Chapter 2 for more on stress and relaxation techniques.) Mind-body practices typically can be used in combination with conventional cancer therapies.

For other types of therapies, the National Cancer Institute suggests that patients and their families consider the following questions when making decisions about cancer treatment:

- *Has the treatment been evaluated in clinical trials?* Advances in cancer treatment are made through carefully monitored clinical trials. If a patient wants to try a new therapy, participation in a clinical trial may be a treatment option. (See For More Information at the end of the chapter for more on clinical trials.)

- *Do the practitioners of an approach claim that the medical community is trying to keep their cure from the public?* No one genuinely committed to finding better ways to treat a disease would knowingly keep an effective treatment secret or try to suppress such a treatment.

- *Does the treatment rely on nutritional or diet therapy as its main focus?* Although diet can be a key risk factor in the development of cancer, there is no evidence that diet alone can get rid of cancerous cells in the body.

- *Do those who endorse the treatment claim that it is harmless and painless and that it produces no unpleasant side effects?* Reputable researchers are working to develop less toxic cancer therapies, but because effective treatments for cancer must be powerful, they frequently have unpleasant side effects.

- *Does the treatment have a secret formula that only a small group of practitioners can use?* Scientists who believe they have developed an effective treatment routinely publish their results in reputable journals so they can be evaluated by other researchers.

Use special caution when evaluating cancer remedies promoted online; one recent study found that as many as one-third of cancer-related alternative medicine sites offered advice that was harmful or potentially dangerous.

One danger of alternative medicine is the very real possibility that proven therapies will be neglected while unproven, faddish alternative approaches are pursued; if alternate therapies delay proven therapies, lives may be lost. Another danger is that complementary therapies may counteract or affect conventional therapies; for example, some herbal supplements have been found to affect how cancer drugs are absorbed and used by the body. It is extremely important for users of complementary therapies to inform their physicians so any side effects or harmful interactions can be prevented.

SOURCES: American Cancer Society. 2005. *Complementary and Alternative Therapies* (http://www.cancer.org/docroot/ETD/ETD_5.asp; retrieved January 26, 2005); National Cancer Institute. 2004. *Complementary and Alternative Medicine in Cancer Treatment: Questions and Answers* (http://cis.nci.hin.gov/fact/9_14.htm; retrieved January 26, 2005); Ernst, E., and K. Schmidt. 2002. "Alternative" cancer cures via the Internet? *British Journal of Cancer* 87(5): 479–480; Aulas, J. 1996. Alternative cancer treatments. *Scientific American,* September.

discovered important new subtypes of tumors for breast cancer, melanoma, leukemia, and lymphomas based on patterns of gene expression. These patterns were revealed through the use of **gene chips,** which lay out thousands of specific DNA sequences on small glass chips for comparison with the sequences found in the tumor cells. Scientists can analyze which genes are present in the tumor, which have suffered mutations, and which are being expressed. Using this approach, researchers hope to develop a variety of powerful, targeted therapies for use in treatment of specific cancers, much as specific antibiotics are now used to treat specific bacterial diseases.

- *Bone marrow and stem cell transplants.* In cancers of the blood-forming cells or lymph cells, a patient's own bone marrow may have to be eliminated by radiation or chemotherapy to rid the body of cancer cells. Bone marrow can then be restored by transplanting healthy bone marrow cells from a compatible donor. Transplant incompatibility can be a problem, but progress on this front has been made recently through the use of **stem cells.** These unique, unspecialized cells can divide and produce more specialized cell types, including bone marrow cells (see Chapter 19). These stem cells can be identified, purified, and grown outside the body and then transplanted back into the cancer patient. This technique would allow for safe repopulation of bone marrow after radiation treatment.

• *Biological therapies.* Biological therapies are based on enhancing the immune system's reaction to a tumor. Techniques include cancer vaccines, genetic modification of the body's immune cells, and the use of genetically engineered **cytokines,** which enhance immune cell function. Melanomas seem particularly susceptible to these biological approaches. Cancer vaccines are also under study for kidney cancer, lymphoma, lung cancer, and other cancers.

• *Protease inhibitors.* To spread, cancer cells must activate a set of enzymes known as proteases, which enable them to dissolve the substances between cells and then migrate through normal tissues. **Protease inhibitors** are being developed to interfere with actions of specific proteases, thereby blocking cancer cells' ability to invade normal tissue and metastasize.

• *Anti-angiogenesis drugs.* To obtain nutrients, cancer cells signal the body to produce new blood vessels, a process called angiogenesis. Drugs that block angiogenesis could keep tumors from growing and spreading.

• *Telomerase inhibitors.* Normal human cells die after a limited number of divisions; cancer cells do not, in part because of the enzyme telomerase. Researchers hope to develop drugs to block the enzyme.

Living with Cancer

Throughout much of the 20th century, a diagnosis of cancer was almost equivalent to a death sentence. Gradually, however, survival has become the norm, and there are, in fact, 8.9 million cancer survivors in the United States today. However, for these people, the fear of cancer never completely disappears, and there is always the risk of a recurrence.

Cancer survivors may suffer economic prejudice from insurers, who can refuse to issue or renew health coverage. This sort of problem can be devastating to a cancer survivor who may be struggling both psychologically and financially to restore a normal existence. Several states have passed legislation to prevent this kind of discrimination, but it still exists.

Psychological support is an important factor during treatment for cancer (see the box "Coping with Cancer" on p. 508). For some patients, family and friends plus a caring physician or nurse provide all the support that is necessary. But often health care providers are busy or aloof, and family members and friends are just as fearful about the outcome as the patient. For many people, an organized support group can help provide needed social and psychological support.

Social support can play a crucial role in cancer treatment for these patients. Studies indicate that support group participants have lower levels of anxiety and depression, and manage pain more successfully.

PREVENTING CANCER

Your lifestyle choices can radically lower your cancer risks, so you *can* take a very practical approach to cancer prevention (Figure 16-7).

Avoiding Tobacco

Smoking is responsible for 80–90% of all lung cancers and for about 30% of all cancer deaths. People who smoke two or more packs of cigarettes a day have lung cancer mortality rates 15–25 times greater than those of nonsmokers. The carcinogenic chemicals in smoke are transported throughout the body in the bloodstream, making smoking a carcinogen for many forms of cancer other than lung cancer. ETS is dangerous to nonsmokers.

Terms

gene chips Small glass chips on which tens of thousands of specific DNA sequences have been laid out in precise grids using a process similar to that used to make silicon chips.

stem cells Unspecialized cells that can divide and produce cells that differentiate into the many different types of specialized cells in the body (brain cells, muscle cells, skin cells, blood cells, and so on).

cytokine A chemical messenger produced by a variety of cell types that helps regulate many cell functions; immune system cells release cytokines that help amplify and coordinate the immune response.

protease inhibitor A drug that inhibits the action of any of the protein-splitting enzymes known as proteases. Because some proteases facilitate metastasis, protease inhibitors are being developed for cancer therapy.

A cancer diagnosis was once viewed as the equivalent of a death sentence, and individuals and families were often left to face their fears alone. People were sometimes reluctant to admit to the diagnosis of cancer or share it with others because of feelings of hopelessness or irrational guilt. Since about the 1970s, a cultural shift has taken place. Improved diagnostic methods and therapies have resulted in longer survival times and an increasing percentage of cures. Media attention on positive developments has created a better understanding of the scientific basis of cancer. Some of the mystery and dread of cancer has begun to abate, leading to a more positive atmosphere for cancer patients and their families.

If You Are the Patient

Each person's experience with cancer is unique, based on his or her own personality and values. Some people turn to their friends and family members for support, whereas others prefer help from other cancer patients, professional counselors, or faith-based groups. If you are a cancer patient, it is important to do what is right for you. Strategies for dealing with difficult emotions such as fear, anxiety, depression, and loss of control include the following:

• Remember that cancer doesn't always mean death. Many cancers are curable or controllable for long periods, and survivors may return to a normal, healthy life. Hope and optimism are important elements in cancer survival.

• Focus on controlling what you can. Be informed and involved with your medical care, keep your appointments, and make healthy changes in your lifestyle.

• Work toward having a positive attitude, but don't feel guilty if you can't maintain it all the time. Having cancer is difficult, and low moods will occur no matter how good you are at coping. If they become frequent or severe, seek help.

• Use strategies that have helped you solve problems and manage your emotions in the past. Some people respond to information gathering, talking with others, and prayer or meditation. Physical activity, music, art, and sharing personal stories may help lessen stress.

• Confide feelings and worries to someone close to you. Don't bottle up

your feelings to spare your loved ones. If you don't feel comfortable sharing with others, consider expressing your emotions in a journal.

• Explore groups that can help you get through this difficult time. There are many support groups for people who have cancer or who have survived it.

Finding a Support Group

Support groups may be led by cancer survivors, group members, or trained professionals. These groups typically present information, teach coping skills, and give cancer patients a place to share common concerns and obtain emotional support. Support groups may focus on education, behavioral training, or group interaction. Behavioral training can involve meditation and other techniques to reduce stress or the effects of chemotherapy or radiation therapy.

Research has shown that support groups can enhance quality of life in very practical ways. For instance, patients in breast cancer support groups were found to have improved psychological symptoms, less pain, and improved family relationships compared with patients in a control group. Some early studies even suggested a longer survival time for cancer patients in support groups, but more recent studies have cast doubt on this result.

Support groups vary in quality, and people with cancer may find that a support group fails to discuss topics relevant to their personal situation. Some people may find a support group upsetting because it stirs up too many uncomfortable feelings or because the leader is not skilled. Find a group that is right for you. Online support groups can be very helpful for people living in rural areas or confined to their homes. However, medical information on the Internet is highly variable in quality, and you should check with your physician before making any treatment changes based on online information.

Supporting a Person with Cancer

There is no one right way to act with a person facing cancer. Reassure the person of your love, and let him or her know that you are available for both practical and emotional support. A person with cancer may want you to be very involved in treatment or coping, or he or she may

want your help in maintaining a more normal routine. Guidelines for visiting a cancer patient include the following:

• Before you visit, call to ask if it's a good time. Surprise visits are often not welcome. Don't overstay your welcome.

• Be a good listener. Allow the person to express all his or her feelings, and don't discount fears or minimize the seriousness of the situation. Let the patient decide whether the two of you talk about the illness. It's human to want to laugh and talk about other things sometimes.

• Ask "What can I get you?" or "How can I help?" instead of saying "Let me know if I can help." Make specific offers: to clean the bathroom, go grocery shopping, do laundry, or give caregivers a break.

• Refrain from offering advice. You may have heard about the latest treatment or hottest physician, but unless you are asked for suggestions, keep them to yourself.

• If you want to take food, ask about dietary restrictions ahead of time. Use a disposable container so the person won't have to return it.

• Don't be put off if your first visit gets a lukewarm reception. Many cancer victims are on an emotional roller coaster, and their feelings and needs will change over time.

If you find yourself struggling with difficult emotions or challenging new roles and responsibilities, remember that support groups also exist for friends and family members of cancer patients. These groups give people a place to express their fears about issues such as relationship changes, financial problems, and providing emotional support for the cancer patient.

SOURCES: Kissane, D. W., et al. 2004. Effect of cognitive-existential group therapy on survival in early-stage breast cancer. *Journal of Clinical Oncology* 22(21): 4255–4260; National Cancer Institute. 2002. *Your Mind and Your Feelings After Cancer Treatment* (http://www.cancer.gov/cancerinfo/life-after-treatment/page4; retrieved August 25, 2002); Goodwin, P. J., et al. 2001. The effect of group psychosocial support on survival in metastatic breast cancer. *New England Journal of Medicine* 345(24): 1719–1726; Life with cancer: How to provide support. 1996. *Women's Health Advocate,* September; Holland, J. C. 1996. Cancer's psychological challenges. *Scientific American,* September.

Do More

- Eat a varied, plant-based diet that is high in fiber-rich foods such as legumes and whole grains

- Eat 7–13 servings of fruits and vegetables every day, favoring foods from the following categories:
  - Cruciferous vegetables
  - Citrus fruits
  - Berries
  - Dark green leafy vegetables
  - Dark yellow, orange, or red fruits and vegetables

- Be physically active

- Maintain a healthy weight

- Practice safer sex (to avoid HPV infection)

- Protect your skin from the sun with appropriate clothing and sunscreen

- Perform regular self-exams (breast self-exam, testicular self-exam, skin self-exam)

- Obtain recommended screening tests and discuss with your physician any family history of cancer.

Do Less

- Don't use tobacco in any form:
  - Cigarettes
  - Spit tobacco
  - Cigars and pipes
  - Bidis and clove cigarettes

- Avoid exposure to environmental tobacco smoke

- Limit consumption of fatty meats and other sources of saturated fat

- Avoid excessive alcohol consumption

- Limit consumption of salt

- Don't eat charred foods, and limit consumption of cured and smoked meats and meat and fish grilled in a direct flame

- Limit exposure to UV radiation from sunlight or tanning lamps or beds

- Avoid occupational exposure to carcinogens

Figure 16-7   Strategies for reducing your risk of cancer.

If you smoke, stop. If you don't smoke, avoid breathing the smoke from other people's cigarettes.

The use of spit tobacco, highly habit-forming because of its nicotine content, is also dangerous because it increases the risk of cancers of the mouth, larynx, throat, and esophagus. Refer to Chapter 11 for tips on breaking the tobacco habit.

Controlling Diet and Weight

Based on hundreds of studies, the National Cancer Institute estimates that about one-third of all cancers are in some way linked to what we eat. Choose a low-fat, plant-based diet containing a wide variety of fruits, vegetables, and whole grains rich in phytochemicals. See the specific suggestions in the Behavior Change Strategy at the end of this chapter.

Drink alcohol only in moderation, if at all. Oral cancer and cancers of the larynx, throat, esophagus, and liver occur more frequently among heavy drinkers of alcohol. The risk is even higher among heavy drinkers who smoke.

The risk of several cancers increases for obese people. Maintaining a healthy weight through a moderate diet and regular exercise lowers the risk. Chapters 12 and 14 provide strategies for improving your diet and maintaining a healthy body weight.

Regular Exercise

Regular exercise is linked to lower rates of colon and other cancers. It also helps control weight. Refer to Chapter 13 for advice on setting up a lifelong program of regular exercise.

Protecting Skin from the Sun

Almost all cases of nonmelanoma skin cancer are considered to be sun-related, and sun exposure is a major factor in the development of melanoma as well. Wear protective clothing when you're out in the sun, and use a sunscreen with an SPF rating of 15 or higher. Don't go to tanning salons; they do not provide safe tans.

Avoiding Environmental and Occupational Carcinogens

Most medical X rays are adjusted to deliver the lowest dose of radiation possible without sacrificing image quality. Radiation from radon may pose a threat in some homes; remedial steps should be taken if tests indicate high levels of radon. A number of industrial agents that some people are exposed to on the job are associated with cancer, including nickel, chromate, asbestos, and vinyl chloride. Try to avoid occupational exposure to carcinogens, and don't smoke; the cancer risks of many of these agents increase greatly when combined with smoking.

Recommended Screening Tests

Your first line of defense against cancer involves the lifestyle changes described above that help you avoid cancer-causing agents. Your second line of defense involves having any cancers that do develop discovered as quickly as possible through regular self-exams and medical screening tests. Stay alert for the signs and symptoms that could indicate cancer (see Figure 16-6), and follow the American Cancer Society screening guidelines listed in Table 16-2. Both lifestyle changes and a program of early detection are important to your long-term health.

SUMMARY

- A malignant tumor can invade surrounding structures and spread to distant sites via the blood and lymphatic system, producing additional tumors.

- A malignant cell divides without regard for normal growth. As tumors grow, they produce signs or symptoms that are determined by their location in the body.

- One in two men and one in three women will develop cancer, but more than half will be cured.

- Lung cancer kills more people than any other type of cancer. Tobacco smoke is the primary cause.

- Colon and rectal cancer is linked to age, heredity, obesity, and a diet rich in red meat and low in fruits and vegetables. Most colon cancers arise from preexisting polyps.

- Breast cancer affects about one in seven women in the United States. Although there is a genetic component to breast cancer, diet and hormones are also risk factors.

- Prostate cancer is chiefly a disease of aging; diet and lifestyle probably are factors in its occurrence. Early detection is possible through rectal examinations, PSA blood tests, and sometimes ultrasound.

- Cancers of the female reproductive tract include cervical, uterine, and ovarian cancer. The Pap test is an effective screening test for cervical cancer.

- Abnormal cellular changes in the epidermis, often a result of exposure to the sun, cause skin cancer, as does chronic exposure to certain chemicals. Skin cancers occur as basal cell carcinoma, squamous cell carcinoma, and melanoma.

- Oral cancer is caused primarily by smoking, excess alcohol consumption, and use of spit tobacco. Oral cancers are easy to detect but often hard to treat.

- Testicular cancer can be detected early through self-examination.

- Mutational damage to a cell's DNA can lead to rapid and uncontrolled growth of cells; mutagens include radiation, viral infection, and chemical substances in food and air.

- Cancer-promoting dietary factors include meat, certain types of fats, and alcohol.

- Diets high in fruits and vegetables are linked to a lower risk of cancer.

- Other possible causes of cancer include inactivity and obesity, certain types of infections and chemicals, and radiation.

- Self-monitoring and regular screening tests are essential to early cancer detection; early signs can be remembered by using the acronym CAUTION.

- Methods of cancer diagnosis include magnetic resonance imaging, computed tomography, and ultrasound.

- Treatment methods usually consist of some combination of surgery, chemotherapy, and radiation. Gene therapy, bone marrow and stem cell transplants, protease inhibitors, biological therapies, and drugs that inhibit angiogenesis or telomerase also hold promise as effective treatments.

- Strategies for preventing cancer include avoiding tobacco; eating a varied, moderate diet and controlling weight; exercising regularly; protecting skin from the sun; avoiding exposure to environmental and occupational carcinogens; and getting recommended cancer screening tests.

Take Action

1. **Try some cancer-fighting foods:** Look through the foods listed in Table 16-1 and the Behavior Change Strategy and choose four or five that you don't typically eat. During the next week, make a point of trying each of the foods you've chosen.

2. **Do a self-exam:** Devise a plan for incorporating regular self-examinations for cancer (breast self-examination or testicle self-examination) into your life. What strategies will help you remember to do your monthly exam? How can you keep yourself motivated?

Incorporating More Fruits and Vegetables into Your Diet

When we think about the health benefits of fruits and vegetables, we usually focus on the fact that they are rich in carbohydrates, dietary fiber, and vitamins and low in fat. A benefit that we may overlook is that they contain specific cancer-fighting compounds, phytochemicals, that help slow, stop, or even reverse the process of cancer. The National Cancer Institute (NCI) reports that people who eat five or more servings a day of fruits and vegetables have half the risk of cancer of those who eat less than two; according to the NCI, seven to nine servings or more per day is optimal. The NCI, along with industry groups, has developed a program to help more Americans increase their intake of fruits and vegetables to health-promoting levels—the "Eat 5 to 9 a Day for Better Health" program.

Most Americans need to double the amount of fruits and vegetables they eat every day. Begin by monitoring your diet for 1–2 weeks to assess your current intake; then look for ways to incorporate these foods into your diet in easy and tasty ways. Here are some tips to get you started.

Breakfast

- Drink 100% juice every morning.
- Add raisins, berries, or sliced fruit to cereal, pancakes, or waffles. Top bagels with tomato slices.
- Try a fruit smoothie made from fresh or frozen fruit and orange juice or low-fat yogurt.

Lunch

- Choose vegetable soup or salad with your meal.

- Replace potato chips or french fries with cut-up vegetables.
- Add extra chunks of fruits or vegetables to salads.
- Try adding vegetables such as roasted peppers, cucumber slices, shredded carrots, avocado, or salsa to sandwiches.
- Drink tomato or vegetable juice instead of soda (watch for excess sodium).

Dinner

- Choose a vegetarian main course, such as stir-fry or vegetable stew. Have at least two servings of vegetables with every dinner.
- Microwave vegetables and sprinkle them with a little bit of Parmesan cheese.
- Substitute vegetables for meat in casseroles and pasta and chili recipes.
- At the salad bar, pile your plate with healthy vegetables and use low-fat or nonfat dressing.

Snacks and On the Go

- Keep ready to eat fruits and vegetables on hand (apples, plums, pears, and carrots).
- Keep small packages of dried fruit in the car (try dried apricots, peaches, and pears and raisins).
- Make ice cubes from 100% fruit juice and drop them into regular or sparkling water.
- Freeze grapes for a cool summer treat.

In the Grocery Store

- Stock up on canned, frozen, and dried fruits and vegetables when they go

on sale. Buy fresh fruits and vegetables in season; they'll taste best and be less expensive.

- To save on preparation time, buy presliced vegetables and fruits and prepackaged salads.
- Try a new fresh fruit or vegetable every week.

The All-Stars

Different fruits and vegetables contribute different vitamins, phytochemicals, and other nutrients, so be sure to get a variety. The following types of produce are particularly rich in nutrients and phytochemicals:

- Cruciferous vegetables (broccoli, cauliflower, cabbage, bok choy, brussels sprouts, kohlrabi, turnips, etc.)
- Citrus fruits (oranges, lemons, limes, grapefruit, tangerines, etc.)
- Berries (strawberries, raspberries, blueberries, etc.)
- Dark green leafy vegetables (spinach, chard, collards, beet greens, kale, mustard greens, romaine and other dark lettuces, etc.)
- Deep yellow, orange, and red fruits and vegetables (carrots, pumpkin, sweet potatoes, winter squash, red and yellow bell peppers, apricots, cantaloupe, mangoes, papayas, etc.)

SOURCES: National Cancer Institute. 2005. *Eat 5 to 9 A Day for Better Health* (http://www.5aday.gov; retrieved March 29, 2005); The produce prescription. 2000. *Consumer Reports on Health*, December; Welland, D. 1999. Fruits and vegetables: Easy ways to five-a-day. *Environmental Nutrition*, June.

---

3. **Construct a family cancer health history:** Interview your parents or grandparents about your family medical history. Are there any cases of cancer in your family, and has anyone died of cancer? Do you see any patterns? Be sure to discuss your family history with your physician.

4. **Participate in a cancer fundraiser:** Many local and national cancer organizations sponsor events such as walkathons to help raise money for cancer research and treatment. Consider volunteering at such an event.

For More Information

Books

American Cancer Society. 2003. *Cancer: What Causes It. What Doesn't.* Atlanta, Ga.: American Cancer Society. *Provides basic background information about cancer and its causes.*

American Institute for Cancer Research. 2005. *The New American Plate Cookbook.* Berkeley, Calif.: U.C. Berkeley Press. *Provides guidelines and recipes for healthy eating to prevent cancer and other chronic diseases.*

Hartmann, L. C., C. L. Loprinzi, and B. S. Gostout. 2005. *Mayo Clinic: Guide to Women's Cancers*. New York: Kensington Publishing. *Provides information about a variety of women's cancers.*

Johns Hopkins Consumer Health. 2005. *Prostate Disorders.* Redding, Conn.: Medletter Associates. *Provides information about the diagnosis and treatment options for benign prostate problems and prostate cancer.*

Rose, S., and R. Hara. 2003. *100 Questions and Answers About Caring for Family or Friends with Cancer.* Sudbury, Mass.: Jones & Bartlett. *Provides helpful practical advice about caring for patients and coping with emotional challenges.*

Runkington, C., and J. J. Straus. 2005. *The Encyclopedia of Cancer.* New York: Facts on File. *Includes entries on a variety of topics relating to cancer causes, prevention, diagnosis, and treatment.*

Ｖ☼Ｗ Organizations, Hotlines, and Web Sites

American Academy of Dermatology. Provides information on skin cancer prevention.
> 888-462-DERM
> http://www.aad.org

American Cancer Society. Provides a wide range of free materials on the prevention and treatment of cancer.
> 800-ACS-2345
> http://www.cancer.org

American Institute for Cancer Research. Provides information on lifestyle and cancer prevention, especially nutrition.
> 800-843-8114
> http://www.aicr.org

Cancer Guide: Steve Dunn's Cancer Information Page. Links to many good cancer resources on the Internet and advice about how to make best use of information.
> http://www.cancerguide.org

Cancer News. Provides links to news and information on many types of cancer.
> http://www.cancernews.com

Centers for Disease Control and Prevention: DES Update. Provides information about drugs containing DES and advice for exposed women and DES daughters and sons.
> http://www.cdc.gov/DES

Clinical Trials. Information about clinical trials for new cancer treatments can be accessed at the following sites:
> http://www.cancer.gov/clinicaltrials
> http://www.centerwatch.com

Dole 5-A-Day/Nutrition Education. Provides resources for parents, children, and educators, including extensive nutrition information about fruits and vegetables.
> http://www.dole5aday.com

EPA/Sunwise. Information about the UV Index and the effects of sun exposure, with links to sites with daily UV Index ratings for cities in the United States and other countries.
> http://www.epa.gov/sunwise/uvindex.html

Food and Drug Administration, Center for Drug Evaluation and Research: Oncology Tools. Provides information about types of cancer, treatments, and clinical trials.
> http://www.fda.gov/cder/cancer

Harvard Center for Cancer Prevention: Your Disease Risk. Includes interactive risk assessments as well as tips for preventing common cancers.
> http://www.yourcancerrisk.harvard.edu

MedlinePlus Cancer Information. Provides news and links to reliable information on a variety of cancers and cancer treatment.
> http://www.nlm.nih.gov/medlineplus/cancers.html

National Cancer Institute. Provides information on treatment options, screening, and clinical trials and on the national "Eat 5 to 9 Servings of Fruits and Vegetables A Day for Better Health Program" that promotes greater consumption of fruits and vegetables.
> 800-4-CANCER
> http://www.cancer.gov
> http://5aday.nci.nih.gov

National Comprehensive Cancer Network (NCCN). Presents treatment guidelines for physicians and patients related to the treatment of various cancers; these guidelines were developed by a group of leading cancer centers.
> http://www.nccn.org

National Toxicology Program. The federal program that creates regular reports listing those substances that are known or reasonably assumed to cause cancer in humans.
> http://ntp-server.niehs.nih.gov

New York Online Access to Health (NOAH)/Cancer. Provides information about cancer—causes, symptoms, types, treatments, clinical trials—and links to related sites.
> http://www.noah-health.org/en/cancer

Oncolink/The University of Pennsylvania Cancer Center Resources. Contains information on different types of cancer and answers to frequently asked questions.
> http://www.oncolink.org

See also the listings in Chapters 10–14.

Selected Bibliography

Abbasi, N. R., et al. 2004. Early diagnosis of cutaneous melanoma. *Journal of the American Medical Association* 292(22): 2771–2776.

American Cancer Society. 2005. *Cancer Facts and Figures, 2005.* Atlanta: American Cancer Society.

Beral, V., E. Banks, and G. Reeves. 2002. Evidence from randomized trials on the long-term effects of hormone replacement therapy. *Lancet* 360(9337): 942–944.

Bjorge, T., S. Tretli, and A. Engeland. 2004. Relation of height and body mass index to renal cell carcinoma in two million Norwegian men and women. *American Journal of Epidemiology* 160(12): 1168–1176.

Brenner, D. J., et al. 2004. Estimated radiation risks potentially associated with full-body CT screening. *Radiology* 232(3): 735–738.

Calle, E. E., et al. 2003. Overweight, obesity, and mortality from cancer in a prospectively studied cohort of U.S. adults. *New England Journal of Medicine* 348: 1625–1638.

Carretero Pelaez, M. A., et al. 2004. Alcohol-containing mouthwashes and oral cancer. Critical Analysis of Literature. *Medicina Oral* 9(2): 120–123, 116–120.

Chao, A., et al. 2005. Meat consumption and risk of colorectal cancer. *Journal of the American Medical Association* 293(2): 172–182.

Chia, K. S., et al. 2005. Profound changes in breast cancer incidence may reflect changes into a Westernized lifestyle: A comparative population-based study in Singapore and Sweden. *International Journal of Cancer* . 113(2): 302–306.

de Vries, S. H., et al. 2004. Prostate cancer characteristics and prostate specific antigen changes in screening detected patients initially treated with a watchful waiting policy. *Journal of Urology* 172(6 Pt 1): 2193–2196.

Dorn, J., et al. 2003. Lifetime physical activity and breast cancer risk in pre- and postmenopausal women. *Medicine and Science in Sports and Exercise* 35(2): 278–285.

Elmore, J. G., et al. 2005. Screening for breast cancer. *Journal of the American Medical Association* 293(10): 1245–1256.

Flood, A., et al. 2005. Calcium from diet and supplements is associated with reduced risk of colorectal cancer in a prospective cohort of women. *Cancer Epidemiology, Biomarkers and Prevention* 14(1): 126–132.

Food and Agriculture Organization and World Health Organization. 2005. *Joint FAO/WHO Expert Committee on Food Additives: Summary and Conclusions* (http://www.who.int/ipcs/food/jecfa/summaries/en; retrieved March 29, 2005).

Fung, T., et al. 2003. Major dietary patterns and the risk of colorectal cancer in women. *Archives of Internal Medicine* 163(3): 309–314.

Genetics and breast cancer. 2004. *Journal of the American Medical Association* 292(4): 522.

Goff, B. A., et al. 2004. Frequency of symptoms of ovarian cancer in women presenting to primary care clinics. *Journal of the American Medical Association* 291(22): 2705–2712.

Harper, D. M., et al. 2004. Efficacy of a bivalent L1 virus-like particle vaccine in prevention of infection with human papillomavirus types 16 and 18 in young women: A randomised controlled trial. *Lancet* 364(9447): 1757–1765.

Hou, L., et al. 2004. Computing physical activity and risk of colon cancer in Shanghai, China. *American Journal of Epidemiology* 160(9): 860–867.

Jee, S. H., et al. 2005. Fasting serum glucose level and cancer risk in Korean men and women. *Journal of the American Medical Association* 293(2): 194–202.

Jemal, A., et al. 2005. Cancer Statistics, 2005. *CA: A Cancer Journal for Clinicians* 55(1): 10–30.

Karagas, M. R., et al. 2002. Use of tanning devices and risk of basal cell and squamous cell skin cancers. *Journal of the National Cancer Institute* 94(3): 224–226.

Knight, J. M., et al. 2002. Awareness of the risks of tanning lamps does not influence behavior among college students. *Archives of Dermatology* 138(10): 1311–1315.

Koutsky, L. A., et al. 2002. A controlled trial of a human papillomavirus type 16 vaccine. *New England Journal of Medicine* 347(12): 1645–1651.

Kroenke, C. H., et al. 2005. Weight, weight gain, and survival after breast cancer diagnosis. *Journal of Clinical Oncology* 23(7): 1370–1378.

Laaksonen, D. E., et al. 2004. Serum linoleic and total polyunsaturated fatty acids in relation to prostate and other cancers: A population-based cohort study. *International Journal of Cancer* 111(3): 444–450.

Li, C. I., K. E. Malone, and J. R. Daling. 2003. Differences in breast cancer stage, treatment, and survival by race and ethnicity. *Archives of Internal Medicine* 163(1): 49–56.

Martinez, M. E. 2005. Primary prevention of colorectal cancer: Lifestyle, nutrition, exercise. *Recent Results in Cancer Research* 166: 177–211.

Meadows, M. 2004. Cancer vaccines: Training the immune system to fight cancer. *FDA Consumer,* September/October.

Melanoma. 2004. *Journal of the American Medical Association* 292(22): 2800.

Mor, G., et al. 2005. Serum protein markers for early detection of ovarian cancer. *Proceedings of the National Academy of Sciences USA,* epub May 12.

Mucci, L. A., et al. 2003. Dietary acrylamide and cancer of the large bowel, kidney, and bladder: Absence of an association in a population-based study in Sweden. *British Journal of Cancer* 88(1): 84–89.

National Toxicology Program. 2005. *Report on Carcinogens,* Eleventh Edition. Research Triangle Park, N. C.: National Toxicology Program.

New treatments for colorectal cancer. 2004. *FDA Consumer,* May/June.

Osborn, N. K., and D. A. Ahlquist. 2005. Stool screening for colorectal cancer: Molecular approaches. *Gastroenterology* 128(1): 192–206.

Paik, S., et al. 2004. A multigene assay to predict recurrence of tamoxifen-treated, node-negative breast cancer. *New England Journal of Medicine* 351(27): 2817–2826.

Pelucchi, C., et al. 2004. Fibre intake and prostate cancer risk. *International Journal of Cancer* 109(2): 278–280.

Prostate cancer: Should you still have a PSA test? 2005. *University of California, Berkeley Wellness Letter,* January.

Rigel, E. G., et al. 2003. Ultraviolet radiation in alpine skiing: Magnitude of exposure and importance of regular protection. *Archives of Dermatology* 139(1): 60–62.

Roden, R. B., et al. 2004. Vaccination to prevent and treat cervical cancer. *Human Pathology* 35(8): 971–982.

Seeff, L. C., et al. 2004. How many endoscopies are performed for colorectal cancer screening? Results from CDC's survey of endoscopic capacity. *Gastroenterology* 127(6): 1670–1677.

Terry, M. B., et al. 2004. Association of frequency and duration of aspirin use and hormone receptor status with breast cancer risk. *Journal of the American Medical Association* 291(20): 2433–2440.

Thompson, I. M., et al. 2004. Prevalence of prostate cancer among men with prostate-specific antigen level < or =4.0 ng per milliliter. *New England Journal of Medicine* 350(22): 2239–2246.

Trimble, C. L., et al. 2005. Active and passive cigarette smoking and the risk of cervical neoplasia. *Obstetrics and Gynecology* 105(1): 174–181.

Van Gils, C. H., et al. 2005. Consumption of vegetables and fruits and risk of breast cancer. *Journal of the American Medical Association* 293(3): 183–193.

Velicer, C. M., et al. 2004. Antibiotic use in relation to the risk of breast cancer. *Journal of the American Medical Association* 291(7): 827–835.

Weinstein, S. J., et al. 2005. Serum alpha-tocopherol and gamma-tocopherol in relation to prostate cancer risk in a prospective study. *Journal of the National Cancer Institute* 97(5): 396–399.

World Health Organization. 2005. *Cancer: Diet and Physical Activity's Impact* (http://www.who.int/dietphysicalactivity/publications/facts/cancer/en/; retrieved January 20, 2005).

17

Looking AHEAD

After reading this chapter, you should be able to

- Describe the step-by-step process by which infectious diseases are transmitted

- List the body's physical and chemical barriers to infection

- Explain how the immune system responds to an invading microorganism

- List the major types of pathogens and describe the common diseases they cause

- Discuss steps you can take to prevent infections and strengthen your immune system

Immunity and Infection

Test Your

Knowledge

1. **A person with an infectious disease is not contagious unless he or she exhibits symptoms.**
   True or false?

2. **First-year college students, particularly those who live in dormitories or residence halls, are at moderately increased risk for contracting meningitis compared with others their age.**
   True or false?

3. **When taking a prescription antibiotic, you should stop taking the medicine as soon as your infection clears up.**
   True or false?

4. **Which of the following is most likely to increase your risk of catching a cold?**
   a. getting chilled or overheated
   b. talking to someone who may have a cold
   c. shaking hands with someone who may have a cold

5. **Because of widespread vaccination, few people now die from vaccine-preventable diseases.**
   True or false?

6. **You can lower your chances of getting sick by doing which of the following?**
   a. washing your hands frequently
   b. obtaining all recommended immunizations
   c. getting adequate sleep

ANSWERS

1. FALSE. A person can be contagious before exhibiting any symptoms and may cease to be contagious before symptoms disappear.

2. TRUE. The Centers for Disease Control and Prevention recommend the meningococcal vaccine for first-year college students living in dormitories and others at risk.

3. FALSE. More than 50% of people fail to take all their medication, leading to relapses and the development of antibiotic-resistant bacteria.

4. C. Most cold viruses are transmitted through hand-to-hand contact; frequent, thorough hand washing can decrease the risk of contracting a cold.

5. FALSE. Vaccine-preventable diseases kill 30,000 Americans each year. Worldwide, nearly 2 million children die of vaccine-preventable diseases each year; a child dies of measles every minute.

6. ALL THREE. Frequent hand washing prevents the transmission of many disease-causing agents. Immunizations prime the body to tackle an invading organism; adequate sleep helps support a healthy immune system.

W W Visit the *Core Concepts in Health* Online Learning Center (www.mhhe.com/insel10e) for study aids and many additional resources.

515

Most of the time, we go about our daily lives thinking of the world as a place inhabited by beings more or less like ourselves. We seldom think of the countless unseen microscopic organisms that live around, on, and in us. Although most microbes are beneficial, many of them can cause human disease. But the constant vigilance of our immune system keeps them at bay and our bodies intact and healthy.

Even without these "invaders," our bodies have a tendency to develop problems and diseases. The natural aging process of the human body is a prime example of the second law of thermodynamics: that all things have a tendency toward disorder or disintegration. The immune system works to keep the body from being overwhelmed not just by external invaders that cause **infections**, but also by internal changes such as cancer.

Most people don't pay much attention to these internal skirmishes unless they become sick and find themselves deprived of their usual feelings of well-being. But many people today are more knowledgeable about the complexities of immunity because they have heard about, or had experience with, HIV infection, which directly attacks the immune system. This chapter provides information that will help you understand immunity, infection, and how to keep yourself well in a world of disease-causing microorganisms.

THE CHAIN OF INFECTION

Infectious diseases are transmitted from one person to another through a series of steps—a chain of infection (Figure 17-1). New infections can be prevented by interfering with any of the steps in this process.

Links in the Chain

The chain of infection has six major links: the pathogen, its reservoir, a portal of exit, a means of transmission, a portal of entry, and a new host.

Terms

V i w

infection Invasion of the body by a microorganism.

pathogen An organism that causes disease.

toxin A poisonous substance produced by a microorganism.

vector An insect, rodent, or other organism that carries and transmits a pathogen from one host to another.

lymphatic system A system of vessels and organs that picks up excess fluid, proteins, lipids, and other substances from the tissues; filters out pathogens and other waste products; and returns the cleansed fluid to the general circulation.

systemic infection An infection spread by the blood or lymphatic system to large portions of the body.

Pathogen The infectious disease cycle begins with a **pathogen**, a microorganism that causes disease. HIV, the virus that causes AIDS, and the tuberculosis bacterium are examples of pathogens. Many pathogens cause illness because they produce **toxins** that harm human tissue; others do so by directly invading body cells.

Reservoir The pathogen has a natural environment in which it typically resides. This reservoir can be a person, an animal, or an environmental component like soil or water. A person who is the reservoir for a pathogen may be ill or may be an asymptomatic carrier who, although having no symptoms, is capable of spreading infection.

Portal of Exit To transmit infection, the pathogen must leave the reservoir through some portal of exit. In the case of a human reservoir, portals of exit include saliva (for mumps, for example), the mucous membranes (for many sexually transmitted diseases), blood (for HIV and hepatitis), feces (for intestinal infections), and nose and throat discharges (for colds and influenza).

Means of Transmission Transmission can occur directly or indirectly. In direct transmission, the pathogen is passed from one person to another without an intermediate component. Direct transmission usually requires fairly close association with an infected host, but not necessarily physical contact. For example, sneezing and coughing can discharge infectious particles into the air, where they can be inhaled by someone nearby. Most common respiratory infections are passed directly: A person with a cold blows her nose and gets some infectious droplets on her hands; she then shakes hands with someone, who later touches his nose and passes the pathogen into his own body. Many intestinal infections are also transmitted hand-to-hand; the initial contamination may result from a failure to wash hands after using the toilet or changing a diaper. Other means of direct transmission include sexual contact and contact with blood.

Transmission can also occur indirectly. Animals or insects such as rats, ticks, and mosquitoes can serve as **vectors**, carrying the pathogen from one host to another. Pathogens can also be transmitted via contaminated soil, food, or water or from inanimate objects, such as eating utensils, doorknobs, and handkerchiefs. Some pathogens float in the air for long periods, suspended on tiny particles of dust or droplets that can travel long distances before they are inhaled and cause infection.

Portal of Entry To infect a new host, a pathogen must have a portal of entry into the body. Pathogens can enter in one of three general ways:

1. Penetration of the skin or direct contact.
2. Inhalation through the mouth or nose.
3. Ingestion of contaminated food or water.

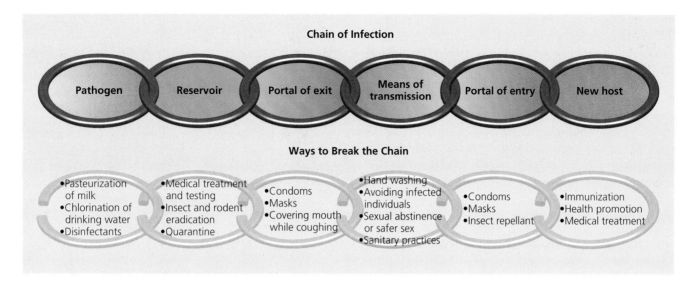

Figure 17-1 The chain of infection. Any break in the chain of infection can prevent disease.

Pathogens that enter the skin or mucous membranes can cause a local infection of the tissue, or they may penetrate into the bloodstream or **lymphatic system,** thereby causing a more extensive **systemic infection.** Agents that cause STDs usually enter the body through the mucous membranes lining the urethra (in males) or the cervix (in females). Organisms that are transmitted via respiratory secretions may cause upper respiratory infections or pneumonia, or they may enter the bloodstream and cause systemic infection. Foodborne and waterborne organisms enter the mouth and travel to the location that will best support their reproduction. They may attack the cells of the small intestine or the colon, causing diarrhea, or they may enter the bloodstream via the digestive system and travel to other parts of the body.

The New Host Once in the new host, a variety of factors determine whether the pathogen will be able to establish itself and cause infection. People with a strong immune system or resistance to a particular pathogen will be less likely to become ill than people with poor immunity (the concept of immunity will be discussed later in the chapter). The number of pathogens that enter the new host is also important; the body's defenses may be able to overcome a few bacteria, for example, but may be overwhelmed by thousands. If conditions are right, the pathogen will multiply and produce disease in the new host. In such a case, the new host may become a reservoir from which a new chain of infection can be started.

Breaking the Chain

Interruption of the chain of infection at any point can prevent disease. Strategies for breaking the chain include a mix of public health measures and individual action. For example, a pathogen's reservoir can be isolated or destroyed, as when a sick individual is placed under quarantine or when insects or animals carrying pathogens are killed. Public sanitation practices, such as sewage treatment and the chlorination of drinking water, can also kill pathogens. Transmission can be disrupted through strategies like hand washing and the use of facemasks. Immunization and the treatment of infected hosts can stop the pathogen from multiplying, producing a serious disease, and being passed on to a new host. Some methods of breaking the chain of infection are given in Figure 17-1.

THE BODY'S DEFENSE SYSTEM

Our bodies have very effective ways of protecting themselves against invasion by foreign organisms, especially pathogens. The body's first line of defense is a formidable array of physical and chemical barriers. When these barriers are breached, the body's immune system comes into play. Together, these defenses provide an effective response to nearly all the challenges and invasions our bodies will ever experience.

Physical and Chemical Barriers

The skin, the body's largest organ, prevents many microorganisms from entering the body. Although many bacterial and fungal organisms live on the surface of the skin, very few can penetrate it except through a cut or break. Wherever there is an opening in the body, or an area without skin, other barriers exist. The mouth, the main entry to the gastrointestinal system, is lined with mucous membranes, which contain cells designed to prevent the passage of unwanted organisms and particles. Body openings and the fluids that cover them (for example, tears, saliva, and vaginal secretions) are rich in antibodies (discussed in detail later in the chapter) and in enzymes that break down and destroy many microorganisms.

The respiratory tract is lined not only with mucous membranes but also with cells having hairlike protrusions called cilia. The cilia sweep foreign matter up and out of the respiratory tract. Particles that are not caught by this mechanism may be expelled from the system by a cough. If the ciliated cells are damaged or destroyed, a cough is the body's only way of ridding the airways of foreign particles. This is one reason smokers generally have a chronic cough—to compensate for damaged airways.

The Immune System

Once the body has been invaded by a foreign organism, an elaborate system of responses is activated. The immune system operates through a remarkable information network involving billions of cellular defenders who rush to protect the body when a threat arises. We discuss here two of the body's responses: the inflammatory response and the immune response. But before we cover these specific defenses, we briefly describe the defenders themselves and the mechanisms by which they work.

Immunological Defenders The immune response is carried out by different types of white blood cells, all of which are continuously being produced in the bone marrow. **Neutrophils,** one type of white blood cell, travel in the bloodstream to areas of invasion, attacking and ingesting pathogens. **Macrophages,** or "big eaters," take up stations in tissues and act as scavengers, devouring pathogens and worn-out cells. **Natural killer cells** directly destroy virus-infected cells and cells that have turned cancerous. **Dendritic cells,** which reside in tissues, eat pathogens and activate lymphocytes. **Lymphocytes,** of which there are several types, are white blood cells that travel in both the bloodstream and the lymphatic system. At various places in the lymphatic system there are lymph nodes (or glands), where macrophages and dendritic cells congregate and filter bacteria and other substances from the lymph (Figure 17-2). When these nodes are actively involved in fighting an invasion of microorganisms, they fill with cells; physicians use the location of swollen lymph nodes as a clue to the location and cause of an infection.

The two main types of lymphocytes are known as **T cells** and **B cells.** T cells are further differentiated into **helper T cells, killer T cells,** and **suppressor T cells.** B cells are lymphocytes that produce **antibodies.** The first time T cells and B cells encounter a specific invader, some of them are reserved as **memory T and B cells,** enabling the body to mount a rapid response should the same invader appear again in the future. These cells and cell products—macrophages, natural killer cells, dendritic cells, T cells, B cells and antibodies, and memory cells—are the primary players in the body's immune response.

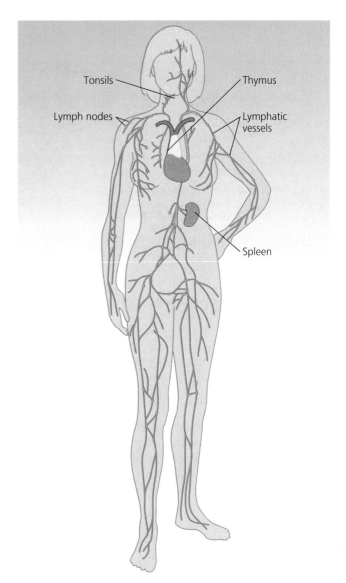

Figure 17-2 The lymphatic system. The lymphatic system consists of a network of vessels and organs, including the spleen, lymph nodes, thymus, and tonsils. The vessels pick up excess fluid and proteins, lipids, and other particles from body tissues. These pass through the lymph nodes, where macrophages and dendritic cells help clear the lymph (fluid) of debris and bacteria and other pathogens. The cleansed lymph is then returned to the bloodstream. The lymphatic organs are production centers for infection-fighting cells and sites for some immune responses.

The immune system is built on a remarkable feature of these defenders: the ability to distinguish foreign cells from the body's own cells. Because lymphocytes are capable of great destruction, it is essential that they not attack the body itself. When they do, they cause **autoimmune diseases,** such as lupus and rheumatoid arthritis.

How do lymphocytes know when they have encountered foreign substances? All the cells of an individual's body display markers on their surfaces—tiny molecular shapes—that identify them as "self" to lymphocytes that encounter them. Invading microorganisms also display markers on their surface; lymphocytes identify these as foreign, or "nonself." Nonself markers that trigger the immune response are known as **antigens.**

Antibodies have complementary surface markers that work with antigens like a lock and key. When an antigen appears in the body, it eventually encounters an antibody with a complementary pattern; the antibody locks onto the antigen, triggering a series of events designed to destroy the invading pathogen. The truly astonishing thing is that the body does not synthesize the appropriate antibody lock after it comes into contact with the antigen key. Rather, antibodies already exist for millions, if not billions, of possible antigens.

The Inflammatory Response When the body has been injured or infected, one of the body's responses is the inflammatory response. Special cells in the area of invasion or injury release **histamine** and other substances that cause blood vessels to dilate and fluid to flow out of capillaries into the injured tissue. This produces increased heat, swelling, and redness in the affected area. White blood cells, including neutrophils, dendritic cells, and macrophages, are drawn to the area and attack the invaders—in many cases, destroying them. At the site of infection there may be pus, a collection of dead white blood cells and debris resulting from the encounter.

The Immune Response The immune system makes two types of responses to invading pathogens: natural (innate) and acquired (adaptive). Neutrophils, macrophages, dendritic cells, and natural killer cells are part of the natural response. They recognize pathogens as "foreign" but have no memory of past infections; they respond the same way no matter how many times a pathogen invades. These cells essentially eat the invaders, destroying them internally. Natural killer cells also destroy infected body cells, breaking the chain of reproduction of a pathogen and helping to stop an infection. T and B cells are part of the acquired response. They change after one contact with the pathogen, developing a memory for the antigen. If the body is invaded again, they recognize the pathogen and mount a much more potent response.

For convenience, we can think of the immune response as having four phases: (1) recognition of the invading pathogen, (2) amplification of defenses, (3) attack, and (4) slowdown (Figure 17-3, p. 520). In each phase, crucial actions occur that are designed to destroy the invader and restore the body to health.

• *Phase 1.* Dendritic cells are drawn to the site of the injury and consume the foreign cells; they then provide information about the pathogen by displaying its antigen on their surfaces. Helper T cells read this information and rush to respond.

• *Phase 2.* Helper T cells multiply rapidly and trigger the production of killer T cells and B cells in the

spleen and lymph nodes. **Cytokines,** chemical messengers secreted by lymphocytes, help regulate and coordinate the immune response; *interleukins* and *interferons* are two examples of cytokines. They stimulate increased production of T cells, B cells, and antibodies; promote the activities of natural killer cells; produce fever; and have special antipathogenic properties themselves.

• *Phase 3.* Killer T cells strike at foreign cells and body cells that have been invaded and infected, identifying them by the antigens displayed on the cell surfaces. Puncturing the cell membrane, they sacrifice body cells in order to destroy the foreign organism within. This type of action is known as a *cell-mediated immune response,* because the attack is carried out by cells. Killer T cells also trigger an amplified inflammatory response and recruit more macrophages to help clean up the site.

Terms Review

neutrophil A type of white blood cell that engulfs foreign organisms and infected, damaged, or aged cells; particularly prevalent during the inflammatory response.

macrophage A large phagocytic (cell-eating) cell that devours foreign particles.

natural killer cell A type of white blood cell that directly destroys virus-infected cells and cancer cells.

dendritic cell A white blood cell specialized to activate T and B cells.

lymphocyte A white blood cell continuously made in lymphoid tissue as well as in bone marrow.

T cell A lymphocyte that arises in bone marrow and matures in the thymus (thus its name).

B cell A lymphocyte that matures in the bone marrow and produces antibodies.

helper T cell A lymphocyte that helps activate other T cells and may help B cells produce antibodies.

killer T cell A lymphocyte that kills body cells that have been invaded by foreign organisms; also can kill cells that have turned cancerous.

suppressor T cell A lymphocyte that inhibits the growth of other lymphocytes.

antibody A specialized protein, produced by white blood cells, that can recognize and neutralize specific microbes.

memory T and B cells Lymphocytes generated during an initial infection that circulate in the body for years, remembering the specific antigens that caused the infection and quickly destroying them if they appear again.

autoimmune disease A disease in which the immune system attacks the person's own body.

antigen A marker on the surface of a foreign substance that immune system cells recognize as nonself and that triggers the immune response.

histamine A chemical responsible for the dilation and increased permeability of blood vessels in allergic reactions.

cytokine A chemical messenger produced by a variety of cell types that helps regulate many cell functions; immune system cells release cytokines that help amplify and coordinate the immune response.

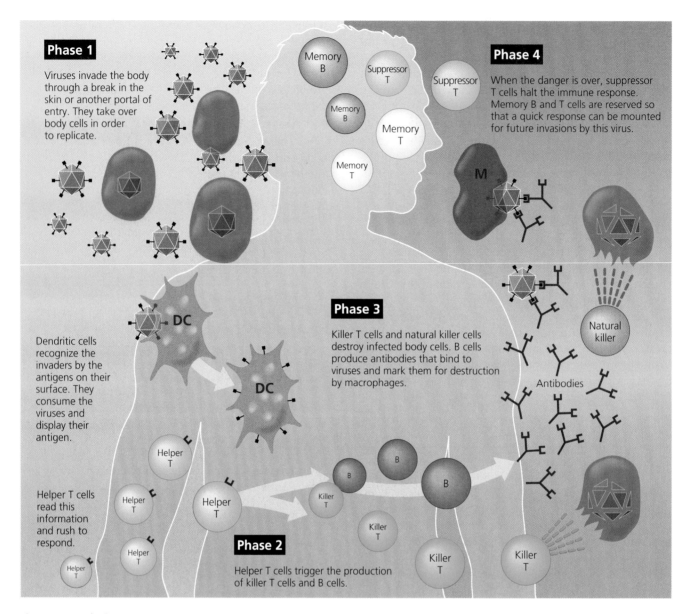

Phase 1

Viruses invade the body through a break in the skin or another portal of entry. They take over body cells in order to replicate.

Memory B

Suppressor T

Memory B

Memory T

Memory T

Phase 4

Suppressor T

When the danger is over, suppressor T cells halt the immune response. Memory B and T cells are reserved so that a quick response can be mounted for future invasions by this virus.

M

Dendritic cells recognize the invaders by the antigens on their surface. They consume the viruses and display their antigen.

Helper T cells read this information and rush to respond.

DC

DC

Phase 3

Killer T cells and natural killer cells destroy infected body cells. B cells produce antibodies that bind to viruses and mark them for destruction by macrophages.

Natural killer

Antibodies

Helper T

Helper T

Helper T

Helper T

Helper T

Killer T

B

B

B

Killer T

Killer T

Killer T

Killer T

Phase 2

Helper T cells trigger the production of killer T cells and B cells.

Figure 17-3   The immune response.   Once invaded by a pathogen, the body mounts a complex series of reactions to eliminate the invader. Pictured here are the principal elements of the immune response to a virus; not shown are the many types of cytokines that help coordinate the actions of different types of defenders.

B cells work in a different way. Stimulated to multiply by helper T cells, they produce large quantities of antibody molecules, which are released in the bloodstream and tissues. Antibodies are Y-shaped protein molecules that bind to antigen-bearing targets and mark them for destruction by macrophages. This type of response is known as an *antibody-mediated immune response.* Antibodies work against bacteria and against viruses and other substances when they are in the body but outside cells. They do not work against infected body cells or viruses that are replicating inside cells.

• *Phase 4.* The last phase of the immune response is a slowdown of activity. When the danger is over, suppressor

T cells halt the immune response and restore homeostasis, or stability. The dead cells, killed pathogens, and other debris that result from the immune response are scavenged by certain types of white blood cells; filtered out of circulation by the liver, spleen, and kidneys; and excreted from the body.

Immunity   After an infection, survival often confers **immunity;** that is, an infected person will never get the same illness again. This is because some of the lymphocytes created during the amplification phase of the immune response are reserved as memory T and B cells. As part of the acquired immune response, they continue to

Dendritic cells are white blood cells that engulf foreign cells and display their antigens, thereby activating T and B cells. The dendritic cell shown in this scanning electron micrograph is magnified 2700 times.

circulate in the blood and lymphatic system for years or even for the rest of the person's life. If the same antigen enters the body again, the memory T and B cells recognize and destroy it before it can cause illness. This subsequent response takes only a day or two, whereas the original response lasted several days, during which time the individual suffered the symptoms of illness. The ability of memory lymphocytes to remember previous infections is known as **acquired immunity.**

Symptoms and Contagion   The immune system is operating at the cellular level at all times, maintaining its vigilance when you're well and fighting invaders when you're sick. How does it all feel to you, the host for these activities? How do your symptoms relate to the course of the infection and the immune response?

During **incubation,** when viruses are multiplying in the body or when bacteria are actively multiplying before the immune system has gathered momentum, you may not have any symptoms of the illness, but you may be contagious. During the second and third phases of the immune response, you may still be unaware of the infection, or you may "feel a cold coming on." Symptoms first appear during the **prodromal period,** which follows incubation. If the infected host has acquired immunity, the infection may be eradicated during the incubation period or the prodromal period. In this case, although you may have felt you were coming down with a cold, for example, it does not develop into a full-blown illness.

Many symptoms of an illness are actually due to the immune response of the body rather than to the actions or products of the invading organism. For example, fever is caused by the release and activation of certain cytokines in macrophages and other cells during the immune response. These cytokines travel in the bloodstream to the brain and cause the body's thermostat to be reset to a higher level. The resulting elevated temperature helps the body in its fight against pathogens by enhancing immune responses. (During an illness, it is necessary to lower a fever only if it is uncomfortably high [over 101.5°F] or if it occurs in an infant who is at risk for seizures from fever.)

Similarly, you get a runny nose when your lymphocytes destroy infected mucosal cells, leading to increased mucus production. You get a sore throat when your lymphocytes destroy infected throat cells, and the malaise and fatigue of the flu may be caused by interferons.

You are contagious when there are infectious microbes in your body and they can gain access to another person. This may be before a vigorous immune response has occurred, so at times you may be contagious before experiencing any symptoms. This means that you can transmit an illness without knowing you're infected or catch an illness from someone who doesn't appear to be sick. On the other hand, your symptoms may continue after the pathogens have been mostly destroyed, when you are no longer infectious.

Immunization

The ability of the immune system to remember previously encountered organisms and retain its strength against them is the basis for immunization. When a person is immunized, the immune system is primed with an antigen similar to the pathogenic organism but not as dangerous. The body responds by producing antibodies, which prevent serious infection when and if the person is exposed to the disease organism itself. These preparations used to manipulate the immune system are known as **vaccines** (Table 17-1, p. 522).

Terms
Vw

immunity Mechanisms that defend the body against infection; specific defenses against specific pathogens.

acquired immunity The body's ability to mobilize the cellular memory of an attack by a pathogen to throw off subsequent attacks; acquired through vaccination as well as the normal immune response.

incubation The period when bacteria or viruses are actively multiplying inside the body's cells; usually a period without symptoms of illness.

prodromal period The stage of an infection, following incubation, during which initial symptoms begin to appear but the host does not feel ill; a highly contagious period.

vaccine A preparation of killed or weakened microorganisms, inactivated toxins, or components of microorganisms that is administered to stimulate an immune response; a vaccine protects against future infection by the pathogen.

Table 17-1 Immunizations for Children and Adults

Vaccine	People for Whom Immunization Is Recommended
Diphtheria	All children; adults need boosters every 10 years
H. influenzae type b (Hib)	All children (protects against meningitis)
Hepatitis A	Children in selected states and regions; injection drug users, men who have sex with men, people with chronic hepatitis, and others at risk
Hepatitis B	All children and unvaccinated adolescents; adults at risk, including health care workers, household contacts and sex partners of infected people, injection drug users, and people with STDs
Influenza	Annual vaccination for adults age 50 and older; nursing home residents; anyone with heart, lung, or other chronic disorders (including asthma and diabetes) and others at high risk; women who will be in the second or third trimester of pregnancy during the influenza season; children age 6–23 months; anyone over age 6 months who wishes to reduce risk of influenza
Measles and mumps	All children; unvaccinated adults born after 1956 who are not immune (those who received only one dose or were vaccinated between 1963 and 1967 may need revaccination)
Meningococcal conjugate	All children at age 11–12 years or at high-school entry, first-year college students living in dormitories, military recruits, and others at increased risk.
Pertussis (whooping cough)	All children; booster shots may be recommended for adolescents
Pneumococcal polysaccharide	Adults age 65 and older; anyone with chronic heart or lung disease or with no functional spleen; others at high risk, including Alaska Natives and certain American Indian groups
Pneumococcal conjugate	All children
Polio	All children; adults at risk, including certain laboratory and health care workers
Rabies	Anyone at risk from a bite, scratch, or mucous membrane exposure to a potentially rabid animal or from any direct contact with a bat (unless the person can be certain that exposure did not occur); people who work with animals may need preexposure immunization
Rubella (German measles)	All children; unvaccinated adults who are not immune, especially women
Tetanus (lockjaw)	All children; adults need boosters every 10 years (sooner if more than 5 years has elapsed since the previous booster and the individual has a contaminated wound)
Varicella (chicken pox)	Children over age 12 months; unvaccinated adolescents and adults who have not had varicella, especially health care workers and others at high risk for exposure

For international travelers, the CDC recommends that all standard childhood immunizations be up to date and that additional vaccines such as hepatitis A and influenza be considered. Travelers to areas where certain diseases are common may need others, including vaccines for yellow fever, typhoid fever, meningococcal meningitis, and Japanese or tickborne encephalitis; a one-time polio booster may also be given. Further information about immunization is available from the CDC's National Immunization Program (800-232-2522; http://www.cdc.gov/nip) and the CDC's Travel Information (877-394-8747; http://www.cdc.gov/travel).

SOURCES: National Immunization Program. 2005. *ACIP Recommends Meningococcal Vaccine for Adolescents and College Freshmen* (http://www.cdc. gov/nip/vaccine/meningitis/mcv4/mcv4_acip.htm; retrieved April 6, 2005). Centers for Disease Control and Prevention. 2005. Recommended childhood and adolescent immunization schedule. *Morbidity and Mortality Weekly Report* 53(51–52): Q1–Q4; Centers for Disease Control and Prevention. 2004. Recommended adult immunization schedule. *Morbidity and Mortality Weekly Report* 53(45): Q1–Q4; Centers for Disease Control and Prevention. 1999. Human rabies prevention—Recommendations of the Advisory Committee on Immunization Practices. *MMWR Recommendations and Reports* 48(RR-1).

Types of Vaccines Vaccines can be made in several ways. In some cases, microbes are cultured in the laboratory in a way that attenuates (weakens) them. These live, attenuated organisms are used in vaccines against diseases such as measles, mumps, and rubella (German measles). In other cases, when it is not possible to breed attenuated organisms, vaccines are made from pathogens that have been killed in the laboratory but that still retain their ability to stimulate the production of antibodies. Vaccines composed of killed viruses are used against influenza viruses, among others.

Vaccines confer what is known as *active immunity*—that is, the vaccinated person produces his or her own antibodies to the microorganism. Another type of injection confers *passive immunity*. In this case, a person exposed to a disease is injected with the antibodies themselves, produced by other human beings or animals who have recovered from the disease. Injections of gamma globulin—a product made from the blood plasma of many individuals containing all the antibodies they have ever made—are sometimes given to people exposed to a disease against which they have not been immunized. Such injections create a rapid but temporary immunity and are useful against certain viruses, such as hepatitis A. Gamma globulin is also sometimes used to treat antibody deficiency syndromes.

Immunization Issues   Potential shortages and safety issues are areas of concern related to vaccines.

VACCINE SHORTAGES IN THE UNITED STATES   The shortage of influenza vaccine during the winter flu season of 2004–2005 made headlines, but it was not the only recent shortage. There have been temporary shortages of most childhood vaccines in the past 5 years. Contributing factors include insufficient vaccine stockpiles, manufacturing and production problems, and the limited number of companies involved in vaccine production. Vaccines are expensive to develop and produce and have high liability and relatively low profits. The influenza vaccine, which must be changed each year to match the viral strains in circulation and takes months to produce, may be particularly vulnerable to supply problems.

DEATHS FROM VACCINE-PREVENTABLE DISEASES WORLDWIDE
The number of illnesses and deaths from vaccine-preventable diseases are at near record low levels in the United States. But worldwide, more than 4 million people—most of them infants and children in developing countries—die each year from vaccine-preventable diseases. Factors such as unsanitary and crowded living conditions, poor nutritional status, and limited access to health care make a child more likely to acquire infections and become seriously ill. The WHO and other organizations and governments are working to vaccinate as many children as possible. Challenges include not only funding for sufficient vaccine supplies but also overcoming problems related to storage, transportation, and delivery of multiple doses of vaccines. Infection rates around the world highlight the importance of immunization in the United States; if vaccination rates fall, an epidemic of measles or diphtheria may be just one airline passenger away.

VACCINE SAFETY   Side effects from immunization are usually mild, such as soreness at the injection site. It is estimated that an allergic reaction may occur in 1 in 1.5 million doses. Any risk from vaccines must be balanced against of the risk posed by the diseases they prevent; for example, the death rate from diphtheria is about 5–10%. The CDC monitors reports of adverse reactions to vaccines, and new formulations or types of vaccines are being developed to increase safety. For example, oral polio vaccine, which contains live but weakened polio

virus, has been replaced by inactivated polio virus, which contains killed virus. The oral vaccine is somewhat more effective, but in about 1 in 2.4 million cases, it causes polio; because of the low risk for polio in the United States, the oral vaccine is no longer used.

A possible link has also been proposed between immunization and autism, a severe developmental disorder characterized by behavioral problems and impaired social and communication skills. However, a 2004 Institute of Medicine report concluded that evidence does not support such a link. Thimerosol, a mercury-containing preservative, was withdrawn from pediatric vaccines beginning in 1999. Although no clear link has been found between thimerosol-containing vaccines and autism, removing thimerosol from vaccines is an appropriate strategy to reduce children's overall exposure to mercury, a known neurotoxin.

Allergy: The Body's Defense System Gone Haywire

Are you among the estimated 50 million Americans affected by **allergies?** Allergies result from a hypersensitive and overactive immune system. The immune system typically defends the body against only genuinely harmful pathogens such as viruses and bacteria. However, in someone with an allergy, the immune system also mounts a response to a harmless substance such as pollen or animal dander. The unpleasant and potentially serious symptoms of an allergy—stuffy nose, sneezing, wheezing, skin rashes, and so on—result primarily from the immune response rather than from the substances that provoke the response.

Allergens   Substances that provoke allergies are known as **allergens**; they may cause a response if they are inhaled or swallowed or if they come in contact with the skin. Different people have allergic reactions to different substances. Common allergens include the following:

- *Pollen:* Referred to as hay fever or allergic rhinitis, pollen allergies are widespread; weeds, grasses, and trees are common producers of allergenic pollen.
- *Animal dander:* People with animal allergies are usually allergic not to fur but to dander (dead skin flakes), urine, or a protein found in saliva; allergies to mice, dogs, and/or cats are common.
- *Dust mites and cockroaches:* The droppings of cockroaches and microscopic dust mites can trigger

Terms

Vw

allergy   A disorder caused by the body's exaggerated response to foreign chemicals and proteins; also called *hypersensitivity*.

allergen   A substance that triggers an allergic reaction.

During sensitization, allergens such as pollen trigger the production of IgE antibodies, which bind to mast cells.

During an allergic reaction, the allergens enter the bloodstream and are recognized and bound by the IgE antibodies.

The IgE-allergen combination causes mast cells to release histamine and other compounds into surrounding tissue, producing allergy symptoms.

Figure 17-4   The allergic response.

allergies; mites live in carpets, upholstered furniture, and bedding.

- *Molds and mildew:* The small spores produced by these fungi can trigger allergy symptoms; molds and mildew thrive in damp areas of buildings.
- *Foods:* The most common food allergens in adults include peanuts, tree nuts, fish, and shellfish.
- *Insect stings:* The venom of insects such as yellow jackets, honeybees, hornets, paper wasps, and fire ants causes allergic reactions in some people.

People may also be allergic to certain medications, plants such as poison oak, latex, metals such as nickel, and compounds found in cosmetics.

The Allergic Response   Most allergic reactions are due to the production of a special type of antibody known as immunoglobulin E (IgE). Initial exposure to a particular allergen may cause little response, but it sensitizes the immune system by causing the production of allergen-specific IgE, which binds to mast cells (Figure 17-4). When the body is subsequently exposed to the allergen, the allergen binds to IgE, causing the mast cells to release large amounts of histamine and other compounds into surrounding tissues.

Histamine has many effects, including increasing the inflammatory response and stimulating mucus production. The precise symptoms depend on what part of the body is affected. In the nose, histamine may cause congestion and sneezing; in the eyes, itchiness and tearing; in the skin, redness, swelling, and itching; in the intestines, bloating and cramping; and in the lungs, coughing,

wheezing, and shortness of breath. In some people, an allergen can trigger an asthma attack (see the box "Poverty, Ethnicity, and Asthma"). Symptoms often occur immediately, within minutes of exposure, but inflammatory reactions may take hours or days to develop and then may persist for several days.

The most serious, but rare, kind of allergic reaction is **anaphylaxis,** which results from a release of histamine throughout the body. Anaphylactic reactions can be life-threatening because symptoms may include swelling of the throat, extremely low blood pressure, fainting, heart arrhythmia, and seizures. Anaphylaxis is a medical emergency, and treatment requires immediate injection of epinephrine. People at risk for anaphylaxis should wear medical alert identification and keep self-administrable epinephrine readily available.

Dealing with Allergies   If you suspect you might have an allergy, visit your physician or an allergy specialist. You may be asked to keep a diary to help identify allergens to which you are susceptible, or you may undergo allergy skin tests or blood tests. Your physician can help you put together a plan for your condition. There are three general strategies for dealing with allergies:

- *Avoidance:* You may be able to avoid or minimize exposure to allergens by making changes in your environment or behavior. For example, removing carpets from the bedroom and using special bedding can reduce dust mite contact. Pollen exposure can be limited by avoiding outdoor activities during peak pollination times, keeping windows shut, and showering and changing clothes following outdoor activities. If you can't part with a pet, keep pets out of bedrooms and frequently vacuum or damp-mop floors.

- *Medication:* A variety of medications are available for allergy sufferers. Many over-the-counter (OTC) antihistamines are effective at controlling symptoms such as blocked nasal, sinus, or middle ear passages.

Term

V w

anaphylaxis A severe systemic hypersensitive reaction to an allergen characterized by difficulty breathing, low blood pressure, heart arrhythmia, seizure, and sometimes death.

Dimensions of Diversity

Poverty, Ethnicity, and Asthma

What Is Asthma?

The symptoms of asthma—wheezing, tightness in the chest, and shortness of breath—may be mild and occur only occasionally, or they may be severe and occur daily. Asthma is caused by both inflammation of the airways and spasm of the muscles surrounding the airways. The spasm causes constriction, and the inflammation causes the airway linings to swell and secrete extra mucus, which further obstructs the passages. The inflammation can become chronic, making airways even more sensitive to triggers.

An attack begins when something sets off inflammation of the bronchial tubes. Usually it's an allergic reaction to an inhaled allergen, most commonly dust mites, mold, animal dander, or pollen. Anything that irritates or overtaxes the bronchial airways can also trigger spasms: exercise, cold air, pollutants, tobacco smoke, infection, or stress. In female asthmatics, hormonal changes that occur as menstruation starts may increase vulnerability to attacks.

Patterns and Prevalence

Asthma can be disabling and even fatal—and the prevalence of asthma is increasing. In the United States, more than 22 million adults and 8 million children have asthma; each year, asthma is responsible for almost 2 million emergency department visits and more than 4000 deaths. Since 1980, the number of Americans with asthma has more than doubled, and despite better treatment options, the death rate has nearly tripled.

The tendency to develop asthma may be hereditary, but some patterns appear to link it to ethnicity and socioeconomic status. Particularly affected are African Americans, American Indians, and Alaska, Natives; people living in inner cities; children; and people older than age 65. Asian and Pacific Islander Americans have a relatively low incidence of asthma. Poor, inner-city, African American and Latino children are more likely to visit emergency departments due to asthma symptoms and are three times more likely to die from asthma than other groups.

Much of the difference between ethnic groups disappears when poverty is factored in. People with low incomes are more often exposed to underlying risk factors and to attack triggers—higher levels of indoor air pollutants and allergens—in part because they may live in poorly ventilated housing and spend more time indoors. Higher levels of outdoor air pollution are also typically found in poor neighborhoods. Cockroach and mouse allergies are important causes of asthma-related illness among children in inner-city areas.

Treatment and Prevention of Attacks

Inhaling a muscle-relaxing medication from a bronchodilator can relieve an asthma attack immediately by opening the bronchial tubes. Inhaling an anti-inflammatory drug can treat the underlying inflammation. Both types of treatments may be needed to get asthma

under control. Other medications for asthma block the actions of molecules involved in the body's inflammatory response. Asthmatics can monitor their condition by self-testing their peak air flow several times a day; a drop in peak air flow can signal an upcoming attack.

It's also a good idea to avoid allergens when possible. A recent study of urban children found that relatively small changes can reduce asthma symptoms and health care visits. In this study, allergen exposures were reduced by covering the mattresses and pillows with special covers; by using HEPA filters in vacuum cleaners and room air purifiers; and by employing professional pest control. Other researchers have found that many children with asthma live in households in which simple allergen-control methods haven't been taken, including closing windows to keep pollen out, avoiding environmental tobacco smoke, and reducing or eliminating exposure to pets.

SOURCES: Morgan, W. J., et al. 2004. Results of a home-based environmental intervention among urban children with asthma. *New England Journal of Medicine* 351: 1068–1080; Centers for Disease Control and Prevention. 2004. Asthma prevalence and control characteristics by race/ethnicity—United States, 2002. *Morbidity and Mortality Weekly Report* 53(7): 145–148; Cabana, M. D., et al. 2004. Parental management of asthma triggers within a child's environment. *Journal of Allergy and Clinical Immunology* 114(2): 352–357; National Institute of Allergy and Infectious Disease. 2001. *Asthma: A Concern for Minority Populations* (http://www.niaid.nih.gov/factsheets/asthma.htm; retrieved January 31, 2005).

Prescription corticosteroids markedly reduce allergy symptoms, but they have significant side effects, including reduced bone density, if used for long periods. Drug manufacturers have designed aerosol delivery systems for corticosteroids that help limit systemic absorption and side effects.

• *Immunotherapy:* Referred to as "allergy shots," immunotherapy desensitizes a person to a particular allergen through the administration of gradually increasing doses of the allergen over a period of months or years. Allergy symptoms often diminish markedly during the period in which the person receives the injections and sometimes for years afterward.

THE TROUBLEMAKERS: PATHOGENS AND DISEASE

Now that we've discussed the intricate system that protects us from disease, let's consider some pathogens, the disease-producing organisms that live within us and around us. When they succeed in gaining entry to body tissue, they can cause illness and sometimes death to the unfortunate host. Worldwide, infectious diseases are responsible for more than 10 million deaths each year (Table 17-2, p. 526).

Pathogens include bacteria, viruses, fungi, protozoa, parasitic worms, and prions (Figure 17-5, p. 527). Infections

Table 17-2   **Top Infectious Diseases Worldwide**

Disease	Approximate Number of Deaths per Year
Pneumonia	3,884,000
HIV/AIDS	2,777,000
Diarrheal diseases	1,798,000
Tuberculosis	1,566,000
Malaria	1,272,000
Measles	611,000
Pertussis (whooping cough)	294,000
Tetanus	214,000
Meningitis	173,000
Syphilis	157,000

Many of the 618,000 deaths from liver cancer each year can be traced to viral hepatitis. Overall, infectious diseases kill more than 11 million people each year, representing nearly 19% of all deaths.

SOURCE: World Health Organization. 2004. *The World Health Report 2004*. Geneva: World Health Organization.

can occur almost anywhere in or on the body; common types of infection include bronchitis, infection of the airways (bronchi); meningitis, infection of the tissue surrounding the brain and spinal cord; conjunctivitis, infection of the layer of cells surrounding the eyes; pharyngitis, or sore throat; pneumonia, infection of the lung; gastroenteritis, infection of the gastrointestinal tract; cellulitis, infection of the soft tissues; osteomyelitis, infection of the bones; and so on, for every tissue and organ.

Bacteria

The most abundant living things on earth are **bacteria,** single-celled organisms that usually reproduce by splitting in two to create a pair of identical cells. Many species of bacteria feed on dead matter and play an important role in the recycling of nutrients for other organisms; other species feed on living things and may cause disease. Bac-

Terms

V\W

bacterium (plural, bacteria) A microscopic single-celled organism; about 100 bacterial species can cause disease in humans.

pneumonia Inflammation of the lungs, typically caused by infection or exposure to chemical toxins or irritants.

mycoplasma A small bacterium with an incomplete cell wall that may cause sore throats, ear infections, and pneumonia.

meningitis Infection of the meninges (membranes covering the brain and spinal cord).

streptococcus Any of a genus (*Streptococcus*) of spherical bacteria; streptococcal species can cause skin infections, strep throat, rheumatic fever, pneumonia, scarlet fever, and other diseases.

teria are often classified according to their shape: they may be bacilli (rod-shaped), cocci (spherical), spirochete (spiral-shaped), or vibrios (comma-shaped).

We harbor both helpful and harmful bacteria on our skin and in our gastrointestinal and reproductive tracts. The human colon contains friendly bacteria that produce certain vitamins and help digest nutrients. (A large portion of feces consists of bacteria.) Friendly bacteria also keep harmful bacteria in check by competing for food and resources and secreting substances toxic to pathogenic bacteria. For example, *Lactobacillus acidophilus* resides in the vagina and produces chemicals that kill yeast and bacteria that cause vaginal infections.

Not all bacteria found in the body are beneficial, however. If they gain access to the gastrointestinal tract via food or drink, unfriendly bacteria can disrupt the normal harmony in the intestines by invading cells or producing damaging toxins. Sexual activity can introduce pathogenic bacteria into the reproductive tract. Within the bloodstream, tissues, and organs, the human body is usually aseptic—devoid of bacteria. If bacteria find their way into these areas, infection may result. It is here that the immune system keeps up its constant surveillance, seeking out and destroying any invaders. Some bacterial infections of concern are described on the following pages.

Pneumonia   Inflammation of the lungs, called **pneumonia,** may be caused by infection with bacteria, viruses, or fungi or by contact with chemical toxins or irritants. Pneumonia can be serious if the alveoli (air sacs) become clogged with fluid, thus preventing oxygen from reaching the bloodstream. Pneumonia often follows another illness, such as a cold or the flu, but the symptoms are typically more severe—fever, chills, shortness of breath, increased mucus production, and cough. Pneumonia ranks seventh among the leading causes of death for Americans; people most at risk for severe infection include those under age 2 and over age 75 and those with chronic health problems such as heart disease, asthma, or HIV. Bacterial pneumonia can be treated with antibiotics.

Pneumococcus bacteria are the most common cause of bacterial pneumonia; a vaccine is available and recommended for all adults age 65 and older and others at risk. Other bacteria that may cause pneumonia include *Streptococcus pneumoniae, Chlamydia pneumoniae*, and **mycoplasmas.** Outbreaks of infection with mycoplasmas are relatively common among young adults, especially in crowded settings such as dormitories.

Meningitis   Infection of the *meninges*, the membranes covering the brain and spinal cord, is called **meningitis.** Viral meningitis is usually mild and goes away on its own; bacterial meningitis, however, can be life-threatening and requires immediate treatment with antibiotics. Symptoms of meningitis include fever, a severe

Type of Organism	Selected Pathogens	Associated Diseases
Bacteria Microscopic single-celled organisms 	*Bordetella pertussis* *Borrelia burgdorferi* *Chlamydia* *Clostridium tetani* *Helicobacter pylori* *Legionella pneumophila* *Mycobacterium tuberculosis* Mycoplasma *Neisseria* Rickettsia Staphylococcus Streptococcus	Pertussis (whooping cough) Lyme disease Pneumonia (*C. pneumoniae*), chlamydia (*C. trachomatis*) Tetanus Peptic ulcers Legionnaire's disease Tuberculosis Pneumonia, ear infections, sore throat, urethritis Gonorrhea (*N. gonorroeae*), meningitis (*N. meningitidis*) Rocky Mountain spotted fever, typhus Boils and other skin infections, toxic shock syndrome Strep throat, skin infections, pneumonia, rheumatic fever and rheumatic heart disease, necrotizing fasciitis
Viruses Infectious agents consisting of a protein shell enclosing DNA or RNA	Coronavirus, rhinovirus Epstein-Barr virus Hepatitis viruses Herpes simplex 1 and 2 Human immunodeficiency virus Human papillomaviruses Influenza viruses A and B Paramyxovirus Rhabdovirus Togavirus Varicella-zoster	Severe acute respiratory syndrome (SARS), common cold Infectious mononucleosis Hepatitis (inflammation of the liver) Cold sores, genital herpes HIV/AIDS Warts, cervical cancer Flu Measles, mumps Rabies Rubella Chicken pox, shingles
Fungi Single- or multicelled organisms (e.g., yeasts, molds)	*Candida albicans* *Cryptococcus neoformans* Dermatophyte fungi *Histoplasma capsulatum* *Coccidioides immitis*	Yeast infections, thrush Pneumonia, meningitis Athlete's foot, jock itch, ringworm, nail infections Histoplasmosis Coccidioidomycosis
Protozoa Single-celled organisms	*Entamoeba histolytica* *Giardia lamblia* *Plasmodia* *Trichomonas vaginalis* *Trypanosoma brucei*	Amoebic dysentery Giardiasis Malaria Trichomoniasis African sleeping sickness
Parasitic worms Worms that feed and live on or in a host	*Ancylostoma duodenale* *Ascaris lumbricoides* Beef, pork, or fish tapeworms *Enterobius vermicularis* *Necator americanus* Schistosoma	Ancylostomiasis (hookworm infection) Ascariasis (roundworm infection) Tapeworm infection Pinworm infection Hookworm infection Cercarial dermatitis (swimmer's itch), schistosomiasis
Prions Proteinaceous infectious particles	PrP^{Sc}	Creutzfeldt-Jakob disease (CJD)

Figure 17-5   Pathogens and associated infectious diseases.

headache, stiff neck, sensitivity to light, and confusion. Before the 1990s, *Haemophilus influenzae* type b (Hib) was the leading cause of bacterial meningitis, but routine vaccination of children has reduced the occurrence of Hib meningitis. Today, *Neisseria meningitidis* and *Streptococcus pneumoniae* are the leading causes of bacterial meningitis.

In the United States, about 2700 cases of meningitis are reported each year, although the actual number is probably higher. The disease is fatal in 10% of cases, and about 10–20% of people who recover have permanent hearing loss or other serious effects. Worldwide, meningitis kills about 170,000 people each year, particularly in the so-called meningitis belt in sub-Saharan Africa.

A vaccine is available, but it is not effective against all strains of meningitis-causing bacteria. The CDC recommends routine vaccination of children 11–12 years old, previously unvaccinated adolescents at high school entry, and first-year college students who live in dormitories.

Strep Throat and Other Streptococcal Infections   The **streptococcus** bacterium is spherical-shaped and often grows in chains. Streptococcal pharyngitis, or strep throat, is characterized by a red, sore throat with white patches on the tonsils, swollen lymph nodes, fever, and headache. It is typically spread through close contact with an infected person via respiratory droplets (sneezing or coughing). If left untreated, strep throat can develop into the more serious rheumatic fever (see Chapter 15). Other streptococcal infections include scarletina (scarlet fever), characterized by a sore throat, fever, bright red tongue, and a rash over the upper body; impetigo, a superficial skin infection most common among children; and erysipelas, inflammation of skin and underlying tissues.

A particularly virulent type of streptococcus can invade the bloodstream, spread to other parts of the body, and produce dangerous systemic illness. It can also cause a serious but rare infection of the deeper layers of the skin, a condition called necrotizing fasciitis, or "flesh-eating strep." This dangerous infection is characterized by tissue death and is treated with antibiotics and removal of the infected tissue or limb. Other species of streptococci are implicated in pneumonia, endocarditis (infection of the heart lining and valves), and serious infections in pregnant women and newborns.

Toxic Shock Syndrome and Other Staphylococcal Infections
The spherical-shaped **staphylococcus** bacterium often grows in small clusters. It is commonly found on the skin and in the nasal passages of healthy people. Occasionally, staphylococci enter the body and cause an infection, ranging from minor skin infections such as boils to very serious conditions such as blood infections and pneumonia.

A particular species of the bacteria, *Staphylococcus aureus*, is responsible for many cases of **toxic shock syndrome (TSS).** The bacteria produce a deadly toxin that causes shock (potentially life-threatening low blood pressure), high fever, a peeling skin rash, and inflammation of several organ systems. TSS was first diagnosed in women using highly absorbent tampons, which appear to allow the growth of staphylococci; however, about half of all cases occur in men and in women not using tampons. The number of cases of TSS dropped dramatically after a particular type of tampon was discontinued.

Terms

V‿w

staphylococcus Any of a genus (*Staphylococcus*) of spherical, clustered bacteria commonly found on the skin or in the nasal passages; staphylococcal species may enter the body and cause conditions such as boils, pneumonia, and toxic shock syndrome.

toxic shock syndrome (TSS) Sudden onset of fever, aches, vomiting, and peeling rash, followed in some cases by shock and inflammation of multiple organs; often caused by a toxin produced by *Staphylococcus aureus*.

tuberculosis (TB) A chronic bacterial infection that usually affects the lungs.

endemic Persistent and relatively widespread in a given population.

rickettsia A bacterium that can reproduce only inside living cells, transmitted by ticks, fleas, and lice; causes Rocky Mountain spotted fever and typhus.

Tuberculosis
Caused by the rod-shaped bacterium *Mycobacterium tuberculosis*, **tuberculosis (TB)** is a chronic bacterial infection that usually affects the lungs. TB is spread via the respiratory route through prolonged contact with someone who has the disease in its active form. Symptoms include coughing, fatigue, night sweats, weight loss, and fever.

Ten to 15 million Americans have been infected with, and therefore continue to carry, *M. tuberculosis*. However, only about 10% of people with latent TB infections actually develop an active case of the disease during their lifetime. Although their skin tests for TB antibodies register positive, the immune system prevents the disease from becoming active. In the United States, active TB is most common among people infected with HIV, recent immigrants from countries where TB is **endemic,** and those who live in the inner cities. Worldwide, about 2 billion people—one-third of the population—are infected with TB, and each year about 8.4 million develop active TB and more than 1.5 million die.

Many strains of tuberculosis respond to antibiotics, but only over a course of treatment lasting 6–12 months. Failure to complete treatment can lead to relapse and the development of strains of antibiotic-resistant bacteria. The increase in recent years in the number of people with multidrug-resistant TB has alarmed public health officials and led to the development of new strategies to help ensure that infected individuals receive and complete appropriate treatment. A promising new treatment for TB is now undergoing human trials; this new compound eliminates the bacteria in about half the time of standard antibiotics. The worrisome growth of drug-resistant TB is due in part to the long treatment time, as patients may stop taking their medication after they start feeling better but before the bacterium is completely eliminated.

Lyme Disease and Other Tickborne Infections
As described earlier, one method of disease transmission is via insect vectors. Lyme disease is one such infection, and it accounts for more than 95% of all reported vector-borne illness in the United States—more than 23,000 cases per year. It is spread by the bite of a tick of the genus *Ixodes* that is infected with the spiral-shaped bacterium *Borrelia burgdorferi*. Ticks acquire the spirochete by ingesting the blood of an infected animal; they may then transmit the microbe to their next host. The deer tick is responsible for transmitting Lyme disease bacteria to humans in the northeastern and north-central United States; on the Pacific Coast, the culprit is the western black-legged tick. Lyme disease has been reported in 48 states, but significant risk of infection is found in only about 100 counties in 10 states located in the northeastern and mid-Atlantic seaboard, the upper north-central region, and parts of northern California.

Symptoms of Lyme disease vary but typically occur in three stages. In the first stage, about 80% of affected

Take Charge

Avoid Tick Habitat

When possible, avoid areas that are likely to be infested with ticks, particularly in spring and summer, when the immature ticks, called nymphs, are most likely to feed. Ticks favor moist, shaded habitats, especially as provided by leaf litter and low-lying vegetation in wooded, brushy, or overgrown grassy habitats. Don't sit on logs or lean against trees. State and local health departments, park personnel, and agricultural extension services can provide information on the distribution of ticks in your area.

Avoid Mosquitoes

Dawn, dusk, and early evening are times of major mosquito activity, so limit your outdoor activities during these periods or take special care to wear appropriate clothing and use insect repellent. Installing or repairing window and door screens can help keep insects outside. Place mosquito netting over infant carriers when you are outdoors with infants.

Eliminate any standing water near your home to prevent mosquitoes from breeding. Drain or upend containers (flower pots, pet dishes, and so on), change birdbath water weekly, and drill holes in the bottom of containers and tire swings that are left outside. Report dead birds to state and local health departments; birds are particularly susceptible to West Nile virus, and dead ones may indicate local infection.

Wear Protective Clothing and Apply Insect Repellent

Wear light-colored clothing so that insects can be spotted more easily. Wear long-sleeved shirts and tuck pants into socks or the tops of boots to help keep ticks from reaching your skin. Ticks are usually located close to the ground, so wearing high boots may provide additional protection. In 2005, the CDC expanded its list of recommended mosquito repellents to include DEET (n,n-diethyl-m-toluamide), picaridin (KBR 3023), and oil of lemon eucalyptus (PMD); the repellent permethrin can be ap-

plied to clothing but not skin. All repellents should be used carefully and as described on the product label.

Remove Attached Ticks

Transmission of an infectious agent is unlikely to occur until a tick has fed on you for several hours (36 hours in the case of Lyme disease), so daily checks for ticks and their prompt removal will help prevent infection. Search your entire body for ticks, using a handheld or full-length mirror; also check children and pets. Ticks are small; in the nymph phase, they may resemble poppy seeds (see figure).

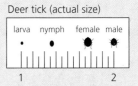

Deer tick (actual size)

To remove a tick, use blunt-tipped tweezers and shield your fingers with rubber gloves or a paper towel. Grasp the tick as close to the skin surface as possible and pull upward (away from the skin) with steady, even pressure. Do not twist or jerk the tick, as this may cause the mouthparts to break off and remain in the skin. If this happens, remove the mouthparts with tweezers. Do not squeeze, crush, or puncture the body of the tick because its fluids may contain infectious organisms. After removing the tick, disinfect the bite site and wash your hands with soap and water. Save ticks for identification in case you become ill. Place the tick in a plastic bag in your freezer, and note the date of the bite.

SOURCES: Centers for Disease Control and Prevention. 2005. *Updated Information Regarding Mosquito Repellents* (http://www.cdc.gov/ncidod/dvbid/westnile/RepellentUpdates.htm; retrieved May 13, 2005). West Nile: Behind the buzz. 2004. *UC Berkeley Wellness Letter,* July; Centers for Disease Control and Prevention. 2003. *West Nile Virus Prevention* (http://www.cdc.gov/ncidod/dvbid/westnile/qa/prevention.htm; retrieved January 31, 2005); Centers for Disease Control and Prevention. 2002. *Lyme Disease: Prevention and Control* (http://www.cdc.gov/ncidod/dvbid/lyme; retrieved December 10, 2002).

---

individuals develop a bull's-eye-shaped red rash expanding from the area of the bite, usually about 2 weeks after the bite occurs. The second stage occurs weeks to months later in 10–20% of untreated patients; symptoms may involve the nervous and cardiovascular systems and can include impaired coordination, partial facial paralysis, and heart rhythm abnormalities. These symptoms usually disappear on their own within a few weeks. The third stage, which occurs in about half of untreated people, can develop months or years after the tick bite and usually consists of chronic or recurring arthritis. Lyme disease can also cause fetal damage or death at any stage of pregnancy. Lyme disease is preventable by avoiding contact with ticks or by removing a tick before it has had the chance to transmit the infection (see the box "Protecting Yourself Against Tickborne and Mosquitoborne Infections"). Lyme disease is treatable at all stages, although arthritis symptoms may not completely resolve.

Rocky Mountain spotted fever and typhus are caused by **rickettsias** and are also transmitted via tick bites. Rocky Mountain spotted fever is characterized by sudden onset of fever, headache, and muscle pain, followed by development of a spotted rash. Prior to the development of antibiotics, as many as 30% of affected individuals died; the death rate has now dropped to 3–5%. Ehrlichiosis, another tickborne disease, typically causes less severe symptoms. As with Lyme disease, the risk of acquiring Rocky Mountain spotted fever and ehrlichiosis is greater in areas where specific bacteria-carrying tick species are common.

Ulcers About 25 million Americans suffer from ulcers, sores or holes in the lining of the stomach or the first part of the small intestine (duodenum). It used to be thought that spicy food and stress were major causes of ulcers, but it is now known that as many as 90% of ulcers are caused by infection with *Helicobacter pylori*. Ulcer symptoms include gnawing or burning pain in the abdomen, nausea, and loss of appetite. If tests show the presence of *H. pylori*, treatment with antibiotics often cures the infection and the ulcers.

Other Bacterial Infections The following are a few of the many other infections caused by bacteria:

- *Tetanus:* Also known as lockjaw, tetanus is caused by the bacterium *Clostridium tetani*, which thrives in deep puncture wounds and produces a deadly toxin. The toxin causes muscular stiffness and spasms, and infection is fatal in about 30% of cases. Due to widespread vaccination, tetanus is rare in the United States. Worldwide, however, more than 200,000 people die from tetanus each year, primarily newborns infected through the unsterile cutting of the umbilical cord.

- *Pertussis:* Also known as whooping cough, pertussis is a highly contagious respiratory illness caused by a toxin produced by the bacterium *Bordetella pertussis*. Pertussis is characterized by bursts of rapid coughing, followed by a long attempt at inhalation that is often accompanied by a high-pitched whoop; symptoms may persist for 2–8 weeks. The number of U.S. cases has risen steadily over the past two decades, to more than 20,000 cases per year. Those at high risk include infants and children who are too young to be fully vaccinated and those who have not completed the primary vaccination series. Adolescents and adults become susceptible when immunity from vaccination decreases over time. New booster shots for adolescents may help reduce U.S. cases.

- *Urinary tract infections (UTIs):* Infection of the bladder and urethra is most common among sexually active women but can occur in anyone. The bacterium *Escherichi coli* is the most common infectious agent, responsible for about 80% of all UTIs. Infection most often occurs when bacteria from the digestive tract that live on the skin around the anus get pushed toward the opening of the urethra during sexual intercourse; then, the bacteria travel up the urethra and into the bladder. Women are more susceptible to UTIs than men because their urethra is much shorter, so it is easier for bacteria to reach the bladder. Women who are particularly susceptible may be given a supply of antibiotics to use after intercourse or at the first sign of infection; urinating before and after intercourse may also help prevent UTIs.

Bacteria responsible for foodborne illness were described in Chapter 12; Chapter 18 discusses sexually transmitted bacterial infections such as chlamydia.

Antibiotic Treatments The body's immune system can fight off many, if not most, bacterial infections. However, while the body musters its defenses, some bac-

One of the dangers of antibiotic overuse is the development of bacteria resistant to drugs. Cultures of *E. coli* (a bacterium normally present in the human intestine) in this laboratory dish are sensitive to four different types of antibiotics, as indicated by the wide circles where no bacteria are growing, but they are resistant to two other types, which have no effect on their growth.

teria can cause a great deal of damage: Inflammation, caused by the gathering of white blood cells, may lead to scarring and permanently damaged tissues. To help the body deal with these infections, science and medicine have made a considerable contribution: antibiotics.

ACTIONS OF ANTIBIOTICS Antibiotics are both naturally occurring and synthetic substances having the ability to kill bacteria. Most antibiotics work in a similar fashion: They interrupt the production of new bacteria by damaging some part of their reproductive cycle or by causing faulty parts of new bacteria to be made. Penicillins inhibit the formation of the cell wall when bacteria divide to form new cells. Other antibiotics inhibit the production of certain proteins by the bacteria, and still others interfere directly with the reading of genetic material (DNA) during the process of bacterial reproduction. Antibiotics are among the most widely prescribed and effective drugs.

ANTIBIOTIC RESISTANCE When antibiotics are misused or overused, the pathogens they are designed to treat can become resistant to their effects. A bacterium can become resistant from a chance genetic mutation or through the transfer of genetic material from one bacterium to another. When exposed to antibiotics, resistant bacteria can grow and flourish, while the antibiotic-sensitive bacteria die off. Eventually, an entire colony of bacteria can become resistant to one or more antibiotics and can become very difficult to treat. Antibiotic-resistant strains of many common bacteria have developed, including strains of gonorrhea (an STD) and salmonellosis (a foodborne illness). One strain of tuberculosis is resistant to seven different antibiotics.

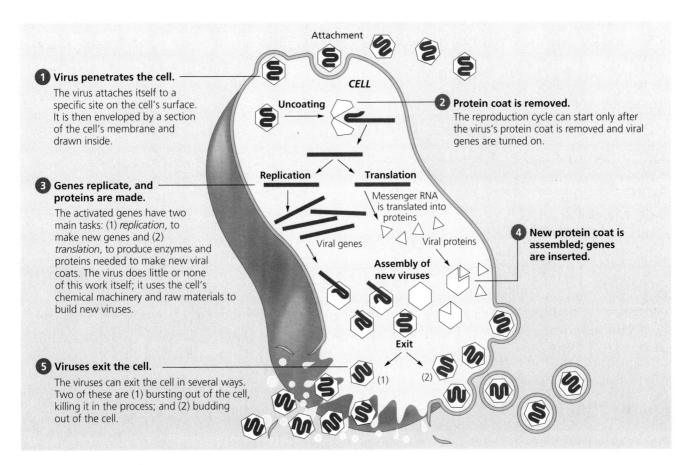

① Virus penetrates the cell.
The virus attaches itself to a specific site on the cell's surface. It is then enveloped by a section of the cell's membrane and drawn inside.

② Protein coat is removed.
The reproduction cycle can start only after the virus's protein coat is removed and viral genes are turned on.

③ Genes replicate, and proteins are made.
The activated genes have two main tasks: (1) *replication*, to make new genes and (2) *translation*, to produce enzymes and proteins needed to make new viral coats. The virus does little or none of this work itself; it uses the cell's chemical machinery and raw materials to build new viruses.

④ New protein coat is assembled; genes are inserted.

⑤ Viruses exit the cell.
The viruses can exit the cell in several ways. Two of these are (1) bursting out of the cell, killing it in the process; and (2) budding out of the cell.

Attachment
CELL
Uncoating
Replication
Translation
Messenger RNA is translated into proteins
Viral genes
Viral proteins
Assembly of new viruses
Exit
(1) (2)

Figure 17-6   Life cycle of a virus.

Antibiotic resistance is a major factor contributing to the recent rise in problematic infectious diseases.

The more often bacteria encounter antibiotics, the more likely they are to develop resistance. Resistance is promoted when people fail to take the full course of an antibiotic or when they inappropriately take antibiotics for viral infections. Another possible source of resistance is the use of antibiotics in agriculture, which is estimated to account for 50–80% of the 25,000 tons of antibiotics used annually in the United States. At least four species of antibiotic-resistant bacteria are documented to have been transmitted from food animals to humans. In 2002, the FDA issued guidelines to the pharmaceutical industry regarding the use of new antibiotics in food-producing animals. Limits may be placed on the use in animals of drugs used in human medicine as last resorts for serious or life-threatening disease.

You can help prevent the development of antibiotic-resistant strains of bacteria by using antibiotics properly:

- Don't take an antibiotic every time you get sick. They are mainly helpful for bacterial infections; they are ineffective against viruses.

- Use antibiotics as directed, and finish the full course of medication even if you begin to feel better. This helps ensure that all targeted bacteria are killed off.

- Never take an antibiotic without a prescription. If you take an antibiotic for a viral infection, take the wrong one, or take an insufficient dose, your illness will not improve, and you'll give bacteria the opportunity to develop resistance.

Viruses

Visible only with an electron (high-magnification) microscope, **viruses** are on the borderline between living and nonliving matter. Viruses lack all the enzymes essential to energy production and protein synthesis in normal animal cells, and they cannot grow or reproduce by themselves. Viruses are **parasites;** they use what they need for growth and reproduction from the cells they invade. Once a virus is inside the host cell, it sheds its protein covering, and its genetic material takes control of the cell and manufactures more viruses like itself (Figure 17-6).

Terms

virus A very small infectious agent composed of nucleic acid (DNA or RNA) surrounded by a protein coat; lacks an independent metabolism and reproduces only within a host cell.

parasite An organism that lives on or within a living host; the relationship benefits the parasite and harms the host.

Prevention

Colds are usually spread by hand-to-hand contact with another person or with objects such as doorknobs and telephones, which an infected person may have handled. The best way to avoid transmission is to wash your hands frequently with warm water and soap. Keeping your immune system strong is another good prevention strategy (see the guidelines provided later in the chapter).

Home Treatments

- Get some extra rest. It isn't usually necessary to stay home in bed, but you will need to slow down a little from your usual routine to give your body a chance to fight the infection.

- Drink plenty of liquids to prevent dehydration. Hot liquids such as herbal tea and clear chicken soup will soothe a sore throat and loosen secretions; gargling with a glass of slightly salty water may also help. Avoid alcoholic beverages when you have a cold.

- Hot showers or the use of a humidifier can help eliminate nasal stuffiness and soothe inflamed membranes.

Over-the-Counter Treatments

Avoid multisymptom cold remedies. Because these products include drugs to treat symptoms you may not even have, you risk suffering from side effects from medications you don't need. It's better to treat each symptom separately:

- *Analgesics*—aspirin, acetaminophen (Tylenol), ibuprofen (Advil or Motrin), and naproxen sodium (Aleve)—all help lower fever and relieve muscle aches. Use of aspirin is asso-

ciated with an increased risk of a serious condition called Reye's syndrome in children and teenagers; for this reason, aspirin should be given only to adults.

- *Decongestants* shrink nasal blood vessels, relieving swelling and congestion. However, they may dry out mucous membranes in the throat and make a sore throat worse. Nasal sprays shouldn't be used for more than 2–3 days to avoid rebound congestion.

- *Cough medicines* may be helpful when your cough is nonproductive (not bringing up mucus) or if it disrupts your sleep or work. Expectorants make coughs more productive by increasing the volume of mucus and decreasing its thickness, thereby helping remove irritants from the respiratory airways. Suppressants (antitussives) reduce the frequency of coughing.

- *Antihistamines* decrease nasal secretions caused by the effects of histamine, so they are much more useful in treating allergies than colds. *Caution:* Many antihistamines can make you drowsy.

Antibiotics will not help a cold unless a bacterial infection such as strep throat is also present, and overuse of antibiotics leads to the development of drug resistance. The jury is still out on whether other remedies, including zinc gluconate lozenges, echinacea, and vitamin C, will relieve symptoms or shorten the duration of a cold. Researchers are also studying antiviral drugs that target the most common types of cold viruses.

Sometimes a cold leads to a more serious complication, such as bronchitis, pneumonia, or strep throat. If a fever of 102°F or higher persists, or if cold symptoms don't get better after 2 weeks, see your physician.

The normal functioning of the host cell is thereby disrupted. In order to fight viruses, the cellular immunity system produces substances such as interferon; unfortunately, these same substances are also responsible for most of the symptoms of a viral illness.

Illnesses caused by viruses are the most common forms of **contagious disease.** Different viruses affect different kinds of cells, and the seriousness of the disease they cause depends greatly on which kind of cell is affected. The viruses that cause colds, for example, attack upper respiratory tract cells, which are constantly cast off and replaced; the disease is therefore mild. Poliovirus, in contrast, attacks nerve cells that cannot be replaced, and the consequences, such as paralysis, are severe. HIV infection, a viral illness that destroys immune system cells, can destroy the body's ability to fight infectious diseases (see Chapter 18).

The Common Cold Although generally brief, lasting only 4–7 days, colds are nonetheless irritating and often interfere with one's normal activities. A cold may be

caused by any of more than 200 different viruses that attack the lining of the nasal passages; rhinoviruses and coronaviruses cause a large percentage of all colds among adults. Cold viruses are almost always transmitted by hand-to-hand contact. To lessen your risk of contracting a cold, wash your hands frequently; if you touch someone else, avoid touching your face until after you've washed your hands. Colds are not caused by exposure to cold weather or by being chilled or overheated; more colds do occur in the fall and winter months, probably because of the opening of school season (children contract more colds than adults) and because people spend more time indoors in the fall and winter months, making person-to-person transmission of viruses more likely.

If you do catch a cold, over-the-counter cold remedies may help treat your symptoms but do not directly attack the viral cause (see the box "Preventing and Treating the Common Cold"). Sometimes it is difficult to determine whether your symptoms are due to a virus (as for colds, flu, and some sinus infections), a bacterium (as for other sinus infections), or an allergy, but this information is

Table 17-3 What's Causing My Symptoms?

Symptoms	Influenza	Common Cold	Allergy	Sinusitis
Headache	Usually	Occasionally	Occasionally	Usually
Muscle aches	Usually (severe)	Usually (mild)	Rarely	Rarely
Fatigue, weakness	Usually (severe; sudden onset; may last several weeks)	Usually (mild)	Rarely	Rarely
Fever	Usually (high, typically 102–104°F; sudden onset; lasts 3–4 days)	Occasionally (mild)	Never	Occasionally
Cough	Usually (often severe)	Occasionally	Occasionally	Usually
Runny, stuffy nose	Occasionally	Usually	Usually	Usually (stuffy)
Nasal discharge	Occasionally	Usually (thick, clear to yellowish green)	Usually (watery, clear)	Usually (thick, yellowish green)
Sneezing	Occasionally	Occasionally	Usually	Rarely
Sore throat	Occasionally	Usually	Occasionally	Rarely
Itchy eyes, nose, throat	Rarely	Rarely	Usually	Never

SOURCE: Is it the flu? 2000. *Consumer Reports*, November. Copyright © 2000 by Consumer Union of U.S., Inc. Yonkers, NY 10703-1057, a nonprofit organization. Reprinted with permission from the November 2000 issue of *Consumer Reports*® for educational purposes only. No commercial use or reproduction permitted. www.ConsumerReports.org, www.ConsumerReportsOnHealth.org.

important for appropriate treatment (Table 17-3). For example, antibiotics will not help treat a cold but will help treat a bacterial sinus infection.

Influenza Commonly called the flu, **influenza** is an infection of the respiratory tract caused by the influenza virus. (Many people use the term "stomach flu" to describe gastrointestinal illnesses, but these infections are actually caused by organisms other than influenza viruses). Compared to the common cold, influenza is a more serious illness, usually including a fever and extreme fatigue. Most people who get the flu recover within 1–2 weeks, but some develop potentially life-threatening complications, such as pneumonia. Influenza is associated with more than 100,000 hospitalizations and 36,000 deaths each year, primarily among people over age 50 and those with chronic health problems. Influenza is highly contagious and is spread via respiratory droplets (see the box "The Next Influenza Pandemic—When, Not If?").

The most effective way of preventing the flu is through annual vaccination. The influenza vaccine consists of killed virus and provides protection against the strains of the virus currently circulating; it is updated each year in response to changes in the virus. Vaccination can be appropriate for anyone age 6 months or older who wants to reduce his or her risk of the flu. Those most at risk from complications or death from influenza are children age 6 to 23 months, people age 65 or older, anyone age 2–64 with long-term health conditions, anyone with a weakened immune system, women who will be pregnant during the flu season, residents of nursing homes and long-term care facilities, people age 6 months to 18 years

on long-term aspirin treatment, health care workers with direct patient contact, and household contacts of persons at high risk. It was to these groups that the CDC gave vaccination priority during the vaccine shortage of 2004–2005.

A number of medications are used to treat influenza, but in most cases they can shorten the duration of illness by little more than a day and then only if treatment begins within 1–2 days after onset of symptoms. Several medications are also effective in reducing the risk of illness from influenza; however, they are less effective than the vaccine.

Measles, Mumps, and Rubella Three childhood viral illnesses that have waned in the United States due to effective vaccines are measles, mumps, and rubella (German measles). Measles and rubella are generally characterized by rash and fever. Measles can occasionally cause more severe illness, including liver or brain infection or pneumonia; worldwide, more than 600,000 people die each year from measles. Measles is a highly contagious disease, and prior to the introduction of vaccines, more than 90% of Americans contracted measles by age 15. Rubella, if it infects a

Terms

contagious disease A disease that can be transmitted from one person to another; most are viral diseases, such as the common cold and flu.

influenza Infection of the respiratory tract by the influenza virus, which is highly infectious and adaptable; the form changes so easily that every year new strains arise, making treatment difficult; commonly known as the flu.

Influenza Virus Basics

There are three main types of influenza viruses, designated A, B, and C. Influenza C usually causes only mild illness and has not been associated with widespread outbreaks. Types A and B, however, are responsible for **epidemics** of respiratory illness that occur almost every winter. Influenza A viruses are further divided into subtypes, based on differences in two surface antigens: hemagglutinin (H) and neuraminidase (N). During a particular flu season, one or more influenza A subtypes and B viruses usually circulate.

Influenza A viruses also differ from types B and C in that they can infect a variety of animals in addition to humans. Aquatic birds, such as ducks, are a natural reservoir for influenza A; they carry and can spread the virus but do not themselves become ill. (Causing no symptoms or only mild illness in an animal reservoir is a good strategy for a virus, because if the original hosts die quickly from the infection, the virus isn't passed along.) Avian strains can infect and cause serious illness in domestic poultry and may also infect pigs, humans, and other mammals.

Antigenic Drift and Shift

Through replication errors and gene sharing, influenza viruses undergo constant change, enabling them to evade the immune system and thereby make people susceptible to influenza throughout life. A person infected with influenza does develop antibodies, but as the H and N antigens change, the antibodies no longer recognize the virus, and reinfection can occur.

Small changes in H and N antigens are referred to as *antigenic drift;* these changes are why the flu vaccine is reformulated each year. Fortunately, if the changes in H and N are small, the immune system may at least partially recognize the virus,

giving many people some immune protection against the new strain.

Occasionally, an influenza A virus undergoes a sudden, dramatic change, called *antigenic shift*. If this occurs and the new virus spreads easily from person to person, a worldwide epidemic, called a **pandemic**, can occur because few people have any antibody protection against the virus. Antigenic shift occurs when an avian influenza virus mixes and exchanges genes with a human virus; this mixing may occur when a human or an animal such as a pig is simultaneously infected by both human and avian strains of influenza A.

Influenza pandemics usually occur about every 30 years or so. During the twentieth century, three major influenza pandemics occurred in humans:

- 1918–1919 ("Spanish flu"): About 20–40% of the world's population became ill, and as many as 40 million people died, including more than 500,000 Americans.

- 1957–1958 ("Asian flu")

- 1968–1969 ("Hong Kong flu")

The Next Pandemic

Many experts believe that an influenza pandemic is overdue, inevitable, and possibly imminent. Conditions that allow the mingling of flu viruses—including wild and domestic birds, humans, and other flu carriers living in crowded conditions and close proximity—exist in many parts of the world.

Scientists have been monitoring the progress of a strain of avian influenza A(H5N1) in Asia that has caused a small but deadly number of cases in humans. The initial outbreak in 1997–1998 killed 6 people in Hong Kong. Local authorities contained the outbreak quickly by tracing its source to infected chickens, ducks,

and geese and then ordering the slaughter of all domestic poultry. Many experts believe that this quick action probably averted a pandemic. Additional outbreaks have occurred in China, Hong Kong, Thailand, Vietnam, and Cambodia.

The H5N1 strain doesn't pass easily to or between humans; the only case of human-to-human transmission involved a mother caring for a dying child. However, when it infects humans, it is deadly—as of April 2005, there had been 79 confirmed cases and 50 deaths.

The more people who are infected, the greater the chance that avian and human strains will mix, producing an influenza virus that is easily transmitted between people. It is hoped that the resulting strain will be less lethal than the avian strain; human strains tend to be less deadly, and, as described earlier, the quick death of hosts prevents the virus from being transmitted. However, one lesson from the 1918–1919 pandemic is that crowded human conditions—such as the army trenches, military hospitals, and troop transport ships associated with World War I—promote the development of lethal human flu strains.

Scientists are studying the virus to determine how many mutations it would take to allow H5N1 to pass easily between humans. Attempts are also being made to develop a vaccine ahead of a pandemic; however, the long lag time in flu vaccine production presents a major challenge. Close monitoring and quick action may be the world's best protection.

SOURCES: Orent, W. 2005. Worrying about killer flu. *Discover*, February; Taubenberger, J. K., A. H. Reid, and T. G. Fanning. 2005. Capturing a killer flu virus. *Scientific American,* January; U.S. Department of Health and Human Services. 2004. *National Vaccine Program Office: Influenza* (http://www.hhs.gov/nvpo/pandemics/fluprint. htm; retrieved February 3, 2005).

pregnant woman, can be transmitted to a fetus, causing miscarriage, stillbirth, and severe birth defects, including deafness, eye and heart defects, and mental impairment. Mumps generally causes swelling of the parotid (salivary) glands, located just below and in front of the ears. This virus can also cause meningitis and, in males, inflammation of the testes.

Chicken Pox, Cold Sores, and Other Herpesvirus Infections The **herpesviruses** are a large group of viruses. Once infected, the host is never free of the virus. The virus lies latent within certain cells and becomes active periodically, producing symptoms. Herpesviruses are particularly dangerous for people with a depressed immune system, as in the case of

Are all diseases infectious? Probably not, although researchers have recently been identifying infectious bases for more and more diseases—even diseases that have long been thought to be caused by other factors. Some scientists feel that the role of infectious agents in the major killers of today—CVD, cancer, diabetes, and so on—has been greatly underestimated. The following are just a few examples:

• **Ulcers.** Although long believed to be caused by spicy food, stress, and smoking, most cases of ulcers are now known to be caused by infection with *Helicobacter pylori*.

• **Type 1 diabetes.** A viral infection is thought to trigger the immune system to destroy insulin-producing cells in the pancreas; when this occurs, the pancreas is no longer able to produce enough insulin to metabolize glucose.

• **Multiple sclerosis (MS).** Infection with a virus, possibly human herpesvirus 6, has been proposed as the precipitating cause of MS, a condition characterized by damage to nerve fiber coverings and progressive muscle weakness.

• **Schizophrenia.** Some studies have found that people with schizophrenia are more likely than unaffected individuals to have elevated antibodies to the Borna virus. The Borna virus may be one of several infectious agents that trigger changes in the brain leading to schizophrenia.

• **Childhood obsessive-compulsive disorder (OCD).** Some cases of OCD that begin in early childhood have been found to follow infection with streptococcus bacteria. It is thought that antibodies produced to fight the infection, rather than the infection itself, may cause OCD.

Some affected children improve when they are given intravenous immunoglobulin or undergo plasma exchange to remove the antibodies from their blood.

• **Heart disease.** Several infectious agents have been implicated in the inflammatory processes underlying atherosclerosis, including *Chlamydia pneumoniae* and *Cytomegalovirus*. Research is under way to determine if antibiotics can lessen the risk of heart attack in infected individuals.

• **Cancer.** A number of infections have been linked to specific types of cancer: human papillomavirus and cervical cancer; Epstein-Barr virus and Burkitt's lymphoma, nasopharyngeal cancer and some B-cell lymphomas; hepatitis B and C viruses and liver cancer; HTLV-1 and T-cell leukemia; *Helicobacter pylori* and stomach cancer; and human herpesvirus 8 and Kaposi's sarcoma.

HIV infection. The family of herpesviruses includes the following:

• *Varicella-zoster virus,* which causes chicken pox and shingles. Chicken pox is a highly contagious childhood disease characterized by an itchy rash made up of small blisters; the infection is usually mild, although complications are more likely to occur in young infants and adults. After the rash resolves, the virus becomes latent, living in sensory nerves. Many years later, the virus may reactivate and cause shingles; symptoms of shingles include pain in the affected nerves and a rash on the skin that follows the pattern of the nerve pathways (often a band over the ribs on one side of the body). A vaccine is available that prevents chicken pox in the majority of cases and results in milder illness if the disease does occur.

• *Herpes simplex virus (HSV) types 1 and 2,* which cause cold sores and the STD herpes. Herpes infections are characterized by small, painful ulcers in the area around the mouth or genitals, at the site where a person first contracts the virus. Following the initial infection, HSV becomes latent and may reactivate again and again over time. Many infected people do not know they are infected, and the virus can be transmitted even when sores are not apparent. Heat and sunlight can trigger recurrences of lip ulcers, so using a lip balm with sunscreen may be a helpful strategy; antiviral medications are available to prevent recurrences of genital herpes. See Chapter 18 for more on sexually transmitted HSV infection.

• *Epstein-Barr virus (EBV),* which causes infectious mononucleosis. Mono, as it is commonly called, is characterized by fever, sore throat, swollen lymph nodes, and fatigue. It is usually spread by intimate contact with the saliva of an infected person—hence the name "kissing disease." Mono most often affects adolescents and young adults; by age 40, nearly 90% of Americans have become infected with EBV. Although EBV does reactivate throughout life, it generally does not cause any further symptoms. In a few people, especially those with HIV infection, EBV is associated with the development of cancers of the lymph system (see the box "Are All Diseases Infectious?").

At one time, EBV was implicated as a cause of *chronic fatigue syndrome (CFS)*, a disorder characterized by severe chronic fatigue, impaired memory or concentration, and physical symptoms such as persistent sore throat or muscle pain. However, CFS has not been linked to any single infectious agent; other possible causes of CFS

Terms

epidemic The occurrence in a particular community or region of more than the expected number of cases of a particular disease.

pandemic A disease epidemic that is unusually severe or widespread; often used to refer to worldwide epidemics affecting a large proportion of the population.

herpesvirus A family of viruses responsible for cold sores, mononucleosis, chicken pox, and the STD known as herpes; frequently causes latent infections.

include abnormalities in immunity, hormone levels, and the regulation of blood pressure.

Two herpesviruses that can cause severe infections in people with a suppressed immune system are cytomegalovirus (CMV), which infects the lungs, brain, colon, and eyes, and human herpesvirus 8 (HHV-8), which has been linked to Kaposi's sarcoma.

Viral Encephalitis HSV type 1 is a possible cause of viral **encephalitis**, inflammation of brain tissue due to a viral infection. Other possible causes include HIV and several mosquitoborne viruses, including Japanese encephalitis virus, equine encephalomyelitis virus, and West Nile virus. Mild cases of encephalitis may cause fever, headache, nausea, and lethargy; severe cases are characterized by memory loss, delirium, diminished speech function, and seizures, and they may result in permanent brain damage or death.

Viral Hepatitis Viral **hepatitis** is a term used to describe several different infections that cause inflammation of the liver. Hepatitis is usually caused by one of the three most common hepatitis viruses. Hepatitis A virus (HAV) causes the mildest form of the disease and is usually transmitted by food or water contaminated by sewage or an infected person. Hepatitis B virus (HBV) is usually transmitted sexually; it is discussed in detail in Chapter 18. Hepatitis C virus (HCV) can also be transmitted sexually, but it is much more commonly passed through direct contact with infected blood via injection drug use or, prior to the development of screening tests, blood transfusions. HBV and, to a lesser extent, HCV can also be passed from a pregnant woman to her child. There are effective vaccines for hepatitis A and B, but more than 150,000 new cases of hepatitis occur in the United States each year.

Symptoms of acute hepatitis infection can include fatigue, **jaundice**, abdominal pain, loss of appetite, nausea, and diarrhea. Most people recover from hepatitis A within a month or so. However, 5–10% of people infected with HBV and 85–90% of people infected with HCV become chronic carriers of the virus, capable of infecting others for the rest of their lives. Some chronic carriers remain asymptomatic, while others slowly develop chronic liver disease, cirrhosis, or liver cancer. An estimated 4 million Americans and 500 million people worldwide may be chronic carriers of hepatitis. Each year in the United States, HBV and HCV are responsible for more than 15,000 deaths, and these numbers are expected to climb as more people infected in the 1970s and 1980s develop problems. HCV infection is already the most frequent reason for liver transplants among U.S. adults, and it is thought to be a major factor in the 70% increase in U.S. liver cancer rates since the 1970s.

The extent of HCV infection has only recently been recognized, and most infected people are unaware of their condition. To ensure proper treatment and prevention, testing for HCV may be recommended for people at risk, including people who have ever injected drugs (even once), who received a blood transfusion or a donated organ prior to July 1992, who have engaged in high-risk sexual behavior, or who have had body piercing, tattoos, or acupuncture involving unsterile equipment. (See the box "Tattoos and Body Piercing" for information on improving safety and satisfaction related to body art.) Antiviral drugs are available to treat chronic hepatitis, but they are not completely effective and may have significant side effects.

Poliomyelitis An infectious viral disease that affects the nervous system, **poliomyelitis** can cause irreversible paralysis and death in some affected individuals. As with other vaccine-preventable diseases, the incidence of polio declined dramatically in the United States following the introduction of the vaccine, and North and South America are now considered free of the disease. In 1998, the WHO set the goal of eradicating polio from the world; cases have significantly declined since this campaign began.

Rabies Caused by a rhabdovirus, rabies is a potentially fatal infection of the central nervous system that is most often transmitted through an animal bite. U.S. rabies-related deaths among humans declined dramatically during the twentieth century due to the widespread vaccination of domestic animals and the development of a highly effective vaccine regimen that provides immunity following exposure (post-exposure prophylaxis, or PEP). Although rabies is rare in the United States, most recent cases have been traced to bats. Unlike bites from larger animals that may carry rabies (raccoons, foxes, skunks, and the like), bat bites or scratches are likely to go unnoticed; thus, people may be unaware of their exposure and fail to seek treatment. The CDC recommends that PEP be considered for anyone who has had direct physical contact with a bat, including someone who has been in the same room with a bat and who might be unaware that contact has occurred (a sleeping child, for example). PEP consists of one dose of immunoglobulin and five doses of rabies vaccine over a 28-day period.

Warts Infection by the human papillomavirus (HPV), which causes cell proliferation, can cause warts (noncancerous skin tumors). The more than 100 different

Careful selection of a body artist and attention to aftercare instructions can help improve safety and satisfaction following tattooing or piercing.

Tattoos

Tattoos are permanent marks or designs applied with an electrically powered instrument that injects dye into the second layer of the skin with an action that resembles that of a sewing machine. Needles in the machine are connected to tubes containing different colors of dye. Depending on the size of the tattoo, it may take several hours or possibly several visits to apply. Pain and a small amount of bleeding are common; a tattoo typically takes a week or two to heal. Tattoos need to be protected from sun exposure until completely healed.

Body Piercing

Piercing is usually done with pliers-like equipment that pushes a needle or other sharp device through the skin; the piercing is kept open by a piece of jewelry. Earlobe piercing is the most common, but people may also pierce the upper ear, eyebrow, tongue, lip, nose, navel, nipples, or genitals. Healing time may vary from several weeks to a year depending on the site of the piercing and other factors. Some pain and swelling are common; there may be prolonged bleeding following oral piercing due to the high degree of vascularization of the tongue.

Potential Health Issues

- **Infection:** There is a risk of transmission of bloodborne infectious agents, including hepatitis B and C and HIV, if instruments are not sterilized properly; however, no cases of HIV infection have been traced to tattooing or piercing. The risk of infection is much higher if body art is applied by untrained individuals or if people fail to follow aftercare instructions. Any unexpected degree of pain or swelling should be promptly evaluated by a physician. Due to the potential risks, people currently cannot donate blood for 12 months following application of body art, including tattoos and some body piercings. People with heart valve problems should check with a physician prior to body piercing to determine if they should take antibiotics in advance of the procedure in order to prevent infection of the heart.

- **Allergic reactions:** Some people may be allergic to pigments used in tattooing or to metals used in body-piercing jewelry. All jewelry should be of noncorrosive materials such as stainless steel or titanium; avoid jewelry that contains nickel.

- **Nodules and scars:** Some people may develop granulomas (nodules) or keloids (a type of scar) following tattooing or body piercing.

- **Problems relating to placement:** Tattoos may become swollen or burned if people undergo magnetic resonance imaging (MRI), and tattoos may also interfere with the quality of MRI images. Oral ornaments may obscure dental problems in dental X rays; they may also damage teeth and fillings and interfere with speech and chewing. Women who breastfeed should remove nipple ornaments before doing so. Navel piercings may become infected more easily because tight-fitting clothes allow moisture to collect in the area.

- **Dissatisfaction:** The most common problem with body art is dissatisfaction. Tattoos are meant to be permanent and so are expensive and very difficult (or impossible) to remove completely. Tattoo removal may involve scraping or cutting off the layers of tattooed skin or using laser surgery to break up the pigment in the tattoo; some scarring can occur. Body piercings may close and heal once the jewelry is removed, but they may leave a permanent scar.

Choosing a Body Artist and Studio

Ask about experience and infection-control procedures. *Remember:* You could be wearing someone else's mistake for the rest of your life. A body art studio should be clean and have an autoclave for sterilizing instruments. Needles should be sterilized and disposable; piercing guns should not be used, as they cannot be adequately sterilized. The body artist should wear disposable latex gloves throughout the procedure. Leftover tattoo ink should be thrown away and not reused. Ask to see references and aftercare instructions beforehand.

Some states and local health departments regulate body art facilities. In addition, you can ask if the studio and/or artist are members of the Alliance for Professional Tattooists (http://www.safe-tattoos.com) or the Association of Professional Piercers (http://www.safepiercing.org); these organizations have developed infection-control and other guidelines for their members to follow.

---

types of HPV cause a variety of warts, including common warts on the hands, plantar warts on the soles of the feet, and genital warts around the genitalia. Depending on their location, warts may be removed using over-the-counter preparations or professional methods such as laser surgery or cryosurgery. Because HPV infection is chronic, warts can reappear despite treatment. Because of the link between HPV infection and cervical cancer, genital warts are of particular concern (see Chapter 18).

Treating Viral Illnesses Although many viruses cannot be treated medically, researchers have recently be-

gun to develop antiviral drugs. These typically work by interfering with some part of the viral life cycle; for example, they may prevent a virus from entering body cells or from successfully reproducing within cells. Antivirals are currently available to fight infections caused by HIV, influenza, herpes simplex, varicella-zoster, HBV, and HCV. Most other viral diseases must simply run their course.

Fungi

A **fungus** is an organism that absorbs food from organic matter. Fungi may be multicellular (like molds) or

Hand washing is one of the best ways to prevent the spread of infectious diseases. Always wash your hands before, during, and after preparing food; before eating; and after using the bathroom. Wet your hands, apply soap, and rub vigorously for 10–20 seconds.

unicellular (like yeasts). Mushrooms and the molds that form on bread and cheese are all fungi. Only about 50 fungi out of many thousands of species cause disease in humans, and these diseases are usually restricted to the skin, mucous membranes, and lungs. Some fungal diseases are extremely difficult to treat because some fungi form spores, an especially resistant dormant stage of the organism.

Candida albicans is a common fungus found naturally in the vagina of most women. In normal amounts, it causes no problems, but when excessive growth occurs, the result is itching and discomfort, commonly known as a yeast infection. Factors that increase the growth of *C. albicans* include the use of antibiotics, clothing that keeps the vaginal area excessively warm and moist, pregnancy, oral contraceptive use, and certain diseases, including diabetes and HIV infection. The most common symptom is usually a thick white or yellowish discharge. Treatment consists of OTC antifungal creams and suppositories or prescription oral antifungal medication. Women should not self-treat unless they are certain from a past medical diagnosis that they have a yeast infection. (Misdiagnosis could mean that a different and more severe infection goes untreated.) *C. albicans* overgrowth can occur in other areas of the body, especially in the mouth in infants (a condition known as thrush).

Other common fungal conditions, including athlete's foot, jock itch, and ringworm, affect the skin. These three mild conditions are usually easy to cure and rarely cause major problems.

Fungi can also cause systemic diseases that are severe, life-threatening, and extremely difficult to treat. Histoplasmosis, or valley fever, causes pulmonary and sometimes systemic disease and is most common in the Mississippi and Ohio River Valleys. Coccidioidomycosis is also known as valley fever because it is most frequent in the San Joaquin Valley of California. Fungal infections can be especially deadly in people with an impaired immune system.

Protozoa

Another group of pathogens is microscopic single-celled organisms known as **protozoa.** Many protozoal diseases are recurrent: The pathogen remains in the body, alternating between activity and inactivity. Hundreds of millions of people in developing countries suffer from protozoal infections.

Malaria, caused by a protozoan of the genus *Plasmodium,* is characterized by recurrent attacks of severe flu-like symptoms (chills, fever, headache, nausea, and vomiting). The protozoan is injected into the bloodstream via a mosquito bite; during its reproductive phase, it breaks down red blood cells and may cause anemia in severe cases. Although relatively rare in the United States, malaria is a major killer worldwide; each year, there are more than 500 million new cases of malaria and more than 1 million deaths, mostly among infants and children. Drugs are available to prevent and treat malaria.

Giardiasis is caused by *Giardia lamblia,* a single-celled parasite that lives in the intestines of humans and animals. Giardiasis is characterized by nausea, diarrhea, bloating, and abdominal cramps, and it is among the most common waterborne diseases in the United States. People may become infected with *Giardia* if they consume contaminated food or water or pick up the parasite from the contaminated surface of an object such as a bathroom fixture, diaper pail, or toy. People at risk include child care workers, children who attend day care, international travelers, and hikers and campers who drink untreated water. Giardiasis is rarely serious and can be treated with prescription medications.

Other protozoal infections include the following:

- *Trichomoniasis,* a common vaginal infection. Although usually mild and treatable, trich may increase the risk of HIV transmission (see Chapter 18).

- *Trypanosomiasis* (African sleeping sickness), which is transmitted through the bite of an infected tsetse fly and causes extreme fatigue, fever, rash, severe headache, central nervous system damage, and death.

- *Amoebic dysentery,* a severe form of amebiasis, infection of the intestines with the parasite *Entamoeba histolytica.* It is characterized by bloody diarrhea, stomach pain, and fever.

Parasitic Worms

The **parasitic worms** are the largest organisms that can enter the body to cause infection. The tapeworm, for example, can grow to a length of many feet. Worms, including intestinal parasites such as the tapeworm and hookworm, cause a great variety of relatively mild infections. Pinworm, the most common worm infection in the United States, primarily affects young children. Pinworms are white and about the size of a staple and live in the rectum of humans; they can cause itching and difficulty sleeping. Smaller worms known as flukes infect organs such as the liver and lungs and, in large numbers, can be deadly. Generally speaking, worm infections originate from contaminated food or drink and can be controlled by careful attention to hygiene.

Prions

In recent years, several fatal degenerative disorders of the central nervous system have been linked to **prions,** or proteinaceous infectious particles. Unlike all other infectious agents, prions appear to lack DNA or RNA and to consist only of protein; their presence in the body does not trigger an immune response. Prions have an abnormal shape and form deposits in the brain. They may spread by triggering normal proteins to change their structure to the abnormal, damaging, form.

Prions are associated with a class of diseases known as *transmissible spongiform encephalopathies (TSEs),* which are characterized by spongelike holes in the brain; symptoms of TSEs include loss of coordination, weakness, dementia, and death. Known prion diseases include Creutzfeldt-Jakob disease (CJD) in humans; bovine spongiform encephalopathy (BSE), or mad cow disease, in cattle; and scrapie in sheep. Some prion diseases are inherited or the result of spontaneous genetic mutations, whereas others are the result of eating infected tissue or being exposed to prions during medical procedures such as organ or tissue transplants. Differences exist between CJD cases that appear to result from spontaneous mutations and those variant cases (vCJD) tied to eating meat contaminated with central nervous system tissue from cows infected with BSE; for example, the average age among people with the former type is 68, compared with 28 for people with vCJD. (Ongoing research is exploring whether prions play a role in more common degenerative brain disorders such as Alzheimer's disease.)

Many countries have reported cows infected with BSE; the first U.S. BSE case was identified in 2003 (see Chapter 12). Several steps have been taken or proposed to reduce the number of BSE-infected cows and the likelihood of meat from an infected animal entering the human food supply. These include increased surveillance, limiting or banning the use of cattle products in feed for other cattle, prohibiting meat imports from countries with BSE-infected cattle, restricting certain people from giving blood, and banning the use of downer (nonambulatory disabled)

cattle for food for human consumption. Prions present special challenges because they are resistant to heat, radiation, and chemicals that kill other pathogens and because the diseases they cause have a long incubation period. Scientists are working to develop new tests that would detect low levels of dangerous prions in asymptomatic cattle.

Emerging Infectious Diseases

The reduction in deaths from infectious diseases in the United States is one of the major public health achievements of the past century. Improvements in sanitation, hygiene, and water quality and the development of antibiotics all contributed to reduced death rates from tuberculosis, pneumonia, diarrhea, and other infections. However, after decades of decline, the U.S. death rate from infectious diseases began to climb in 1981, largely due to the HIV/AIDS epidemic. Globally, infectious diseases remain a major killer, and new concerns such as antibiotic resistance and bioterrorism have emerged in the past 20 years. Emerging infectious diseases are those infections whose incidence in humans has increased or threatens to increase in the near future. They include both known diseases that have experienced a resurgence, such as tuberculosis and cholera, and diseases that were previously unknown or confined to specific areas, such as the Ebola and West Nile viruses.

Selected Infections of Concern Although the chances of the average American contracting an exotic infection are very low, emerging infections are a concern to public health officials and represent a challenge to all nations in the future. Some emerging infections, including avian influenza and mad cow disease, were discussed earlier; other infections of concern include the following.

WEST NILE VIRUS A mini-outbreak of encephalitis in New York in 1999 led to identification of this virus, which had previously been restricted to Africa, the Middle East, and parts of Europe. Since that time, the virus has spread across the United States and caused more than 17,000 illnesses

---

Terms

protozoan (plural, protozoa) A microscopic single-celled organism that often produces recurrent, cyclical attacks of disease.

malaria A severe, recurrent, mosquitoborne infection caused by the protozoan *Plasmodium*.

giardiasis An intestinal disease caused by the protozoan *Giardia lamblia*.

parasitic worm A pathogen that causes intestinal and other infections; includes tapeworms, hookworms, pinworms, and flukes.

prion Proteinaceous infectious particles thought to be responsible for a class of neurodegenerative diseases known as transmissible spongiform encephalopathies; Creutzfeldt-Jakob disease (CJD) in humans and bovine spongiform encephalopathy (BSE, or mad cow disease) are prion diseases.

and 650 deaths. West Nile virus is carried by birds and then passed to humans when mosquitoes bite first an infected bird and then a person. A few cases have also been traced to blood transfusions from infected donors. Most people who are bitten have few or no symptoms, but the virus can cause permanent brain damage or death in some. Vaccines are being developed for West Nile virus, but it is important to protect yourself from mosquito bites.

SEVERE ACUTE RESPIRATORY SYNDROME (SARS) In late 2002, SARS appeared in southern China and quickly spread to more than 15 countries; it is a form of pneumonia that is fatal in about 5–15% of cases. SARS is caused by a new type of coronavirus found in wildlife that may have crossed the species barrier when certain wildlife species were consumed as delicacies. It has reemerged several times since 2002, and by 2005 had been responsible for more than 8000 illnesses and 800 deaths.

MONKEYPOX The first U.S. cases of this cousin of smallpox were reported in 2003. Although less dangerous than smallpox, monkeypox is a potentially deadly infection, causing fever and a blistered rash. The virus was previously found only in Africa, but it came to the United States in an infected African rat, which in turn infected a group of prairie dogs with which it shared a cage. Sold as pets, the prairie dogs infected their owners through bites or other close contact.

ESCHERICHIA COLI O157:H7 This potentially deadly strain of *E. coli*, transmitted in contaminated food, can cause bloody diarrhea and kidney damage. The first major outbreak occurred in 1993, when over 600 people became ill and 4 children died after eating contaminated and undercooked fast-food hamburgers. Additional outbreaks have been linked to lettuce, alfalfa sprouts, unpasteurized juice, petting zoos, and contaminated public swimming pools. An estimated 70,000 cases and 6 deaths occur in the United States each year.

HANTAVIRUS Since first being recognized in 1993, over 300 cases of hantavirus pulmonary syndrome (HPS) have been reported in the United States. HPS is caused by the rodentborne Sin Nombre virus (SNV) and is spread primarily through airborne viral particles from rodent urine, droppings, or saliva. It is characterized by a dangerous fluid buildup in the lungs and is fatal in about 45% of cases.

EBOLA So far, outbreaks of the often fatal Ebola hemorrhagic fever (EHF) in humans have occurred only in Africa. The Ebola virus is transmitted by direct contact with infected blood or other body secretions, and many cases of EHF have been linked to unsanitary conditions in medical facilities. Because symptoms appear quickly and 70% of victims die, usually within a few days, the virus tends not to spread widely (unlike HIV or hepatitis, which can infect a person for years before any symptoms appear). Also of concern is the potential use of the Ebola virus by bioterrorists.

Factors Contributing to Emerging Infections

What's behind this rising tide of infectious diseases? Contributing factors are complex and interrelated.

DRUG RESISTANCE New or increasing drug resistance has been found in organisms that cause malaria, tuberculosis, gonorrhea, influenza, AIDS, and pneumococcal and staphylococcal infections. Infections caused by drug-resistant organisms prolong illness, and—if not treated in time with more effective, expensive drugs—they can cause death. Some bacterial strains now appear to be resistant to all available antibiotics. The cost of drug resistance exceeds $25 billion each year and is increasing.

POVERTY More than 1 billion people live in extreme poverty, and half the world's population have no regular access to essential drugs. Population growth, urbanization, overcrowding, and migration (including the movement of refugees) also spread infectious diseases.

BREAKDOWN OF PUBLIC HEALTH MEASURES A poor public health infrastructure is often associated with poverty and social upheaval, but problems such as contaminated water supplies can occur even in industrial countries. Inadequate vaccination has led to the reemergence of diseases such as diphtheria and pertussis. Natural disasters such as the 2004 tsunami also disrupt the public health infrastructure, leaving survivors with contaminated water and food supplies and no shelter from disease-carrying insects.

ENVIRONMENTAL CHANGES Changes in land use—deforestation, the damming of rivers, the spread of ranching and farming—alter the distribution of disease vectors and bring people into contact with new pathogens. A shift in rainfall patterns caused by global warming may allow mosquitoborne diseases such as malaria to spread from the tropics into the temperate zones.

TRAVEL AND COMMERCE More than 500 million travelers cross national borders each year, and international tourism and trade open the world to infectious agents. SARS was quickly spread throughout the world by infected air travelers. The reintroduction of cholera into the Western Hemisphere is thought to have occurred through the discharge of bilge water from a Chinese freighter into the waters off Peru.

MASS FOOD PRODUCTION AND DISTRIBUTION Food now travels long distances to our table, and microbes are transmitted along with it. Mass production of food increases the likelihood that a chance contamination can lead to mass illness.

HUMAN BEHAVIORS Changes in patterns of human behavior also influence the spread of infectious diseases. The widespread use of injectable drugs rapidly transmits HIV infection and hepatitis. Changes in sexual behavior over the past 30 years have led to a proliferation of old and new STDs. The use of day-care facilities for children has led to increases in the incidence of several infections that cause diarrhea.

Although the immune systems of men and women are essentially the same, women have much higher rates of many autoimmune diseases. The reason is somewhat of a mystery. One clue may come from pregnancy: In order to conceive and carry a baby to term, a woman's body must temporarily suppress its immune response so it doesn't attack the sperm or the fetus. Another factor seems to be related to estrogen. Estrogen receptors have been found on suppressor T cells, pointing to a possible link between the glands controlling immunity and those controlling sex hormones. The expression of certain kinds of immune response genes is also linked to some autoimmune diseases, as are certain infections. Women also appear to have somewhat enhanced immunity compared to men, a factor that could be linked to both longer life spans and higher rates of autoimmune disorders.

Systemic lupus erythematosus is an autoimmune disease in which the immune system attacks the body's normal tissue, causing inflammation of the joints, blood vessels, heart, lungs, brain, and kidneys. Its symptoms include painful swollen joints, a rash on the nose and cheeks, sensitivity to sunlight, chest pain, fatigue, and dizziness. There are about 1.4–2.0 million Americans with lupus, 80% of them women; the disorder is especially common among Native American and African American women. Lupus usually begins before menopause and may flare up during pregnancy; for some women, symptoms also increase in severity during menstruation or with the use of oral contraceptives. A link between these exacerbating factors is increased levels of estrogen, but this connection is not well understood. Researchers have also identified genetic mutations that may be associated with lupus.

In rheumatoid arthritis, the body's immune system attacks the membranes lining the joints, causing pain and swelling. Among the estimated 1% of American adults with rheumatoid arthritis, women outnumber men 3 to 1. The causes of the disease are not well understood. Re-

searchers have hypothesized that an as-yet-unidentified virus may stimulate the immune system and trigger the disease. When the disease is present in younger women, symptoms often improve during pregnancy, when estrogen levels are higher, the opposite of what is seen in the case of lupus. Therefore, although estrogen levels may play a role in these disorders, its effects appear to be influenced by many other factors.

Other autoimmune disorders more common among women than men include multiple sclerosis, a neurological disease caused by the destruction of the protective coating around nerves; scleroderma, a connective tissue disease characterized by thickening, hardening, and tightening of the skin; and Graves' disease, characterized by an increase in the production of thyroid hormone, which affects metabolism and many body systems. Continued scientific investigation will help pinpoint the causes and triggers of autoimmune disorders and explain their higher incidence among women.

BIOTERRORISM The deliberate release of deadly infectious agents is an ongoing concern. In 2001, infectious anthrax spores sent through the mail sickened 11 and killed 5 people in the United States. Potential bioterrorism agents that the CDC categorizes as a highest concern are those that can be easily disseminated or transmitted from person to person and that have a high mortality rate and the potential for a major public health impact; these include anthrax, smallpox, plague, botulism, and viral hemorrhagic fevers such as Ebola.

International efforts at monitoring, preventing, and controlling the spread of emerging infections are under way. Microbes do not respect national borders, so only a global response can make the world a safer and healthier place for everyone.

Other Immune Disorders: Cancer and Autoimmune Diseases

The immune system has evolved to protect the body from invasion by foreign microorganisms. Sometimes, as in the case of cancer, the body comes under attack by its own cells. As explained in Chapter 16, cancer cells cease to cooperate normally with the rest of the body and multiply uncontrollably. The immune system can often detect cells

that have recently become cancerous and then destroy them just as it would a foreign microorganism. But if the immune system breaks down, as it may when people get older, when they have certain immune disorders (including HIV infection), or when they are receiving chemotherapy for other diseases, the cancer cells may multiply out of control before the immune system recognizes the danger. By the time the immune system gears up to destroy the cancerous cells, it may be too late.

Another immune disorder occurs when the body confuses its own cells with foreign organisms. As described earlier, the immune system must recognize many thousands of antigens as foreign and then be able to recognize the same antigens again and again. Our own tissue cells also are antigenic; that is, they would be recognized by another person's immune system as foreign. A delicate balance must be maintained to ensure that one's immune system recognizes only truly foreign antigens as enemies; erroneous recognition of one's own cells as foreign produces havoc.

This is what happens in autoimmune diseases such as rheumatoid arthritis and systemic lupus erythematosus. In this type of malady, the immune system seems to be a bit too sensitive and begins to misapprehend itself as nonself. For reasons not well understood, these conditions are much more common in women than in men (see the box "Women and Autoimmune Diseases").

Many people believe that stress makes them more vulnerable to illness. Studies have shown that rates of illness are higher for weeks or even months in people who have experienced the severe emotional trauma of divorce or the death of a loved one. Can more commonplace anxieties and stresses also cause measurable changes in the immune system? And can common stress-management techniques actually boost the immune system? The answer to these questions appears to be yes. Consider the following research findings:

• Medical students taking final exams showed a much weaker immune response to a hepatitis vaccination than unstressed students. In other studies, stress was associated with lower T-cell responses and antibody levels following influenza vaccinations.

• Individuals who had higher levels of stress and who had a negative or pessimistic outlook developed more colds over the course of a yearlong study than individuals with lower levels of stress and a more positive outlook.

• In a study of caregivers, relaxation sessions were associated with increased secretion of cytokines in minor wounds, thus speeding healing. Relaxation and imagery have also been shown to increase T-cell levels in some people.

• A study comparing parents of children with cancer (who presumably had high stress levels) with parents of healthy children found that stress appears to interfere with the body's ability to shut down the inflammatory response after it gets started. Continuing high levels of cytokines and inflammation could harm health. The same study found that social support improves the immune response.

In seeking to explain these effects, researchers are looking at the connections between stress, hormones, and immunity. Some hormones, such as cortisol, appear to impair the ability of immune cells to multiply and function. Others, such as prolactin, seem to give immune cells a boost. By matching stress levels and hormonal changes to the ups and downs of immune function, researchers hope to gain a better grasp of the shifting chemistry of mind and immunity.

SOURCES: Miller, G. E., S. Cohen, and A. .K. Ritchey. 2002. Chronic psychological stress and the regulation of pro-inflammatory cytokines: A glucocorticoid-resistance model. *Health Psychology* 21(6): 531–541; Takkouche, B., et al. 2001. A cohort study of stress and the common cold. *Epidemiology* 12: 345–349; Bauer, M. E., et al. 2000. Chronic stress in caregivers of dementia patients is associated with reduced lymphocyte sensitivity to glucocorticoids. *Journal of Neuroimmunology* 103(1): 84–92; Cohen, S., W. J. Doyle, and D. P. Skoner. 1999. Psychological stress, cytokine production, and severity of upper respiratory illness. *Psychosomatic Medicine* 61(2): 175–180.

GIVING YOURSELF A FIGHTING CHANCE: HOW TO SUPPORT YOUR IMMUNE SYSTEM

Pathogens pose a formidable threat to wellness, but you can take many steps to prevent them from getting control of your body and compromising your health. Public health measures protect people from many diseases that are transmitted via water, food, or insects. A clean water supply and adequate sewage treatment help control typhoid fever and cholera, for example, and mosquito eradication programs control malaria and encephalitis. Proper food inspection and preparation prevent illness caused by foodborne pathogens (see Chapter 12).

What can you do as an individual to strengthen your immune system to help prevent infection? The most important thing you can do is to take good care of your body, with adequate nutrition, exercise, rest, and moderation in lifestyle. Medical science has not come up with anything that can improve on the millions of years of evolution that have culminated in your immune system. Of course, once infection has begun, some diseases can be fought with the aid of antibiotics and antiviral drugs. But these medications are not helpful in *preventing* infection, except in circumstances where normal immunity is breached, such as in surgery.

Scientists have discovered, however, that even the strongest immune system (as measured by the number of helper T cells) fluctuates throughout a person's life. You are most susceptible to disease at the extremes of life—when first born, before you have developed active immunity against most pathogens, and in old age, when the immune system, like the rest of the body, starts to deteriorate. You can't avoid being young or old, but you can make sure you get appropriate vaccinations to help the immune system in case of invasion by specific pathogens (see Table 17-1).

Stress, affected by lifestyle and attitudes, influences the immune response. Research has shown that the actual number of helper T cells rises and falls inversely with stress; that is, the higher the stress, the lower the T-cell count (see the box "Immunity and Stress"). As described in Chapter 2, stress encompasses many variables, ranging from emotional stressors, such as anger, anxiety, depression, and grief, to physical stressors, such as poor nutrition, sleep deprivation, overexertion, and substance abuse. Developing effective ways of coping with stress can improve many of the dimensions of wellness.

In addition to managing the stress in your life and getting all your immunizations, you can help your body defend itself against disease by following the guidelines in the box "How to Keep Yourself Well." As is the case with all your body systems, your immune system works best when you support it with a healthy lifestyle.

Take Charge

- Eat a balanced diet, and maintain a healthy weight. Consume a variety of nutrient-dense foods to obtain the recommended amount of nutrients every day (see Chapter 12).

- Get enough sleep, 6–8 hours every night. Sleep is extremely important in helping the body replenish itself. Adequate sleep allows the proper production and performance of all immune system cells and functions. Insufficient sleep predisposes you to a great number of illnesses and more severe infections.

- Exercise (but not while you're sick). Moderate endurance exercise is an excellent way to reduce stress and strengthen the body, thereby preventing infection. However, exercising vigorously while you are sick may actually decrease your immunity and can prolong the infection, probably by facilitating the replication of the viruses.

- Don't smoke, and drink alcohol only in moderation. Smoking decreases the levels of some immune cells, and heavy and long-term drinking interferes with the normal functioning of the immune system.

- Wash your hands frequently. Remove your rings, and rub all surfaces of your hands with lather for at least 10–20 seconds; rinse thoroughly. Antibacterial soaps have not been found to reduce the risk of infection, and some experts are concerned that widespread use of antibacterial products may contribute to the development of drug-resistant bacteria. The most important thing is to wash your hands well

and often. (One study found that although 95% of adults claim they wash their hands after using a public restroom, only about 67% actually do.)

- Avoid contact with people who are contagious with infectious diseases transmitted via the respiratory route, such as influenza, chicken pox, and tuberculosis.

- Handle and prepare foods safely (see Chapter 12); don't drink water from streams or lakes, even in seemingly pristine wilderness areas.

- Avoid contact with mosquitoes and ticks. (See p. 530)

- Avoid contact with rodents and other disease carriers. Don't touch or feed wild rodents or any wild animals. Air out unused cabins before occupying them, and avoid stirring up dust when cleaning rodent-infested areas by first wetting the areas with disinfectant.

- Practice safer sex (see Chapter 18) and don't inject drugs.

- Get all appropriate immunizations, and use antibiotics appropriately. If you have a heart valve disorder and are at increased risk for infection (see Chapter 15), check with your physician about antibiotic use before dental or surgical procedures and before body piercing.

- If you do become ill, allow yourself time to recover. Be courteous to others by washing your hands frequently and covering your nose and mouth when you sneeze or cough.

Tips for Today

The immune system is a remarkable information network; it operates continuously on the cellular level to keep you well. You can support your immune system by practicing a wellness lifestyle—getting enough sleep, managing stress, eating well, exercising, and protecting yourself against infectious agents.

Right now you can

- Go wash your hands, and count out 20 seconds while doing so; you can estimate 20 seconds by singing "Twinkle, Twinkle, Little Star" slowly or "Happy Birthday" twice.

- Plan to move up your bedtime by 15 minutes, starting tonight.

- Put a small pack of tissues in your bag or coat pocket to use when you sneeze or cough, to avoid transmitting infection to others.

- Contribute a bar of soap or liquid hand soap to a public washroom you use frequently, such as in a common living area, in an academic building, or at work.

SUMMARY

- The step-by-step process by which infections are transmitted from one person to another involves the pathogen, its reservoir, a portal of exit, a means of transmission, a portal of entry, and a new host.

- Infection can be prevented by breaking the chain at any point. Strategies include public health measures such as treatment of drinking water and individual actions such as hand washing.

- Physical and chemical barriers to microorganisms include skin, mucous membranes, and the cilia lining the respiratory tract.

- The immune response is carried out by white blood cells that are continuously produced in the bone marrow. These include neutrophils, macrophages, dendritic cells, natural killer cells, and lymphocytes.

- The immune response has four stages: recognition of the invading pathogen; rapid replication of killer T cells and B cells; attack by killer T cells and macrophages; suppression of the immune response.

- Immunization is based on the body's ability to remember previously encountered organisms and retain its strength against them.
- Allergic reactions occur when the immune system responds to harmless substances as if they were dangerous antigens.
- Bacteria are single-celled organisms; some cause disease in humans. Bacterial infections include pneumonia, meningitis, strep throat, toxic shock syndrome, tuberculosis, Lyme disease, and ulcers.
- Most antibiotics work by interrupting the production of new bacteria; they do *not* work against viruses. Bacteria can become resistant to antibiotics.

- Viruses cannot grow or reproduce themselves; different viruses cause the common cold, influenza, measles, mumps, rubella, chicken pox, cold sores, mononucleosis, encephalitis, hepatitis, polio, and warts.
- Other diseases are caused by certain types of fungi, protozoa, parasitic worms, and prions.
- Autoimmune diseases occur when the body identifies its own cells as foreign.
- The immune system needs little help other than adequate nutrition and rest, a moderate lifestyle, and protection from excessive stress. Vaccinations also help protect against disease.

Take Action

1. **Create an immunization record:** Find out from your parents or your health records which immunizations you have had, including when you last had a tetanus shot. Are your immunizations up to date? If they aren't, or if you're not sure, check with your school health center for recommendations.

2. **Compare cold remedies:** Go to your local pharmacy and examine the cold and cough remedies. Exactly which symptoms does each one claim to alleviate and with what active ingredient? If possible, ask the pharmacist which ones he or she recommends for various symptoms.

For More Information

Books

Barry, J. 2005. *The Great Influenza: The Epic Story of the Deadliest Plague in History*. New York: Penguin. *A compelling account of the medical, social, and political aspects of the influenza epidemic of 1918–1919.*

Bollet, A. J. 2004. *Plagues and Poxes: The Impact of Human History on Epidemic Disease*. New York: Demos Medical. *Describes how human activity affects diseases.*

Karlen, A. 2001. *Biography of a Germ*. New York: Knopf. *An entertaining look at the natural history and life cycle of* Borrelia burgdorferi, *the bacterium that causes Lyme disease, from the microbe's point of view.*

Preston, R. 2002. *The Demon in the Freezer*. New York: Random House. *A look at the recent history of smallpox, including its eradication in nature and its potential use as a bioweapon.*

Sompayrac, L. M. 2003. *How the Immune System Works*. 2nd ed. Malden, Mass.: Blackwell Science. *A highly readable overview of basic concepts of immunity.*

Organizations, Hotlines, and Web Sites

Alliance for the Prudent Use of Antibiotics. Provides information on the proper use of antibiotics and tips for avoiding infections.
  http://www.tufts.edu/med/apua

American Academy of Allergy, Asthma, and Immunology. Provides information and publications; pollen counts are available from the Web site.
  800-822-2762
  http://www.aaaai.org

American Autoimmune-Related Diseases Association. Provides background information, coping tips, and an online knowledge quiz about autoimmune diseases.
  http://www.aarda.org

American College of Allergy, Asthma, and Immunology. Provides information for patients and physicians; Web site includes an extensive glossary of terms related to allergies and asthma.
  http://www.acaai.org

American Society for Microbiology. Includes a library of images and an introduction to microbes.
  http://www.microbeworld.org (Microbe World online)
  http://www.washup.org (Clean Hands Campaign)

Bugs in the News! Provides information about microbiology—allergies, antibodies, antibiotics, mad cow disease, and more—in easy-to-understand language.
  http://people.ku.edu/~jbrown/bugs.html

CDC National Center for Infectious Diseases. Provides extensive information on a wide variety of infectious diseases.
  http://www.cdc.gov/ncidod

CDC National Immunization Program. Information and answers to frequently asked questions about immunizations.
  800-CDC-SHOT
  877-FYI-TRIP (international travel information)
  http://www.cdc.gov/nip; http://www.cdc.gov/travel

Cells Alive! Includes micrographs of immune cells and pathogens at work.
  http://www.cellsalive.com

National Foundation for Infectious Diseases. Provides information about a variety of diseases and disease issues.
http://www.nfid.org

National Institute of Allergy and Infectious Diseases. Includes fact sheets about many topics relating to allergies and infectious diseases, including tuberculosis and STDs.
http://www.niaid.nih.gov

World Health Organization: Infectious Diseases. Provides fact sheets about many emerging and tropical diseases as well as information about current outbreaks.
http://www.who.int/topics/en

See also the listings in Chapter 12 (food safety), Chapter 18, and Appendix B.

Selected Bibliography

Andries, K., et al. 2005. A diarylquinoline drug active on the ATP synthetase of *Mycobacterium tuberculosis. Science* 307(5707): 223–227.

Cashman, N. R., and B. Caughey. 2004. Prion diseases—Close to an effective therapy? *Nature Reviews: Drug Discovery* 3(12): 874–884.

Centers for Disease Control and Prevention. 2004. *Basic Facts About Asthma* (http://www.cdc.gov/asthma/faqs.htm; retrieved January 31, 2005).

Centers for Disease Control and Prevention. 2004. Bovine spongiform encephalopathy in a dairy cow—Washington state, 2003. *Morbidity and Mortality Weekly Report* 52(53): 1280–1285.

Centers for Disease Control and Prevention. 2004. Trends in tuberculosis—United States, 1998–2003. *Morbidity and Mortality Weekly Report* 53(10): 209–214.

Centers for Disease Control and Prevention. 2004. Update: West Nile virus screening of blood donations and transfusion-associated transmission. *Morbidity and Mortality Weekly Report* 53(13): 281–284.

Centers for Disease Control and Prevention. 2005. *West Nile Virus Statistics, Surveillance, and Control* (http://www.cdc.gov/ncidod/dvbid/westnile/surv&controlCaseCount04_detailed.htm; retrieved January 31, 2005).

Cieslak, P. R., K. Hedberg, and L. E. Lee. 2004. Chickenpox outbreak in a highly vaccinated school population: In reply. *Pediatrics* 114(4): 1131.

Fairweather, D., and N. R. Rose. 2004. Women and autoimmune diseases. *Emerging Infectious Diseases* 10(11): 2005–2011.

Fauci, A. S. 2004. Emerging infectious diseases: A clear and present danger to humanity. *Journal of the American Medical Association* 292(15): 1887–1888.

Food and Drug Administration. 2005. *First Combination Vaccine Approved to Help Protect Adolescents Against Whooping Cough* (http://www.fda.gov/bbs/topics/ANSWERS/2005/ANS01354.html; retrieved May 13, 2005.)

Immunization Safety Review Committee. 2004. *Immunization Safety Review: Vaccines and Autism.* Washington, D.C.: National Academy Press.

Keene, W. E., A. C. Markum, and M. Samadpour. 2004. Outbreak of *Pseudomonas aeruginosa* infections caused by commercial piercing of upper ear cartilage. *Journal of the American Medical Association* 291(8): 981–985.

Ksiazek, T. G., et al. 2003. A novel coronavirus associated with severe acute respiratory syndrome. *New England Journal of Medicine* Online Article NEJMoa030781.

Larson, E. L., et al. 2004. Effect of antibacterial home cleaning and hand-washing products on infectious disease symptoms: A randomized, double-blind trial. *Annals of Internal Medicine* 140(5): 321–329.

Lee, G. M., et al. 2005. Illness transmission in the home: A possible role for alcohol-based hand gels. *Pediatrics* 115(4): 852–860.

Levy, S. B., and B. Marshall. 2004. Antibacterial resistance worldwide: Causes, challenges, and responses. *Nature Medicine* 10(12 Suppl): S122–S129.

National Immunization Program. 2005. *ACIP Recommends Meningococcal Vaccine for Adolescents and College Freshmen* (http://www.cdc.gov/nip/vaccine/meningitis/mcv4/mcv4_acip.htm; retrieved April 6, 2005).

National Immunization Program. 2005. *Epidemiology and Prevention of Vaccine-Preventable Diseases,* 8th ed. Rev. Waldorf, Md.: Public Health Foundation.

Parker, S. K., et al. 2004. Thimerosal-containing vaccines and autistic spectrum disorder: A critical review of published original data. *Pediatrics* 114(3): 793–804.

Prusiner, S. B. 2004. Detecting mad cow disease. *Scientific American,* July.

Samandari, T., B. P. Bell, and G. L. Armstrong. 2004. Quantifying the impact of hepatitis A immunization in the United States, 1995–2001. *Vaccine* 22(31–32): 4342–4350.

Simon, P. A., et al. 2003. Prevalence of childhood asthma and associated morbidity in Los Angeles County: Impacts of race/ethnicity and income. *Journal of Asthma* 40(5): 535–543.

Smeeth, L., et al. 2004. MMR vaccination and pervasive developmental disorders: A case-control study. *Lancet* 364(9438): 963–969.

Snow, R. W., et al. 2005. The global distribution of clinical episodes of *Plasmodium falciparum* malaria. *Nature* 434: 214–217.

Tanaka, M., et al. 2003. Trends in pertussis among infants in the United States. *Journal of the American Medical Association* 290(22): 2968–2975.

Vazquez, M., et al. 2004. Effectiveness over time of varicella vaccine. *Journal of the American Medical Association* 291(7): 851–855.

World Health Organization. 2004. *WHO Guidelines for the Global Surveillance of Severe Acute Respiratory Syndrome (SARS), Updated Recommendations, October 2004.* Geneva: World Health Organization.

World Health Organization. 2004. *The World Health Report 2004: Changing History.* Geneva: World Health Organization.

18

AHEAD

After reading this chapter, you should be able to

- Explain how HIV infection affects the body and how it is transmitted, diagnosed, and treated

- Discuss the symptoms, risks, and treatments for the other major STDs

- List strategies for protecting yourself from STDs

Sexually Transmitted Diseases

1. **If you have a sexually transmitted disease (STD), you will know it.**
   True or false?

2. **Worldwide, HIV infection is spread primarily via which of the following?**
   a. injection drug use
   b. sex between men
   c. mother-to-child transmission
   d. heterosexual sex

3. **About _____ Americans are infected with HIV, the virus that causes AIDS; and about _____ Americans are infected with HSV 2, the virus that causes most cases of genital herpes.**
   a. 1 in 30,000 (HIV); 1 in 20 (HSV 2)
   b. 1 in 3,000 (HIV); 1 in 10 (HSV 2)
   c. 1 in 300 (HIV); 1 in 5 (HSV 2)

4. **A man with an STD is more likely to transmit the infection to a female partner than vice versa.**
   True or false?

5. **After you have had an STD once, you become immune to that disease and cannot get it again.**
   True or false?

ANSWERS

1. FALSE. Many people with STDs have no symptoms and do not know they are infected; however, they can still pass an infection to their partners.

2. D. The vast majority of HIV infection cases worldwide result from heterosexual contact, and nearly two-thirds of all new cases occur in teenage girls and young women.

3. C. Worldwide, about 1 in 100 people is infected with HIV. Most of the approximately 1 in 5 Americans infected with HSV 2 are asymptomatic and unaware they are infected.

4. TRUE. For many STDs, infected men are at least twice as likely as infected women to transmit an STD to their partner. And many STDs are more physically damaging to women than to men.

5. FALSE. Reinfection with STDs is very common. For example, if you are treated and cured of chlamydia and then you have sex with your untreated partner, the chances are very good that you will be infected again.

Visit the *Core Concepts in Health* Online Learning Center
(www.mhhe.com/insel10e) for study aids and many additional resources.

547

Acquired immunodeficiency syndrome (AIDS) is a leading cause of death in many parts of the world. Most of the nearly 40 million people around the world who are infected with **human immunodeficiency virus (HIV)**, the virus that causes AIDS, will likely die within the next 10 years. Although the death rate from AIDS in the United States began to decline in 1996, more than 500,000 of the approximately 1.5 million Americans who have been infected with HIV have died from the disease, and it remains a major killer of Americans. Worldwide, AIDS is the leading cause of death for people age 15–59.

Although recent public education campaigns have focused primarily on HIV infection, all the **sexually transmitted diseases (STDs)**—gonorrhea, HPV infection (genital warts), chlamydia, herpes, syphilis, and others—continue to have a high incidence among Americans (Table 18-1). The United States has the highest rate of STDs of any developed nation; at current U.S. rates, half of all young people will acquire an STD by age 25. Worldwide, more than 340 million people are affected by STDs each year.

STDs are a particularly insidious group of diseases because a person can be infected and be able to transmit the disease to others yet not look or feel sick. The cost of unprotected sex may not become apparent for many years. Then a person may find that an undiagnosed STD has led to infertility, contributed to the development of cancer, or caused a birth defect in a child. In the case of HIV infection, the immune system becomes weakened and can no longer provide protection against disease.

It is important that everyone have a clear understanding of what STDs are, how they are transmitted, and—most important—how they can be prevented. The crucial message is that they *can* be prevented. And many can also be cured if they are treated early and properly. This chapter is designed to provide information about healthy, safer sexual behavior and to help you understand what you can do to reduce the further spread of these diseases.

THE MAJOR STDS

In general, seven different STDs pose major health threats: HIV/AIDS, hepatitis, syphilis, chlamydia, gonorrhea, herpes, and HPV infection (genital warts). These diseases are considered major because they are serious in themselves, cause serious complications if left untreated, and/or pose risks to a fetus or newborn. In addition, pelvic inflammatory disease (PID) is a common complication of gonorrhea and chlamydia and merits discussion as a separate disease. The pathogens responsible for these and other STDs are listed in Table 18-2.

VITAL STATISTICS

Table 18-1

Estimated Incidence and Prevalence of STDs in the United States

	Estimated Annual Incidence	Estimated Prevalence[a]
Trichomoniasis	7,400,000	n/a
HPV infection	6,200,000	20,000,000
Chlamydia	2,800,000	1,900,000
Genital herpes	1,600,000	45,000,000
Gonorrhea	718,000	n/a
Hepatitis B[b]	81,000	1,250,000
Syphilis (all stages)[c]	61,000	n/a
HIV infection[b]	40,000	900,000

n/a = not available.

[a]Because the viral STDs are persistent and incurable, the number of currently infected people capable of transmitting the infection (prevalence) greatly exceeds the annual number of new cases (incidence) of the viral STDs. Chlamydia prevalence remains high because most cases are asymptomatic and undiagnosed.

[b]Hepatitis B and HIV infection can be transmitted in a variety of ways; about half of all cases of HIV and 30–60% of cases of hepatitis B are transmitted sexually.

[c]Total includes about 8,000 cases of primary- and secondary-stage syphilis, the stages of the disease during which it can be easily transmitted to others.

SOURCES: Weinstock; H., S. Berman, and W. Cates. 2004. Sexually transmitted diseases among American youth: Incidence and prevalence estimates, 2000. *Perspectives on Sexual and Reproductive Health* 36(1): 6–10. Additional data from the Centers for Disease Control and Prevention and the Kaiser Family Foundation.

The bacterial STDs, including chlamydia, gonorrhea, and syphilis, are curable with antibiotics. Unfortunately, previous infection does not confer immunity, so a person can be reinfected despite treatment. The viral STDs—herpes, genital HPV infection (warts), hepatitis, and HIV infection—are not curable with current therapies. Although antiviral drugs and other medications can reduce the effects of these STDs, the virus remains in the body and may cause chronic or recurrent infection. A further risk of all STDs is that they can substantially contribute to the spread of HIV. The sores and inflammation caused by STDs allow HIV to pass more easily from one person to another.

HIV Infection and AIDS

HIV infection is one of the most serious and challenging problems facing the United States and the world today. Worldwide, it is estimated that more than 60 million people have been infected since the epidemic began—nearly 1% of the world's population—and that more than 20 million have died (see the box "HIV Infection Around the World" on p. 550). About 10 people are infected

Table 18-2 Sexually Transmitted Pathogens and Associated Diseases

Bacteria[a]

Chlamydia trachomatis	Chlamydia, pelvic inflammatory disease, epididymitis, urethritis
Gardnerella vaginalis[b]	Bacterial vaginosis
Haemophilus ducreyi	Chancroid
Neisseria gonorrhoeae	Gonorrhea, pelvic inflammatory disease, epididymitis, urethritis
Treponema pallidum	Syphilis

Viruses[c]

Hepatitis B virus (HBV)	Hepatitis, cirrhosis, liver cancer
Herpes simplex viruses (HSV)	Genital herpes, oral-labial herpes (cold sores)
Human immunodeficiency virus (HIV)	HIV infection/AIDS
Human papillomavirus (HPV)	Genital warts, cervical cancer

Protozoa[a]

Trichomonas vaginalis	Trichomoniasis

Ectoparasites[a]

Phthirus pubis	Pubic lice
Sarcoptes scabiei	Scabies

[a]Treatable with antibiotics or topical medications.
[b]Other organisms associated with bacterial vaginosis include *Mycoplasma hominis, Bacteroides,* and *Mobiluncus.*
[c]Incurable with current treatment methods, although medications may reduce symptoms and limit the damage from infection; viral STDs are usually chronic/recurrent.

every minute—5 million per year—and half of these new infections are in people age 15–24. By 2004, nearly 1million Americans were believed to be living with HIV—about 1 in 160 males and 1 in 800 females over age 12. Although the death rate from AIDS among Americans has declined, new infections have held steady at about 40,000 per year since the 1990s, meaning the number of Americans living with HIV infection is growing. More than one-quarter of HIV-infected Americans are unaware they are infected.

HIV is a relatively new disease in humans. Experts believe that the virus initially spread from chimpanzees to people during the middle of the twentieth century as a result of the trapping, butchering, or eating of infected chimps. Initially, HIV infection was relatively rare, but the disease began to spread rapidly in the 1970s and 1980s. Despite the best efforts of health professionals around the world, HIV infection continues to spread, and a cure is yet to be found.

What Is HIV Infection? **HIV infection** is a chronic disease that progressively damages the body's immune system, making an otherwise healthy person less able to resist a variety of infections and disorders. Normally, when a virus or other pathogen enters the body, it is targeted and destroyed by the immune system. But the human immunodeficiency virus (HIV) attacks the immune system itself, invading and taking over **CD4 T cells,** monocytes, and macrophages, which are essential elements of the immune system. HIV enters a human cell

and converts its own genetic material, RNA, into DNA. It then inserts this DNA into the chromosomes of the host cell. The viral DNA takes over the CD4 cell, causing it to produce new copies of HIV; it also makes the CD4 cell incapable of performing its immune functions. HIV primarily affects the T-cell part of the immune system (see Chapter 17).

Immediately following infection with HIV, billions of infectious particles are produced every day. For a time, the immune system keeps pace, also producing billions of new cells. Unlike the virus, however, the immune system cannot make new cells indefinitely; as long as the virus keeps replicating, it wins in the end. The destruction of the immune system is signaled by the loss of CD4 T cells

Terms

acquired immunodeficiency syndrome (AIDS) A generally fatal, incurable, sexually transmitted viral disease.

human immunodeficiency virus (HIV) The virus that causes HIV infection and AIDS.

sexually transmitted disease (STD) A disease that can be transmitted by sexual contact; some STDs can also be transmitted by other means.

HIV infection A chronic, progressive viral infection that damages the immune system.

CD4 T cell A type of white blood cell that helps coordinate the activity of the immune system; the primary target for HIV infection. A decrease in the number of these cells correlates with the risk and severity of HIV-related illness.

Although first detected among heterosexuals in Africa, AIDS captured world attention in the early 1980s as a disease occurring primarily among homosexual men in the United States and Europe. Since then, AIDS has spread around the world. More than 60 million people worldwide have been infected with HIV since the epidemic began, and more than 20 million have died. The United Nations has declared the spread of HIV infection a threat to world peace.

The vast majority of cases—95%—have occurred in developing countries, where heterosexual contact is the primary means of transmission, responsible for 85% of all adult infections. In the developed world, HIV is increasingly becoming a disease that disproportionately affects the poor and ethnic minorities. Worldwide, women are the fastest-growing group of newly infected people, and more than half the new cases of HIV infection in 2004 occurred in women and children. In addition, an estimated 2.2 million children are living with HIV infection and about 15 million children are AIDS orphans.

Sub-Saharan Africa remains the hardest hit of all areas of the world; in some countries, 20–40% of adults carry the virus, and overall life expectancy has begun to decline dramatically. However, because the epidemic started about 10 years later in Asia than in Africa, experts expect an explosion of new cases in Asia. And because Asia accounts for more than 50% of the world's population, the pool of people at risk is much larger than in Africa. HIV is also spreading rapidly in Eastern Europe, where injection drug use and commercial sex are increasing. The former Soviet countries have seen a fifty-fold increase in HIV infection in 8 years.

Efforts to combat AIDS are complicated by political, economic, and cultural barriers. Education and prevention programs are often hampered by resistance from social and religious institutions and by the taboo on openly discussing sexual issues. Condoms are unfamiliar in many countries, and women in many societies do not have sufficient control over their lives to demand that men use condoms during sex. Prevention approaches that have had success include STD treatment and education, public education campaigns about safer sex, and syringe exchange programs for injection drug users.

In countries where there is a substantial imbalance in the social power of men and women, focusing prevention efforts on men is an essential step. In some cultures, older men choose very young women and children as sexual partners, believing that they are less likely to be infected or that an HIV carrier who rapes a virgin will be cured, an unfortunately prevalent myth. Sexual violence and traditional practices such as very early marriage and widows being inherited by their husband's male relatives increase women's exposure to HIV.

International efforts are under way to make condoms more available by lowering their price and to develop effective antiviral creams that women can use without the knowledge of their partners. Education and other public health measures have been successful in slowing rates of new infection in some countries. In developed nations such as the United States, new drugs are easing AIDS symptoms and lowering viral levels dramatically for some patients. In the past few years, a small but growing number of people in poor countries have gained access to antiviral drugs because of the introduction of inexpensive generic drugs and increasing international funding for HIV treatment. Still, the vast majority of people with HIV remain untreated. Ultimately what we need is an effective vaccine. But until vaccines or a low-cost cure is developed, efforts must continue to focus on prevention through widespread educational campaigns and behavior change.

SOURCE: Joint United Nations Programme on HIV/AIDS (UNAIDS). 2004. *AIDS Epidemic Update: December 2004.* Geneva: UNAIDS/WHO.

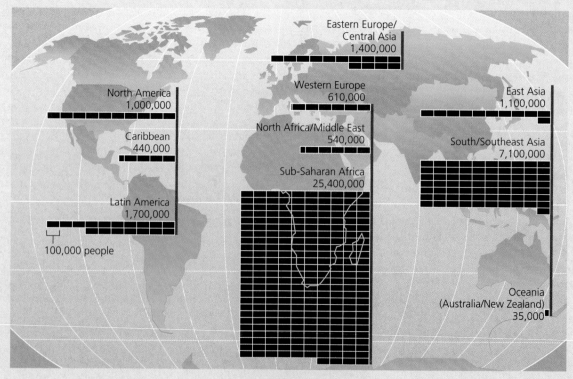

Approximate number of people living with HIV/AIDS at the beginning of 2005.

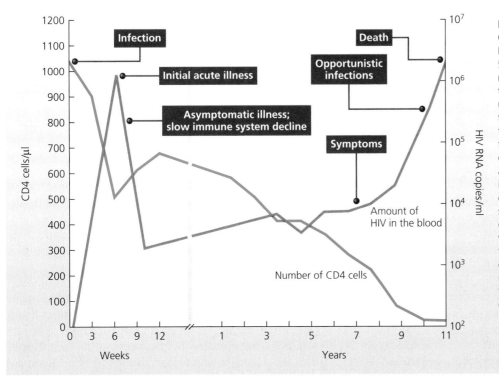

During the initial acute illness, CD4 levels fall sharply and HIV RNA levels increase; more than 50% of infected people experience flulike symptoms during this period. Antibodies to HIV usually appear 2–12 weeks after the initial infection. During the asymptomatic phase that follows, CD4 levels gradually decline, and HIV RNA levels again increase. Due to declines in immunity, infected individuals eventually begin to experience symptoms; when CD4 levels drop very low, people become vulnerable to serious opportunistic infections characteristic of full-blown AIDS. Chronic or recurrent illnesses continue until the immune system fails and death results.

Figure 18-1 The general pattern of untreated HIV infection. The purple line represents the number of CD4 cells in the blood, a marker for the status of the immune system. The orange line shows the amount of HIV RNA in the blood. SOURCE: Adapted from Fauci, A. S., et al. 1996. Immunopathogenic mechanisms of HIV infection. *Annals of Internal Medicine* 124: 654–663. Reprinted with permission of the American College of Physicians.

(Figure 18-1). As the number of CD4 cells declines, an infected person may begin to experience mild to moderately severe symptoms. A person is diagnosed with full-blown AIDS when he or she develops one of the conditions defined as a marker for AIDS or when the number of CD4 cells in the blood drops below a certain level (200/μl). People with AIDS are vulnerable to a number of serious—often fatal—secondary, or **opportunistic, infections.** The infections that most often prove deadly for people with HIV are seldom serious in people with a healthy immune system. In fact, opportunistic infections are usually caused by organisms that are very common in the environment and generally do not cause illness in healthy people.

The first weeks after being infected with HIV are called the *primary infection* phase. About half of infected people develop flulike symptoms during this time. During primary HIV infection, people have large amounts of HIV in the bloodstream, making them much more infectious than they will be several months later when they enter the chronic infection stage. Experts believe that about half of all cases of HIV infection are acquired from people who are in the primary infection stage. The vast majority of people with primary infection have no idea they are infected, and even if they suspect infection and get tested, the most commonly used tests for HIV will be negative in this stage. Special tests (see below) can detect primary infection, and

experts believe that increasing detection of primary infection could help reduce the spread of the virus.

The next phase of HIV infection is the chronic **asymptomatic** (symptom-free) stage. This period can last from 2 to 20 years, with an average of 11 years in untreated adults. During this time the virus progressively infects and destroys the cells of the immune system. People infected with HIV can transmit the disease to others, even if they are symptom-free. Even if they receive treatment, they remain infectious to a varying degree throughout their lives.

Transmitting the Virus HIV lives only within cells and body fluids, not outside the body. It is transmitted by blood and blood products, semen, vaginal and cervical secretions, and breast milk. It cannot live in air, in water, or on objects or surfaces such as toilet seats, eating utensils, or telephones. The three main routes of HIV transmission are (1) from specific kinds of sexual contact, (2) from direct exposure to infected blood, and (3) from

Terms

Vⁱw

opportunistic infection An infection caused when organisms take the opportunity presented by a primary (initial) infection to multiply and cause a secondary infection.

asymptomatic Showing no signs or symptoms of a disease.

Chapter 18 Sexually Transmitted Diseases 551

an HIV-infected woman to her fetus during pregnancy or childbirth or to her infant during breastfeeding.

SEXUAL CONTACT   HIV is more likely to be transmitted by unprotected anal or vaginal intercourse than by other sexual activities. Being the receptive partner during unprotected anal intercourse is the riskiest of all sexual activities. Oral-genital contact carries some risk of transmission, although less than anal or vaginal intercourse. Still, oral sex is responsible for a small but significant number of cases of HIV transmission. HIV can be transmitted through tiny tears in the fragile lining of the vagina, cervix, penis, anus, and mouth and through direct infection of cells in some of these areas.

The presence of lesions, blisters, or inflammation from other STDs in the genital, anal, or oral areas makes it two to nine times easier for the virus to be passed. In addition, any trauma or irritation of tissues, such as might occur from rough or unwanted intercourse or the use of enemas prior to anal intercourse, increases the risk. Spermicides may also cause irritation and increase the risk of HIV transmission. Recent studies of the widely used spermicide nonoxynol-9 (N-9) found that frequent use may cause vaginal and rectal irritation, increasing the risk of transmission of HIV and other STDs. The World Health Organization (WHO) recommends that spermicides containing N-9 not be used for protection against HIV and STDs. Condoms or lubricants with N-9 should never be used during anal intercourse because N-9 damages the lining of the rectum, providing an entry point for HIV and other STDs.

The risk of HIV transmission during oral sex increases if a person has poor oral hygiene, has oral sores, or has brushed or flossed just before or after oral sex. Some evidence suggests that recent consumption of alcohol may make the cells that line the mouth more susceptible to infection with HIV. During vaginal intercourse, male-to-female transmission is more likely to occur than female-to-male transmission. HIV has been found in preejaculatory fluid, so transmission can occur before ejaculation.

Studies in developing nations with high rates of HIV infection have found that circumcised males have a lower risk of HIV infection than uncircumcised males. Studies are ongoing to determine the magnitude of protection offered by circumcision, but most experts doubt whether circumcision, which is uncommon in most parts of the world, would ever be a practical preventive measure. In the United States, where circumcision is common and HIV infection rates are much lower, circumcision does not appear to offer any significant protection against HIV.

Term

V w

hemophilia A hereditary blood disease in which blood fails to clot and abnormal bleeding occurs, requiring transfusions of blood products with a specific factor to aid coagulation.

The odds that an infected person will transmit HIV to an uninfected person depend on a variety of factors. Let's look at an example of a heterosexual couple: Joe is HIV positive, Jane is not. Joe has a strain of HIV that is particularly infectious. He acquired the infection only 3 weeks ago and has no idea he is infected. The viral levels in Joe's blood and semen are extremely high because he is in the primary stage of infection. He also has genital herpes, which increases the likelihood that he will infect Jane with HIV. Jane is HIV-negative, but she also has genital herpes, although she doesn't know it. They have vigorous, unprotected vaginal intercourse. Will Jane acquire HIV? No one can accurately predict, but Jane's risk is substantially increased because of the strain of HIV involved, because Joe has very high viral levels, and because they both have another STD.

DIRECT CONTACT WITH INFECTED BLOOD   Direct contact with the blood of an infected person is the second major route of HIV transmission. Needles used to inject drugs (including heroin, cocaine, and anabolic steroids) are routinely contaminated by the blood of the user. If needles are shared, small amounts of one person's blood are directly injected into another person's bloodstream. HIV may be transmitted through subcutaneous and intramuscular injection as well, from needles or blades used in acupuncture, tattooing, ritual scarring, and piercing of the earlobes, nose, lip, nipple, navel, or other body part.

Nearly half of all new U.S. cases of HIV are caused, directly or indirectly, by sharing drug injection equipment contaminated with HIV. Drug users, their sex partners, and their children are all at extremely high risk for HIV infection. Most experts agree that syringe exchange programs combined with increased substance abuse treatment and prevention could significantly reduce the spread of HIV.

HIV has been transmitted in blood and blood products used in the medical treatment of injuries, serious illnesses, and **hemophilia**, resulting in about 14,000 cases of AIDS in the United States. Nearly all of these cases occurred in the early days of the AIDS epidemic, before effective screening tests were available. All blood in licensed U.S. blood banks and plasma centers is now thoroughly screened for HIV. The American Blood Bank Association estimates that fewer than 1 in 2 million units of blood products is capable of transmitting HIV. Unfortunately, the blood supply is much less safe in the rest of the world. In the developing world in particular, blood is not adequately tested and blood donors are not appropriately screened. In these countries, the risk of contracting HIV or another serious infection from a blood transfusion is very high. The WHO estimates that about 5% of all cases of HIV infection worldwide have resulted from the transfusion of infected blood and blood products.

A small number of health care workers have acquired HIV on the job; most of these cases involve needle sticks, in which a health care worker is accidentally stuck with a needle used on an infected patient. The only reported cases of possible transmission *to* patients are those of 6 patients of a Florida dentist, 1 patient of a nurse in France, and 1 patient of a French orthopedic surgeon. A method of transmission was never determined with certainty in the first two cases; in the third, an injury to the hand of the surgeon during an operation may have exposed the patient to infected blood. Intensive investigations of over 22,000 patients of 63 HIV-infected health care workers showed no other cases of HIV transmission from health care workers to patients in the United States. The likelihood of a patient acquiring HIV infection from a health care worker is almost negligible; the risk to health care workers from infected patients is much greater.

What about contact with other body fluids? Trace amounts of HIV have been found in the saliva and tears of some infected people. However, researchers believe that these fluids do not carry enough of the virus to infect another person. (In the rare cases of HIV infection linked to deep kissing or biting, the virus is thought to have been transmitted in blood from oral sores rather than in saliva.) Contact with the urine or feces of an infected person may carry some risk, but contact with sweat is not believed to carry any risk. There is absolutely no evidence that the virus can be spread by insects such as mosquitoes.

MOTHER-TO-CHILD TRANSMISSION The final major route of HIV transmission is mother-to-child, also called *vertical,* or *perinatal, transmission,* which can occur during pregnancy, childbirth, or breastfeeding. About 25–30% of infants born to untreated HIV-infected mothers are also infected with the virus; treatment can dramatically lower this infection rate. Worldwide, about two-thirds of vertical transmission occurs during pregnancy and childbirth and one-third through breastfeeding.

HIV-infected children rarely appear ill at birth, but they begin to develop health problems over the first months and years of life. About 20% of infected children become very ill and progress to AIDS or death by age 4; the remaining 80% develop problems more slowly. By 2004, over 8500 cases of AIDS in American children had been reported; worldwide, about 600,000 infants are infected each year. In the United States and other developed countries, new treatments to reduce vertical transmission are in use, and the number of new cases of HIV infection has declined more than 90% since 1992. The situation worldwide, however, is bleak: In developing countries, as many as 1 in 3 children born to HIV-positive women become infected. The lack of HIV testing and treatment and common breastfeeding account for this disparity.

NOT THROUGH CASUAL CONTACT A person is not at risk of getting HIV infection by being in the same classroom, dining room, or even household with someone who is infected. Before this was generally known, many people with HIV infection, including children, were the targets of

ostracism, hysteria, and outright violence. Today, it is an acknowledged responsibility of everyone to treat people with HIV infection with respect and compassion, regardless of their age or how they became infected.

Populations of Special Concern for HIV Infection Among Americans with AIDS, the most common means of exposure to HIV has been sexual activity between men; injection drug use (IDU) and heterosexual contact are the next most common (Figure 18-2, p. 554). Although the transmission of HIV occurs through specific individual behaviors, disproportionately high rates of infection in certain groups are tied to social, cultural, and economic factors. HIV in the United States is increasingly becoming a disease that affects ethnic minorities, women, and the poor. The U.S. pattern of HIV infection has changed over time: Heterosexual transmission accounts for a growing proportion of new cases, whereas the share caused by sex between men and injection drug use is falling. Women, especially African American women and Latinas, make up an increasingly large proportion of all U.S. AIDS cases. Overall, African American men and women are vastly overrepresented among people newly diagnosed with AIDS. See the box "HIV/AIDS Among African Americans and Latinos" on page 555 for more on these trends.

Another group of people at increased risk for HIV infection are young men who have sex with men. HIV infection has increased in recent years among this group, primarily because more young men are engaging in unsafe sexual practices such as unprotected anal intercourse. There are probably several factors underlying this trend. Young gay men are less likely than older men to have experienced watching friends die from AIDS and thus are more removed from the reality of the disease. They may be less afraid of acquiring HIV because of advances in treatment and a false belief that a cure is just around the corner. Drug use, especially use of crystal methamphetamine or club drugs, and the practice of meeting sex partners over the Internet are also associated with increased rates of unsafe sex and HIV infection among men who have sex with men.

There also appears to be a growing number of cases among men who acquire HIV through sex with other men but who do not identify themselves as gay. Particularly among minorities, many men who have sex with men also have sex with women, and they identify themselves as heterosexual, not gay or bisexual. Men who have sex with men and still identify themselves as heterosexual are just as likely to be infected with HIV as are gay and bisexual men who are out, but they are much less likely to know their HIV status and so may be more likely to transmit HIV to a male or female partner. Public health efforts directed toward gay men may not reach men in this group, and negative cultural attitudes toward homosexuality may make it difficult for gay and bisexual men to be

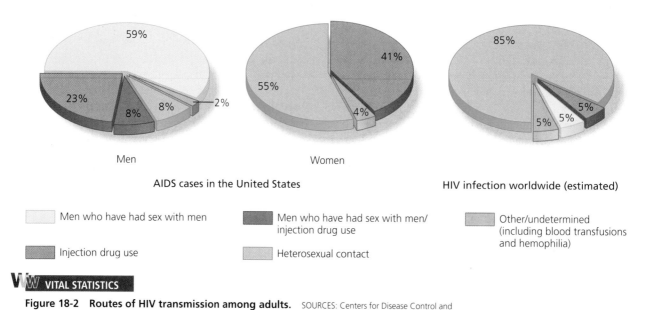

Men

Women

AIDS cases in the United States

HIV infection worldwide (estimated)

Men who have had sex with men

Men who have had sex with men/ injection drug use

Other/undetermined (including blood transfusions and hemophilia)

Injection drug use

Heterosexual contact

VITAL STATISTICS

Figure 18-2   Routes of HIV transmission among adults. SOURCES: Centers for Disease Control and Prevention. 2004. *HIV/AIDS Surveillance Report* 15; Joint United Nations Programme on HIV/AIDS (UNAIDS). 2004. *AIDS Epidemic Update, December 2004.* Geneva: UNAIDS; World Health Organization. 2001. Global AIDS surveillance. *Weekly Epidemiological Record* 76(50): 389–400.

honest with their partners. This trend endangers not only the men but also their male and female partners.

These patterns of HIV infection reflect complex social, economic, and behavioral factors. Reducing the rates of HIV transmission and AIDS death in minorities, women, and other groups at risk will require dealing with the difficult problems of drug abuse, poverty, and discrimination. HIV prevention programs must be tailored to meet the special needs of minority communities.

Increased testing is one of the most important aspects of HIV prevention, but knowledge of HIV status may not be enough to change behavior. Studies show that up to one-third of people who have been diagnosed with HIV continue to have unprotected sex. Testing must be coupled with strategies not only to encourage HIV-positive people to take the steps necessary to avoid infecting others but also to encourage HIV-negative people to consistently practice safer sex.

Symptoms of HIV Infection   Within a few days or weeks of infection with HIV, about half of people will develop symptoms of primary HIV infection. These can include fever, fatigue, rashes, headache, swollen lymph nodes, body aches, night sweats, sore throat, nausea, and diarrhea. Because the symptoms of primary HIV infection are similar to those of many common viral illnesses, the condition often goes undiagnosed, even if an infected individual sees a physician.

Term

HIV RNA assay A test used to determine the viral load (the amount of HIV in the blood).

Diagnosis of HIV at this very early stage of infection, although uncommon, is extremely beneficial. Immediate treatment is sometimes given to help preserve immune function, slow the progress of the disease, and reduce transmission of HIV to others. Studies are under way to evaluate the potential benefits and risks of starting treatment during primary HIV infection. It is critical for people who have engaged in behavior that places them at risk for HIV infection and who then experience symptoms of primary HIV infection to immediately inform their physician of their risk status. Standard tests for HIV will usually be negative in the very early stages of infection, so specialized tests such as the **HIV RNA assay,** which directly measures the amount of virus in the body, must be used.

Other than the initial flulike symptoms associated with primary HIV infection, most people in the first months or years of HIV infection have few if any symptoms. As the immune system weakens, however, a variety of symptoms can develop—persistent swollen lymph nodes; lumps, rashes, sores, or other growths on or under the skin or on the mucous membranes of the eyes, mouth, anus, or nasal passages; persistent yeast infections; unexplained weight loss; fever and drenching night sweats; dry cough and shortness of breath; persistent diarrhea; easy bruising and unexplained bleeding; profound fatigue; memory loss; difficulty with balance; tremors or seizures; changes in vision, hearing, taste, or smell; difficulty in swallowing; changes in mood and other psychological symptoms; and persistent or recurrent pain. Obviously, many of these symptoms can also occur with a variety of other illnesses.

Because the immune system is weakened, people with HIV infection are highly susceptible to infections, both common and uncommon. The infection most often seen

African Americans and Latinos have been disproportionately affected by HIV/AIDS since the start of the epidemic, and the disparity has grown over time.

- African Americans represent 12.6% of the U.S. population but account for 40% of all AIDS cases diagnosed since the start of the epidemic and nearly 50% of new cases diagnosed in 2003 (see figure).

- Latinos represent 13.2% of the U.S. population but account for about 20% of all AIDS cases and about 20% of new cases.

- AIDS is the third leading cause of death among African Americans age 25–34; it is the sixth leading cause among Latinos and whites in the same age group. AIDS deaths have declined among most groups of Americans since 1996. Among African Americans, the decline in AIDS deaths was smaller than among whites and has now leveled off. AIDS deaths among Latinos increased between 1999 and 2003; Latinos were the

only group to experience an increase during this period.

- Among AIDS cases diagnosed in women in 2003, African American women accounted for 67%; Latinas, 16%; and white women, 15%.

- Among teens (age 13–19), African Americans represent 15% of the total population but account for about 65% of newly diagnosed AIDS cases.

- Among AIDS cases diagnosed in men, a greater proportion of cases among African Americans and Latinos are due to heterosexual sex and injection drug use compared with white men. However, the most common means of HIV transmission among men from all groups is sex with other men (78% of cases among white men, 50% among Latinos, and 43% among black men).

What are some of the factors contributing to disparities in HIV incidence?

- *Poverty, drug use, and associated problems:* Low income is linked to lack of information about safer sex and HIV testing and treatment, higher rates of injection drug use, and lack of access to health care. Women who are poor and unemployed are more likely to be financially dependent on a male partner and less likely to use condoms; they are more likely to trade sex for money or drugs. Higher rates of incarceration among minorities also contribute to the spread of HIV. Overall, HIV prevention is likely to be a lower priority among people of low income because they are dealing with many immediate problems.

- *Distrust of physicians and public health campaigns:* Surveys suggest that a substantial proportion of blacks believe that HIV information is being withheld from the public and that a cure exists but is being withheld from the poor. These types of beliefs may deter some people from using condoms; they also highlight the need to tailor HIV prevention programs for different groups.

- *Social patterns and perception of risk:* High prevalence of infection in a group, combined with a low perception of risk, contributes to the spread of HIV as people are more likely to encounter an in-

fected sex partner if they choose partners from a group with a high prevalence.

A recent study of young African American men who have sex with men found that despite high rates of risky behavior, most did not perceive themselves at risk for HIV infection and many thought that HIV status could be determined from someone's appearance or whether they identify themselves as straight or gay. Many of the men in this study did not identify as gay and/or were not open about their sexual identity, and nearly 20% had had recent female sex partners. It is unclear how large a role this pattern plays in the transmission of the virus, but it is a risky pattern for the men and their male and female sexual partners.

New approaches to prevention and treatment will likely be needed to combat the high incidence of HIV/AIDS among African Americans and Latinos. HIV prevention messages need to communicate effectively with the populations most at risk. Programs stressing ethnic and gender pride have been found effective for some groups. To overcome conspiracy beliefs, researchers recommend acknowledging the origin of such beliefs in the context of current and historical discrimination. For those who are already HIV-positive, resources such as peer networks, legal assistance, and on-site child-care at clinics may help improve treatment access and success.

The Department of Health and Human Services' Minority HIV/AIDS Initiative Web site (www.hiv.omhrc.gov) has information about HIV/AIDS among minority populations and extensive links to relevant organizations.

SOURCES: Centers for Disease Control and Prevention. 2005. HIV transmission among black women—North Carolina, 2004. *Morbidity and Mortality Weekly Report* 54(4): 89–94; Kaiser Family Foundation. 2005. *Policy Fact Sheet: African Americans and HIV/AIDS.* Menlo Park, Calif.: Kaiser Family Foundation; Bogart, L. M., and S. Thorburn. 2005. Are HIV/AIDS conspiracy beliefs a barrier to HIV prevention among African Americans? *Journal of Acquired Immune Deficiency Syndromes* 38(2): 213–218; Centers for Disease Control and Prevention. 2004. HIV transmission among black college student and non-student men who have sex with men—North Carolina, 2003. *Morbidity and Mortality Weekly Report* 53(32): 731–734; Centers for Disease Control and Prevention. 2004. *HIV/AIDS Surveillance Report* 15.

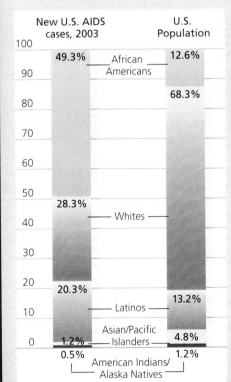

Distribution of U.S. AIDS cases by ethnicity compared to the ethnic distribution of the U.S. population.

in the United States among people with HIV is *Pneumocystis carinii* **pneumonia,** a protozoal infection. **Kaposi's sarcoma,** a previously rare form of cancer, is common in HIV-infected men. Women with HIV infection often have frequent and difficult-to-treat vaginal yeast infections. Cases of tuberculosis (TB) are increasingly being reported in people with HIV, and the CDC recommends TB testing for anyone with HIV infection. In Africa, drug-resistant strains of TB are now the most deadly infection among people with AIDS.

Diagnosing HIV Infection   Early diagnosis of HIV infection is important to minimize the impact of the disease and reduce the risk of infecting others. The most common tests for HIV check for the presence of antibodies to the virus. As described earlier, HIV infection primarily disrupts T-cell immunity; B cells are still able to produce antibodies to HIV, which will show up in tests. Unfortunately, these antibodies do not protect against the spread of the virus. For most other diseases, the presence of an antibody to a particular pathogen may indicate protective immunity. In the case of HIV, however, the presence of the antibody indicates an active case of the disease. **HIV antibody tests** are used for screening because they are accurate and relatively inexpensive. Standard testing involves an initial test called an **ELISA**; if it is positive, a second test called a **Western blot** is done to confirm the results (see the box "Getting an HIV Test").

Not everyone with HIV infection will test positive on antibody tests, however. Antibodies may not appear in the blood for weeks or months after infection, so people who are newly infected are likely to have a negative antibody test. The infection can be detected with a more expensive test that directly measures the presence of the virus, such as an HIV RNA test. The reverse situation is seen in babies born to HIV-infected mothers: They may carry HIV anti-

bodies, passed from their mother, without being infected with HIV. Antibodies can pass through the placenta to a fetus, but in the majority of cases, even without treatment, an infant does not acquire HIV. Thus, an infant may test positive on an HIV antibody test but actually be uninfected. Further tests such as the HIV RNA assay must be done to determine if an infant is actually infected.

If a person is diagnosed as **HIV-positive,** the next step is to determine the current severity of the disease in order to plan appropriate treatment. The status of the immune system can be gauged by taking CD4 T-cell measurements every few months. The infection itself can be monitored by tracking the viral load (the amount of virus in the body) through HIV RNA assay. Keeping track of viral load changes helps physicians evaluate the effects of treatment and can also help predict the likelihood of long-term survival in a person infected with HIV.

A 2004 survey of Americans indicates that nearly half of adults in the United States have been tested for HIV. About 20% of those had been tested in the previous year. Among those who have never been tested, nearly three-fourths say that they haven't been tested because they don't think they are at risk. About 10% say they are afraid of having their blood drawn, 6% say they are worried about confidentiality, and another 6% say they don't know where to go to be tested. Many people are not aware that rapid HIV tests, home tests, and tests that do not require a blood sample are now available.

A new diagnostic test that may help guide treatment decisions is called HIV Replication Capacity. This test shows how fast HIV from a patient's blood sample can reproduce itself. It is a measure of viral fitness, and may be helpful when used in conjunction with CD4 and viral load tests in predicting how quickly a given person may progress to more serious disease.

Diagnosing AIDS   As mentioned earlier, AIDS is the most severe form of HIV infection. The CDC's criteria for a diagnosis of AIDS reflect the stage of HIV infection at which a person's immune system becomes dangerously compromised. Since January 1993, a diagnosis of AIDS has been made if a person is HIV-positive and either has developed an infection defined as an AIDS indicator or has a severely damaged immune system (as measured by CD4 T-cell counts).

Reporting   All diagnosed cases of AIDS must be reported to public health authorities. Before effective treatments for HIV infection were available, officials could use AIDS statistics to track the epidemic because nearly everyone with HIV eventually developed AIDS within a fairly predictable time frame. However, the advent of more effective treatments has lengthened the time between infection and the onset of full-blown AIDS for many patients, making it more difficult to track the U.S. epidemic based on AIDS statistics alone. For this reason,

Terms

Vw

Pneumocystis carinii **pneumonia** A protozoal infection that is common in people infected with HIV.

Kaposi's sarcoma A form of cancer characterized by purple or brownish lesions that are generally painless and occur anywhere on the skin; usually appears in men infected with HIV.

HIV antibody test A blood test to determine whether a person has been infected by HIV; becomes positive within weeks or months of exposure.

ELISA (enzyme-linked immunosorbent assay) A blood test that detects the presence of antibodies to HIV.

Western blot A blood test that detects the presence of HIV antibodies; a more accurate and more expensive test used to confirm positive results from an ELISA test.

HIV-positive A diagnosis resulting from the presence of HIV in the bloodstream; also referred to as *seropositive.*

seroconversion The appearance of antibodies to HIV in the blood of an infected person; usually occurs 1–6 months after infection.

Critical Consumer

Some experts recommend HIV testing for all Americans. An individual should strongly consider being tested if any of the following apply to him or her or to any past or current sexual partner:

- You have had unprotected sex (vaginal, anal, or oral) with more than one partner or with a partner who was not in a mutually monogamous relationship with you.

- You have used or shared needles, syringes, or other paraphernalia for injecting drugs (including steroids).

- You received a transfusion of blood or blood products between 1978 and 1985.

- You have been diagnosed with an STD.

Testing Options

If you decide to get an HIV test, either you can visit a physician or health clinic or you can take a home test. A big advantage to having the test performed by a physician or clinician is that you will get one-on-one counseling about the test, your results, and ways to avoid future infection or spreading the disease. If you have good reason to think you may test positive, it is probably best to be tested by a physician or clinic, where follow-up counseling and medical care will be intensive. The home test is a good alternative for people at low risk who just want to be sure. Home tests can be done privately and anonymously and may be attractive to people who would not otherwise get tested.

Physician or Clinic Testing

Your physician, student health clinic, Planned Parenthood, public health department, or local AIDS association can arrange your HIV test. It usually costs $50–$100, but public clinics often charge little or nothing. The standard test involves drawing a sample of blood that is sent to a laboratory for analysis for the presence of antibodies; if the first stage of testing is positive, a confirmatory test is done. This standard test takes 1–2 weeks, and you'll be asked to phone or come in personally to obtain your results, which should also include appropriate counseling.

Alternative tests are available at some clinics. The Orasure test uses oral fluid, which is collected by placing a treated cotton pad in the mouth; urine tests are also available. Oral fluid and urine tests may be helpful for people who avoid blood tests due to fear of needles; they also protect health care workers from needlestick exposure to potentially infected blood. If you suspect you have been recently exposed to HIV and might have primary infection, see your physician and ask about an HIV RNA test.

New rapid tests are now also available at some locations. These tests involve the use of blood or oral fluid and can provide results in as little as 20 minutes. If a rapid test is positive for HIV infection, a confirmatory test will be performed.

Before you get an HIV test, be sure you understand what will be done with the results. Results from confidential tests may still become part of your medical record and/or be reported (with your name or some other identifier) to state and federal public health agencies. If you decide you want to be tested anonymously—in which case the results will not be reported to anyone but yourself—check with your physician or counselor about how to obtain an anonymous test or use a home test.

Home Testing

Home test kits for HIV are now available; they cost about $40–60. (Take care to avoid testing kits that are not FDA-approved; many such unapproved kits are being sold over the Internet.) To use a home test, you prick a finger with a supplied lancet, blot a few drops of blood onto blotting paper, and mail it to the company's laboratory. In about a week, you call a toll-free number to find out your results. Anyone testing positive is routed to a trained counselor, who can provide emotional and medical support. The results of home test kits are completely anonymous.

Understanding the Results

A negative test result means that no antibodies were found in your sample. However, it usually takes at least a month (and possibly as long as 6 months in some people) after exposure to HIV for antibodies to appear, a process called **seroconversion.** Therefore, an infected person may get a false-negative result. If you think you've been exposed to HIV, get a test immediately; if it's negative but your risk of infection is high, ask about obtaining an HIV RNA assay, which allows very early diagnosis, and about the appropriateness of retesting in a few months. If you test negative, you'll also receive information about how to avoid infection.

A positive result means that you are infected. It is important to seek medical care and counseling immediately. You need to know more about your medical options; the possible psychological, social, and financial repercussions; and how to avoid spreading the disease. Rapid progress is being made in treating HIV, and treatments are potentially much more successful when begun early.

For more information about HIV testing and a national directory of testing sites, visit the CDC National HIV Testing Resources site (www.hivtest.org).

the CDC recommended in 1999 that states require reporting of both HIV infection and AIDS.

Despite efforts to safeguard confidentiality and prohibit discrimination, mandatory reporting of HIV infection remains controversial. If people believe they are risking their jobs, friends, or social acceptability, they may be less likely to be tested. At the same time, it is essential that enough information be disclosed to monitor the epidemic. The CDC recommends that states continue to provide opportunities for people to be tested anonymously; home HIV tests also allow anonymous testing.

Treatment   Although there is no known cure for HIV infection, medications can significantly alter the course of

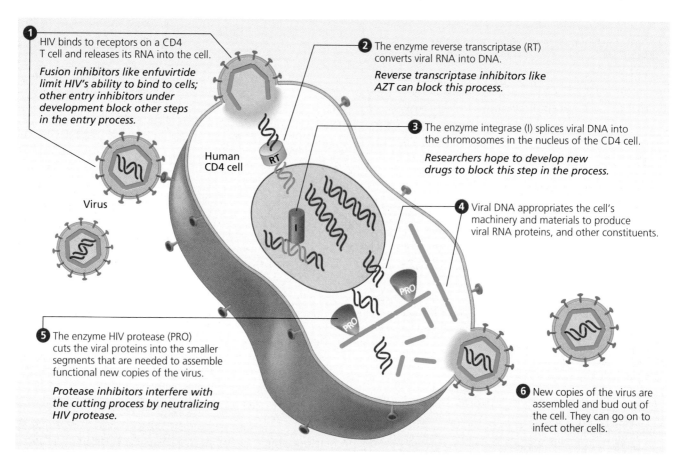

① HIV binds to receptors on a CD4 T cell and releases its RNA into the cell.

Fusion inhibitors like enfuvirtide limit HIV's ability to bind to cells; other entry inhibitors under development block other steps in the entry process.

Virus

Human CD4 cell

② The enzyme reverse transcriptase (RT) converts viral RNA into DNA.

Reverse transcriptase inhibitors like AZT can block this process.

③ The enzyme integrase (I) splices viral DNA into the chromosomes in the nucleus of the CD4 cell.

Researchers hope to develop new drugs to block this step in the process.

④ Viral DNA appropriates the cell's machinery and materials to produce viral RNA proteins, and other constituents.

⑤ The enzyme HIV protease (PRO) cuts the viral proteins into the smaller segments that are needed to assemble functional new copies of the virus.

Protease inhibitors interfere with the cutting process by neutralizing HIV protease.

⑥ New copies of the virus are assembled and bud out of the cell. They can go on to infect other cells.

Figure 18-3   The life cycle of HIV: How antiviral drugs work.   Different classes of drugs block the replication of HIV at different points in the virus's life cycle.   SOURCES: A virus in action. 2001. *Scientific American,* November; Dickinson, G., et al. 1998. The latest recommendations for antiretroviral therapy. *Patient Care,* 15 August.

the disease and extend life. The drop in the number of U.S. AIDS deaths that has occurred since 1996 is in large part due to the increasing use of combinations of new drugs. However, progress in the treatment of HIV infection is irrelevant to the vast majority of AIDS sufferers around the world, because the medications are financially far beyond their reach.

ANTIVIRAL DRUGS   Antiviral drugs in current use to combat HIV fall into several categories based on how they block HIV replication. One category is **reverse transcriptase inhibitors,** which include the widely used drug zidovudine (AZT). These drugs work by inhibiting the enzyme reverse transcriptase, which is used by HIV to integrate its genetic material into human cells (Figure 18-3). Another category of antivirals is the **protease inhibitors;** these target the enzyme HIV protease, which is used by the virus to create a protein coat for each new copy of the virus. In 2003, the FDA approved enfuvirtide (Fuzeon), the first available medication from a category of drugs known as **fusion inhibitors;** these drugs inhibit the fusion of viral and cell membranes and can block HIV from entering and infecting cells. Enfuvirtide can be used

for advanced HIV infection in conjunction with other antivirals. Treatment with combinations of drugs, referred to as highly active antiretroviral therapy, or HAART, can reduce HIV in the blood to undetectable levels in some people. However, research indicates that latent virus is still present in the body and that HIV-infected men on HAART carry potentially transmissible HIV in their semen.

Other antiviral drugs are under development, including entry inhibitors targeting the CCR-5 receptor, one of several receptors on human CD4 cells that interact with HIV and serve as doors through which the virus enters the cell. People who have a particular genetic mutation in one copy of the CCR-5 gene have half the normal number of CCR-5 receptors. Because of this, these individuals are less likely than average to become infected with HIV, and if they do become infected, they tend to stay healthy much longer. People with mutations in both CCR-5 genes are even more resistant to HIV infection, although a few have developed AIDS and died. Researchers are developing drugs that block the CCR-5 receptor as well as other cell entry components. Other expected treatment advances include drugs that stop HIV from integrating its genetic material into human DNA and improved versions of current drugs.

New findings that may someday influence HIV prevention and treatment include the discovery that a person infected with both HIV and the virus GBV-C is more likely to do well than someone who is infected with only HIV. This may be because GBV-C somehow blocks HIV entry into CD4 cells. This information may prove useful in developing a vaccine or new treatments for HIV infection. An intriguing recent study found that Trim5-alpha, a protein produced by nonhuman primates, can block cell entry of HIV and may explain why these animals do not become infected with HIV. Perhaps future research will utilize this protein for drugs that can help prevent or treat HIV.

Care for people with HIV has become increasingly complicated over the years as the number of treatment options has increased dramatically. Studies show that HIV-infected people do better and live longer if they are cared for by a doctor who is very experienced in treating HIV.

For more on treatment, refer to the resources listed in For More Information at the end of the chapter.

POSTEXPOSURE PROPHYLAXIS (PEP) Antiviral medications are being used in some cases in an attempt to prevent infection in people who have been exposed to HIV. The CDC has long recommended that health care workers who have significant exposure to HIV-infected blood or body fluids via a needle stick or other mishap consider starting antiviral medication as soon as possible (preferably within a few hours of exposure) to decrease the risk of infection. PEP is also often recommended for victims of sexual assault. In 2005, the CDC for the first time recommended PEP for people who are at risk for HIV infection from recent nonoccupational exposure to blood, genital secretions, or other potentially infectious body fluids of a person known to have HIV. Nonoccupational exposure refers to situations such as unprotected sex or contact with a contaminated needle. PEP consists of 28 days of HAART, which should begin as soon as possible after exposure, but always within 72 hours.

TREATMENTS FOR OPPORTUNISTIC INFECTIONS In addition to antiviral drugs, most patients with low CD4 T-cell counts also take a variety of antibiotics to help prevent opportunistic infections such as *Pneumocystis carinii* pneumonia and tuberculosis. A person with advanced HIV infection may need to take 20 or more pills every day. Medication side effects can become severe when so many drugs are used in combination.

HIV AND PREGNANCY Early-stage HIV infection does not appear to significantly affect a woman's chance of becoming pregnant. Without treatment, 25–30% of infants born to HIV-infected women are themselves infected with the virus. The risk of an infected mother transmitting HIV to her baby can be reduced to less than 2% by treating the mother during her pregnancy and labor, giving the baby

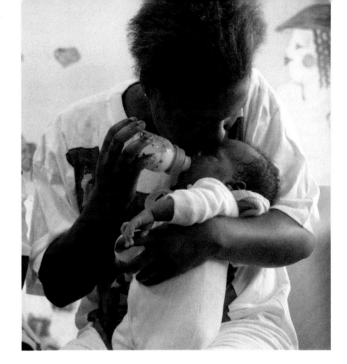

Early diagnosis and treatment of HIV infection are important for everyone, but particularly so for pregnant women. Currently available treatments can significantly increase the chance that this baby, born to an HIV-infected mother, will be free of the virus.

antiretroviral drugs during the first weeks of life, avoiding breastfeeding, and delivering the baby by cesarean section if necessary. Cesarean delivery can lower the risk of infection in women who have high blood levels of HIV; women who have undergone antiviral treatment and have very low levels of HIV can usually deliver vaginally. Because treatment can make such a dramatic difference in the health of the baby, HIV testing is strongly recommended for all pregnant women.

HIV-infected women are usually advised not to breastfeed, because this has been shown to transmit HIV. In developed countries, women infected with HIV generally have the support and resources to bottlefeed their infants. However, this is often not the case in developing countries: Infant formula is often unavailable and/or unaffordable, and many regions lack a supply of safe water with which to mix formula. In addition, bottlefeeding is socially unacceptable in some cultures and may be seen as a

Term V\w

reverse transcriptase inhibitor An antiviral drug used to treat HIV infection that works by inhibiting reverse transcriptase, the enzyme that converts viral RNA to DNA.

protease inhibitor A drug that inhibits the action of any of the protein-splitting enzymes known as proteases. Protease inhibitors have been developed to block the action of HIV protease and thus prevent the replication of HIV.

fusion inhibitor An antiviral drug that blocks the entry of HIV into cells by inhibiting the fusion of viral and cell membranes; part of a broader class of drugs known as *entry inhibitors*.

sign that the mother has AIDS. Many infants in Africa whose mothers do receive treatment during pregnancy and delivery are born uninfected but then acquire the infection later, through breastfeeding.

Testing and the use of antiviral drugs by pregnant HIV-positive women has had a dramatic effect in the United States. Unfortunately, long-term combination antiviral therapy is very expensive and is out of reach for most of the world's HIV-positive women. As newer and less expensive drugs against HIV become available, there is hope that more pregnant women and infants will be treated, resulting in lower vertical transmission rates worldwide. Currently, some resource-poor nations are reducing the spread of HIV to infants by giving a single dose of a relatively inexpensive antiretroviral drug to mother and newborn. Although not as effective as more extensive treatment, this is a major advance in HIV prevention for many developing countries.

TREATMENT CHALLENGES The cost of treatment for HIV continues to be an area of major concern. A recent study revealed an average cost of $14,000–35,000 per year to treat an HIV-infected person in the United States. These costs are tremendous even for relatively wealthy countries. But 95% of people with HIV infection live in developing countries, where these treatments are unlikely to be available to anyone except the wealthiest few. The average per-person health expenditure in many developing countries is only about $10 per year. Pharmaceutical companies and the World Bank are working to develop combination pills and to lower drug costs in developing regions, and international aid is gradually increasing; however, it is still not nearly enough to counteract the devastating impact of AIDS on these countries.

Toxicity of antiretroviral drugs is another concern. Long-term use of HAART can cause a number of serious effects, including bone loss and dangerously high levels of cholesterol. For this reason, the National Institutes of Health issued new HIV treatment guidelines in 2001 that recommend that asymptomatic patients hold off on treatment until they are at a more advanced stage of the disease. However, immediate treatment is still recommended for anyone who is experiencing symptoms. Treatment for primary stage (very recent) infection remains controversial.

Even for those who have access to the drugs and can tolerate the side effects, treatment is difficult. The drug combinations often require people to take many pills every day at precise times. If the drugs are not taken on schedule, their effectiveness is reduced and the virus is much more likely to develop drug resistance. Some people cannot tolerate the toxic side effects of these powerful drugs, and the drugs are

much more effective for some people than for others. Currently available antiviral drugs do not appear able to completely eliminate the virus from the body, even if viral levels in the blood become undetectable. The optimal duration of drug therapy is not currently known, but many scientists feel that lifelong drug therapy will be necessary. It is also unclear to what degree a damaged immune system can rebound from the effects of long-term HIV infection even if the virus is brought under control with antiviral medication.

What About a Vaccine? If an effective, safe, affordable vaccine against HIV could be developed, it might be possible to stop the worldwide HIV epidemic in its tracks. Many different approaches to the development of an AIDS vaccine are currently under investigation, and human trials have begun on several vaccines. Unfortunately, making a vaccine against HIV is proving to be exceedingly difficult. Methods that have been used to produce vaccines against other diseases are often ineffective or unsafe when used against HIV. Adding to the challenge is the fact that HIV comes in numerous subtypes, mutates rapidly, and destroys the very cells that normally protect the body against infectious diseases. It is possible that numerous vaccines will be needed because of the variety of HIV subtypes found around the world and the virus's ability to mutate. Vaccines are currently being tested in humans, but no vaccine is likely to be ready for widespread use within the next 5 years. Vaccines are also being tested as therapy for people already infected with HIV.

Although an effective and safe vaccine is still quite a long way from being a reality, researchers are making relatively rapid progress in producing a **microbicide** that could be used to prevent HIV and other STDs. A microbicide in the form of a cream, gel, sponge, or suppository that could be inserted into the vagina or rectum could function as a kind of chemical condom. Researchers are hoping to develop a product that kills HIV and other STD organisms, is pleasant and easy to use, and can also protect against pregnancy. A microbicide could fill the urgent need for a prevention method that can be used by a woman without requiring cooperation from her partner. Several microbicides are currently undergoing human testing for safety and effectiveness.

Another approach is the use of preexposure treatment as prevention. HIV-negative individuals at high risk for infection would take an anti-HIV medication prior to an activity that might expose them to HIV. This approach is controversial but might be effective in stopping the spread of HIV in highly vulnerable populations such as sex workers. Unlike a vaccine, this form of prevention could be tested and put into practice in a relatively short period of time, especially if an existing HIV drug is used.

How Can You Protect Yourself? Although AIDS is currently incurable, it is preventable. You can protect yourself by avoiding behaviors that may bring you into

Term

V&w

microbicide An agent that destroys microorganisms; also known as an antiseptic.

contact with HIV. This means making careful choices about sexual activity and not sharing needles if you inject drugs.

MAKE CAREFUL CHOICES ABOUT SEXUAL ACTIVITY In a sexual relationship, the current and past behaviors of you and your partner determine the amount of risk involved. If you are uninfected and in a mutually monogamous relationship with another uninfected person, you are not at risk for HIV. Of course, it is often hard to know for sure whether your partner is completely faithful and is truly uninfected. Having a series of monogamous relationships is not a safe prevention strategy.

For anyone not involved in a long-term, mutually monogamous relationship, abstinence from any sexual activity that involves the exchange of body fluids is the only sure way to prevent HIV infection (Figure 18-4). Safer sex includes many activities that carry virtually no risk of HIV infection, such as hugging, massaging, closed-lip kissing, rubbing clothed bodies together, kissing your partner's skin, and mutual masturbation.

Anal and vaginal intercourse are the sexual activities associated with the highest risk of HIV infection. If you have intercourse, always use a condom. Use of a lubricated condom reduces the risk of transmitting HIV during all forms of intercourse. Condoms are not perfect, and they do not provide risk-free sex; however, used properly, a condom provides a high level of protection against HIV. One study of 124 couples in which one partner was infected showed that with consistent condom use, none of the uninfected partners acquired the virus during the 20-month study period. Condoms should also be worn during oral sex. Most condoms are made of latex. If you or your partner is allergic to latex, polyurethane condoms are a good substitute. Do not use natural condoms (made from lamb membranes) because pores in this material can allow STD organisms to pass through.

Remember that you should avoid using nonoxynol-9 lubricants because of the risk of tissue irritation, which can make HIV and STD transmission more likely. It is especially important to not use condoms and lubricants that contain N-9 for anal sex; rectal tissues are thin and delicate and are more prone to irritation and tearing than is vaginal tissue. Experts also suggest the use of latex squares and dental dams, rubber devices that can be used as barriers during oral-genital or oral-anal sexual contact.

Limiting the number of partners you have—particularly those who have engaged in risky sexual behaviors in the past—can also lower your risk of exposure to HIV. Take the time to talk with a potential new partner about HIV and safer sex. Talking about sex may seem embarrassing and uncomfortable, but good communication is critical for your health. Asking a partner about past sexual experiences can be helpful, but you cannot always depend on that information. Recent surveys of HIV-positive people found that about one-third failed to reveal their

High Risk

Unprotected anal sex is the riskiest sexual behavior, especially for the receptive partner.

Unprotected vaginal intercourse is the next riskiest, especially for women, who are much more likely to be infected by an infected male partner than vice versa.

Oral sex is probably considerably less risky than anal and vaginal intercourse but can still result in HIV transmission.

Sharing of sex toys can be risky because they can carry blood, semen, or vaginal fluid.

Use of a condom reduces risk considerably but not completely for any type of intercourse. Anal sex with a condom is riskier than vaginal sex with a condom; oral sex with a condom is less risky, especially if the man does not ejaculate.

Hand-genital contact and deep kissing are less risky but could still theoretically transmit HIV; the presence of cuts or sores increases risk.

Sex with only one uninfected and totally faithful partner is without risk, but effective only if both partners are uninfected and completely monogamous.

Activities that don't involve the exchange of body fluids carry no risk: hugging, massage, closed-mouth kissing, masturbation, phone sex, and fantasy.

Abstinence is completely without risk. For many people, it can be an effective and reasonable method of avoiding HIV infection and other STDs during certain periods of life.

No Risk

Figure 18-4 What's risky and what's not: The approximate relative risk of HIV transmission of various sexual activities. Safer sex strategies that reduce the risk of HIV infection will also help protect you against other STDs. The main point to remember is that any activity that involves contact with blood, semen, or vaginal fluid can transmit HIV.

HIV status to sexual partners; of these, nearly two-thirds failed to always use a condom. Take precautions with every partner. Don't agree to have intercourse or give up precautions as a way to show your love or commitment to a relationship. Your specific sexual practices can be just as important as the number of partners you have.

Removing alcohol and other drugs from sexual activity is another crucial component of safer sex. The use of alcohol and mood-altering drugs may lower inhibitions and affect judgment, making you more likely to engage in unsafe sex. The use of drugs is also associated with sexual activity with multiple partners. Some experts attribute much of the recent increase in rates of syphilis and HIV infection among U.S. gay and bisexual men to the nonmedical use of anti-impotence drugs such as Viagra in combination with crystal methamphetamine. This combination of drugs impairs judgment, increases sexual drive, and allows men to perform sexually with multiple partners for many hours. Unprotected sex in association with abuse of these drugs is common, even among men who are normally more cautious. Studies show that men who use this drug combination are at very high risk for acquiring HIV and other STDs.

Remember, you can't tell if someone is infected by looking at him or her. Researchers believe that HIV has been in the United States since the mid- to late 1970s; anyone who has engaged in an unsafe behavior since that time is potentially at risk for HIV infection. Consider in advance what you will say and do in particular situations. Be assertive, and negotiate for safer sex practices.

Surveys of college students indicate that the majority of students are not engaging in safer sex. Although most students know that condom use can protect against HIV infection, this knowledge is often not translated into action. Many students also report a willingness to lie about past sexual activity in order to obtain sex. In addition, many students believe their risk of contracting HIV depends on who they are rather than on their sexual behavior. These attitudes and behaviors place college students at continued high risk for contracting HIV.

If you are sexually active, take responsibility for undergoing testing for HIV and other STDs at least once a year—more often if you have a new sexual partner or multiple partners. Remember that having any other STD makes you much more likely to acquire HIV infection. Prompt detection and treatment of other STDs can help decrease your risk of HIV infection.

DON'T SHARE DRUG NEEDLES People who inject drugs should avoid sharing needles, syringes, or anything that might have blood on it. Any injectable drug, legal or illegal, can be associated with HIV transmission. Needles can be decontaminated with a solution of bleach and water, but it is not a foolproof procedure, and HIV can survive in a syringe for a month or longer. (Boiling needles and syringes does not necessarily destroy HIV either.) As described in Chapter 9, obtaining sterile syringes through a syringe exchange program is much more effective than attempting to sterilize used syringes. Many prominent health organizations, including the United Nations AIDS Program and the American Medical Association, support syringe exchange programs, but these programs are unavailable and/or illegal in many parts of the world.

If you are an injection drug user, your best protection against HIV is to obtain treatment and refrain from using drugs. (See Chapter 9 for more on drug abuse.)

PARTICIPATE IN AN HIV EDUCATION PROGRAM Many schools and colleges have peer education programs about preventing the transmission of HIV. These programs give you a chance to practice communicating with potential sex partners and negotiating safer sex, to engage in role playing to build self-confidence, and to learn how to use condoms. Studies show that educational programs in which

Accurate information about HIV/AIDS, including where to go for testing and treatment, is available from many sources, including health professionals, community-based organizations, and national hotlines.

students learn from their peers and then try out what they've learned through role playing are more likely to result in real behavior change.

Many young people still believe that they are invulnerable to most kinds of harm and persist in thinking of themselves as not being at risk for HIV. The attitude of "It won't happen to me" is pervasive among high school and college students and is a major stumbling block to HIV/AIDS prevention. Until an effective vaccine and a cure are found, HIV infection will remain one of the biggest challenges of this generation. Education and individual responsibility can lead the way to controlling this devastating epidemic (see the box "Preventing HIV Infection and Other STDs").

Chlamydia

Chlamydia trachomatis causes **chlamydia,** the most prevalent bacterial STD in the United States. About 3 million new cases occur each year, down from a high of about 4 million; the drop is likely due to increased screening and treatment. An estimated 5–15% of all sexually active young American women are infected with chlamydia; rates among men are similar. The highest rates of infection occur in single people between ages 18 and 24. African American men and women have higher rates of infection than other groups for both chlamydia and gonorrhea. Up to 70% of people who are diagnosed with gonorrhea also have chlamydia. *C. trachomatis* can be transmitted by oral sex as well as by other forms of sexual intercourse.

For those who don't have a long-term monogamous relationship with an uninfected partner, abstinence is the only truly safe option. Individuals should remember that it's OK to say no to sex and drugs.

Safer sexual activities that allow close person-to-person contact with almost no risk of contracting STDs or HIV include fantasy, hugging, massage, rubbing clothed bodies together, self-stimulation by both partners, and kissing with lips closed.

If you choose to be sexually active, talk with potential partners about HIV, safer sex, and the use of condoms before you begin a sexual relationship. The following behaviors will help lower your risk of exposure to HIV during sexual activities:

- Don't drink alcohol or use drugs in sexual situations. Mood-altering drugs can affect your judgment and make you more likely to engage in risky behaviors. Having sex when intoxicated significantly increases the risk of STDs.

- Limit the number of partners. Avoid sexual contact with people who have HIV or an STD or who have engaged in risky behaviors in the past, including unprotected sex and injection drug use.

- Use condoms during every act of intercourse and oral sex. Many STDs are not easy to diagnose in their asymptomatic stage, which can last for years, and asymptomatic individuals can still infect others. Even if your partner claims to have been tested for HIV and STDs, you have no guarantee that you will not contract an STD during any sexual encounter. If you choose to have intercourse, your best protection is to *always* use a condom. Condoms do not provide perfect protection, but they greatly reduce your risk of contracting an infection.

- Use condoms properly to obtain maximum protection (refer to the instructions for condom use in Chapter 6). Use a water-based lubricant; don't use oil-based lubricants such as petroleum jelly or baby oil or any vaginal product containing mineral or vegetable oil. Avoid using lubricants or condoms containing nonoxynol-9, particularly for anal intercourse. Unroll condoms gently to avoid tearing them, and smooth out any air bubbles.

- Avoid sexual contact that could cause cuts or tears in the skin or tissue. Using extra lubricant (water-based) can help prevent damage to delicate tissues.

- Get periodic screening tests for STDs and HIV. Young women need yearly pelvic exams and Pap tests.

- Get vaccinated for hepatitis B. Take advantage of this safe and effective vaccine.

- Get prompt treatment for any STDs you contract.

If you inject drugs of any kind, don't share needles, syringes, or anything that might have blood on it. If your community has a syringe exchange program, use it. Seek treatment; stop using injectable drugs.

If you are at risk for HIV infection, don't donate blood, sperm, or body organs. Don't have unprotected sex or share needles or syringes. Get tested for HIV soon, and get treated. HIV-infected people who get early treatment generally feel better and live longer than those who delay.

Both men and women are susceptible to chlamydia, but, as with most STDs, women bear the greater burden because of possible complications and consequences of the disease (see the box "Women Are Hit Hard by STDs"). In most women, chlamydia produces no early symptoms. If left untreated, it can lead to pelvic inflammatory disease (PID), a serious infection involving the oviducts (fallopian tubes) and uterus. PID, discussed later in this chapter, is a leading cause of infertility, and even an infection that produces no symptoms can cause significant scarring of the oviducts. Chlamydia also greatly increases a woman's risk for ectopic (tubal) pregnancy. Because rates of infection are high and most women with chlamydia have no symptoms, many physicians screen sexually active women at the time of their routine pelvic exam. The U.S. Preventive Services Task Force currently recommends routine screening for all sexually active women age 25 or younger and for older women who are at increased risk (such as those who have multiple sex partners).

Chlamydia can also lead to infertility in men, although not as often as in women. In men under age 35, chlamy-dia is the most common cause of **epididymitis**, inflammation of the sperm-carrying ducts. And up to half of all cases of **urethritis**, inflammation of the urethra, in men are caused by chlamydia. Despite these statistics, many infected men have no symptoms. Screening for chlamydia in heterosexual men currently is not routine, but some experts feel that screening young sexually active men in addition to young women would be effective in reducing chlamydia rates.

Infants of infected mothers can acquire the infection through contact with the pathogen in the birth canal

Terms

chlamydia An STD transmitted by the pathogenic bacterium *Chlamydia trachomatis.*

epididymitis An inflammation of the small body of sperm-carrying ducts that rests on the testes.

urethritis Inflammation of the tube that carries urine from the bladder to the outside opening.

Sexually transmitted diseases cause suffering for all who are infected, but in many ways, women and girls are the hardest hit, for both biological and social reasons. Among Americans, 62% of all cases of adverse health problems from STDs occur in women. Worldwide, as many women as men now die from AIDS each year, and in the hardest-hit regions of Africa, nearly 60% of HIV-positive adults are women.

Male-to-female transmission of many infections is more likely to occur than female-to-male transmission. This is particularly true of HIV: Studies show that it is three to eight times easier for an HIV-positive man to transmit the virus to a woman than it is for an HIV-positive woman to infect a man.

Young women are even more vulnerable to STDs than older women because the less-mature cervix is more susceptible to injury and infection. As a woman ages, the type of cells at the opening of the cervix gradually changes so that the tissue becomes more resistant to infection. If an 18-year-old woman and a 30-year-old woman are exposed to the same pathogen, the younger woman is far more likely to develop a serious STD. Young women are also more vulnerable for social and emotional reasons: Lack of control in relationships, fear of discussing condom use, and having an older sex partner are all linked to increased STD risk.

Once infected, women tend to suffer more consequences of STDs than men.

For example, gonorrhea and chlamydia can cause PID and permanent damage to the oviducts in women, but these infections tend to have less serious effects in men. HPV infection causes nearly all cases of cervical cancer. HPV infection is also associated with penile cancer in men, but penile cancer is much less common than cervical cancer. Women also have the added concern of the potential effects of STDs during pregnancy.

Between 1985 and 2003, the proportion of new U.S. AIDS cases in women increased from 7% to 28%. Women with HIV infection often face tremendous challenges when they are ill because they may be caring for family members who are also infected and ill. Many women are dealing with substance-abuse problems in themselves or in family members. In addition, women may become sicker at lower viral loads compared with men. Women and men with HIV do about equally well if they have similar access to treatment, but in many cases women are diagnosed later in the course of HIV infection, receive less treatment, and die sooner.

Worldwide, social and economic factors play a large role in the transmission and consequences of AIDS and other STDs for women. Violence against women is spreading AIDS, as are such practices as very early marriage for women, often to much older men who have had many sexual partners. For many women, being vulnerable to HIV can simply mean being married. Cultural gender norms that pro-

mote premarital and extramarital relationships for men, combined with women's lack of power to negotiate safer sex, make HIV a risk even for women who are married and monogamous. In addition, lack of education and limited economic opportunities can force women into commercial sex work, placing them at high risk for all STDs.

In some parts of the world, the stigma of AIDS hits women harder. Men with HIV are typically cared for by female family members, without being questioned about the source of their infection. Women, in contrast, may be accused of having had extramarital sex and receive less help and support. It is women who typically provide care to relatives with HIV as well as support the household financially when other earners are too ill to work. But if husbands die, women often do not inherit property and can be thrown deeper into poverty. Solutions to the STD crisis in women must include empowerment in the social sphere in addition to direct health care.

SOURCES: Ebrahim, S. H., M. T. McKenna, and J. S. Marks. 2005. Sexual behaviour: Related adverse health burden in the United States. *Sexually Transmitted Infection* 81(1): 38–40; Dunkle, K. M., et al. 2004. Gender-based violence, relationship power, and risk of HIV infection in women attending antenatal clinics in South Africa. *Lancet* 363(9419): 1415–1421; Joint United Nations Programme on HIV/AIDS. 2004. *AIDS Epidemic Update, December 2004.* Geneva: UNAIDS; World Health Organization. 2003. *Gender and HIV/AIDS.* Geneva: World Health Organization.

during delivery. Every year, over 150,000 newborns suffer from eye infections and pneumonia as a result of untreated maternal chlamydial infections.

Symptoms In men, chlamydia symptoms include painful urination, a slight watery discharge from the penis, and sometimes pain around the testicles. Although most women with chlamydia are asymptomatic, some notice increased vaginal discharge, burning with urination, pain or bleeding with intercourse, and lower abdominal pain. Less common symptoms in both men and women include arthritis, conjunctivitis, sore throat, and rectal inflammation and pain (in people who become infected during receptive anal intercourse). Symptoms in both

men and women can begin within 5 days of infection. However, most people experience few or no symptoms, increasing the likelihood that they will inadvertently spread the infection to their partners.

Diagnosis Chlamydia is typically diagnosed through laboratory tests on a urine sample or a small amount of fluid from the urethra or cervix. The lab test may involve growing the organism in culture, using special dyes to detect bacterial proteins, or a process that quickly copies and detects genetic material from the bacteria. Testing pregnant women and treating those with chlamydia is a highly effective way to prevent infection of newborns. A home test is currently being studied.

Treatment Once chlamydia has been diagnosed, the infected person and his or her partner(s) are given antibiotics—usually doxycycline, erythromycin, or a newer drug, azithromycin, which can cure infection in one dose. Treatment of partners is important because people who have been treated for chlamydia are susceptible to getting the disease again if they have sexual contact with an infected person. The CDC now recommends that women who have been treated for chlamydia be retested 3–4 months after treatment is completed. Chlamydia is an expensive disease, with costs running higher than $2 billion annually in the United States. For an individual, the physical and emotional costs—damaged reproductive organs, infertility, or an infected infant—can be devastating.

Gonorrhea

In the United States, an estimated 700,000 new cases of **gonorrhea** are diagnosed every year. The highest incidence is among 15–24-year-olds. Like chlamydia, untreated gonorrhea can cause PID in women and urethritis and epididymitis in men. It can also cause arthritis, rashes, and eye infections, and it occasionally involves internal organs. Being infected with gonorrhea increases the likelihood that HIV will be transmitted. A woman who is infected during pregnancy is at risk for preterm delivery and for having a baby with life-threatening gonorrheal infection of the blood or joints. An infant passing through the birth canal of an infected mother may contract **gonococcal conjunctivitis,** an infection in the eyes that can cause blindness if not treated. In most states, all newborn babies are routinely treated with antimicrobial eyedrops to prevent eye infection.

Gonorrhea is caused by the bacterium *Neisseria gonorrhoeae*, which flourishes in mucous membranes, including the moist linings of the mouth, throat, vagina, cervix, urethra, and anal canal. The microbe cannot thrive outside the warm, moist environment of the human body and dies within moments of exposure to light and air. Consequently, gonorrhea cannot be contracted from toilet seats, towels, or other objects.

Symptoms In males, the incubation period for gonorrhea is brief, generally 2–7 days. The first symptoms are due to urethritis, which causes urinary discomfort and a thick, yellowish white or yellowish green discharge from the penis. The lips of the urethral opening may become inflamed and swollen. In some cases, the lymph glands in the groin become enlarged and swollen. Up to half of males have very minor symptoms or none at all.

Most females with gonorrhea are asymptomatic. Those who do have symptoms often experience pain with urination, increased vaginal discharge, and severe menstrual cramps. Up to 40% of women with untreated gonorrhea develop PID. Women may also develop painful abscesses in the Bartholin's glands, a pair of glands located on either side of the opening of the vagina.

Gonorrhea can also infect the throat or rectum of people who engage in oral or anal sex. Gonorrhea symptoms in the throat may be a sore throat or pus on the tonsils, and those in the rectum may be pus or blood in the feces or rectal pain and itching.

Diagnosis Several tests—gram stain, detection of bacterial genes or DNA, or culture—may be performed; depending on the test, samples of urine or cervical, urethral, throat, or rectal fluids may be collected.

Treatment A variety of new and relatively expensive antibiotics are usually effective in curing gonorrhea. Older, less expensive antibiotics such as penicillin and tetracycline are not currently recommended for treating gonorrhea because of widespread drug resistance. People with gonorrhea often also have chlamydia, so additional antibiotics are typically given to treat chlamydia. Follow-up tests are sometimes performed to make sure the infection has been eradicated. If you have had gonorrhea and have been treated, you can still get the disease again if you have sexual contact with an infected partner.

Pelvic Inflammatory Disease

A major complication in 10–40% of women who have been infected with either gonorrhea or chlamydia and have not received adequate treatment is **pelvic inflammatory disease (PID)**. PID occurs when the initial infection with gonorrhea and/or chlamydia travels upward, often along with other bacteria, beyond the cervix into the uterus, oviducts, ovaries, and pelvic cavity. PID is often serious enough to require hospitalization and sometimes surgery. Even if the disease is treated successfully, about 25% of affected women will have long-term problems such as a continuing susceptibility to infection, ectopic pregnancy, infertility, and chronic pelvic pain.

PID is the leading cause of infertility in young women, often going undetected until the inability to become pregnant leads to further evaluation. Infertility occurs in 8% of women after one episode of PID, 20% after two episodes, and 40% after three episodes. The risk of ectopic pregnancy increases significantly in women who have had PID.

Young women under age 25 are much more likely to develop PID than are older women. As with all STDs, the

Terms

gonorrhea A sexually transmitted bacterial infection that usually affects mucous membranes.

gonococcal conjunctivitis An inflammation of the mucous membrane lining of the eyelids, caused by the gonococcus bacterium.

pelvic inflammatory disease (PID) An infection that progresses from the vagina and cervix to the uterus, oviducts, and pelvic cavity.

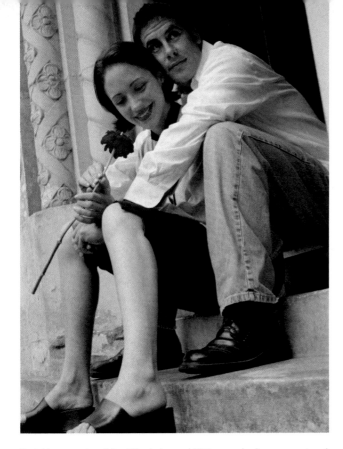

By taking a responsible attitude toward STDs, people show respect and concern for themselves and their partners. This couple's plans for the future could be seriously disrupted if one of them contracted an STD like gonorrhea or chlamydia. Either of these diseases, if untreated, could result in PID, the leading cause of infertility in young women.

more sex partners a woman has had, the greater her risk of PID. Smokers have twice the risk of PID as nonsmokers. Using IUDs for contraception also increases the risk of PID. Research into whether the use of other contraceptives protects against PID has yielded mixed results; OC use may reduce the severity of PID symptoms.

Symptoms Symptoms of PID vary greatly. Some women, especially those with chlamydia, may be asymptomatic; others may feel very ill with abdominal pain, fever, chills, nausea, and vomiting. Early symptoms are essentially the same as those described earlier for chlamydia and gonorrhea. Symptoms often begin or worsen during or soon after a woman's menstrual period. Many women have abnormal vaginal bleeding—either bleeding between periods or heavy and painful menstrual bleeding.

Terms

Vīw

human papillomavirus (HPV) The pathogen that causes human warts, including genital warts.

genital warts A sexually transmitted viral infection characterized by growths on the genitals; also called *genital HPV infection* or *condyloma.*

Diagnosis Diagnosis of PID is made on the basis of symptoms, physical examination, ultrasound, and laboratory tests. Laparoscopy may be used to confirm the diagnosis and obtain material for cultures. Cultures from the rectum or cervix may also be taken to help identify the specific organism. The symptoms of PID, ectopic pregnancy, and appendicitis can be quite similar, so careful evaluation is required to make the correct diagnosis.

Treatment Starting treatment of PID as quickly as possible is important in order to minimize damage to the reproductive organs. Antibiotics are usually started immediately; in severe cases, the woman may be hospitalized and antibiotics given intravenously. It is especially important that an infected woman's partners be treated. As many as 60% of the male contacts of women with PID are infected but asymptomatic.

Human Papillomavirus Infection (Genital Warts)

Human papillomavirus (HPV) infection is one of the most common STDs in the United States (see the box "Half of Americans Will Have an STD by Age 25"). All human warts, including **genital warts,** as well as almost all cases of cervical cancer are caused by HPV infection. HPV is also a major risk factor for penile cancer. The CDC estimates that more than 20 million people in the United States have this persistent genital viral infection, and another 6.2 million people are infected each year. Nearly 20% of Americans age 15–59 years have genital HPV infection and are potentially contagious. The vast majority of these people have no visible warts and have no idea that they are infected. Rates are even higher among college students. HPV infection is the most common STD for which diagnosis and treatment are sought in student health services (see the box "College Students and STDs"). Many young women contract HPV infection within 3 months of becoming sexually active.

HPV infection presents a challenge to the medical community because of its known relationship to cervical cancer. A precancerous condition known as cervical dysplasia often occurs among women with genital HPV infection (see Chapter 16). If untreated, women with this condition sometimes develop cervical cancer. (Other factors that increase a woman's chance of getting cervical cancer include smoking, sexual activity at a young age, multiple sex partners, and infection with genital herpes.) Recent evidence suggests that HPV infection also increases the risk of HIV transmission.

Human papillomaviruses cause many types of human warts. There are more than 100 different strains of HPV, and different strains infect specific locations. More than 30 types are likely to cause genital infections, and 5 of these are often implicated in cervical cancer; other strains are linked to anal, penile, and other genital cancers. The

The United States has the highest STD rate of any industrialized country. Estimates released in 2004 showed that half of all Americans will have at least one STD by age 25, and nearly half of all STDs that occur each year are in people age 15–24. The direct lifetime medical cost of STDs, including HIV, is estimated at $10–15 billion for the new STDs acquired each year. STDs are public health challenges for many reasons.

• *STDs are stealth diseases.* Many STDs, including chlamydia, genital herpes, trichomoniasis, and HPV infection have few, if any, recognizable symptoms. The large number of disease carriers who are unaware of their infection makes these diseases extremely difficult to control. Experts believe that in most cases, HIV is transmitted very early in the disease, before people are aware of the infection. The fact that most people are symptom-free for the first several years of HIV infection highlights the need to test people at risk often.

• *Viral STDs are persistent and incurable.* Even if detected, most viral STDs—genital herpes, HPV infection, and HIV infection—are not curable with current therapies. This means that the number of people capable of infecting others continues to grow. The best hope for

controlling viral STDs is the development and widespread use of effective vaccines. The hepatitis B vaccine provides a positive example: In the years since introduction of the vaccine, the rate of new cases of hepatitis B has dropped by more than 50%, and further declines are expected.

• *Screening tests may be underutilized.* Nationwide, too many physicians and clinics fail to follow the CDC recommendations for screening, especially for chlamydia in young women. In addition, too many individuals are too unaware of or too embarrassed to request STD screening. Testing more people for STDs could potentially bring STD rates down; it would at least provide an opportunity to counsel people about risky sexual behavior. In surveys, up to 75% of people support offering STD testing in schools. Also potentially helpful would be media messages about the benefits and availability of confidential STD screening services.

• *Young people are particularly vulnerable to STDs.* Young adults are more likely to be ignorant about STDs and safer sex, embarrassed to ask for information, and unaware of how to access appropriate STD testing and treatment services. Nearly all young adults are

sexually active by age 25, but young people are more likely to be unmarried, have more than one partner over time, and/or have a partner who has an STD. Young people need medically accurate information about abstinence, condoms, and other contraceptive methods—and open communication and encouragement from family, friends, and the community to behave responsibly.

Until STDs are controllable with vaccines or effective screening and treatment, the only way to reduce your risk is to limit the number of sexual partners and to use condoms consistently (see guidelines presented earlier in the chapter). For those who choose abstinence or a mutually monogamous relationship with one uninfected partner, there is no risk of STDs.

SOURCES: Cates, J. R., et al. 2004. *Our Voices, Our Lives, Our Futures: Youth and Sexually Transmitted Diseases.* Chapel Hill, N.C.: School of Journalism and Mass Communication, University of North Carolina at Chapel Hill; Weinstock, H., S. Berman, and W. Cates. 2004. Sexually transmitted diseases among American youth: Incidence and prevalence estimates, 2000. *Perspectives on Sexual and Reproductive Health* 36(1): 6–10; Chesson, H. W., et al. 2004. The estimated direct medical cost of sexually transmitted diseases among American youth, 2000. *Perspectives on Sexual and Reproductive Health* 36(1): 11–19.

HPV strains that cause most visible genital warts are less likely to cause cancer than some of the other HPV strains. A person can be infected with several different strains.

Genital HPV infection is quite contagious. Condoms and other barrier methods can help prevent the transmission of HPV, but HPV infection frequently occurs in areas where condoms are not fully protective. These areas are the labia in women, the base of the penis and the scrotum in men, and around the anus in both men and women.

Controlling the current genital HPV epidemic is difficult for several reasons. First, many people who carry HPV have no visible warts or symptoms. And although people with visible genital warts may be more likely to transmit the disease, asymptomatic people can also infect others. Second, although current treatments can often (but not always) eliminate visible warts, HPV continues to infect healthy tissue nearby. So even after treatment, a person can still transmit HPV to someone else. Third, as

mentioned above, condoms do not provide complete protection against the transmission of HPV.

The good news about HPV is that a vaccine may soon prevent many cases of genital warts and cervical cancer. Human trials are under way for several new vaccines that protect against HPV, and preliminary results are very encouraging. Researchers are hopeful that these vaccines will be available for general use within a few years.

Symptoms HPV-infected tissue often appears normal; it may also look like anything from a small bump on the skin to a large, warty growth. Depending on location and size, genital warts are sometimes painful. Untreated warts can grow together to form a cauliflower-like mass. In males, they appear on the penis and often involve the urethra, appearing first at the opening and then spreading inside. The growths may cause irritation and bleeding, leading to painful urination and a urethral discharge. Warts may also appear around the anus or within the rectum.

College Students and STDs

Why Do College Students Have High Rates of STDs?

- Risky sexual behavior is common. One study of college students found that fewer than half used condoms consistently and one-third had had ten or more sex partners. Another study found that 19% of male students and 33% of female students had consented to sexual intercourse simply because they felt awkward refusing.

- College students underestimate their risk of STDs and HIV. Although students may have considerable knowledge about STDs, they often feel the risks do not apply to them—a dangerous assumption. One study of students with a history of STDs showed that more than half had unprotected sex while they were infected, and 25% of them continued to have sex without ever informing their partner(s).

- As described earlier in the chapter, young women are more vulnerable to STDs than older women because the less-mature cervix is more easily infected.

What Effect Does Alcohol or Drug Use Have on My Likelihood of Getting an STD?

- Between one-third and one-half of college students report participating in sexual activity as a direct result of being intoxicated. All too often, sexual activity while intoxicated leads to unprotected intercourse.

- Students who binge-drink are more likely to have multiple partners, use condoms inconsistently, and delay seeking treatment for STDs than students who drink little or no alcohol. Sexual assaults occur more frequently when either the perpetrator or the victim has been drinking.

What Can Students Do to Protect Themselves Against STDs?

- Limit the number of sex partners. Even people who are always in a monogamous relationship can end up with extensive potential exposure to STDs if, over the years, they have numerous relationships.

- Use condoms consistently, and don't assume it's safe to stop after you've been with a partner for several months. HIV infection, HPV infection, herpes, and chlamydia can be asymptomatic for months or years and can be transmitted at any time. If you haven't been using condoms with your current partner, start now.

- Think about how you use alcohol or other drugs. If alcohol or drug use is causing problems in your life, get help.

- Enjoy sexuality on your own terms. Don't let the expectations of friends and partners cause you to ignore your own feelings. Let your own wellness be your first priority. If you choose to be sexually active, learn about safer sex practices.

- Get to know your partner, and talk to him or her before becoming intimate. Be honest about yourself, and encourage your partner to do the same. Unfortunately, studies show that many people lie about their sexual past and that, in general, people significantly underestimate their partners' sexual experience and risk for STDs. So practice safer sex no matter what.

In women, warts may appear on the labia or vulva and may spread to the perineum, the area between the vagina and the rectum. They may also appear on the cervix. If warts occur only on the cervix, the woman will generally have no symptoms or awareness that she has HPV.

The incubation period ranges from 1 month to 2 years from the time of contact. People can be infected with the virus and be capable of transmitting it to their sex partners without having any symptoms at all. The vast majority of people with HPV infection have no visible warts or symptoms of any kind.

Genital warts sometimes grow very large during pregnancy and can occasionally be large enough to make vaginal delivery difficult. However, most pregnant women with HPV infection can deliver vaginally. HPV infection is infrequently transmitted to an infant during delivery but can occasionally cause warts to form on the infant's vocal cords.

Diagnosis Genital warts are usually diagnosed based on the appearance of the lesions. Sometimes examination with a special magnifying instrument or biopsy is done to evaluate suspicious lesions. HPV infection of the cervix is often detected on routine Pap tests. Special tests are now available to detect the presence of HPV infection and to distinguish among the more common strains of HPV, including those that cause most cases of cervical cancer.

Treatment Treatment of genital warts focuses on reducing the number and size of warts. The currently available treatments do not eradicate HPV infection. Warts may be removed by cryosurgery (freezing), electrocautery (burning), or laser surgery. Direct applications of podophyllin or other cytotoxic acids may be used. Two treatments may be applied by patients at home: imiquimod, an immune system enhancer, and podofilox, a drug that destroys warts. The success rates of methods vary, and warts often recur despite initial improvement.

HPV infection often resolves on its own after a number of months, although this is unpredictable. Even after treatment and the disappearance of visible warts, the individual may continue to carry HPV in healthy-looking tissue and can probably still infect others. Anyone who has ever had HPV infection should inform all partners. Condoms should be used, even though they do not provide total protection. Because of the relationship between HPV and cervical cancer, women who have had genital warts should have Pap tests at least every 12 months. Treatment for cervical dysplasia and cervical cancer is discussed in Chapter 16.

Genital Herpes

Genital herpes affects about 45 million people in the United States and is also very common worldwide. Genital herpes is a major factor in the transmission of HIV worldwide. Most people with HIV are also infected with HSV 2, and herpes lesions contain large amounts of HIV, making it more likely that the virus is transmitted. The presence of herpes lesions in an HIV-negative person increases the likelihood that she or he will be infected by an HIV-positive partner. Genital herpes may also interact with HPV infection to increase the risk of cervical cancer.

Two types of herpes simplex viruses, HSV 1 and HSV 2, cause genital herpes and oral-labial herpes (cold sores). Genital herpes is usually caused by HSV 2, and oral-labial herpes is usually caused by HSV 1, although both virus types can cause either genital or oral-labial lesions. The proportion of U.S. genital herpes cases caused by HSV 1 has increased dramatically over the past several decades and now stands at about 20% of cases. Genital herpes due to HSV 1 is usually acquired through oral-genital contact. Many people wrongly assume that they are unlikely to pick up an STD if they limit their sexual activity to oral sex, but this is not true, particularly in the case of genital herpes. HSV can also cause rectal lesions, usually transmitted through anal sex. (Other types of herpesviruses cause different illnesses; see Chapter 17.) Infection with HSV is generally lifelong; after infection, the virus lies dormant in nerve cells and can reactivate at any time.

HSV 1 infection is so common that 50–80% of U.S. adults have antibodies to HSV 1 (indicating previous exposure to the virus); most were exposed to HSV 1 during childhood. HSV 2 infection usually occurs during adolescence and early adulthood, often between ages 18 and 25. Approximately 22% of adults—nearly one in four—have antibodies to HSV 2; about a million are infected each year.

HSV 2 is almost always sexually transmitted. It is theoretically possible, but much less common, to become infected through contaminated clothing, towels, or other objects. The infection is more easily transmitted when people have active sores, but HSV 2 can be transmitted to a sex partner even when no obvious lesions are present. A recent study of women with HSV-2 showed the presence of the virus in genital secretions more than one-fourth of the time when the women were symptom-free. Because HSV is asymptomatic in 80–90% of people, the infection is often acquired from a person who has no awareness that he or she is infected. This makes controlling the spread of genital herpes very difficult. If you have ever had an outbreak of genital herpes, you must consider yourself always contagious and inform your partners. Avoid intimate contact when any sores are present, and use condoms during all sexual contact.

Newborns can occasionally be infected with HSV, usually during passage through the birth canal of an infected mother or due to HSV infection acquired by the mother during the third trimester of pregnancy. Without treatment, 65% of newborns with HSV will die, and most who survive will have some degree of brain damage. The risk of mother-to-child HSV transmission during pregnancy and delivery is low (less than 1%) in women with long-standing herpes infection. However, a woman who acquires the infection during pregnancy, especially in the third trimester, has a much higher risk of transmitting the infection to her infant. Some experts believe that the use of new herpes blood tests to screen pregnant women and their sexual partners could substantially reduce the number of neonatal herpes infections. If an uninfected pregnant woman's partner carries HSV, abstinence or the use of condoms could prevent infection during pregnancy.

Pregnant women who have been exposed to genital herpes should inform their physician so that appropriate precautions can be taken to protect the baby from infection. These precautions sometimes include a cesarean section if active lesions are present at the time of delivery. Fortunately, most babies born to mothers with a history of genital herpes do not acquire the infection, and most women are able to have normal vaginal deliveries.

Symptoms Up to 90% of people who are infected with HSV have no symptoms. Those that do develop symptoms often first notice them within 2–20 days of having sex with an infected partner. (However, it is not unusual for the first outbreak to occur months or even years after initial exposure.) The first episode of genital herpes frequently causes flulike symptoms in addition to genital lesions. The lesions usually heal within 3 weeks, but the virus remains alive in an inactive state within nerve cells. A new outbreak of herpes can occur at any time. On average, newly diagnosed people will experience five to eight outbreaks per year, with a decrease in the frequency of outbreaks over time. Recurrent episodes are usually less severe than the initial one, with fewer and less painful sores that heal more quickly. Outbreaks can be triggered by stress, illness, fatigue, sun exposure, sexual intercourse, and menstruation (see the box "Stress and Genital Herpes").

Diagnosis Genital herpes is often diagnosed on the basis of symptoms; a sample of fluid from the lesions may also be sent to a laboratory for evaluation. A new blood test that can determine if a person is infected with HSV 1 or HSV 2 is now available and may potentially alert many asymptomatic people to the fact that they are infected. This knowledge may help prevent transmission of HSV in

Term

genital herpes A sexually transmitted infection caused by the herpes simplex virus.

Patients and health care workers alike have long suspected that stress and genital herpes outbreaks are related. Research into this potential link has yielded mixed results. There is no doubt that having genital herpes is a considerable stress to many people, but does stress itself make a person with herpes infection more likely to have an outbreak? A recent study of women with genital herpes found that persistent stressors (those lasting more than a week) and persistent high levels of anxiety were associated with increased outbreaks. Short-term stress, mood changes, and brief negative life experiences did not influence the rate of herpes outbreaks.

Why should persistent stress make a person with genital herpes have more frequent outbreaks? No one knows for sure, but experts suspect that stress has a negative impact on the immune system. Studies have shown that cell-mediated immune function and antibody levels may drop in response to psychological stress. Perhaps herpesviruses that are usually dormant in nervous system tissue become activated when immune function declines due to stress.

The next logical step is to investigate whether stress-reduction techniques such as meditation or exercise result in reduced rates of herpes outbreaks. Until such research becomes available, it makes sense for people who suffer recurrent genital herpes outbreaks to do what they can to reduce stress, especially long-term stress and anxiety (see Chapter 2). If you have herpes, joining a support group may help reduce your stress and improve your ability to cope with this chronic disease (see

For More Information at the end of the chapter). If you have several outbreaks a year, or if you have recently had your first episode of genital herpes, talk to your health care provider about suppressive antiviral medication, which can reduce outbreaks substantially. Keep in mind that regardless of stress level, genital herpes outbreaks naturally tend to become less and less frequent over time. Knowing that your outbreaks are likely to diminish can, in and of itself, help reduce your feelings of stress.

SOURCES: Gupta, R., et al. 2004. Valacyclovir and acyclovir for suppression of shedding of herpes simplex virus in the genital tract. *Journal of Infectious Diseases* 190(8): 1374–1381; Rein, M. 2000. Stress and genital herpes recurrences in women: Commentary. *Journal of the American Medical Association* 283(11): 1394.

---

couples where one partner is infected and the other is not (particularly important for uninfected women who are pregnant).

Treatment   There is no cure for herpes. Once infected, a person carries the virus for life. Antiviral drugs such as acyclovir can be taken at the beginning of an outbreak to shorten the severity and duration of symptoms. People who have frequent outbreaks can take acyclovir or similar drugs on a daily basis to suppress outbreaks. Suppressive treatment significantly reduces the number of painful outbreaks and decreases viral shedding between outbreaks. Anyone diagnosed with a first episode of genital herpes should talk with a health care provider about suppressive treatment. A person on suppressive therapy can still transmit HSV to an uninfected partner, but the risk is probably reduced by about half. Using condoms consistently and taking suppressive medication is a reasonable way to reduce the risk of passing herpes to an uninfected sexual partner. It is always important to inform a sexual partner if you have genital herpes.

The psychological aspects of genital herpes often cause more suffering than the disease itself. Support groups are available to help people learn to cope with herpes (see For More Information at the end of the chapter). Vaccines for genital herpes are currently in development.

Hepatitis B

Hepatitis (inflammation of the liver) can cause serious and sometimes permanent damage to the liver, which can result in death in severe cases. One of the many types of hepatitis is caused by hepatitis B virus (HBV). HBV is somewhat similar to HIV; it is found in most body fluids, and it can be transmitted sexually, by injection drug use, and during pregnancy and delivery. However, HBV is much more contagious than HIV, and it can also be spread through nonsexual close contact. Health care workers who are exposed to blood are frequently infected, as are people who live in close contact with each other, such as prisoners and residents of mental health care facilities. In the Far East and in developing countries, hepatitis B is extremely common, and the virus is primarily transmitted from the mother to child during pregnancy or delivery.

Hepatitis B is a potentially fatal disease with no cure, but fortunately there is an effective vaccine. The number of cases of acute hepatitis B in the United States has dropped by more than 50% in the past decade, primarily as a result of the vaccine. In addition, mother-to-child transmission has been greatly reduced because of routine HBV screening of pregnant women. Vaccination is recommended for everyone under age 19 and for all adults at increased risk for hepatitis B.

Other forms of viral hepatitis can also be sexually transmitted. Hepatitis A is of particular concern for people who engage in anal sex; a vaccine is available and is recommended for all people at risk. Less commonly, hepatitis C can be transmitted sexually. Experts believe that traumatic sexual activity that causes tissue damage is most likely to transmit HCV. See Chapter 17 for more on these and other forms of hepatitis.

Transmission HBV is found in all body fluids, including blood and blood products, semen, saliva, urine, and vaginal secretions. It is easily transmitted through any sexual activity that involves the exchange of body fluids, the use of contaminated needles, and any blood-to-blood contact, including the use of contaminated razor blades, toothbrushes, and eating utensils. The primary risk factors for acquiring HBV are sexual exposure and injection drug use; having multiple partners greatly increases risk. As mentioned, a pregnant woman can transmit HBV to her unborn child.

Symptoms Many people infected with HBV never develop symptoms; they have what are known as silent infections. The normal incubation period is 30–180 days. Mild cases of hepatitis cause flulike symptoms such as fever, body aches, chills, and loss of appetite. As the illness progresses, there may be nausea, vomiting, dark-colored urine, abdominal pain, and jaundice. Some people with hepatitis also develop a skin rash and joint pain or arthritis. Acute hepatitis B can sometimes be severe, resulting in prolonged illness or even death.

People with hepatitis B sometimes recover completely, but they can also become chronic carriers of the virus, capable of infecting others for the rest of their life. Some chronic carriers remain asymptomatic, while others develop chronic liver disease. Chronic hepatitis can cause cirrhosis of the liver, liver failure, and a deadly form of liver cancer. Hepatitis kills some 5000 Americans each year; worldwide, the annual death toll exceeds 600,000.

Diagnosis and Treatment Blood tests can be used to diagnose hepatitis through analysis of liver function and detection of the specific organism causing the infection. There is no cure for hepatitis B and no specific treatment for acute infections; antiviral drugs may be used for cases of chronic HBV infection. For people exposed to HBV, treatment with hepatitis B immunoglobulin can provide protection against the virus.

Prevention Preventive measures for hepatitis B are similar to those for HIV infection: Avoid sexual contact that involves sharing body fluids, including saliva; use condoms during sexual intercourse; and don't share needles. If you choose to have tattooing or body piercing done, make sure all needles and equipment are sterile. The vaccine for hepatitis B is safe and highly effective.

Syphilis

Syphilis, a disease that once caused death and disability for millions, can now be effectively treated with antibiotics. Each year, there are about 7000–10,000 new cases of early syphilis in the United States, and about 70,000 people are diagnosed at all stages of the disease. The number of new cases hit an all-time low in 1999 but rose by 19% between 2000 and 2003. The increase was seen mainly in homosexual and bisexual men, prompting health officials to call for increased education in safer sex practices among these groups. Studies have found an association between syphilis infection and the use of the Internet as a means to meet sex partners among men who have sex with men. Another recent trend is an increase in the proportion of cases of syphilis from oral sex; in nearly 15% of recent cases among gay men and 7% of cases among heterosexual men and women, the means of transmission was through oral sex. People with syphilis in the mouth may not have symptoms, or they may mistake the sores for another illness. The sores associated with syphilis, regardless of their location, dramatically increase the risk of acquiring HIV or transmitting it to someone else.

Syphilis is caused by a spirochete called *Treponema pallidum*, a thin, corkscrew-shaped bacterium. The disease is usually acquired through sexual contact, although infected pregnant women can transmit it to the fetus. The pathogen passes through any break or opening in the skin or mucous membranes and can be transmitted by kissing, vaginal or anal intercourse, or oral-genital contact. Although easy to treat, syphilis can be difficult to recognize, and if left untreated the disease can cause devastating damage to almost any system of the body.

Symptoms Syphilis progresses through several stages. *Primary syphilis* is characterized by an ulcer called a **chancre** that appears within 10–90 days after exposure. The chancre is usually found at the site where the organism entered the body, such as the genital area, but it may also appear in other sites such as the mouth, breasts, or fingers. Chancres contain large numbers of bacteria and make the disease highly contagious when present; they are often painless and typically heal on their own within a few weeks. If the disease is not treated during the primary stage, about a third of infected individuals progress to chronic stages of infections.

Secondary syphilis is usually marked by mild, flulike symptoms and a skin rash that appears 3–6 weeks after the chancre. The rash may cover the entire body or only a few areas, but the palms of the hands and soles of the feet are usually involved. Areas of skin affected by the rash are highly contagious but usually heal within several weeks or months.

Terms

hepatitis Inflammation of the liver, which can be caused by infection, drugs, or toxins; some forms of infectious hepatitis can be transmitted sexually.

syphilis A sexually transmitted bacterial infection caused by the spirochete *Treponema pallidum*.

chancre The sore produced by syphilis in its earliest stage.

If the disease remains untreated, the symptoms of secondary syphilis may recur over a period of several years; affected individuals may then lapse into an asymptomatic latent stage in which they experience no further consequences of infection. However, in about a third of cases of untreated secondary syphilis, the individual develops *late,* or *tertiary, syphilis.* Late syphilis can damage many organs of the body, possibly causing severe dementia, cardiovascular damage, blindness, and death.

In infected pregnant women, the syphilis bacterium can cross the placenta. If the mother is not treated, the probable result is stillbirth, prematurity, or congenital deformity. In many cases, the infant is also born infected (*congenital syphilis*) and requires treatment.

Diagnosis and Treatment Syphilis is diagnosed by examination of infected tissues and with blood tests. All stages can be treated with antibiotics, but damage from late syphilis can be permanent.

OTHER STDS

Although less serious than the diseases already described, a few other diseases are transmitted sexually or linked to sexual activity. They include trichomoniasis, bacterial vaginosis, chancroid, pubic lice, and scabies.

Trichomoniasis, often called "trich," is a common STD, with about 5 million new cases per year. The single-celled organism that causes trich, *Trichomonas vaginalis,* thrives in warm, moist conditions, making women particularly susceptible to these infections in the vagina. This protozoan can remain alive on external objects for as long as 60–90 minutes, in urine for 3 hours, and in seminal fluid for 6 hours. Thus it is possible, although rare, to contract trich by nonsexual means.

Women who become symptomatic with trich develop a greenish, foul-smelling vaginal discharge 5–28 days after the time of contact with the organism. The discharge can cause severe itching and irritation of the vagina and vulva, causing redness and pain. Although most males do not have any symptoms, some may experience slight itching, clear discharge, and sometimes painful urination.

Diagnosis of trich can be done through microscopic examination of the discharge. The drug of choice is metronidazole (Flagyl). Partners should also be treated, to prevent the Ping-Pong effect that occurs when partners pass infection back and forth. Treatment is important because studies suggest that trich may increase the risk of HIV transmission. *Trichomonas* infection may also increase a pregnant woman's risk of premature delivery.

Bacterial vaginosis (BV) is the most common cause of abnormal vaginal discharge in women of reproductive age. BV involves a shift in the makeup of the bacteria that normally inhabit the vagina: Instead of *Lactobacillus* being most numerous, there is an overgrowth of anaerobic mi-croorganisms and bacteria such as *Gardnerella vaginalis.* BV is clearly associated with sexual activity, often occurring after a change in partners. However, research on the degree to which BV is sexually transmitted is ongoing. Recent research suggests that a sexually transmitted virus that infects and kills *Lactobacillus* may be the underlying cause of BV. Douching also substantially increases the risk of BV. Topical and oral antibiotics are used to treat BV, but BV often recurs after treatment.

Symptoms of BV include a vaginal discharge with a fishlike odor and, in some cases, vaginal irritation; many women with BV have no symptoms. Some studies have shown an association between BV and increased risk of PID, HIV transmission, infection following childbirth or gynecological surgery (including abortion), and, in pregnant women, premature delivery. The CDC recommends that any pregnant woman who has symptoms of BV or who is at risk for premature delivery be screened and, if necessary, treated for BV. The recognition that BV may contribute to more serious conditions has led to an increase in screening and treatment.

Chancroid is a sexually transmitted bacterial infection caused by *Haemophilus ducreyi.* Prevalent in some parts of the world, chancroid is relatively uncommon in the United States, although there are periodic outbreaks. The infection is characterized by painful open sores in the genital area that may resemble the sores associated with herpes or syphilis; other symptoms may include painful urination and vaginal discharge. As with any STD that causes genital sores, chancroid can increase the risk of HIV transmission. Chancroid is treated with antibiotics.

Pubic lice, commonly known as crabs, are highly contagious, both sexually and nonsexually. They are often difficult to see but are the color and size of small freckles until they have fed, and then they become dark brown in color. Like mosquitoes, lice feed on human blood. Although usually found attached to pubic hair, they have been known to attach themselves to hair on the head, eyelashes, underarm hair, and even mustaches and beards. (Head lice are a different species than pubic lice.) Separated from their human hosts, lice can survive for about 24 hours.

Easily passed from person to person, lice can also be transmitted via infested bedding, towels, clothing, sleeping bags, and even toilet seats. Intense itching is the usual symptom, and with careful examination, both the parasite and its eggs, or nits, can be seen. Treatment is generally easy, although the infestation can require repeated applications of nonprescription medications. These preparations are in lotion or shampoo form and include a fine comb for removing any remaining lice or nits from body hair. Carefully washing clothing and linen is also essential for preventing reinfestation. If the infestation persists, other medications are available by prescription.

Scabies is another fairly common infestation. A burrowing parasite, the scabies mite deposits eggs beneath

All sexually transmitted diseases are preventable. You have control over the behaviors and attitudes that place you at risk for contracting STDs and for increasing their negative effects on your health. To identify your risk factors, read the following list of statements and identify whether they're true or false for you.

True or False

1. I have never been sexually active. (If false, continue. If true, you are not at risk; respond to the remaining statements based on how you realistically believe you would act.)

2. I am in a mutually monogamous relationship with an uninfected partner or am not currently sexually active. (If false, continue. If true, you are at minimal risk now; respond to the remaining statements according to your attitudes and past behaviors.)

3. I have only one sex partner.

4. I always use a condom for each act of intercourse, even if I am fairly certain my partner has no infections.

5. I do not use oil-based lubricants or other products with condoms.

6. I discuss STDs and prevention with new partners before having sex.

7. I do not use alcohol or another mood-altering drug in sexual situations.

8. I would tell my partner if I thought I had been exposed to an STD.

9. I am familiar with the signs and symptoms of STDs.

10. I regularly perform genital self-examination.

11. When I notice any sign or symptom of any STD or if I engage in risky sexual behavior, I consult my physician immediately.

12. I obtain screening for HIV and STDs regularly. In addition (if female), I obtain yearly pelvic exams and Pap tests.

13. When diagnosed with an STD, I inform all recent partners.

14. When I have a sign or symptom of an STD that goes away on its own, I still consult my physician.

15. I do not use drugs prescribed for friends or partners or left over from other illnesses to treat STDs.

16. I do not share syringes or needles to inject drugs.

False answers indicate attitudes and behaviors that may put you at risk for contracting STDs or for suffering serious medical consequences from them. (For a more detailed self-assessment, take the quiz at www.thebody.com/surveys/sexsurvey.html).

the skin, especially in the creases of the body. The eggs hatch in a few days, and the new mites congregate around hair follicles. This burrowing parasite produces intense itching, especially at night. The usual sites of infestation are between the fingers, on wrists, in armpits, underneath the breasts, along the inner surfaces of the thighs, on the penis and scrotum, and occasionally on the female genitals. Scabies is easily spread from person to person, not only through sexual contact but also through any direct or close contact. Diagnosis is made by actual identification of the mite, the eggs, or the larvae in scrapings taken from the burrows in the skin of the human host. Scabies is generally treated with prescription permethrin cream. Clothing and bedding must be washed to prevent reinfestation with the scabies mite.

WHAT YOU CAN DO

You can take responsibility for your health and contribute to a general reduction in the incidence of STDs in three major areas: education, diagnosis and treatment, and prevention. To assess your current level of responsibility for STD prevention, complete the quiz in the box "Do Your Attitudes and Behaviors Put You at Risk for STDs?"

Education

Since the AIDS epidemic began, public and private agencies have grown more serious about educating the public and increasing their awareness of all STDs. This campaign may already be paying off in changing attitudes and sexual behaviors, at least among certain segments of the population. Recent surveys indicate that condom use is increasing, and the number of new cases of HIV infection in the gay population has been smaller in recent years. Most gay men with HIV practice safer sex. However, many younger gay men are participating in very high risk behaviors, and a second wave of the AIDS epidemic among homosexual

Terms

trichomoniasis A protozoal infection caused by *Trichomonas vaginalis,* transmitted sexually and externally.

bacterial vaginosis (BV) A condition linked to sexual activity; caused by an overgrowth of certain bacteria inhabiting the vagina.

chancroid A sexually transmitted bacterial infection caused by *Haemophilus ducreyi.*

pubic lice Parasites that infest the hair of the pubic region, commonly called *crabs.*

scabies A contagious skin disease caused by a type of burrowing parasitic mite.

men can be expected if younger men fail to use preventive measures. Also discouraging is the fact that the number of cases of HIV infection among harder-to-reach groups, such as injection drug users and their partners and children, is still increasing. In particular, more educational efforts are needed among U.S. ethnic minorities.

Education efforts targeted at increasing public awareness about AIDS through the media have included public service announcements, dramatic presentations, and support from well-known public figures. Colleges offer courses in human sexuality. Free pamphlets and other literature are available from public health departments, health clinics, physicians' offices, student health centers, and Planned Parenthood, and easy-to-understand books are available in libraries and bookstores. Several national hotlines have been set up to provide free, confidential information and referral services to callers anywhere in the country (see the For More Information section at the end of the chapter).

Although information about STDs is widely disseminated, learning about STDs is still up to every person individually. You must assume responsibility for learning about the causes and nature of STDs and their potential effects on you, those with whom you have sexual relationships, and the children you may have. Once you know about STDs—their symptoms, how they're transmitted, how they can be prevented—you are in a position to educate others. Providing information to your friends and partners, whether in casual conversation or in more serious decision-making discussions, is an important way that you can make a difference in both your own wellness and that of others.

Diagnosis and Treatment

Early diagnosis and treatment of STDs can help you and your sex partner(s) avoid unnecessary complications and help prevent the spread of STDs.

Get Vaccinated   Every young, sexually active person should be vaccinated for hepatitis B. Men who have sex with men should also be vaccinated for hepatitis A. In the next 5–10 years, vaccines for HPV, HSV, and possibly even some strains of HIV may become available. Vaccines offer the possibility that these common, incurable viral infections can be controlled.

Be Alert for Symptoms   If you are sexually active, be alert for any sign or symptom of disease, such as a rash, a discharge, sores, or unusual pain, and don't hesitate to have a professional examination if you notice such a symptom. Although only a physician can make a proper diagnosis of an STD, you can perform *genital self-examination* between checkups to look for early warning signs of infection. Women should examine the entire genital area, including the area covered by pubic hair, the outer and inner lips of the vagina, the clitoris, and the area around the urinary and vaginal openings. Men should look at the entire head, shaft,

and base of the penis and the scrotum. (A mirror may be helpful for checking difficult-to-see areas.)

Throughout the exam, look for bumps, sores, blisters, or warts on the skin. Bumps or blisters may be red or light colored; they may look like pimples, or they may develop into open sores. Genital warts may appear as very small bumpy spots, or they may have a fleshy, cauliflower-like appearance. Also stay alert for other signs of STDs, including pain or burning upon urination, itchiness in the genital area, abnormal discharge from the vagina or penis, pelvic pain, and, in women, bleeding between menstrual periods. Be alert for these signs or symptoms in your partner, too, and don't hesitate to question him or her if you notice something unusual.

Get Tested   Remember that almost all STDs—including HIV infection—can be completely asymptomatic for long periods of time. If you are sexually active, be sure to get periodic STD and HIV checks, even if you have no symptoms. If you have a risky sexual encounter, see a physician as soon as possible (see the box "Don't Wait—Early Treatment of STDs Really Matters"). Sexually active young women should have pelvic exams and Pap tests at least once a year, with chlamydia and gonorrhea screening in most cases. Sexually active men, especially if they have had more than one partner, should have periodic STD and HIV screening.

Men who have sex with men are at especially high risk for HIV and other STDs. The CDC currently recommends that sexually active men who have sex with men be tested annually for HIV, chlamydia (anal and urethral), syphilis, and gonorrhea (anal, urethral, and pharyngeal). Men who have multiple anonymous partners or who are injection drug users should be screened more frequently. All sexually active gay and bisexual men should be vaccinated for hepatitis A and B.

Testing for STDs is done through private physicians, public health clinics, community health agencies, and most student health services. If you are diagnosed as having an STD, you should begin treatment as quickly as possible. Inform your partner(s), and avoid any sexual activity until your treatment is complete and testing indicates that you are cured. If your partner tells you that he or she has contracted an STD, get tested immediately, even if you don't have any symptoms. Asymptomatic partners are often treated to ensure that an infection will not spread or recur.

Inform Your Partners   Telling a partner that you have exposed him or her to an STD isn't easy. You may be afraid your partner will be angry or resentful, or you may worry that your partner will think less of you or reject you. At the same time, you may be feeling afraid, ashamed, embarrassed, or angry yourself. Despite the awkwardness and difficulty, it is crucial that your sex partner or partners be informed and urged to seek testing and/or treatment as quickly as possible.

You can't take back an unwise sexual choice, but quickly owning up to the fact that you are at risk for infection and taking action right away can make a big difference. Treating STDs like chlamydia and gonorrhea within a few days of infection is very likely to prevent complications such as PID and infertility. You will also be much less likely to pass the infection on to anyone else. If you have had a recent risky sexual encounter, visit your physician, student health center, or local STD clinic and ask for testing. Don't wait for symptoms to develop—you may never have any. Permanent damage from STDs, including infertility, can occur even if you have no symptoms.

If you feel a recent sexual encounter puts you at high risk for HIV, see a physician immediately. Unsafe sex with a person who is infected with HIV meets the criteria for PEP treatment described earlier in the chapter; if you are treated within 72 hours of possible exposure, PEP will significantly reduce your risk of HIV infection. If you develop flulike symptoms in the days or weeks following risky sexual or drug-taking behavior, see your physician and ask for an HIV RNA test in addition to standard STD tests. (HIV antibody tests may not register primary HIV infection.) If HIV treatment is begun within the first weeks of the infection, there is a good chance that damage to the immune system can be reduced or even prevented. Many physicians will not think of primary HIV infection when you describe flulike symptoms, so be sure to speak up about your recent risky activities and your concerns about HIV.

If tests come back positive for a particular STD, you need to be tested for others, including HIV infection. Infection with any STD means that you are at higher risk for all others. Women should also have a pelvic exam and a Pap test. If you are given medication to treat an STD, take all of it as directed. Incomplete treatment can result in an incomplete cure, thereby contributing to the development of drug-resistant organisms. Do not share your medication with a partner; he or she should see a physician for testing and treatment.

Do not have sexual intercourse until your treatment—and your partner's treatment—is complete. If your partner still carries the infection, you are likely to be reinfected when you resume sexual activity. If you have an incurable STD such as herpes or HPV infection, always use a condom and make sure your partner is fully informed of the potential risks of being intimate with you, even if you are using condoms.

Avoiding risky sexual encounters is by far the best course of action. But if you do make a mistake, improve your odds of staying healthy by getting tested and treated as soon as possible. And think seriously about what steps you can take to protect yourself in the future.

You can get help telling your partner if you need it. Public health departments will notify sex partners of their possible exposure while maintaining your confidentiality and anonymity. Peer counseling and student health programs often help students with practice in role playing in these circumstances, and concerned health care personnel can provide assistance.

As emphasized throughout this chapter, undetected and untreated STDs can lead to serious medical complications and even death. In asymptomatic cases, the only way infected people can find out they have a disease is by being tested. Uninformed, untested, partners can go on to spread the disease, contributing to anguish for others as well as spiraling public health problems. The responsibility of informing partners is an ethical task too important to shirk.

Get Treated   With the exception of AIDS treatments, treatments for STDs are safe and generally inexpensive. If you are being treated, follow instructions carefully and complete all the medication as prescribed. Don't stop taking the medication just because you feel better or your symptoms have disappeared. Above all, don't give any of your medication to your partner or to anyone else. Doing so will only make your treatment incomplete and reinfection more likely. Being cured of an STD does not mean that you will not get it again, and exposure does not confer lasting immunity, nor does it prevent you from getting any other STD—all the more reason to be informed, to inform your partners, and to practice safer sex.

Prevention

STDs *are* preventable. As discussed earlier, the only sure way to avoid exposure to STDs is to abstain from sexual activity. But if you do choose to be sexually active, the key

The use of condoms declined as more advanced methods of contraception, such as birth control pills and IUDs, became available. But condoms are once again gaining in popularity because of the protection they provide against STDs.

The only sure way to prevent STDs, including HIV infection, is to abstain from sexual activity. If you choose to be sexually active, you should do everything possible to protect yourself from STDs. This includes good communication with your sex partner(s).

The time to talk about safer sex is before you begin a sexual relationship. However, even if you've been having unprotected sex with your partner, it is still worth it to start practicing safer sex now. If you're nervous about initiating a conversation about safer sex, rehearse what you will say first. Practice in front of a mirror or with a friend.

There are many ways to bring up the subject of safer sex and condom use with your partner. Be honest about your concerns and stress that protection against STDs means that you care about yourself and your partner. Here are a few suggestions:

- "I heard on the news that more and more people are buying and using condoms. I think it shows that people are being more responsible about sex. What do you think?"

- "I'm worried about the diseases we can get from having sex because so many don't have symptoms. I want to protect both of us by using condoms whenever we have sex."

- "I've been thinking about making love with you. But first we need to talk about how to have safer sex and be protected."

You may find that your partner shares your concerns and also wants to use condoms. He or she may be happy and relieved that you have brought up the subject of safer sex. However, if he or she resists the idea of using condoms, you may need to negotiate. Stress that you both deserve to be protected and that sex will be more enjoyable when you aren't worrying about STDs (see the suggestions to the right). If you and your partner haven't used condoms before, buy some and familiarize yourselves with how to use them. Once you feel more comfortable handling condoms, you'll be able to use them correctly and incorporate them into your sexual activity in fun ways. Consider trying the female condom.

If your partner still won't agree to use condoms, think carefully about whether you want to have a sexual relationship with him or her. Safer sex is part of a responsible, caring sexual relationship, and it's smart to say no to a partner who won't use a condom. It's up to you to protect yourself.

If your partner says . . .	Try saying . . .
"They're not romantic."	"Worrying about AIDS isn't romantic, and with condoms we won't have to worry." OR "If we put one on together, a condom could be fun."
"You don't trust me."	"I do trust you, but how can I trust your former partners or mine?" OR "It's important to me that we're both protected."
"I don't have any diseases. I've been tested."	"I'm glad you've been tested, but tests aren't foolproof for all diseases. To be safe, I always use condoms."
"I forgot to bring a condom. But it's OK to skip it just this once."	"I'd really like to make love with you, but I never have sex without a condom. Let's go get some."
"I don't like the way they feel."	"They might feel different, but let's try." OR "Sex won't feel good if we're worrying about diseases." OR "How about trying the female condom?"
"I don't use condoms."	"I use condoms every time." OR "I don't have sex without condoms."
"But I love you."	"Being in love can't protect us from diseases." OR "I love you, too. We still need to use condoms."
"But we've been having sex without condoms."	"I want to start using condoms now so we won't be at any more risk." OR "We can still prevent infection or reinfection."

SOURCE: Dialogue from San Francisco AIDS Foundation. 1998. *Condoms for Couples* (IMPACT AIDS, 3692 18th Street, San Francisco, CA 94110). Copyright © 1998 San Francisco AIDS Foundation. All rights reserved. Used with permission.

is to think about prevention *before* you have a sexual encounter or find yourself in the heat of the moment. Find out what your partner thinks before you become sexually involved. Remember, you can become infected with an STD from just one unprotected encounter.

All your good intentions are likely to fly out the window if you enter into a sexual situation when you are intoxicated. If you or your partner (or both of you) is drunk, you are likely to be less cautious about sex than you would be if you were sober. Many people use alcohol and drugs as a way to deal with their anxiety in social and sexual situations. However, being intoxicated leaves you vulnerable to sexual assault and greatly increases your risk of acquiring a serious STD.

Most people don't want to think, talk, or ask questions about STDs for a variety of reasons. They may think it detracts from the appeal and excitement of the moment, that it takes away from the spontaneity of the experience, or that it will be perceived as a personal insult. For others, simply not knowing how to talk about STDs and safer sex may prevent them from bringing up the issue with a partner. (For advice on communicating with potential sex partners, see the box "Talking About Condoms and Safer Sex.")

Plan ahead for safer sex. Know what sexual behaviors are risky. Find out about your partner's sexual history and practices. Be honest, and ask your partner to do the same, but don't stake your health and life on assumptions about your partner's honesty. Even if your partner's past seems low-risk, still insist on using a condom every time you have sex. Any sexual activity exposes partners to everyone from their partner's sexual past as well everyone from those people's pasts. In one recent study, researchers mapped the sexual relationships of a group of high school students and found a chain of 288 one-to-one sexual relationships, meaning the teen at the end of the chain may have had direct sexual contact with only 1 person—but was indirectly exposed to 286 others. In addition, many honest people are simply unaware that they have an STD.

You may find that your partner is just as concerned as you are. By thinking and talking about responsible sexual behavior, you are expressing a sense of caring for yourself, your potential partner, and your future children. Taking STDs seriously is practical, courageous, and loving; it means giving yourself the respect you deserve.

Everyone can reduce the risk of infection by behaving responsibly. Aside from abstinence, the next most effective approach to preventing STDs is having sex only with one mutually monogamous, uninfected partner. If you are sexually active, use a condom during every act of intercourse to reduce your risk of contracting a disease. Although not foolproof, a properly used condom provides an effective barrier against pathogens, including HIV. A disease can be transmitted if there is contact with an infected area that isn't protected by the condom, however. The use of a barrier over the cervix (diaphragm or cervical cap) in addition to a condom may provide women with some additional protection against the organisms that cause gonorrhea, genital warts, and chlamydia (see Chapter 6).

Approaches to STD prevention that do not work include urinating or douching after intercourse, engaging in oral sex, and genital play without full penetration. Birth control pills and sterilization protect you against conception and unwanted pregnancy but not against STDs.

The decision to have a sexual relationship is accompanied by uncertainties and risks, both physical and emotional. It also carries the responsibility of safeguarding your own health and that of others. You and your partner must have mutual respect and honesty in order to make good decisions together. Caring about yourself and your partner means asking questions and being aware of signs and symptoms. It may be a bit awkward, but the temporary embarrassment of asking intimate questions is a small price to pay to avoid contracting or spreading disease. If your partner thinks less of you for being concerned, you may want to reconsider the relationship in terms of your personal values. Concern about STDs is part of a sexual relationship, not an intrusion into it, just as sexuality is part of life, not separate from it.

Tips for Today

STDs are among the most common infections you can contract—and some are among the most dangerous. Because they can have serious, long-term effects, it's important to be vigilant about exposure, treatment, and, most critically, prevention.

Right now you can

- Make an appointment with a school health clinic, Planned Parenthood, a public health department, or your personal physician if you are sexually active and have not recently been screened for STDs, including HIV.

- If you are sexually active and have not been using condoms, go to your student health clinic or a local pharmacy and buy some.

- Inform a friend or roommate that people can have an STD and not have any symptoms.

- Resolve to discuss condom use with your partner if you are sexually active and are not already using condoms.

SUMMARY

- HIV affects the immune system, making an otherwise healthy person less able to resist a variety of infections.

- HIV is carried in blood and blood products, semen, vaginal and cervical secretions, and breast milk. HIV is transmitted through the exchange of these fluids.

- There is currently no cure or vaccine for HIV infection. Drugs have been developed to slow the course of the disease and to prevent or treat certain secondary infections.

- HIV infection can be prevented by making careful choices about sexual activity, not sharing drug needles, and learning about how to protect oneself from contracting HIV.

- Chlamydia causes epididymitis and urethritis in men; in women, it can lead to PID and infertility if untreated.

- Untreated, gonorrhea can cause PID in women and epididymitis in men, leading to infertility. In infants, untreated gonorrhea can cause blindness.

- Pelvic inflammatory disease (PID), a complication of untreated gonorrhea or chlamydia, is an infection of the uterus and oviducts that may extend to the ovaries and pelvic cavity. It can lead to infertility, ectopic pregnancy, and chronic pelvic pain.

- Human papillomavirus (HPV) is the cause of both genital warts and cervical cancer. Treatment does not eradicate the virus, which can be passed on even by asymptomatic people.

- Genital herpes is a common incurable infection that can be fatal to newborns. After an initial infection, outbreaks may recur at any time.

- Hepatitis B is a viral infection of the liver transmitted through sexual and nonsexual contact. Following an initial infection, most people recover; but some become chronic carriers of the virus who may develop serious, potentially fatal, complications.

- Syphilis is a highly contagious bacterial infection that can be treated with antibiotics. If left untreated, it can lead to deterioration of the central nervous system and death.

- Less serious diseases that can be transmitted sexually or are linked to sexual activity include trichomoniasis, bacterial vaginosis, chancroid, pubic lice, and scabies.

Any STD that causes sores or inflammation can increase the risk of HIV transmission.

- Successful diagnosis and treatment of STDs involve being alert for symptoms, getting tested, informing partners, and following treatment instructions carefully.

- All STDs are preventable; the key is practicing responsible sexual behaviors. Those who are sexually active are safest with one mutually monogamous, uninfected partner. Using a condom properly with every act of sexual intercourse helps protect against STDs.

Take Action

1. **Check out OTC contraceptives:** Go to a drugstore and examine the OTC contraceptives. Which ones provide protection against STDs? Are both male and female condoms available? Can you find, select, and purchase condoms in your local pharmacy without undue embarrassment? If not, why not? If you are sexually active, make sure you use the best protection available.

2. **Consider being a volunteer:** More and more communities have treatment and support programs for people with HIV infection. Look in the yellow pages or contact local health agencies to find out what services are available where you live. If any of these agencies use volunteers, consider donating some of your time to help.

3. **Visit a health care provider:** If you have ever engaged in unprotected sex or another behavior that puts you at risk for STDs, talk with your health care provider about being screened for common STDs. What tests are available and useful for your situation?

For More Information

Books

Alcamo, I. E. 2003. *AIDS: The Biological Basis.* Sudbury, Mass.: Jones & Bartlett. *A review of current information, including biological, medical, and social implications of HIV/AIDS.*

Ebel, C., and A. Wald. 2002. *Managing Herpes: How to Live and Love with a Chronic STD.* Research Triangle Park, N.C.: American Social Health Association. *Describes the medical and emotional issues related to genital herpes.*

Hayden, D. 2004. *Pox: Genius, Madness, and the Mysteries of Syphilis.* New York: Basic Books. *Presents the history, symptoms, and course of syphilis, along with accounts of key historical figures who suffered from the disease.*

Henderson, G., A. Warshowsky, and B. W. Yasgur. 2002. *Women at Risk: The HPV Epidemic and Your Cervical Health.* New York: Avery Penguin Putnam. *Describes the disorders caused by HPV infection and provides advice for women who have abnormal Pap tests.*

King, J. L. 2004. *On the Down Low: A Journey into the Lives of "Straight" Black Men Who Sleep with Men.* New York: Broadway. *A controversial look at black men who have sex with other men but don't consider themselves to be gay; based on the author's personal experiences.*

McIlvenna, T. 2005. *The Complete Guide to Safer Sex.* Fort Lee, N.J.: Barricade Books. *Provides practical advice for STD prevention.*

Moore, E. A. 2004. *Encyclopedia of Sexually Transmitted Diseases.* Jefferson, N.C.: McFarland. *Includes a variety of information about STDs in an easy-to-use format.*

Organizations, Hotlines, and Web Sites

American College Health Association. Offers free brochures on STDs, alcohol use, acquaintance rape, and other health issues.
410-859-1500
http://www.acha.org

American Social Health Association (ASHA). Provides written information and referrals on STDs; sponsors support groups for people with herpes and HPV.
919-361-8400
919-361-8488 (herpes hotline)
http://www.ashastd.org

Black AIDS Institute. Provides public health information about a variety of topics including testing, treatment, vaccines, and health care access.
http://www.blackaids.org

The Body/A Multimedia AIDS and HIV Information Resource. Provides basic information about HIV—prevention, testing, treatment—and links to related sites.
http://www.thebody.com

CDC National Prevention Information Network. Provides extensive information and links on HIV/AIDS and other STDs.
800-458–5231
http://www.cdcnpin.org

ASHA/CDC STD and AIDS Hotlines. Callers can obtain information, counseling, and referrals for testing and treatment. The hotlines offer information on more than 20 STDs and include Spanish and TTY service.
800-342-AIDS or 800-227-8922
800-344-SIDA (Spanish); 800-243-7889 (TTY, deaf access)

HIV InSite: Gateway to AIDS Knowledge. Provides information about prevention, education, treatment, statistics, clinical trials, and new developments.
http://hivinsite.ucsf.edu

Joint United Nations Programme on HIV/AIDS (UNAIDS). Provides statistics and information on the international HIV/AIDS situation.
http://www.unaids.org

Latex Love. Sponsored by the makers of Trojan condoms, this site includes directions for condom use and sample dialogues for overcoming excuses for not using condoms.

http://www.trojancondoms.com/quizzes/safer_sex

The NAMES Project Foundation AIDS Memorial Quilt. Includes the story behind the quilt, images of quilt panels, and information and links relating to HIV infection.

http://www.aidsquilt.org

National Institute of Allergies and Infectious Disease/STDs Information. Provides up-to-date fact sheets and brochures.

http://www.niaid.nih.gov/publications/stds.htm

Planned Parenthood Federation of America. Provides information on STDs, family planning, and contraception.

http://www.plannedparenthood.org

WHO: Sexually Transmitted Infections. Provides information on international statistics and prevention efforts.

http://www.who.int/topics/sexually_transmitted_infections/en

See also the listings for Chapters 6 and 17.

Selected Bibliography

Agot, K. E., et al. 2004. Risk of HIV-1 in rural Kenya: A comparison of circumcised and uncircumcised men. *Epidemiology* 15(2): 157–163.

American Association of Blood Banks. 2004. *Facts About Blood and Blood Banking* (http://www.aabb.org/All_About_Blood/FAQs/aabb_faqs.htm; retrieved December 2, 2004).

AVERT. 2005. *Origins of AIDS and HIV* (http://www.avert.org/origins.htm; retrieved February 7, 2005).

Baeten, J. M., et al. 2005. Female-to-male infectivity of HIV-1 among circumcised and uncircumcised Kenyan men. *Journal of Infectious Diseases* 191(4): 546–553.

Brown, D. R., et al. 2005. A longitudinal study of genital human papillomavirus infection in a cohort of closely followed adolescent women. *Journal of Infectious Diseases* 191(2): 182–192.

Centers for Disease Control and Prevention. 2002. 2002 guidelines for treatment of sexually transmitted diseases. *MMWR Recommendations and Reports* 51(RR-6).

Centers for Disease Control and Prevention. 2003. *Are Patients in a Health Care Setting at Risk of Getting HIV?* (http://www.cdc.gov/hiv/pubs/faq/faq29.htm; retrieved December 2, 2004).

Centers for Disease Control and Prevention. 2003. Internet use and early syphilis infection among men who have sex with men. *Morbidity and Mortality Weekly Report* 52(50): 1229–1232.

Centers for Disease Control and Prevention. 2003. HIV/STD risks in young men who have sex with men who do not disclose their sexual orientation. *Morbidity and Mortality Weekly Report* 52(5): 81–85.

Centers for Disease Control and Prevention. 2004. Chlamydia screening among sexually active young female enrollees of health plans. *Morbidity and Mortality Weekly Report* 53(42): 983–985.

Centers for Disease Control and Prevention. 2004. Increases in fluoroquinolone-resistant *Neisseria gonorrhoeae* among men who have sex with men, and revised recommendations for gonorrhea treatment, 2004. *Morbidity and Mortality Weekly Report* 53(16): 335–338.

Centers for Disease Control and Prevention. 2004. Transmission of primary and secondary syphilis by oral sex. *Morbidity and Mortality Weekly Report* 53(41): 966–968.

Centers for Disease Control and Prevention. 2005. Antiretroviral postexposure prophylaxis after sexual, injection-drug use, or other nonoccupational exposure to HIV in the United States. *MMWR Recommendations and Reports* 54(RR02): 1–20.

Cohen, Myron. 2004. HIV and sexually transmitted diseases: A lethal synergy. *Topics in HIV Medicine* 12(4):104–107.

Crosby, R., and R. J. DiClemente. 2004. Use of recreational Viagra among men having sex with men. *Sexually Transmitted Infections* 80(6): 466–468.

Erbelding, E. J., and J. M. Zenilman. 2005. Toward better control of sexually transmitted diseases. *New England Journal of Medicine* 352(7): 720–721.

Food and Drug Administration. 2004. *FDA Approves First Oral Fluid Based Rapid HIV Test Kit* (http://www.fda.gov/bbs/topics/news/2004/NEW01042.html; retrieved February 7, 2005).

Fox, M. 2005. Sex map shows chain of almost 300 high school lovers. *Reuters Health* (http://www.nlm.nih.gov/medlineplus/news/fullstory_22551.html; retrieved February 3, 2005).

Gupta, R., et al. 2004. Valacyclovir and acyclovir for suppression of shedding of herpes simplex virus in the genital tract. *Journal of Infectious Diseases* 190(8): 1374–1381.

Harrigan, P. R., et al. 2005. Predictors of HIV drug-resistance mutations in a large antiretroviral-naive cohort initiating triple antiretroviral therapy. *Journal of Infectious Diseases* 191(3): 339–347.

Hightow, L. B., et al. 2005. The unexpected movement of the HIV epidemic in the Southeastern United States: Transmission among college students. *Journal of Acquired Immune Deficiency Syndrome* 38(5): 531–537.

Kaiser Family Foundation. 2004. *Survey of Americans on HIV/AIDS: Testing* (http://www.kff.org/hivaids/loader.cfm?url=/commonspot/security/getfile.cfm&PageID=37451; retrieved December 12, 2004).

Kimberlin, D., and D. Rouse. 2004. Genital herpes. *New England Journal of Medicine* 350(19): 1970–1977.

Miller, W. C., et al. 2004. Prevalence of chlamydial and gonococcal infections among young adults in the United States. *Journal of the American Medical Association* 291(18): 2229–2236.

Ness, R. B., et al. 2005. Douching, pelvic inflammatory disease, and incident gonococcal and chlamydial genital infection in a cohort of high-risk women. *American Journal of Epidemiology* 61(2): 186–195.

Sanders, G. D., et al. 2005. Cost-effectiveness of screening for HIV in the era of highly active antiretroviral therapy. *New England Journal of Medicine* 352(6): 570–585.

Wang, C., et al. 2004. Mortality in HIV-seropositive versus -seronegative persons in the era of highly active antiretroviral therapy: Implications for when to initiate therapy. *Journal of Infectious Diseases* 190(6): 1046–1054.

Weinstock, H., S. Berman, and W. Cates. 2004. Sexually transmitted diseases among American youth: Incidence and prevalence estimates, 2000. *Perspectives on Sexual and Reproductive Health* 36(1): 6–10.

World Health Organization. 2004. *Antiretroviral Drugs for Treating Pregnant Women and Preventing HIV Infection in Infants* (http://www.who.int/hiv/pub/mtct/en/arvdrugswomenguidelinesfinal.pdf; retrieved December 6, 2004).

Yap, M. W., S. Nisole, and J. P. Stoye. 2005. A single amino acid change in the SPRY domain of human Trim5alpha leads to HIV-1 restriction. *Current Biology* 15(1): 73–78.

Yeni, P. G., et al. 2004. Treatment for adult HIV infection. *Journal of the American Medical Association* 292(2): 251–265.

Zheng, J., et al. 2004. Ethanol stimulation of HIV infection of oral epithelial cells. *Journal of Acquired Immune Deficiency Syndromes* 37(4): 1445–1453.

Zou, S., et al. 2004. Probability of viremia with HBV, HCV, HIV, and HTLV among tissue donors in the United States. *New England Journal of Medicine* 351(8): 751–759.

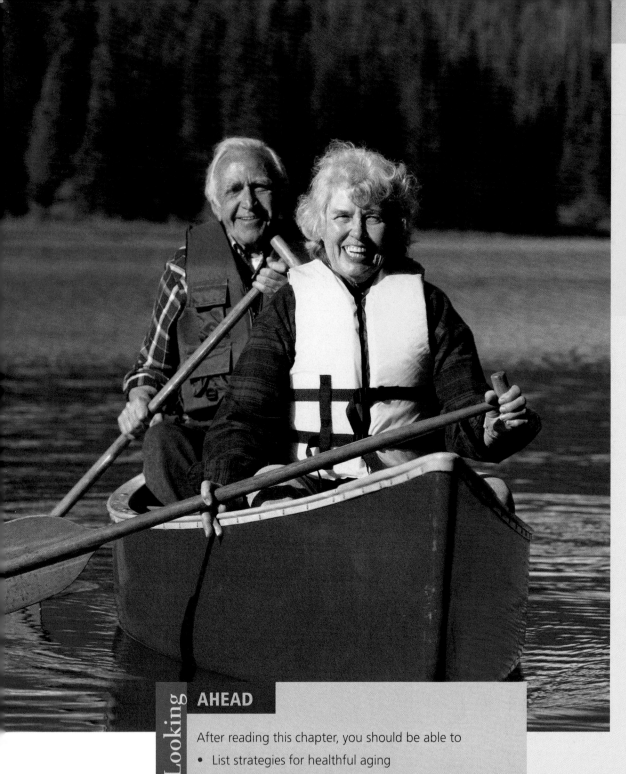

19

After reading this chapter, you should be able to

- List strategies for healthful aging

- Explain the physical, social, and mental changes that may accompany aging and discuss how people can best confront these changes

- Compare different theories on the causes of aging

- Describe practical considerations of older adults and caregivers, including housing, finances, health care, communication, and transportation

Aging: A Vital Process

1. **Women do not need to take preventive measures against osteoporosis until after menopause.**
   True or false?

2. **Medicare and private insurers pay for what percentage of nursing home costs overall?**
   a. 3%
   b. 33%
   c. 66%

3. **On average, a woman will spend more time caring for an aging relative than raising children.**
   True or false?

4. **Exercise is beneficial for older people because it**
   a. protects against osteoporosis.
   b. maintains alertness and intelligence.
   c. prevents falls.

5. **Alcohol abuse is rare among older adults.**
   True or false?

6. **About how many Americans over age 65 have been prescribed medications that are inappropriate and unsafe when used by older adults?**
   a. 1 in 20
   b. 1 in 10
   c. 1 in 5

ANSWERS

1. FALSE. Everyone—but especially women—needs to pay attention to diet and exercise in younger years in order to build bone mass.

2. A. Medicare pays less than 2% of costs, and private insurers pay less than 1% for the more than 1 million older Americans currently living in nursing homes.

3. TRUE. The average woman will spend 17 years raising children and 18 years caring for an aging relative.

4. ALL THREE. Even for people over 80, exercise can improve physical functioning and balance and reduce falls and injuries.

5. FALSE. Alcohol abuse affects about 10% of elderly people. It often goes undetected because its symptoms may mimic those of other conditions, such as Alzheimer's disease.

6. C. An estimated 20% of Americans over age 65 have been prescribed drugs that have potentially dangerous side effects for older adults. Education about inappropriate medications is needed for both physicians and patients.

WW Visit the *Core Concepts in Health* Online Learning Center (www.mhhe.com/insel10e) for study aids and many additional resources.

581

Many people would like to live for a long time and never grow old. When we see that old age has taken us in its grip, we're stunned. We regard old age as something foreign: Can I become a different person while I still remain myself? Yes. And no. Life is like a river. The flow is continuous, and you can never step in the same place twice. Aging does not begin at age 65, and there is no precise age at which a person becomes "old." Rather, aging is a normal process of development that occurs over the entire lifetime. It happens to everyone, but at different rates for different people. Some people are "old" at 25, and others are still "young" at 75.

Although youth is not entirely a state of mind, your attitude toward life and your attention to your health significantly influence the satisfaction you will derive from life, especially when new physical, mental, and social challenges occur in later years. If you optimize wellness during young adulthood, you can exert great control over the physical and mental aspects of aging, and you can better handle your response to events that might be out of your control. With foresight and energy you can shape a creative, graceful, and even triumphant old age.

GENERATING VITALITY AS YOU AGE

As we age, we experience both gains and losses. Physical and mental changes occur gradually, over a lifetime. Biological aging includes all the normal, progressive, irreversible changes to one's body that begin at birth and continue until death. Psychological aging and social aging usually involve more abrupt changes in circumstance and emotion: relocating, changing homes, losing a spouse and friends, retiring, having a lower income, and changing roles and social status. These changes represent opportunities for growth throughout life.

Not all of them happen to everybody, and their timing varies, partly depending on how we have prepared for our later days. Some people never have to leave their homes and appear to be in good health until the day they die. Others have tremendous adjustments to make—to entirely new surroundings with fewer financial resources, to new acquaintances, to the changing physical condition of their bodies and new health problems, and possibly to loneliness and loss of self-esteem.

Successful aging requires preparation. People need to establish good health habits in their teens and twenties. During their twenties and thirties, they usually develop important relationships and settle into a particular lifestyle. By their mid-forties, they generally know how much money they need to support the lifestyle they've chosen. At this point, they must assess their financial status and perhaps adjust their savings in order to continue enjoying that lifestyle after retirement. In their mid-fifties, they need to reevaluate their health insurance plans and may want to think about retirement housing. In their seventies and beyond, they need to consider ways of sharing their legacy with the next generation. Throughout life, people should cultivate interests and hobbies they enjoy, both alone and with others, so they can continue to live an active and rewarding life in their later years.

What Happens as You Age?

Many of the characteristics associated with aging are not due to aging at all. Rather, they are the result of neglect and abuse of our bodies and minds. These assaults lay the foundation for later psychological problems and chronic conditions like arthritis, heart disease, diabetes, hearing loss, and hypertension. We sacrifice our optimal health by smoking, having poor nutrition, overeating, abusing alcohol and drugs, bombarding our ears with excessive noise, and exposing our bodies to too much ultraviolet radiation from the sun. We also jeopardize our bodies through inactivity, encouraging our muscles and even our bones to wither and deteriorate. And we endure abuse from the toxic chemicals in our environment.

But even with the healthiest behavior and environment, aging inevitably occurs. It results from biochemical processes we don't yet fully understand. The physiological changes in organ systems are caused by a combination of gradual aging and impairment from disease. Because of redundancy in most organ systems, the body's ability to function is not affected until damage is fairly extensive. Studies of healthy people indicate that functioning remains essentially constant until after age 70. Further research may help pinpoint the causes of aging and aid in the development of therapies to repair damage to aging organs (see the box "Stem Cells"). Figure 19-1 (p. 584) shows some of the changes that are a part of aging.

Life-Enhancing Measures: Age-Proofing

You can prevent, delay, lessen, or even reverse some of the changes associated with aging through good habits. Simple things you can do daily will make a vast difference to your level of energy and vitality—your overall wellness. The following suggestions have been mentioned throughout this text. But because they are profoundly related to health in later life, we highlight them here.

Challenge Your Mind Creativity and intelligence remain stable in healthy individuals. Develop interests and hobbies you can enjoy throughout your life. Staying involved in learning as a lifelong process can help you remain alert and keep your mental abilities.

What Are Stem Cells?

Nearly all the cells in our body are differentiated, meaning they are committed to specific functions. We have heart cells, skin cells, nerve cells—over 260 cell types in all. Stem cells, in contrast, are undifferentiated; they can renew themselves by continuing to divide in their undifferentiated state for long periods, and they can develop into specialized cells. The ability of stem cells to develop into almost any type of tissue is referred to as *plasticity*, and it is plasticity that gives stem cells great therapeutic potential.

Stem cells theoretically could be used to generate replacement cells for a wide array of diseased or injured tissues and organs—for example, insulin-producing cells to treat type 1 diabetes, cardiac muscle cells for repair of a damaged heart, or healthy brain cells for people with Parkinson's disease. Donated organs and tissues are sometimes used to replace damaged tissue, but the need far outstrips the available supply. It is hoped that stem cells could be widely produced and matched to an individual's cellular makeup. But before this can occur, both technical and ethical problems must be addressed.

Embryonic Stem Cells

As their name suggests, embryonic stem cells are derived from embryos. About 4–5 days after fertilization, an embryo is a microscopic hollow ball of cells referred to as a blastocyst (see Chapter 8). The inner cell mass contains about 30 stem cells; researchers can remove these cells and grow them in culture for a fairly long period, producing millions of embryonic stem cells. Currently, most embryonic stem cells used in research are derived from eggs that have been fertilized in vitro and then donated for research purposes; they are not derived from embryos fertilized within a woman's body.

Stem cells from embryos are *pluripotent,* that is, they can develop into virtually any cell type. Researchers hope to learn how to initiate cell differentiation and then use the resulting cells to repair or replace tissues and organs damaged by disease or injury. Although stem cells can become many different types of cells, they are not capable of forming a new embryo and cannot give rise to a whole person. Only a complete fertilized egg is *totipotent,* with the potential to generate all the cells and tissues that make up an embryo and its developmental support (placenta, umbilical cord, and so on).

Adult Stem Cells

Some organs and tissues in the adult body can replace cells, while others do not seem to have this ability. Researchers now believe that cellular repair is carried out by stem cells that may lie dormant in tissues until they are needed. These cells are rare—perhaps only 1 adult stem cell for every 100,000 specialized tissue cells in the body.

Adult stem cells appear to have some degree of plasticity; for example, hematopoietic stem cells in bone marrow can differentiate into all the different types of blood cells. However, evidence that adult stem cells from one tissue can develop into fully functional cells of another type of tissue is limited. Adult stem cells can be more challenging for researchers to work with than embryonic stem cells because they are more difficult to locate, identify, and produce in large numbers.

The most studied type of adult stem cell, and the only type of stem cell widely used in clinical applications, is the hematopoietic stem cell. These cells are used in transplants to restore blood and immune components to the bone marrow of people being treated for cancer and other diseases. (Although commonly referred to as bone marrow transplants, many such transplants actually involve white blood cells drawn from peripheral circulation rather than bone marrow.) Hematopoietic stem cells for transplant can be collected from a donor, but they are also sometimes derived from umbilical cord blood.

Although transplant success rates have improved, rejection remains a major problem, and success depends on finding a close cellular match between donor and recipient. Another avenue of stem cell research—and one possible way around the rejection problem—is somatic cell nuclear transfer. In this technique, the nucleus from a somatic (body) cell is transferred into an egg from which the nucleus has been removed. The egg is then allowed to develop in the lab into a blastocyst, and the resulting stem cells are removed and cultured. This technique, also known as *therapeutic cloning,* produces a line of stem cells that are genetically matched to the cell donor; using these cells for transplant should eliminate problems with rejection. (This technique is distinct from so-called *reproductive cloning,* in which an embryo is created in the lab using somatic cell transfer but then is implanted in a uterus and allowed to develop in order to produce an offspring who is genetically identical to the donor of the original somatic cell.)

The Future: Potential and Controversy

Stem cell research is in its infancy, and both technical difficulties and major ethical questions remain. For example, it is still unclear how stem cells remain undifferentiated for long periods or how they can be made to differentiate in desired ways.

Many scientists believe that research into both embryonic and adult stem cells will be needed to advance the therapeutic potential of stem cell research. However, the use (and destruction) of human embryos for this research is controversial. Some people advocate a complete ban; others would permit the use of existing stem cell lines, the use of extra embryos produced by in vitro fertilization, and/or the use of embryos created specifically for research from eggs and sperm donated by volunteers. The NIH has established a group of scientists, ethicists, and others to oversee research on human stem cells.

In 2001, President Bush banned the use of federal funds for any research related to the creation of new embryonic stem cell lines, thus limiting research to a small number of existing cell lines. Researchers believe that there are problems with this limitation, highlighted by the announcement in 2005 that all existing stem cell lines may have become contaminated with nonhuman compounds via the technique used to maintain them. A number of private institutions and individual states are now providing funds for the creation of new embryonic stem cell lines.

Despite the many problems and unknowns, researchers are optimistic. Results from early tests of adult stem cells used to treat heart failure have been promising, and trials on treatments for other conditions may begin soon. The hope is that stem cell research will lead to beneficial therapies for common conditions that are currently difficult or impossible to treat.

Blood flow to the brain decreases and nerve cells atrophy. Neuron loss does not necessarily mean a decline in mental ability.

The ability to focus on objects close to you declines, and night driving may become more difficult.

Many of the sensory receptors in the nose die; long-term exposure to smoke also lessens the ability to smell.

Teeth can last a lifetime; however, a buildup of plaque can lead to tooth loss if brushing and flossing are neglected.

About two-thirds of the taste buds in the mouth die by age 70; some medications can interfere with taste.

Body fat increases and muscle mass decreases as activity levels drop and calorie needs decline. Regular exercise helps maintain a healthy body composition

Men take longer to attain an erection and it may not be as firm or as large as when they were younger. Enlargement of the prostate gland is common. In women, menopause occurs and estrogen levels drop.

Women in particular are prone to bone loss, especially after menopause, when bones become weaker, more porous, and more likely to fracture. Calcium intake and weight-bearing exercise in younger years can slow bone loss later.

Cells at the base of hair follicles produce progressively less pigment and eventually die, causing hair to turn gray and some men to go bald. Hair also becomes finer.

Ability to hear high-pitched and sibilant (hissing) sounds such as *s*, *z*, *sh*, and *ch* declines. Some losses may be due to damage from loud music or machinery.

The heart pumps less blood with each beat; this is particularly noticeable during exercise. A healthy diet and regular exercise can often counteract potential cardiovascular problems.

Lung capacity stays steady or even increases with regular exercise. Colds are fewer and less severe due to a buildup in immunity.

Kidneys filter waste more slowly, affecting drug clearance and increasing frequency of urination.

Decreases in acid production and digestive enzymes make digestion take longer; constipation may become more common unless fiber intake increases.

Long-term sun exposure produces wrinkles and spotty pigmentation ("age spots"). Skin gets looser, stretches more easily, and is less resilient.

Muscle fibers atrophy and lose their ability to contract as more protein is broken down and less is synthesized. Regular exercise can slow this process. Muscles are also less flexible and more susceptible to injury.

Figure 19-1 Age-related changes in the body. The body changes in predictable ways as we age. Many of these changes can be slowed by choices we make throughout our lives.

Develop Physical Fitness Exercise significantly enhances both psychological and physical health. The positive effects of exercise include

- Lower blood pressure and healthier cholesterol levels
- Better protection against heart attacks and an increased chance of survival should one occur
- Sustained capacity of the lungs
- Weight control through less accumulation of fat
- Maintenance of strength, flexibility, and balance
- Protection against osteoporosis and type 2 diabetes
- Increased effectiveness of the immune system
- Maintenance of mental agility and flexibility, response time, memory, and hand-eye coordination

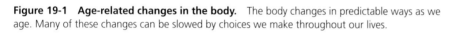

Terms

V W **fluid intelligence** The ability to develop a solution when confronted with a new problem.

glaucoma A disease in which fluid inside the eye is under abnormally high pressure; can lead to the loss of peripheral vision and blindness.

The stimulus that exercise provides also seems to protect against the loss of **fluid intelligence**, the ability to find solutions when confronted with a new problem. Fluid intelligence depends on rapidity of responsiveness, memory, and alertness. Individuals who exercise regularly are also less susceptible to depression than those whose level of physical activity has declined.

Find a variety of activities that you enjoy and can do regularly. Accumulate at least 30–60 minutes of moderate-intensity physical activity every day, and begin a formal exercise program to develop cardiorespiratory endurance, muscular strength and endurance, and flexibility (see Chapter 13). Older individuals who have been sedentary should be encouraged to become more active. It's never too late to start exercising. Even in people over 80, endurance and strength training can improve balance, flexibility, and physical functioning and reduce the potential for dangerous falls. A recent study of seniors in a tai chi program found that the exercises reduced the risk of falls even among those who used assistive devices for mobility.

Eat Wisely Good health at any age is enhanced by eating a varied diet full of nutrient-rich foods. Follow the recommendations in the 2005 Dietary Guidelines for

Regular exercise throughout life is an important key to successful aging. By keeping fit, this couple has maintained a high level of physical functioning. Regular exercise also helps prevent depression, boredom, and losses in fluid intelligence typically associated with aging.

Americans to obtain adequate amounts of all essential nutrients while maintaining a healthy weight. For many adults, that means increasing intake of fruits, vegetables, and whole grains while decreasing intake of foods high in saturated and trans fats and added sugars. Special guidelines for older adults include the following:

- Consume vitamin B-12 and extra vitamin D from fortified foods or supplements.
- To help control blood pressure, limit consumption of sodium to 1500 mg per day and consume adequate potassium (4700 mg per day). Older adults tend to have higher blood pressure and to be salt-sensitive.
- Consume foods rich in dietary fiber and adequate fluids to help prevent constipation, which may occur in up to 20% of older adults. A diet rich in whole grains, vegetables, and fruits can meet the recommended goals for fiber.
- Focus on nutrient-dense foods to obtain adequate nutrients while keeping energy intake at a level that doesn't lead to unhealthy weight gain.
- Pay special attention to food safety; older adults tend to be more susceptible to foodborne illness. Take special care not to eat or drink raw (unpasteurized) milk or any products made from unpasteurized milk (such as some soft cheeses), raw or partially cooked

eggs or foods containing raw eggs, raw or undercooked meat and poultry, unpasteurized juices, and raw sprouts. In addition, avoid raw or undercooked fish or shellfish, and reheat leftover deli meats and frankfurters until they are steaming hot.

Refer to Chapter 12 for more on the Dietary Guidelines for Americans. Tufts University has developed a special food pyramid for older adults (http://nutrition.tufts.edu).

Maintain a Healthy Weight Weight management is especially difficult if you have been overweight most of your life. A sensible program of expending more calories through exercise, cutting calorie intake, or a combination of both will work for most people who want to lose weight, but there is no magic formula. Obesity is not physically healthy, and it leads to premature aging (see Chapter 14).

Control Drinking and Overdependence on Medications Alcohol abuse ranks with depression as a common hidden mental health problem, affecting about 10% of older adults. (The ability to metabolize alcohol decreases with age.) The problem is often not identified because the effects of alcohol or drug dependence can mimic disease, such as Alzheimer's disease. Signs of potential alcohol or drug dependence include unexplained falls or frequent injuries, forgetfulness, depression, and malnutrition. Older people who retire or lose a spouse are especially at risk. Problems can be avoided by not using alcohol to relieve anxiety or emotional pain and not taking medication when safer forms of treatment are available.

Don't Smoke The average pack-a-day smoker can expect to live about 13–14 years less than a nonsmoker. Furthermore, smokers suffer more illnesses that last longer, and they are subject to respiratory disabilities that limit their total vigor for many years before their death. Premature balding, skin wrinkling, and osteoporosis have been linked to cigarette smoking. Smokers at age 50 often have wrinkles resembling those of a person of 60.

Schedule Physical Examinations to Detect Treatable Diseases When detected early, many diseases, including hypertension, diabetes, and many types of cancer, can be successfully controlled by medication and lifestyle changes. Regular testing for **glaucoma** after age 40 can prevent blindness from this eye disease. Recommended immunizations, including those for influenza and pneumococcus, can protect you from preventable infectious diseases. (See Chapters 14–17 for screening and immunization guidelines.)

Recognize and Reduce Stress Stress-induced physiological changes increase wear and tear on your body. Cut down on the stresses in your life. Don't wear yourself out through lack of sleep, substance abuse or misuse, or overwork. Practice relaxation, using the techniques described in Chapter 2. If you contract a disease, consider it your body's attempt to interrupt your life pattern; reevaluate your lifestyle, and perhaps slow down.

The health behaviors you practice *now* are more influential in determining how long and how well you will live than your behaviors at a later age. Retiring from your life's occupation with a physically healthy body will allow far more options for enjoying yourself than will retiring with frail health or disabilities. Preventable poor health drains finances, emotions, and energy and contributes to poor psychological health. By enhancing your wellness today, you're ensuring some wellness for the future.

CONFRONTING THE CHANGES OF AGING

The changes that occur with aging have repercussions that must be grappled with and resolved. Just as you can act now to prevent or limit the physical changes of aging, you can also begin preparing yourself psychologically, socially, and financially for changes that may occur later in life. If you have aging parents, grandparents, and friends, the following information may give you insight into their lives and encourage you to begin cultivating appropriate and useful behaviors now.

Planning for Social Changes

Retirement marks a major change in the second half of life. As the longevity of Americans has increased, people spend a larger proportion of their lives in retirement: 17 years or more. This has implications for reestablishing important relationships, developing satisfying interests outside work, and saving for an adequate retirement income. People who have well-developed leisure pursuits adjust better to retirement than those with few interests outside work.

Changing Roles and Relationships Changes in social roles are a major feature of middle age. Children become young adults and leave home, putting an end to daily parenting. Parents experiencing this empty-nest syndrome must adapt to changes in their customary responsibilities and personal identities. And although retirement may be a desirable milestone for most people, it may also be viewed as a threat to prestige, purpose, and self-respect—the loss of a valued or customary role—and will probably require a period of adjustment.

Retirement and the end of child rearing also bring about changes in the relationship between marriage part-

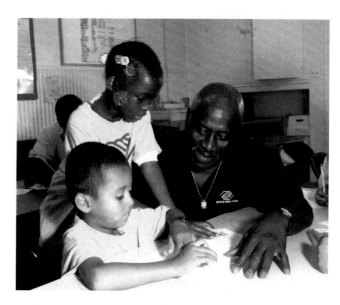

One of the challenges of aging is finding satisfying activities that provide meaningful connections with others. This retired man provides homework assistance and learning activities as part of an afterschool program.

ners. The amount of time a couple spends together will increase and activities will change. Couples may need a period of adjustment, in which they get to know each other as individuals again. Discussing what types of activities each partner enjoys can help couples set up a mutually satisfying routine of shared and independent activities.

Increased Leisure Time Planning ahead for retirement is crucial. What kinds of things do you enjoy doing? How will you spend your days? Although retirement confers the advantages of leisure time and freedom from deadlines, competition, and stress, many people do not know how to enjoy their free time. If you have developed diverse interests, retirement can be a joyful and fulfilling period of your life. It can provide opportunities for expanding your horizons by giving you the chance to try new activities, take classes, and meet new people. Volunteering in your community can enhance self-esteem and allow you to be a contributing member of society (see the box "Help Yourself by Helping Others").

The Economics of Retirement Retirement is usually accompanied by a new economic situation. It may mean a severely restricted budget or possibly even financial disaster if you don't take stock of your finances and plan ahead. Financial planning for retirement should begin early in life. People in their twenties and thirties should estimate how much money they need to support their standard of living, calculate their projected income, and begin a savings program. The earlier people begin such a program, the more money they will have at retirement.

Help Yourself by Helping Others

Mind/Body/Spirit

Choosing to help others—whether as a volunteer for a community organization or through spontaneous acts of kindness—can enhance emotional, social, spiritual, and physical wellness. Surveys and studies indicate that the sense of purpose and service and the feelings of generosity and kindness that go with helping others may be as important a consideration for wellness as good nutrition and regular exercise. Older adults who volunteer have higher levels of emotional and social wellness and lower rates of death.

In a national survey of volunteers from all fields, helpers reported the following benefits:

- Helper's high—physical and emotional sensations such as sudden warmth, a surge of energy, and a feeling of euphoria that occur immediately after helping

- Feelings of increased self-worth, calm, and relaxation

- A perception of greater physical health

- Fewer colds and headaches, improved eating and sleeping habits, and some relief from the pain of chronic diseases such as asthma and arthritis

Just how might helping benefit the health of the helper? By helping others, we may relieve our own distress and guilt over their problems. We focus on things other than our own problems, and we get a special kind of attention from the people we help. Helping others can be effective at banishing a bad mood or a case of the blues. Helping may block physical pain because we can pay attention to only a limited number of things at a given time. Helping others can also expand our perspective and enhance our appreciation for our own lives. Helping may benefit physical health by providing a temporary boost to the immune system and by combating stress and hostile feelings linked to the development of chronic diseases.

Helping others doesn't require a huge time commitment or a change of career. To get the most out of helping, keep the following guidelines in mind:

- *Make contact.* Choose an activity that involves personal contact.

- *Help as often as possible.* If your schedule allows, volunteer at least once a week. But, as with many parts of a wellness lifestyle, any amount of time helping is better than none.

- *Make helping voluntary.* Voluntary helping has positive results, whereas obligatory helping situations can actually increase stress.

- *Volunteer with others.* Working with a group enables you to form bonds with other helpers who can support your interests and efforts. Studies have found that the health benefits of volunteering are strongest for people who otherwise have low levels of social interaction.

- *Focus on the process, not the outcome.* We can't always measure or know the results of our actions.

- *Practice random acts of kindness.* Smile, let people go ahead of you in line, pick up litter, and so on.

- *Adopt a pet.* Several studies suggest that pet owners enjoy better health, perhaps by feeling needed or by having a source of unconditional love and affection.

- *Avoid burnout.* Recognize your own limits, pace yourself, and try not to feel guilty or discouraged. Take pride in being a volunteer or caregiver.

You can experience "helper's high" and the other personal rewards of volunteering as soon as you begin helping others. In addition to the benefits for you, volunteering has the added bonus of having a positive impact on the wellness of others. It fosters a sense of community and can provide some practical help for many of the problems facing our society today.

SOURCES: Shmotkin, D., T. Blumstein, and B. Modan. 2003. Beyond keeping active: Concomitants of being a volunteer in old-old age. *Psychological Aging* 18(3): 602–607; adapted with permission from Sobel, D. S., M.D., and R. Ornstein, Ph.D. 1996. *The Healthy Mind, Healthy Body Handbook.* Los Altos, Calif.: DRx.

Financial planning for retirement is especially critical for women. American women are much less likely than men to be covered by pension plans, reflecting the fact that many women have lower-paying jobs or work part-time during their childbearing years. They tend to have less money vested in other types of retirement plans as well. Although the gap is narrowing, women currently outlive men by about 5–6 years, and they are more likely to develop chronic conditions that impair their daily activities later in life. The net result of these factors is that older women are almost twice as likely as older men to live in poverty. Women should investigate their retirement plans and take charge of their finances to be sure they will be provided for as they get older.

Adapting to Physical Changes

As described earlier in the chapter, there are many things a person can do to avoid or minimize the effects of the physical changes associated with aging. However, some changes in physical functioning are inevitable, and successful aging involves anticipating and accommodating these changes.

Decreased energy and changes in health mean that older people have to develop priorities for how to use their energy. Rather than curtailing activities to conserve energy, they need to learn how to generate energy. This usually involves saying yes to enjoyable activities and paying close attention to the need for rest and sleep.

Adapting, rather than giving up, favorite activities may be the best strategy for dealing with physical limitations. For example, if **arthritis** interferes with playing an instrument, a person can continue to enjoy music by attending concerts or checking out music from the local library.

Hearing Loss The loss of hearing is a common physical change that can have a particularly strong effect on the lives of older adults. Hearing loss affects a person's ability to interact with others and can lead to a sense of isolation and depression. If someone you know complains that words are difficult to understand, that another person's speech sounds slurred or mumbled, or that people are not speaking loudly enough, that person may have suffered some hearing loss. You may also notice that the person sets the volume of a radio or TV very high.

Hearing loss should be assessed and treated by a health care professional; in some cases, hearing can be completely restored by dealing with the underlying cause of hearing loss. In other cases, hearing aids may be prescribed.

Vision Changes Vision usually declines with age. For some individuals this can be traced to conditions such as glaucoma or **age-related macular degeneration (AMD)** that can be treated medically. For others, the effects of a decline in vision can be managed using strategies to make the most of remaining vision.

Glaucoma is caused by increased pressure within the eye due to built-up fluid. The optic nerve can be damaged by this increased pressure, resulting in a loss of side vision and, if untreated, blindness. Medication can relieve the pressure by decreasing the amount of fluid produced or by helping it drain more efficiently. Laser and conventional surgery are other options. Of the 3 million Americans with glaucoma, only half know that they have it; others lose the opportunity to control it and preserve their sight. People over 60, African Americans over 40, and anyone with a family history of glaucoma are at risk.

AMD is a slow disintegration of the macula, the tissue at the center of the retina where fine, straight-ahead detail is distinguished. Losing this vision makes it difficult to read, drive, or perform other close-up activities. It is not known what causes the 85% of AMD cases known as "dry," in which usually one eye is gradually affected. About 15% of AMD cases are the more serious "wet" type, in which new blood vessels in the eye grow toward the macula and leak fluid, quickly causing serious damage. Risk factors for AMD are age, gender (women may be at higher risk than men), smoking, elevated cholesterol levels, and family history. Although dry AMD cannot be treated, it progresses so gradually that many people can adjust to it. Some cases of wet AMD can be treated with laser surgery. Both glaucoma and AMD can be detected with regular screening.

Vision can also be affected by conditions that are products of aging. By the time they reach their forties, many people have developed **presbyopia**, a gradual decline in the ability to focus on objects close to them. This occurs because the lens of the eye no longer expands and contracts as readily. **Cataracts**, a clouding of the lens caused by lifelong oxidation damage (a by-product of normal body chemistry), may dim vision by the sixties.

Arthritis Half of people over age 65 have some form of arthritis. This degenerative disease causes joint inflammation leading to chronic pain, swelling, and loss of mobility. Its warning signs include swelling, pain, redness, warmth, tenderness, changes in joint mobility, early-morning stiffness, and unexplained weight loss, fever, or weakness in combination with joint pain.

There are more than 100 different types of arthritis; osteoarthritis (OA) is by far the most common. (Rheumatoid arthritis and lupus, both autoimmune disorders that affect the joints, are described in Chapter 17.) In a person with OA, the cartilage that caps the bones in joints wears away, forming sharp spurs (Figure 19-2). It most often affects the hands and weight-bearing joints of the body—knees, ankles, and hips. OA is second only to heart disease in disabling people so that they cannot work; 74% of those it affects are women.

Strategies for reducing the risk of arthritis and, for those who already have OA, for managing it include exercise, weight management, and avoidance of heavy or repetitive muscle use. Exercise lubricates joints and strengthens the muscles around them, protecting them from further damage. Swimming, walking, and tai chi are good low-impact exercises; knitting and crocheting are excellent ways to exercise the hands. Maintaining an appropriate weight is important to avoid placing stress on the hips, knees, and ankles. Assistive devices such as kitchen utensils and repair tools with large handles can help people with arthritis maintain independence.

It is also important to visit a physician as soon as arthritis symptoms occur so appropriate treatment can be started to reduce pain and swelling, keep joints moving safely, and prevent further joint damage. If joints are severely damaged and activity is limited, surgery to repair or replace joints may be considered, but medication is usually the first treatment. Many people with OA take medication to relieve inflammation and reduce pain. Because arthritis is a chronic condition, researchers are trying to find medications that are effective and safe when used over the long term. Nonsteroidal anti-inflammatory drugs like ibuprofen can help but can irritate the digestive tract; prescription drugs that relieve pain without damaging the stomach have been found to have other dangerous side effects (see Chapter 21). Acetaminophen can also reduce pain without upsetting the stomach, but exceeding the recommended dosage can cause liver damage. Balancing the benefits and risks of medications is an important consideration for people at any age. Acupuncture is being studied as an addition to conventional therapy, and

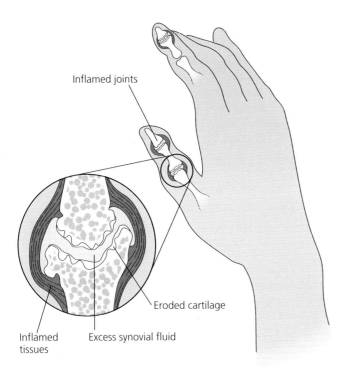

Figure 19-2 Osteoarthritis. When cartilage wears away within a joint, sharp spurs form and the amount of fluid increases, causing pain and swelling.   SOURCE: Clayman, C., ed. 1995. The Human Body: An Illustrated Guide to Its Structure, Function, and Disorders. New York: DK.

Inflamed joints

Eroded cartilage

Excess synovial fluid

Inflamed tissues

preliminary studies have shown that it helps reduce pain and improve function in the affected joints.

Some studies suggest that two dietary supplements, glucosamine and chondroitin sulfate, do have a mild anti-inflammatory effect that eases some OA symptoms. It is not clear if the two compounds need to be taken together to be effective or even exactly how they work. Glucosamine is extracted from crustacean shells and thus should not be taken by people with shellfish allergies; neither supplement should be taken in combination with blood-thinning medications. A health care provider should be consulted before either compound is taken.

Menopause   A special concern for women is the natural process of menopause and the changes accompanying it. During their forties or fifties, women's ovaries gradually stop functioning; estrogen levels drop, and eventually menstruation ceases. Several years before a woman stops menstruating, her periods usually become irregular. Hot flashes, vaginal dryness, sleep disturbances, and mood swings may start around this time.

During the 1990s, about one-third of menopausal women used hormone replacement therapy (HRT) to alleviate the symptoms of menopause and possibly prevent chronic diseases such as CVD and osteoporosis. Many experts believed that HRT would substantially reduce a woman's risk for CVD because estrogen has favorable effects on blood lipids, clotting, and other factors known to influence cardiovascular health. However, several recent large, well-designed studies have shown that HRT may actually increase a woman's risk for CVD, as well as her risk for breast cancer, gallbladder disease, and blood clots. The risks are slight but significant, and experts now recommend that women use HRT only for the control of severe menopausal symptoms and for as brief a time as possible. HRT has been shown to significantly reduce the risk of fractures and to lower the risk of colon cancer. Researchers are studying variations in the timing, duration, and composition of HRT to see if these changes will improve its effects on health. The bottom line is that decisions about HRT may be difficult and are best made by taking into account an individual woman's overall health.

As described in earlier chapters, drugs called selective estrogen-receptor modulators (SERMs) mimic estrogen's effects on some body tissues while blocking its effects on others. Researchers hope to develop SERMs that provide all estrogen's beneficial effects without the risks associated with HRT. Raloxifene (Evista), for example, protects bone density and improves cholesterol levels; however, it does increase the occurrence of hot flashes. Some antidepressants and blood pressure medications may reduce hot flashes, and some dietary supplements are also being investigated for their potential to ease the effects of menopause. Phytoestrogens, plant-based substances similar to estrogen, are found as isoflavones in soy protein and as lignans in whole grains and some fruits and vegetables. They may provide the protective effects of estrogen without its drawbacks. Black cohosh and vitamin E are also being studied.

Lifestyle strategies to reduce menopause-related problems include many of the healthy habits discussed throughout the text: stop smoking, exercise, eat a healthy diet, lose excess weight, and perform relaxation techniques regularly.

Osteoporosis   As described in Chapter 12, **osteoporosis** is a condition in which bones become dangerously thin and fragile over time. Fractures are the most

Terms

arthritis Inflammation of a joint or joints, causing pain and swelling.

age-related macular degeneration (AMD) A deterioration of the macula (the central area of the retina) leading to blurred vision and sensitivity to glare; some cases can lead to blindness.

presbyopia The inability of the eyes to focus sharply on nearby objects, caused by a loss of elasticity of the lens that occurs with advancing age.

cataracts Opacity of the lens of the eye that impairs vision and can cause blindness.

osteoporosis The loss of bone density, causing bones to become weak, porous, and more prone to fractures.

serious consequence of osteoporosis; up to 20% of all people who suffer a hip fracture die within a year. Other problems associated with osteoporosis are loss of height and a stooped posture due to vertebral fractures, severe back and hip pain, and breathing problems caused by changes in the shape of the skeleton.

Women are at greater risk than men for osteoporosis because they have 10–25% less bone in their skeleton. As they lose bone mass with age, women's bones become dangerously thin sooner than men's bones (although more men will probably develop osteoporosis in the future as they live into their eighties and nineties). Bone loss accelerates in women during the first 5–10 years after the onset of menopause because of the drop in estrogen production. (Estrogen improves calcium absorption and reduces the amount of calcium the body excretes.) Black women have higher bone density and fewer fractures than white or Asian women. Other risk factors include a family history of osteoporosis, early menopause (before age 45), abnormal or irregular menstruation, a history of anorexia, and a thin, small frame. Thyroid medication, corticosteroid drugs for arthritis or asthma, and long-term use of the contraceptive Depo-Provera can also have a negative effect on bone mass.

Preventing osteoporosis requires building as much bone as possible during your young years and then maintaining it as you age. Diet and exercise play key roles; see Chapter 12 for recommendations for calcium, vitamin D, and vitamin K intake. Weight-bearing aerobic activities must be performed regularly throughout life to have lasting effects. Strength training improves bone density, muscle mass, strength, and balance, protecting against both bone loss and falls, a major cause of fractures. Even for people in their seventies, low-intensity strength training has been shown to improve bone density.

Two other lifelong strategies for reducing the effects of osteoporosis are avoiding tobacco use and managing depression and stress. Smoking reduces the body's estrogen levels and is linked to earlier menopause and more rapid postmenopausal bone loss. Some women with depression experience significant bone loss. Researchers have not identified the reason, but it may be linked to increases in the stress hormone cortisol.

Bone mineral density testing can be used to gauge an individual's risk of fracture and help determine if any treatment is needed. It is recommended for all women over age 65 and for younger postmenopausal women who have a fracture or one or more risk factors. Below-normal bone density may be classified as *osteopenia,* which is usually treated with exercise and nutrition. A greater loss of bone mass is classified as full-blown osteoporosis and is often treated with medications. Possible drug treatments include bisphosphonates such as alendronate (Fosamax), SERMS such as raloxifene (Evista), calcitonin (Miacalcin), HRT, and injections of teriparatide (Forteo), a compound derived from parathyroid hormone.

Handling Psychological and Mental Changes

Many people associate old age with forgetfulness, and slowly losing one's memory was once considered an inevitable part of growing old. However, we now know that most older adults in good health remain mentally alert and retain their full capacity to learn and remember new information. Slight confusion and occasional forgetfulness may indicate only a temporary information overload, fatigue, or response to medications. Many people become smarter as they become older and more experienced.

Dementia Severe and significant brain deterioration in elderly individuals, termed **dementia,** affects about 7% of people under age 80 (the incidence rises sharply for people in their eighties and nineties). Early symptoms include slight disturbances in a person's ability to grasp the situation he or she is in. As dementia progresses, memory failure becomes apparent, and the person may forget conversations, the events of the day, or how to perform simple tasks. It is important to have any symptoms evaluated by a health care professional because some of the over 50 known causes of dementia are treatable (for example, depression, dehydration, malnutrition, vitamin B-12 deficiency, alcoholism, misuse of medications, and thyroid gland problems). The two most common forms of dementia among older people—**Alzheimer's disease** and multi-infarct dementia—are irreversible. Alzheimer's disease is characterized by changes in brain nerve cells. Multi-infarct dementia results from a series of small strokes or changes in the brain's blood supply that destroy brain tissue. Even for the incurable forms of dementia, however, appropriate treatment may greatly improve an affected person's quality of life (see the box "Alzheimer's Disease").

Repeatedly telling stories about the past—something older people often do—doesn't necessarily indicate dementia. Reminiscence is a normal part of development and allows an older person to integrate life by making past events meaningful in the present. Reminiscing can be of great significance to members of the younger generations because it is a rich source of social, cultural, and family history.

Terms

V w

dementia Deterioration of mental functioning (including memory, concentration, and judgment) resulting from a brain disorder; often accompanied by emotional disturbances and personality changes.

Alzheimer's disease A disease characterized by a progressive loss of mental functioning (dementia), caused by a degeneration of brain cells.

In Focus

Alzheimer's Disease

Alzheimer's disease (AD) is a fatal brain disorder that causes physical and chemical changes in the brain. As the brain's nerve cells are destroyed, the system that produces the neurotransmitter acetylcholine breaks down, and communication among parts of the brain deteriorates. Autopsies reveal that the interiors of the affected neurons are filled with clusters of proteins known as tangles: the spaces between the neurons are filled with protein deposits called amyloid plaques. More than 4 million Americans have Alzheimer's disease, and that number is expected to quadruple in the next 50 years, as more people live into their eighties and nineties. AD usually occurs in people over 60 but can occur in people as young as 40.

Symptoms

The first symptoms of AD are forgetfulness and inability to concentrate. A person may have difficulty performing familiar tasks at home and work and have problems with abstract thinking. As the disease progresses, people experience severe memory loss, especially for recent events. They may vividly remember events from their childhood but be unable to remember the time of day or their location. Depression and anxiety are also common. In the later stages, people with AD are disoriented and may even hallucinate; some experience personality changes—becoming very aggressive or very docile. Eventually, they lose control of physical functioning and are completely dependent on caregivers. On average, a person will survive 8 years after the development of the first symptoms.

Causes

Scientists do not yet know what causes Alzheimer's disease. Age is the main risk factor, although about 10% of cases seem tied to inherited gene mutations. Inherited familial AD generally strikes people before age 65, while the more common late-onset AD occurs in people 65 and older. Some evidence suggests that many of the same factors that affect heart disease risk also apply to AD. High blood pressure, excess body weight, inactivity, smoking, unhealthy cholesterol levels, high homocysteine and CRP levels, metabolic syndrome, diabetes, depression, stress, and diets high in saturated and trans fats all seem to be associated with increased risk for AD.

People who regularly take nonsteroidal anti-inflammatory drugs (NSAIDs) like ibuprofen (often to control arthritis) and people who regularly consume fish rich in omega-3 fatty acids appear to have lower rates of AD, indicating a possible protective effect of substances that reduce inflammation. Some studies indicate that vitamin E and other antioxidants may reduce risk for AD or slow the progress of the disease, suggesting that oxidative stress caused by free radicals may also play a role.

Diagnosis and Treatment

Currently, the only certain way to diagnose AD is to examine brain tissue during an autopsy. In most cases, physicians use a combination of medical history, neurological and psychological tests, physical exams, blood and urine tests, and a brain-imaging scan. Good early results have also been seen using a test that measures levels of a specific protein in spinal fluid. A behavior diary can also aid in diagnosis.

For people with mild to moderate AD, there are several drugs that provide modest improvements in memory. Several medications help maintain cognitive function by inhibiting the breakdown of the neurotransmitter acetylcholine but do not alter the course of the disease. These so-called cholinesterase inhibitors include Aricept (donepezil), Cognex (tacrine), Exelon (rivastigmine), and Reminyl (galantamine). People with AD may also be prescribed antidepressant or antianxiety medications. As scientists gain more insight into Alzheimer's disease, they hope to develop more effective treatments that will ease the burden of AD for both families and society.

Grief Another psychological and emotional challenge of aging is dealing with grief and mourning. Aging is associated with loss—the loss of friends, peers, physical appearance, possessions, and health. Grief is the process of getting through the pain of loss, and it can be one of the loneliest and most intense times in a person's life. It can take a year or two or more to completely come to terms with the loss of a loved one. (See Chapter 20 for more information about responses to loss and how to support a grieving person.)

Unresolved grief can have serious physical and psychological or emotional health consequences and may require professional help. Signs of unresolved grief include hostility toward people connected with the death (physicians or nurses, for example), talking about the death as if it occurred yesterday, and unrealistic or harmful behavior (such as giving away all of one's own belongings). Many people become depressed after the loss of a loved one or when confronted with retirement or a chronic illness. But after a period of grieving, people are generally able to resume their lives.

Depression Unresolved grief can lead to depression, a common problem in older adults (see Chapter 3). If you notice the signs of depression in yourself or someone you know, consult a mental health professional. A marked loss of interest in usually pleasurable activities, decreased appetite, insomnia, fatigue, and feelings of worthlessness are signs of depression. Listen carefully when an older friend or relative complains about being depressed; it may be a request for help. Suicide rates are relatively high among the elderly, and depression should be taken seriously (see the box "Suicide Among Older Men" on p. 592).

It is a mistake to think that a depressed person will snap out of it or that people are too old to be helped. Both professional treatment and support groups can help people deal successfully with major life changes, such as

Suicide Among Older Men

One group of Americans is more than twice as likely to commit suicide than any other. From mass media accounts, you might imagine this group to be adolescents; however, suicide is much more common among the elderly—especially white males over age 65. Among men over age 65, the rate of suicide among whites is more than double that of any other group. Women and minorities of all ages have much lower rates of suicide than older white men.

Why is this so? One explanation is that because white men generally have greater power and status in our society, aging and retirement represent a relatively greater loss for them. Women, more accustomed to lesser status, are not as threatened by the loss of economic and social power. Another theory is that white men tend to have weaker social ties than women or than men from other cultural groups and as they retire their increasing social isolation leads to depression and suicide. Indeed, depression is probably the single most significant factor associated with suicidal behavior in older adults. Men who commit suicide are more likely to have a physical illness and be widowed or divorced.

Why are rates for other groups lower? In general, women are more likely than men to attempt suicide, but men are more likely to succeed, due in large part to their choice of more lethal methods. Some cultural groups, particularly Latinos and African Americans, afford greater respect and status to older people, who are valued for their wisdom and experience. Cultural groups that emphasize family and social ties also seem to have lower rates of suicide. See Chapter 3 for more on risk and protective factors for suicide.

The high rate of suicide among the elderly often fails to receive much attention. As a society, we are less disturbed about the deaths of older Americans from any cause than the deaths of younger people. What does it say about our society if, after a lifetime of contributions, an older person finds himself or herself in a position where suicide seems to be the best option?

---

retirement, moving, health problems, or loss of a spouse. If someone refuses help, be reassuring and emphasize that treatment helps make people feel better; in some cases, a mental health professional can make a home visit.

One of the most important ways of dealing with the changes associated with aging is to adopt a flexible attitude toward whatever life brings you. Self-acceptance can help make the later years more meaningful and enjoyable. Accepting limitations, having an optimistic outlook, and having a sense of humor are tools that can help you cope with all of life's changes.

AGING AND LIFE EXPECTANCY

Life expectancy is the average length of time we can expect to live. It is calculated by averaging mortality statistics, the ages at death of a group of people over a certain period. Current life expectancy is 77.3 years for someone born in 2002, but those who reach age 65 can expect to live even longer—18 more years or longer—because they have already survived hazards to life in the younger years. Women have a longer life expectancy than men (see the box "Why Do Women Live Longer?"). Life expectancy also varies among ethnic groups; reasons for these differences include socioeconomic, genetic, and lifestyle factors.

Terms

life expectancy The average length of time a person is expected to live.

life span A theoretically projected length of life based on the maximum potential of the human body in the best environment.

Factors Influencing Life Expectancy

Life expectancy in the United States increased dramatically in the twentieth century, as described in Chapter 1. This does not mean that every American lives longer now than in 1900; rather, far fewer people die young now, because childhood and infectious diseases are better controlled and diet and sanitation are much improved. Only 30% of people born in 1900 would live to age 70; of those born in 2004, closer to 77% can expect to live that long.

How long can humans expect to live in the best of circumstances? It now seems possible that our maximum potential **life span** is 100–120 years. (A woman in France died in 1997 at the age of 122 years, 164 days.) Failure to achieve that span in good health results to some degree from destructive environmental and behavioral factors—factors over which we can exert considerable control. Long life does not necessarily mean a longer period of disability, either. People often live longer because they have been well longer. A healthy, productive old age is very often an extension of a healthy, productive middle age. However, behavior changes cannot extend the maximum human life span, which seems to be built into our genes.

Theories on Aging

Throughout history, people have searched in vain for ways to preserve youth. Now scientists are studying the aging process and looking for ways to help people live longer and maintain much of their youthful vigor. What causes the eventual breakdown of the body? No existing theory on aging accommodates all the facts. Perhaps aging is caused by a variety of different processes and

Gender Matters

Why Do Women Live Longer?

Women live longer than men in most countries around the world, even in places where maternal mortality rates are high. In the United States, women on average can expect to live about 5 years longer than men (see table). Worldwide, among people over age 100, women outnumber men about 9 to 1.

The reason for the gender gap in life expectancy is not entirely understood but may be influenced by biological, social, and lifestyle factors. Estrogen production and other factors during a woman's younger years may protect her from early heart disease and from age-related declines in the pumping power of the heart. Women may have lower rates of stress-related illnesses because they cope more positively with stress by seeking social support.

The news for women is not all good, however, because not all their extra years are likely to be healthy years. They are more likely than men to suffer from chronic conditions like arthritis and osteoporosis. Women's longer life spans, combined with the facts that men tend to marry younger women and that widowed men remarry more often than widowed women, means there are many more sin-

gle older women than men. Older men are more likely to live in family settings, whereas older women are more likely to live alone. Older women are also less likely to be covered by a pension or to have retirement savings, so they are more likely to be poor.

Increased male mortality can be traced in part to higher rates of behaviors such as smoking and alcohol and drug abuse. Testosterone production may be partly responsible in that it is linked to aggressive and risky behavior and to unhealthy cholesterol levels. Men have much higher rates of death than women from car crashes and other unintentional injuries, firearm-related deaths, homicide, suicide, AIDS, and early heart attack. Gender roles that promote risky behavior among young men are a factor in many of these causes of death. Indeed, among people who have made it to age 65, the gender longevity gap is smaller.

Social and behavioral factors may be more important than physiological causes in explaining the gender gap; for example, among the Amish, a religious sect that has strict rules against smoking and drinking, men usually live as long as women. This suggests that the longevity

gap could be substantially narrowed through lifestyle changes.

Life Expectancy

Year	Men	Women
At birth		
1900	46.3	48.3
1950	65.6	71.1
2000	74.3	79.7
2050*	79.7	84.3
At age 65		
1900	11.5	12.2
1950	12.8	15.0
2000	16.2	19.3
2050*	20.3	22.4

*projected

SOURCES: U.S. Census Bureau. 2005. *We the People: Women and Men in the United States.* Washington, D.C.: U.S. Census Bureau; Aging: The stronger sex. 2005. *Economist,* January 13; National Centers for Health Statistics. 2004. *Health, United States, 2004.* Hyattsville, Md.: National Center for Health Statistics; World Health Organization. 2003. *Gender, Health, and Aging.* Geneva: World Health Organization.

---

affected by a multitude of factors, both environmental and biological.

A cellular theory of aging based on the genetic makeup of cells suggests that a cell contains aging genes that specify the exact number of times the cell can duplicate itself. The limiting number varies from species to species: The maximum life span for fruit flies is about 100 days, for dogs 25–30 years, for humans about 110 years, and for giant tortoises about 180 years.

Another cellular theory is that the body generates free radicals, which undermine the integrity of cell membranes, damage DNA, and inactivate many enzymes and proteins required for normal cellular functioning. Environmental pollution also promotes free radical activity, but a diet rich in antioxidants can reduce it (see Chapter 12). As scientists map the human genome, a number of genes are being identified as playing a role in the aging process.

A theory of aging involving the immune system suggests that the body begins to make errors in protein synthesis, producing proteins that the immune system cannot recognize. The immune system then attacks them as it would any foreign substance, destroying cells and

impairing body functions (see Chapter 17). Also, the immune system itself may weaken as we age, producing fewer antibodies to fight disease. Researchers are testing drugs that would reinforce faltering immune systems.

A theory of aging that focuses on metabolic function helps explain the immobility seen in old age. Connective tissue all over the body is given structural support by fibers of a class of proteins called collagen. Collagen becomes stiffer and chemically immobilized with age. This is because by-products of metabolism, called cross-links, form between parallel collagen fibers, making it impossible for the two fibers to slip past each other or stretch. Lowering the metabolic rate by not overeating has been shown to reduce age-related diseases such as diabetes.

LIFE IN AN AGING AMERICA

As life expectancy increases, a larger proportion of the population will be in their later years. This change will necessitate new government policies and changes in our general attitudes toward older adults.

America's Aging Minority

People over 65 are a large minority in the American population—over 35 million people, about 13% of the total population in 2000 (Figure 19-3). As birth rates drop, the percentage increases dramatically. Many older people are happy, healthy, and self-sufficient. Changes that come with age, including negative ones, normally occur so gradually that most people adapt, some even gracefully.

Today the status of older adults is improving more than ever before. The enormous increase in the over-55 population is markedly affecting our stereotypes of what it means to grow old. The misfortunes associated with aging—frailty, forgetfulness, poor health, isolation—occur in fewer people in their sixties and seventies and are shifting instead to burden the very old, those over 85.

The "younger" elderly who are in good physical and psychological health are gaining status in our society; politicians are listening to them, and advertisers have targeted them as a valuable market. In general, today's older adults are better off than they have ever been in the past. They have more money than they did 20 years ago. The poverty rate of the elderly has dropped from 28.5% to 10% since the 1960s, largely from the effects of Social Security payments and health care benefits from Medicare.

About 81% of older Americans own their homes. Their living expenses are lower after retirement because they no longer support children and have fewer work-related expenses; they consume and buy less food. They are more likely to continue practicing their expertise for years after retirement: Thousands of retired consultants, teachers, technicians, and craftspeople work until their middle and late seventies. They receive greater amounts of assistance, such as Medicare, pay proportionately lower taxes, and have greater net worth from lifetime savings.

As the aging population increases proportionately, however, the number of older people who are ill and dependent rises. Health care remains the largest expense for older adults. On average, they visit a physician 10–12 times a year and are hospitalized more frequently and require twice as many prescription drugs as the general population. Tens of thousands of older Americans live in poverty, particularly minorities and women living alone. These elderly—poverty-stricken, isolated, lonely—are just as ignored as they ever were, and their numbers are increasing.

Retirement finds many older people with their incomes reduced to subsistence levels. This is especially true of the very old and women. The majority of older Americans live with fixed sources of income, such as pensions, that are eroded by inflation. Expenses tend to increase more rapidly, especially those due to circumstances over which people have little or no control, such as deteriorating health. Many Americans rely on Social Security payments as their only source of income; they are not covered by other types of retirement plans. **Social Security** was intended to serve as a supplement to personal

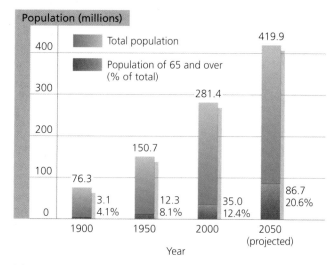

(a) Population growth over age 65 as a proportion of the total population.

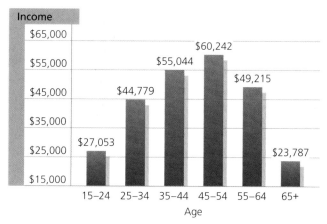

(b) Median household income by age of the household head.

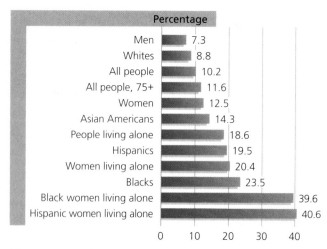

(c) Percentages of groups over age 65 below the poverty level.

Figure 19-3 A statistical look at older Americans. SOURCE: U.S. Bureau of the Census. U.S. Administration on Aging.

savings and private pensions, not as a sole source of income. It is vital that people plan early for an adequate retirement income.

Family and Community Resources for Older Adults

With help from friends, family members, and community services, people in their later years can remain active and independent. About 66% of noninstitutionalized older Americans live with a spouse or other family member; the other 34% live alone or with a nonrelative. Overall, only 4% live in nursing homes or other institutional settings at any point in time, but among those over age 85, about 20% live in a nursing home.

Family Involvement in Caregiving
Most families do not abandon their aging relatives when they need help. Studies show that in about three out of four cases, a grown daughter or daughter-in-law assumes a caregiving role for elderly relatives. This may mean bringing them into the home, helping them remain in their own homes, or arranging for alternative housing. With more parents living into their eighties and with fewer children per family, many people, especially women, will face the dilemma of how best to care for an aging relative. Recent surveys indicate that the average woman will spend about 17 years raising children and 18 years caring for an aging relative.

Caregiving can be rewarding, but it is also hard work. If the experience is stressful and long-term, family members may become emotionally exhausted. Caregivers should use available community services and consider their own needs for relaxation and relief from caregiving duties. Corporations are increasingly responsive to the needs of their employees who are family caregivers by providing services such as referrals, flexible schedules and leaves, and on-site adult care. Professional health care advice is another critical part of successful home care. An aging relative who is mentally impaired by Alzheimer's disease or another form of dementia poses special challenges for caregivers (see the box "Communication and Care for the Older Adults in Your Life" on p. 596).

The best thing a family can do to prepare for the task of caring for aging parents is to talk frankly about the future. What does everyone expect will happen? What living and caring options are available, and which ones do family members prefer? What community resources are available? Planning ahead can reduce the stress on everyone involved and help ease difficult transitions.

Other Living and Care Options
If living together is not possible for aging parents and adult children, other living and care options are available. There are agencies that specialize in recruiting and matching like-minded individuals for shared living situations. Home-sharing, as this is called, offers older adults who are in fairly good health the opportunity for new relationships, either with peers or with a younger family. Intergenerational homesharing may relieve elders of transportation problems and demanding physical tasks, which can be taken care of by younger household members. Conversely, elders in good health can help busy, working families with child care and household chores.

Retirement communities are an option for individuals in good health and with a good income who want to maintain home ownership. Other types of facilities are available for people who need more assistance with daily living (see the box "Choosing a Place to Live" on p. 597).

Community Resources
Different kinds of community resources are available to help older adults remain active and in their own homes. The key to success is matching services with the needs of the individual person. Typical services include the following:

- *Senior citizens' centers or adult day-care centers,* which may provide meals, social activities, and health care services for those unable to be alone during the day
- *Homemaker services,* which may include light housekeeping, cooking, running errands, shopping, and providing escort service
- *Visiting nurses,* who provide some basic health care services
- *Household services,* which may include basic household repairs and seasonal work
- *Friendly visitor or daily telephone reassurance services,* which provide daily contacts for older people who live alone and may feel isolated
- *Home food delivery services,* which provide daily meals to homebound people
- *Adult day hospital care,* which provides day care plus physical therapy and treatment for chronic illnesses
- *Low-cost legal aid,* which can help in managing finances and health care
- *Transportation,* which includes buses with special senior rates for visits to doctors' offices, hospitals, or grocery stores
- *Case management,* which helps seniors navigate through complex and confusing health care services

Services can usually be located by looking in the phone book under local government agencies or in the yellow pages under Senior Citizens' Services.

Term

Social Security A government program that provides financial assistance to people who are unemployed, disabled, or retired (and over a certain age); financed through taxes on business and workers.

Take Charge

At some point in your life, you are likely to find yourself caring for an aging relative. You may be sharing a residence, providing assistance via long-distance caregiving, or just trying to stay in close touch. Key considerations include keeping an older adult connected with others and physically safe. The following are just a few suggestions for communicating with, and caring for, older adults with specific health concerns.

Hearing Loss

Don't leave people suffering from hearing loss out of the conversation—including them not only prevents them from becoming socially and emotionally isolated but can also improve their ability to communicate. Speak more slowly and at a slightly louder level, and lower the pitch of your voice. Talking too loudly raises your pitch and distorts your speech, making it more difficult for the other person to follow visual cues. Stand or sit in good light that allows your lip movements, facial expressions, and gestures to be seen clearly. Reduce background noise as much as possible.

Vision Loss

Older people and those with vision loss need more light, so increase the number and strength of light sources and paint rooms in a lighter color. Improving light in dark areas like stairwells can reduce falls and injuries from the slower light-to-dark accommodation that occurs with age. Wearing a hat and sunglasses outside helps reduce glare. If visual losses are more severe, large-print books, talking clocks, magnifying mirrors, large numbers on telephone keypads, and a variety of electronic devices are available to help seniors safely maintain independence.

Not every person with low vision needs assistance, so take care to help people preserve their independence. For example, when walking with a person with vision problems, ask if she needs help. If she does, offer your arm (don't take her arm unasked) and walk a half step in front of her. Warn quietly as you approach steps, ramps, curbs, and corridors.

For additional information and resources, contact your state association for the blind or visually impaired.

Dementia

In some ways, caring for someone with dementia can be like caring for a small child—safety is a key concern, and the person may need help or supervision for many of the tasks of daily living such as dressing, bathing, and eating. Hazardous objects should be placed out of reach, and medication use should be supervised. A structured routine for daily tasks can be helpful; for example, lay clothes out in sequence to help with dressing. The person may need to wear an identification bracelet in case she or he wanders away from the residence.

Allow the person as much independence as possible, and don't take over activities that she or he can do without assistance. Although communication skills are likely to be affected, it is important that the person feel connected with others and, as abilities allow, participate in favorite activities. Caregivers can improve communication by reducing distractions, speaking slowly and calmly, using common words, keeping sentences short, and asking two-choice (either-or) rather than open-ended questions. Don't make corrections; the person can't help making mistakes in memory or cognition, and you will not be able to talk sense into her or him. Reassure and support the person if she or he feels confused, disoriented, frustrated, fearful, lost, or abandoned.

Medication Issues

Problems related to medications are an important issue for older adults and caregivers. Patients, caregivers, physicians, and pharmacists need to work together to help ensure that medications are prescribed and used appropriately. Older adults are more likely to be taking multiple medications, increasing the risk for side effects and drug interactions. Older adults may have problems scheduling multiple doses that may need to occur at specific intervals or times of day; they may also have difficulty remembering to take medications, reading small print on labels, opening bottles, and so on.

Caregivers can help older adults take medications on schedule. They can also be alert for side effects, which may be mistaken for signs of aging or dementia. For example, medications can cause drowsiness, confusion, depression, tremors, muscle weakness, loss of appetite, and memory impairment. Any mental or physical change in an older adult should be evaluated as possibly related to medication use.

Caring for the Caregiver

Caregiving is difficult and stressful, and caregivers need help and support. Adult day-care programs and respite care programs can provide important breaks. Call on family and friends for help, and consider joining a support group. See For More Information for a few of the organizations providing information and resources for caregivers.

Transportation Older drivers usually have safe driving records compared with young adults because they tend to be more cautious; however, crashes in the older age group are more likely to be fatal. Many states require special driver's testing for people over age 70 and may restrict some drivers as to the time, area, and distances they may drive. Because of changes in vision or other health problems, some older drivers may be required to give up their license before they feel ready. Elderly people report that the loss of a driver's license, and the loss of independence it brings, is one of the most severe hardships they face.

Critical Consumer

Later in life many older people need help with everyday activities like shopping, cooking, walking, or bathing. Help from family and friends may be all some people need to stay active and healthy in their own homes, while others may choose to move to a place that offers more services. A variety of options are available:

- *Retirement communities* allow maximum independence with very little supervision. They may offer transportation, activities, and other services but do not routinely offer assistance with basic needs.

- *Residential care homes* are licensed to provide services to three or more residents in a smaller environment, typically in a private home. They may provide assistance with medications, bathing, dressing, transportation, daily laundry, daily housekeeping, and meals.

- *Assisted living facilities* allow independence with supervision and are licensed by the state. They provide some meals, housekeeping and laundry, transportation, and activities.

- *Nursing homes* provide 24-hour medical care and rehabilitation for residents, who are mostly very frail or suffer from the later stages of dementia.

Some providers offer all levels of care at one site. These continuing-care communities allow people to move from one level to another as their needs change.

Finding the right place to live takes some investigation. Because the best homes often have a waiting list, plan ahead. Don't wait until your family member is too sick to function. Once you have an initial list of facilities in your area start visiting the homes, keeping the following evaluation points in mind:

- Ask questions about specific facilities. Doctors, friends, relatives, local hospital discharge planners, social workers, and religious organizations can help. The ombudsperson at your state's office of long-term care can let you know if there have been problems in a particular nursing home. Residential care homes and assisted living facilities do not follow the same licensing requirements as nursing homes. Talk to people in the community to find out about these options.

- Contact the places that interest you. Ask basic questions about vacancies, number of residents, cost, and any services of interest to you, such as transportation and meals.

- Visit several places. Talk to the staff, residents, and, if possible, family members of residents. Set up an appointment, but also go unannounced and at different times of the day. Make sure residents are clean, well groomed, involved in activities, and treated with respect.

- Evaluate the facility's financial agreements. Have a lawyer look them over before you sign. Nursing homes may accept Medicare or Medicaid, but most other facilities are private-pay only. Costs can range from $1500 per month to $5500 per month or more.

- Moving is a big change that affects the whole family. Talk about how you feel. Once a family member has moved to a new home, visit often and pay attention to the quality of care. Say something nice when care is good, and speak up when care is poor. If you have trouble resolving a complaint, your local ombudsperson or citizen advocacy groups may be able to help.

Whatever their circumstances, older adults have the same needs as people at any other stage of life, including the need to feel that their lives have meaning. Becoming dependent on others for daily care and transportation is difficult for many people to accept. Most caregivers are motivated by love and responsibility and want to do the best they can for their aging friend or relative. However, some situations can lead to physical or economic abuse. Assistance is available, including respite care for caregivers and legal and protective services for abused elders.

Government Aid and Policies

The federal government helps older Americans through several programs, such as food stamps, housing subsidies, Social Security, Medicare, and Medicaid. Social Security, the life insurance and old-age pension plan, has saved many from destitution, although it is intended not as a sole source of income but as a supplement to other income. Social Security funds have been used to cover other government financial deficits, so the future solvency of the program is uncertain.

Medicare is a major health insurance program for the elderly and the disabled. It has two parts: Part A is financed by part of the payroll (FICA) tax that also pays for Social Security; Part B is financed by monthly premiums paid by people who choose to enroll. Part A helps pay for inpatient hospital care, some inpatient care in a skilled nursing facility, and some types of home and hospice care. Medicare Part B helps pay for physicians' services and other services not covered by Part A.

Medicare pays about 30% of the medical costs of older Americans. It provides basic health care coverage for acute episodes of illness that require skilled professional care; it pays for some preventive services, including an

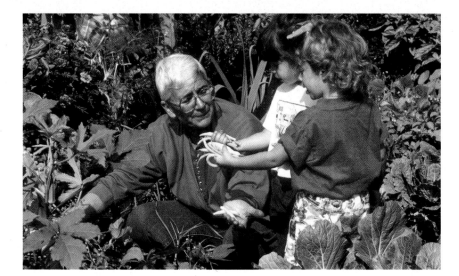

Some individuals defy all preconceived ideas about age and continue to live vigorous and productive lives into their seventies, eighties, and beyond.

initial physical exam, vaccinations, and screenings for CVD, certain cancers, osteoporosis, diabetes, and glaucoma. It does not pay for many office visits, dental care, and dentures. In the past, Medicare did not cover prescription drug costs, but programs involving discount cards and drug benefits are being phased in. Over 1 million older people currently live in nursing homes, but Medicare pays less than 2% of nursing home costs, and private insurers pay less than 1%, creating a tremendous financial burden for nursing home residents and their families. Because of these gaps in coverage, many older people are joining managed health care plans to get more care for their money. See Chapter 21 for more information on insurance options.

When their financial resources are exhausted, people may apply for Medicaid. A 1965 amendment to the Social Security Act, Medicaid provides medical insurance to low-income people of any age. Funded by state and federal contributions, the services vary from state to state but typically include hospital, nursing home and home health care, physician services, and some medical supplies and services. The portion of federal Medicaid spending attributed to the elderly has declined since 1980 from about 37% to about 30%.

A crucial question regarding aid for the elderly is Who will pay for it? The government picks up many of the health care expenses, primarily through Medicare and Medicaid. Total health care expenditures are about 15.7%

of the U.S. gross national product; about one-third of these expenditures go to care for older Americans.

Health care policy planners hope that rising medical costs for older adults will dwindle dramatically through education and prevention. Health care professionals, including **gerontologists** and **geriatricians,** are beginning to practice preventive medicine, just as pediatricians do. They advise older people about how to avoid and, if necessary, how to manage disabilities. They try to instill an ethic of physical and psychological maintenance that will prevent chronic disease and enable older people to live long, healthy, vigorous lives.

Changing the Public's Idea of Aging

Aging people may be one of our least used and least appreciated resources. (For another view, see the box "Multicultural Wisdom About Aging.") How can we use the knowledge and productivity of our growing numbers of older citizens, particularly those now leaving the work force through mandatory early retirement?

To start, we must change our thinking about what aging means. We must learn to judge productivity rather than age. Capacity to function should replace age as a criterion for usefulness. Instead of singling out 65 as a magic number, we could consider ages 50–75 as the third quarter of life. Changes occur around 50 that signal a new era: Children are usually grown and gone, and a person has often achieved a level in career, earnings, and accomplishments that meets his or her ambitions. The upper end of the quarter is determined by the fact that most people today are vigorous, in good health, mentally alert, and capable of making a productive contribution until they are at least in their seventies.

However we define old age, the costs of losing what these people can contribute to our national productivity

Terms

gerontologist One who studies the biological, psychological, and social phenomena associated with aging and old age.

geriatrician A physician specializing in the diseases, disabilities, and care of older adults.

Multicultural Wisdom About Aging

Dimensions of Diversity

The following is excerpted from an article written by Dr. Robert Coles, a professor of psychiatry and medical humanities at Harvard Medical School.

Why are so many Americans afraid of growing old? This question occurred to me often during the three years my wife and I lived in New Mexico and Arizona. Not a day went by when we weren't reminded of how much Native American and Hispanic families value old age. These are cultures that grant dignity and authority to their elders.

One young Hispanic woman described to us her relationship with her parents, both in their seventies, in this way: "When I am wondering what to do about a problem, I turn to my mother or my father. Even if they are not here, I still turn to them. I picture them in my mind and I hear them saying words that make good sense." One day, this woman's father made a show of his humorous and practical good sense before his young grandson. "You know what my son said to me that night when he was going to bed?" the woman asked. "He told me he wished he could be old like his grandpapa!"

To be old is to "last" oneself—to go through ups and downs, to survive bad luck and avoid all sorts of hazards. To be old is to be blessed by fate, by chance and circumstance. Pueblo Indians know that. One Hopi child drew me a picture of an old woman shaking hands with the moon. Then she explained, "When you're old, you're a full moon; you make the night a little less dark." For Hopi children, an older person is a source of encouragement, instruction, inspiration, a part of nature's awesome presence.

For many young people living in other parts of America, old age is regarded not as a major achievement but rather as a last, sad, brief way station. One boy in Boston commented, "It's no fun to be old; it's the worst thing in the world, except to die." To many of us, old age means abandonment, rejection, loneliness, a loss of respect from others, and subsequently a loss of self-respect. This is not the case, though, in Hispanic and Native American cultures. The elders we met in New Mexico and Arizona showed a great deal of self-confidence, and in general they seemed contented with their lives. In their contentment and harmony with nature lies a lesson for all of us.

SOURCE: Adapted from Coles, R. 1989. Full-moon wisdom. *New Choices for the Best Years,* September. Reprinted with permission of Robert Coles, James Agee Professor of Social Ethics, Harvard University.

---

and quality of life are too high. Through their early retirement, we forfeit substantial income tax and Social Security tax revenues on their earnings. Those who retire at 62 start using their Social Security benefits earlier than otherwise.

A far better arrangement would be to make available full-time and part-time volunteer and paid employment. We would benefit by providing retraining programs for both occupational and leisure time activities. Volunteer opportunities, such as preparing recordings for the blind, helping with activities for the disabled, and performing necessary tasks in hospitals, could be expanded. At the same time, we could possibly change both public and private pension programs to make partial retirement possible. In such cases we could allow people to borrow against their Social Security benefits to finance retraining or enrollment in new educational programs.

There can be benefits to aging, but they don't come automatically. They require planning and wise choices earlier in life. One octogenarian, Russell Lee, founder of a medical clinic in California, perceived the advantages of aging as growth: "The limitations imposed by time are compensated by the improved taste, sharper discretion, sounder mental and esthetic judgment, increased sensitivity and compassion, clearer focus—which all contribute to a more certain direction in living. . . . The later years can be the best of life for which the earlier ones were preparation."

Tips for Today

Aging is a natural process that we all face. How we age—gracefully or painfully—is largely an outgrowth of how we live. You can help ensure a high quality of life in your later years by cultivating healthy habits in your earlier years.

Right now you can

- Decide to learn a challenging new skill, such as chess or a foreign language

- Start a list of the books you'd like to read for pleasure and get one of them from the library or bookstore

- Resolve to quit smoking, if you smoke, and to get at least 30 minutes of exercise nearly every day

- Get in the habit of volunteering by contacting a nonprofit group in your community and offering your time and talent; consider a literacy campaign, a soup kitchen, a youth mentoring program, or Habitat for Humanity

- Review your finances, and determine if you are saving as much as possible toward retirement.

SUMMARY

- People who take charge of their health during their youth have greater control over the physical and mental aspects of aging.

- Biological aging takes place over a lifetime, but some of the other changes associated with aging are more abrupt.

- A lifetime of interests and hobbies helps maintain creativity and intelligence.

- Exercise and a healthy diet throughout life enhances physical and psychological health.

- Alcohol abuse is a common but often hidden problem, as is overdependence on medications. Tobacco use not only shortens life but also may cause severe health impairment for many years.

- Regular physical examinations help detect conditions that can shorten life and make old age less healthy.

- Stress increases wear and tear on the body; getting enough sleep, avoiding drugs, and practicing relaxation help reduce stress.

- Retirement can be a fulfilling and enjoyable time of life for those who adjust to their new roles, enjoy participating in a variety of activities, and have planned ahead for financial stability.

- Successful aging involves anticipating and accommodating physical changes and limitations.

- Slight confusion and forgetfulness are not signs of a serious illness; however, severe symptoms may indicate Alzheimer's disease or another form of dementia.

- Resolving grief and mourning and dealing with depression are important tasks for older adults.

- Theories on aging examine the influences of cellular changes, free radicals, inappropriate immune responses, and changes in metabolism.

- Older adults can be role models for the successful integration of life's experiences and the ability to adapt to challenges.

- People over 65 form a large minority in the United States, and their status is improving. But older adults who are ill and dependent—often those who were already poor—experience major social and economic problems.

- Family and community resources can help older adults stay active and independent.

- Government aid to the elderly includes food stamps, housing subsidies, Social Security, Medicare, and Medicaid.

Take Action

1. **Interview family members:** Talk with your parents or grandparents to find out how they want to spend their later years. Do they want to live at home, in a retirement community, with a relative? Do they plan to live on a pension, a retirement account, Social Security? Have they made any concrete plans, or have they not yet confronted those decisions?

2. **Be a volunteer:** Develop a project that benefits you and a facility for the elderly in your community. For example, teach an older adult how to send e-mail. Have an older adult teach you how to repair a leaky faucet or make bread. Organize a group of friends or coworkers to volunteer at a nursing home.

3. **Investigate cultural attitudes about aging:** Interview several people from different cultural backgrounds about their attitudes toward aging and older people. How do they view the aging process? How are elderly people treated or viewed in their culture? What family stories do they have about older members of the family? Do you notice any significant differences between their attitudes and stories and yours?

For More Information

Books

Beers, M. H. 2004. *Merck Manual of Health and Aging: The Complete Home Guide to Healthcare and Healthy Aging for Older People and Those Who Care About Them.* New York: Pocket. *Provides information on fundamentals of aging and preventive care.*

King, J. E., ed. 2003. *Mayo Clinic on Healthy Aging.* Broomall, Penn.: Mason Crest Publishers. *A practical guide to healthy aging for all wellness dimensions.*

Lazarus, R. S., and B. N. Lazarus. 2005. *Coping with Aging.* New York: Oxford. *Explores the experience of aging from the standpoint of the individual.*

National Institute on Aging. 2003. *Fitness Over Fifty: An Exercise Guide from the National Institute on Aging.* New York: Hatherleigh Press. *A practical guide to physical activity and exercise, with specific guidelines for safe exercise for older adults.*

Vaillant, G. E. 2003. *Aging Well: Surprising Guideposts to a Happier Life from the Landmark Harvard Study of Adult Development.* New York: Little, Brown. *Provides information on quality-of-life issues from three longevity studies that followed people for more than 50 years.*

Organizations and Web Sites

AARP. Provides information on all aspects of aging, including health promotion, health care, and retirement planning.
888-OUR-AARP
http://www.aarp.org

Access America for Seniors. A gateway to government resources on the Internet for older Americans.
http://www.seniors.gov

Aging Well. A practical resource for seniors that includes information on diet, exercise, safety, and medical care.
http://agingwell.state.ny.us

Alzheimer's Association. Offers tips for caregivers and patients and information on the causes and treatment of Alzheimer's disease.
800-272-3900
http://www.alz.org

American Association of Homes and Services for the Aging (AAHSA). Provides information about living and care arrangements available for older adults.
http://www.aahsa.org

Arthritis Foundation. Provides information about arthritis, including free brochures, referrals to local services, and research updates.

    800-568-4045

    http://www.arthritis.org

ElderWeb. A gateway to aging resources on the Internet, with information about health, housing, and financial issues.

    http://www.elderweb.com

Exercise: A Guide from the National Institute on Aging. Provides practical advice on fitness for seniors; includes animated instructions for specific exercises.

    http://weboflife.ksc.nasa.gov/exerciseandaging/toc.html

Medicare. Provides information about Medicare.

    http://Medicare.gov

National Council on Aging. Provides helpful information on retirement planning, health promotion, and lifelong learning.

    http://www.ncoa.org

National Institute on Aging. Provides fact sheets and brochures on aging-related topics.

    http://www.nih.gov/nia

    http://nihseniorhealth.gov

National Osteoporosis Foundation. Provides information on the causes, prevention, detection, and treatment of osteoporosis.

    http://www.nof.org

U.S. Administration on Aging. Provides fact sheets, statistical information, and Internet links to other resources on aging.

    http://www.aoa.gov

Selected Bibliography

Abbott, R. D., et al. 2004. Walking and dementia in physically capable elderly men. *Journal of the American Medical Association* 292(12): 1447–1453.

Americans over 50 at risk for bone fractures. 2005. *FDA Consumer,* January/February.

Anderson, K., et al. 2005. Depression and the risk of Alzheimer's disease. *Epidemiology* 16(2): 233–238.

Arthritis Foundation. 2004. *Alternative Therapies: Glucosamine and Chondroitin Sulfate* (http://www.arthritis.org/conditions/alttherapies/Glucosamine.asp; retrieved February 6, 2005).

Banks, E., et al. 2004. Fracture incidence in relation to the pattern of use of hormone therapy in postmenopausal women. *Journal of the American Medical Association* 291(18): 2212–2220.

Berman, B. M., et al. 2004. Effectiveness of acupuncture as adjunctive therapy in osteoarthritis of the knee: A randomized, controlled trial. *Annals of Internal Medicine* 141(12): 901–910.

Beyond menopause: Life after estrogen. 2005. *Mayo Clinic Health Letter Supplement,* February.

Bischoff-Ferrari, H. A., et al. 2004. Effect of vitamin D on falls. *Journal of the American Medical Association* 291(16): 1999–2006.

Centers for Disease Control and Prevention. 2005. Racial/ethnic differences in the prevalence and impact of doctor-diagnosed arthritis—United States, 2002. *Morbidity and Mortality Weekly Report* 54(5): 119–123.

Centers for Disease Control and Prevention. 2004. *Suicide: Fact Sheet* (http://www.cdc.gov/ncipc/factsheets/suifacts.htm; retrieved February 6, 2005).

Cirillo, D., et al. 2005. Effect of estrogen therapy on gallbladder disease. *Journal of the American Medical Association* 293(3): 330–339.

Congdon, N., et al. 2004. Causes and prevalence of visual impairment among adults in the United States. *Archives of Ophthalmology* 144(4): 477–485.

Curtis, L. H., et al. 2004. Inappropriate prescribing for elderly Americans in a large outpatient population. *Archives of Internal Medicine* 164(15): 1621–1625.

Cushman, M., et al. 2004. Estrogen plus progestin and risk of venous thrombosis. *Journal of the American Medical Association* 292: 1573–1580.

Espeland, M. A., et al. 2004. Conjugated equine estrogens and global cognitive function in postmenopausal women. *Journal of the American Medical Association* 291: 2959–2968.

Ettinger, B., et al. 2004. Effects of ultralow-dose transdermal estradiol on bone mineral density: A randomized clinical trial. *Obstetrics and Gynecology* 104(3): 443–451.

Evans, M. L., et al. 2004. Management of postmenopausal hot flushes with venlafaxine hydrochloride: A randomized, controlled trial. *Obstetrics and Gynecology* 105(1): 161–166.

Food and Drug Administration. 2003. *Fact Sheet: FDA Approves New Labeling and Provides New Advice to Postmenopausal Women Who Use or Who Are considering Using Estrogen and Estrogen with Progestin* (http://www.fda.gov/bbs/topics/factsheets/2003/fs1.html; retrieved March 8, 2003).

Kado, D. M., et al. 2005. Homocysteine versus the vitamins folate, B(6), and B(12) as predictors of cognitive function and decline in older high-functioning adults: MacArthur Studies of Successful Aging. *American Journal of Medicine* 118(2): 161–167.

Kronenberg, F., and A. Fugh-Berman. 2002. Complementary and alternative medicine for menopausal symptoms: A review of randomized, controlled trials. *Annals of Internal Medicine* 137(10): 805–813.

Lanza, R., and N. Rosenthal. 2004. The stem cell challenge. *Scientific American,* June.

Martin, M. J., et al. 2005. Human embryonic stem cells express an immunogenic nonhuman sialic acid. *Nature Medicine* 11(2): 228–232.

Medicare. 2004. *Stay Healthy* (http://www.medicare.gov/health/overview.asp; retrieved February 10, 2005).

National Institutes of Health. 2004. *Stem Cell Basics* (http://stemcells.nih.gov/info/basics; retrieved February 6, 2005).

National Research Council. 2002. *Stem Cells and the Future of Regenerative Medicine.* Washington, D.C.: National Academy Press.

Nelson, H. D. 2004. Commonly used types of postmenopausal estrogen for treatment of hot flashes. *Journal of the American Medical Association* 291(13): 1610–1620.

Rosengren, A., et al. 2005. Body mass index, other cardiovascular risk factors, and hospitalization for dementia. *Archives of Internal Medicine* 165(3): 321–326.

Stepping into the Vioxx void. 2005. *Harvard Health Letter,* January.

Tsang, W. W., and C. W. Hui-Chan. 2005. Comparison of muscle torque, balance, and confidence in older tai chi and healthy adults. *Medicine and Science in Sports and Exercise* 37(2): 280–289.

U.S. Department of Health and Human Services. 2004. *Bone Health and Osteoporosis: A Report of the Surgeon General.* Washington, D.C.: U.S. Department of Health and Human Services.

Whitmer, R. A., et al. 2005. Midlife cardiovascular risk factors and risk of dementia in late life. *Neurology* 64(2): 277–281.

Wilson, R. S., et al. 2005. Proneness to psychological distress and risk of Alzheimer disease in a biracial community. *Neurology* 64(2): 380–382.

Yaffe, K., et al. 2004. The metabolic syndrome, inflammation, and risk of cognitive decline. *Journal of the American Medical Association* 292(18): 2237–2242.

Yoon, Y. S., et al. 2005. Clonally expanded novel multipotent stem cells from human bone marrow regenerate myocardium after myocardial infarction. *Journal of Clinical Investigation* 115(2): 326–338.

Zhan, C., et al. 2001. Potentially inappropriate medication use in the community-dwelling elderly. *Journal of the American Medical Association* 286(22): 2823–2829.

Looking **AHEAD**

After reading this chapter, you should be able to

- Identify the physical, mental, social, behavioral, and spiritual dimensions of dying and death

- Describe various ways of defining death and the components of a mature concept of death

- Understand personal considerations in preparing for death, including making a will, assessing choices for end-of-life care, and making arrangements for a funeral or memorial service

- Describe the experience of living with a life-threatening illness and list ways to support a person who is dying

- Explain the grieving process and how support can be offered to adults and children who have experienced a loss

Dying and Death

Test Your

Knowledge

1. **If you die in a car crash, your organs will automatically be donated to people waiting for transplants.**
   True or false?

2. **How many Americans die without leaving a will?**
   a. 1 in 10
   b. 4 in 10
   c. 7 in 10

3. **Terminally ill patients can more accurately predict their own survival time than physicians using clinical measures of health.**
   True or false?

4. **Physician-assisted suicide is considered murder and is illegal in all 50 states.**
   True or false?

5. **The best way to help a friend who is grieving is to distract her or him from the loss by talking about sports, gossip, or other lighthearted topics.**
   True or false?

ANSWERS

1. FALSE. For your organs to be donated, you must have authorized it prior to your death (such as by completing an organ donor card), or the donation must be authorized by relatives at the time of your death.

2. C. In such cases, the estate is distributed according to state law, which may not reflect what the individual would have wanted.

3. TRUE. Studies have found that patients' own ratings of health status are better predictors of survival time than clinical indicators and other, more objective, measures.

4. FALSE. Physician-assisted suicide is legal in Oregon, where the Death with Dignity Act was approved in 1997. By 2005, more than 200 terminally ill people participating in PAS had died from lethal doses of prescription medication.

5. FALSE. Most people who are grieving need to talk about their loss, and a friend who will let them talk freely is very valuable. The best strategy is simply to be a good listener.

Visit the *Core Concepts in Health* Online Learning Center (www.mhhe.com/insel10e) for study aids and many additional resources.

603

From a tsunami devastating a fishing village in South-east Asia to a man in a crowded restaurant having a heart attack to an elderly woman dying peacefully with her family close by, images of death pervade our consciousness. Nevertheless, very rarely do we think about the inevitability of death in our own lives. Accepting and dealing with death are important tasks that present unique challenges to our sense of self and relationship to others and our understanding of the meaning of life itself.

Although times of pain and distress may accompany the dying process, facing death also presents opportunity for growth as well as affirmation of the preciousness of simple aspects of our daily lives. If you suddenly discovered that you had a terminal illness, how would you want to spend your last year or months? What would you want to say to your loved ones, and how would you want to experience those close to you during this final period? Would you want extraordinary measures taken in an attempt to preserve your life even if it meant living in a vegetative state? What kind of final ceremony would you want to mark your passing? How would you want to dispose of your possessions? Have you discussed such issues with your family? The manner we choose to confront death can greatly influence how we live our lives.

WHY IS THERE DEATH?

Ultimately, no answer to the question of why death exists is completely satisfying. When we look at the big picture, we see that death promotes variety through the evolution of species. The average human life span is long enough to allow us to reproduce ourselves and ensure that the lineage of our species continues. Yet it is brief enough to allow for new genetic combinations, thereby providing a means of adaptation to changing conditions in the environment. From the perspective of species survival, the cycle of life and death makes sense.

From a personal point of view, however, death challenges our emotional and intellectual security. We may acknowledge the fact that all living things eventually die, that this is nature's way of renewal, but this recognition offers little comfort when death touches our own lives. Questions about the meaning of death and what happens when we die are central concerns of the great religions and philosophies. Some promise a better life after death. Others teach that everyone is evolving toward perfection or divinity, a goal reached after successive rounds of death and rebirth. There are also those who suggest that it is not possible to know what happens—if anything—after death, that any judgment about whether life is worth living must be made on the basis of satisfactions or rewards that we create for ourselves in this life.

It is worth noting that, even in modern secular societies, religion plays a major role in shaping our attitudes and behaviors toward death. Religion offers solace to the

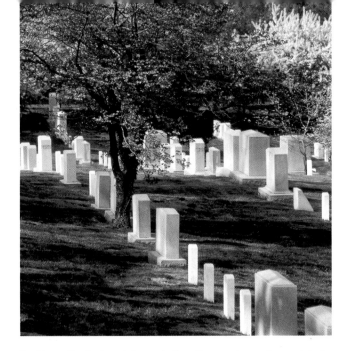

Death awaits all of us at the end of our lives, and accepting and dealing with death are difficult but important tasks. Some people have found that facing the prospect of death makes them more aware of the preciousness of life.

extent that it suggests some meaning in dying. The mourning ceremonies associated with various religious practices ease the pangs of grief for many people. Dying and death are more than biological events; they have social and spiritual dimensions. Our beliefs—religious or philosophical—can be a key to how we relate to the prospect of our own death as well as the deaths of others.

UNDERSTANDING DEATH AND DYING

Death forces us to puzzle out an understanding of its meaning in our lives. We may choose not to think about some issues, such as the possibility of an afterlife, but we cannot keep from facing the reality of dying and death. Regardless of our explanations or efforts to minimize its effects, death can be challenging and painful—both to the person who is dying and to those left behind. However, it also offers opportunity for remarkable growth and a deepening appreciation of relationships and the myriad aspects of life itself.

Defining Death

Traditionally, death has been defined as cessation of the flow of vital bodily fluids. This occurs when the heart stops beating and breathing ceases. These traditional signs are adequate for determining death in most cases. However, the use of respirators and other **life-support systems** in modern medicine allows some body functions to be artificially sustained. To make a determination of death in such cases requires investigating the presence or absence of a physical response other than heartbeat or breathing. The concept of **brain death** has been developed to determine whether a person is alive or dead when the traditional signs are inadequate because of supportive medical technology.

According to the standards published in 1968 by a Harvard Medical School committee, brain death involves the following four characteristics: (1) lack of receptivity and response to external stimuli, (2) absence of spontaneous muscular movement and spontaneous breathing, (3) absence of observable reflexes, and (4) absence of brain activity, as signified by a flat **electroencephalogram (EEG)**. The Harvard criteria require a second set of tests to be performed after 24 hours has elapsed, and they exclude cases of hypothermia (body temperature below 90°F), as well as situations involving central nervous system depressants, such as barbiturates.

In contrast to **clinical death**, which is determined by either the cessation of heartbeat and breathing or the criteria for establishing brain death, **cellular death** refers to a gradual process that occurs when heartbeat, respiration, and brain activity have stopped. It encompasses the breakdown of metabolic processes and results in complete nonfunctionality at the cellular level. In a biological sense, therefore, death can be defined as the cessation of life due to irreversible changes in cell metabolism.

The way in which death is defined has potential legal and social consequences in a variety of areas, including criminal prosecution, inheritance, taxation, treatment of the corpse, and even mourning. It also affects the practice of organ transplantation, because some organs—hearts, most obviously—must be harvested from a human being who is legally determined to be dead. Timing is critical in removing a heart from someone who has been declared dead and transplanting it into a person whose life can thereby be saved. Safeguards are necessary to ensure that the determination of death occurs without regard to any plans for subsequent transplantation of the deceased's organs.

Learning About Death

Our understanding of death changes as we grow and mature, as do our attitudes toward it. Very young children view death as an interruption and an absence, but their lack of a mature time perspective means that they do not understand death as final and irreversible. A child's understanding of death evolves greatly from about age 5 to age 9. During this period, most children come to understand that death is final, universal, and inevitable. A child who consciously recognizes these facts is said to possess a **mature understanding of death.** This understanding of death is further refined during the years of adolescence and young adulthood by considering the impact of death

on close relationships and contemplating the value of religious or philosophical answers to the enigma of death.

Based on work done by Mark Speece and Sandor Brent, a formal statement of the empirical, or observable, facts about death includes four components:

1. *Universality.* All living things eventually die. Death is all-inclusive, inevitable, and unavoidable (although unpredictable with respect to its exact timing).

2. *Irreversibility.* Organisms that die cannot be made alive again.

3. *Nonfunctionality.* Death involves the cessation of all physiological functioning, or signs of life.

4. *Causality.* There are biological reasons for the occurrence of death.

It is important to add, however, that individuals who possess a mature understanding of death commonly hold nonempirical ideas about it as well. Such nonempirical ideas—that is, ideas not subject to scientific proof—deal mainly with the notion that human beings survive in some form beyond the death of the physical body. What happens to an individual's personality after he or she dies? Does the self or soul continue to exist after the death of the physical body? If so, what is the nature of this afterlife? Developing personally satisfying answers to such questions, which involve what Speece and Brent term **noncorporeal continuity,** is also part of the process of acquiring a mature understanding of death.

Denying Versus Welcoming Death

Understanding death in a mature fashion does not imply that we never experience anxiety about the deaths of those we love or about the prospect of our own death. The news

Terms V̇i̇w

life-support systems Medical technologies, such as the respirator, that allow vital body functions to be artificially sustained.

brain death A medical determination of death as the cessation of brain activity indicated by various diagnostic criteria, including a flat EEG reading.

electroencephalogram (EEG) A record of the electrical activity of the brain (brain waves).

clinical death A determination of death made according to accepted medical criteria.

cellular death The breakdown of metabolic processes at the level of the cell.

mature understanding of death The recognition that death is universal and irreversible, that it involves the cessation of all physiological functioning, and that there are biological reasons for its occurrence.

noncorporeal continuity The notion that human beings survive in some form after the death of the physical body.

Día de los Muertos in Mexico is characterized by a mixture of reverent remembrance of the departed, festivity to make them happy on their return, and irony and mockery to defy the fear of death itself. Customary decorations and offerings for the graveyards include candles, marigolds, fruit, round loaves of bread marked with a cross, and decorated skulls made from sugar.

of a friend's or loved one's serious illness can shock us into an encounter with mortality that creates a need to cope not only with the painful reality of our friend's or loved one's illness, but also with our own eventual death. Our ability to find meaning and comfort in the face of mortality depends not only on our having an understanding of the facts of death, but also on our attitudes toward it.

Many people seek to avoid any thought or mention of death. The sick and old are often isolated in hospitals and nursing homes. Relatively few Americans have been present at the death of a loved one. Where the reality of death is concerned, "out of sight, out of mind" often appears to be the rule of the day. Instead of facing death directly, we tend to amuse ourselves with unrealistic portrayals on television and movie screens. The fictitious deaths of characters we barely know do not cause us to confront the reality of death as it is experienced in real life. Moreover, such faked death is often presented as reversible. Children watch a daily fare of superhuman heroes, invincible to bullets and other weapons. In their games, they reenact these false ideas about death—falling down dead and jumping up again unharmed. Cartoons and video games present death in a two-dimensional world where one can die and then be reborn to play another day.

Although some commentators characterize the predominant attitude toward death in the United States as "death denying," others are reluctant to paint society as a whole with such a broad brush. Individuals often maintain conflicting or ambivalent attitudes toward death. Those who come to view death as a relief or release from insufferable pain may have at least a partial sense of welcoming death. Few people wholly avoid or wholly welcome death. Problems can arise, however, when avoidance or denial fosters the notion that death happens to others, but not to you or me. (For another perspective, see the box "Día de los Muertos: The Day of the Dead.")

PLANNING FOR DEATH

Acknowledging the inevitability of death allows us to plan for it. Adequate planning can help ensure that a sudden, unexpected death is not made even more difficult for survivors. Even when death is not sudden, individuals with a debilitating illness may become unable to make decisions that could have been made before the onset of crisis. Although some decisions cannot be made until one is actually in a particular situation, many decisions relating to dying and death can be anticipated, considered, and discussed with close relatives and friends.

Basic tasks in planning for death include making a will, anticipating medical care needs and expressing preferences for end-of-life care, considering whether to become an organ donor, and helping survivors plan tasks that will be carried out after we die. It is reasonable to begin such planning and decision making during the college years and to periodically review and revise one's choices throughout life.

Making a Will

Surveys indicate that about seven out of ten Americans die without leaving a will. Perhaps the failure to plan ahead for death by making a will is attributable to the

Terms

Vw

will A legal instrument expressing a person's intentions and wishes for the disposition of his or her property after death.

estate The money, property, and other possessions belonging to a person.

testator The person who makes a will.

intestate Referring to the situation in which a person dies without having made a legal will.

Dimensions of Diversity

Día de los Muertos: The Day of the Dead

In contrast to the solemn attitude toward death so prevalent in the United States, a familiar and even ironic attitude is more common among Mexicans and Mexican Americans. In the Mexican worldview, death is another phase of life, and those who have passed into it remain accessible. Ancestors are not forever lost, nor is the past dead. This sense of continuity has its roots in the culture of the Aztecs, for whom regeneration was a central theme. When the Spanish came to Mexico in the sixteenth century, their beliefs about death, along with symbols such as skulls and skeletons, were absorbed into the native culture.

Mexican artists and writers confront death with humor and even sarcasm, depicting it as the inevitable fate that all—even the wealthiest—must face. At no time is this attitude toward death livelier than at the beginning of each November on the holiday known as Día de los Muertos, "the Day of the Dead." This holiday coincides with All Souls' Day, the Catholic commemoration of the dead, and represents a unique blending of indigenous ritual and religious dogma.

Festive and gay, the celebration in honor of the dead typically spans two days—one day devoted to dead children, one to adults. It reflects the belief that the dead return to Earth in spirit once a year to rejoin their families and partake of holiday foods prepared especially for them. The fiesta usually begins at midday on October 31, with flowers and food—candies, cookies, honey, milk—set out on altars in each house for the family's dead. The next day, family groups stream to the graveyards, where they have cleaned and decorated the graves of their loved ones, to celebrate and commune with the dead. They bring games, music, and special food—chicken with *mole* sauce, enchiladas, tamales, and *pan de muertos*, the "bread of the dead," sweet rolls in the shape of bones. People sit on the graves, eat, sing, and talk with the departed ones. Tears may be shed as the dead are remembered, but mourning is tempered by the festive mood of the occasion.

During the season of the dead, graveyards and family altars are decorated with yellow candles and yellow marigolds—the "flower of death." In some Mexican villages, yellow flower petals are strewn along the ground, connecting the graveyard with all the houses visited by death during the year.

As families cherish memories of their loved ones on this holiday, the larger society satirizes death itself—and political and public figures. The impulse to laugh at death finds expression in what are called *calaveras,* a word meaning "skeletons" or "skulls" but also referring to humorous newsletters that appear during this season. The *calaveras* contain biting, often bawdy, verses caricaturing well-known public figures, often with particular reference to their deaths. Comic skeletal figures march or dance across these pages, portraying the wealthy and influential as they will eventually become.

Wherever Mexican Americans have settled in the United States, Día de los Muertos celebrations keep the traditions alive, and the cultural practices associated with the Day of the Dead have found their way into the nation's culture. Books and museum exhibitions have brought to the public the art of the dead, with its striking blend of skeletons and flowers, bones and candles. Even the schools in some areas celebrate the holiday. Students create paintings and sculptures depicting skeletons and skulls with the help of local artists.

Does this more familiar attitude toward death help people accept death and come to terms with it? Keeping death in the forefront of consciousness may provide solace to the living, reminding them of their loved ones and assuring them that they themselves will not be forgotten when they die. Yearly celebrations and remembrances may help people keep in touch with their past, their ancestry, and their roots. The festive atmosphere may help dispel the fear of death, allowing people to look at it more directly. Although it is possible to deny the reality of death even when surrounded by images of it, such practices as Día de los Muertos may help people face death with more equanimity.

SOURCES: Adapted from DeSpelder, L., and A. Strickland. 2005. *The Last Dance,* 7th ed. New York: McGraw-Hill; Azcentral. 2000. *Día de los Muertos* (http://www.azcentral.com/rep/dead; retrieved March 8, 2001); Puente, T. 1991. Día de los Muertos. *Hispanic,* October; Milne, J. 1965. *Fiesta Time in Latin America.* Los Angeles: Ward Ritchie Press.

---

discomfort people feel about their own mortality. Whatever the reason, dying without having made a will can lead to unnecessary hardships for survivors, even when an estate is modest in size. If an estate is substantial, the complications can be formidable.

A **will** is a legal instrument expressing a person's intentions and wishes for the disposition of his or her property after death. It is a declaration of how one's **estate**—that is, money, property, and other possessions—will be distributed after death. During the life of the **testator** (the person making the will), a will can be changed, replaced, or revoked. Upon the testator's death, it becomes a legal instrument governing the distribution of the testator's estate.

When a person dies **intestate**—that is, without having left a valid will—property is distributed according to rules set up by the state. The failure to execute a will may result in a distribution of property that is not compatible with a person's wishes nor best suited to the interests and needs of heirs. If you haven't yet made a will, start thinking about how you'd like your property distributed in the case of your death. If you have a will, consider whether it needs to be updated in response to a key life event such as marriage, the birth of a child, or the purchase of a home. In making a will, it is generally advisable to involve close family members to prevent problems that can arise when actions are taken without the knowledge of those who will be affected.

Considering Options for End-of-Life Care

If you were facing the prospect of dying soon, would you prefer to spend your last days or weeks at home, cared for by relatives and friends? Or would you rather have access to the sophisticated medical technologies available in a hospital? An appropriate balance in end-of-life care may involve a combination of home care, hospital stays, and hospice or palliative care. By becoming aware of our options, we and our families are empowered to make informed, meaningful choices.

Home Care   Many people express a preference to be cared for at home during the end stage of a terminal illness. An obvious advantage of home care is the fact that the dying person is in a familiar setting, ideally in the company of family and friends. For home care to be an option, however, support generally must be provided not only by family and friends, but also by skilled, professional caregivers.

Home care is a full-time job, and it is not always possible to provide a sufficient level of care in the home. Success depends on adequate preparation and commitment. When a patient requires sophisticated medical procedures, does not have access to qualified caregivers, or intends to be an organ donor, institutional care may be more appropriate. When suitable, however, home care is arguably the most satisfying option for care as a person's life comes to a close. Currently, about 25% of Americans die at home (about 25% die in nursing facilities, and about 50% die in hospitals, including more than 20% in intensive care units).

Hospital-Based Palliative Care   Although hospitals are primarily organized to provide short-term intensive treatment for acute injury and illness, they are also adopting the principles of **palliative care** for patients who require comprehensive care at the end of life. Unlike acute care, which involves taking active measures to sustain life, palliative care focuses on controlling pain and relieving suffering by caring for the physical, psychological, spiritual, and existential needs of the patient. Although the emphasis is generally placed on comfort care, palliative therapies can be combined with cure-oriented treatment approaches in some cases. In all cases, the goal of

palliative care is to achieve the best possible quality of life for patients and their families.

Hospice Programs   As a comprehensive program of care offering a set of services designed to support terminally ill patients and their families, **hospice** is a well-known form of palliative care. Although the term *hospice* sometimes refers to a freestanding medical facility to which terminally ill patients are admitted, most hospice care takes place in patients' homes with family members as primary caregivers. Entering hospice care usually means affiliating with a hospice program—that is, arranging to receive the services of a local hospice. Such hospices are generally community-based organizations that coordinate a range of palliative care services that may be provided in nursing homes and hospitals, as well as in patients' homes. (For more on the history and development of hospice, see the box "Hospice: Comfort and Care for the Dying.") Qualifying for hospice care usually requires a doctor's certification that a patient's life expectancy is 6 months or less, and both patient and physician agree to forgo treatment aimed at prolonging life.

Hospice (and palliative care generally) involves a team-oriented approach to care that typically includes physicians, nurses, social workers, home health aides, pharmacists, chaplains, physical and occupational therapists, and trained volunteers. This team-oriented approach seeks to provide state-of-the-art care to prevent or relieve pain and other distressing symptoms, as well as to offer emotional and spiritual support to both patient and family. The notion that hospice is appropriate only when there is no hope is a myth. Much can be done even when recovery or cure is not a realistic possibility.

The primary aim of hospice and palliative care is to help people live as fully as possible until the end of their lives. In addition to its goal of helping patients achieve a good or peaceful death, an important gift of such care is the potential to help patients and families discover how much can be shared at the end of life through personal and spiritual connections that might not have been possible otherwise.

Deciding to Prolong Life or Hasten Death

If you were given a prognosis of only a very short time to live and told that any further treatment toward a cure was useless, would you want aggressive treatment to keep you alive, even if it meant that your vital bodily functions were maintained on life-support systems? The decision to limit treatment, to stop doing everything that can be done, is often a difficult one for patients and their families. Many people owe their lives to the advanced medical technologies now available. Yet a medical stance that strives to keep people alive by all means and at any cost is increasingly being questioned.

Terms

ViW

palliative care A form of medical care aimed at reducing the intensity or severity of a disease by controlling pain and other discomforting symptoms.

hospice A program of care for dying patients and their families.

persistent vegetative state A condition of profound unconsciousness in which a person lacks normal reflexes and is unresponsive to external stimuli, lasting for an extended period with no reasonable hope of improvement.

In Focus

Hospice: Comfort and Care for the Dying

Hospice is a special kind of care for people in the final phase of a terminal illness. Instead of being in a hospital, where the emphasis is on curing disease, most hospice patients stay in their home or another homelike setting surrounded by family and friends. The goals of hospice care include the following:

- To make every terminally ill patient as pain-free as possible
- To support the patient and family as a unit
- To respect the feelings and beliefs about death held by patients and their families
- To involve patients in decision making regarding their care
- To help patients and family members deal with feelings of loneliness and fears of abandonment
- To counsel family members after a patient's death

Although institutions dedicated to the care of the dying have existed throughout history, the modern hospice movement began in 1967, when Dr. Cicely Saunders founded St. Christopher's Hospice near London. The first hospice program in the United States began in 1974. Today there are more than 3300 such programs, serving an estimated 950,000 terminally ill patients and their families each year. Once a patient can no longer benefit from medical treatment based on curing disease,

the primary physician may refer the patient to hospice. Referrals can also be made by family members, friends, clergy, or health professionals.

Most patients receive care at home, with the primary caregiver often a partner or family member. Providing medical care and other types of support to the patient, family, and caregivers is a team of trained professionals—physicians, nurses, counselors, therapists, social workers, home health aides, and volunteers. The emphasis of care is on enhancing the quality of life rather than extending its length. Most hospice patients have a life expectancy of 6 months or less at the time they enter hospice, and about 65% of them are over 75 years old. The median length of hospice service is about 20–25 days.

Hospice care can be less expensive than conventional care—high-cost technology is much less likely to be used, and family, friends, and volunteers provide much of the day-to-day patient care at home. Because a principle of hospice is to offer services based on need rather than the ability to pay, many hospices rely on grants, donations, and a large volunteer staff. At the same time, hospice has grown into a more formal, regulated industry. Hospice care is a covered benefit under most private insurance plans, Medicare, and, in many states, Medicaid. Medicare-certified hospice programs meet quality standards set by the federal government, including 24-hour access to professional care.

Some experts believe hospice could serve many more patients than it does. There are several stumbling blocks, however. Physicians may be reluctant to stop treatment and tell patients and their families that nothing further can be done to effect a cure. Establishing a specific timeline for a patient's expected death is difficult. Patients and family members may be reluctant to face an imminent death.

In addition, under Medicare rules, a physician must certify that the patient will likely die in 6 months or less. Although the rules do provide for extensions, many hospices feel pressured to accept only patients near death, turning away those who may linger beyond the half-year cutoff. The 6-month rule is supposed to be based on life expectancy at the time of the physician's certification, not an absolute deadline by which the patient must die. Nevertheless, some hospices have been subjected to audits that have left them feeling bitter and suspicious about how Medicare benefits are administered. Nearly everyone agrees that there is a need for eligibility criteria that are not time-dependent, so that hospice services can be extended to more patients and their families.

SOURCES: National Hospice and Palliative Care Organization (NHPCO). 2004. *Hospice Facts and Figures* (http://www.nhpco.org; retrieved February 15, 2005); Hospice: A healthy way to let go. 2004. *Consumer Reports on Health*, May; Hospice care. 1997. *Mayo Clinic Health Letter*, July.

Modern medicine can keep the human organism alive despite the cessation of normal heart, brain, respiratory, or kidney function. But should a patient without any hope of recovery be kept alive by means of artificial life support? At what point does such treatment become futile? What if a patient has fallen into a **persistent vegetative state,** a state of profound unconsciousness, lacking any sign of normal reflexes and unresponsive to external stimuli, with no reasonable hope of improvement?

Ethical questions about a person's right to die have become prominent since the landmark case of Karen Ann Quinlan in 1975. At age 22, she was admitted in a comatose state to an intensive care unit, where her breathing was sustained by a respirator. When she remained unresponsive,

in a persistent vegetative state, her parents asked that the respirator be disconnected, but the medical staff responsible for Karen's care denied their request. The request to withdraw treatment eventually reached the New Jersey Supreme Court, which ruled that artificial respiration could be discontinued.

Since then, courts have ruled on removing other types of life-sustaining treatment, including artificial feeding mechanisms that provide nutrition and hydration to permanently comatose patients who are able to breathe on their own. Most notable was the case of Nancy Beth Cruzan, heard before the U.S. Supreme Court in 1990. As a result of injuries she received in 1983, Cruzan was in a persistent vegetative state. To provide nourishment, Nancy's physicians implanted a feeding tube, the only form of life support she was receiving. When Nancy's parents requested that the feeding tube be taken out, hospital personnel refused, arguing that the state had an inherent interest in preserving life.

In the Cruzan case, the U.S. Supreme Court ruled that the right to refuse unwanted treatment, even if it is life-sustaining, is constitutionally protected. However, the court said that states are justified in requiring that only the patient can decide to withdraw treatment. Because Nancy apparently had not provided a clear expression of her wishes prior to her injury, the state of Missouri was not bound to honor her parents' request. A few months later, however, in light of new testimony from several of Nancy's friends that she had expressed a wish "not to live like a vegetable," a state court ruled that the legal standard of "clear and convincing" evidence of Nancy's wishes had been met, and therefore permission was granted for removal of the feeding tube. The question of whether to remove an implanted feeding tube was also at the heart of the high-profile case of Terri Schiavo. These cases emphasized the importance of expressing one's preferences about life-sustaining treatment—preferably in writing—before the need arises.

Withholding or Withdrawing Treatment The right of a competent patient to refuse unwanted treatment is now generally established in both law and medical practice. The consensus is that there is no medical or ethical distinction between withholding (not starting) a treatment and withdrawing (stopping) a treatment once it has been started. The choice to forgo life-sustaining treatment involves refusing treatments that would be expected to extend life. The right to refuse treatment remains constitutionally protected even when a patient is unable to communicate. Although specific requirements vary, all of the states authorize some type of written advance directive to honor the decisions of individuals unable to speak for themselves but who have previously recorded their wishes in an appropriate legal document. (Advance directives are discussed later in this chapter.)

The practice of withholding or withdrawing a treatment that could potentially sustain life is sometimes termed **passive euthanasia**, although many people consider this term a misnomer because it tends to confuse the widely accepted practice of withholding or withdrawing treatment with the generally unacceptable and unlawful practice of taking active steps to cause death. It can be argued that passive euthanasia is not euthanasia at all, but rather letting nature take its course. This distinction is sometimes phrased as the difference between "killing" and "allowing to die."

Assisted Suicide and Active Euthanasia In contrast to withdrawing or withholding treatment, assisted suicide and active euthanasia refer to practices that intentionally hasten the death of a person. Although some ethicists argue that the constitutional basis for the right to refuse treatment provides the same basis for a right to active euthanasia, this argument has not been accepted

by the Supreme Court or by the majority of health care practitioners.

Assisted suicide refers to providing someone with the means to commit suicide, knowing that the recipient intends to use them to end his or her life. In **physician-assisted suicide (PAS),** a physician provides lethal drugs or other interventions—at the patient's explicit request—with the understanding that the patient plans to use them to end his or her life. The patient, not the doctor, administers the fatal dose.

In 1997, the Supreme Court reviewed two cases relating to physician-assisted suicide. The decisions in these cases (*Washington v. Glucksberg* and *Vacco v. Quill*) are important for several reasons. First, the Court upheld the distinction between, on the one hand, withholding or withdrawing treatment and, on the other hand, physician-assisted suicide. In doing so, the Court clarified its ruling in the Cruzan case, noting that the right to refuse treatment is based on the right to *maintain one's bodily integrity,* not on a right to *hasten one's death.* When treatment is withheld or withdrawn, the Court said, the intent is to honor the patient's wishes, not cause death, unlike with PAS, where the patient dies from the lethal medication. Second, the Court affirmed the rights of states to craft policy concerning physician-assisted suicide, either prohibiting it, as most states now do, or permitting it under some regulatory system, as is now happening in Oregon.

Oregon is currently the only state where PAS is permitted. The Death with Dignity Act, a ballot initiative, was passed by Oregon voters in 1994 and, after surviving judicial challenges, was reaffirmed in 1997. During its first 7 years of implementation, 208 people were reported to have legally committed suicide with the assistance of their physicians. These patients exhibited strong beliefs in personal autonomy and a determination to control the end of their lives. The decision to request a prescription for lethal medication was associated mainly with concerns about loss of autonomy and control. Specific quality-of-life concerns included decreasing ability to participate in activities that make life enjoyable, losing control of bodily functions, and physical suffering.

A third finding of importance in the Supreme Court's 1997 rulings about PAS relates to the concept of **double effect** in the medical management of pain. The doctrine of double effect states that a harmful effect of treatment, even if it results in death, is permissible if the harm is not intended and occurs as a side effect of a beneficial action. Sometimes the dosages of medication needed to relieve a patient's pain (especially those in the end stage of some diseases) must be increased to levels that can cause respiratory depression, resulting in the patient's death. Thus, the relief of suffering, the intended good effect, may have a potential bad effect, which is foreseen but is not the primary intention. The Court said that such medication for pain, even if it hastens death, is not physician-assisted suicide if the intent is to relieve pain.

Unlike physician-assisted suicide, **active euthanasia** involves a deliberate act to end another person's life. Generally, it is understood as the intentional act of killing someone who would otherwise suffer from an incurable and painful disease. It is important, however, to recognize that active euthanasia can be involuntary, nonvoluntary, or voluntary. Involuntary euthanasia (or involuntary active euthanasia) refers to the ending of a patient's life by a medical practitioner *without* the patient's consent. The most notorious example of this is the medical killing programs of the Nazi regime. Nonvoluntary euthanasia occurs when a surrogate decision maker (not the patient) asks a physician for assistance to end another person's life.

Voluntary euthanasia (also known as voluntary active euthanasia, or VAE) is the intentional termination of life at the patient's request by someone other than the patient. In practice, this generally means that a competent patient requests direct assistance to die, and he or she receives assistance from a qualified medical practitioner.

At present, active euthanasia has found greatest acceptance in the Netherlands, where physicians are permitted to give lethal injections to patients who request death. The guidelines for VAE in the Netherlands include the presence of a terminal diagnosis, the patient's unwavering desire to die, the presence of suffering that the patient finds unbearable, and a second medical opinion. Voluntary active euthanasia is currently unlawful in the United States, and it is for this practice that Michigan physician Dr. Jack Kevorkian was convicted of second-degree murder in 1999. Taking active steps to end someone's life is a crime— even if the motive for doing so results from good intentions as an act of mercy.

Many people believe that the emphasis on a right to die, along with the movement to legalize physician-assisted suicide and active euthanasia, results from inattention to the needs of the dying by the health care system. Inadequate pain management has been called "the shame of American medicine." The advocates of hospice and palliative care have highlighted the need for adequate pain management, not only for patients with terminal illness, but for all patients with untreated or undertreated pain and suffering. Increasingly, pain is being viewed as a "fifth vital sign," one that should be added to the four vital signs—temperature, pulse, respiration, and blood pressure—now recorded and assessed as a standard part of patient care. Unfortunately, there is tremendous variation among health care providers with respect to assessing and managing pain adequately.

Completing an Advance Directive

To make your preferences known about medical treatment to health care providers and others who should be aware of them, it is important to document them through a written **advance directive.** In a general sense, an advance directive is any statement made by a competent person about choices for medical treatment should he or she become unable to make such decisions or communicate them at some time in the future.

Two forms of advance directives are legally important. First is the **living will,** which enables individuals to provide instructions about the kind of medical care they wish to receive if they become incapacitated or otherwise unable to participate in treatment decisions (Figure 20-1). Many people believe that living wills are appropriate only for stating a desire to forgo life-sustaining procedures or to avoid medical heroics when death is imminent; indeed, most standard forms for completing a living will reflect this purpose. In fact, however, a living will can be drafted to express very different ideas about the kinds of treatment a person would or would not want, and they can be written to cover various contingencies.

The second important form of advance directive is the **health care proxy,** which is also known as a durable power of attorney for health care. This document makes it possible to appoint another person to make decisions about medical treatment if you become unable to do so. This decision maker, also known as a **surrogate,** may be a family member, close friend, or attorney with whom you have discussed your treatment preferences. The proxy is

Terms

passive euthanasia The practice of withholding (not starting) or withdrawing (stopping) treatment that could potentially sustain a person's life, with the recognition that, without such treatment, death is likely to occur.

physician-assisted suicide (PAS) The practice of a physician intentionally providing, at the patient's request, lethal drugs or other means for a patient to hasten death with the understanding that the patient plans to use them to end his or her life.

double effect A situation in which a harmful effect occurs as an unintended side effect of a beneficial action, such as when medication intended to control a patient's pain has the unintended result of causing the patient's death.

active euthanasia A deliberate act intended to end another person's life; voluntary active euthanasia involves the practice of a physician administering—at the request of a patient—medication or some other intervention that causes death.

advance directive Any statement made by a competent person about his or her choices for medical treatment should he or she become unable to make such decisions or communicate them in the future.

living will A type of advance directive that allows individuals to provide instructions about the kind of medical care they wish to receive if they become unable to participate in treatment decisions.

health care proxy A type of advance directive that allows an individual to appoint another person as an agent in making health care decisions in the event he or she becomes unable to participate in treatment decisions; also known as a durable power of attorney for health care.

surrogate The agent or substitute decision maker appointed by a person to act on his or her behalf by means of a health care proxy.

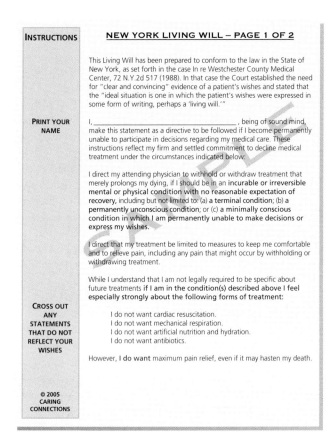

INSTRUCTIONS

PRINT YOUR NAME

CROSS OUT ANY STATEMENTS THAT DO NOT REFLECT YOUR WISHES

© 2005 CARING CONNECTIONS

NEW YORK LIVING WILL – PAGE 1 OF 2

This Living Will has been prepared to conform to the law in the State of New York, as set forth in the case In re Westchester County Medical Center, 72 N.Y.2d 517 (1988). In that case the Court established the need for "clear and convincing" evidence of a patient's wishes and stated that the "ideal situation is one in which the patient's wishes were expressed in some form of writing, perhaps a 'living will.'"

I, _____, being of sound mind, make this statement as a directive to be followed if I become permanently unable to participate in decisions regarding my medical care. These instructions reflect my firm and settled commitment to decline medical treatment under the circumstances indicated below:

I direct my attending physician to withhold or withdraw treatment that merely prolongs my dying, if I should be in an incurable or irreversible mental or physical condition with no reasonable expectation of recovery, including but not limited to: (a) a terminal condition; (b) a permanently unconscious condition; or (c) a minimally conscious condition in which I am permanently unable to make decisions or express my wishes.

I direct that my treatment be limited to measures to keep me comfortable and to relieve pain, including any pain that might occur by withholding or withdrawing treatment.

While I understand that I am not legally required to be specific about future treatments if I am in the condition(s) described above I feel especially strongly about the following forms of treatment:

I do not want cardiac resuscitation.
I do not want mechanical respiration.
I do not want artificial nutrition and hydration.
I do not want antibiotics.

However, **I do want** maximum pain relief, even if it may hasten my death.

ADD PERSONAL INSTRUCTIONS (IF ANY)

SIGN AND DATE THE DOCUMENT AND PRINT YOUR ADDRESS

WITNESSING PROCEDURE

YOUR WITNESSES MUST SIGN AND PRINT THEIR ADDRESSES

© 2005 CARING CONNECTIONS

NEW YORK LIVING WILL – PAGE 2 OF 2

Other directions:

These directions express my legal right to refuse treatment, under the law of New York. I intend my instructions to be carried out, unless I have rescinded them in a new writing or by clearly indicating that I have changed my mind.

Signed _____ Date _____

Address _____

I declare that the person who signed this document appeared to execute the living will willingly and free from duress. He or she signed (or asked another to sign for him or her) this document in my presence.

Witness 1 _____

Address _____

Witness 2 _____

Address _____

Courtesy of Caring Connections
1700 Diagonal Road, Suite 625, Alexandria, VA 22314
www.caringinfo.org, 800/658-8898

Figure 20-1 Sample living will. Because of differences in state law, each state has its own format for advance directives. SOURCE: Valid copies of this and other state specific advance directives can be found at www.caringinfo.org. Reprinted with permission of The National Hospice and Palliative Care Organization. Copyright © 2005 National Hospice and Palliative Care Organization. All rights reserved. Reproduction and distribution by an organization or organized group without the written permission of the National Hospice and Palliative Care Organization is expressly forbidden.

expected to act in accordance with your wishes as stated in an advance directive or as otherwise made known.

For advance directives to be of value, you must do more than merely complete the paperwork. Discuss your wishes ahead of time with caregivers and family members as well as with your physician. If you have completed an advance directive in one state and subsequently move elsewhere, find out if you need to complete a new one. Indeed, it is a good idea to revisit the issue occasionally to be sure the preferences expressed in the directive continue to match your wishes. (See Take Action at the end of the chapter for information on obtaining an advance directive form for your state.)

Becoming an Organ Donor

A human body is a valuable resource. Of all the advances in medical techniques for helping patients who were formerly beyond recovery, perhaps the best known is the transplantation of human organs. Yet the demand for organs continues to drastically outpace the number of organ donations. Each day about 74 people receive an organ transplant while another 17 people on the waiting list die because not enough organs are available (Figure 20-2).

Figure 20-2 The need for organ donors. As organ transplants have become an option for more and more patients, the number of people waiting for transplants has increased. The number of actual donations has not grown nearly as significantly. SOURCE: United Network for Organ Sharing (http://www.unos.org).

Since the first organ, a kidney, was successfully transplanted in 1954, the transplanting of organs into people whose organs have failed has become almost commonplace. As transplant techniques and other medical care have improved, however, an acute shortage of available organs has developed. The number of people on the waiting list for organ transplants more than tripled between 1990 and 2000, and the shortage of organs for transplant is blamed for over 6000 deaths annually.

Sources of Organs and Tissues

Organs and tissues for transplant have several sources, each with its associated challenges.

- *Self-donation (autograft).* This type of transplant involves taking part of the patient's own tissue and using it to replace damaged tissue in another area. An example of an autograft is moving skin from the thigh to replace skin elsewhere that has been burned. Autografts are free from rejection problems (described below) but obviously are not a source of replacement organs.

- *Deceased donor (cadaveric transplant).* A typical scenario for cadaveric transplant involves a young injury victim who is brain-dead but whose other organs are still functioning. Rejection is a serious problem, and attempts are made to match donors and recipients in terms of blood and immune factors.

- *Living donor.* Organs from siblings, parents, and other close relatives are less likely than cadaveric transplants to be rejected by the body of the recipient. Because of their own need, living donors can donate only bone marrow, liver lobes, lung lobes, and kidneys.

- *Animal donor (xenotransplantation).* There is a potentially much greater supply of animal organs than human organs, but xenotransplantation has both ethical and scientific problems. Organ rejection is very likely, and scientists fear the introduction of animal viruses into humans.

Except in cases of self-donation, rejection is a major problem associated with organ transplants. Rejection occurs when a patient's body recognizes a transplanted organ as foreign and the immune system attacks and destroys it. Thus, the more similar the transplanted tissue is to the patient's tissue, the less likely it is that immediate rejection will occur. Autografts are almost always successful, and tissues or organs transplanted from close relatives are the next best alternative. To help prevent rejection, transplant recipients often must take powerful drugs to suppress their immune systems.

Causes of the Organ Shortage

There are many reasons for the current shortage of donor organs. First, more people are now waiting for transplants because new technologies and drugs are keeping people with serious health problems alive longer. Another reason is good for most of us: Fewer brain-dead donors are available because the introduction of safety belts and motorcycle helmets has reduced the number of injury deaths.

The current consent system used to obtain donor organs may also contribute to shortages. Families of recently deceased patients are required to give their consent for the patient's organs to be donated to a representative of an organ procurement organization. Families often do not know the wishes of their loved ones regarding organ donation and are not likely to allow the donation if they are unsure. In addition, families may not understand or trust the medical system or the system of organ procurement.

Possible Solutions to the Organ Shortage

Several possible solutions to the donor organ shortage have been adopted or are being considered:

- Education initiatives to encourage people to talk with their families and complete organ donor cards.

- Financial or other incentives for families of donors.

- Adoption of a system of presumed consent, in which organs are donated unless the family denies permission.

- Development of transgenic animals (those that have been genetically engineered to carry human proteins instead of animal proteins) to allow broader use of xenotransplantation.

- Greater use of synthetic devices such as heart pacemakers and insulin pumps that replace specific organ functions.

- Development of bioartifical organs, which are made up of both genetically engineered living cells and mechanical components.

- Stem cells, which could eventually be used to replace cells in damaged or diseased organs.

The process of donating and receiving organs is both complex and ethically sensitive. Given the many people in need, however, the hope is that many of these potential solutions can help alleviate the organ shortage crisis in the near future. For now, individuals can increase the likelihood that their own organs will be donated by completing an organ donor card and making their wishes known to their family members.

There are currently over 85,000 Americans waiting for organ transplants, including more than 12,000 people under age 35. For more information about organ donation, see the box "What Can Be Done About the Shortage of Organ Donors?"

If you decide to become a donor, the first step is to indicate your wish by completing a **Uniform Donor Card**

Term

Uniform Donor Card A consent form authorizing the use of the signer's body parts for transplantation or medical research upon his or her death.

Organ/Tissue Donor Card

I wish to donate my organs and tissues. I wish to give:

☐ any needed organs and tissues ☐ only the following organs and tissues:

_____

Donor
Signature _____ Date _____
Witness _____
Witness _____

Figure 20-3   A sample organ/tissue donor card.   SOURCE: U.S. Department of Health and Human Services (http://www.organdonor.gov/signup1.html; retrieved February 15, 2005).

(Figure 20-3); alternatively, you can indicate your wish on your driver's license. Because relatives are called on to make decisions about organ and tissue donation at the time of a loved one's death, your second step is to discuss your decision with your family. Decisions about whether to become an organ donor are often based on both personal and cultural values.

Planning a Funeral or Memorial Service

Just as people gather to commemorate other major transitions in a person's life, such as birth and marriage, funerals and memorial services are rites of passage that commemorate a person's life in a community and acknowledge his or her passing from that community. Funerals and memorial services provide a framework that allows survivors to support one another as they cope with the fact of their loss and express their grief. The presence of death rites in every human culture suggests that they serve innate human needs.

Disposition of the Body   When a death occurs, one of the immediate concerns of survivors is the disposition of the corpse. Although corpses must be disposed of for sanitary reasons, the disposition of a body is surrounded by a web of social, cultural, religious, psychological, and interpersonal considerations that influence how this basic human task is accomplished.

People generally have a preference about the final disposition of their body. For most Americans, the choice is either burial or cremation. *Burial* usually involves a grave dug into the soil or entombment in a mausoleum. *Cremation* involves subjecting a body to intense heat, thereby reducing its organic components to a mineralized skeleton. The remaining bone fragments are then usually put through a cremulator, which reduces them to a granular state, often referred to as ashes (which actually resemble coarse coral sand). Cremated remains can be buried, placed in a columbarium niche, put into an urn kept by the family or interred in an urn garden, or scattered at sea or on land. A body destined for burial or cremation may or may not be embalmed. If the body is to be viewed during a wake or will be present at the funeral, **embalming** is generally done.

Arranging a Service   In commemorating a person's life and death, the choice of last rites may involve a traditional funeral ceremony or a simple memorial service. Whereas the casketed body is typically present at a funeral, it is not at a memorial service. In some cases, both a funeral and a memorial service are held, the former occurring within a few days after death and the latter being held sometime later (perhaps in a different town where the deceased had a large social network). Although it is

Funeral or memorial services give friends and relatives of the deceased the opportunity to mark their grief through ritual and ceremony.

A Consumer Guide to Funerals

Funerals are a consumer product. They are also among the most expensive purchases many consumers will ever make. A traditional funeral with a casket costs about $6,000, and many funerals run to $10,000 or more. When no preplanning has been done, as often occurs, family members have to make decisions under time pressure and in the grip of strong feelings. As a result, they may make poor decisions and spend more than they need to.

To avoid these problems, millions of consumers are now making funeral arrangements in advance, comparing prices and services so they can make well-informed purchasing decisions. Many people see funeral planning as an extension of will and estate planning. It is also possible to prepay some or all of the expenses involved.

A federal law called the Funeral Rule, enforced by the Federal Trade Commission, regulates the funeral provider business. It includes many requirements designed to protect consumers from unprofessional business practices. To ensure that you make the best possible decisions, follow these guidelines:

- Plan ahead. Think about what type of funeral you want—simple or elaborate, public or private, religious or secular. Do you want your funeral to be held in a house of worship, a funeral home, or a private setting? Also think about the disposition of the body—do you want your remains to be buried or cremated?

- Shop around. Look for a funeral home that belongs to the National Funeral Directors Association (NFDA), and compare prices from at least two funeral homes. You are not legally required to use a funeral home, but many people find it makes arrangements easier.

- Ask for a price list. The Funeral Rule requires funeral directors to give you an itemized price list when you ask either in person or over the telephone. Many funeral homes offer package funerals that cost less than individual items, but you may not need or want everything included in the package.

- Decide on the goods and services you want. Basic services include planning the funeral and coordinating arrangements with the cemetery or crematory. Embalming is not necessary or legally required if the body is buried or cremated shortly after death. The casket is usually the single most expensive item; an average casket costs slightly more than $2,000, but some caskets sell for as much as $10,000. You do not have to buy the casket from the funeral home you use. The Funeral Rule prohibits funeral directors from claiming that some caskets can preserve a body indefinitely; they can't.

- Resist pressure to buy goods and services you don't really want or need. Funeral directors are required to inform you that you need buy only those goods and services you want.

- In choosing a cemetery, take into consideration its location; its religious affiliation, if any; the types of monuments allowed; and cost. Visit the cemetery ahead of time to make sure it's suitable.

- Once you have made decisions, put them in writing, give copies to family members, and keep a copy accessible. It's a good idea to review your decisions every few years and revise them if necessary.

- Know the facts, including which goods and services are required by law in your state and which are optional. Many organizations provide information about making funeral arrangements; see the For More Information section at the end of the chapter.

- If you need help dealing with a funeral home, contact consumer protection agencies listed in the telephone book, the Funeral Consumer's Alliance (800-458-5563 or http://www.funerals.org), or the Funeral Service Consumer Assistance Program (800-662-7666). To file a complaint about a funeral home, contact the Federal Trade Commission at 877-FTC-HELP or http://www.ftc.gov.

SOURCES: Federal Trade Commission. 2000. *Funerals: A Consumer Guide* (http://www.ftc.gov/bcp/conline/pubs/services/funeral.htm; retrieved July 14, 2000); National Funeral Directors Association. 2000. *Ensure Wise Decision-Making: Know the Facts* (http://www.nfda.org/resources/ensure.html; retrieved July 14, 2000).

becoming more common for individuals and families to express a preference for no services, bereaved relatives and friends can derive important benefits from having an opportunity to honor the deceased and express their grief through ceremony.

Decisions about your last rites are ideally made with a view to the needs and wishes of your survivors. It can be worthwhile to consider such decisions early in life, so you can gather information about options and discuss plans with family members (see the box "A Consumer Guide to Funerals"). Religious and cultural or ethnic traditions play a major role in shaping the way people honor their dead. The diversity of life and death in the United States calls for a diversity of rites. A meaningful funeral or memorial service can be designed in many ways.

Term

embalming The process of removing blood and other fluids and replacing them with chemicals to disinfect and temporarily retard deterioration of a corpse.

Tasks for Survivors

Some of the following tasks must be attended to soon after a death occurs, whereas others take weeks or months to complete. Many of these tasks, especially those that need to be dealt with in the first hours and days following the death, can be taken care of by friends and relatives of the immediate survivors.

- Prepare a list of relatives, close friends, and business colleagues, and arrange to telephone them about the death as soon as possible. Friends can help with the notification process.

- Find out whether the deceased left instructions or made plans for disposition of the body or for a funeral or memorial service.

- If no prior plan exists, contact a mortuary or memorial society for help in making arrangements. Clergy, friends, and other family members can be asked to help decide what is most appropriate.

- If flowers are to be omitted from the funeral or memorial service, choose an appropriate charity or other memorial to which gifts can be made.

- Write the obituary. Include the deceased's age, place of birth, cause of death, occupation, academic degrees, memberships, military service record, accomplishments, names and relationships of nearest survivors, and an announcement of the time and place of the funeral or memorial service.

- Arrange for family members or close friends to take turns welcoming those who come to express their condolences in person and responding to those who telephone their condolences.

- Ask friends to help coordinate the supplying of meals for the first few days following the death, as well as the management of other household tasks and child care, if necessary.

- Arrange hospitality for relatives and friends who are visiting from out of town.

- If a funeral ceremony is planned, choose the individuals who are to be pallbearers, and notify them that you would like their participation.

- Notify the lawyer, accountant, and other personal representatives who will be helping to settle the deceased's estate.

- Send handwritten or printed notes of acknowledgment to the people who have provided assistance or who have sent flowers, contributions, or their condolences.

- With the help of a lawyer or an accountant, review all insurance policies as well as other sources of potential death benefits, such as Social Security, military service, fraternal organizations, and unions.

- Review all debts, mortgages, and installment payments. Some may carry clauses that cancel debt in the event of death. If payments must be delayed, contact creditors to arrange for a grace period.

Costs also may influence the choices people make for last rites. The typical cost of a funeral, not including cemetery costs, is about $5000–$7000. More than $2000 of this cost can go toward purchase of a casket, which people usually feel is the centerpiece of a funeral due to its symbolic and emotional significance in honoring the deceased. Less expensive options for disposal of the body include direct cremation or immediate burial, both of which involve no viewing and no funeral ceremony. Although both of these options are generally available from mortuaries that also offer traditional funeral services, people who prefer a no-frills approach may have the option of arranging economic burial or cremation through a nonprofit **memorial society.** Veterans are eligible for burial in a national cemetery, an option that can also reduce costs.

The bottom line is that a wide range of options is available to meet consumers' diverse needs and wishes. Making at least some plans ahead of time and discussing the options with family members can help reduce the burden on survivors who find themselves facing a number of tasks and decisions once death occurs (see the box "Tasks for Survivors").

COPING WITH DYING

There is no one right way to live with or die of a life-threatening illness. Every disease has its own set of problems and challenges, and each person copes with these problems and challenges in his or her own way. It is said that doctors treat *disease;* people suffer from *illness.* Much of the suffering experienced by people with a life-threatening illness comes from overwhelming feelings of loss on all levels. Besides the emotional havoc accompanying news of a potentially life-ending disease, there are usually concerns about costly medical care, loss of income, repeated and perhaps lengthy hospitalization, and physical pain. How a person copes with such an experience is likely to reflect his or her personality and life history, as well as the nature of family relationships and patterns of interaction in the person's wider social environment.

Awareness of Dying

Living with an illness that is life-threatening and incurable can be described as a living-dying experience. From the time discomforting symptoms are first noticed and a person's worst fears confirmed by a diagnosis, through the ups and downs of treatment, and on to the final days or hours of life, hope and honesty are often delicately balanced—honesty to face reality as it is, hope for a positive outcome. The object of hope changes. The early hope that the symptoms are not really serious gives way to hope that a cure is possible. When the illness is deemed incurable, there is hope for more time. As time begins to run out, one hopes for a pain-free death, a "good death."

Psychiatrist Avery Weisman described this process of coping as involving **middle knowledge,** with patients and their families seeking a balance between sustaining hope and acknowledging the reality. Maintaining a sense of self-worth, setting goals and striving to reach them, engaging in fruitful interactions with one's environment—all of these reflect a coping strength that sustains the will to live fully despite a bleak prognosis.

The Tasks of Coping

In her 1969 book *On Death and Dying,* Elisabeth Kübler-Ross suggested that the response to an awareness of imminent death involves five psychological stages: denial, anger, bargaining, depression, and acceptance. The notion that these five stages occur in a linear progression has since become a kind of modern myth of how people *ought* to cope with dying. Unfortunately, this can lead to the idea that it is a person's task to move sequentially through these stages, one after another, and that if this is not accomplished, the person has somehow failed. In fact, however, Kübler-Ross said that individuals go back and forth among the stages during the course of an illness and different stages can occur simultaneously.

The stage-based model devised by Kübler-Ross more than three decades ago has been a stimulus toward a better understanding of how people cope with dying. The notion of stages, however, has been deemphasized in favor of highlighting the tasks that deserve attention in coping with a life-threatening illness. Charles Corr, for example, distinguishes four primary dimensions in coping with dying:

1. *Physical:* Satisfying bodily needs and minimizing physical distress
2. *Psychological:* Maximizing a sense of security, self-worth, autonomy, and richness in living
3. *Social:* Sustaining significant relationships and addressing the social implications of dying
4. *Spiritual:* Identifying, developing, or reaffirming sources of meaning and fostering hope

Contemplating these dimensions gives us a framework for considering the specific tasks that need to be addressed in coping with dying. In addition to an *acute* phase initiated by the diagnosis, a *chronic* phase of living with the disease, and a *terminal* phase that involves coping with

impending death, there are sometimes two other phases: first, a *prediagnostic* phase, during which a person suspects the illness and may seek medical attention; and, second, a *recovery* phase following a cure or remission of a previously life-threatening disease. Even as the threat of dying recedes into the background, however, there can be a need to cope with the fact that one has had a potentially terminal illness.

In addition, though, we must remember that a person's death is as unique as his or her life. Thus, although models can help us gain understanding, they need to be balanced by paying attention to the dying person's own unfolding *life* story. Each person's pathway through life-threatening illness is determined by factors such as the specific disease and its course, his or her personality, and the available supportive resources (see the box "In Search of a Good Death" on p. 618).

People who apparently cope best with life-threatening illness often exhibit a fighting spirit that views the illness not only as a threat but also as a challenge. These people strive to inform themselves about their illness and take an active part in treatment decisions. They are optimistic and have a capacity to discover positive meaning in ordinary events. Holding to a positive outlook despite distressing circumstances involves creating a sense of meaning that is bigger than the threat. In the context of life-threatening illness, this encompasses a person's ability to comprehend the implications an illness has for the future, as well as for his or her ability to accomplish goals, maintain relationships, and sustain a sense of personal vitality, competence, and power. Although life-threatening illness disrupts virtually all aspects of a person's life, there is a vital link between finding meaning and achieving a sense of mastery.

The Trajectory of Dying

Our expectations about dying may be quite different from what most people actually experience. The concept of a **trajectory of dying** is useful for understanding patients' experiences as they near death. Although sudden death from an unexpected cause—a massive heart attack or an accident, for example—is one type of dying trajectory, our focus here is on deaths that occur when there is forewarning. Among

Mind/Body/Spirit

What does it mean to die a "good death"? Participants in a recent study were asked to discuss the deaths of family members, friends, or patients and reflect on what made those deaths good or bad. From these discussions and interviews, six major themes emerged as components of a good death.

The first component was pain and symptom management. Many people fear dying in pain, and portrayals of bad deaths usually included inadequate pain management. Every health care provider in the study told regret-filled stories of patients who died in pain. Patients were concerned with both current and future pain control; when reassured that pain could be managed with drugs, they were less anxious.

The second component of a good death was clear decision making. Both providers and families feared entering a medical crisis without knowledge of patient preferences. Patients and families who had good communication with health care providers and had discussed treatment decisions ahead of time felt empowered, and providers felt they were giving good care. Researchers noted that although all uncertainty about end-of-life decisions cannot be eliminated, tolerance for uncertainty may increase if values and preferences are clarified.

The third component was preparation for death. Patients expressed satisfaction when they had adequate time to prepare

their wills and help plan the events that would follow their death, such as funeral arrangements. Many times, providers avoided end-of-life discussions to prevent their patients from losing hope, thus depriving them of the opportunity to plan ahead. Patients and families also wanted to know what to expect during the course of the illness and what physical and psychosocial changes would take place as death approached. It was important for providers and families to have reached some personal comfort with death so they felt prepared when death occurred.

The fourth component was completion, the opportunity to review one's life, to resolve conflicts, to spend time with loved ones, and to say good-bye. Participants confirmed the deep importance of spirituality or meaningfulness at the end of life. Many times, patients were able to view their experience of dying as part of a broader life trajectory and thus continue to grow emotionally and spiritually in their last days. Issues of faith were often mentioned as important to healing, but participants emphasized that the cues about the particular expression of faith must be taken from the patient.

The fifth component was contributing to others. Patients wanted to know that they still had something to offer to others, whether it was making someone laugh or lightening the load of someone closer to death. Many patients found that as they

reflected on their lives, what they valued most was their personal relationships with family and friends, and they were anxious to impart this wisdom to others.

The sixth component of a good death was affirmation of the whole person. Patients appreciated empathic health care providers, and family members were comforted by those who treated their loved ones as unique and whole people, rather than as a disease. The quality of dying is related to the acknowledgment that people die in character, that is, as an extension of who they have been in their lives. Health care providers also focused on their personal relationships with patients and family members as important to a satisfying death.

The study affirmed that most people think of death as a natural part of life, not as a failure of technology. Although the biomedical aspects of end-of-life care are crucial, they merely provide a point of departure toward a good death. When pain is properly managed and the practical aspects of dying are taken care of, patients and their families have the opportunity to address the important emotional, psychological, and spiritual issues that all human beings face at the end of life.

SOURCE: Steinhauser, K. S., et al. 2000. In search of a good death: Observations of patients, families, and providers. *Annals of Internal Medicine* 132(10): 825–832.

these, some trajectories involve a steady and fairly predictable decline. This is the case with many cancers, which tend to follow the course of a progressive disease with a terminal phase. Other kinds of advanced, chronic illness involve a long period of slow decline marked by episodes of crisis, the last of which proves to be "suddenly" fatal.

We can also distinguish between different stages in a dying trajectory, namely, a period when a person is known to be terminally ill but is living with a life expectancy of perhaps weeks or months, possibly years and a later period when dying is imminent and the person is described as actively dying. The way in which such trajectories are estimated—their duration and expected course—can affect both patients and caregivers and influence their actions. Deaths that occur out of time (too quickly or too slowly) may pose special difficulties.

When a person is actively dying, his or her death is expected to occur within hours or, at most, a few days. During the last phase of a fatal illness, a dying person may exhibit irregular breathing or shortness of breath, decreased appetite and thirst, nausea and vomiting, incontinence, restlessness and agitation, disorientation and confusion, and diminished consciousness. These symptoms usually can be managed by skilled palliative care. Pain, if it is present, should be treated aggressively as part of a comprehensive approach to comfort care. Since most patients are more comfortable without eating or drinking at the end of life, forcing food or liquids is usually not beneficial. The stopping of eating and drinking has always been part of the last phase of a terminal condition. Near the time of death, relaxation of the throat muscles or secretions in the throat may cause the person's breathing to become noisy, resulting in a sound called the death rattle. Most dying patients are not aware of this noisy breathing. If it unnerves family or caregivers, giving medication or repositioning the person can help. Just before death, the person may take a breath and sigh or shudder.

When a family member or close friend is dying, people often feel that they should be at the bedside at the very moment of death. This is not always possible, however, because the exact timing of death is difficult to predict. Sometimes people keep a deathwatch for days. Then, when they step out briefly for a break, the person dies. Perhaps this phenomenon is just a matter of chance, or perhaps it is the case that the dying person was waiting for a moment to be on her own before letting go.

Supporting a Dying Person

People often feel uncomfortable in the presence of a person who is close to dying. What can we say? How should we act? It may seem that any attempt to be comforting could result only in words that are little more than stale platitudes. Yet we want to express concern and establish meaningful contact with the person who is facing death. In such circumstances, the most important gift we can bring is that of listening. Offering the dying person opportunities to speak openly and honestly about his or her experience can be crucial, even when such conversation is initially painful.

We tend to place dying people in a special category, but the reality is that their needs are not fundamentally different from anyone else's, although their situation is perhaps more urgent. Dying people need to know that they are valued, that they are not alone, that they are not being unfairly judged, and that those closest to them are also striving to come to terms with a difficult situation. As with any relationship, there are opportunities for growth on both sides.

Besides friends and family, the dying person may need other supportive resources. These may include counselors and clergy. Many hospitals, hospices, and other health care providers sponsor programs for dying patients and their families, offering opportunities for them to share their concerns in a supportive and validating atmosphere. Programs of this kind can be located by asking hospital staff or other medical personnel. Local chapters of support groups affiliated with organizations such as the American Cancer Society and Make Today Count also can be found in many cities.

In supporting someone who is facing the prospect of dying from a terminal illness, the most important thing is simply to be there for the person and his or her family. Listen more than talk. At the same time, remember to take care of yourself. Especially if you are a member of the caregiving team, be sure to make time for yourself. To accomplish this, it may be necessary to find others to help you. It can be important to strengthen your own support system even as you offer support.

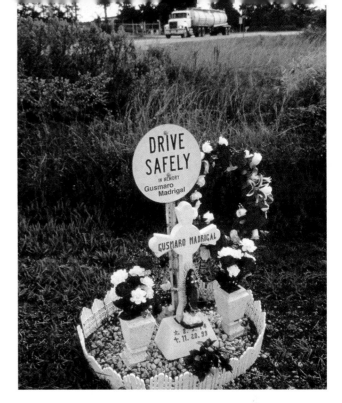

Death, particularly the sudden death of a young person, can challenge our sense of emotional and intellectual security. This roadside marker was placed in memory of a young man killed in an automobile crash at this site.

COPING WITH LOSS

Even if we have not experienced the death of someone close, we are all survivors of losses that occur in our lives because of changes and endings. The loss of a job, the ending of a relationship, transitions from one school or neighborhood to another—these are examples of the kinds of losses that occur in all our lives. Such losses are sometimes called little deaths, and, in varying degrees, they all involve grief.

Experiencing Grief

Grief is the reaction to loss. It encompasses thoughts and feelings, as well as physical and behavioral responses. Mental distress may involve disbelief, confusion, anxiety, disorganization, and depression. The emotions that can be present in normal grief include not only sorrow and sadness, but also relief, anger, and self-pity, among others. Bereaved people experience a range of feelings, even conflicting ones. Recognizing that grief can involve many

Term

V∤w

grief A person's reaction to loss as manifested physically, emotionally, mentally, and behaviorally.

Chapter 20   Dying and Death   619

Loss of a loved one can be a challenging and difficult process that generates for nearly everyone a broad range of reactions—physical, emotional, and behavioral. But, we might ask ourselves, do women and men typically react differently to the loss of someone close to them? Some clinicians say yes, and studies now support the idea that there can be different gender patterns in grief.

Data suggest that a greater proportion of women may be vulnerable to the more distressing and disruptive symptoms characteristic of severe grief reactions. It is important to note that, in general, women have a higher lifetime incidence and prevalence of depressive and anxiety disorders (see Chapter 3). It is thus not surprising that at times of great stress, such as the loss of a loved one, these gender differences in vulnerabilities to depression and anxiety would be present.

In a study of gender differences in grief among parents who have lost a child, researchers found that compared with fathers, mothers showed greater feelings of being hurt, cheated, and depressed,

while also revealing greater irritability and anger. The women also cried more, experienced greater numbness and confusion, were more preoccupied with thoughts of the deceased, and felt more guilt both for having failed to prevent the death and for having survived. Compared with men, they also experienced more physical symptoms such as insomnia and loss of appetite.

In another study that involved people who had lost a spouse, researchers similarly found that women had a higher level of emotional distress in reaction to loss. Women who lost a husband had higher levels of traumatic grief, depression, and anxiety than men who had lost a wife. These findings persisted through at least the first 2 years following the death of the spouse.

It is difficult and controversial to speculate on the basis of such gender differences in grief, although it is likely that many factors contribute. Physiological factors might include hormonal differences, subtle differences in brain chemistry or function, or genetic influences.

Gender roles and cultural expectations also likely play a role. Despite some change over recent decades, it is still probably not as accepted for men to reveal strong emotions or vulnerability as it is for women to do so. Women are often readier to express emotion and seek out social support and opportunities to talk about loss, whereas men may be more reticent to admit to any psychological distress or allow the appearance of excessive emotionality.

Are these differences primarily related to biology, or do cultural and social influences play a greater role? These questions need to be studied further. It is clear, however, that gender can play an important role in the reaction to loss.

SOURCES: Cole, M. G., et al. 2003. Risk factors for depression among elderly community subjects: A systematic review and meta-analysis. *American Journal of Psychiatry* 160: 1147–1156; Chen, J. H., et al. 1999. Gender differences in the effects of bereavement-related psychological distress in health outcomes. *Psychological Medicine* 29: 367–380; Schwab, R. 1996. Gender differences in parental grief. *Death Studies* 20(2): 103–113.

different feelings—not just sadness—makes us more able to cope with it. Common behaviors associated with grief include crying, searching for the deceased, and talking incessantly about the deceased and the circumstances of the death. Bereaved people may be restless, as if not knowing what to do with themselves. Physically, grief may involve frequent sighing, insomnia, and loss of appetite. Grief may also evoke a reexamination of religious or spiritual beliefs as a person struggles to make meaning of the loss. All such manifestations of grief can be present as part of one's total response to **bereavement**—that is, the event of loss.

Mourning is closely related to grief and is often used as a synonym for it. However, mourning refers not so much to the *reaction* to loss but to the *process* by which a bereaved person adjusts to loss and incorporates it into his or her life. How this process is managed is determined, at least partly, by cultural and gender norms for the expression of grief (see the box "Grief and Gender"). Considered jointly, grief and mourning are the means to healing the pain of loss.

Tasks of Mourning   Experiencing grief is part of the process by which a bereaved person integrates a signifi-

cant loss into his or her life. Psychologist William Worden has identified four tasks that must be attended to:

1. *Accepting the reality* of the loss
2. *Working through the pain* of grief
3. *Adjusting to a changed environment* in which the deceased is absent
4. *Emotionally relocating the deceased and moving on with life*

Accomplishing the fourth task does not mean dishonoring the deceased's memory or denying normal feelings of connection that persist beyond death. Finding healthy ways to maintain bonds with the deceased is a testimony to the enduring strength of love. When this task is managed successfully, however, the bereaved is not stuck in the past. Making the journey of grief and attending to the various tasks along the way, we come to a place where we learn how to keep a special place for the deceased in our hearts and memories while moving forward with our lives.

The Course of Grief   Grieving, like dying, is highly individual. In the first hours or days following a death, a bereaved person is likely to experience overwhelming shock and numbness, as well as a sense of disbelief. There is often a period of denial—"No! This can't be true!"—especially if the death was unexpected. Consider the ways in which people die: the aged grandmother, dying quietly in her sleep; the young child pronounced DOA after a bicycle crash; the despondent executive who commits suicide; a young soldier killed in battle; the chronically ill person who dies a lingering death. The cause or mode of death—natural, accidental, homicide, or suicide—has an influence on how grief is experienced (see the box "Profound Trauma and Loss" on p. 622). Even when a death is anticipated, grief is not necessarily diminished when the loss becomes real.

The sense of disorganization experienced by survivors during the early period of grief is set against the need to attend to decisions and actions surrounding the disposition of the deceased's body. As family and friends gather to offer mutual support, funeral ceremonies are held. Engaging in such activities promotes accepting the reality of the death and moving beyond the initial shock and numbness.

In its middle phase, the course of grief is characterized by anxiety, apathy, and pining for the deceased. The pangs of grief are felt as the bereaved person deeply experiences the pain of separation. There is often a sense of despair as a person repeatedly goes over the events surrounding the loss, perhaps fantasizing that somehow everything could be undone and be as it was before. During this period, the bereaved also begins looking toward the future and taking the first steps toward building a life without the deceased.

This can be a difficult time in grieving. Yet the bereaved often find themselves without the social support of the relatives and friends who were present during the initial period. Grief occurs within a particular social or cultural context, and individual grievers differ in their particular styles of grieving. This leads to the recognition that there is no standard way of coping with loss. Colin Murray Parkes points to three main influences on a person's course of grieving:

1. The urge to look back, cry, and search for what is lost

2. The urge to look forward, explore the world that emerges out of the loss, and discover what can be carried forward from the past into the future

3. The social and cultural pressures that influence how the first two urges are inhibited or expressed

As these influences interact in various ways, at times the bereaved tries to avoid the pain of grief and at other times confronts it. The goal is to achieve a balance between avoidance and confrontation that facilitates coming to terms with the loss. Attaining this goal can be seen as an oscillation between what Margaret Stroebe and Henk Schut call loss-oriented and restoration-oriented mourning. From this perspective, looking at old photographs and yearning for the deceased are examples of loss-oriented coping, whereas doing what is needed to reorganize life in the wake of the loss—for example, learning to do tasks that the deceased had always managed, such as finances or cooking—is part of restoration-oriented coping.

There is no predetermined timetable for completing this mourning process. In moving toward the restoration of one's well-being, however, the last phase of active grief involves coming to a sense of resolution. The acute pain and emotional turmoil of grief subside. Physical and mental balance is reestablished. The bereaved becomes increasingly reintegrated into his or her social world. Sadness doesn't go away completely, but it recedes into the background. Although reminders of the loss stimulate active grieving from time to time, the main focus is the present, not the past. Adjusting to loss may sometimes feel like a betrayal of the deceased loved one, but it is healthy to engage again in ongoing life and the future (see the box "Coping with Grief" on p. 623).

Coming to terms with loss doesn't mean forgetting the loved one or minimizing the significance of the lost relationship. Rather, making the journey of grief allows us to incorporate the loss into our lives. We learn to maintain connections with deceased loved ones through memories and other means that sustain relationships beyond the grave. The course of grief has no absolute end point as long as we keep the deceased alive in our memories.

Supporting a Grieving Person

In experiencing a significant loss, a person initially may feel and behave much like a frightened, helpless child. He or she may respond best to the kind of loving support that is given by a parent. A hug may be more comforting than any words. Also, because talking about a loss is an important way that survivors cope with the changed reality, simply listening can be very helpful. The key to being a good listener is to refrain from making judgments about whether the feelings expressed by a survivor are right or wrong, good or bad. The emotions, thoughts, and behaviors evoked by loss may not be the ones we expect, but they can nonetheless be valid and appropriate within a survivor's experience of loss.

Terms

Vìw

bereavement The objective event of loss.

mourning The process whereby a person actively copes with grief in adjusting to a loss and integrating it into his or her life.

Profoundly traumatic events such as the devastation caused by the tsunami in Southeast Asia, the terrorist attacks on the World Trade Center, or the ongoing deaths in combat in the war in Iraq all represent a category of loss far beyond normal comprehension. Experiencing traumatic loss in such extraordinary circumstances can cause severe and disruptive reactions in emotion and behavior.

World War I soldiers fighting in brutal trench warfare witnessed multiple horrific deaths and suffered through persistent fear of sudden, unexpected, painful death. Significant numbers of veterans of such traumatic events developed psychological symptoms that collectively were described as shell shock. However, it was not until after the Vietnam War that the medical community became fully aware of how disruptive and enduring the psychological effects could be for those experiencing profound traumatic loss.

It is now widely recognized that significant psychological symptoms can follow the experiencing of loss in traumatic circumstances. Elements commonly seen in a customary reaction to grief, such as sadness, disbelief, crying, insomnia, and loss of appetite, are frequently exaggerated in the aftermath of profoundly traumatic events and will often include more pronounced symptoms, such as overwhelming distress, numbness, doubt, despair, guilt, and disabling depression and anxiety.

Depending on the severity of exposure and a person's underlying vulnerability, the symptoms can persist long after the original trauma. Memories and images of the event may suddenly pop into the victim's mind, causing anxiety, depression, and anger. Insomnia and nightmares can disrupt the sleep-wake cycle. The person may start avoiding everything that serves as a reminder of the event and, as a kind of self-protection, may begin to become numb, to lose all feelings. Such people may startle easily and have difficulty concentrating. Their work life, social life, and intimate relationships may become markedly impaired. People experiencing these severe symptoms are said to have post-traumatic stress disorder (PTSD), which can persist for months or years.

The events of September 11, 2001, are an example of a profound trauma that caused PTSD in affected people. As described in Chapter 3, PTSD symptoms occurred among survivors, rescue workers, passersby, residents of Manhattan, and some people exposed to the events through repeated television images. Researchers who interviewed residents of Manhattan found that about 7.5% reported symptoms consistent with a diagnosis of PTSD and 9.7% reported symptoms consistent with new onset of depression; these numbers are about twice as high as the expected rates in surveys of this type. Among people who lived closest to the World Trade Center, the prevalence of PTSD was as high as 20%.

Another dramatic example, which bears similarities to the 2004 tsunami in Southeast Asia, is the flood that devastated the 17 communities of Buffalo Creek, West Virginia, on February 26, 1972. Following several days of rain, a dam owned by a coal company burst and released millions of gallons of black water—a wall of water described by some to be 30 feet high. Survivors of the flood described scenes similar to the 2004 tsunami—houses pushed from their foundations and thrown against one another, railroad tracks torn from the ground, and children swept from the arms of parents. Nearly 60% of survivors of the tragedy developed PTSD; and in 25% of survivors, PTSD persisted at least 14 years after the flood.

It is important to note that these statistics do not include all the psychological damage such events may cause. Many people experience disabling depression or anxiety but do not meet the full criteria for PTSD. More persistent and severe grief reactions, unexplained physical symptoms, and the increased use of alcohol and drugs are frequent occurrences for people who have undergone such trauma. In addition, family and interpersonal conflict and financial strain are commonly seen. All too frequently, in war or natural disasters, the primary wage earner of the family dies or the family's house and belongings are destroyed.

How long will an individual's symptoms last after experiencing an event like September 11 or witnessing a friend killed by a roadside bomb in Iraq? Factors such as the severity of the trauma, the individual's proximity to the event, and his or her emotional closeness to those who have died can all play important roles in the magnitude and duration of the reaction to traumatic loss. In general, though, symptoms will diminish with time, especially in the absence of new threats and traumatic losses. Studies of those who have developed full-blown PTSD suggest that approximately half of the cases resolve within 2 years but that nearly a third never fully recover.

Psychological support and treatment can greatly help many of those who suffer from disabling emotional symptoms in reaction to traumatic loss. Building on research and work done with Vietnam veterans in the 1970s and 1980s, clinicians have developed multiple therapeutic strategies involving group therapy, individual psychological support, and pharmacologic intervention to treat persistent symptoms.

What to do in the immediate aftermath of a profoundly traumatic event is more controversial. Some studies suggest that early debriefing by well-trained clinicians can be helpful in reducing the risk of disabling symptoms; others argue that premature therapeutic intervention can actually increase the likelihood of PTSD. However, it is clear that for individuals who develop significant and enduring emotional reactions to traumatic loss, treatment by mental health professionals can help alleviate symptoms and restore well-being to their lives.

SOURCES: Galea, S., and H. Resnick. 2005. Posttraumatic stress disorder in the general population after mass terrorist incidents: Considerations about the nature of exposure. *CNS Spectrums* 10(2): 107–115; Galea, S., et al. 2002. Psychological sequelae of the September 11 terrorist attacks in New York City. *New England Journal of Medicine* 346(13): 982–987; Shuster, M., et al. 2001. A national survey of stress reactions after the September 11, 2001, terrorist attacks. *New England Journal of Medicine* 345(20): 1507–1512; Ornstein, R. D., and R. K. Pitman, section eds. 2000. Trauma and post-traumatic stress disorder. In *Massachusetts General Hospital Psychiatry Update and Board Preparation*, 2nd ed., eds. T. A. Stern and J. B. Herman. New York: McGraw-Hill; Gorman, J. M., section ed. 2000. Anxiety disorders. In *Kaplan and Sadock's Comprehensive Textbook of Psychiatry*, 7th ed., eds. B. J. Sadock and V. A. Sadock. Baltimore: Lippincott Williams and Wilkins. *Buffalo Creek Flood Disaster February 26, 1972* (http://www. rootsweb.com/~wvlogan/buffalo.htm; retrieved January 5, 2005).

Coping with Grief

- Recognize and acknowledge the loss.
- React to grief by accepting and expressing it.
- Take time for nature's process of healing.
- Know that powerful, overwhelming feelings will change with time.
- Review and remember the relationship with the deceased.
- Share your pain by accepting support from others.
- Surround yourself with life: plants, animals, friends.
- Make use of mementos to promote your mourning, not to live in the past.

- Avoid major decisions, if possible, and give yourself time to readjust.
- Adapt to a new world without forgetting the old.
- Prepare for change, new interests, new friends, creativity, and growth.
- Reinvest in life.

SOURCES: The Centre for Living with Dying (554 Mansion Park Dr., Santa Clara, CA 95054; 408-980-9801); Rando, T. A. 1993. *The Treatment of Complicated Mourning*. Champaign, Ill.: Research Press.

Talking and crying, even yelling in rage, are among the ways of coping with intense feelings of grief. Bereaved persons should not be urged to hold back their feelings or to be strong and brave. Expressions of grief are healing. On the other hand, if strong emotions aren't expressed, the bereaved need not pretend to grieve or exaggerate his or her feelings to satisfy others' expectations. Funerals and other leave-taking ceremonies generally help survivors gain a sense of closure and begin to integrate a loss into their lives. For some, funerals are occasions of weeping and wailing; for others, stoic and subdued emotions are the rule. Different styles of mourning behavior can be equally valid and appropriate.

Social support is as critical during the later course of grief as it is during the first days after a loss. Bereaved people need the reliable support of those they trust. In offering support, we can reassure them that grief is normal and confirm that it is permissible and appropriate to express grief. They may also need permission to occasionally give themselves a break from grieving. As they move forward in life, the bereaved may need encouragement from others to face the world confidently. An extended need for support often continues through the first year or two of mourning. The first anniversary following a significant loss can be a time of renewed grieving when the support of others is important and appreciated. Knowing that others remember and acknowledge the loss and that they take time to touch base is usually perceived as very helpful.

Besides the support from individuals who are part of their social network, bereaved people may want to share their stories and concerns through organized support groups, such as those intended for widowed persons. Many support groups are organized around a focus for some specific type of bereavement. Compassionate Friends, for example, is a nationwide organization composed of parents who have experienced a child's death.

Referrals to support groups for bereaved people are available through community service organizations.

Helping Children Cope with Loss

Children tend to cope with loss in a healthier fashion when they are included as part of their family's experience of grief and mourning. Although adults may be uncomfortable about sharing potentially disturbing or painful news with children, a child's natural curiosity usually negates the option of withholding information. Sudden changes in family communication patterns without any explanation can alarm a child and create anxiety. When children are asked about their experiences of family crises involving death, many say that the most difficult times occurred when they did not know what was happening. Thus, the question is How should we offer our help to a child who is bereaved?

In talking about death with children, the most important guideline is to be honest. Set the explanation you are offering at the child's level of understanding. Children generalize from familiar concepts to make new experiences fit. We don't want to overwhelm a child with excessive detail, but we must beware of talking down to the child as if he or she were incapable of any comprehension. In general, it's advisable to keep the explanation simple, stick to basics, and verify what the child has understood from your explanation. A child's readiness for more details can usually be assessed by paying attention to his or her questions.

COMING TO TERMS WITH DEATH

We may wish we could keep death out of view and not make a place for it in our lives. But this wish cannot be fulfilled. With the death of a beloved friend or relative, we are confronted with emotions and thoughts that relate not only to the immediate loss but also to our own mortality.

Our encounters with dying and death teach us that relationships are more important than things and that life offers no guarantees. In discovering the meaning of death in our own lives, we find that life is both precious and precarious.

Allowing ourselves to make room for death, we discover that it touches not only the dying or bereaved person and his or her family and friends, but also the wider community of which we are all part. We recognize that dying and death offer opportunities for extraordinary growth in the midst of loss. Denying death, it turns out, results in denying life.

SUMMARY

- Although death makes rational sense in terms of species survival and evolution, there may be no completely satisfying answer to the question of why death exists from a personal point of view.

- Dying and death are more than biological events; they have social and spiritual dimensions.

- The traditional criteria for determining death focus on vital signs such as breathing and heartbeat. Brain death is characterized by a lack of physical responses other than breathing and heartbeat.

- Between ages 5 and 9, most children develop a mature understanding of death; that is, they come to understand death as final, universal, and inevitable.

- A mature understanding of death can include ideas about the survival of the human personality after death.

- Problems arise when avoidance or denial of death fosters the notion that it happens only to others.

- Many basic tasks in preparing for death can and should be accomplished while one is young.

- A will is a legal instrument that governs the distribution of a person's estate after death.

- End-of-life care may involve a combination of home care, hospital stays, and hospice or palliative care.

- Palliative care is devoted to making dying patients comfortable by controlling pain and relieving suffering.

- Hospice programs apply a team-oriented approach to caring for dying patients and their families with the goal of helping people live as fully as possible until the end of their lives.

- Exercising choices about end-of-life care can involve making decisions about prolonging life or hastening death.

- The practice of withholding or withdrawing potentially life-sustaining treatment is sometimes termed passive euthanasia.

- Physician-assisted suicide occurs when a physician provides lethal drugs or other interventions, at a patient's request, with the understanding that the patient plans to use them to end his or her life. Voluntary active euthanasia refers to the intentional ending of a patient's life, at his or her request, by someone other than the patient.

- Advance directives, such as living wills and health care proxies, are used to express one's wishes about the use of life-sustaining treatment.

- People can donate their bodies or specific organs for transplantation and other medical uses after death.

- For Americans, the decision about what to do with the body after death usually involves either burial or cremation.

- Bereaved people usually benefit from participating in a funeral or memorial service to commemorate a loved one's death.

- Coping with dying involves physical, psychological, social, and spiritual dimensions.

- It is useful for patients and caregivers to understand the trajectory, or course, of dying.

- In offering support to a dying person, the gift of listening can be especially important.

- Grief encompasses thoughts and feelings, as well as physical and behavioral responses.

- Mourning, the process by which a person integrates a loss into his or her life, is determined partly by social and cultural norms for expressing grief.

- Children tend to cope with death in a healthier fashion when they are included in their family's experience of grief and mourning.

- Dying and death offer opportunities for growth in the midst of loss.

1. **Consider organ donation:** In most states, the Department of Motor Vehicles provides organ donor forms. You can also request a donor form or download one from the National Kidney Foundation (800-622-9010; http://www.kidney.org), the Coalition on Donation (800-355-7427; http://www.shareyourlife.org), or the Department of Health and Human Services (http://www.organdonor.gov). When you receive your donor form, consider the advantages and disadvantages of becoming a donor. If you decide to be a donor, fill out the card and keep it with your driver's license. Discuss your decision with members of your family. If your state has an organ donor registry, sign up.

2. **Review an advance directive:** Obtain sample copies of advance directives that are appropriate for the state you live in. Check with your local hospital or health services organization for these forms, or request them from the National Hospice and Palliative Care Organization (800-658-8898; http://www.nhpco.org). Review the forms and consider the advantages and disadvantages of using them. If you decide to execute a living will or health care proxy, discuss your decision with members of your family and anyone else who might become involved in your health care.

3. **Discuss end-of-life care:** Talk with your parents, grandparents, spouse, or other family members about their wishes for care at the end of their lives. Ask if they have made wills or completed advance directives. If they do not wish to discuss these matters, let them know that you are open to such a discussion in the future.

4. **Visit a hospice:** Visiting a hospice or speaking with someone who works in a hospice is a good way to learn more about the process of death and dying and how such a setting can support patient and family in making a more peaceful and meaningful death where dignity and connection with loved ones is carefully preserved. To find a hospice close to you, visit the Web site for the National Hospice and Palliative Care Organization (www.nhpco.org). Click on "Find a Provider" and then "Hospice Program." After you enter your zip code, the site will provide contact information for the hospices nearest to you.

For More Information

Books

Albom, M. 2002. *Tuesdays with Morrie: An Old Man, A Young Man, and Life's Greatest Lesson.* New York: Broadway Books. *A young man reconnects with an old professor in his last months of life and learns some of the greatest lessons that life has to offer.*

Armstrong, L., and S. Jenkins. 2001. *It's Not About the Bike: My Journey Back to Life.* New York: Berkley. *An inspirational story about a world champion athlete battling cancer to go on to win the most celebrated bicycle race in the world.*

Batuello, J. T. 2003. *End of Life Decisions: A Practical Guide.* College Station, Tx.: Virtualbookworm. *A guide to end-of-life decisions, including those related to pain relief and palliative and hospice care.*

Callanan, M., and P. Kelly. 1997. *Final Gifts: Understanding the Special Awareness, Needs, and Communication of the Dying.* New York: Bantam. *A moving book that uses case stories to show how approaching death can give clarity and meaning to how we relate to one another; also gives many practical suggestions about how we can respond to the needs of the dying.*

Colby, W. H. 2003. *Long Goodbye: The Deaths of Nancy Cruzan.* Carlsbad, Calif.: Hay House. *A close-up look at a key case that helped define medical and legal issues related to brain death.*

DeSpelder, L. A., and A. L. Strickland. 2005. *The Last Dance: Encountering Death and Dying,* 7th ed. New York: McGraw-Hill. *A comprehensive and readable text highlighting a broad range of topics related to dying and death.*

Doka, K. J. 1998. *Living with Life-Threatening Illness: A Guide for Patients, Their Families, and Caregivers.* San Francisco: Jossey-Bass. *Sheds light on coping with life-threatening illness, from diagnosis through treatment to eventual recovery or impending death.*

Kübler-Ross, E., and D. Kessler. 2001. *Life Lessons: Two Experts on Death and Dying Teach Us About the Mysteries of Life and Living.* New York: Scribner. *Essays and personal accounts about lessons the living can learn from the dying.*

Mitford, J. 2000. *The American Way of Death Revisited.* Reprint Edition. New York: Vintage. *A scathing, witty exposé of the funeral industry, updated from the 1963 classic.*

Silverman, P. R. 2000. *Never Too Young to Know: Death in Children's Lives.* New York: Oxford University Press. *A compassionate book that challenges mistaken beliefs about how children cope with grief and loss.*

Williams, H., ed. 2003. *Archaeologies of Remembrance: Death and Memory in Past Societies.* New York: Plenum. *An interesting look at the treatment of death and remembrance in past societies.*

Organizations and Web Sites

Association for Death Education and Counseling (ADEC). Provides resources for education, bereavement counseling, and care of the dying.
    860-586-7503
    http://www.adec.org

Caregiver Survival Resources. Designed to help people cope with the demands of caregiving.
    http://www.caregiver911.com

The Dougy Center. Offers education about childhood bereavement and support groups for bereaved children.
    866-775-5683
    http://www.dougy.org

Dying Well. A Web site focused on wellness through the end of life.
    http://www.dyingwell.com

GriefNet. A site where you can communicate with others via e-mail support groups in the areas of death, grief, and major loss.
    http://www.griefnet.org

Growth House. Offers an extensive directory of Internet resources relating to life-threatening illness and end-of-life care.

http://www.growthhouse.org

Hospice Foundation of America. Promotes the hospice concept of care through education and leadership.

800-854-3402

http://www.hospicefoundation.org

Longwood College Library: Doctor Assisted Suicide—A Guide to Web Sites and the Literature. Information on physician-assisted suicide and links to related sites.

http://web.lwc.edu/administrative/library/suic.htm

National Funeral Directors Association (NFDA). Provides resources related to funerals and funeral costs, body disposition, and bereavement support.

800-228-6332

http://www.nfda.org

National Hospice and Palliative Care Organization (NHPCO). Provides information about hospice care and advance directives, including an online national directory of hospices listed by state and city.

800-658-8898

http://www.nhpco.org

National Public Radio: The End of Life—Exploring Death in America. Download transcripts of this 1998 NPR series on end-of-life issues, as well as resources, a bibliography, and readings.

http://www.npr.org/programs/death

Nolo Press: Wills and Estate Planning. Provides answers to questions about planning for death, from writing a basic will to organ donation.

http://www.nolo.com

On Our Own Terms: Public Broadcasting System. A companion Web site to the Bill Moyers PBS series on improving end-of-life care.

http://www.pbs.org/wnet/onourownterms

Oregon Department of Health and Human Services. Provides information about Oregon's Death with Dignity Act.

http://egov.oregon.gov/DHS/ph/pas

Soros Foundation: Project on Death in America. A Web site focusing on different approaches to achieving a good death.

http://www.soros.org/initiatives/pdia

The following organizations provide information about organ donation and donor cards.

Coalition on Donation

http://www.donatelife.net

National Kidney Foundation

800-622-9010

http://www.kidney.org

Organ Procurement and Transplantation Network

http://www.optn.org

U.S. Department of Health and Human Services

http://www.organdonor.gov

Selected Bibliography

Abouna, G. M. 2003. Ethical issues in organ transplantation. *Medical Principles in Practice* 12(1): 54–69.

Angus, D. C., et al. 2004. Use of intensive care at the end of life in the United States: An epidemiologic study. *Critical Care Medicine* 32(3): 638–643.

Annas, G. J. 2005. "Culture of life" politics at the bedside—the case of Terri Schiavo. *New England Journal of Medicine*, epub March 23.

Attig, T. 1996. *How We Grieve: Relearning the World.* New York: Oxford University Press.

BBC. 2001. *Transplantation—a Summary* (http://www.bbc.co.uk/dna/h2g2/A619436; retrieved September 25, 2002).

Byock, I. 2000. Palliative care. In *On Our Own Terms: Moyers on Dying,* ed. Public Affairs Television, 10–11. New York: WNET.

Capron, A. M. 2001. Brain death—well settled yet still unresolved. *New England Journal of Medicine* 344(16): 1244–1246.

Casarett, D., et al. 2005. Making difficult decisions about hospice enrollment: What do patients and families want to know? *Journal of the American Geriatrics Society* 53(2): 249–254.

Choice in Dying. 1999. *Issue: Background on the Right to Die* (http://www.choices.org/issues.htm; retrieved September 9, 2000).

Comarow, A. 2003. Transplant trauma. New tactics fight the growing organ donor deficit. *US News & World Report* 134(1): 42–44.

Delmonico, F. L., et al. 2002. Ethical incentives—not payment—for organ donation. *New England Journal of Medicine* 346(25): 2002–2005.

Ditto, P. H., et al. 2001. Advance directives as acts of communication: A randomized controlled trial. *Archives of Internal Medicine* 161(3): 421–430.

Folkman, S., and J. T. Moskowitz. 2000. Positive affect and the other side of coping. *American Psychologist* 55: 647–654.

Ganzini, L., et al. 2001. Oregon physicians' attitudes about and experiences with end-of-life care since passage of the Oregon Death with Dignity Act. *Journal of the American Medical Association* 285(18): 2363–2369.

Ganzini, L., et al. 2002. Experiences of Oregon nurses and social workers with hospice patients who requested assistance with suicide. *New England Journal of Medicine* 347(8): 582–588.

Kirsch, B. 2002. Salve for the body and mind. *Scientific American,* October.

Kohara, H., et al. 2005. Sedation for terminally ill patients with cancer with uncontrollable physical distress. *Journal of Palliative Medicine* 8(1): 20–25.

Kübler-Ross, E. 1997. *On Death and Dying.* Reprint Edition. New York: Simon & Schuster.

Lo, B., et al. 2002. Discussing religious and spiritual issues at the end of life. *Journal of the American Medical Association* 287(6): 749–754.

Lynn, J. 2001. Serving patients who may die soon and their families. The role of hospice and other services. *Journal of the American Medical Association* 285(7): 925–932.

Making end-of-life medical decisions ahead of time. 2002. *Tufts University Health and Nutrition Letter,* September.

McGrath, P. 2003. Spiritual pain: A comparison of findings from survivors and hospice patients. *American Journal of Hospice and Palliative Care* 20(1): 23–33.

Melhem, N. M., et al. 2004. Traumatic grief among adolescents exposed to a peer's suicide. *American Journal of Psychiatry* 161(8): 1411–1416.

Merboth, M. K., and S. Barnason. 2000. Managing pain: The fifth vital sign. *Nursing Clinics of North America* 35: 375–383.

Moskop, J. 2000. Increasing the supply of transplant organs: Prospects and problems. *Bioethics Center Newsletter* 3(1).

National Funeral Directors Association. 2002. *Funeral Service Facts* (http://nfda.atlantistech.net/nfdafactsheets.php; retrieved December 14, 2002).

National Hospice and Palliative Care Organization. 2004. *Hospice Facts and Figures* (http://www.nhpco.org; retrieved February 15, 2005).

Niklason, L. E., and R. Langer. 2001. Prospects for organ and tissue replacement. *Journal of the American Medical Association* 285(5): 573–576.

O'Brien, C. N., G. A. Madek, and G. R. Ferrera. 2000. Oregon's guidelines for physician-assisted suicide: A legal and ethical analysis. *University of Pittsburgh Law Review* 61: 329–365.

Oregon Health Division. 2005. *Seventh Annual Report on Oregon's Death with Dignity Act* (http://egov.oregon.gov/DHS/ph/pas/ar-index.shtml; retrieved April 11, 2005).

Organ transplants. 2004. *Mayo Clinic Health Letter Supplement,* October.

Palliative care. 2002. *Journal of the American Medical Association* 287(7): 938.

Patel, K. 2004. Euthanasia and physician-assisted suicide policy in the Netherlands and Oregon: A comparative analysis. *Journal of Health and Social Policy* 19(1): 37–55.

Persson, M. O., et al. 2003. Xenotransplantation public perceptions: Rather cells than organs. *Xenotransplantation* 10(1): 72–79.

Pivar, I. L., and N. P. Field. 2004. Unresolved grief in combat veterans with PTSD. *Journal of Anxiety Disorders* 18(6): 745–755.

Quill, T. E. 2005. Terri Schiavo—A tragedy compounded. *New England Journal of Medicine,* epub March 23.

Rabow, M. W., J. M. Hauser, and J. Adams. 2004. Supporting family caregivers at the end of life. *Journal of the American Medical Association* 291(4): 483–491.

Rietjens, J. A., et al. 2004. Physician reports of terminal sedation without hydration or nutrition for patients nearing death in the Netherlands. *Annals of Internal Medicine* 141(3): 178–185.

Saunders, C. 2000. The evolution of palliative care. *Patient Education and Counseling* 41: 7–13.

Searight, H. R., and J. Gafford. 2005. Cultural diversity at the end of life: Issues and guidelines for family physicians. *American Family Physician* 71(3): 515–522.

Shadbolt, B., J. Barresi, and P. Craft. 2002. Self-rated health as a predictor of survival among patients with advanced cancer. *Journal of Clinical Oncology* 20(10): 2514–2519.

Speece, M. W., and S. B. Brent. 1996. The development of children's understanding of death. In *Handbook of Childhood Death and Bereavement,* ed. C. A. Corr and D. M. Corr. New York: Springer.

Stroebe, M., and H. Schut. 1995. *The Dual Process Model of Coping with Bereavement.* Paper presented at the meeting of the International Work Group on Death, Dying, and Bereavement, Oxford, England, June 29, 1995.

Tierney, W. M., et al. 2001. The effect of discussions about advance directives on patients' satisfaction with primary care. *Journal of General Internal Medicine* 16(1): 32–40.

United Network for Organ Sharing. 2002. *Donors Recovered in the U.S. by Donor Type* (http://www.optn.org/latestData/rptData.asp; retrieved December 14, 2002).

Vastag, B. 2002. Need for donor organs spurs thought and action. *Journal of the American Medical Association* 287(19): 2491.

Walsh, K., et al. 2002. Spiritual beliefs may affect outcome of bereavement: Prospective study. *British Medical Journal* 324(7353): 1551.

Weisman, A. D. 1984. *The Coping Capacity: On the Nature of Being Mortal.* New York: Human Sciences Press.

Weithman, P. J. 1999. Of assisted suicide and "the philosophers' brief." *Ethics* 109: 548–578.

Wenrich, M. D., et al. 2003. Dying patients' need for emotional support and personalized care from physicians. Perspectives of patients with terminal illness, families, and health care providers. *Journal of Pain and Symptom Management* 25(3): 236–246.

Wicks, M. 2000. Biotechnological solutions to the organ crisis. *Medscape Transplantation* 1(1).

Windler, D., and N. Dickert. 2001. The consent process for cadaveric organ procurement. How does it work? How can it be improved? *Journal of the American Medical Association* 285(3): 329–333.

Worden, J. W. 1991. *Grief Counseling and Grief Therapy: A Handbook for the Mental Health Practitioner,* 2nd ed. New York: Springer.

21

AHEAD

After reading this chapter, you should be able to

- Explain the self-care decision-making process and discuss options for self-treatment

- Describe the basic premises, practices, and providers of conventional medicine

- Describe the basic premises, practices, and providers of complementary and alternative medicine

- Explain how to communicate effectively with a health care provider and to evaluate different forms of treatment

- Discuss different types of health insurance plans

Conventional and Complementary Medicine: Skills for the Health Care Consumer

Knowledge

1. **The people most likely to use complementary and alternative medicine are those without a regular primary care physician.**
   True or false?

2. **Which practice or interest is shared by both conventional Western medicine and complementary and alternative medicine?**
   a. careful observation of symptoms
   b. treatment with remedies derived from plants
   c. concern with the patient-physician relationship

3. **Herbal remedies and dietary supplements like ginkgo and St. John's wort must meet FDA standards for safety and effectiveness before they can be put on the market.**
   True or false?

4. **Generic drugs are generally less effective than brand-name drugs.**
   True or false?

5. **Most Americans who do not have insurance can obtain adequate health care through emergency rooms or charity care at hospitals.**
   True or false?

ANSWERS

1. FALSE. The more often a person visits a primary care physician, the more likely he or she is to use complementary and alternative medicine.

2. ALL THREE. Although there are profound philosophical differences between the approaches, they share many characteristics.

3. FALSE. Manufacturers are responsible for the safety of the dietary supplements they sell; the FDA has the power to restrict a product if it is found to pose a health risk after it is on the market. Manufacturers do not have to prove that their products are effective.

4. FALSE. Price is often the only difference. The generic version of a drug has the same active ingredient as the brand-name drug, but it may have different inactive ingredients.

5. FALSE. Research has shown that uninsured people are less than half as likely as the insured to get needed care for serious medical conditions. It's estimated that each year more than 18,000 Americans age 25–64 die because they lack health insurance.

VW Visit the *Core Concepts in Health* Online Learning Center (www.mhhe.com/insel10e) for study aids and many additional resources.

629

Today, people are becoming more confident of their ability to solve personal health problems on their own. People who manage their own health care gather information and learn skills from physicians and other health care providers, friends, classes, books, magazines, Web sites, or self-help groups. They solicit opinions and advice, make decisions, and take action. They know how to practice safe, effective self-care, and they know how to make decisions about professional medical care, whether conventional Western medicine or complementary and alternative medicine. This chapter will help you develop the skills both to identify and manage medical problems and to make the health care system work effectively for you.

SELF-CARE: MANAGING MEDICAL PROBLEMS

Effectively managing medical problems involves developing several skills. First, you need to learn how to be a good observer of your own body and assess your symptoms. You also must be able to decide when to seek professional advice and when you can safely deal with the problem on your own. You need to know how to safely and effectively self-treat common medical problems. Finally, you need to know how to develop a partnership with physicians and other health care providers and how to carry out treatment plans.

Self-Assessment

Symptoms are often an expression of the body's attempt to heal itself. For example, the pain and swelling that occur after an ankle injury immobilize the injured joint to allow healing to take place. A fever may be an attempt to make the body less hospitable to infectious agents. A cough can help clear the airways and protect the lungs. Understanding what a symptom means and what is going on in your body helps reduce anxiety about symptoms and enables you to practice safe self-care that supports your body's own healing mechanisms.

Carefully observing symptoms also lets you identify those signals that suggest you need professional assistance. You should begin by noting when the symptom began, how often and when it occurs, what makes it worse, what makes it better, and whether you have any associated symptoms. You can also monitor your body's vital signs, such as temperature and heart rate. Medical self-tests for such things as blood pressure, blood sugar, pregnancy detection, and urinary tract infections can also help you make a more informed decision about when to seek medical help and when to self-treat.

Decision Making: Knowing When to See a Physician

In general, you should check with a physician for symptoms that are described as follows:

1. *Severe.* If the symptom is very severe or intense, medical assistance is advised. Examples include severe pains, major injuries, and other emergencies.

2. *Unusual.* If the symptom is peculiar and unfamiliar, it is wise to check it out with your physician. Examples include unexplained lumps, changes in a mole, problems with vision, difficulty swallowing, numbness, weakness, unexplained weight loss, and blood in sputum, urine, or stool.

3. *Persistent.* If the symptom lasts longer than expected, seek medical advice. Examples in adults include fever for more than 5 days, a cough lasting longer than 2 weeks, a sore that doesn't heal within a month, and hoarseness lasting longer than 3 weeks.

4. *Recurrent.* If a symptom tends to return again and again, medical evaluation is advised. Examples include recurrent headaches, stomach pains, and backache.

Sometimes a single symptom is not a cause for concern, but when the symptom is accompanied by other symptoms, the combination suggests a more serious problem. For example, a fever with a stiff neck suggests meningitis. If you evaluate your symptoms and think that you need professional help, you must decide how urgent the problem is. If it is a true emergency, you should go (or call someone to take you) to the nearest emergency room (ER). Emergencies would include

- Major trauma or injury, such as head injury, suspected broken bone, deep wound, severe burn, eye injury, or animal bite
- Uncontrollable bleeding or internal bleeding, as indicated by blood in the sputum, vomit, or stool
- Intolerable and uncontrollable pain or severe chest pain
- Severe shortness of breath
- Persistent abdominal pain, especially if associated with nausea and vomiting
- Poisoning or drug overdose
- Loss of consciousness or seizure
- Stupor, drowsiness, or disorientation that cannot be explained
- Severe or worsening reaction to an insect bite or sting or to a medication, especially if breathing is difficult

If your problem is not an emergency but still requires medical attention, call your physician's office. Often you can be given medical advice over the phone without the

The act of writing down feelings and thoughts about stressful life events has been shown to help people with chronic conditions improve their health. In one recent study, people with asthma or rheumatoid arthritis were asked to write down their feelings about the most stressful event in their lives; they wrote for 20 minutes a day over a 3-day period. In follow-up exams 4 months later, nearly half of the patients who engaged in expressive writing experienced positive changes in their condition, such as improved lung function or reduced joint pain. Only about a quarter of the control group, who wrote about their daily plans, experienced a positive change in health.

Investigators remain unsure why writing about one's feelings has beneficial effects. It is possible that expressing feelings about a traumatic event helps people work through the event and put it behind them. The resulting sense of release and control may reduce stress levels and have positive physical effects such as reduced heart rate and blood pressure and improved immune function. Alternatively, expressive writing may change the way people think about previous stressful events in their lives and help them cope with new stressors. Whatever the cause, it's clear that expressive writing can be a safe, inexpensive, and effective supplement to standard treatment of certain chronic illnesses.

What about the effects of expressive writing on otherwise healthy individuals? Other studies have, in fact, found a similar benefit: People who wrote about traumatic experiences reported fewer symptoms, fewer days off work, fewer visits to the doctor, improved mood, and a more positive outlook.

If you'd like to try expressive writing to help you deal with a traumatic event, set aside a special time—15 minutes a day for 4 consecutive days, for example, or 1 day a week for 4 weeks. Write in a place where you won't be interrupted or distracted. Explore your very deepest thoughts and feelings and why you feel the way you do. Don't worry about grammar or coherence or about what someone else might think about what you're writing; you are writing just for yourself. You may find the writing exercise to be distressing in the short term—sadness and depression are common when dealing with feelings about a stressful event—but most people report relief and contentment soon after writing for several days.

SOURCES: Pennebaker, J. W. 2004. *Writing to Heal: A Guided Journal for Recovering from Trauma and Emotional Upheaval.* Oakland, Calif.: New Harbinger; Smyth, J. M., et al. 1999. Effects of writing about stressful experiences on symptom reduction in patients with asthma or rheumatoid arthritis: A randomized trial. *Journal of the American Medical Association* 281(14): 1304–1309; Spiegel, D. 1999. Healing words: Emotional expression and disease outcome. *Journal of the American Medical Association* 281(14): 1328–1329.

inconvenience of a visit. To help you make wise medical decisions, a Self-Care Guide for Common Medical Problems is provided in Appendix B.

Self-Treatment: Many Options

When confronted with a new symptom, many people try to find some pill or potion that will relieve or cure it. However, other self-treatment options are available.

Watchful Waiting In most cases, your body itself can relieve your symptoms and heal the disorder. The prescriptions filled by your body's internal pharmacy are frequently the safest and most effective treatment, so patience and careful self-observation are often the best choices in self-treatment.

Nondrug Options Nondrug options are often easy, inexpensive, safe, and highly effective. For example, massage, ice packs, and neck exercises may at times be more helpful than drugs in relieving headaches and other pains. Getting adequate rest, increasing exercise, drinking more water, eating more or less of certain foods, using humidifiers, changes in ergonomics when working at a desk, and so on are just some of the hundreds of nondrug options for preventing or relieving many common health problems. For a variety of disorders caused or aggravated by stress, the treatment of choice may be relaxation, visualization, humor, assertive communication, changing negative thoughts, or other stress-management strategies (see Chapter 2 and the box "Expressive Writing and Chronic Conditions").

Self-Medication Self-treatment with nonprescription medications is an important part of our health care system. Nonprescription or **over-the-counter (OTC) medications** are medicines that the Food and Drug Administration (FDA) has determined are safe for use without a physician's prescription. There are more than 100,000 OTC drugs on the market; about 60% of all medications are sold over the counter. Within every 2-week period, nearly 70% of Americans use one or more OTC drugs.

Many OTC drugs are highly effective in relieving symptoms and sometimes in curing illnesses. In fact, many OTC drugs were formerly prescription drugs. More than 600 products sold over the counter today use ingredients or dosage strengths available only by prescription

Term

over-the-counter (OTC) medication A medication or product that can be purchased by the consumer without a prescription.

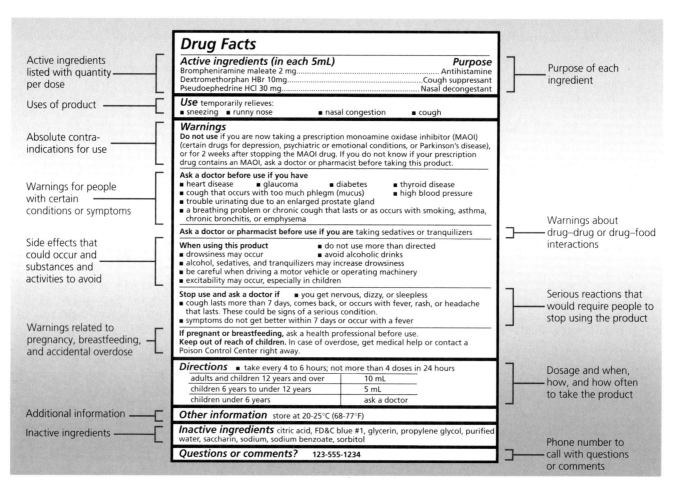

Figure 21-1 Reading and understanding OTC drug labels. SOURCE: Food and Drug Administration. 1999. Over-the-counter human drugs; labeling requirements; final rule. *Federal Register* 64, no. 51(17 March): 13254–13303.

20 years ago. With this increased consumer choice, however, comes increased consumer responsibility for using OTC drugs safely.

Consumers also need to be aware of the barrage of OTC drug advertising aimed at them. The implication of such advertising is that every symptom can and should be relieved by a drug. Although many OTC products are effective, others are unnecessary or divert attention from better ways of coping. Many ingredients in OTC drugs—perhaps 70%—have not been proven to be effective, a fact the FDA does not dispute. And any drug may have risks and side effects.

Follow these simple guidelines to self-medicate safely:

1. Always read labels, and follow directions carefully. The information on most OTC drug labels now appears in a standard format developed by the FDA (Figure 21-1). Ingredients, directions for safe use, and warnings are clearly indicated; but, if you have any questions, ask a pharmacist or physician before using a product.

2. Do not exceed the recommended dosage or length of treatment unless you discuss this change with your physician.

3. Use caution if you are taking other medications or supplements, because OTC and prescription drugs and herbs can interact. If you have questions about drug interactions, ask your physician or pharmacist *before* you mix medicines.

4. Try to select medications with one active ingredient rather than combination products. A product with multiple ingredients is likely to include drugs for symptoms you don't even have. Why risk the side effects of medications you don't need? Using single-ingredient products also allows you to adjust the dosage of each medication separately for optimal symptom relief with minimal side effects.

5. When choosing medications, try to buy **generic drugs,** which contain the same active ingredient as the brand-name product but generally at a much lower cost. (Brand-name and generic drugs are discussed in more detail later in the chapter.)

6. Never take or give a drug from an unlabeled container or in the dark when you can't read what the label says.

Closet	Medicine Cabinet
• Analgesic (relieves pain)	• Adhesive bandages
• Antacid (relieves upset stomach)	• Adhesive tape
• Antibiotic ointment (reduces risk of infection)	• Alcohol wipes
• Antihistamine (relieves allergy symptoms)	• Calibrated measuring spoon
• Antiseptic (helps stop infection)	• Disinfectant
• Fever reducer (adult and child)	• Gauze pads
• Hydrocortisone (relieves itching and inflammation)	• Thermometer
• Decongestant (relieves stuffy nose and other cold symptoms)	• Tweezers

Figure 21-2   Your home medical care kit.   A cool, dark, and dry place such as the top of a linen closet, preferably in a locked container and out of a child's reach, is best for storing medicines. Showers and baths create heat and humidity that can cause some drugs to deteriorate rapidly. Use your bathroom medicine cabinet for supplies that aren't affected by heat and humidity.   SOURCE: Lewis, C. 2000. Your medicine cabinet needs an annual checkup, too. *FDA Consumer,* March/April.

7.   If you are pregnant or nursing or have a chronic condition such as kidney disease, consult your physician before self-medicating.

8.   The expiration date marked on many medications is an estimate of how long the *unopened* medication is likely to be potent. Once the package is opened, the medication will probably be potent for about a year if stored properly. Mark the date on the package when you open it, and dispose of it safely after a year by taking it to a pharmacy or hospital.

9.   Store your medications in a cool, dry place that is out of the reach of children (Figure 21-2).

10.   Use special caution with aspirin. Because of an association with a rare but serious problem known as Reye's syndrome, aspirin should not be used by children or adolescents who may have the flu, chicken pox, or any other viral illness.

PROFESSIONAL MEDICAL AND HEALTH CARE: CHOICES AND CHANGE

When self-treatment is not appropriate or sufficient, you need to seek professional medical care, whether by going to a hospital emergency room, by scheduling an appointment with your physician, or by accessing some other part of the American medical and health care system. This system is a broad network of individuals and organizations, including independent practitioners, allied health care providers, hospitals, clinics, and public and private insurance programs.

In recent years, many Americans have also sought health care from practitioners of **complementary and alternative medicine (CAM)**, defined as those therapies and practices that do not form part of conventional, or mainstream, health care and medical practices as taught

in most U.S. medical schools and offered in most U.S. hospitals. The most commonly used CAM therapies are relaxation techniques, herbal medicine, massage, and chiropractic (Table 21-1). People often use CAM therapies in addition to their conventional medical treatments, but many do not tell their physicians about it.

Consumers turn to CAM for a large variety of purposes related to health and well-being, such as boosting their immune system, lowering their cholesterol levels, losing weight, quitting smoking, or enhancing their memory. There are indications that people with chronic conditions, including cancer, asthma, autoimmune diseases, and HIV infection, are particularly likely to try CAM therapies. Despite their growing popularity, many CAM practices remain controversial, and individuals need to be critically aware of safety issues. In the next sections of this chapter, we examine the principles and providers of both **conventional medicine**—the dominant medical system in the United States and Europe, also referred to as standard Western medicine or biomedicine—and of complementary and alternative medicine, with particular attention to consumer issues.

Terms

generic drug A drug that is not registered or protected by a trademark; a drug that does not have a brand name.

complementary and alternative medicine (CAM) Therapies or practices that are not part of conventional or mainstream health care and medical practice as taught in most U.S. medical schools and available at most U.S. health care facilities; examples of CAM practices include acupuncture and herbal remedies.

conventional medicine A system of medicine based on the application of the scientific method; diseases are thought to be caused by identifiable physical factors and characterized by a representative set of symptoms; also called *biomedicine* or *standard Western medicine.*

Table 21-1	Use of Complementary and Alternative Therapies in the United States	

	Percent Who Ever Used Therapy
Prayer	55.3
Natural products (nonvitamin, nonmineral)	25.0
Chiropractic care	19.9
Deep breathing exercises	14.6
Meditation	10.2
Massage	9.3
Yoga	7.5
Diet-based therapies	6.8
Progressive relaxation	4.2
Acupuncture	4.0
Megavitamin therapy	3.9
Homeopathic treatment	3.6
Guided imagery	3.0
Tai chi	2.5
Hypnosis	1.8
Energy healing therapy/Reiki	1.1
Biofeedback	1.0
Any therapy	**74.6**

SOURCE: Barnes, P. M., et al. 2004. Complementary and alternative medicine use among adults: United States, 2002. *Advance Data from Vital and Health Statistics* No. 343. Hyattsville, Md.: National Center for Health Statistics.

CONVENTIONAL MEDICINE

Referring to conventional medicine as standard Western medicine draws attention to the fact that it differs from the various medical systems that have developed in China, Japan, India, and other parts of the world. Calling it "biomedicine" reflects conventional medicines basis in the findings of a variety of biological sciences.

Premises and Assumptions of Conventional Medicine

One of the important characteristics of Western medicine is the belief that disease is caused by identifiable physical factors. This belief can be traced back to Hippocrates, the Greek physician of the fourth century B.C. who is credited with placing the practice of medicine on a scientific footing. In Hippocrates' time, the causes of disease were thought to include the interplay of various forces and elements; today, Western medicine identifies the causes of disease as pathogens, such as bacteria and viruses, genetic factors, and unhealthy lifestyles that result in changes at the molecular and cellular levels. In most cases, however, the focus is primarily on the physical causes of the illness rather than mental or spiritual imbalance.

Another feature that distinguishes Western biomedicine from other medical systems is the concept that every disease is defined by a certain set of symptoms and that these symptoms are similar in most patients suffering from this disease. Western medicine tends to treat illness as an isolated biological disturbance that can occur in any human being, rather than as integral in some way to the individual with the illness.

Related to the idea of illness as the result of invasion by outside factors is the strong orientation toward methods of destroying pathogens or preventing them from causing serious infection. The public health measures of the nineteenth and twentieth centuries—chlorination of drinking water, sewage disposal, food safety regulations, vaccination programs, education about hygiene, and so on—are an outgrowth of this kind of orientation. (As described in Chapter 1, these public health measures are largely responsible for the 25-year increase in life expectancy that Americans experienced in the twentieth century.)

The implementation of public health measures is one way to control pathogens; another is the use of drugs. The discovery and development of sulfa drugs, antibiotics, and steroids in the twentieth century, along with advances in chemistry that made it possible to identify the active ingredients in common herbal remedies, paved the way for the current close identification of Western medicine with **pharmaceuticals** (medical drugs, both prescription and over-the-counter). Western medicine also relies heavily on surgery and on advanced medical technology to discover the physical causes of disease and to remove or destroy them.

Further, Western medicine is based on scientific ways of obtaining knowledge and explaining phenomena. Scientific explanations result from the application of the scientific method to a question or problem; they have a blend of characteristics that set them apart from other types of explanation, such as those based on common sense, faith, belief, or authority. Scientific explanations are

- *Empirical*—they are based on the evidence of the senses and on objective and systematic observation, often carried out under carefully controlled conditions; they must be capable of verification by others.
- *Rational*—they follow the rules of logic and are consistent with known facts.
- *Testable*—either they are verifiable through direct observation or they lead to predictions about what should occur under conditions not yet observed.
- *Parsimonious*—they explain phenomena with the fewest number of assumptions.
- *General*—they have broad explanatory power.
- *Rigorously evaluated*—they are constantly evaluated for consistency with the evidence and known principles, for parsimony, and for generality.

Conventional Western medicine is firmly grounded in scientific explanations resulting from the application of the scientific method to a question or problem. The identification of bacteria and other microorganisms as a key cause of disease led to many public health measures and treatments that reduced U.S. deaths from infectious diseases.

- *Tentative*—scientists are willing to entertain the possibility that their explanations are faulty.

The scientific method is both a way of acquiring knowledge and a way of thinking that involves approaching a problem by carefully defining its parameters, seeking out relevant information, and subjecting proposed solutions to rigorous testing.

Western medicine translates the scientific method into practice through the research process, a highly refined and well-established approach to exploring the causes of disease and ensuring the safety and efficacy of treatments. Research studies range from case studies—descriptions of a single patient's illness and treatment—to clinical trials conducted on large populations and carried out under carefully controlled conditions over a period of many years. The process of drug development is equally rigorous. Drugs are developed and tested through an elaborate course that begins with preliminary research in the lab and continues through trials with human participants, review and approval by the FDA, and monitoring of the drug's effects after it is on the market. The process may take 12 years or more, and only about 20% of drugs are eventually approved.

When results of research studies are published in medical journals, a community of scientists, physicians, researchers, and scholars has the opportunity to share the findings and enter a dialogue about the subject. Publication

of research often prompts further research designed to replicate and confirm the findings, challenge the conclusions, or pursue a related line of thought or experiment. (For guidelines on how to interpret research when it is reported in the popular press, see the box "Evaluating Health News" on p. 636.)

The Providers of Conventional Medicine

Conventional medicine is practiced by a wide range of health care professionals in the United States. Several kinds of professionals are permitted to practice medicine independently, including medical doctors, osteopaths, podiatrists, optometrists, and dentists.

- **Medical doctors** are practitioners who hold a doctor of medicine (M.D.) degree from an accredited medical school. In the United States, an education in medicine has several stages: 4 years of premedical education in a college or university, with an emphasis on the sciences; 4 years of medical school, which teaches basic medical skills and awards the M.D. degree; graduate medical study, called a residency and lasting from 3 to 8 years, during which a specialty is chosen and studied and a medical license is obtained; and continuing medical education to keep abreast of advances in medical science. Twenty-four medical specialties are currently approved by the American Board of Medical Specialties, each with its own rule-making and certifying body. The larger specialties are further divided into subspecialties; for example, internal medicine includes subspecialties such as cardiology and gastroenterology. Visit the Web site for the American Board of Medical Specialties (www.abms.org) for a complete list. Becoming a subspecialist generally requires several more years of formal training after the completion of a residency.

- **Doctors of osteopathic medicine** (D.O.) receive a medical education similar to that of medical doctors, but their training places special emphasis on musculoskeletal problems and manipulative therapy. M.D.s and D.O.s are the two types of "complete" physicians in the United States, meaning they are trained and licensed to perform surgery and prescribe medication. D.O.s are graduates of osteopathic medical schools, which

Terms

V w

pharmaceuticals Medical drugs, both prescription and over-the-counter.

medical doctor An independent practitioner who holds a doctor of medicine degree from an accredited medical school.

doctor of osteopathic medicine A medical practitioner who has graduated from an osteopathic medical school; osteopathy incorporates the theories and practices of scientific medicine but focuses on musculoskeletal problems and manipulative therapy.

Critical Consumer

Health-related research is now described in popular newspapers and magazines rather than just medical journals, meaning that more and more people have access to the information. Greater access is certainly a plus, but news reports of research studies may oversimplify or exaggerate both the results and what those results mean to the average person. Researchers do not set out to mislead people, but they must often strike a balance between reporting promising preliminary findings to the public, thereby allowing people to act on them, and waiting 10–20 years until long-term studies confirm (or disprove) a particular theory.

All this can leave you in a difficult position. You cannot become an expert on all subjects, capable of effectively evaluating all the available health news. However, the following questions can help you better assess the health advice that appears in the popular media:

1. *Is the report based on research or on an anecdote?* Information or advice based on one or more carefully designed research studies has more validity than one person's experiences.

2. *What is the source of the information?* A study published in a respected peer-reviewed journal has been examined by editors and other researchers in the field, people who are in a position to evaluate the merits of a study and its results. Many journal articles also include information on the authors and funders of research, alerting readers to any possible conflicts of interest. Research presented at medical meetings should be considered very preliminary because the results have not yet undergone a thorough prepublication review; many such studies are never published. It is also wise to ask who funded a study to determine whether there is any potential for bias. Information from government agencies and national research organizations is usually considered fairly reliable.

3. *How big was the study?* A study involving many subjects is more likely to yield reliable results than a study involving only a few subjects. Another important indication that a finding is meaningful is if several studies yield the same results.

4. *Who were the participants involved in the study?* Research findings are more likely to apply to you if you share important characteristics with the participants of the study. For example, the results of a study on men over age 50 who smoke may not be particularly meaningful for a 30-year-old nonsmoking woman. Even less applicable are studies done in test tubes or on animals. Such research should be considered very preliminary in terms of its applicability to humans. Promising results from laboratory or animal research frequently cannot be replicated in human study subjects.

5. *What kind of study was it?* Epidemiological studies involve observation or interviews in order to trace the relationships among lifestyle, physical characteristics, and diseases. While epidemiological studies can suggest links, they cannot establish cause-and-effect relationships. Clinical or interventional studies or trials involve testing the effects of different treatments on groups of people who have similar lifestyles and characteristics. They are more likely to provide conclusive

evidence of a cause-and-effect relationship. The best interventional studies share the following characteristics:

- *Controlled.* A group of people who receive the treatment is compared with a matched group of people who do not receive the treatment.

- *Randomized.* The treatment and control groups are selected randomly.

- *Double-blind.* Researchers and participants are unaware of who is receiving the treatment.

- *Multicenter.* The experiment is performed at more than one institution.

A third type of study, meta-analysis, involves combining the results of individual studies to get an overall view of the effectiveness of a treatment.

6. *What do the statistics really say?* First, are the results described as statistically significant? If a study is large and well designed, its results can be deemed statistically significant, meaning there is less than a 5% chance that the findings resulted from chance. Second, are the results stated in terms of relative or absolute risk? Many findings are reported in terms of relative risk—how a particular treatment or condition affects a person's disease risk. Consider the following examples of relative risk:

- According to some estimates, taking estrogen without progesterone can increase a postmenopausal woman's risk of dying from endometrial cancer by 233%.

- Giving AZT to HIV-infected pregnant women reduces prenatal transmission of HIV by about 90%.

The first of these findings seems far more dramatic than the second—until you also consider absolute risk, the actual risk of the illness in the population being considered. The absolute risk of endometrial cancer is 0.3%; a 233% increase based on the effects of estrogen raises it to 1%, a change of 0.7%. Without treatment, about 25% of infants born to HIV-infected women will be infected with HIV; with treatment, the absolute risk drops to about 2%, a change of 23%. Because the absolute risk of an HIV-infected mother passing the virus to her infant (25%) is so much greater than a woman's risk of developing endometrial cancer compared with (0.3%), a smaller change in relative risk translates into a much greater change in absolute risk.

7. *Is new health advice being offered?* If the media report new guidelines for health behavior or medical treatment, examine the source. Government agencies and national research foundations usually consider a great deal of evidence before offering health advice. Above all, use common sense, and check with your physician before making a major change in your health habits based on news reports.

SOURCES: Woloshin, S., and L. M. Schwartz. 2002. Press releases: Translating research into news. *Journal of the American Medical Association* 287(21): 2856–2858; Medicine and the media. 1999. *Harvard Women's Health Watch,* February; Medical hype: How to read between the lines. 1998. *Consumer Reports on Health,* October; Making sense of health research. 1998. *Healthline,* May.

emphasize training students to be primary care physicians and to practice a whole-person approach to medicine.

• **Podiatrists** are practitioners who specialize in the medical and surgical care of the feet. They hold a doctor of podiatric medicine (D.P.M.) degree; the length of training is similar to that of M.D.s. They can prescribe drugs and perform surgery on the feet.

• **Optometrists** are practitioners trained to examine the eyes, detect eye diseases, and treat vision problems. They hold a doctor of optometry (O.D.) degree. All states permit optometrists to use drugs for diagnostic purposes, and most permit them to use drugs to treat minor eye problems. (Ophthalmologists are M.D. eye specialists who care for all types of eye problems and can perform eye surgery.)

• **Dentists** specialize in the care of the teeth and mouth. They are graduates of 4-year dental schools and hold the doctor of dental surgery (D.D.S.) or doctor of medical dentistry (D.M.D.) degree; specialists receive additional education. Dentists can perform surgery and prescribe drugs within the scope of their training.

In addition to these practitioners, there are millions of other trained health care professionals, known as **allied health care providers**, working in the United States. Some of them are licensed to work independently; others are permitted to work under medical supervision or medical referral. They include registered nurses (R.N.s), licensed vocational nurses (L.V.N.s), physical therapists, social workers, registered dietitians (R.D.s), physician assistants (P.A.s), nurse practitioners, and certified nurse midwives.

Choosing a Primary Care Physician

Most experts believe it is best to have a primary care physician, someone who gets to know you, who coordinates your medical care, and who refers you to specialists when you need them. Primary care physicians include those certified in family practice, internal medicine, pediatrics, and obstetrics-gynecology. These physicians are able to diagnose and treat the vast majority of common health problems; they also provide many preventive health services. The best time to look for a physician is before you are sick (see the box "Health Care Visits and Gender" on p. 638).

To select a physician, begin by making a list of possible choices. If your insurance limits the health care providers you can see, check the plan's list first. Ask for recommendations from family, friends, coworkers, local medical societies, and the physician referral service at a local clinic or hospital. Some clinics provide brief biographies of physicians on staff who are taking new patients. If you have a particular health problem, you may want to identify physicians who are board-certified in appropriate specialties. Once you have a list of possible physicians, find out if a consumer or other independent group has

rated doctors in your area; this will help you check on the quality of care they provide.

Once you have the names of a few physicians you might want to try, call their offices to find out information such as the following:

• Is the physician covered by your health plan and accepting new patients?

• What are the office hours, and when is the physician or office staff available? What do patients do if they need urgent care or have an emergency?

• Which hospitals does the physician use?

• How many other physicians are available to cover when he or she isn't available, and who are they?

• How long does it usually take to get a routine appointment?

• Does the office send reminders about preventive tests such as Pap tests?

• Does the physician (or a nurse or physician assistant) give advice over the phone for common problems?

Schedule a visit with the physician you think you would most like to use. During that first visit, you'll get a sense of how well matched you are and how well he or she might meet your medical needs. After the visit, consider the following:

• Do you feel you were listened to, and did you have a chance to ask questions?

• Do you feel you were treated with respect and made to feel comfortable?

• Do you understand what the physician told you, and did he or she spend enough time with you?

• Do you feel that the physician addressed your health problems or concerns, and do you feel comfortable with the recommended course of action?

Although you may want to give the relationship some time to develop, you should trust your own reactions when deciding whether a particular health care provider is the right one for you.

Terms

podiatrist A practitioner who holds a doctor of podiatric medicine degree and specializes in the medical and surgical care of the feet.

optometrist A practitioner who holds a doctor of optometry degree and is trained to examine the eyes, detect eye diseases, and prescribe corrective lenses.

dentist A practitioner who holds a doctor of medical dentistry or doctor of dental surgery degree and who specializes in the prevention and treatment of diseases and injuries of the teeth, mouth, and jaws.

allied health care providers Health care professionals who typically provide services under the supervision or control of independent practitioners.

Gender Matters

Among Americans age 15 and over, females are more likely than males to visit a health care provider (see figure). The difference is most pronounced among adults age 25–44; in this age group, women make nearly twice as many physician visits as do men. Women are also more likely to report use of complementary and alternative therapies.

What are some of the factors underlying this difference? Reproductive health care needs may be one key factor, with women making doctor visits related to prenatal care and childbirth. Women of reproductive age may also need to make health care visits in order to obtain prescription contraceptives and have the pelvic exams and Pap tests required to obtain certain contraceptives.

But even when physician visits related to reproductive care are discounted, women are more likely than men to see a health care provider, especially for preventive care. Male gender roles may play a role in this trend, with men being socialized to be strong and tough, to ignore pain or symptoms of illness, or to feel that physician visits for preventive care (when no symptoms are present) are unnecessary. And without preventive-care visits, men may be unaware of such asymptomatic conditions as high cholesterol levels or high blood pressure, which, once diagnosed, would require regular visits for monitoring and treatment.

At all ages, it is important for both men and women to obtain recommended health care screenings and immunizations. Preventive care throughout life is important to maximize wellness. Don't wait until you are ill before you see a physician.

SOURCES: Centers for Disease Control and Prevention. 2004. National ambulatory medical care survey: 2002 summary. *Advance Data from Vital and Health Statistics* No. 346. Hyattsville, Md.: National Center for Health Statistics; Centers for Disease Control and Prevention. 2004. Complementary and alternative medicine use among adults: United States, 2002. *Advance Data from Vital and Health Statistics* No. 343. Hyattsville, Md.: National Center for Health Statistics.

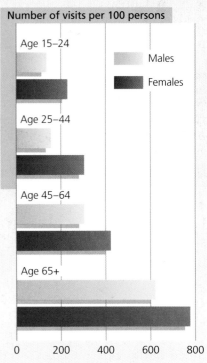

Health care visits by age and gender

Getting the Most Out of Your Medical Care

The key to making the health care system work for you lies in good communication with your physician and other members of the health care team. Studies show that patients who interact more with physicians and ask more questions enjoy better health outcomes.

The Physician-Patient Partnership The physician-patient relationship is undergoing an important transformation. The image of the all-knowing physician and the passive patient is slowly fading. What is emerging is more of a physician-patient *partnership,* in which the physician acts more like a consultant and the patient participates more actively. You should expect your physician to be attentive, caring, and able to listen and clearly explain things to you. You also must do your part. You need to be assertive in a firm but not aggressive manner. You need to express your feelings and concerns, ask questions, and, if necessary, be persistent. If your physician is unable to communicate clearly with you despite your best efforts, you probably need to change physicians.

Your Appointment with Your Physician Physicians are often pressed for time, so prepare for your visit ahead of time. Make a written list of your key concerns and questions, along with notes about your symptoms (when they started, how long they last, what makes them better or worse, what treatments you have already tried, and so on). If there are questions you're uncomfortable about asking, practice discussing them ahead of time. Bring a list of all the medications you're taking—prescription, nonprescription, and herbal. Also bring any medical records or test results your physician may not already have.

Present your concerns at the beginning of the visit, to set the agenda. Be specific and concise about your symptoms, and be open and honest about your concerns. Share your hunches with your physician—your guesses can provide vital clues. Ask questions if you don't understand something. Let your physician know if you are taking any drugs, are allergic to any medications, are breastfeeding, or may be pregnant.

At the end of the visit, briefly repeat the physician's diagnosis, prognosis, and instructions, and make sure you understand your next steps, such as making another appointment, phoning for test results, watching for new symptoms, and so on. You may also want to ask about the possibility of using e-mail for follow-up.

The Diagnostic Process The first step in the diagnostic process is the medical history, which includes

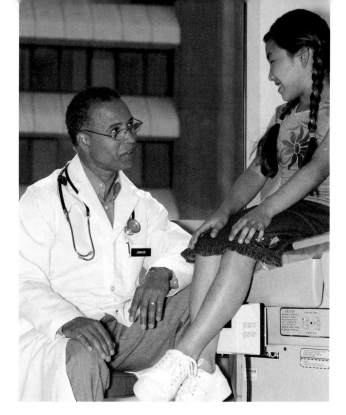

Good communication is a crucial factor in an effective physician-patient partnership.

your primary reason for the visit, your current symptoms, your past medical history, and your social history (job, family life, major stressors, living conditions, and health habits). Keeping up-to-date records of your medical history can help you provide your physician with key facts about your health (see the box "Personal Health Profile" on p. 640).

The next step is the physical exam, which usually begins with a review of vital signs: blood pressure, heart rate (pulse), breathing rate, and temperature. Depending on your primary complaint, your physician may give you a complete physical, or the exam may be directed to specific areas, such as your ears, nose, and throat.

Additionally, your physician may order medical tests to complete the diagnosis. Diagnostic testing provides a wealth of information to help solve medical problems; such testing now accounts for nearly one-third of our national health bill. Physicians can order X rays, biopsies, blood and urine tests, scans of various types, and a wide array of **endoscopies** to view, probe, or analyze almost any part of the body.

If your physician orders a test for you, be sure you know why you need it, what the risks and benefits of the test are for you, how you should prepare for it (for example, by fasting or discontinuing medications or herbal remedies), and what the test will involve. Also ask what the test results mean, because no test is 100% accurate—**false positives** and **false negatives** do occur—and interpretation of some tests is subjective. Sometimes it is

important to get an experienced second opinion on a diagnosis.

Medical and Surgical Treatments   Once the diagnosis is made, you and your physician can consider treatment options. Many conditions can be treated in a variety of ways; in some cases, lifestyle changes should be considered along with other options. Make sure you know the possible risks and side effects of each treatment option, as well as the likelihood that it will improve your condition.

PRESCRIPTION MEDICATIONS   Each month, about 40–50% of Americans use at least one prescription medication; among those 65 and older, more than 80% are current prescription drug users. Thousands of lives are saved each year by **antibiotics,** heart medications, insulin, and scores of other drugs, but we pay a price for having such powerful tools. A report from the Institute of Medicine (IOM) estimated that preventable medication errors result in more than 7000 deaths each year in hospitals alone, with tens of thousands more in outpatient facilities. Problems and issues related to prescription drug use include the following:

• *Medication errors:* Physicians may overprescribe drugs, sometimes in response to pressure by patients (see the box "Prescription Drug Use and Regulation: Lessons from Vioxx" on p. 641). Adverse effects can occur if a physician prescribes the wrong drug or a dangerous combination of drugs; such problems are especially prevalent for older adults, who typically take more medications. At the pharmacy, patients may receive the wrong drug or may not be given complete information about drug risks, side effects, and interactions. Problems can occur because of a physician's poor handwriting, misinterpretation of an abbreviated drug name, or similarities between the names and packaging of different drugs. In 2004, the FDA mandated the addition of bar codes with drug names and dosages to prescription drugs to help eliminate medication errors.

Terms

Vw

endoscopy A medical procedure in which a viewing instrument is inserted into a body cavity or opening. Specific procedures are named for the area viewed: inside joints (arthroscopy), inside airways (bronchoscopy), inside the abdominal cavity (laparoscopy), and inside the lower portion of the large intestine, or sigmoid colon (sigmoidoscopy).

false positive A test result that incorrectly detects a disease or condition in a healthy person.

false negative A test result that fails to correctly detect a disease or condition.

antibiotic A substance derived from a mold or bacterium that inhibits the growth of other microorganisms.

General Information

Age: _____   Total cholesterol: _____   Blood pressure: ___/___   Other: _____

Height: _____   HDL: _____   Triglycerides: _____   _____

Weight: _____   LDL: _____   Glucose: _____   _____

Medical Conditions

Check any of the following that apply to you and add other conditions that might affect your health and well-being.

_____ heart disease   _____ back pain   _____ depression, anxiety, or another psychological disorder

_____ lung disease   _____ arthritis

_____ diabetes   _____ other injury or joint problem   _____ eating disorder

_____ allergies   _____ other: _____

_____ asthma   _____ substance abuse problem   _____ other: _____

Medications/Treatments

List any drugs you are taking or any medical treatments you are undergoing. Include the name of the substance or treatment and its purpose. Include both prescription and OTC drugs and any vitamin, mineral, or other dietary supplement you are taking.

_____   _____   _____

_____   _____   _____

Health Care Providers

Primary care physician: name _____ phone _____

Specialist physician: name _____ phone _____

   Condition treated: _____

Other health care provider: name _____ phone _____

   Condition treated: _____

Health insurance provider and policy number: _____

To ensure that you get the most out of your medical care, you should also keep a record of your vaccinations and medical screening tests. Chapters 15–18 describe recommended vaccinations and screening tests for CVD, cancer, and STDs.

• *Off-label drug use:* Another potential problem is off-label use of drugs. Once a drug is approved by the FDA for one purpose, it can legally be prescribed (although not marketed) for purposes not listed on the label. For example, the problems caused by the prescription weight-loss medications removed from the market in the 1990s were mainly the result of off-label use: They were prescribed in combination and for long periods, a pattern of use that was not part of preapproval testing. Many off-label uses are safe and supported by some research, but both consumers and health care providers need to take special care with off-label use of medications.

• *Online pharmacies:* A recent area of concern is the advent of online pharmacies. Although convenient, some online pharmacies may sell products or engage in practices that are illegal in the offline world, putting consumers at risk for receiving adulterated, expired, or counterfeit drugs. The FDA recommends that consumers avoid sites that prescribe drugs for the first time without a physical exam, sell prescription drugs without a prescription, or sell drugs not approved by the FDA. You should also avoid sites that do not provide access to a registered pharmacist to answer questions or that do not provide a U.S. address and phone number to contact if there's a problem. The National Association of Boards of Pharmacy sponsors a voluntary certification program for Internet pharmacies. To be certified, a pharmacy must have a state license and allow regular inspections. Many experts recommend that consumers

In February 2005, the FDA announced plans for changes designed to enhance its oversight of prescription drugs. Pressure on the agency had been growing following several high-profile problems with approved drugs. These cases included the risk of suicide associated with use of certain antidepressants among children and teenagers (see Chapter 3), and, more recently, the risk of heart problems among people taking certain anti-inflammatory drugs for arthritis.

The Vioxx Story in Brief

Many people with arthritis take medications to reduce pain and inflammation. Traditional nonsteroidal anti-inflammatory drugs (NSAIDs) like aspirin and ibuprofen are effective, but they carry the risk of stomach irritation and even ulcers—especially if taken over long periods, as is common for a chronic condition like arthritis. Newer NSAIDs known as COX-2 inhibitors are designed to reduce pain and inflammation while causing less stomach irritation. COX-2 inhibitors include Vioxx (rofecoxib), Celebrex (celecoxib), and Bextra (valdecoxib).

Vioxx, approved in 1999, was heavily advertised and widely used. As early as 2000, studies began to find increased rates of cardiovascular problems among Vioxx users. Results of a large-scale study in 2004 found that Vioxx users were more likely to suffer a heart attack or sudden cardiac death than people using Celebrex or older NSAIDs. In response to this study, Vioxx was removed from the market. (Due to risks related to CVD and a serious skin condition, Bextra was pulled from the market in April 2005.)

The rise and fall of Vioxx has inspired debate on a number of issues relating to how drugs are marketed, prescribed, and regulated. Why weren't the risks identified before the drug was approved? Why didn't the FDA act earlier? Should such widespread drug marketing be allowed?

New Drugs and Postapproval Monitoring

Although pharmaceutical companies carry out extensive preapproval trials on new drugs, even the most extensive studies involve just a few thousand people. A large natural experiment begins when the drug is approved and physicians start prescribing it to people in the general population. Side effects and risks that did not show up in studies often become apparent when more people begin taking a drug. Problems can also develop when certain drugs are used in combination with other drugs or dietary supplements.

Preapproval studies may exclude certain groups for safety reasons. For example, initial studies of Vioxx did not include people with preexisting heart conditions, who may have been more at risk for the problems identified after the drug was approved. In addition, the increased risk from Vioxx did not show up until people had been taking the drug for at least 18 months—a longer period than most preapproval drug studies.

Part of the FDA's 2005 proposal is for greater postapproval surveillance, including an independent review board and a Web site with emerging drug safety data accessible to both physicians and consumers. Consumers should be especially alert for adverse effects if they are taking a drug that is new to the market. Consider older, more widely used drugs first.

Direct-to-Consumer Advertising

The pharmaceutical industry spends up to 20% of its marketing budget on direct-to-consumer (DTC) advertising, which has grown rapidly since 1995. Most of these ads are for a small number of the most popular drugs.

Proponents of DTC advertising claim that it enhances public health by providing educational information about under-diagnosed conditions such as diabetes, high cholesterol, and depression and by motivating people to seek care. DTC advertising may be particularly useful in getting health information to people who have no regular source of health care. It may also provide patients with an opportunity to discuss medical conditions that they might otherwise be hesitant to bring up, such as depression.

Opponents claim that DTC advertising is more promotional than educational, is misleading and omits important precautions, is designed to create consumer demand by creating problems and needs, and causes patients to pressure physicians to prescribe particular drugs. One recent study found that most DTC ads fail to provide information about how a drug works, its success rate, how long it must be taken, alternative treatments, or helpful lifestyle changes.

There is also concern that DTC advertising leads patients to request heavily advertised drugs when older, less expensive medications may be equally effective. Many people equate "newer" with "better,"

but that is not always the case. The COX-2 inhibitors were designed for people at risk for stomach irritation from traditional NSAIDs, but most people who used Vioxx were actually at low risk for problems from traditional NSAIDs. For most people, older NSAIDs, which have an established safety record, are just as effective as the newer drugs and much less expensive.

Selective Publication of Study Results

Many drug studies are carried out by the pharmaceutical industry, which has little incentive to publish the results of trials in which medications are found to be ineffective. In the case of antidepressants, manufacturers did not publicize studies that raised safety questions and failed to show drugs were effective for treating pediatric depression. Selective publication provides an inaccurate picture of the risks and benefits of a particular drug.

In response to criticism, pharmaceutical companies have set up a voluntary Web-based clearinghouse that will contain both positive and negative research findings (www.clinicalstudyresults.org). Major medical journals have pledged not to publish results of any clinical trial that is not preregistered. That is, researchers must register all trials when they begin, so unflattering or conflicting findings cannot be covered up. The U.S. Congress has also proposed legislation on this issue.

Balancing Risks and Benefits

All medications have risks and benefits. When choosing a particular medication, work with your physician to balance the risks and benefits of the drug to your own personal health. Apply critical thinking skills to drug ads, recognizing them for what they are, and use special caution when taking recently approved medications.

SOURCES: Food and Drug Administration. 2005. *FDA Improvements in Drug Safety Monitoring* (http://www.fda.gov/oc/factsheets/drugsafety.html; retrieved February 28, 2005); Beardsley, S. 2005. Avoiding another Vioxx. *Scientific American*, February; Kimmel, S. E., et al. 2005. Patients exposed to rofecoxib and celecoxib have different odds of nonfatal myocardial infarction. *Annals of Internal Medicine* 142(3): 157–164; Dai, C., R. S. Stafford, and G. C. Alexander. 2005. National trends in cyclooxygenase-2 inhibitor use since market release: Nonselective diffusion of a selectively cost-effective innovation. *Archives of Internal Medicine* 165(2): 171–177.

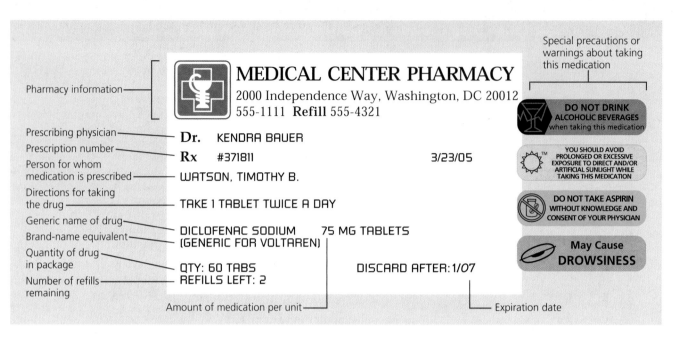

Pharmacy information

MEDICAL CENTER PHARMACY
2000 Independence Way, Washington, DC 20012
555-1111 **Refill** 555-4321

Special precautions or
warnings about taking
this medication

Prescribing physician — **Dr.** KENDRA BAUER

Prescription number — **Rx** #371811   3/23/05

Person for whom
medication is prescribed — WATSON, TIMOTHY B.

Directions for taking
the drug — TAKE 1 TABLET TWICE A DAY

Generic name of drug — DICLOFENAC SODIUM   75 MG TABLETS
Brand-name equivalent — (GENERIC FOR VOLTAREN)

Quantity of drug
in package — QTY: 60 TABS   DISCARD AFTER: 1/07
Number of refills
remaining — REFILLS LEFT: 2

Amount of medication per unit ——   Expiration date

DO NOT DRINK ALCOHOLIC BEVERAGES when taking this medication

YOU SHOULD AVOID PROLONGED OR EXCESSIVE EXPOSURE TO DIRECT AND/OR ARTIFICIAL SUNLIGHT WHILE TAKING THIS MEDICATION

DO NOT TAKE ASPIRIN WITHOUT KNOWLEDGE AND CONSENT OF YOUR PHYSICIAN

May Cause DROWSINESS

Figure 21-3   Reading and understanding prescription medication labels.

use online pharmacies only to obtain medicines prescribed by their usual health care provider.

• *Costs:* Spending on prescription drugs is rising faster than the rate of inflation and is now the fastest-growing portion of U.S. health care spending. Many Americans have no or limited insurance coverage for prescription drug costs. Consumers may be able to lower their drug costs by using generic versions of medications; by joining a drug discount program sponsored by a company, organization, or local pharmacy; and by investigating mail-order or Internet pharmacies.

There is ongoing controversy about the importation of lower-cost drugs from Canada. Canada imports U.S. drugs and regulates Canadian-produced drugs, so safety should theoretically not be a concern for drugs from Canada. However, companies in Canada may make drugs for export only, thus avoiding regulation; and online pharmacies may claim they are operating in Canada but may be located in another country where there is little or no regulation. U.S. regulators have found online sites advertising Canadian drugs but shipping fake or substandard versions of medications. In addition, shipping costs can be high, and U.S. generic drugs are often less expensive than Canadian drugs.

Patients also share some responsibility for problems with prescription drugs. Many people don't take their medications properly, skipping doses, taking incorrect doses, stopping too soon, or not taking the medication at all. An estimated 30–50% of the more than 3 billion prescriptions dispensed annually in the United States are not taken correctly and thus do not produce the desired results. Consumers can increase the safety and effectiveness of their treatment by asking the following questions:

• *Do I really need this prescription, or are there non-drug alternatives?*

• *What is the name of the medication, and what is it supposed to do, within what period of time?*

• *How and when do I take the medication, how much do I take, and for how long? What should I do if I miss a dose?*

• *What other medications, foods, drinks, or activities should I avoid?* Other drugs, including alcohol, herbs, and OTC drugs, can interact with medications, diminishing or increasing their effect (Figure 21-3). For example, certain antibiotics, including ampicillin and tetracycline, may prevent oral contraceptives from working. Others may increase the effects of sunlight on the skin.

• *What are the side effects, and what do I do if they occur?* If you have a drug allergy or other medical condition, such as epilepsy or diabetes, that may require special attention in case of an emergency, wear a medical ID necklace or bracelet or carry a medical ID card. For comprehensive emergency medical service, consider joining Medic Alert (www.medicalert.org); call 1-800-ID-ALERT for more information.

• *Can I take a generic drug rather than a brand-name one?* Generic drugs contain the same active ingredients as the original brand-name drug, but they may contain different inactive ingredients. They are usually substantially less expensive, but sometimes physicians have reasons for preferring a particular brand.

• *Is there written information about the medication?* There are many sources of information, including the FDA-approved inserts in drug packaging and books.

Remember to store your medications in a cool, dry place, out of direct light. Never share your prescription medications with anyone else, and never use an old prescription for a new ailment.

SURGERY Surgical procedures are performed more often in the United States than anywhere else in the world. Each year, more than 70 million operations and related procedures are performed. About 20% are in response to an emergency such as a severe injury, and 80% are **elective surgeries,** meaning the patient can generally choose when and where to have the operation, if at all. Some key questions include the following:

• *Why do I need surgery at this time?* Your physician should be able to explain the reason for the surgery and what is likely to happen if you don't have it. Getting a second opinion about surgery is recommended and may be required by your health insurance plan.

• *What are the risks and complications of the surgery?* Overall risk depends on the type of operation performed, the surgeon, and your general state of health. Ask about the *mortality rate* (risk of death) and the *morbidity rate* (risk of nonlethal complications).

• *Can the operation be performed on an outpatient basis?* **Outpatient** (ambulatory) surgery has many advantages, including lower costs and fewer opportunities for hospital-associated complications.

• *What can I expect before, during, and after surgery?* Knowing what to expect can help you prepare for the surgery and speed your recovery.

COMPLEMENTARY AND ALTERNATIVE MEDICINE

Where conventional Western medicine tends to focus on the body, on the physical causes of disease, and on ways to eradicate pathogens in order to restore health, traditional medicine tends to focus on an integration of mind, body, and spirit and to seek ways to restore the whole person to harmony so that he or she can regain health. Where conventional medicine is based on science, traditional medicine tends to be based on accumulated experience.

Many alternative medical systems with long-standing traditions have concepts and theories of medicine that are very different from those of current Western medical thought. Some people consider all of CAM quackery and tell you that you can recognize a quack by his or her use of pseudoscientific language. However, the use of phrases like "bringing into harmony with nature" or "enhancing the flow of vital energy" does not necessarily mean that a practitioner is a quack; rather, it may reflect this practitioner's different concept of health and healing.

You might have heard that there are only anecdotal testimonials to support the value of many forms of CAM and that because such reports do not constitute scientific proof of effectiveness, they are therefore meaningless. Although it is correct that anecdotes and testimonials are not scientifically reliable evidence, that does not mean that they are meaningless. What is called anecdotal evidence may actually be a form of case report, a valuable and standard form of study in which a researcher describes a single patient, his or her medical history, the treatments administered, and the outcome of the case. Still, case reports alone are not sufficient to scientifically prove the effectiveness of a medical treatment. Caution is in order when choosing any mode of treatment that has not been scientifically evaluated for safety and effectiveness (see the box "Avoiding Health Fraud and Quackery").

The NIH National Center for Complementary and Alternative Medicine (NCCAM) groups CAM practices into five domains: alternative medical systems, mind-body interventions, biological-based therapies, manipulative and body-based methods, and energy therapies (Figure 21-4, p. 645). It is impossible to discuss all of these forms fully in a single chapter. Instead, what follows is a general introduction to the types of CAM available and a brief description of some of the more widely used ones. To learn more about any of these approaches, consult the For More Information section at the end of the chapter.

Alternative Medical Systems

Many cultures elaborated complete systems of medical philosophy, theory, and practice long before the current biomedical approach was developed. The complete systems that are best known in the United States are probably traditional Chinese medicine (TCM), also known as traditional Oriental medicine, and homeopathy. Traditional medical systems have also been developed in many other regions of the world, including North, Central, and South America; the Middle East; India; Tibet; and Australia. In many countries, these medical approaches continue to be used today—frequently alongside Western medicine and quite often by physicians trained in Western medicine.

Alternative medical systems tend to have concepts in common. For example, the concept of life force or energy exists in many cultures. In traditional Chinese medicine, the life force contained in all living things is called *qi* (sometimes spelled chi). Qi resembles the *vis vitalis* (Latin for "life force") of Greek, Roman, and European medical systems, and *prana* of ayurveda, the traditional medical system of India. Most traditional medical systems think of

According to the Federal Trade Commission, consumers waste billions of dollars on unproven, fraudulently marketed, and sometimes useless health care products and treatments. In addition, those with serious medical problems may waste valuable time before seeking proper treatment. Worse yet, some of the products they're buying may cause serious harm. Health fraud is a business that sells false hope. It preys on people with diseases that have no medical cure and on people who want shortcuts to weight loss or improvements to personal appearance.

The first rule of thumb for evaluating any health claim is that if it sounds too good to be true, it probably is. Also be on the lookout for the typical phrases and marketing techniques fraudulent promoters use to deceive consumers:

- The product is advertised as a quick and effective cure-all or diagnostic tool for a wide range of ailments.

- The promoters use words like *scientific breakthrough, miraculous cure, exclusive product, secret ingredient,* or *ancient remedy.* Also remember that just because a product is described as natural or unprocessed does not necessarily mean it's safe.

- The text is written in medicalese—impressive-sounding terminology to disguise a lack of good science.

- The promoter claims the government, the medical profession, or researchers have conspired to suppress the product.

- The advertisement includes undocumented case histories claiming amazing results.

- The product is advertised as in limited supply or available from only one source, and payment is required in advance.

- The promoter promises a no-risk money-back guarantee. Be aware that many fly-by-night operators are not around to respond to your request for a refund.

To check out a particular product, talk to a physician or another health care professional and to family members and friends. Be wary of treatments offered by people who tell you to avoid talking to others. Check with the Better Business Bureau or local attorney general's office to see whether other consumers have lodged complaints about the product or the product's mar-

keter. You can also check with the appropriate health professional group. For example, check with the American Diabetes Association or the National Arthritis Foundation if the products are promoted for diabetes or arthritis. Take special care with products and devices sold online; the broad reach of the Internet, combined with the ease of setting up and removing Web sites, makes online sellers particularly difficult to regulate.

If you think you have been a victim of health fraud or if you have an adverse reaction that you think is related to a particular supplement, you can report it to the appropriate agency:

- *False advertising claims:* Contact the FTC by phone (877-FTC-HELP), by mail (Consumer Response Center, Federal Trade Commission, Washington, DC 20580), or online (http://www.ftc.gov; click on File a Complaint). You can also contact your state attorney general's office, your state department of health, or the local consumer protection agency (check your local telephone directory).

- *False labeling on a product:* Contact the FDA district office consumer complaint coordinator for your geographic area. (The FDA regulates safety, manufacturing, and product labeling.)

- *Adverse reaction to a supplement:* Call a doctor or another health care provider immediately. You may also report your adverse reaction to FDA MedWatch by calling 800-FDA-1088 or by visiting the MedWatch Web site (http://www.fda.gov/medwatch).

- *Unlawful Internet sales:* If you find a Web site that you think is illegally selling drugs, medical devices, dietary supplements, or cosmetics, report it to the FDA. Problems can be reported to MedWatch or via the FDA Web site (http://www.fda.gov/oc/buyonline/buyonlineform.htm).

SOURCES: Meadows, M. 2005. Use caution buying medical products online. *FDA Consumer,* January/February; Federal Trade Commission. 2001. *"Miracle" Health Claims: Add a Dose of Skepticism* (http://www.ftc.gov/bcp/conline/pubs/health/frdheal.htm; retrieved December 14, 2002); Food and Drug Administration. 1999. *How to Report Adverse Reactions and Other Problems with Products Regulated by FDA* (http://www.fda.gov/opacom/backgrounders/problem.html; retrieved July 19, 2000); Kurtzweil, P. 1999. How to spot health fraud. *FDA Consumer,* November/December.

disease as a disturbance or imbalance not just of physical processes but also of forces and energies within the body, the mind, and the spirit. In traditional Chinese medicine, for example, the principle of balance is expressed as yin and yang, which are opposites yet complement each other. Disease is a disturbance of qi reflecting an imbalance between yin and yang. Treatment aims at reestablishing equilibrium, balance, and harmony.

Because the whole patient, rather than an isolated set of symptoms, is treated in most comprehensive alternative medical systems, it is rare that only a single treatment

approach is used. Most commonly, multiple techniques and methods are employed and are continually adjusted according to the changes in the patient's health status that occur naturally or are brought about by the treatment.

Traditional Chinese Medicine Traditional Chinese medicine (TCM) is based on highly abstract concepts; a sophisticated set of techniques and methods; and individualized diagnosis, treatment, and prevention. No identical diseases exist in TCM. Two patients with the same diagnosis in Western medicine will get

Domain	Characteristics	Examples
Alternative Medical Systems	Involve complete systems of theory and practice that have evolved independently of and often long before the conventional biomedical approach	Traditional Chinese medicine; Kampo; ayurveda (India); Native American, Aboriginal, African, Middle-Eastern, Tibetan, Central and South American medical systems; homeopathy; naturopathy
Mind-Body Interventions	Employ a variety of techniques designed to make it possible for the mind to affect bodily function and symptoms	Meditation, certain uses of hypnosis, prayer, mental healing
Biological-Based Therapies	Include natural and biologically based practices, interventions, and products, many of which overlap with conventional medicine's use of dietary supplements	Herbal, special dietary, orthomolecular,* and individual biological therapies
Manipulative and Body-Based Methods	Include methods that are based on manipulation and/or movement of the body	Chiropractic, osteopathy, massage therapy
Energy Therapies	Focus on energy fields within the body (biofields) or from other sources (electromagnetic fields)	Qi gong, Reiki, therapeutic touch, bioelectromagnetic-based therapies

*Orthomolecular therapies are treatments of diseases with varying, but usually high, concentrations of chemicals, including minerals (e.g., magnesium), hormones (e.g., melatonin), or vitamins.

Figure 21-4   The five domains of CAM practices.

different diagnoses in TCM and will be given different treatments.

In TCM, the free and harmonious flow of qi produces health—a positive feeling of well-being and vitality in body, mind, and spirit. Illness occurs when the flow of qi is blocked or disturbed. TCM works to restore and balance the flow of blocked qi; the goal is not only to treat illnesses but also to increase energy, prevent disease, and support the immune system.

Two of the primary treatment methods in TCM are herbal remedies and **acupuncture.** Chinese herbal remedies number about 5800 and include plant products, animal parts, and minerals. Herbal remedies, like everything else, have yin and yang properties. When a disease is perceived to be due to a yin deficiency, remedies with more yin characteristics might be used for treatment. The use of a single medicinal botanical is rare in Chinese herbal medicine; rather, several different plants are combined in very precise proportions, often to make a tea or soup. For example, a remedy might include a primary herb that targets the main symptom, a second herb that enhances the effects of the primary herb, a third that lessens side effects, and a fourth that helps deliver ingredients to a particular body site.

Acupuncture works to correct disturbances in the flow of qi through the insertion of long, thin needles at appropriate points in the skin. Qi is believed to flow through the body along several meridians, or pathways, and there

are approximately 360 acupuncture points located along these meridians. Acupuncturists use a variety of diagnostic techniques to identify the nature of the imbalance in a patient and to choose the points at which acupuncture needs to be applied. The traditional method consists of inserting the needle and then manipulating it manually, but other means of manipulation, such as heat, pressure, friction, suction, or electric stimulation, can also be used. The points chosen for acupuncture are highly individualized for each patient, and they change over the course of treatment as the patient's health status changes.

The World Health Organization has compiled a list of over 40 conditions in which acupuncture may be beneficial. At a conference called by the National Institutes of Health (NIH), a panel of experts recently analyzed the available information on the scientific evidence for the efficacy of

Terms

traditional Chinese medicine (TCM) The traditional medical system of China, which views illness as the result of a disturbance in the flow of qi, the life force; therapies include acupuncture, herbal medicine, and massage.

acupuncture Insertion of long, thin needles into the skin at points along meridians, pathways through which qi is believed to flow; needles correct imbalances in qi; a practice common in traditional Chinese medicine.

Acupuncture is one of the key treatment methods in traditional Chinese medicine. It involves the insertion of long, thin needles at appropriate points in the skin to restore balance to the flow of qi.

acupuncture in many of these conditions. These experts found evidence that acupuncture was effective in relieving nausea and vomiting after chemotherapy and pain after surgery, including dental surgery. They added, however, that there is not yet enough evidence to show conclusively that acupuncture is effective for headaches, menstrual cramps, tennis elbow, back pain, carpal tunnel syndrome, asthma, or other conditions. Western researchers typically use a different framework for understanding the effects of acupuncture. For example, they might explain pain relief not in terms of qi but in terms of stimulation of the nervous system and release of hormones and neurotransmitters.

Although more than 1 million Americans receive acupuncture each year, there have been few adverse events (negative effects) associated with it in the United States. Nonetheless, problems can occur from the improper insertion and manipulation of needles and from the use of unsterile needles. The FDA regulates acupuncture needles like other standard medical devices and requires that they be sterile. Most acupuncture practitioners follow these regulations, but, if you consider acupuncture, you should ask your practitioner about the relative risks of the procedure and the safety practices he or she observes. A majority of states require some form of licensing or credentialing for practitioners of acupuncture, but the requirements for licensure vary widely.

Homeopathy An alternative medical system of Western origin, **homeopathy** was developed about 200 years ago by the German physician Samuel Hahnemann (1755–1843) and is based on two main principles: "Like cures like," and remedies become more effective with greater dilution. "Like cures like" summarizes the concept that a substance that produces the symptoms of an illness or disease in a healthy person can cure the illness when given in very minute quantities. Remedies containing very small quantities of a particular substance are ob-

tained by repeatedly diluting the original solution. The extent of dilution varies, but the final extract is often so dilute that few, if any, of the original molecules are left in it. According to homeopathic thinking, such highly diluted extracts not only retain some form of biological activity but actually become more potent.

Over 1000 different substances (plant and animal parts, minerals, and chemicals) can be used to prepare homeopathic remedies, and each of these substances is thought to have different effects at different dilutions. That means a homeopath must not only choose the correct remedy for a particular patient but also decide on the specific dilution of that remedy in order to achieve the desired effect.

Like other traditional systems of medicine, homeopathy constitutes a highly individualized form of therapy; that is, the treatment of each patient is determined by the overall condition of the patient rather than by specific symptoms. In order to assess a patient's condition, homeopaths generally spend quite a bit of time talking with a patient and assessing his or her physical, psychological, and emotional health before deciding on the correct remedy at the proper dilution. This intensive interaction between the practitioner and the patient might play an important role in the success of the therapy. Indeed, critics of homeopathy often attribute its reported effectiveness to this nonspecific placebo effect (see the box "The Power of Belief: The Placebo Effect").

However, when the results of 185 homeopathic trials were analyzed recently, it was concluded that the clinical effects of homeopathy could not be completely explained by the placebo effect. At the same time, homeopathy was not found to be effective for any single clinical condition. Homeopathy remains one of the most controversial forms of CAM.

Because of the extremely dilute nature of homeopathic remedies, it is generally assumed that they are safe. To date, the FDA has not found any serious adverse events associated with the use of homeopathy, with the possible exception of situations in which a patient might have been successfully treated with standard medical approaches but chose to rely solely on homeopathy. The FDA regulates homeopathic remedies, but they are subject to many fewer restrictions than prescription or over-the-counter drugs. Remedies designed to treat conditions such as colds and headaches can be sold over the counter; products that claim to treat serious conditions such as heart disease can be sold only by prescription. A few states require practitioners to have special licenses, but most providers practice homeopathy as a specialty under another medical license, such as medical doctor or nurse practitioner.

Mind-Body Interventions

Mind-body interventions make use of the integral connection between mind and body and the effect each can have on the other. They include many of the stress-management techniques discussed in Chapter 2, including

The Power of Belief: The Placebo Effect

A placebo is a chemically inactive substance or ineffective procedure that a patient believes is an effective medical therapy for his or her condition. Researchers frequently give placebos to the control group in an experiment testing the efficacy of a particular treatment. By comparing the effects of the actual treatment with the effects of the placebo, researchers can judge whether the treatment is effective. The placebo effect occurs when a patient improves after receiving a placebo. In such cases, the effect of the placebo on the patient cannot be attributed to the specific actions or properties of the drug or procedure.

Researchers have consistently found that 30–40% of all patients given a placebo show improvement. This result has been observed for a wide variety of conditions or symptoms, including coughing, seasickness, depression, migraines, and angina. For some conditions, placebos have been effective in up to 70% of patients. In some cases, people given a placebo even report having the side effects associated with an actual drug. Placebos are particularly effective when they are administered by a physician whom the patient trusts.

A clear demonstration of the placebo effect occurred in a recent study that examined the effectiveness of a drug used to treat benign enlargement of the prostate. The men who participated in the study were randomly assigned to one of two groups: One group received the medication; the other received a placebo, a look-alike dummy pill. More than half the men who got the placebo pills reported significant relief from their symptoms, including faster urine flow—despite the fact that men on the placebo actually experienced an *increase* in the size of their prostates. How did the men in the study experience fewer symptoms despite no actual improvement in their condition? Researchers hypothesize that the patients' positive expectations of the medication's effects may have resulted in decreased nerve activity and muscle relaxation affecting the bladder, prostate, and urethra. Studies on patients with depression and people with Parkinson's disease have found that treatment with an inactive placebo results in changes in brain function. Such changes in the electrical or chemical activity of the brain may help explain the placebo effect.

The placebo effect can be exploited by unscrupulous people who sell worthless medical treatments to the scientifically unsophisticated public. But placebo power can also be harnessed for its beneficial effects. When a skilled and compassionate medical practitioner provides a patient with a sense of confidence and hope, the positive aspects of placebo power can boost the benefits of standard medical treatment. Whenever you swallow a pill, you swallow your expectations right along with the medication or herb; imagining how the pill is helping you can stimulate a positive placebo effect. Getting well, like getting sick, is a complex process. Anatomy, physiology, mind, emotions, and the environment are all inextricably intertwined. But the placebo effect does show that belief can have both psychological and physical effects.

SOURCES: Leuchter, A. F., et al. 2002. Changes in brain function of depressed subjects during treatment with placebo. *American Journal of Psychiatry* 159(1): 122–129; Nordenberg, T. 2000. The healing power of placebos. *FDA Consumer*, January/February; The powerful placebo: An effect without a cause. 2000. *Harvard Men's Health Watch,* June.

---

meditation, yoga, visualization, taijiquan, and biofeedback. Psychotherapy, support groups, prayer, and music, art, and dance therapy can also be thought of as mind-body interventions. Obviously, there is no clear line between these forms of CAM and conventional medicine. The placebo effect is one of the most widely known examples of mind-body interdependence.

Some forms of **hypnosis** are considered to be CAM therapies, although the use of hypnotherapy for certain conditions was accepted more than 40 years ago by the American Medical Association. Hypnosis involves the induction of a state of deep relaxation during which the patient is more suggestible (more easily influenced). While the patient is in such a hypnotic trance, the practitioner tries to help him or her change unwanted behavior or deal with pain and other symptoms. An NIH-sponsored report found strong evidence for the effectiveness of relaxation techniques and hypnosis in reducing chronic pain stemming from a variety of medical conditions, although subsequent studies have cast some doubt on this conclusion. Hypnosis is sometimes used in smoking cessation programs and as a nondrug approach to anxiety

disorders such as phobias and chronic conditions such as irritable bowel syndrome.

Hypnosis can be used by medical professionals (M.D.s, D.O.s, D.D.S.s) but is also offered by hypnotherapists. Physicians are certified by their own associations; many states require hypnotherapists to be licensed, but the requirements for licensing vary substantially. There is little regulation of practitioners of other relaxation techniques, but it is very rare that adverse events result from such techniques. Many studies have shown that support groups, friendships, strong family relationships, and prayer can all have a positive impact on health.

Terms

V w

homeopathy An alternative medical system of Western origin in which illnesses are treated by giving very small doses of drugs that in larger doses in a healthy person would produce symptoms like those of the illness.

hypnosis The process by which a practitioner induces a state of deep relaxation in which an individual is more suggestible; commonly used in cases of pain, phobia, and addiction.

Biological-Based Therapies

Biological-based therapies consist primarily of herbal therapies or remedies, botanicals, and dietary supplements. Herbal therapies are sometimes referred to as *materia medica,* Latin for "medical matter," a term that can include a much larger variety of compounds than just herbs (which are plants that die down at the end of a growing season and do not produce woody tissue). Some herbal remedies are not technically herbs, such as the leaves of the *Ginkgo biloba* tree, and some are not even from plants, such as shark cartilage and bear gallbladder. Other items that constitute *materia medica* are algae, bacteria, fungi, and minerals. For traditional remedies that are of plant origin, many scientists prefer to use the term *botanicals.* Nonetheless, because even official government definitions use the word *herbs* to designate substances from the categories of herbs, botanicals, and other *materia medica,* the terms are used somewhat interchangeably in this chapter.

Herbal remedies are a major component of all indigenous forms of medicine; prior to the development of pharmaceuticals at the end of the nineteenth century, people everywhere in the world relied on materials from nature for pain relief, wound healing, and treatment of a variety of ailments. Herbal remedies are also a common element in most systems of traditional medicine. Much of the **pharmacopoeia** of modern scientific medicine originated in the folk medicine of native peoples, and many drugs used today are derived from plants.

A majority of botanical products are sold as dietary supplements, that is, in the form of tablets, pills, capsules, liquid extracts, or teas. Like foods, dietary supplements must carry ingredient labels (see Chapter 12). As with food products, it is the responsibility of the manufacturers to ensure that their dietary supplements are safe and properly labeled prior to marketing. The FDA is responsible for monitoring the labeling and accompanying literature of dietary supplements and for overseeing their safety once they are on the market.

Well-designed clinical studies have been conducted on only a small number of botanicals. A few other commonly used botanicals, their uses, and the evidence supporting their efficacy are presented in Table 21-2. Participants in clinical trials with St. John's wort, ginkgo, and echinacea experienced only minor adverse events. However, most clinical trials of this type last for only a few weeks, so the tests did not indicate whether it is safe to take these botanicals for longer periods of time. They also didn't examine the effects of different dosages or how the botanicals interact with other drugs.

For the vast majority of other botanicals, there are almost no reliable research findings on efficacy or safety. That is extremely worrisome because, of all the CAM approaches, the consumption of botanical supplements has the greatest potential to result in serious and even life-threatening consequences. For more information, see the box "Herbal Remedies: Are They Safe?" on p. 650.

Manipulative and Body-Based Methods

Touch and body manipulation are long-standing forms of health care. Manual healing techniques are based on the idea that misalignment or dysfunction in one part of the body can cause pain or dysfunction in another part; correcting these misalignments can bring the body back to optimal health.

Manual healing methods are an integral part of osteopathic medicine, now considered a form of conventional medicine. Other physical healing methods include massage, acupressure, Feldenkrais, Rolfing, and numerous other techniques. The most commonly accepted of the CAM manual healing methods is **chiropractic,** a method that focuses on the relationship between structure, primarily of joints and muscles, and function, primarily of the nervous system, to maintain or restore health. An important therapeutic procedure is the manipulation of joints, particularly those of the spinal column. However, chiropractors also use a variety of other techniques, including physical therapy, exercise programs, patient education and lifestyle modification, nutritional supplements, and orthotics (mechanical supports and braces) to treat patients. They do not use drugs or surgery.

Chiropractors, or doctors of chiropractic, are trained for a minimum of four full-time academic years at accredited chiropractic colleges and can go on to postgraduate training in many countries. Although specifically listed by NCCAM as one of the manipulative and body-based methods of CAM, chiropractic is accepted by many health care and health insurance providers to a far greater extent than the other types of CAM therapies. Based on research showing the efficacy of chiropractic

Terms

V w

biological-based therapies CAM therapies that include natural and biologically based practices, interventions, and products; examples include herbal remedies and dietary supplements.

pharmacopoeia A collection of drugs and medicinal preparations.

chiropractic A system of manual healing most frequently used to treat musculoskeletal problems; the primary treatment is manipulation of the spine and other joints. Practitioners hold a doctor of chiropractic degree and are licensed.

energy therapies Forms of CAM treatment that use energy fields originating either within the body or from outside sources to promote healing.

qigong A component of traditional Chinese medicine that combines movement, meditation, and regulation of breathing to enhance the flow of qi, improve blood circulation, and enhance immune function.

Table 21-2 — Commonly Used Botanicals, Their Uses, Evidence for Their Effectiveness, and Contraindications

Botanical	Use	Evidence	Examples of Adverse Effects and Interactions
Echinacea (*Echinacea purpurea, E. angustifolia, E. pallida*)	Stimulation of immune functions; to prevent colds and flulike diseases; to lessen symptoms of colds and flus	Some trials showed that it prevents colds and flus and helps patients recover from colds faster, but others found it ineffective	Might cause liver damage if taken over long periods of time (more than 8 weeks); since it is an immune stimulant, it is not advisable to take it with immune suppressants (e.g., corticosteroids)
Evening primrose oil* (*Oenothera biennis L.*)	Reduction of inflammation	Long-term supplementation effective in reducing symptoms of rheumatoid arthritis	None known
Feverfew (*Tanacetum parthenium*)	Prevention of headaches and migraines	The majority of trials indicate that it is more effective than placebo, but the evidence is not yet conclusive	Should not be used by people allergic to other members of the aster family; has the potential to increase the effects of warfarin and other anticoagulants
Garlic (*Allium sativum*)	Reduction of cholesterol	Short-term studies have found a modest effect; long-term studies are needed	May interact with some medications, including anticoagulants, cyclosporine, and oral contraceptives
Ginkgo (*Ginkgo biloba*)	Improvement of circulation and memory	Improves cerebral insufficiency and slows progression of Alzheimer's disease and other types of senile dementia in some patients; improves blood flow in legs	Could increase bleeding time; should not be taken with nonsteroidal anti-inflammatory drugs or anticoagulants; gastrointestinal disturbance
Ginseng** (*Panax ginseng*)	Improvement of physical performance, memory, immune function, and glycemic control in diabetes; treatment of herpes simplex 2	No conclusive evidence exists for any of these uses	Interacts with warfarin and alcohol in mice and rats, hence should probably not be used with these drugs; may cause liver damage
St. John's wort (*Hypericum perforatum*)	Treatment of depression	There is strong evidence that it is significantly more effective than placebo, is as effective as some standard antidepressants for mild to moderate depression, and causes fewer adverse effects	Known to interact with a variety of pharmaceuticals and should not be taken together with digoxin, theophylline, cyclosporine, indinavir, and serotonin-reuptake inhibitors
Saw palmetto (*Serenoa repens*)	Improvement of prostate health	Appears to be moderately effective, but the evidence is not yet considered conclusive	Has no known interactions with drugs, but should probably not be taken with hormonal therapies
Valerian (*Valeriana officinalis*)	Treatment of insomnia	Appears to help with sleep disorders, but further trials are needed	Interacts with thiopental and pentobarbital and should not be used with these drugs

*Similar results have been obtained with borage oil (*Borago officinalis L.*).

**There are two other species of ginseng, *Panax quinquefolium* (American ginseng) and *Eleutherococcus senticosus* (Siberian ginseng), but in clinical trials for cerebral insufficiency and dementia only *Panax ginseng* has been tested.

---

management in acute low-back pain, spinal manipulation has been included in the federal guidelines for the treatment of this condition. Promising results have also been reported with the use of chiropractic techniques in neck pain and headaches. However, there are no well-controlled studies to support manipulation for asthma, gastrointestinal problems, infectious diseases, or other nonmechanical problems.

A caution is in order regarding chiropractic: Spinal manipulation performed by a person without proper chiropractic training can be extremely dangerous. There are several organizations, in particular the American Chiropractic Association, that can help you locate a licensed chiropractor near you.

Energy Therapies

Energy therapies are forms of treatment that use energy fields originating either within the body (biofields) or from other sources (electromagnetic fields). Biofield therapies are based on the idea that energy fields surround and penetrate the body and can be influenced by movement, touch, pressure, or the placement of hands in or through the fields. **Qigong**, a component of traditional Chinese

Consider the following research findings and FDA advisories:

• St. John's wort interacts with drugs used to treat HIV infection and heart disease; the herb may also reduce the effectiveness of oral contraceptives, antirejection drugs used with organ transplants, and some medications used to treat infections, depression, asthma, and seizure disorders.

• Chinese herbs contaminated through a manufacturing error with the powerful carcinogen aristolochic acid caused kidney damage and bladder cancer in patients at a weight-loss clinic in Belgium.

• Supplements containing kava have been linked to severe liver damage, and anyone who has liver problems or takes medications that can affect the liver are advised to consult a physician before using kava-containing supplements.

• In a sample of ayurvedic herbal medicine products, 20% were found to contain potentially harmful levels of lead, mercury, and/or arsenic.

These findings highlight growing safety concerns about dietary supplements, which now represent annual sales of more than $15 billion in the United States.

Drug Interactions

As in the case of St. John's wort, the chemicals in botanicals can interact dangerously with prescription and over-the-counter drugs. Botanicals may decrease the effects of drugs, making them ineffective, or increase their effects, in some cases making them toxic. Alarmingly, most patients fail to tell their physicians about their use of herbal substances. Botanicals can also interact with alcohol, usually heightening alcohol's effects. There

are also complex interactions among the constituents of a single herbal preparation. And many manufacturers are offering new combinations of botanical preparations without empirical or scientific information about the interactions of the individual ingredients.

Lack of Standardization

A related problem is the lack of standardization in the manufacturing of herbal products. The Dietary Supplement Health and Education Act of 1994 requires that dietary supplement labels list the name and quantity of each ingredient. However, confusion can result because different plant species—with distinct chemical compositions and effects—may have the same common name. The content of herbal preparations is also variable. A 2003 study of echinacea supplements found that only about half contained the species and amount listed on the label; 10% of the samples contained no echinacea at all. Part of the reason for such variation is the difficulty of identifying the active ingredients in botanicals and isolating and standardizing their concentrations. The chemical composition of a supplement is also affected by the growing, harvesting, processing, and storage conditions of plants.

Contamination, Adulteration, and Toxicity

A variety of traditional Chinese and ayurvedic remedies contain heavy metals such as lead, mercury, and arsenic as part of the formula, all of which can be highly toxic and can cause irreversible damage. Some Chinese herbal remedies have been found to contain pharmaceutical drugs, including tranquilizers and steroids. Others contain herbs not listed on the label, sometimes substitute herbs that have toxic effects, as in the case of the weight-

loss pills used in the Belgian clinic. Furthermore, many plants are poisonous or can cause damage to the liver or kidneys if taken over long periods of time. Experts have also advised against taking supplements that contain raw animal parts, particularly central nervous system tissue, out of concern that disease may be transmissible this way.

The Role of Government in Safety Issues

Some European governments assume greater responsibility in regulating botanicals than the U.S. government. In Germany, herbal medicine has a long history, but herbs are considered medicines rather than supplements; they are usually prescribed by physicians. Manufacturing is standardized so that content, quantity, quality, and purity are guaranteed. Botanicals do not have to be proven effective to be marketed, but they do have to be proven safe.

In the United States, because herbs are considered supplements rather than food or drug products, they do not have to meet FDA food and drug standards for safety or effectiveness, nor do they currently have to meet any manufacturing standards. The manufacturer is responsible for ensuring that a supplement is safe before it is marketed; the FDA has the power to restrict a substance if it is found to pose a health risk after it is on the market. Because U.S. manufacturers can put almost anything into an herbal supplement, American consumers are at risk for buying and using products that may be not just useless but harmful as well. Part of the reasoning behind this situation is that herbal products are considered safer than conventional medicines. As the incidents with St. John's wort, aristolochic acid, kava, and ayurvedic products demonstrate, this is not always the case.

medicine, combines movement, meditation, and regulation of breathing to enhance the flow of qi, improve blood circulation, and enhance immune function. **Therapeutic touch** is derived from the ancient technique of laying-on of hands; it is based on the premise that healers can identify and correct energy imbalances by passing their hands over the patient's body. **Reiki** is one form of therapeutic

touch; it is intended to correct disturbances in the flow of life energy (ki is the Japanese form of the Chinese qi) and enhance the body's healing powers through the use of 13 specific hand positions on the patient.

Bioelectromagnetics is the study of the interaction between living organisms and electromagnetic fields, both those produced by the organism itself and those produced by outside sources. The recognition that the body produces electromagnetic fields has led to the development of many diagnostic procedures in Western medicine, including electroencephalography (EEG), electrocardiography (ECG), and nuclear magnetic resonance (NMR) scans. **Bioelectromagnetic-based therapies** involve the use of electromagnetic fields to manage pain and to treat conditions such as asthma. There are some indications that the use of electromagnetic fields might be useful in the areas of bone repair, wound healing, nerve stimulation, immune system stimulation, and modulation of the neuroendocrine (nerve and hormonal) system. Although promising, the available research is still very limited and does not allow firm conclusions about the efficacy of these therapies. Most scientists believe that consumer products containing small magnets have no significant effect on the human body.

Evaluating Complementary and Alternative Therapies

Because there is less information available about complementary and alternative therapies, as well as less regulation of associated products and providers, it is important for consumers to take an active role when they are thinking about using them.

Working with Your Physician If you are considering a CAM therapy, your first source of information should be your physician or primary health care provider. The NCCAM advises consumers not to seek complementary therapies without first visiting a conventional health care provider for an evaluation and diagnosis of their symptoms. It's usually best to discuss and try conventional treatments that have been shown to be beneficial for your condition. If you are thinking of trying any alternative therapies, it is critically important to tell your physician in order to avoid any dangerous interactions with conventional treatments you are receiving. Areas to discuss with your physician include the following:

- *Safety:* Is there something unsafe about the treatment in general or for you specifically? Are there safety issues you should be aware of, such as the use of disposable needles in acupuncture?

- *Effectiveness:* Is there any research about the use of the therapy for your condition?

- *Timing:* Is the immediate use of a conventional treatment indicated?

- *Cost:* Is the therapy likely to be very expensive, especially in light of the potential benefit?

If you are not comfortable discussing CAM therapies with your physician, ask yourself why. Are you embarrassed about it? Do you think your doctor will think less of you? Do you think he or she doesn't know enough

Good communication between consumers and health care providers is important in both conventional and complementary medicine. It is important for consumers who choose to use CAM to discuss their choice with their physician to prevent any dangerous interactions with conventional treatments.

about the therapy you are considering? You have the right to expect your physician to take you and your concerns seriously, to respect your interest in a CAM therapy, to be informed about CAM approaches or at least make an effort to find out about them, and to be willing to discuss the evidence for and against them with you.

If appropriate, schedule a follow-up visit with your physician to assess your condition and your progress after a certain amount of time using a complementary therapy. Keep a symptom diary to more accurately track your symptoms and gauge your progress. (Symptoms such as pain and fatigue are very difficult to recall with accuracy, so an ongoing symptom diary is an important tool.) If you plan to pursue a therapy against your physician's advice, you need to tell him or her.

For supplements, particularly botanicals, pharmacists can also be an excellent source of information, especially if they are familiar with other medications you are taking.

Terms

therapeutic touch A CAM practice based on the premise that healers can identify and correct energy imbalances by passing their hands over the patient's body.

Reiki A CAM practice intended to correct disturbances in the flow of life energy and enhance the body's healing powers through the use of 13 hand positions on the patient.

bioelectromagnetic-based therapies CAM therapies based on the notion that electromagnetic fields can be used to promote healing and manage pain.

Questioning the CAM Practitioner You can also get information from individual practitioners and from schools, professional organizations, and state licensing boards. Ask about education, training, licensing, and certification. If appropriate, check with local or state regulatory agencies or the consumer affairs department to determine if any complaints have been lodged against the practitioner. Some guidelines for talking with a CAM practitioner include the following:

- Ask the practitioner why he or she thinks the therapy will be beneficial for your condition. Ask for a full description of the therapy and any potential side effects.

- Describe in detail any conventional treatments you are receiving.

- Ask how long the therapy should continue before it can be determined if it is beneficial.

- Ask about the expected cost of the treatment. Does it seem reasonable? Will your health insurance pay some or all of the costs?

If anything an alternative practitioner says or recommends directly conflicts with advice from your physician, discuss it with your physician before making any major changes in any current treatment regimen or in your lifestyle.

Doing Your Own Research You can investigate CAM therapies on your own by going to the library or doing research online, although caution is in order when using Web sites for the various forms of CAM. A good place to start is the Web sites of government agencies like the FDA or NCCAM and of universities and similar organizations that conduct government-sponsored research on CAM approaches (see For More Information).

If possible, also talk to people with the same condition you have who have received the same treatment. Remember, though, that patient testimonials shouldn't be used as the sole criterion for choosing a therapy or assessing its safety and efficacy. Controlled scientific trials usually provide the best information and should be consulted whenever possible. The absence of documented danger is not the same thing as proof of safety. Quite often, people working in health food stores are only too willing to give advice and make recommendations, particularly about botanical supplements. Many of these people are not qualified to give this kind of advice. Ask about qualifications (training or education) before accepting recommendations from anyone. Perhaps more so than for any other consumer products and services, the use of CAM calls for consumer skills, critical thinking, and caution.

Why Do Consumers Use Complementary Medicine?

Why are American consumers attracted to complementary and alternative medicine? Numerous reasons have been proposed. CAM often offers hope to people who have been disappointed by conventional medical therapies or who have chronic conditions that are incurable with conventional medical treatments. People with cancer, AIDS, and arthritis are among the heaviest users of CAM. Those most likely to use CAM are elderly people, approximately 80% of whom have at least one chronic health problem, and teenagers, who are concerned about their appearance and respond to a variety of appeals. Both these groups may be particularly susceptible to fraudulent claims for products promising new, quick, or easy ways to stay thin, strong, or attractive. A major source of CAM's appeal is that CAM practitioners often spend much more time listening and touching their patients than conventional physicians. Patients may find CAM practitioners to be warmer, more empathetic, and less rushed than their conventional counterparts.

Some experts speculate that the persuasive appeal of complementary and alternative medicine may come from the power of its underlying beliefs and cultural assumptions, which offer patients an experience they are missing in conventional medicine. People using CAM may feel they are connecting to nature or a more natural version of society; they may also feel a connection to vital energy or a life force, such as qi. They may view CAM as operating from a more holistic, person-centered body of knowledge than Western science, and they may find their quest for health imbued with an almost sacred quality. According to this view, CAM is attractive because of what it offers people when their sense of intactness and connection with the world is threatened by illness: empowerment, participation, authenticity, connection to nature and the universe, a renewed sense of purpose and meaning, and a new set of behavioral options. The assumptions of CAM can redefine the experience of illness in ways that inspire and empower the individual.

Despite many profound and irreconcilable philosophical differences between conventional medicine and CAM, there are abundant opportunities for learning, collaborating, and providing parallel care. Conventional medicine has already adopted many principles prevalent in complementary and alternative disciplines, including the ideas of health promotion, of personal responsibility for health, and of wellness as a multidimensional ideal. Western medicine is looking at the soaring use of CAM to discover what patients are missing in conventional care—perhaps more information, interest, or time from their physicians. At the same time, practitioners of CAM are looking to Western methods to modernize and optimize some of their practices, such as the preparation and standardization of herbal remedies. Within each is an enormous amount of time-tested information that has its own logic and use. In the future, greater understanding and collaboration across boundaries will certainly benefit the patient-consumer.

PAYING FOR HEALTH CARE

The American health care system is one of the most advanced and comprehensive in the world, but it is also the most expensive. The United States currently spends more than $1.7 trillion on health care, or $6000 per person. Health care costs are expected to reach $2.8 trillion, or about $9000 per person, by 2010. Numerous factors contribute to the high cost of health care in the United States, including the cost of advanced equipment and new technology; expensive treatments for some illnesses and conditions, such as cancer, heart disease, HIV infection, injuries, and low birth weight in infants; the aging of the population; and high earnings by some people in the health care industry and, in some cases, the demand for profits by investors.

The Current System

Health care is currently financed by a combination of private and public insurance plans, patient out-of-pocket payments, and government assistance (Figure 21-5). Currently, private insurance and individual patients pay about 55% of the total; the government pays the remaining 45%, mainly through Medicare and Medicaid (discussed below). Most nonelderly Americans receive their health insurance through their employers.

Despite high spending, not everyone is included in this financing system. More than 40 million people, the vast majority of them employed, have no health care insurance at all (see the box "Who Are the Uninsured?"). Many more are underinsured, meaning they may be uninsured for periods of time, have health insurance that does not cover all needed services, and/or have high out-of-pocket costs. People who are underinsured may skip physician visits and not take all prescribed medications. New government health insurance programs for children have reduced the number of Americans under age 18 who lack health insurance; however, the uninsured include almost 8 million children—10% of all American children—most in working, low-income families. Among Americans age 18–64, about 18% are without health insurance.

Lack of insurance affects both access to care and quality of care. People without insurance use health services less often and receive poorer care when they do use the services. Children without insurance are less likely to have screening tests and immunizations. They have fewer checkups, are less likely to be treated for injuries and for chronic conditions such as asthma, and are more likely to go without eyeglasses and prescribed drugs.

Another problem is that national health spending is growing faster than the rest of the economy, consuming an ever-increasing share of the U.S. gross domestic product (GDP). Health care spending represented 13.1% of the GDP in 2000 and is projected to reach 17.4% by 2010. Health care costs soared in the 1980s and then

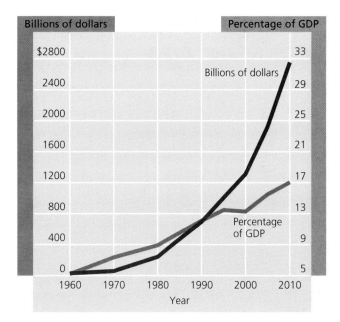

(a) National health care expenditures

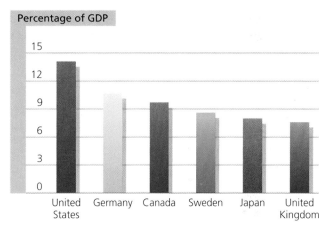

(b) Health care expenditures as a percentage of GDP

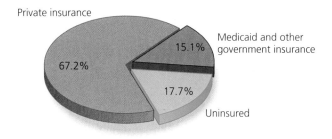

(c) Health insurance coverage of nonelderly Americans (age 0–64)

VITAL STATISTICS

Figure 21-5 A statistical look at health care expenditures and health insurance. SOURCES: National Center for Health Statistics. 2004. *Health, United States, 2004*. Hyattsville, Md.: U.S. Public Health Service; Centers for Medicare and Medicaid Services (http://cms.hhs.gov).

Despite high national levels of spending on health care, many Americans under age 65—almost 17% or nearly 1 in 5—do not have health insurance. (Americans age 65 and over are often covered by government programs.) This overall statistic about the uninsured hides some important differences among groups (see table).

- *Low income:* The factor most closely associated with lack of health insurance is low income. People who are at 200% or more of the federal poverty level are significantly more likely to be insured than those in low-income brackets.

- *Age:* Young adults are less likely to be insured than older adults. Younger adults may not be regularly employed and so may not be covered by an insurance plan through work.

- *Ethnicity:* Ethnic minorities are less likely to be insured than whites. Native Americans and Alaska Natives and Latinos are the groups with the lowest rates of insurance coverage. Much of the ethnic variations are explained by

socioeconomic status. However, other factors may also contribute, including language barriers, differing cultural attitudes toward medical care, and living in medically underserved communities.

People without health insurance receive less health care and lower quality of care. They have fewer physician visits and less preventive care. To help overcome the health gap between ethnic minorities and the general population, the U.S. Department of Health and Human Services sponsors "Take a Loved One to the Doctor Day." Held on the third Tuesday in September, this event is designed to encourage people to obtain preventive care. People are encouraged to make an appointment for themselves or for a friend or family member who hasn't seen a health care provider recently.

People who don't have a regular health care provider or who don't have health insurance can contact a local health department or local community center to find out more about free or low-cost care. For more information, visit the Closing the Health Gap Web site (www.healthgap.omhrc.gov).

	Uninsured Americans Under Age 65 (Percent)
Total	16.6
Income (percent of poverty level)	
Below 100%	31.4
100–149%	32.8
150–199%	25.6
200% or more	10.9
Age (years)	
Under 18	10.7
18–24	28.2
25–34	23.8
35–44	17.8
45–54	14.1
55–64	11.6
Ethnicity	
White	12.6
Asian American	17.2
African American	19.2
Latino	33.8
American Indian/ Alaska Native	38.7

SOURCES: Office of Minority Health Resource Center. 2005. *Fact Sheet: Take a Loved One to the Doctor Day 2005* (http://www.healthgap.omhrc. gov/2005factsheetdrday.htm; retrieved February 25, 2005); National Center for Health Statistics. 2004. *Health, United States, 2004.* Hyattsville, Md.: National Center for Health Statistics.

were contained to some extent in the 1990s by a large-scale switch from private insurance to managed care (discussed below), which is designed to achieve cost economies. But the savings from this switch were likely a one-time phenomenon, as more than 90% of working Americans are now covered by managed-care plans. Experts predict that health costs will increase drastically in the near future, with much of the increase borne by the government and individuals.

Health Insurance

Health insurance enables people to receive health care they might not otherwise be able to afford. Hospital care costs hundreds of dollars a day, and surgical fees can cost thousands. Health insurance is important for everyone, especially as health care costs continue to rise.

Health insurance plans are either fee-for-service (indemnity) or managed care. With both types the individual or the employer pays a basic premium, usually on a monthly basis; there are often other payments as well. In-

surance policies are sold to both groups and individuals; group plans tend to cover more services and cost less. Group coverage is often available through employers to workers and their families. People who are self-employed or whose employers don't offer group policies may need to buy individual plans. Americans who are 65 or older, have disabilities, or have a low income may receive health insurance through government programs.

Traditional Fee-for-Service (Indemnity) Plans

In a fee-for-service, or indemnity, plan, you can use any medical provider (such as a physician or a hospital) you choose. You or the provider sends the bill to your insurance company, which pays part of it. Usually you have to pay a deductible amount each year, and then the plan will pay a percentage—often 80%—of what they consider the "usual and customary" charge for covered services. You pay the remaining 20%, which is known as coinsurance. Freedom of choice is a major benefit of indemnity plans. You can see any physician you choose, including specialists. Your physician is paid based on the services he or she provides. Critics point to the fee-for-service payment system as a contributing factor in the rapid growth of U.S. health care costs because physicians have a financial incentive to order more tests and treatments for their patients. However, the vast majority of working Americans are now covered by managed-care plans.

Managed-Care Plans Managed-care plans have agreements with certain physicians, hospitals, and health care providers to offer a range of services to plan members at reduced cost. In general, you have lower out-of-pocket costs and less paperwork with a managed-care plan than with an indemnity plan, but you also have less freedom in choosing health care providers. Most Americans with job-based insurance are covered by managed-care plans, which may follow several different models:

- **Health maintenance organizations (HMOs)** offer members a range of services for a set monthly fee. You choose a primary care physician who manages your care and refers you to specialists if you need them. If you go outside the HMO, you have to pay for the service yourself. Physicians in the HMO agree to accept a monthly per-patient fee, or **capitation**, or to charge less than standard fees for services.

- **Preferred provider organizations (PPOs)** plans have arrangements with physicians and other providers who have agreed to accept lower fees. If you go outside the PPO, you have to pay more.

- **Point-of-service (POS) plans** are options offered by many HMOs in which you can see a physician outside the plan and still be partially covered (for example, for a specialist outside the network).

Many managed-care plans try to reduce costs over the long term by paying for routine preventive care, such as regular checkups and screening tests and prenatal care; they may also encourage prevention by offering health education and lifestyle modification programs for members. Other cost-cutting measures are less consumer-oriented. Consumers' choice of physicians is limited, and they may have to wait longer for appointments and travel farther to see participating doctors. Managed-care plans may also try to discourage overtreatment through the use of gatekeepers: In many plans, patients must get preapproval from their primary care physician or a plan representative for diagnostic tests, referrals to specialists, or hospital treatments. If a patient violates the rules for obtaining services, the plan typically will not cover the cost of the services in question. Nonemergency visits to emergency rooms are also frequently not covered.

Plans based on a capitation system give physicians a financial incentive to limit the number of tests and treatments they offer patients, the reverse of the financial incentive in indemnity plans. Critics claim that physicians in managed-care plans deny patients needed services in their efforts to keep costs down.

Health Savings Accounts Health savings accounts (HSAs) are a new form of health insurance coverage that became available in 2004. An HSA includes two parts: a health plan with a high deductible, and a tax-exempt personal savings account that is used for qualified medical expenses. The individual makes pre-tax contributions to the savings account, and later uses these funds or other cash payments to cover medical expenses until the plan's deductible is met. Once the deductible is met, the plan pays remaining medical costs according to the type of policy. The savings account can also be used for certain other types of expenses not covered by the plan. The benefit of an HSA is that it gives the consumer more control over health care spending; it can also potentially lower insurance premiums for some people because health plans with high deductibles tend to have lower premiums. Consumers are advised to carefully compare health insurance options, taking into account anticipated expenses and current and future finances.

Government Programs Americans who are 65 or older and younger people with certain disabilities can be covered by **Medicare,** a federal health insurance program that helps pay for hospitalization, physician services, and prescription drugs. As a result of limits placed on payments, however, some physicians and managed-care programs have stopped accepting Medicare patients. **Medicaid** is a joint federal-state health insurance program that covers some low-income people, especially children, pregnant

Terms

V w

managed-care plan A health care program that integrates the financing and delivery of services by using designated providers, utilization review, and financial incentives for following the plan's policies; HMOs, PPOs, and POS plans are examples of managed-care plans.

health maintenance organization (HMO) A prepaid health insurance plan in which patients receive health care from designated providers.

capitation A payment to health care providers according to the number of patients they agree to serve, rather than the amount of service rendered.

preferred provider organization (PPO) A prepaid health insurance plan in which providers agree to deliver services for discounted fees; patients can go to any provider, but using nonparticipating providers results in higher costs to the patient.

point-of-service (POS) plan A managed-care plan that covers treatment by an HMO physician but permits patients to seek treatment elsewhere with a higher copayment.

health savings account (HSA) Health insurance coverage that includes a health plan with a high deductible and a tax-exempt personal savings account that is used for qualified medical expenses.

Medicare A federal health insurance program for people 65 or older and for younger people with certain disabilities.

Medicaid A federally subsidized state-run plan of health care for people with low income.

Critical Consumer

Choosing a Health Care Plan

Before you choose a health plan, it's important that you understand your options and how they affect your choice of providers and services, costs, and quality of care. The following questions can help guide you in evaluating each of the health plans you are considering:

• *How is the plan rated for quality?* Find out if consumer ratings or consumer satisfaction information is available. Possible sources include the Consumer Assessment of Health Plans (CAHPS), the Health Plan Employer Data and Information Set (HEDIS), or your state health insurance commissioner (check the phone book for contact information).

• *Is the plan accredited?* Many health plans choose to be reviewed and accredited (given a "seal of approval") by the National Committee for Quality Assurance (NCQA), the Joint Commission on Accreditation of Healthcare Organizations (JCAHO), or the American Accreditation HealthCare Commission/URAC.

• *Does the plan include the doctors and hospitals you want?* If you are happy with your current physician, find out which plans he or she is in. If going to a certain hospital is important to you, investigate where a particular physician has privileges and whether a hospital is covered by the plan.

• *Does the plan provide the benefits you need?* Determine which health care services are most important to you and your family and then check to see if the plan covers them. Possible services to consider include physician office visits, preventive services, diagnostic tests and X rays, outpatient prescription medications, inpatient medical and hospital costs, physical therapy, drug and alcohol counseling, prenatal and well baby care, eye exams and glasses or contact lenses, mental health services, complementary therapies such as acupuncture, home health care, and care for preexisting or chronic conditions.

• *Do the doctors, pharmacies, and other services in the plan have convenient times and locations?* Find out about such things as after-hours care and parking as well.

• *Does the plan fit your budget?* Consider all the applicable costs of a plan: monthly premiums, annual deductibles, and copayments for doctor and hospital visits and prescription drugs. Also find out about how much more you will need to pay if you go outside the health plan's network of physicians, hospitals, and other providers to obtain services.

SOURCE: Agency for Health Care Policy and Research. 2001. *Your Guide to Choosing Quality Health Care* (http://www.ahcpr.gov/consumer/qnt; retrieved March 18, 2003).

women, and people with certain disabilities. The number of people and the number and cost of services covered by government programs has grown in recent years, challenging the ability of these programs to make all payments. The fund that pays Medicare hospital costs is currently expected to become insolvent in 2019.

Choosing a Policy

Choosing health insurance can be complicated; it's important to evaluate the coverage provided by different plans and decide which one is best for you (see the box "Choosing a Health Care Plan"). Colleges typically provide medical services through a student health center; some require students to purchase additional insurance if they are not covered by family policies. It's usually economical to remain on a family policy as long as possible.

After college, most people secure group coverage through their place of employment or through membership in an organization. If group coverage is not available, individuals should contact several different insurance companies for information about policies. Managed-care plans tend to have lower premiums and fewer out-of-pocket costs, an advantage for young adults and families with young children. Traditional fee-for-service plans tend to cost more and involve more paperwork, but they offer a wider choice of providers. If you are choosing insurance, consider a number of different plans and use your critical thinking skills to find the one that best suits your needs.

Tips for Today

Most of the time, you can take care of yourself without consulting a health care provider. You can eat sensibly, get enough exercise, manage stress, minimize your chances of getting an infection, and so on. When you do need professional care, you can continue to take responsibility for yourself by making informed, reasoned decisions about the care you obtain, whether conventional or CAM.

Right now you can

• Make sure you have enough on hand of any prescription medication that you take and that your prescription is up to date.

• Make sure you have basic first aid supplies at home and prepare or buy a small first aid kit for your car or office.

• Research any alternative or complementary practice or product you are using, either at the library or online, to find out if it is considered safe.

• Sit back in your chair and practice relaxation through breathing: Inhale slowly and deeply, imagining warm air flowing to all parts of your body; exhale from your abdomen, imagining tension flowing out of your body; continue for 5 or 10 minutes or until you feel relaxed.

Complying with Physicians' Instructions

Even though we sometimes have to entrust ourselves to the care of medical professionals, that doesn't mean we give up responsibility for our own behavior. Following medical instructions and advice often requires the same kind of behavioral self-management that's involved in quitting smoking, losing weight, or changing eating patterns. For example, if you have an illness or injury, you may be told to take medication at certain times of the day, do special exercises or movements, or change your diet.

The medical profession recognizes the importance of patient adherence, or compliance, and encourages different strategies to support it, such as the following:

1. Use reminders placed at home, in the car, at work, on your computer screensaver, or elsewhere that improve follow-through in taking medication and keeping scheduled appointments. To help you remember to take medications:

   - Link taking the medication with some well-established routine, like brushing your teeth or eating breakfast.

   - Use a medication calendar, and check off each pill.

   - Use a medication organizer or pill dispenser.

   - Plan ahead; don't wait until the last pill to get a prescription refilled.

2. Use a journal and other forms of self-monitoring to keep a detailed account of health-related behaviors, such as pill taking, diet, exercise, and so on.

3. Use self-reward systems so that desired behavior changes are encouraged, with a focus on short-term rewards.

4. Develop a clear image or explanation of how the medication or behavior change will improve your health and well-being.

If these strategies don't help you stick with your treatment plan, you may need to consider other possible explanations for your lack of adherence. For example, are you confused about some aspect of the treatment? Do you find the schedule for taking your medications too complicated, or do the drugs have bothersome side effects that you'd rather avoid? Do you feel that the recommended treatment is unnecessary or unlikely to help? Are you afraid of becoming dependent on a medication or that you'll be judged negatively if people know about your condition and treatment? An examination of your attitudes and beliefs about your condition and treatment plan can also help improve your compliance.

SUMMARY

- Informed self-care requires knowing how to evaluate symptoms. It's necessary to see a physician if symptoms are severe, unusual, persistent, or recurrent.

- Self-treatment doesn't necessarily require medication, but OTC drugs can be a helpful part of self-care.

- Conventional medicine is characterized by a focus on the external, physical causes of disease; the identification of a set of symptoms for different diseases; the development of public health measures to prevent disease and of drugs and surgery to treat them; the use of rational, scientific thinking to understand phenomena; and a well-established research methodology.

- Conventional practitioners include medical doctors, doctors of osteopathic medicine, podiatrists, optometrists, and dentists, as well as allied health care providers.

- The diagnostic process involves a medical history, a physical exam, and medical tests. Patients should ask questions about medical tests and treatments recommended by their physicians.

- Safe use of prescription drugs requires knowledge of what the medication is supposed to do, how and when to take it, and what the side effects are.

- All surgical procedures carry risk; patients should ask about alternatives and get a second opinion from another physician.

- Complementary and alternative medicine (CAM) is defined as those therapies and practices that do not form part of conventional or, mainstream, health care and medical practice as taught in most U.S. medical schools and offered in most U.S. hospitals.

- CAM is characterized by a view of health as a balance and integration of body, mind, and spirit; a focus on ways to restore the individual to harmony so that he or she can fight disease and regain health; and a body of knowledge based on accumulated experience and observations of patient reactions.

- Alternative medical systems such as traditional Chinese medicine and homeopathy are complete systems of medical philosophy, theory, and practice.

- Mind-body interventions include meditation, yoga, group support, hypnosis, and prayer.

- Biological-based therapies consist of herbal remedies, botanicals, and dietary supplements.

- Manipulative and body-based methods include massage and other physical healing techniques; the most commonly accepted is chiropractic.

- Energy therapies are designed to influence the flow of energy in and around the body; they include qigong, therapeutic touch therapies, and Reiki.

- Because there is less information available about CAM and less regulation of its practices and providers, consumers must be proactive in researching and choosing treatments, using critical thinking skills and exercising caution.

- Health insurance plans are usually described as either fee-for-service (indemnity) or managed-care plans. Indemnity plans allow consumers more choice in medical providers, but managed-care plans are less expensive.

- Government programs include Medicaid, for the poor, and Medicare, for those age 65 and over or chronically disabled.

Take Action

1. **Prepare for a health care visit:** Before your next visit to your physician, prepare a written list of your concerns. Be prepared to ask questions. After the visit, review how it went. Were your concerns satisfactorily addressed? Were you able to communicate your needs? Did you feel involved and in control? What aspects would you like to handle better the next time?

2. **Compare supplements:** Visit a local drugstore and compare different brands of the same herbal remedy or dietary supplement. How similar are the supplements in terms of ingredients, recommended dosages, and price? What aspect of health do the supplements claim to benefit, and how do they make the claim? Research any unfamiliar ingredients using the resources listed in For More Information and in Chapter 12.

3. **Consider special health risks:** Ask your physician whether you have any medical condition that may require special attention in an emergency. If you do, complete a medical ID card for your wallet, or obtain a medical ID bracelet or necklace. More complete emergency service can be obtained by joining Medic Alert (800-ID-ALERT; www.medicalert.org.)

4. **Make a preventive-care appointment for yourself or someone you know:** Promote wellness in yourself and those around you by participating in "Take a Loved One to the Doctor Day." Make an appointment for preventive care for yourself and/or a friend or family member (see p. 654 for more information). If needed, help someone keep an appointment by volunteering to provide transportation or child care.

For More Information

Books

Brody, H. 2000. *The Placebo Response.* New York: Cliff Street Books. *Describes the placebo effect and how it may be used to benefit health.*

Committee on the Use of Complementary and Alternative Medicine by the American Public. 2005. *Complementary and Alternative Medicine in the United States.* Washington, D.C.: National Academy Press. *Outlines ways of integrating conventional and complementary therapies, and proposes changes to dietary supplement laws.*

Howard Hughes Medical Institute, ed. 2000. *Exploring the Biomedical Revolution.* Baltimore: Johns Hopkins University Press. *Explores biomedical research and its effects on the fight against human disease.*

Medical Economics Staff. 2005. *PDR for Nonprescription Drugs and Dietary Supplements, 2005.* Montvale, N.J.: Medical Economics. *A reference covering the safety and efficacy of over-the-counter drugs and dietary supplements available today.*

Spencer, J. W., and J. Jacobs. 2003. *Complementary and Alternative Medicine: An Evidence-Based Approach.* St. Louis, Mo.: Mosby. *Provides background information and the current state of evidence for the efficacy of a wide variety of CAM therapies.*

Whorton, J. C. 2002. *Nature Cures: The History of Alternative Medicine in America.* New York: Oxford University Press. *Provides a history of alternative medicine in the United States, including background information on many CAM therapies.*

VW Organizations, Hotlines, and Web Sites

Agency for Healthcare Research and Quality (AHRQ). Provides practical, evidence-based information on health care treatments and outcomes for consumers and practitioners.
   http://www.ahrq.gov

American Board of Medical Specialties. Provides information on board certification, including information on specific physicians.
   866-275-2267
   http://www.abms.org

American Chiropractic Association. Provides information on chiropractic care, consumer tips, and a searchable directory of certified chiropractors.
   http://www.amerchiro.org

American Medical Association (AMA). Provides information about physicians, including their training, licensure, and board certification.
   http://www.ama-assn.org

American Osteopathic Association. Provides information on osteopathic physicians, including board certification.
   800-621-1773
   http://www.osteopathic.org

ConsumerLab.com. Provides information on the results of tests of dietary supplements, including information on actual ingredients and concentrations.
   http://www.consumerlab.com

Food and Drug Administration: Information for Consumers. Provides materials on dietary supplements, foods, prescription and OTC drugs, and other FDA-regulated products.
   888-INFO-FDA
   http://www.fda.gov/opacom/morecons.html

National Center for Complementary and Alternative Medicine (NCCAM). Provides general information packets, answers to frequently asked questions about CAM, consumer advice for safer use of CAM, research abstracts, and bibliographies.
   888-644-6226
   http://nccam.nih.gov

National Council Against Health Fraud. Provides news and information about health fraud and quackery and links to related sites.

http://www.ncahf.org

Quackwatch. Provides information on health fraud, quackery, and health decision making.

http://www.quackwatch.org

U.S. Treasury Department: Health Savings Accounts. Provides information about HSAs and links to relevant IRS forms.

http://www.treas.gov/offices/public-affairs/hsa/

See also the listings for Chapters 2 and 12; the box on dietary supplements in Chapter 12 (p. 361) suggests Web sites with more information on supplements.

Selected Bibliography

Allais, G., et al. 2002. Acupuncture in the prophylactic treatment of migraine without aura: A comparison with flunarizine. *Headache* 42(9): 855–861.

American Medical Association. 2004. *Health Savings Accounts at a Glance.* Chicago: American Medical Association.

Bach, P. B., et al. 2004. Primary care physicians who treat blacks and whites. *New England Journal of Medicine* 351(6): 575–584.

Bell, R. A., R. L. Kravitz, and M. S. Wilkes. 2000. Direct-to-consumer prescription drug advertising, 1989–1998. A content analysis of conditions, targets, inducements, and appeals. *Journal of Family Practice* 49(4): 329–335.

Bordens, K. S., and B. B. Abbott. 2005. *Research Design and Methods: A Process Approach,* 6th ed. New York: McGraw-Hill.

Bren, L. 2004. Study: U.S. generic drugs cost less than Canadian drugs. *FDA Consumer,* July/August.

Brobst, D. E., et al. 2004. Guggulsterone activates multiple nuclear receptors and induces CYP3A gene expression through the pregnane X receptor. *Journal of Pharmacology and Experimental Therapeutics* 310(2): 528–535.

Budetti, P. P. 2004. 10 years beyond the health security act failure: Subsequent developments and persistent problems. *Journal of the American Medical Association* 292(16): 2000–2006.

Centers for Disease Control and Prevention. 2004. Complementary and alternative medicine use among adults: United States, 2002. *Advance Data from Vital and Health Statistics* No. 343. Hyattsville, Md.: National Center for Health Statistics.

Centers for Medicare and Medicaid Services. 2004. *National Health Expenditures and Selected Economic Indicators, Levels and Average Annual Percent Change: Selected Calendar Years 1990–2013* (http://www.cms.hhs.gov/statistics/nhe/projections-2003/t1.asp; retrieved February 23, 2005).

Cherkin, D. C., et al. 2002. Characteristics of visits to licensed acupuncturists, chiropractors, massage therapists, and naturopathic physicians. *Journal of the American Board of Family Practice* 15(6): 463–472.

Eisenberg, D. M. 1997. Advising patients who seek alternative medical therapies. *Annals of Internal Medicine* 127: 61–69.

Ernst, E. 2004. Prescribing herbal medications appropriately. *Journal of Family Practice* 53(12): 985–988.

Fontanarosa, P. B., D. Rennie, and C. D. DeAngelis. 2003. The need for regulation of dietary supplements—lessons from ephedra. *Journal of the American Medical Association* 289(12): 1568–1570.

Free rein for drug ads? 2003. *Consumer Reports,* February.

Gan, T. J., et al. 2004. A randomized controlled comparison of electro-acupoint stimulation or ondansetron versus placebo for the prevention of postoperative nausea and vomiting. *Anesthesia and Analgesia* 99(4): 1070–1075.

Gilroy, C. M., et al. 2003. Echinacea and truth in labeling. *Archives of Internal Medicine* 163.

Institute of Medicine, Committee on the Consequences of Uninsurance. 2003. *A Shared Destiny: Community Effects of Uninsurance.* Washington, D.C.: National Academy Press.

Kaiser Family Foundation. 2005. *Trends and Indicators in the Changing Health Care Marketplace.* Menlo Park, Calif.: Kaiser Family Foundation.

Linde, K., et al. 1998. Are the clinical effects of homeopathy placebo effects? A meta-analysis of placebo-controlled trials. *Lancet* 350(9081): 834–843.

Miller, F. G., et al. 2004. Ethical issues concerning research in complementary and alternative medicine. *Journal of the American Medical Association* 291(5): 599–604.

National Center for Health Statistics. 2005. Trends in health insurance and access to medical care for children under age 19 years. *Advance Data from Vital Health Statistics* No. 355.

National Center for Complementary and Alternative Medicine. 2002. *Are You Considering Complementary and Alternative Therapies?* (http://nccam.nih.gov/health/decisions/index.htm; retrieved February 28, 2005).

Rados, C. 2004. FDA reiterates warning against online drug buying. *FDA Consumer,* September/October.

Rosenthal, M. B., et al. 2002. Promotion of prescription drugs to consumers. *New England Journal of Medicine* 346(7): 498–505.

Saper, R. B., et al. 2004. Heavy metal content of ayurvedic herbal medicine products. *Journal of the American Medical Association* 292(23): 2868–2873.

Solomon, P. R., et al. 2002. Ginkgo for memory enhancement: A randomized controlled trial. *Journal of the American Medical Association* 288(7): 835–840.

Taseng, C., et al. 2004. Cost-lowering strategies used by Medicare beneficiaries who exceed drug benefit caps and have a gap in drug coverage. *Journal of the American Medical Association* 292(8): 952–960.

The uninsured: Americans at risk. 2004. *Consumer Reports,* January.

Weissman, J. S., et al. 2003. *Health Affairs: Forum on Prescription Drug Promotion* (http://www.healthaffairs.org/WebExclusives/Pharma_Web_Excl_022603.htm; retrieved March 18, 2003).

22

After reading this chapter, you should be able to

- Discuss factors that contribute to unintentional injuries.

- List the most common types of unintentional injuries and strategies for preventing them

- Describe factors that contribute to violence and intentional injuries

- Discuss different forms of violence and how to protect yourself from intentional injuries

- List strategies for helping others in an emergency situation

Personal Safety: Protecting Yourself from Unintentional Injuries and Violence

Test Your Knowledge

1. **More people are injured each year through intentional acts of violence than through unintentional injuries (accidents).**
   True or false?

2. **It is dangerous to be wearing a safety belt if your car catches on fire or is submerged in water.**
   True or false?

3. **About how many students have a working firearm with them at college?**
   a. 1 in 23
   b. 1 in 53
   c. 1 in 103

4. **Talking on a cell phone while driving increases the risk of motor vehicle crashes.**
   True or false?

5. **About what percentage of sexual assaults against women are committed by strangers?**
   a. 20%
   b. 40%
   c. 80%

ANSWERS

1. FALSE. Far more people are injured and killed each year through unintentional injuries than through violence. Your lifetime odds of dying from an unintentional injury are 1 in 36, while the odds of your being murdered are 1 in 182.

2. FALSE. Safety belts will help prevent you from being knocked unconscious, so you'll have a better chance of escaping the car. (Only 0.5–1.0% of motor vehicle crashes involve fire or submersion.)

3. A. For male students, the number is 1 in 12. Students from states with high rates of gun ownership are more likely to have brought guns to college and to have been threatened by a firearm at college than students from states where gun ownership is rare.

4. TRUE. Using a handheld or hands-free cell phone while driving decreases attentiveness and reaction time. A 20-year-old using a phone has the reaction time of a 70-year-old not using a phone.

5. A. The vast majority of sexual assaults against women are committed by friends, acquaintances, or intimate partners.

Visit the *Core Concepts in Health* Online Learning Center (www.mhhe.com/insel10e) for study aids and many additional resources.

661

Each year, about 150,000 Americans die from injuries, and many more are temporarily or permanently disabled. Injuries can be intentional or unintentional. An **intentional injury** is one that is purposely inflicted, by either oneself or another person; examples are homicide, suicide, and assault. If an injury occurs when no harm is intended, it is considered an **unintentional injury.** Motor vehicle crashes, falls, and fires often result in unintentional injuries. (Public health officials prefer not to use the word *accidents* to describe unintentional injuries because it suggests events beyond human control. *Injuries* are predictable outcomes of factors that can be controlled or prevented.) Although Americans tend to express more concern about intentional injuries, unintentional injuries are actually more common. The following occur on an average day in the United States:

- 45 homicides
- 85 suicides
- 280 deaths from unintentional injuries
- 1500 suicide attempts
- 20,000 interpersonal assaults
- 55,000 disabling injuries
- 110,000 unintentional injury–related emergency room visits

Unintentional injuries are the fifth leading cause of death among all Americans and the leading cause of death and disability among children and young adults. Heart disease, cancer, stroke, and chronic lower respiratory diseases are responsible for more deaths each year than injuries, but because unintentional injuries are so common among people, they account for more **years of potential life lost** than any other cause of death. Suicide and homicide rank eleventh and sixteenth respectively on the list of leading causes of death among Americans; because they often affect young people, they also account for many years of potential life lost. Injuries affect all segments of the population, but they are particularly common among men, minorities, and people with low incomes, primarily due to social, environmental, and economic factors. Although rates of both unintentional and intentional injuries have fallen in recent years, they remain a major area of concern.

The economic cost of injuries is high, with more than $600 billion spent each year for medical care and rehabilitation of injured people. Injuries also cause emotional suffering for injured people and their families, friends, and colleagues. Luckily, there are many steps that can be taken to reduce the risk of injuries. Engineering strategies such as safety belts can help lower injury rates, as can the passage and enforcement of safety-related laws, such as those requiring tamper-proof containers for OTC medications. Public education campaigns about risky behaviors such as driving under the influence of alcohol or smoking in bed can also help prevent injuries.

Ultimately, though, it is up to each individual to take responsibility for his or her actions and make wise choices about safety behaviors. Many of the same sensible attitudes, responsible behaviors, and informed decisions that optimize your wellness can improve your chances of avoiding injuries. This chapter explains how you can protect yourself and those around you from becoming the victims of unintentional and intentional injuries.

UNINTENTIONAL INJURIES

Unintentional injuries are the leading cause of death in the United States for people under age 35. Injury situations are generally categorized into four general classes, based on where they occur: motor vehicle injuries, home injuries, leisure injuries, and work injuries. The greatest number of deaths occur in motor vehicle crashes, but the greatest number of disabling injuries occur in the home (Table 22-1). In all of these arenas, the action you take can mean the difference between injury or death and no injury at all.

What Causes an Injury?

Most injuries are caused by a combination of human and environmental factors. Human factors are inner conditions or attitudes that lead to an unsafe state, whether physical,

VₗW **VITAL STATISTICS**

Table 22-1	Unintentional Injuries in the United States	
	Deaths	**Disabling Injuries**
Motor vehicle	44,800	2,400,000
Home	33,100	900,000
Leisure	21,300	7,100,000
Work	4,500	3,400,000
All classes*	101,500	20,700,000

*Deaths and injuries for the four separate classes total more than the "All classes" figures because of rounding and because some deaths and injuries are included in more than one class.

SOURCE: National Safety Council. 2004. *Injury Facts, 2004 Edition.* Itasca, Ill.: National Safety Council.

Gender Matters

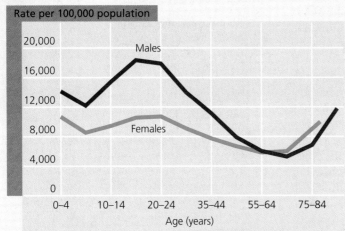

Males **Females**

Rate per 100,000 population

Males

Females

Age (years)

Figure 1 Nonfatal injury rate by age and sex.

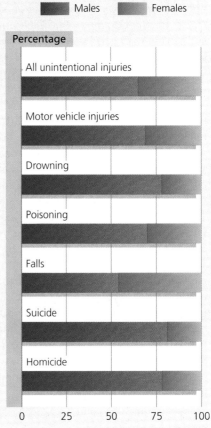

Percentage

All unintentional injuries

Motor vehicle injuries

Drowning

Poisoning

Falls

Suicide

Homicide

0   25   50   75   100

Figure 2 Injury deaths: Percentage of victims by sex.

Overall, rates of injury are highest among young adults and seniors over age 85. Except among the oldest group of adults, the nonfatal injury rate is substantially higher in males than in females—and it peaks among young adult males (Figure 1). Males also significantly outnumber females in injury deaths—whether unintentional or intentional (Figure 2).

Why do men, especially young men, have such high rates of injury? Gender roles may play a key role: Traditional gender roles for males may associate masculinity with risk-taking behavior and a disregard for pain and injury, and risk-taking behavior may be particularly common among young men. Men are more likely to drive dangerously, drink and drive, binge drink, and use aggressive behavior to control situations—all of which can lead to higher rates of fatal and nonfatal injury. Men may also have a lower perception of risk of dangerous behaviors compared with women.

Traditional gender roles may also make it more difficult for men to admit to injury or emotional vulnerability. Physical injuries may worsen or become chronic if

care is not sought promptly. Untreated depression can lead to suicide.

In addition, men may have greater exposure to some injury situations. Compared with women, men may drive more miles, have greater access to firearms, and be more likely to ride motorcycles, operate machinery, and have jobs associated with high rates of workplace injuries. They may be more likely to be engage in sports and other recreational activities associated with high rates of injuries. Greater access and use of firearms plays a role in higher rates of deaths among men from assault and suicide; as described in Chapter 3, women are more likely than men to attempt suicide, but men are much more likely to succeed, primarily because they are more likely to use firearms.

Some researchers suggest that the male hormone testosterone may play a role in risky and aggressive behavior. Differences in brain structure and activity may also influence how men and women respond to stressors and how quickly and to what degree they become verbally or physically aggressive in response to anger.

Further studies are needed to identify all the factors underlying excessive risk-taking among men and how these risk behaviors can be changed to lower the rates of fatal and nonfatal injury among men.

SOURCES: Centers for Disease Control and Prevention. 2004. Surveillance for fatal and nonfatal injuries—United States, 2001. *MMWR Surveillance Summaries* 53(SS7): 1–57; World Health Organization. 2002. *Gender and Road Traffic Injuries.* Geneva: World Health Organization; Courtenay, W. 1998. College men's health: An overview and a call to action. *Journal of American College Health* 46(6): 279–290.

emotional, or psychological. Environmental factors are external conditions and circumstances, such as poor road conditions, a slippery surface, or the undertow of the ocean at the beach.

A common human factor that leads to injuries is risk-taking behavior. People vary in the amount of risk they tend to take in life; young men are especially prone to

taking risks (see the box "Injuries Among Young Men"). Some people take risks to win the admiration of their peers; other people simply overestimate their physical abilities. Using alcohol or drugs is another common risk factor that leads to many injuries and deaths.

Psychological and emotional factors can also play a role in injuries. People sometimes act on the basis of inadequate or inaccurate beliefs about what is safe or unsafe. For example, a person who believes that safety belts trap people in cars when a crash occurs and who therefore decides not to wear a safety belt is acting on an inaccurate belief. However, many people who have accurate information still decide to engage in risky behavior. Young people often have unsafe attitudes, such as "I won't get hurt" or "It won't happen to me." Attitudes like this can lead to risk taking and ultimately to injuries.

Environmental factors leading to injury may be natural (weather conditions), social (a drunk driver), work-related (defective equipment), or home-related (faulty wiring). Making the environment safer is an important aspect of safety. Laws are often passed to try to make our environment safer; examples include speed limits on roads and highways and workplace safety requirements.

When unsafe human states and unsafe environmental factors interact, an injury is often the result. A good example might be an inexperienced person borrowing a rifle to go hunting with his friends on a cold, rainy afternoon. Those in the group drink alcohol because they mistakenly believe it will keep them warmer. It is not difficult to imagine how these human and environmental factors could lead to an injury. Again, it is important to realize that injuries do not "just happen." With hindsight, we can almost always pinpoint the internal and external factors that combined to cause an injury situation.

Motor Vehicle Injuries

Motor vehicle crashes are the leading cause of death for Americans between the ages of 1 and 34. Worldwide, motor vehicle crashes kill 1.2 million and injure up to 50 million people each year, making motor vehicle injuries the eleventh leading cause of death overall. The groups most affected by motor vehicle crashes are people age 15–24 and over 75. It is more likely that your death will be caused by a motor vehicle crash than by any other type of unintentional or intentional injury (Table 22-2). **Motor vehicle injuries** also result in the majority of cases of paralysis due to spinal injuries, and they are the leading cause of severe brain injury in the United States.

Factors Contributing to Motor Vehicle Injuries
Common causes of motor vehicle injuries are speeding, aggressive driving, fatigue, inexperience, cell phones and other distractions, the use of alcohol and

Ww VITAL STATISTICS

Table 22-2 | Lifetime Odds of Death Due to Injury

All unintentional injuries	**1 in 36**
Motor vehicle	1 in 77
Fall	1 in 246
Poisoning	1 in 262
Fire	1 in 1,116
Drowning	1 in 1,126
Choking	1 in 1,222
Air and space transport	1 in 4,023
Struck by falling object	1 in 4,329
Firearms discharge	1 in 4,605
Exposure to natural cold	1 in 6,165
Electric current	1 in 8,568
Exposure to natural heat	1 in 12,310
Cataclysmic storm	1 in 68,388
Lightning	1 in 89,930
Earthquake/volcano	1 in 131,890
Suicide	**1 in 121**
Homicide (assault)	**1 in 182**

SOURCE: National Safety Council. 2003. *What Are the Odds of Dying?* (http://www.nsc.org/lrs/statinfo/odds.htm; retrieved December 16, 2004).

other drugs, and the incorrect use of safety belts and other safety devices.

SPEEDING Nearly 60% of all motor vehicle crashes are caused by bad driving, especially speeding. As speed increases, momentum and the force of impact increase, and the time allowed for the driver to react (reaction time) decreases. Speed limits are posted to establish the safest maximum speed limit for a given area under ideal conditions; if visibility is limited or the road is wet, the safe maximum speed may be considerably lower. Many states have raised their highway speed limits since the 1995 repeal of the National Maximum Speed Limit, and overall motor vehicle fatalities have since increased. Raising speed limits on rural interstates has caused a 35% increase in crash death rates.

AGGRESSIVE DRIVING Speeding is also a hallmark of aggressive drivers—those who operate a motor vehicle in an unsafe and hostile manner. Aggressive driving, also known as road rage, has increased more than 50% since 1990, and one in four U.S. drivers admits to driving aggressively at least some of the time. Other characteristics of aggressive driving include frequent, erratic, and abrupt lane changes; tailgating; running red lights or stop signs; passing on the shoulder; and blocking other cars trying to change lanes or pass. Aggressive drivers increase the risk of crashes for themselves and others; injuries may also occur if aggressive drivers stop their vehicles and confront each other following an incident. For more on aggressive

Term

Ww

motor vehicle injuries Unintentional injuries and deaths involving motor vehicles in motion, both on and off the highway or street; incidents causing motor vehicle injuries include collisions between vehicles and collisions with objects or pedestrians.

To find out if you are an aggressive driver, check any of the following statements that are true for you:

_____ I consistently exceed the speed limit; I'm often unaware of both my speed and the speed limit.

_____ I frequently follow closely behind the car in front of me.

_____ If I feel the car in front of me is going too slowly, I tailgate.

_____ I change lanes frequently to pass people.

_____ I seldom use my turn signal when changing lanes or turning.

_____ I often run red lights or roll through stop signs.

_____ I react to what I feel is another driver's mistake by cursing, shouting, or making rude gestures; by blocking a car from passing or changing lanes; by using high beams; or by braking suddenly in front of a tailgater.

_____ My personality changes and I become more competitive when I get behind the wheel.

_____ I often get angry or impatient with other drivers and with pedestrians.

_____ I would consider pulling over for a personal encounter with a bad driver.

Each of these statements is characteristic of aggressive drivers; the more items you checked, the greater your road rage. If you checked even one statement, consider taking some of the following steps to reduce your hostility behind the wheel:

• Allow enough time for your trip to reach your destination without speeding.

• Avoid driving during periods of heavy traffic.

• Don't drive when you are angry, tired, or intoxicated.

• Imagine that the other drivers are all people that you know and like. Be courteous and forgiving.

• Listen to soothing music or a book on tape, or practice a relaxation technique such as deep breathing (see Chapter 2).

• Take a course in anger management.

Even if you are successful at controlling your own aggressive driving inpulses, you may still encounter an aggressive driver on the road. The AAA Foundation for Traffic Safety recommends the following strategies to avoid being the victim of an aggressive driver:

• Avoid behaviors that may enrage an aggressive driver; these include cutting off cars when merging, driving slowly in the left lane, tailgating, and making rude gestures.

• If you make a mistake while driving, apologize. In surveys, the most popular and widely understood gestures for apologies include raising or waving a hand and touching or knocking the head with the palm of your hand (to indicate "What was I thinking?").

• Refuse to join in a fight. Avoid eye contact with an angry driver, and put distance between your car and his or her vehicle. If you think another driver is following you or trying to start a fight, call the police on a cell phone or drive to a public place.

SOURCES: New York State Department of Motor Vehicles. 2000. *Aggressive Driving* (http://www.nysgtsc.state.ny.us/aggr-ndx.htm; retrieved December 27, 2000); AAA Foundation for Traffic Safety. 1997. *Road Rage: How to Avoid Aggressive Driving*. Washington, D.C.: AAA Foundation for Traffic Safety.

---

driving, take the quiz and review the strategies in the box "Are You an Aggressive Driver?"

FATIGUE AND SLEEPINESS Driving requires mental alertness and attentiveness. Many fatal crashes occur on the weekend, late on Saturday night or early on Sunday morning. Studies have shown that sleepiness causes slower reaction time, reduced coordination and vigilance, and delayed information processing. Drowsiness can be caused by not getting enough hours of sleep, by sleep disorders that prevent sleep from being refreshing, or by disruptions caused by shift work that force people to sleep at odd hours. Research shows that even mild sleep deprivation causes a deterioration in driving ability comparable to that caused by a 0.05% blood alcohol concentration—a level considered hazardous when driving. Being awake for 18 hours can impair driving ability as much as drinking two alcoholic beverages.

CELL PHONES AND OTHER DISTRACTIONS Anything that distracts a driver—a bad mood, pets or children in the car—can increase the risk of a motor vehicle injury. Several common causes of crashes, including failing to yield and disregarding traffic signals and stop signs, have been linked to driver distraction, and it is estimated that distraction is a contributing factor in 25–50% of all crashes. As the use of cell phones has spread, their potential to distract drivers has been recognized. Studies have documented a higher rate of crashes among cell phone users compared to nonusers; see the box "Cellular Phones and Distracted Driving" for strategies on using a phone more safely.

ALCOHOL AND OTHER DRUGS Alcohol is involved in about 40% of all fatal crashes. Alcohol-impaired driving is illegal in all states; the legal limit for blood alcohol concentration (BAC) is 0.08%, but people are impaired at much lower BACs. A driver with a BAC between 0.05%

At any given moment, nearly 8% of drivers—about 1 in 12—are talking on a cell phone. In 2001, New York became the first state to ban the use of handheld cellular phones while driving; drivers there must use hand-free equipment or face fines of up to $100. In 2004, New Jersey and the District of Columbia passed similar bans, and many other states have bans under consideration. Around the world, many countries have laws against the use of handheld cell phones while driving.

Available evidence indicates that use of a cell phone while driving can increase the risk of motor vehicle crashes. In a study using a driver-training simulator, cell phone users were about 20% slower to respond to sudden hazards than were other drivers, and they were about twice as likely to rear-end a braking car in front of them. Among young adult drivers who used a cell phone, reaction time was reduced to the level of a 70-year-old driver who was not using a phone. Another study found a fourfold increase in the risk of collision among motorists who talk on the phone while driving. It is unclear, however, if bans such as those in New York will help reduce the risk: Studies have not found much, if any, benefit in the use of headsets. It appears that the mental distraction of talking is a factor in crashes rather than that one hand is holding the phone.

The safest strategy is not to use your phone while driving. For people who live in areas where cell phone use is legal while driving and who choose to use a phone, the following strategies may help increase safety:

- Be very familiar with your phone and its functions, especially speed dial and redial.

- Store frequently called numbers on speed dial so you can place calls without looking at the phone.

- Use a hands-free device so that you can keep both hands on the steering wheel.

- Let the person you are speaking to know you are driving and be prepared to end the call at any time.

- Don't place or answer calls in heavy traffic or hazardous weather conditions.

- Don't take notes or look up phone numbers while driving.

- Time calls so that you can place them when you are at a stop.

- Never engage in stressful or emotional conversations while on the road. If you are discussing a complicated or emotional matter, pull over to the side of the road or into a parking lot to complete your conversation.

Remember that, as a driver, your primary obligation is to pay attention to the road—for your own safety and the safety of others.

SOURCES: National Traffic Safety Administration. 2005. *Traffic Safety Facts Research Note: Driver Cell Phone Use in 2004—Overall Results.* Washington, D.C.: National Traffic Safety Administration; Strayer, D. L., and F. A. Drews. 2004. Profiles in driver distraction: Effects of cell phone conversations on younger and older drivers. *Human Factors* 46(4): 640–649; World of Wireless Communications. 2000. *Consumer Resources: Driving Safety Tips* (http://www.wow-com/consumer/driving/safetyold.cfm; retrieved December 16, 2000); Redelmeier, D. A., and R. J. Tibshirani. 1997. Association between cellular-telephone calls and motor vehicle collisions. *New England Journal of Medicine* 336(7): 453–458.

and 0.09% is nine times more likely to have a crash than a person who has not been drinking. The combination of fatigue and alcohol use increases the risk even further. Because alcohol affects reason and judgment as well as the ability to make fast, accurate, and coordinated movements, a person who has been drinking will be less likely to recognize that he or she is impaired.

Other substances also affect judgment and driving ability. A recent study found that hay fever sufferers who had taken diphenhydramine (an antihistamine found in over-the-counter allergy medications such as Benadryl) were as impaired as if they were legally drunk. Use of many over-the-counter and all psychoactive drugs is potentially dangerous if you plan to drive. (For a full discussion of the effects of alcohol and other drugs on users, refer to Chapters 9 and 10.)

SAFETY BELTS, AIR BAGS, AND CHILD SAFETY SEATS   The improper use of safety belts, air bags, and child safety seats contributes to injuries and deaths in motor vehicle crashes. Although some type of mandatory safety belt law is in effect in 49 states (excluding New Hampshire) and the District of Columbia, only about 80% of motor vehicle occupants use safety belts even though they are the single most effective way to reduce the risk of crash-related death. Of drivers not wearing a safety belt who have been killed in automobile crashes, an estimated 60–70% would have survived if they had been wearing one. If you wear a combination lap and shoulder belt, your chance of surviving a crash is three to four times better than those of a person who doesn't wear one. And ask others in the vehicle to buckle up; unrestrained passengers increase the risk of injury and death to others in the car should a crash occur. The National Highway Traffic Safety Administration (NHTSA) has mandated that, starting in 2008, all motor vehicles must have safety belts installed in the rear center seat; it is estimated that this measure will prevent about 25 deaths and 500 injuries each year.

Some people think that if they are involved in a crash they are better off being thrown free of their vehicle. In fact, the chances of being killed are 25 times greater if you are thrown from a vehicle, whether it is due to injuries caused by hitting a tree or the pavement or by being hit by another vehicle. Safety belts not only prevent you from being thrown from the car at the time of the crash but also provide protection from the second collision: If a car is traveling at 65 mph and hits another vehicle, the car stops first; then the occupants stop because they are traveling at the same speed. The second collision occurs when the occupants of the car hit something inside the car, such as the steering column, dashboard, or windshield. The safety belt stops the second collision from occurring and spreads the stopping force of the collision over the body.

Since 1998, all new cars have been equipped with dual air bags—one for the driver and one for the front passenger. Many vehicles also offer optional side air bags, which further reduce the risk of injury. Although air bags provide supplementary protection in the event of a collision, most are useful only in head-on collisions. They also deflate immediately after inflating and therefore do not provide protection in collisions involving multiple impacts. Air bags are not a replacement for safety belts; everyone in a vehicle should buckle up.

Air bags deploy forcefully and can injure a child or short adult who is improperly restrained or sitting too close to the dashboard. To ensure that air bags work safely, always follow these basic guidelines: Place infants in rear-facing infant seats in the back seat, transport children age 12 and under in the back seat, always use safety belts or appropriate safety seats, and keep 10 inches between the air bag cover and the breastbone of the driver or passenger. If necessary, adjust the steering wheel or use seat cushions to ensure that an inflating air bag will hit a person in the chest and not in the face. Another adjustment should be made for children who have outgrown child safety seats but are still too small for adult safety belts alone (usually age 4–8). These children should be secured using booster seats that ensure that the safety belt is positioned low across the waist.

In the rare event that a person cannot comply with air bag guidelines, permission to install an on-off switch that temporarily disables the air bag can be applied for from the National Highway Traffic Safety Administration (NHTSA). Air bags currently prevent far more injuries than they cause and are expected to save at least 3200 lives each year once they are installed in all vehicles. Advanced air bag systems are slowly being introduced that include risk-reduction technologies such as sensors to detect and respond to crash severity, seat position, passenger size, and whether a passenger is wearing a safety belt.

Preventing Motor Vehicle Injuries   About 75% of all motor vehicle collisions occur within 25 miles of home and at speeds lower than 40 mph. Strategies for preventing motor vehicle injuries include the following:

- Obey the speed limit. If you have to speed to get somewhere on time, you're not allowing enough time.
- Always wear a safety belt. Fasten the lap belt, even if the vehicle has automatic shoulder belts. The shoulder strap should cross the collarbone, and the lap belt should fit low and snug across the hips and pelvic area. The shoulder strap should never be slipped under the arm or behind the back. Pregnant women should position the lap belt as low as possible on the pelvic area.
- Never drive under the influence of alcohol or other drugs. Never ride with a driver who has been drinking or using drugs.
- Keep your car in good working order. Regularly inspect the tires, oil and fluid levels, windshield wipers, spare tire, and so on.
- Always allow enough following distance. Use the 3-second rule: When the vehicle ahead passes a reference point, count out 3 seconds. If you pass the reference point before you finish counting, drop back and allow more following distance.
- Always increase your following distance and slow down if weather or road conditions are poor.
- Choose interstate highways rather than rural roads. Highways are much safer because of better visibility, wider lanes, fewer surprises, and other factors.
- Always signal when turning or changing lanes.
- Stop completely at stop signs. Follow all traffic laws.
- Take special care at intersections. Always look left, right, and then left again. Make sure you have plenty of time to complete your maneuver in the intersection.
- Don't pass on two-lane roads unless you're in a designated passing area and have a clear view ahead.
- Children under the age of 12 should ride in the back seat of a motor vehicle. Young children and infants should ride in approved child safety seats or booster seats appropriate for their age and size.

Motorcycles and Mopeds   About one out of every ten traffic fatalities among people age 15–34 involves someone riding a motorcycle. In more than two-thirds of crashes involving a car and a motorcycle, the driver of the car is at fault. Injuries from motorcycle collisions are generally more severe than those involving automobiles because motorcycles provide little, if any, protection. Because head injuries are the major cause of death, the use of a helmet is critical for rider safety. Learning the skills to operate the motorcycle safely is another key injury-prevention strategy; operator error is a factor in 75% of fatal crashes involving motorcycles.

Moped riders face additional challenges. Mopeds usually have a maximum speed of 30–35 mph and have less power for maneuverability, especially in an emergency. Moped riders should use caution and take the time to develop the skills needed to handle the vehicle in traffic.

Additional strategies for preventing motorcycle and moped injuries include the following:

- Maximize your visibility by wearing light-colored clothing, driving with your headlights on, and correctly positioning yourself in traffic.
- Develop the necessary skills. Lack of skill, especially when evasive action is needed to avoid a collision, is a major factor in motorcycle and moped injuries. Skidding from improper braking is the most common cause of loss of control.
- Wear a helmet. Helmets should be marked with the symbol DOT, certifying that they conform to federal safety standards established by the Department of Transportation. Helmet use is required by law in nearly half of the states.
- Protect your eyes with goggles, a face shield, or a windshield.
- Drive defensively, particularly when changing lanes and at intersections, and never assume that you've been seen by other drivers.

Bicycles   Injuries to bicyclists and pedestrians are considered motor-vehicle-related because they are usually caused by motor vehicles. Bicycle injuries result primarily from riders not knowing or understanding the rules of the road, failing to follow traffic laws, not having sufficient skill or experience to handle traffic conditions, or being intoxicated. Bicycles are considered vehicles; bicyclists must obey all traffic laws that apply to automobile drivers, including stopping at traffic lights and stop signs.

Head injuries are involved in about two-thirds of all bicycle-related deaths. Wearing a helmet reduces the risk of head injury by 85%, but fewer than 50% of cyclists wear helmets (see the box "Choosing a Bicycle Helmet"). Safe cycling strategies include the following:

- Wear safety equipment, including a helmet, eye protection, gloves, and proper footwear. Secure the bottom of your pant legs with clips, and secure your shoelaces so they don't get tangled in the chain.
- Maximize your visibility by wearing light-colored, reflective clothing. Equip your bike with reflectors, and use lights, especially at night or when riding in wooded or other dark areas.
- Ride with the flow of traffic, not against it, and follow all traffic laws. Use bike paths when they are available.

Term

home injuries Unintentional injuries and deaths that occur in the home and on home premises to occupants, guests, domestic servants, and trespassers; falls, burns, poisonings, suffocations, unintentional shootings, drownings, and electrical shocks are examples.

- Ride defensively; never assume that drivers have seen you. Be especially careful when turning or crossing at corners and intersections. Watch for cars turning right.
- Stop at all traffic lights and stop signs. Know and use hand signals.
- Continue pedaling at all times when moving (no coasting) to help keep the bike stable and to maintain your balance.
- Properly maintain the working condition of your bicycle.

Pedestrians   Pedestrians are no match for the speed, size, and weight of motor vehicles, particularly the popular sport utility vehicles. About one in seven motor vehicle deaths involves pedestrians, and more than 80,000 pedestrians are injured each year. The highest rates of death and injury occur among the very young and the elderly. Nearly 45% of pedestrian deaths occur when people cross or enter the roadway between intersections. Alcohol intoxication plays a significant role in up to half of all adult pedestrian fatalities.

The following strategies can help prevent injuries when you're walking or jogging:

- Walk or jog in daylight.
- Maximize your visibility by wearing light-colored, reflective clothing.
- Face traffic when walking or jogging along a road, and follow traffic laws.
- Avoid busy roads or roads with poor visibility.
- Cross only at marked crosswalks and intersections.
- Don't listen to a radio, tape, or CD on headphones while walking.
- Don't hitchhike; it places you in a potentially dangerous situation.

Home Injuries

A person's place of residence, whether a house, an apartment, a trailer, or a dormitory, is considered home. People spend a great deal of time at home and feel that they are safe and secure there. However, home can be a dangerous place. The most common fatal **home injuries** are the result of falls, fires, poisoning, suffocation, and unintentional shootings.

Falls   About 90% of fatal falls involve people age 45 and over, but falls are the fifth leading cause of unintentional death for people under 25. Most deaths occurring from falls involve falling on stairs or steps or from one level to another. Falls also occur on the same level, from tripping, slipping, or stumbling. Alcohol is a contributing

Critical Consumer

Wearing a bicycle helmet can help you avoid serious head injury, brain damage, or even death in the event of a collision or fall. Helmets have a layer of stiff foam, which absorbs shock and cushions a blow to your head, covered by a thin plastic shell that will skid along the ground. For maximum protection, it's important to select a correctly fitting helmet. When you go shopping, remember the four S's: size, strap, straight, and sticker.

• *Size:* Try on several different sizes before making your selection; it may take several tries before you find the most comfortable fit. The helmet should be very snug but not overly tight on your head. Pads are usually provided to help adjust the fit. A good salesperson can also help you get the right fit. When the helmet is strapped onto your head, it should not move more than an inch in any direction, and you should not be able to pull or twist it off no matter how hard you try.

• *Strap:* Be sure that the chin strap fits snugly under your chin and that the V in the strap meets under your ear. Avoid thin straps, which can be uncomfortable. Check to be sure that

the buckle is strong and won't pop open and that the straps are sturdy.

• *Straight:* The helmet should sit straight on your head, not tilted back or forward (see the figure). A rule of thumb is that the rim should be about two finger widths above your eyebrows (depending on the height of your forehead).

• *Sticker:* Since March 1999, helmets sold in the United States must meet uniform safety standards established by the U.S. Consumer Product Safety Commission (CPSC). Look for a sticker or label that says the helmet meets the CPSC standard. If a helmet does not have one, it does not meet federal safety standards and should not be used.

You are more likely to wear your helmet if it is comfortable, so be sure that vents on the helmet provide airflow to promote cooling and sweat control. You will be safer with a brightly colored helmet that makes you more visible to drivers, especially in rainy, foggy, or dark conditions. Reflective tape will also increase your visibility. Finally, a helmet is a good place to put emergency information (your name, address, and phone number, plus any emergency medical conditions and an emergency contact). Tape change inside the helmet for a phone call.

If you are involved in a crash, replace your helmet. Even if the helmet doesn't have any visible signs of damage, its ability to protect your head may be compromised. As the Bicycle Helmet Safety Institute says, "No one ever complains about the cost of their second bike helmet."

Hard plastic shell

Stiff foam liner

Strap and buckle

SOURCES: Bicycle Helmet Safety Institute. 2005. *A Consumer's Guide to Bicycle Helmets* (http://www.helmets.org/guide.htm; retrieved March 3, 2005); Bicycle Helmet Safety Institute. 2004. *How to Fit a Bicycle Helmet* (http://www.bhsi.org/fit.htm; retrieved December 10, 2004); National Safety Council. 2000. *Choose the Right Helmet for Your Favorite Summer Sport* (http://www.nsc.org/pubs/fsh/archive/summr00/helmet.htm; retrieved July 26, 2000).

---

factor in many falls. Strategies for preventing falls include the following:

• Install handrails and nonslip applications in the shower and bathtub.

• Keep floors, stairs, and outside areas clear of objects or conditions that could cause slipping or tripping, such as ice, snow, electrical cords, and toys.

• Put a light switch by the door of every room so no one has to walk across a room to turn on a light. Use night lights in bedrooms, halls, stairs, and bathrooms.

• When climbing a ladder, use both hands. Never stand higher than the third step from the top. When using a stepladder, make sure the spreader brace is in the locked position. With straight ladders, set the base out 1 foot for every 4 feet of height.

• Don't use chairs to reach things; they are meant to be sat on, not stood on.

• If there are small children in the home, place gates at the top and bottom of stairs. Never leave a baby unattended on a bed or table. Install window guards to prevent children from falling out of windows.

Fires   Each year in the United States, approximately 80% of fire deaths and 65% of fire injuries occur in the home; a death caused by a residential fire occurs every 2 hours. Most fires begin in the kitchen, living room, or bedroom. Cooking is now the leading cause of home fire injuries; careless smoking is the leading cause of fire deaths, followed by problems with heating equipment and arson. To prevent fires, it's important to dispose of all cigarettes in ashtrays and to never smoke in bed. Other strategies include proper maintenance of fireplaces, furnaces, heaters, chimneys, and electrical outlets, cords, and appliances. If you use a portable heater, keep it at least 3 feet away from curtains, bedding, or

The risk of dying in a fire is reduced by half if you use a smoke detector. Install detectors on every floor, check them monthly, and replace the batteries at least once a year.

anything else that might catch fire. Never leave heaters on unattended.

It's important to be adequately prepared to handle fire-related situations. Plan at least two escape routes out of each room, and designate a location outside the home as a meeting place. For practice, stage a home fire drill; do it at night, as that's when most deadly fires occur.

Install smoke detectors on every level of your home. Your risk of dying in a fire is almost twice as high if you do not use them. Clean the detectors and check the batteries once a month, and replace the batteries at least once a year. More than 90% of U.S. homes have at least one smoke alarm, but about half are no longer functioning a year after installation, most commonly because batteries need to be replaced or dust and debris need to be cleaned out of the unit. Be sure that all residents are familiar with the sound of the smoke detector's alarm; when it goes off, take it seriously.

If a fire does occur, following these strategies can help prevent injuries:

- Get out as quickly as possible, and go to the designated meeting place. Don't stop for a keepsake or a pet. Never hide in a closet or under a bed. Once outside, count heads to see if everyone is out. If you think someone is still inside the burning building, tell the firefighters. Never go back inside a burning building.

- If you're trapped in a room, feel the door. If it is hot or if smoke is coming in through the cracks, don't open it; use the alternative escape route. If you can't get out of a room, go to the window and shout or wave for help.

- Smoke inhalation is the largest cause of death and injury in fires. To avoid inhaling smoke, crawl along the floor away from the heat and smoke. Cover your mouth and nose, ideally with a wet cloth, and take short, shallow breaths.

- If your clothes catch fire, don't run. Drop to the ground, cover your face, and roll back and forth to smother the flames. Remember: stop-drop-roll.

Although house fires cause the most deaths, hot water causes the most nonfatal burns. Young children are particularly at risk. Place barriers around stoves and radiators, and keep young children out of the kitchen, where they might be burned by spills. Put pans on rear burners, and turn pot handles toward the back of the stove. Keep hot foods away from the edge of counters and tables, and don't put them on a tablecloth that a small child can pull. Set your water heater no higher than 120°F. Always test the contents of a baby bottle; when bottles are heated in microwave ovens, the liquid can become scalding before the outside of the bottle gets very hot.

Poisoning More than 2.4 million poisonings and over 14,000 poison-related deaths occur every year in the United States. Poisons come in many forms, some of which are not typically considered poisons. For example, medications are safe when used as prescribed, but overdosing and incorrectly combining medications with another substance may result in poisoning. Other poisonous substances in the home include cleaning agents, petroleum-based products, insecticides and herbicides, cosmetics, nail polish and remover, and many houseplants. All potentially poisonous substances should be used only as directed and stored carefully, out of the reach of children.

The most common type of poisoning by gases is carbon monoxide poisoning. Carbon monoxide gas is emitted by motor vehicle exhaust and some types of heating equipment. The effects of exposure to this colorless, odorless gas include headache, blurred vision, and shortness of breath, followed by dizziness, vomiting, and unconsciousness. Carbon monoxide detectors similar to smoke detectors are available for home use; they should be used according to the manufacturer's instructions. To prevent poisoning by gases, never operate a vehicle in an enclosed space, have your furnace inspected yearly, and use caution with any substance that produces potentially toxic fumes.

A key strategy for preventing serious poisoning injuries is to keep the national poison control hotline number (800-222-1222) in a convenient location. A call to the national hotline will be routed to a local Poison Control Center, which provides expert emergency advice 24 hours a day. If a poisoning does occur, it's important that you act quickly. Remove the poison from contact with the victim's eyes, skin, or mouth, or move the victim away from contact with poisonous gases. Call the Poison Control Center immediately for instructions; do not follow the emergency instructions on product labels because they may be incorrect. Depending on the situation, you may be instructed to give the victim water to drink, or to flood affected parts of the skin or eyes with water. Do not induce vomiting. If you are advised to go to an emergency room, take the poisonous substance or container with you.

Suffocation and Choking Suffocation and choking account for about 3500 deaths annually in the United States. Children can suffocate if they put small items in their mouth, get tangled in their crib bedding, or get trapped in airtight appliances like old refrigerators. Keep small objects out of reach of children under age 3, and don't give them raw carrots, hot dogs, popcorn, gum, or hard candy. Examine toys carefully for small parts that could come loose; don't give plastic bags or balloons to small children.

Adults can also become choking victims, especially if they fail to chew food properly, eat hurriedly, or try to talk and eat at the same time. Many choking victims can be saved with the **Heimlich maneuver.** The American Red Cross recommends abdominal thrusts as the easiest and safest thing to do when an adult is choking (refer to the inside back cover of your text). Back blows administered in conjunction with abdominal thrusts are an acceptable procedure for dislodging an object from the throat of an infant.

Firearms About 40% of all unintended firearm deaths occur among people age 5–29. People who use firearms should remember the following:

- Never point a loaded gun at something you do not intend to shoot.
- Store unloaded firearms under lock and key, in a place separate from the ammunition.
- Always inspect firearms carefully before handling.
- Behave in the safe and responsible manner advocated in firearms safety courses.

Proper storage is critical. Do not assume that young children cannot fire a gun. About 25% of 3–4-year-olds and 70% of 5–6-year-olds have enough finger strength to pull a trigger. Every year, about 120 Americans are unintentionally shot to death by children under 6. About 8.3 million children live in households with unlocked guns, including 2.6 million who live in households where guns are stored loaded or with ammunition nearby.

Probably the best advice for anyone who picks up a gun is to assume it is loaded. Too many deaths and injuries occur when someone unintentionally shoots a friend while under the impression that the gun he or she is handling is not loaded. If you plan to handle a gun, you should also avoid the use of alcohol and drugs, which affect judgment and coordination. (Firearms and intentional injuries are discussed later in the chapter.)

Leisure Injuries

Leisure activities encompass a large part of our free time, so it is not surprising that **leisure injuries** are a significant health-related problem in the United States. Key factors in leisure injuries include misuse of equipment, lack of experience and skill, use of alcohol or other drugs, and failure to use appropriate safety equipment. Specific safety strategies for activities associated with leisure injuries include the following:

- Don't swim alone, in unsupervised places, under the influence of alcohol, or for an unusual length of time; use caution when swimming in unfamiliar surroundings or in water colder than 70°F. Check the depth of water before diving. Make sure that residential pools are fenced and that children are never allowed to swim unsupervised.
- Always use a **personal flotation device,** life jacket, when on a boat.
- For all sports and recreational activities, make sure facilities are safe, follow the rules, and practice good sportsmanship. Develop adequate skill in the activity, and use proper safety equipment, including, where appropriate, a helmet, eye protection, correct footwear, and knee, elbow, and wrist pads.
- If using equipment such as skateboards, snowboards, mountain bikes, or all-terrain vehicles, wear a helmet and other safety equipment, and avoid excessive speeds and unsafe stunts. Playground equipment should be used only for those activities for which it is designed.
- If you are active in excessively hot and humid weather, drink plenty of fluids, rest frequently in the shade, and slow down or stop if you feel uncomfortable. Danger signals of heat stress include excessive perspiration, dizziness, headache, muscle cramps, nausea, weakness, rapid pulse, and disorientation.
- Do not use alcohol or other drugs during recreational activities—such activities require coordination and sound judgment. To avoid choking, don't chew gum or eat while active.

Terms

V w

Heimlich maneuver A maneuver developed by Henry J. Heimlich, M.D., to help force an obstruction from the airway.

leisure injuries Unintentional injuries and deaths that occur in public places or places used in a public way, not involving motor vehicles; includes most sports and recreation deaths and injuries; falls, drownings, burns, and heat and cold stress are examples.

personal flotation device A device designed to save a person from drowning by buoying up the body while in the water; also called a *life jacket.*

Leisure activities injure more than 6 million people each year, including 250,000 in-line skaters. The use of proper safety equipment—helmet, wrist guards, and elbow and knee pads—is critical for injury prevention.

For more on exercise safety, refer to Chapter 13. Two activities that have recently become popular and that are associated with many leisure injuries are in-line skating and the use of nonmotorized scooters.

In-Line Skating Injuries More than 26 million Americans use in-line skates, and more than 250,000 are injured badly enough each year to wind up in an emergency room. Injuries to the wrist and head are most common; many occur because users do not wear appropriate safety gear. Researchers estimate that more than one-third of all serious injuries could be prevented if all skaters wore helmets and wrist and elbow protection.

To reduce your risk of being injured while rollerblading, wear a helmet, elbow and knee pads, wrist guards, a long-sleeved shirt, and long pants. Alcohol use appears to be a significant factor in in-line skating injuries that occur on college campuses. Because in-line skating involves skill, judgment, and coordination, it makes sense not to mix skating and drinking.

Scooter Injuries Scooters are lightweight and have low-friction wheels for quickness and portability. Along with their skyrocketing popularity have come scooter-related injuries. Over 30,000 people are treated for scooter-related injuries in hospital emergency rooms each year, and several deaths related to scooter use have been reported. The most common injuries are arm or hand fractures and dislocations, cuts and bruises, and sprains; 85% of injuries involve children under the age of 15. Viewing scooters as toys more than transportation may lead riders to ignore important safety precautions:

- Wear a helmet that meets bicycle helmet standards, along with knee and elbow pads.
- Be sure that handlebars, the steering column, and all nuts and bolts are securely fastened.
- Ride on smooth, paved surfaces away from motor vehicle traffic. Avoid streets and surfaces with water, sand, gravel, or dirt.
- Don't ride after dark.
- Closely supervise young children.

Work Injuries

Since 1912, when industrial records were first kept in the United States, the work site has become a much safer place, as evidenced by a nearly 90% reduction in the unintentional death rate. That figure becomes even more impressive when you realize that the size of the labor force has more than doubled and production has increased more than tenfold. One very significant factor to account for such a marked decline in **work injuries** has been the Occupational Safety and Health Act of 1970. As a result of that act, the Occupational Safety and Health Administration (OSHA) was created within the U.S. Department of Labor to ensure a safer and healthier environment for workers.

Despite improvements, more than 3 million Americans suffer disabling injuries on the job each year, and certain types of injuries, including skin disorders and repetitive strain injuries, are increasing. Although laborers make up less than half of the workforce, they account for more than 75% of all work-related injuries and illnesses. Their jobs usually involve extensive manual labor and lifting, neither of which is addressed in OSHA safety standards. Skin disorders account for nearly 40% of reported occupational illnesses; the introduction of more hazardous chemicals at the work site means that these disorders are of increasing concern. Most fatal occupational injuries involve crushing injuries, severe lacerations, burns, and electrocutions; among women, the leading cause of workplace injury deaths is homicide.

Back Injuries Back problems account for about 25% of work injuries; many of these could be prevented through proper lifting technique (Figure 22-1).

- Avoid bending at the waist. Remain in an upright position and crouch down if you need to lower yourself to grasp the object. Bend at the knees and hips.

Figure 22-1 Correct lifting technique. Stay upright, bending at the knees and hips.

- Place feet securely about shoulder-width apart; grip the object firmly.
- Lift gradually, with straight arms. Avoid quick, jerky motions. Lift by standing up or pushing with your leg muscles. Keep the object close to your body.
- If you have to turn, change the position of your feet. Twisting is a common and dangerous cause of injury. Plan ahead so that your pathway is clear and turning can be minimized.
- Put the object down gently, reversing the steps for lifting.

Repetitive Strain Injuries Musculoskeletal injuries and disorders in the workplace include **repetitive strain injuries (RSIs)**. RSIs are caused by repeated strain on a particular part of the body. Twisting, vibrations, awkward postures, and other stressors may contribute to RSIs. **Carpal tunnel syndrome** is one type of RSI that has increased in recent years due to increased use of computers, both at work and in the home (see the box "Carpal Tunnel Syndrome" on p. 674 for more information).

General strategies for preventing work-related injuries include following the safety instructions associated with the job, finding out where first aid equipment is located and knowing how to use it, watching for and reporting safety hazards, and using any safety equipment that is provided by the employer. Whatever the working conditions, employees should make a conscious effort to avoid hazardous situations.

VIOLENCE AND INTENTIONAL INJURIES

Violence—the use of physical force with the intent to inflict harm, injury, or death upon oneself or another—is a major public health concern in the United States. More

than 2 million Americans are victims of violent injury each year; about three violent crimes occur every minute. Worldwide, interpersonal violence is the third leading cause of death among people age 15–44. Examples of types of violence are assault, homicide, sexual assault, domestic violence, suicide, and child abuse.

It is difficult to determine the overall level of violence in our society because the major sources of data, police reports and victim surveys, are often at odds. In general, the overall violent crime rate increased between the 1950s and 1970s and then leveled off until the mid-1980s, when it again began to rise until 1992. The rate fell steadily from 1993 to 2000 and then rose slightly in 2001 and 2002—although it remained well below the 1992 rate and declined again in 2003. Possible factors cited for the general decline in violent crime include the aging of the population, reduced unemployment, the decline of the crack cocaine trade, law enforcement strategies to get guns off the street, violence prevention programs for youth, and longer prison sentences. In comparison to other industrialized countries, U.S. rates of violence are abnormally high in only two areas—homicide and firearm-related deaths. The U.S. homicide death rate is four to ten times that of similar countries, and the firearm death rate in the United States is eight times that of other developed countries.

Factors Contributing to Violence

Everyone gets angry sometimes, but few people translate their angry and aggressive impulses into action. Most intentional injuries and deaths are associated with an argument or the committing of another crime. However, there are a great many forms of violence, and no single factor can explain all of them.

Social Factors Rates of violence are not the same throughout society; they vary by geographic region, neighborhood, socioeconomic level, and many other factors. In the United States, violence is highest in the West, followed by the South, and among those who are disadvantaged in some way. Neighborhoods that are disadvantaged in

Terms

work injuries Unintentional injuries and deaths that arise out of and in the course of gainful work, such as falls, electrical shocks, exposure to radiation and toxic chemicals, burns, cuts, back sprains, and loss of fingers or other body parts in machines.

repetitive strain injury (RSI) A musculoskeletal injury or disorder caused by repeated strain on the hand, arm, wrist, or other part of the body; also called *cumulative trauma disorder (CTD)*.

carpal tunnel syndrome Compression of the median nerve in the wrist, often caused by repetitive use of the hands, such as in computer use; characterized by numbness, tingling, and pain in the hands and fingers; can cause nerve damage.

In Focus

Carpal Tunnel Syndrome

Carpal tunnel syndrome (CTS) is a repetitive strain injury characterized by pressure on the median nerve in the wrist. It is the most commonly reported work-related medical problem, accounting for about half of all work-related injuries. Women are about twice as likely as men to be affected by CTS.

The median nerve travels from the forearm to the hand through a tunnel in the wrist formed by the carpals (wrist bones) and associated tendons and cov-

Carpal tunnel

Ligament

Tendon
sheath

Tendons

Median nerve

Carpals

ered by a ligament (see the figure). The median nerve can become compressed for a variety of reasons, including swelling of the surrounding tendons caused by pregnancy, diabetes, arthritis, or repetitive wrist motions during activities such as typing, cutting, or carpentry work. Symptoms of CTS include numbness, tingling, burning, and/or aching in the hand, particularly in the thumb and the first three fingers. The pain may worsen at night and may shoot up from the hand as far as the shoulder.

Many cases of carpal tunnel syndrome clear up on their own or with minimal treatment. Modification of the movement that is causing the problem is critically important. For example, adjusting the height of a computer keyboard so that the wrists can be held straight during typing can help relieve pressure on the wrists. CTS is often first treated by immobilizing the wrist with a splint during the night. People may also be given anti-inflammatory drugs or injections of cortisone in the wrist to reduce swelling. In a small percentage of severe cases, surgery to cut the ligament and reduce the pressure on the nerve may be recommended.

If you engage in activities like typing or cutting that involve repetitive motions, there are some strategies you can try to reduce your risk of developing carpal tunnel syndrome. Begin by modifying your work environment to reduce the

stress on your wrists. Alternate activities to avoid spending long stretches of time engaged in the same motion. Warm up your wrists before you begin any repetitive motion activity, and take frequent breaks to stretch and flex your wrists and hands:

- Extend your arms out in front of you and stretch your wrists by pointing your fingers to the ceiling; hold for a count of five. Then straighten your wrists and relax your fingers for a count of five.

- With arms extended, make a tight fist with both hands and then bend your wrists so your knuckles are pointed toward the floor; hold for a count of five. Then straighten your wrists and relax your fingers for a count of five.

Repeat these stretches several times, and finish by letting your arms hang loosely at your sides and shaking them gently for several seconds.

SOURCES: Ly-Pen, D., et al. 2005. Surgical decompression versus local steroid injection in carpal tunnel syndrome: A one-year, prospective, randomized, open, controlled clinical trial. *Arthritis and Rheumatism* 52(2): 612–619; Carpal tunnel syndrome. 2002. *Journal of the American Medical Association* 288(10): 1310; American Academy of Orthopaedic Surgeons. 2000. *Exercises to Do at Work to Prevent Carpal Tunnel Syndrome* (http://orthoinfo.aaos.org/fact/thr_report.cfm?Thread_ID=5&topcategory=Hand; retrieved March 11, 2001).

---

status, power, and economic resources are typically the ones with the most violence. Rates of violence are highest among young people and minorities, groups that have relatively little power. People under age 25 account for nearly half the arrests for violent crime in the United States and about 40% of the arrests for homicide.

People who feel a part of society (have strong family and social ties), who are economically integrated (have a reasonable chance at getting a decent job), and who grow up in areas where there is a feeling of community (good schools, parks, and neighborhoods) are significantly less likely to engage in violence. American society, where more than one-third of all children live in poverty and where the gap between rich and poor keeps growing, should be expected to breed violence. Many criminologists feel we have a growing underclass of people who cannot expect to

have even the worst permanent jobs. That absence of hopes and dreams, combined with family devastation and poverty, certainly contributes to violent behavior:

Studies have shown that the environment on college campuses can contribute to violence. The nature of college campuses—transitory communities rather than permanent places where people work and live together over the long term—means that there is less incentive for people to cooperate and coexist amicably. Some campus groups even promote the ideas of bigotry and bias toward others, particularly toward individuals about whom they know little or with whom they have had little contact. Ignorance and insensitivity to differences can be precursors to acts of violence. College students must become more familiar with concepts such as inclusion, tolerance, and diversity if the problem is to be addressed.

Violence in the Media   The mass media play a major role in exposing audiences of all ages to violence as an acceptable and effective means of solving problems. Children may view as many as 10,000 violent acts on television and in movies each year. Computer and video games may also include many violent acts, creating concern that children's exposure to violence will make them more accepting or tolerant of it. The consequences of violence, for both perpetrator and victim, are shown much less frequently.

A 2005 study linked TV viewing to bullying among children. Researchers found that the more hours per day that a 4-year-old spent watching TV, the more likely the child was to engage in bullying behavior in school in later years. Factors that reduced the rate of bullying included cognitive stimulation, such as parents reading to a child, and emotional support and attention. It is thought that emotional support from parents helps children develop empathy, social competence, and self-regulation—skills that make them better able to deal with peers without resorting to aggressive or bullying behavior.

The role of media violence in violent behavior is an area of controversy. Researchers have found that exposure to media violence at least temporarily increases aggressive feelings in children, making them more likely to engage in violent or fearful behavior; the direct, short-term effects on teens and adults are less clear. It makes sense for parents to be aware of the potential influence of the media on their children. A child may not clearly understand the distinctions between the fantasy world portrayed in the media and the complexities of the real world. Parents should monitor the TV shows, movies, video games, music, and other forms of media to which children are exposed. Watching programs with children gives parents the opportunity to talk to children about violence and its consequences, to explain that violence is not the best way to resolve conflicts or solve problems, and to point out examples of positive behaviors such as kindness and cooperation.

Gender   In most cases, violence is committed by men (Figure 22-2). Males are more than nine times more likely than females to commit murder, and three times more likely than females to be murdered. Some researchers have suggested that the male hormone testosterone is in some way linked to aggressive behavior. Others point to prevailing cultural attitudes about male roles (men as dominant and controlling) as an explanation for the high rate of violence among men. However, these theories do not explain why it is that violent men are more likely to live in the West, belong to minorities, be poor, and be young.

Women do commit acts of violence, including a small but substantial proportion of murders of spouses. This fact has been used to argue that women have the same ca-

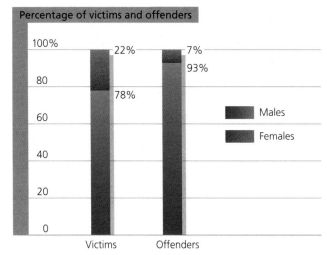

(a) Homicide victims and offenders by sex

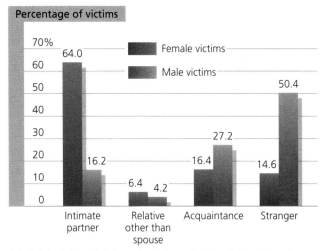

(b) Adult victims of violence by victim-offender relationship and sex of victim

VITAL STATISTICS

Figure 22-2   Facts about violence in the United States.   SOURCES: Federal Bureau of Investigation. 2004. *Crime in the United States. Uniform Crime Reports, 2003.* Washington, D.C.: U.S. Department of Justice; Tjaden, P., and N. Thoennes. 2000. *Full Report of the Prevalence, Incidence, and Consequences of Violence Against Women.* Washington, D.C.: U.S. Department of Justice.

pacity to commit violence as men, but most researchers note substantial differences. Men often kill their wives as the culmination of years of violence or after stalking them; they may kill their entire family and themselves at the same time. Women virtually never kill in such circumstances; rather, they kill their husbands after repeated victimization or while being beaten.

Interpersonal Factors   Although most people fear attack from strangers, the majority of victims are acquainted with their attacker (see Figure 22-2). Approximately 60% of murders of women and 80% of sexual

For every violent death that occurs in the United States, there are at least 100 nonfatal injuries caused by violence. The victims of most types of violence are statistically likely to be young (under age 25), poor, in a minority, urban, and—except for rape and domestic violence—male.

assaults are committed by someone the woman knows. In many cases, the people we need to fear the most live in our own household. Crime victims and violent criminals tend to share many characteristics—that is, they are likely to be young, male, in a minority, and poor.

Alcohol and Other Drugs Substance abuse and dependence are consistently associated with interpersonal violence and suicide. Intoxication affects judgment and may increase aggression in some people, causing a small argument to escalate into a serious physical confrontation. On college campuses, alcohol is involved in about 95% of all violent crimes.

Firearms Many criminologists feel that the high rate of homicide in the United States is directly related to the fact that we are the only industrialized country in which handguns are widespread and easily available. Simply put, most victims of assaults with other weapons don't die, but the death rate from assault by handgun is extremely high. The possession of a handgun can change a suicide attempt to a completed suicide and a violent assault to a murder. Every hour, guns are used to kill four people in the United States.

Over 100,000 deaths and injuries occur in the United States each year as a result of the use of firearms. Firearms are used in more than two-thirds of homicides, and studies reveal a strong correlation between the incidence of gun ownership and homicide rates for a given area of the country. Over half of all suicides involve a firearm, and people living in households in which guns are kept have a risk of suicide that is five or more times greater than that of people living in households without guns. Men between ages 15 and 34 have the highest risk of death from homicide and suicide when guns are the weapon used.

Research indicates that of all firearms, handguns are the murder weapon of choice, used in about 80% of homicides involving firearms. Teenagers and young adults are at particularly high risk for being murdered by handguns.

Assault

Assault is the use of physical force by a person or persons to inflict injury or death on another; homicide, aggravated assault, and robbery are examples of assault. Research indicates that the victims of assaultive injuries and their perpetrators tend to resemble one another in terms of ethnicity, educational background, psychological profile, and reliance on weapons. In many cases, the victim actually magnifies the confrontation through the use of a weapon.

Homicide

Men, teenagers, young adults, and members of minority groups, particularly African Americans and Latinos, are most likely to be murder victims. Although homicide rates for African Americans have declined dramatically in the past 25 years, no other cause of death so greatly differentiates African Americans from other Americans: Among black males, the rate of death from homicide is about six times higher than the rate for the U.S. population as a whole. Poverty and unemployment have been identified as key factors in homicide, and this may account for the high rates of homicide among blacks and other minority groups.

Most homicides are committed with a firearm, occur during an argument, and occur among people who know one another. Intrafamilial homicide, where the perpetrator and victim are related, accounts for about one out of every eight homicides. About 40% of family homicides are committed by spouses, usually following a history of physical and emotional abuse directed at the woman. Wives are more likely to be murdered than husbands, and when a wife kills her husband, it is usually in self-defense.

Gang-Related Violence

Violence results from more than just the acts of individuals, as evidenced by the number of injuries and deaths resulting from gang activities. Gangs are most frequently associated with large cities, but gang activity also extends to the suburbs and even to rural areas. It is estimated that more than 800,000 Americans belong to gangs; the average age for joining a gang is 14. Most gangs control a particular territory and will oppose other gangs, as well as police and community efforts to eliminate them. Gangs may be involved in illegal drug trade, extortion, and protection schemes. Gang members are more likely than non–gang members to possess weapons, and violence may result from conflicts over territory or illegal activities.

Gangs are more common in areas that are poor and suffer from high unemployment, population density, and crime. In these areas, an individual may feel that his or her hope of legitimate success in life is out of reach and know that involvement in the drug market makes some gang members rich. Often, gangs serve as a mechanism for companionship, self-esteem, support, and security; indeed, in some areas gang membership may be viewed as the only possible means of survival.

To prevent gang violence, individuals, communities, and lawmakers must work together to address factors linked to gang membership and activities. A successful program for combating gangs in Los Angeles includes mediators to help handle disputes or negotiate truces between gangs, job skill development for ex–gang members, and programs for at-risk youths that incorporate tutoring, counseling, and recreational activities. The program helps create an anti-gang community infrastructure by promoting neighborhood watch groups, community-based anti-gang activities, and economic development.

Hate Crimes

When bias against another person's race or ethnicity, national origin, religion, sexual orientation, or disability motivates a criminal act, the offense is classified as a hate crime. Hate crimes may be committed against people or property. Those against people may include intimidation, assault, and even rape or murder. Crimes against property most frequently involve graffiti, the desecration of churches or synagogues, cross burnings, and other acts of vandalism or property damage.

About 7500 hate crimes are reported every year; many more go unreported. Crimes against people make up about 70% of all incidents; intimidation and assault are the most common offenses. Racial or ethnic bias was cited as the motivating bias in 51% of the hate crimes reported in 2003; national origin was cited in 14% of the cases, religion in 18%, and sexual orientation in 17%.

Hate crimes may be extremely brutal acts perpetrated at random on total strangers by multiple offenders. Suspects frequently are not identified, but research indicates that a substantial number of hate crimes are committed by males under age 20. Hate crimes are frequently, but not always, associated with fringe groups that have extremist ideologies, such as the Ku Klux Klan and neo-Nazi groups. The Southern Poverty Law Center tracks more than 700 hate groups and group chapters currently active in the United States; the rapid growth of hate sites on the Internet is another area of concern.

A variety of factors lead to the prejudice and intolerance that are a major force behind hate crimes. A social context of unemployment and hard economic times, an influx of immigrants, and the growth of visible minority rights movements have been associated with the recent increases in hate crimes in the United States. To combat hate crimes, individuals and communities must foster tolerance, understanding, and an appreciation of differences among people.

School Violence

Tragedies like the shootings at Columbine High School in Colorado and Red Lake Senior High School in Minnesota have brought national attention to the problem of school violence. According to the National School Safety Center, more than 400 school-associated violent deaths of students, faculty, and administrators have occurred since 1992. A majority of these deaths occurred in urban areas and involved use of a firearm; as with other types of violence, both victims and offenders were predominantly young men. Homicide and suicide are the most serious and least common types of violence in schools; an estimated 400,000 less serious incidents of violence and crime occur each year, including theft, vandalism, and fights not involving weapons.

How risky is the school environment for students? Children are actually much safer at school than away from it. Less than 1% of all homicides among youths age 5–19 occur at school, and 90% of schools report no incidents of serious violence. Children and adolescents are far more likely to be killed by an adult in their own home or away from school than they are to die as a result of school-associated violence. According to the CDC, the overall number of violent incidents has decreased steadily since 1992; however, the number of multiple-victim events may have increased. Recent school shootings received so much attention in part because they were unusual—they took place in predominantly suburban or rural schools and involved multiple victims. Despite declines in violence-related behaviors, about 17% of high school students in a national survey reported carrying a weapon (gun, knife, club) to school at least once in the month before the survey, and 9% reported being threatened with a weapon on school grounds in the past year.

Although schools are basically safe places overall, there are steps that can be taken to identify at-risk youths and improve safety for all students. Characteristics associated with youths who have caused school-associated violent deaths include a history of uncontrollable angry outbursts, violent and abusive language and behavior, isolation from peers, depression and irritability, access to and preoccupation with weapons, and lack of support and supervision from adults. Being a victim of teasing, bullying, or social exclusion (rejection) may lead to aggressive behavior and violence. Recommendations for reducing school violence include offering classroom training in anger management, social skills, and improved self-control; providing mental health and social services for students in need; developing after-school programs that help students build self-esteem and make friends; and keeping guns out of the hands of children and out of schools.

Workplace Violence

Each year U.S. workers experience an average of 1.5 million minor assaults, 400,000 serious assaults, 85,000 robberies, 50,000 sexual assaults, and 700 homicides. In about 60% of cases, workplace violence is committed by strangers; acquaintances account for nearly 40% of cases, and intimates for 1%. Police and corrections officers have the most dangerous jobs, followed by taxi drivers, security guards, bartenders, mental health professionals, and workers at gas stations and convenience and liquor stores. Most of the perpetrators of workplace violence are white males over age 21. Firearms are used in more than 80% of workplace homicides, and the majority of these homicides occur during the commission of a robbery or other crime.

General crime prevention strategies, including use of surveillance cameras and silent alarms and limiting the amount of cash on hand, can help reduce workplace violence related to robberies. A highly stressed workplace is a risk factor in cases of violence between acquaintances or coworkers; clear guidelines about acceptable behavior and prompt action after any threats or incidents of violence can help control this type of workplace violence. The OSHA Web site (www.osha.gov/SLTC/workplaceviolence) has violence prevention tips for workers in some of the jobs with high rates of workplace violence.

Terrorism

In 2001, more Americans died as a result of terrorism than in any prior year; the attacks on September 11 killed more than 3000 people, including citizens of 78 countries. The FBI defines terrorism as the unlawful use of force or violence against persons or property to intimidate or coerce a government, the civilian population, or any segment thereof in furtherance of political or social objectives. Terrorism is one form of what the World Health Organization calls collective violence (see the box "Violence and Health: A Global View"). Terrorism can be either domestic, carried out by groups based in the United States, or international. It comes in many forms, including biological (see Chapter 17), chemical, nuclear, and cyber. Its intent is to promote helplessness by instilling fear of harm or destruction.

Most of the terrorism-prevention activities occur at the federal, state, and community levels. U.S. government efforts include close work with the diplomatic, law-enforcement, intelligence, economic, and military communities. The mission of the Department of Homeland Security is to help prevent, protect against, and respond to acts of terrorism on U.S. soil. It is coordinating efforts to protect electric and water supply systems, transportation, gas and oil, emergency services, the computer infrastructure, and other systems. The Patriot Act was designed to give law-enforcement agencies additional tools and improved interagency cooperation for the purpose of investigating and preventing terrorism.

One step individuals can take is to put together an emergency plan and kit for their family or household that can serve for any type of emergency or disaster (see the box "Emergency Preparedness" on p. 680). As described in Chapters 2 and 3, the impact of terrorism can extend beyond the attack itself; refer to those chapters for advice on coping with the stress of terrorism and mass violence and for guidelines for recognizing and treating post-traumatic stress disorder.

Family and Intimate Violence

Violence in families challenges some of our most basic assumptions about the family. Family violence generally refers to any rough and illegitimate use of physical force, aggression, or verbal abuse by one family member toward another. Such abuse may be physical and/or psychological in nature. Based on reported cases, an estimated 5–7 million women and children are abused each year in the United States.

Battering Studies reveal that 95% of domestic violence victims are women; 20–35% of women who visit medical emergency rooms are there for injuries related to ongoing abuse. Violence against wives or intimate partners, or battering, occurs at every level of society but is more common at lower socioeconomic levels. It occurs more frequently in relationships with a high degree of conflict—an apparent inability to resolve arguments through negotiation and compromise. About 25% of women report having been physically assaulted or raped by an intimate partner, and more than 50% report having experienced some type of abuse—physical or psychological—in a relationship.

At the root of much of this abusive behavior is the need to control another person. Abusive partners are controlling partners. They not only want to have power over another person, but also believe they are entitled to it, no matter what the cost to the other person. Abuse includes behavior that physically harms, arouses fear, prevents a person from doing what she wants, or compels her to behave in ways she does not freely choose. Controlling people use a variety of psychological, emotional, and physical tactics to keep their partners bound to them. Early in a relationship, a person's tendency to be controlling may not be obvious. If you are concerned about whether a person you are dating has the potential to be abusive, review the guidelines in the box "Recognizing the Potential for Abusiveness in a Partner" on p. 681.

In 2002, the World Health Organization (WHO) issued its *World Report on Violence and Health,* which examines the magnitude and impact of violence throughout the world. Each year, more than 1.6 million people die from violent acts: Suicide claims a life every 40 seconds, homicide every minute, and armed conflict every 2 minutes. Violence is among the leading causes of death for people age 15–44, accounting for 14% of deaths among males and 7% of deaths among females. Millions more victims of violence survive but are left with physical, psychological, and reproductive problems, including lost limbs, paralysis, depression, alcohol and drug abuse, sexual dysfunction, and STDs and other reproductive health problems. Beyond individual misery, violence has devastating social and economic consequences.

Interpersonal Violence

WHO defines *interpersonal violence* as the intentional use of physical force or power, threatened or actual, against another person that is likely to result in injury, death, psychological harm, or deprivation. Each year, more than 500,000 people die from interpersonal violence, and more than 60 million children and elderly adults are maltreated. It's estimated that 10–70% of women experience physical violence at the hands of an intimate partner during their lifetime; in addition, forced prostitution, child marriage, sexual trafficking, and female genital mutilation are prevalent in some areas of the world.

Worldwide, adolescents and young adults are the primary victims and perpetrators of interpersonal violence. Individual risk factors for violence highlighted in the WHO report include being young, male, and poor; being intoxicated; and having easy access to firearms. At the community and social levels, risk factors include low social capital (norms and networks that promote coordination and cooperation), high crime rates, rapid social change, poverty, poor rule of law and corruption, gender inequality, firearm availability, and armed conflict. Rates of violence are particularly high among the poorest sectors of the population in countries with high levels of economic inequality (a wide gap between rich and poor).

Collective Violence

WHO applies the term *collective violence* to violence inflicted by one group against another group to achieve political, economic, or social objectives. Collective violence includes armed conflict within or between states; genocide, repression, and other human rights abuses; terrorism; and organized violent crime. Characteristics of countries with increased risk of violent conflict include long-standing tensions between groups, a lack of democratic processes, unequal access to power, unequal distribution and control of resources, and rapid demographic changes.

In the twentieth century, an estimated 191 million people—well over half of them civilians—lost their lives directly or indirectly as a result of armed conflict, and many more were injured. In some conflicts, civilians were mutilated or raped as part of a deliberate strategy to humiliate and demoralize communities. In addition to directly causing deaths and injuries, collective violence destroys infrastructure and disrupts trade, food production, and vital services, thus setting the stage for famine, increased rates of infectious diseases, and mass movements of refugees. The resulting social turmoil also increases rates of interpersonal violence.

What Can Be Done?

The WHO report emphasizes that violence is neither an inevitable part of the human condition nor an intractable social problem. Rather, the wide variation in violence within and among nations over time suggests that violence is the product of a complex but modifiable set of social and environmental factors. Potential strategies to reduce violence include the following:

- Individual and relationship approaches to encourage healthy attitudes and behaviors, such as training in social, parenting, and relationship skills and conflict resolution; mentoring programs; and treatment for people who suffer from depression or who have inflicted abuse on partners or children

- Community-based efforts to raise public awareness and address local social and material causes of violence, such as creating safe places for children to play and adopting community policing

- Societal approaches to change underlying cultural, social, and economic factors, such as new laws and international treaties, policy changes to reduce poverty and inequality, efforts to change harmful social and cultural norms (for example, ethnic discrimination or gender inequality), and disarmament and demobilization programs in countries emerging from conflict

Tackling the problem of violence will require public investment and a collective consensus on what should be done. Only a global response can make the world a safer and healthier place for all.

SOURCES: World Health Organization. 2002. *The World Health Report 2002: Reducing Risks, Promoting Healthy Life.* Geneva: World Health Organization; World Health Organization. 2002. *World Report on Violence and Health.* Geneva: World Health Organization.

In abusive relationships, the abuser (in most cases a man) usually has a history of violent behavior, traditional beliefs about gender roles, and problems with alcohol abuse. He has low self-esteem and seeks to raise it by dominating and imposing his will on another person. Research has revealed a three-phase cycle of battering, consisting of a period of increasing tension, a violent explosion and loss of control, and a period of contriteness in which the man begs forgiveness and promises it will never happen again. The batterer is drawn back to this cycle over and over again, but he never succeeds in changing his feelings about himself.

Battered women often stay in violent relationships for years. They may be economically dependent on their

Recent incidents of terrorism, mass violence, and natural disasters have highlighted the need for individuals to plan ahead for emergencies. Although you usually cannot predict when a disaster situation will occur, there are things you can do to be better prepared.

Emergency Supplies

Your kit of emergency supplies should include everything you'll need to make it on your own for at least 3 days. You'll need nonperishable food, water, first aid supplies, essential medications, a battery-powered radio, toiletries, clothing, a flashlight or candles and matches, cash, keys, copies of important documents, and supplies for sleeping outdoors in any season/weather (blankets, sleeping bags, tent, and so on). Don't forget about special-needs items for infants, seniors, and pets.

In the case of certain types of terrorist attacks or industrial disasters, you may need supplies to "shelter in place"—to create a barrier between yourself and any dangerous airborne materials. These supplies might include filter masks or folded cotton towels that can be placed over the mouth and nose. Plastic sheeting and duct tape can be used to seal windows and doors.

You may want to create several kits of emergency supplies. The primary one would contain supplies for home use. Put together a smaller, lightweight version that you can take with you if you are forced to evacuate your residence. Smaller kits for your car and your office are also recommended.

A Family or Household Plan

You and your family or the members of your household may or may not be together when a disaster strikes. You should have a plan about where to meet and how to communicate. Choose at least two potential meeting places—one in your neighborhood and one or more in other areas. Your community may also have set locations for community shelters.

Where you go may depend on the circumstances of the emergency situation. Use your common sense, and listen to the radio or television to obtain instructions from emergency officials about whether to evacuate or stay in place. In addition, know all the transportation options in the vicinity of your home, school, and workplace; roadways and public transit may be affected, so a sturdy pair of walking shoes is a good item to keep in your emergency kit.

Everyone in the household should also have the same emergency contact person to call, preferably someone who lives outside the immediate area. Local phone service may be significantly disrupted, so long-distance calls may be more likely to go through. Everyone should carry the relevant phone numbers and addresses at all times.

It is also important to check into the emergency plans at any location where you or family members spend time, including schools and workplaces. For each location, know the safest place to be for different types of emergencies—for example, load-bearing interior walls during an earthquake or the basement during a tornado. Also know how to turn off water, gas, and electricity in case of damaged utility lines; keep the needed tools next to the shutoff valves.

Other steps you can take to help prepare for emergencies include taking a first aid class and setting up an emergency response group in your neighborhood or building. More complete information about emergency preparedness is available from the following organizations and agencies:

American Academy of Pediatrics (www.aap.org)

American Red Cross (www.redcross.org)

Federal Emergency Management Agency (www.fema.gov)

U.S. Department of Homeland Security (www.ready.gov)

SOURCES: U.S. Department of Homeland Security. 2005. *Ready America* (http://www.ready.gov/index.html; retrieved March 4, 2005); Your preparedness guide for any emergency. 2004. *Consumer Reports,* September.

---

partners, feel trapped or fear retaliation if they leave, believe their children need a father, or have low self-esteem themselves. They may love or pity their husband, or they may believe they'll eventually be able to stop the violence. They usually leave the relationship only when they become determined that the violence must end. Battered women's shelters offer physical protection, counseling, support, and other assistance.

Many batterers are arrested, prosecuted, and imprisoned. Treatment programs are helpful in some cases but not all. Programs focus on stress management, communication and conflict-resolution skills, behavior change, and individual and group therapy. A crucial factor in changing violent behavior seems to be a partner's adamant insistence that the abuse stop.

Stalking and Cyberstalking Battering is closely associated with **stalking**, characterized by harassing behaviors such as following or spying on a person and making verbal, written, or implied threats. In the United States, it is estimated that 1 million women and 400,000 men are stalked each year; about 87% of stalkers are men. About half of female victims are stalked by current or

Terms

stalking Repeatedly harassing or threatening a person through behaviors such as following a person, appearing at a person's residence or workplace, leaving written messages or objects, making harassing phone calls, or vandalizing property; frequently directed at a former intimate partner.

cyberstalking The use of e-mail, chat rooms, bulletin boards, or other electronic communications devices to stalk another person.

Recognizing the Potential for Abusiveness in a Partner

There are no sure ways to tell whether someone will become abusive or violent toward an intimate partner, but there are warning signs that you can look for. (Remember that, although most abusive relationships involve male violence directed at a woman, women can also be abusive, as can partners in a same-sex relationship. Because most abusers are male, the following material refers to the abuser as "he.") If you are concerned that a person you are involved with has the potential for violence, observe his or her behavior, and ask yourself these questions:

- What is this person's attitude toward women? How does he treat his mother and his sister? How does he work with female students, female colleagues, or a female boss? How does he treat your women friends?

- What is his attitude toward your autonomy? Does he respect the work you do and the way you do it? Or does he put it down, tell you how to do it better, or encourage you to give it up? Does he tell you he'll take care of you?

- How self-centered is he? Does he want to spend leisure time on your interests or his? Does he listen to you? Does he remember what you say?

- Is he possessive or jealous? Does he want to spend every minute with you? Does he cross-examine you about things you do when you're not with him?

- What happens when things don't go the way he wants them to? Does he blow up? Does he always have to get his way?

- Is he moody, mocking, critical, or bossy? Do you feel as if you're walking on eggshells when you're with him?

- Do you feel you have to avoid arguing with him?

- Does he drink too much or use drugs?

- Does he refuse to use condoms or take other precautions for safer sex?

Listen to your own uneasiness, and stay away from any man who disrespects women, who wants or needs you intensely and exclusively, and who has a knack for getting his own way almost all the time.

If you are in a serious relationship with a controlling person, you may already have experienced abuse. Consider the following questions:

- Does your partner constantly criticize you, blame you for things that are not your fault, or verbally degrade you?

- Does he humiliate you in front of others?

- Is he suspicious or jealous? Does he accuse you of being unfaithful or monitor your mail or phone calls?

- Does he track all your time? Does he discourage you from seeing friends and family?

- Does he prevent you from getting or keeping a job or attending school? Does he control your shared resources or restrict your access to money?

- Has he ever pushed, slapped, hit, kicked, bitten, or restrained you? Thrown an object at you? Used a weapon on you?

- Has he ever destroyed or damaged your personal property or sentimental items?

- Has he ever forced you to have sex or to do something sexually you didn't want to do?

- Does he anger easily when drinking or taking drugs?

- Has he ever threatened to harm you or your children, friends, pets, or property?

- Has he ever threatened to blackmail you if you leave?

If you answered yes to one or more of these questions, you may be experiencing domestic abuse. If you believe you or your children are in imminent danger, look in your local telephone directory for a women's shelter, or call 9-1-1. If you want information, referrals to a program in your area, or assistance, contact one of the organizations listed in For More Information at the end of the chapter.

SOURCES: Family Violence Prevention Fund. 1996. *Take Action Against Domestic Violence*. San Francisco, Calif.: Family Violence Prevention Fund; How to tell if you're in an abusive situation. 1994. *San Francisco Chronicle*, 24 June; Jones, A. 1994. *Next Time She'll Be Dead*. Boston: Beacon Press.

former intimate partners; of these, 80% had been physically or sexually assaulted by that partner during the relationship. A stalker's goal may be to control or scare the victim or to keep her or him in a relationship. Most stalking episodes last a year or less, but victims may experience social and psychological effects long after the stalking ends.

The use of the Internet, e-mail, chat rooms, and other electronic communications devices to stalk another person is known as **cyberstalking**. As with offline stalking, the majority of cyberstalkers are men, and the majority of victims are women, although there have been same-sex cyberstalking incidents. Online incidents of harassment or abuse are becoming more common and more serious, and the U.S. Department of Justice estimates that nearly one-half million people each year experience cyberstalking. As the seriousness of the crime is being recognized, several states have passed cyberstalking or related laws, and a federal law is under consideration. There is concern that the impersonal nature of electronic communication may lower the barriers to harassment and threats, because a cyberstalker does not have to physically confront the victim, and thus may result in making stalking more common. The popularity of online dating sites may also increase cyberstalking.

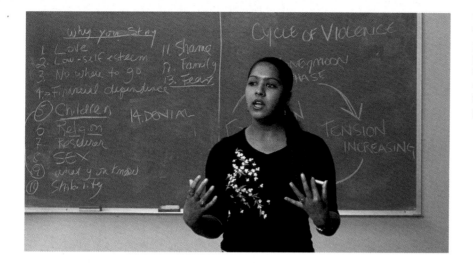

Battering and stalking are related forms of intimate violence, often involving verbal or physical abuse directed at controlling another person. Education, counseling, and support can help the victims of family violence. This college workshop helps people identify the signs of battering and the reasons why people may stay in abusive relationships.

Cyberstalkers may send harassing or threatening e-mails or chat room messages to the victim, or they may encourage others to harass the victim—for example, by impersonating the victim and posting inflammatory messages and personal information on bulletin boards or in chat rooms. Guidelines for staying safe online include the following:

- Never use your real name as an e-mail username or chat room nickname. Select an age- and gender-neutral identity.

- Avoid filling out profiles for accounts related to e-mail use or chat room activities with information that could be used to identify you.

- Do not share personal information in public spaces anywhere online or give it to strangers.

- Learn how to filter unwanted e-mail messages.

- If you do experience harassment online, do not respond to the harasser. Log off or surf elsewhere.

If you receive unwanted online contact, make it clear to that person that you want all contact to stop. If harassment continues, contact the harasser's Internet service provider (ISP) by identifying the domain of the stalker's account (after the "@" sign); most ISPs have an e-mail address for complaints. Often, an ISP can try to stop the conduct by direct contact with the harasser or by closing his or her account. Save all communications for evidence, and contact your ISP and your local police department. Many states have laws against cyberstalking. (See Chapter 4 for more on safely interacting with people online.)

Violence Against Children   Violence is also directed against children. Every year, at least 1 million American children are physically abused by their parents, and another 1 to 2 million are victims of neglect. Parental violence is one of the five leading causes of death for children age 1–18. Parents who abuse children tend to have low self-esteem, to believe in physical punishment, to

have a poor marital relationship, and to have been abused themselves (although many people who were abused as children do not grow up to abuse their own children). Poverty, unemployment, and social isolation are characteristics of families in which children are abused. External stressors related to socioeconomic and environmental factors are most closely associated with neglect, whereas stressors related to interpersonal issues are more closely associated with physical abuse. Single parents, both men and women, are at especially high risk for abusing their children. Very often one child, whom the parents consider different in some way, is singled out for violent treatment.

When government agencies intervene in child-abuse situations, their goals are to protect the victims and to assist and strengthen the families. The most successful programs are those that emphasize education and early intervention, such as home visits to high-risk first-time mothers. Educational efforts focus on stress management, money management, job-finding skills, and information about child behavior and development. Parents may also receive counseling and be referred to substance-abuse treatment programs. Support groups like Parents Anonymous are effective for parents committed to changing their behavior.

Elder Abuse   Each year, at least 500,000 older persons are abused; only one in six incidents is reported. Most abusers are family members who are serving as caregivers. Elder abuse can take different forms: physical, sexual, or emotional abuse; financial exploitation; neglect; or abandonment. Neglect is the most common form of abuse, accounting for about 55% of reported cases. Elders who have lost some mental or physical functions and must rely on others for care are most at risk and may suffer malnutrition, dehydration, mismanaged medication, or infection due to poor hygiene. Physical abuse accounts for about 15% of reported cases, and financial exploitation for about 13%.

Abuse often occurs when caring for a dependent adult becomes too stressful for the caregiver, especially if the elder is incontinent, has suffered mental deterioration, or is violent. Abuse may become an outlet for frustration. Many believe that the solution to elder abuse is support in the form of greater social and financial assistance, such as adult day-care centers and education and public care programs.

Sexual Violence

The use of force and coercion in sexual relationships is one of the most serious problems in human interactions. The most extreme manifestation of sexual coercion—forcing a person to submit to another's sexual desires—is rape, but sexual coercion occurs in many subtler forms, including sexual harassment.

Sexual Assault: Rape   Sexual coercion that relies on the threat and use of physical force or takes advantage of circumstances that render a person incapable of giving consent (such as when drunk) constitutes **sexual assault** or **rape.** When the victim is younger than the legally defined age of consent, the act constitutes **statutory rape,** whether or not coercion is involved. Coerced sexual activity in which the victim knows or is dating the rapist is often referred to as **date rape,** or *acquaintance rape.* Most victims know their assailant, but less than one-third of all sexual crimes are reported.

Any woman—or man—can be a rape victim. It is estimated that more than 3.5 million women are raped each year and that 1 in 6 women and 1 in 33 men has experienced an attempted or completed rape at some point in their lives. A study of college students found that between 1 in 4 and 1 in 5 college women experience a completed or attempted rape during their college years. The majority of male victims of rape are not in prison.

WHO COMMITS RAPE?   Men who commit rape may be any age and come from any socioeconomic group. Some rapists are exploiters in the sense that they rape on the spur of the moment and mainly want immediate gratification. Some attempt to compensate for feelings of sexual inadequacy and an inability to obtain satisfaction otherwise. Others are more hostile and sadistic and are primarily interested not in sex but in hurting and humiliating a particular woman or women in general.

Most women are in much less danger of being raped by a stranger than of being sexually assaulted by a man they know or date. Surveys suggest that as many as 25% of women have had experiences in which the men they were dating persisted in trying to force sex despite pleading, crying, screaming, or resisting. Surveys have also found that more than 60% of all rape victims were raped by a current or former spouse, boyfriend, or date.

Most cases of date rape are never reported to the police, partly because of the subtlety of the crime. Usually no weapons are involved, and direct verbal threats may not have been made. Rather than being terrorized, the victim usually is attracted to the man at first. Victims of date rape tend to shoulder much of the responsibility for the incident, questioning their own judgment and behavior rather than blaming the aggressor.

Sometimes husbands rape their wives. Strong evidence suggests that 15% of American women who have ever married have been raped by their husbands or ex-husbands; as many as 60% of battered women may have been raped by their husbands. A charge of spousal rape can now be taken to court in all states.

FACTORS CONTRIBUTING TO DATE RAPE   One factor in date rape appears to be the double standard about appropriate sexual behavior for men and women. Although the general status of women in society has improved, it is still a commonly held cultural belief that nice women don't say yes to sex (even when they want to) and that real men don't take no for an answer.

There are also widespread differences between men and women in how they perceive romantic encounters and signals. In one study, researchers found that men tend to interpret women's actions on dates, such as smiling or talking in a low voice, as indicating an interest in having sex, whereas the women interpreted the same actions as just being friendly. Men's thinking about forceful sex also tends to be unclear. One psychologist reports that men find "forcing a woman to have sex against her will" more acceptable than "raping a woman," even though the former description is the definition of rape.

Aside from the double standard and unclear perceptions and thinking about sex, men who rape their dates tend to have certain attributes, including hostility toward women, a belief that dominance alone is a valid motive for sex, and an acceptance of sexual violence. They may feel that force is justified in certain circumstances, such as if they are sexually involved with a woman and she refuses to have sex, if the woman is known to have had sex with other men, or if the woman shows up at a party where people are drinking and taking drugs. The man often primes himself to force himself sexually on his date by drinking, which lowers his ordinary social inhibitions. Many college men who have committed date rape tried to seduce their dates by plying them with alcohol first.

Terms

sexual assault or **rape** The use of force to have sex with someone against that person's will.

statutory rape Sexual interaction with someone under the legal age of consent.

date rape Sexual assault by someone the victim knows or is dating; also called *acquaintance rape.*

www.mhhe.com/insel10e   Chapter 22   Personal Safety: Protecting Yourself from Unintentional Injuries and Violence   683

Preventing Date Rape

Take Charge

Guidelines for Women

- Believe in your right to control what you do. Set limits, and communicate these limits clearly, firmly, and early. Say no when you mean no.

- Be assertive with someone who is sexually pressuring you. Men often interpret passivity as permission.

- If you are unsure of a new acquaintance, go on a group date or double date. If possible, provide your own transportation.

- Remember that some men assume sexy dress and a flirtatious manner mean a desire for sex.

- Remember that alcohol and drugs interfere with clear communication about sex.

- Use the statement that has proven most effective in stopping date rape: "This is rape, and I'm calling the police."

Guidelines for Men

- Be aware of social pressure. It's OK to not score.

- Understand that no means no. Don't continue making advances when your date resists or tells you she wants to stop. Remember that she has the right to refuse sex.

- Don't assume sexy dress and a flirtatious manner are invitations to sex, that previous permission for sex applies to the current situation, or that your date's relationships with other men constitute sexual permission for you.

- Remember that alcohol and drugs interfere with clear communication about sex.

DATE-RAPE DRUGS Recently there has been an increase in the reported use of date-rape drugs other than alcohol. Also called predator drugs, the drugs used in date rapes include flunitrazepam (Rohypnol), gamma hydroxybutyrate (GHB), and ketamine hydrochloride ("Special K"). As described in Chapter 9, these drugs have a variety of effects, including sedation; if slipped surreptitiously into a drink, they can incapacitate a person within about 20 minutes and make her or him more vulnerable to assault. Rohypnol, GHB, and other drugs also often cause anterograde amnesia, meaning victims have little memory of what happened while they were under the influence of the drug. (See Chapter 9 for more on the effects of these and other psychoactive drugs.)

The Drug-Induced Rape Prevention and Punishment Act of 1996 adds up to 20 years to the prison sentence of any rapist who uses a drug to incapacitate a victim. Supporters of the law likened dropping a drug in a victim's drink to putting a knife to her throat. The makers of Rohypnol are modifying the pills so they will be a more noticeable color and will dissolve more slowly, thereby reducing the likelihood that Rohypnol can be used as a date-rape drug; however, other drugs in powdered or liquid form can be slipped into drinks unnoticed. Strategies such as the following can help ensure that your drink is not tampered with at a bar or party:

- Check with campus or local police to find out if drug-facilitated sexual assault has occurred in your area and, if so, where.

- Drink moderately and responsibly. Avoid group drinking and drinking games.

- Be wary of opened beverages—alcoholic or nonalcoholic—offered by strangers. When at an unfamiliar bar, watch the bartender pour your drink.

- Let your date be the first to drink from the punchbowl at a bar, club, or rave.

- If an opened beverage tastes, looks, or smells strange, do not drink it. If you leave your drink unattended, such as when you dance or use the restroom, obtain a fresh drink when you return to your table.

- If you go to a party, club, or bar, go with friends. Have a prearranged plan for checking on each other visually and verbally. If you feel giddy or light-headed, get assistance.

Date rape is largely a result of sexual socialization in which the man develops an exaggerated sexual impulse and puts a premium on sexual conquests. Sex and violence are linked in our society, and coercion is accepted by some adolescents as an appropriate form of sexual expression. Both males and females can take actions that will reduce the incidence of acquaintance rape; see the box "Preventing Date Rape" for specific suggestions.

DEALING WITH A SEXUAL ASSAULT Experts disagree about whether a woman who is faced with a rapist should fight back or give in quietly to avoid being injured or to gain time in the hope of escaping. Some rapists say that if a woman had screamed or resisted loudly, they would have run; others report they would have injured or killed her. (If a rapist is carrying a weapon, most experts advise against fighting unless absolutely necessary.) A woman who is raped by a stranger is more likely to be physically injured than a woman raped by someone she knows. Each situation is unique, and a woman should respond in whatever way she thinks best. If a woman chooses not to resist, it does not mean that she has not been raped.

If you are threatened by a rapist and decide to fight back, here is what Women Organized Against Rape (WOAR) recommends:

- Trust your gut feeling. If you feel you are in danger, don't hesitate to run and scream. It is better to feel foolish than to be raped.
- Yell—and keep yelling. It will clear your head and start your adrenaline going; it may scare your attacker and also bring help. Don't forget that a rapist is also afraid of pain and afraid of getting caught.
- If an attacker grabs you from behind, use your elbows for striking his neck, his sides, or his stomach.
- Try kicking. Your legs are the strongest part of your body, and your kick is longer than his reach. Kick with your rear foot and with the toe of your shoe. Aim low to avoid losing your balance.
- His most vulnerable spot is his knee; it's low, difficult to protect, and easily knocked out of place. Don't try to kick a rapist in the crotch; he has been protecting this area all his life and will have better protective reflexes there than at his knees.
- Once you start fighting, keep it up. Your objective is to get away as soon as you can.
- Remember that ordinary rules of behavior don't apply. It's OK to vomit, act crazy, or claim to have a sexually transmitted disease.

If you are raped, tell what happened to the first friendly person you meet. Call the police, tell them you were raped, and give your location. Try to remember as many facts as you can about your attacker; write down a description as soon as possible. Don't wash or change your clothes, or you may destroy important evidence. The police will take you to a hospital for a complete exam; show the physician any injuries. Tell the police simply, but exactly, what happened. Be honest, and stick to your story.

If you decide that you don't want to report the rape to the police, be sure to see a physician as soon as possible. You need to be checked for pregnancy and STDs.

THE EFFECTS OF RAPE Rape victims suffer both physical and psychological injury. For most, physical wounds heal within a few weeks. Psychological pain may endure and be substantial. Even the most physically and mentally strong are likely to experience shock, anxiety, depression, shame, and a host of psychosomatic symptoms after being victimized. These psychological reactions following rape comprise rape trauma syndrome, which is characterized by fear, nightmares, fatigue, crying spells, and digestive upset. (Rape trauma syndrome is a form of post-traumatic stress disorder; see Chapter 3.) Self-blame is very likely; society has contributed to this tendency by perpetuating the myths that women can actually defend themselves and that no one can be raped if she doesn't want to be. Fortunately, these false beliefs are dissolving in the face of evidence to the contrary.

Many organizations offer counseling and support to rape victims. Look in the telephone directory under Rape or Rape Crisis Center for a hotline number to call. Your campus may have counseling services or a support group.

Child Sexual Abuse Child sexual abuse is any sexual contact between an adult and a child who is below the legal age of consent. Adults and older adolescents are able to coerce children into sexual activity because of their authority and power over them. Threats, force, or the promise of friendship or material rewards may be used to manipulate a child. Sexual contacts are typically brief and consist of genital manipulation; genital intercourse is much less common.

Sexual abusers are usually male, heterosexual, and known to the victim. The abuser may be a relative, a friend, a neighbor, or another trusted adult acquaintance. Child abusers are often pedophiles, people who are sexually attracted to children. They may have poor interpersonal and sexual relationships with other adults and feel socially inadequate and inferior.

One highly traumatic form of sexual abuse is **incest**, sexual activity between people too closely related to legally marry. The most common forms of incest are father-daughter (which includes stepfather-stepdaughter) abuse, brother-sister abuse (usually an adolescent boy abusing a preadolescent girl), and uncle-niece abuse; mother-son sexual activity is rare. Adults who commit incest may be pedophiles, but very often they are simply sexual opportunists or people with poor impulse control and emotional problems.

Most sexually abused children are between ages 8 and 12 when the abuse first occurs. More girls are sexually abused than boys. The degree of trauma for the child can be very serious, but it varies with the type of encounters, their frequency, the child's age and relationship to the abuser, and the parents' response. Father-daughter abuse may be the most traumatic form, in part because it is a violation of the basic parent-child relationship and because the abuse tends to be more frequent. Abused children may be depressed or moody, exhibit hyperactivity, play violently with others or with inanimate objects, talk nonsense, or unintentionally injure themselves.

Child sexual abuse is often unreported. Surveys suggest that as many as 27% of women and 16% of men were sexually abused as children. An estimated 150,000–200,000

Term

incest Sexual activity between close relatives, such as siblings or parents and their children.

new cases of child sexual abuse occur each year. It can leave lasting scars; victims are more likely to suffer as adults from low self-esteem, depression, anxiety, eating disorders, self-destructive tendencies, sexual problems, and difficulties in intimate relationships.

If you were a victim of sexual abuse as a child and feel it may be interfering with your functioning today, you may want to address the problem. A variety of approaches can help, such as joining a support group of people who have had similar experiences, confiding in a partner or friend, or seeking professional help.

Sexual Harassment   Unwelcome sexual advances, requests for sexual favors, and other verbal, visual, or physical conduct of a sexual nature constitute **sexual harassment** if such conduct explicitly or implicitly does any of the following:

- Affects academic or employment decisions or evaluations

- Interferes with an individual's academic or work performance

- Creates an intimidating, hostile, or offensive academic, work, or student living environment

Extreme cases of sexual harassment occur when a manager, professor, or other person in authority uses his or her ability to control or influence jobs or grades to coerce people into having sex or to punish them if they refuse. A hostile environment can be created by conduct such as sexual gestures, displaying of sexually suggestive objects or pictures, derogatory comments and jokes, sexual remarks about clothing or appearance, obscene letters, and unnecessary touching or pinching. Sexual harassment can occur between people of the same or opposite sex. Although sexual harassment is forbidden by law, many cases go unreported. In a survey of 17,000 federal employees, 42% of women and 15% of men reported having been sexually harassed.

If you have been the victim of sexual harassment, you can take action to stop it. Be assertive with anyone who uses language or actions you find inappropriate. If possible, confront your harasser either in writing, over the telephone, or in person, informing him or her that the situa-tion is unacceptable to you and you want the harassment to stop. Be clear. "Do not *ever* make sexual remarks to me" is an unequivocal statement. If assertive communication doesn't work, assemble a file or log documenting the harassment, noting the details of each incident and information about any witnesses who may be able to support your claims. You may discover others who have been harassed by the same person, which will strengthen your case. Then file a grievance with the harasser's supervisor or employer, such as someone in the dean's office if you are a student or someone in the human resources office if you are an employee.

If your attempts to deal with the harassment internally are not successful, you can file an official complaint with your city or state Human Rights Commission or Fair Employment Practices Agency, or with the federal Equal Employment Opportunity Commission. You may also wish to pursue legal action under the Civil Rights Act or under local laws prohibiting employment discrimination. Very often, the threat of a lawsuit or other legal action is enough to stop the harasser.

What You Can Do About Violence

It is obvious that violence in our society is not disappearing and that it is a serious threat to our collective health and well-being. This is especially true on college campuses, which in a sense are communities in themselves but sometimes lack the authority or guidance to tackle the issue of violence directly (see the box "Staying Safe on Campus"). Although government and law enforcement agencies are working to address the problem of violence, individuals must take on a greater responsibility to bring about change. New programs are being developed at the grass-roots level to deal with problems of violence directly. Schools are now providing training for conflict resolution and are educating people about the diverse nature of our society, thereby encouraging tolerance and understanding.

Looking at the problem of violence from a public health perspective points to the importance of the social environment. As with any public health problem, one potential approach is to identify and target high-risk groups for intervention. Violence prevention programs currently focus on conflict-resolution training and the development of social skills. These measures have proven effective, but for behavior change to be lasting, the focus of such programs must expand beyond individual intervention to include social and environmental factors.

Reducing gun-related injuries may require changes in the availability, possession, and lethality of the 8–12 million firearms sold in the United States each year. As part of the Brady gun control law, computerized instant background checks are performed for most gun sales to prevent purchases by convicted felons, people with a history of mental instability, and certain other

Terms

V i**w**

sexual harassment Unwelcome sexual advances, requests for sexual favors, and other conduct of a sexual nature that affects academic or employment decisions or evaluations; interferes with an individual's academic or work performance; or creates an intimidating, hostile, or offensive academic, work, or student living environment.

first aid Emergency care given to an ill or injured person until medical care can be obtained.

Take Charge

College campuses can be the site of criminal activity and violence just as any other environment or living situation can be—and so they require the same level of caution and awareness that you would use in other situations. Two key points to remember: 80% of campus crimes are committed by a student against a fellow student, and alcohol or drug use is involved in 90% of campus felonies. Drinking or drug use can affect judgment and lower inhibitions, so be aware if you or another person is under the influence. Here are some suggestions for keeping yourself safe on campus:

- Don't travel alone after dark. Many campuses have shuttle buses that run from spots on campus such as the library and the dining hall to residence halls and other locations. Escorts are often available to walk with you at night.

- Be familiar with well-lit and frequently traveled routes around campus if you do need to walk alone.

- If you have a car, follow the usual precautions about parking in well-lit areas, keeping the doors locked while you are driving, and never picking up hitchhikers.

- Always have your keys ready as you approach your residence hall, room, and car. Don't lend your keys to others.

- Let friends and family members know your schedule of classes and activities to create a sort of buddy system.

- Be sure the doors and windows of your dorm room have sturdy locks, and use them.

- Don't prop open doors or hold doors open for nonstudents or nonresidents trying to enter your dorm. Be aware of

nonresidents around your dorm. If someone says that he or she is meeting a friend inside, that person should be able to call the friend from outside the building.

- Keep valuables and anything containing personal information—credit cards, wallets, jewelry, and so on—hidden. Secure expensive computer and stereo equipment with cables so that it can't be easily stolen. Use a quality U-shaped lock whenever you leave a bicycle unattended.

- Be alert when using an ATM, and don't display large amounts of cash.

- Stay alert and trust your instincts. Don't hesitate to call the police or campus security if something doesn't seem or feel right.

The Jeanne Clery Disclosure of Campus Security Policy and Campus Crime Statistics Act, named for a Lehigh University student who was murdered in her residence hall in 1986, requires colleges and universities to collect and report campus crime statistics. You can now review this information online at the Crime Statistics Web site of the U.S. Department of Education's Office of Postsecondary Education (http://ope.ed.gov/security/Search.asp).

SOURCES: Security on Campus, Inc. 2001. *Campus Safety: Tips and Evaluation Brochure* (http://www.campussafety.org/students/tips.html; retrieved December 16, 2002); U.S. Department of Education, Office of Postsecondary Education. 2000. *Campus Security* (http://www.ed.gov/offices/OPE/PPI/security. html; retrieved December 16, 2000).

groups. In some states, waiting periods are required in addition to the background checks. Some groups advocate a complete and universal federal ban on the sale of all handguns.

Safety experts also advocate the adoption of consumer safety standards for guns, including features such as childproofing and indicators to show if a gun is loaded. Technologies are now available to personalize handguns to help prevent unauthorized use. Magnetic encoding, touch memory, radio frequency, and fingerprint reading are ways to identify the owner and prevent use by others. Although surveys indicate that the public may be willing to pay the increased costs for personalizing a handgun, firearms manufacturers have been hesitant to redesign their products for safety purposes. Education about proper storage is also important. Surveys indicate that more than 40% of homes with children contain guns; in about 23% of gun-owning households, the weapon is stored loaded, and in 28% the gun is kept hidden but not locked. To be effective, any approach to firearm injury prevention must have the support of law enforcement and the community as a whole.

PROVIDING EMERGENCY CARE

By following the safety guidelines described in this chapter and being aware of the potential risks associated with different activities, you can avoid many injuries on the road, at home, at work, and in public places. However, some injuries will inevitably occur. Therefore, it is also important to prepare for situations when you may need to provide emergency care for yourself or others. If you are prepared to help, you can improve someone else's chances of surviving or of avoiding permanent disability.

A course in **first aid** can help you respond appropriately when someone is injured. One important benefit of first aid training is learning what *not* to do in certain situations. For example, a person with a suspected neck or back injury should not be moved unless other life-threatening conditions exist. A trained person can assess emergency situations accurately before acting.

Emergency rescue techniques can save the lives of people who are choking, who have stopped breathing, or whose hearts have stopped beating. As described earlier, the Heimlich maneuver is used when a victim is choking. Pulmonary resuscitation (also known as rescue breathing, artificial respiration, or mouth-to-mouth resuscitation) is used when a person is not breathing. **Cardiopulmonary resuscitation (CPR)** is used when a pulse cannot be found. Training is required before a person can perform CPR. Courses are offered by the American Red Cross and the American Heart Association. A new feature of some of these courses is training in the use of automatic external defibrillators (AEDs), which monitor the heart's rhythm and, if appropriate, deliver an electrical shock to restart the heart. Because of the importance of early use of defibrillators in saving heart attack victims, these devices are being installed in public places, including casinos, airports, and certain office buildings.

As a person providing assistance, you are the first link in the **emergency medical services (EMS) system.** Your responsibility may be to render first aid, provide emotional support for the victim, or just call for help. It is important to remain calm and act sensibly. The basic pattern for providing emergency care is check-call-care:

- *Check the situation:* Make sure the scene is safe for both you and the injured person. Don't put yourself in danger; if you get hurt too, you will be of little help to the injured person.

- *Check the victim:* Conduct a quick head-to-toe examination. Assess the victim's signs and symptoms, such as level of responsiveness, pulse, and breathing rate. Look for bleeding and any indications of broken bones or paralysis.

- *Call for help:* Call 9-1-1 or a local emergency number. Identify yourself and give as much information as you can about the condition of the victim and what happened.

- *Care for the victim:* If the situation requires immediate action (no pulse, shock, etc.), provide first aid if you are trained to do so.

Like other kinds of behavior, avoiding and preventing injuries and acting safely involve choices you make every day. Ultimately, your goal is healthy, safe behavior. Take responsibility for your safety behaviors. You can motivate yourself to act in the safest way possible by increasing your knowledge and level of awareness,

by examining your attitudes to see if they're realistic, by knowing your capacities and limitations, by adjusting your responses when environmental hazards exist, and, in general, by taking responsibility for your actions. You can't eliminate all risks and dangers from your life—no one can do that—but you can improve your chances of avoiding injuries and living to a healthy old age.

Tips for Today

Although people worry about violence, unintentional injuries—such as those resulting from car crashes, falls, and fires—are much more common. In fact, unintentional injuries are the leading cause of death for people under the age of 35. To protect yourself from injuries, learn to incorporate sensible safety precautions into your daily life.

Right now you can

- Pick up anything on the floor of your home that could cause tripping or slipping.

- Make sure the electrical outlets in your home are not overloaded and that extension cords do not run under rugs or where people walk.

- Test the batteries in the smoke detectors in your home and replace them if they aren't working.

- Check your bike helmet to make sure it fits properly and meets the requirements described in the box "Choosing a Bicycle Helmet." Wear it the next time you go for a ride.

SUMMARY

- Injuries are caused by a dynamic interaction of human and environmental factors. Risk-taking behavior is associated with a high rate of injury.

- Key factors in motor vehicle injuries include aggressive driving, speeding, a failure to wear safety belts, alcohol and drug intoxication, fatigue, and distraction.

- Motorcycle, moped, and bicycle injuries can be prevented by developing appropriate skills, driving or riding defensively, and wearing proper safety equipment, especially a helmet.

- Most fall-related injuries are a result of falls at floor level, but stairs, chairs, and ladders are also involved in a significant number of falls.

- Careless smoking and problems with cooking or heating equipment are common causes of home fires. Being prepared for fire emergencies means planning escape routes and installing smoke detectors.

- The home can contain many poisonous substances, including medications, cleaning agents, plants, and fumes from cars and appliances.

- Performing the Heimlich maneuver can prevent someone from dying from choking.

Terms

V⁝w

cardiopulmonary resuscitation (CPR) An emergency first aid procedure that combines artificial respiration and artificial circulation; used in first aid emergencies where breathing and blood circulation have stopped.

emergency medical services (EMS) system A system designed to network community resources for providing emergency care.

Adopting Safer Habits

Why do you get injured? What human and environmental factors contribute to injuries? Identifying those factors is one step toward making your lifestyle safer. Changing unsafe behaviors *before* they lead to injuries is an even better way of improving your chances.

For the next 7–10 days, keep track of any mishaps you are involved in or injuries you receive, recording them on a daily behavior record like the one shown in Chapter 1. Count each time you cut, burn, or injure yourself, fall down, run into someone, or have any other potentially injury-causing mishap, no matter how trivial. Also record any risk-taking behaviors, such as failing to wear your safety belt or bicycle helmet, drinking and driving, exceeding the speed limit, putting off home or bicycle repairs, and so on. For each entry (injury or incidence of unsafe behavior), record the date, the time, what you were doing, who else was there and how you were influenced by him or her, what your motivations were, and what you were thinking and feeling at the time.

At the end of the monitoring period, examine your data. For each incident, determine both the human factors and the environmental factors that contributed to the injury or unsafe behavior. Were you tired? Distracted? Did you not realize this situation was dangerous? Did you take a chance? Did you think this incident couldn't happen to you? Was visibility poor? Were you using defective equipment? Then consider each contributing factor carefully, determining why it existed and how it could have been avoided or changed. Finally, consider what preventive actions you could take to avoid such incidents or to change your behaviors in the future.

As an example, let's say that you usually don't use a safety belt when you run local errands in your car and that several factors contribute to this behavior: You don't really think you could be involved in a crash so close to home, you only go on short trips, you just never think to use it, and so on. One of the contributing factors to your unsafe behavior is inadequate knowledge. You can change this factor by obtaining accurate information about auto crashes (and their usual proximity to a victim's home) from this chapter and from library or Internet research. Just acquiring information about auto crashes and safety belt use may lead you to examine your beliefs and attitudes about safety belts and motivate you to change your behavior.

Once you're committed, you can use behavior change techniques described in Chapter 1, such as completing a contract, asking family and friends for support, and so on, to build a new habit. Put a note or picture reminding you to buckle up in your car where you can see it clearly. Recruit a friend to run errands with you and to remind you about using your safety belt. Once your habit is established, you may influence other people—especially people who ride in your car—to use safety belts all the time. By changing this behavior, you have reduced the chances that you or your passengers will suffer a serious injury or even die in a vehicle crash.

- The proper storage and handling of firearms can help prevent injuries; assume that any gun is loaded.

- Many injuries during leisure activities result from the misuse of equipment, lack of experience, use of alcohol, and a failure to wear proper safety equipment.

- Most work-related injuries involve extensive manual labor; back problems are most common. More recent common problems include repetitive strain injuries.

- Factors contributing to violence include poverty, the absence of strong social ties, the influence of the mass media, cultural attitudes about gender roles, problems in interpersonal relationships, alcohol and drug abuse, and the availability of firearms.

- Types of violence include assault, homicide, gang-related violence, hate crimes, school violence, workplace violence, and terrorism.

- Battering and child abuse occur at every socioeconomic level. The core issue is the abuser's need to control other people.

- Most rape victims are women, and most know their attackers. Factors in date rape include different standards of appropriate sexual behavior for men and women and different perceptions of actions.

- Child sexual abuse often results in serious trauma; usually the abuser is a trusted adult.

- Sexual harassment is unwelcome sexual advances or other conduct of a sexual nature that affects academic or employment performance or evaluations or that creates an intimidating, hostile, or offensive academic, work, or student living environment.

- Strategies for reducing violence include conflict-resolution training, social skills development, and education programs that foster tolerance and understanding among diverse groups.

- Steps in giving emergency care include making sure the scene is safe for you and the injured person, conducting a quick examination of the victim, calling for help, and providing emergency first aid.

Take Action

1. **Take a course:** Contact the American Red Cross or American Heart Association in your area, and ask about first aid and CPR classes. These courses are usually given frequently and at a variety of times and locations. They can be invaluable in saving lives. Consider taking one or both of the courses.

2. **Investigate local resources:** Find out what resources are available on your campus or in your community for victims of rape, hate crimes, or other types of violence. Does your campus sponsor any violence prevention programs or activities? If so, consider participating in one.

3. **Prepare for a fire:** Contact your local fire department and obtain a checklist of fire safety procedures. What would you do if a fire started in your home? What types of evacuation procedures would be necessary? Carry out a practice fire drill at home to see what problems might arise in a real emergency.

4. **Prepare for a poisoning injury:** Post the number for the national poison control hotline (800-222-1222) near your telephone. Obtain information on poisonings from a Poison Control Center, and read it carefully so you know what to do in case of poisoning.

5. **Create a public education campaign:** Choose a key behavior that prevents injuries, and develop a campaign that you think will help convince people of your age and gender to engage in that behavior—for example, use a safety belt, avoid using a cell phone while driving, wear a bicycle helmet, or change smoke alarm batteries. Consider what types of information and emotional appeals would be most effective for your campaign.

6. **Volunteer in your neighborhood or community:** Contact your local police or civic organization to find out about setting up a neighborhood watch or emergency response team. Talk with your neighbors to find out more about what you can do to help prevent crime and prepare for emergencies.

For More Information

Books

Home Emergency Guide. 2003. New York: DK. *Provides background information on first aid and flowcharts with advice for dealing with many emergency situations.*

Lindquist, S. 2000. *The Date Rape Prevention Book: The Essential Guide for Girls and Women.* Naperville, Ill.: Sourcebooks. *How to avoid problem situations and what to do when confronted with danger.*

MacPherson, J. 2003. *AAA Auto Guide: Driving Survival. How to Stay Safe on the Road.* Heathrow, Fl: AAA Publishing. *Provides helpful strategies for choosing and maintaining a safe vehicle and for handling a variety of driving situations.*

McGrew, J. 2005. *Think Safe: Practical Measures to Increase Security at Home, at Work, and Throughout Life.* Hilton Head Island, S.C.: Cameo Publications. *A general guide to safety and crime and violence prevention.*

Ropeik, D., and G. Gray. 2002. *Risk: A Practical Guide for Deciding What's Really Safe and What's Really Dangerous in the World Around You.* New York: Mariner Books. *A practical guide designed to help individuals assess the relative threat posed by various factors.*

World Health Organization *World Reports. Visit the WHO Web site (www.who.int) to review the recent* World Reports *focusing on violence (2002) and motor vehicle injuries (2004).*

VW Organizations, Hotlines, and Web Sites

American Automobile Association Foundation for Traffic Safety. Provides consumer information about all aspects of traffic safety; Web site has online quizzes and extensive links.
800-305-SAFE
http://www.aaafts.org

American Bar Association: Domestic Violence. Provides information on statistics, research, and laws relating to domestic violence.
http://www.abanet.org/domviol/home.html

Consumer Product Safety Commission. Provides information and advice about safety issues relating to consumer products.
http://www.cpsc.gov

CyberAngels. Provides information on online safety and help and advice for victims of cyberstalking.
http://www.cyberangels.org

Insurance Institute for Highway Safety. Provides information about crashes on the nation's highways, as well as reports on topics such as speeding and crashworthiness of vehicles.
http://www.highwaysafety.org

National Center for Injury Prevention and Control. Provides consumer-oriented information about unintentional injuries and violence.
http://www.cdc.gov/ncipc

National Center for Victims of Crime. An advocacy group for crime victims; provides statistics, news, safety strategies, tips on finding local assistance, and links to related sites.
800-FYI-CALL
http://www.ncvc.org

National Highway Traffic Safety Administration. Supplies materials about reducing deaths, injuries, and economic losses from motor vehicle crashes.
888-327-4236
http://www.nhtsa.dot.gov

National Safety Council. Provides information and statistics about preventing unintentional injuries.
630-285-1121
http://www.nsc.org

National Violence Hotlines. Provide information, referral services, and crisis intervention.
800-799-SAFE (domestic violence);
800-422-4453 (child abuse);
800-656-HOPE (sexual assault)

Occupational Safety and Health Administration. Provides information about topics related to health and safety issues in the workplace.
http://www.osha.gov

Prevent Child Abuse America. Provides statistics, information, and publications relating to child abuse, including parenting tips.
http://www.preventchildabuse.org

Rape, Abuse, and Incest National Network (RAINN). Provides guidelines for preventing and dealing with sexual assault and abuse.
http://www.rainn.org

SafeUSA. Provides information about safety at home, in schools, at work, on the road, and in communities.
http://www.safeusa.org

Tolerance.Org: 10 Ways to Fight Hate on Campus. Offers suggestions for fighting hate and promoting tolerance; sponsored by the Southern Poverty Law Center.

http://www.tolerance.org/campus/index.jsp

World Health Organization: Violence and Injury Prevention. Provides statistics and information about the consequences of intentional and unintentional injuries worldwide.

http://www.who.int/violence_injury_prevention

The following sites provide statistics and background information on violence and crime in the United States:

Bureau of Justice Statistics: http://www.ojp.usdoj.gov/bjs
Federal Bureau of Investigation: http://www.fbi.gov
Justice Information Center: http://www.ncjrs.org

Selected Bibliography

Browne, K. D., and C. Hamilton-Giachritsis. 2005. The influence of violent media on children and adolescents: A public-health approach. *Lancet* 365(9460): 702–710.

Centers for Disease Control and Prevention. 2004. Impact of primary laws on adult use of safety belts—United States, 2002. *Morbidity and Mortality Weekly Report* 53(12): 257–260.

Centers for Disease Control and Prevention. 2004. Surveillance for fatal and nonfatal injuries—United States, 2001. *MMWR Surveillance Summaries* 55(SS7): 1–57.

Centers for Disease Control and Prevention. 2004. Violence-related behaviors among high school students—United States, 1991–2003. *Morbidity and Mortality Weekly Report* 53(29): 651–655.

Centers for Disease Control and Prevention. 2005. Increase in poisoning deaths caused by nonillicit drugs. *Morbidity and Mortality Weekly Report* 54(2): 33–36.

Centers for Disease Control and Prevention. 2005. Unintentional non-fire-related carbon monoxide exposures—United States, 2001–2003. *Morbidity and Mortality Weekly Report* 54(2): 36–39.

Connor, J., et al. 2002. Driver sleepiness and risk of serious injury to car occupants. *British Medical Journal* 324(7346): 1125.

Connor, S. M., and K. L. Wesolowski. 2003. "They're too smart for that": Predicting what children would do in the presence of guns. *Pediatrics* 111(2): E109–E114.

Coyne-Beasley, T., et al. 2002. The association of handgun ownership and storage practices with safety consciousness. *Archives of Pediatric and Adolescent Medicine* 156(8): 763–768.

Cummings, P., and F. P. Rivara. 2004. Car occupant death according to the restraint use of other occupants. *Journal of the American Medical Association* 291(3): 343–349.

D'Ovidio, R. D., and J. Doyle. 2003. A study on cyberstalking: Understanding investigative hurdles. *FBI Law Enforcement Bulletin* 72(3): 10–17.

Federal Bureau of Investigation. 2004. *Crime in the United States. Uniform Crime Reports, 2003.* Washington, D.C.: U.S. Department of Justice.

Federal Bureau of Investigation. 2004. *Hate Crime Statistics, 2003.* Washington, D.C.: U.S. Department of Justice.

Graffunder, C. M., et al. 2004. Through a public health lens. Preventing violence against women: An update from the U.S. Centers for Disease Control and Prevention. *Journal of Women's Health* 13(1): 5–15.

Gray-Vickrey, P. 2004. Combating elder abuse. *Nursing* 34(10): 47–51.

Grossman, D. C., et al. 2005. Gun storage practices and risk of youth suicide and unintentional firearm injuries. *Journal of the American Medical Association* 293(6): 707–714.

Guns, lies, and video: Does violent TV breed violence? Do video games breed more of it? 2003. *Discover,* April.

Insurance Institute for Highway Safety. 2003. Faster travel and the price we pay. *Status Report* 38(10).

Iudice, A., et al. 2005. Effects of prolonged wakefulness combined with alcohol and hands-free cell phone divided attention tasks on simulated driving. *Human Psychopharmacology* 20(2): 125–132.

Johnson, J. G., et al. 2002. Television viewing and aggressive behavior during adolescence and adulthood. *Science* 295(5564): 2468–2471.

Kilpatrick, D. 2004. Interpersonal violence and public policy: What about the victims? *Journal of Law, Medicine, and Ethics* 32(1): 73–81.

Krug, E. G. 2004. Injury surveillance is key to preventing injuries. *Lancet* 364(9445): 1563–1566.

McGwin, G., et al. 2003. The association between occupant restraint systems and risk of injury in frontal motor vehicle collisions. *Journal of Trauma* 54: 1182–1187.

Miller, M., D. Azrael, and D. Hemenway. 2002. Rates of household firearm ownership and homicide across U.S. regions and states. *American Journal of Public Health* 92(12).

Miller, M., D. Hemenway, and H. Wechsler. 2002. Guns and gun threats at college. *Journal of American College Health* 51(2): 53–56.

National Center for Health Statistics. 2005. Deaths: Preliminary data for 2003. *National Vital Statistics Reports* 53(15).

National Center for Injury Prevention and Control. 2005. *Sexual Violence Fact Sheet* (http://www.cdc.gov/ncipc/factsheets/svfacts.htm; retrieved April 16, 2005.)

National Center for Injury Prevention and Control. 2004. *Intimate Partner Violence Fact Sheet* (http://www.cdc.gov/ncipc/factsheets/ipvfacts.htm; retrieved January 26, 2005).

National Safety Council. 2004. *Injury Facts.* Itasca, Ill.: National Safety Council.

National School Safety Center. 2005. *Report on School Associated Violent Deaths* (http://www.nssc1.org/savd/savd.pdf; retrieved March 2, 2005).

National Traffic Safety Administration. 2005. *Traffic Safety Facts Research Note: Driver Cell Phone Use in 2004—Overall Results.* Washington, D.C.: National Traffic Safety Administration.

Quinlan, K. P., et al. 2005. Alcohol-impaired driving among U.S. adults, 1993–2002. *American Journal of Preventive Medicine* 28(4): 346–350.

Rosenfeld, R. 2004. The case of the unsolved crime decline. *Scientific American,* February.

Silverman, J. G., A. Raj, and K. Clements. 2004. Dating violence and associated sexual risk and pregnancy among adolescent girls in the United States. *Pediatrics* 114(2): e220–225.

U.S. Department of State. 2002. *Patterns of Global Terrorism* (http://www.state.gov/s/ct/rls/pgtrpt/2001/html/10220.htm; retrieved December 16, 2002).

Windle, M. 2003. Alcohol use among adolescents and young adults. *Alcohol Research and Health* 27(1): 79–85.

World Health Organization. 2004. *World Report on Road Traffic Injury Prevention.* Geneva: World Health Organization.

Zimmerman, F. J., et al. 2005. Early cognitive stimulation, emotional support, and television watching as predictors of subsequent bullying among grade-school children. *Archives of Pediatrics and Adolescent Medicine* 59(4): 384–388.

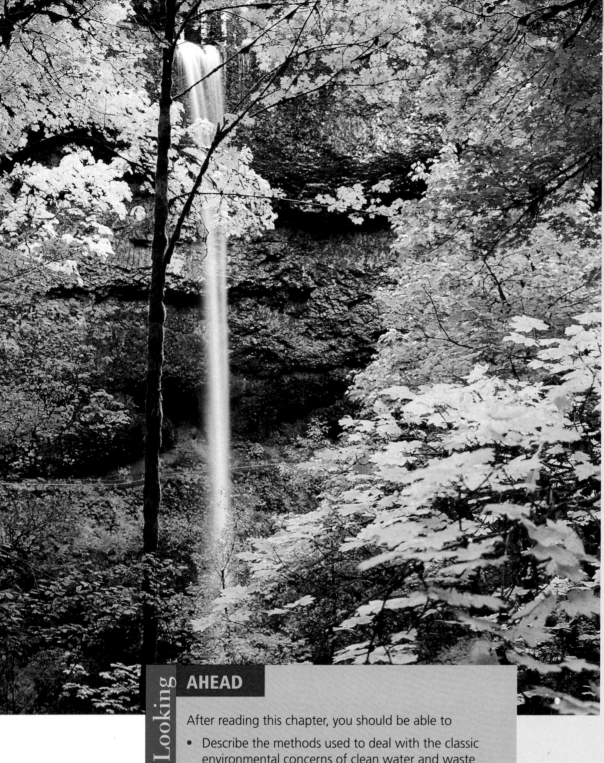

23

Environmental Health

Knowledge

1. **The world's population, currently at about 6.5 billion, is increasing by about ____ people every minute**
   a. 50
   b. 100
   c. 150

2. **Where ozone gas occurs naturally in the upper atmosphere, it benefits human health by protecting Earth from harmful UV radiation; when created from pollutants released at ground level, ozone gas harms human health by negatively affecting respiratory function.**
   True or false?

3. **Which of the following statements about sport utility vehicles is true?**
   a. They currently account for about half of all new vehicles sold.
   b. They get relatively poor gas mileage.
   c. They currently have weaker pollution standards than cars and so pollute more.

4. **Food in the United States typically travels about 500 miles from farm to table.**
   True or false?

5. **Most of the energy used by a standard incandescent lightbulb is converted into light.**
   True or false?

ANSWERS

1. C. Although birth rates are declining, the world's population is expected to nearly double by 2200.

2. TRUE. "Good up high, bad nearby" is how the U.S. Environmental Protection Agency characterizes ozone. The primary source of ground-level ozone precursors is motor vehicle exhaust.

3. ALL THREE. Sport utility vehicles use more nonrenewable fuels and release more pollutants than more energy-efficient vehicles.

4. FALSE. Food typically travels 1500–2500 miles from farm to table, making the food supply vulnerable to disruption and requiring large amounts of fossil fuels. Foods from a chain store may require up to 17 times more fuel for transportation than foods produced locally.

5. FALSE. About 90% of the energy used by a standard bulb is wasted because it is given off as heat, not light. If each American replaced one incandescent bulb with a compact fluorescent, the yearly energy savings would equal the total production of four nuclear power plants.

Visit the *Core Concepts in Health* Online Learning Center (www.mhhe.com/insel10e) for study aids and many additional resources.

693

We are constantly reminded of our intimate relationship with all that surrounds us—our environment. Although the planet provides us with food, water, air, and everything else that sustains life, it also provides us with natural occurrences—earthquakes, tsunamis, hurricanes, drought, climate changes—that destroy life and disrupt society. In the past, humans frequently had to struggle against the environment to survive. Today, in addition to dealing with natural disasters, we also have to find ways to protect the environment from the byproducts of our way of life.

Environmental health has historically focused on preventing infectious diseases spread by water, waste, food, rodents, and insects. Although these problems still exist, the focus of environmental health has expanded and become more complex, for several reasons. We now recognize that environmental pollutants contribute not only to infectious diseases but to many chronic diseases as well. In addition, technological advances have increased our ability to affect and damage the environment. Also, rapid population growth, which has resulted partly from past environmental improvements, means that far more people are consuming and competing for resources than ever before, magnifying the effect of humans on the environment.

Environmental health is therefore seen as encompassing all the interactions of humans with their environment and the health consequences of these interactions. Fundamental to this definition is a recognition that we hold the world in trust for future generations and for other forms of life. Our responsibility is to pass on to the next generation an environment no worse, and preferably better, than the one we enjoy today (see the box "Nature and the Human Spirit"). Although many environmental problems are complex and seem beyond the control of the individual, there are ways that people can make a difference to the future of the planet.

CLASSIC ENVIRONMENTAL HEALTH CONCERNS

The field of environmental health originally grew out of efforts to control communicable diseases. When certain insects and rodents were found to carry microorganisms that cause disease in humans, campaigns were undertaken to eradicate or control these animal vectors. It was also recognized that pathogens could live and be transmitted in sewage, drinking water, and food. These discoveries led to the development of practices such as systematic garbage collection, sewage treatment, filtration and chlorination of drinking water, food inspection, and the establishment of public health enforcement agencies.

These successful efforts to control and prevent communicable diseases changed the health profile of the developed world (see Chapter 1). Although Americans rarely contract cholera, typhoid fever, plague, diphtheria, or other diseases that once killed large numbers of people, it doesn't mean these diseases have been eradicated worldwide. For example, there are more than 250,000 cases of cholera each year.

In the United States, a huge, complex, public health system is constantly at work behind the scenes attending to the details of these critical health concerns. Every time the system is disrupted, danger recurs. After any disaster situation that damages a community's public health system—whether a natural disaster such as the 2004 Asian tsunami or a humanmade disaster such as a terrorist attack—prompt restoration of basic health services becomes crucial to human survival. Every time we venture beyond the boundaries of our everyday world, whether traveling to a less-developed country or camping in a wilderness area, we are reminded of the importance of these basics: clean water, sanitary waste disposal, safe food, and insect and rodent control.

We often take for granted the well-organized system responsible for environmental health in our society, but natural disasters remind us of its fragility. In addition to forcing people from their homes, flooding such as that caused by the 2004 Asian tsunami can cause widespread disruption in essential services such as the delivery of electricity, gas, and clean drinking water, which increases the probability of disease transmission.

Nature and the Human Spirit

Mind/Body/Spirit

In this excerpt from her book *The Sense of Wonder*, noted scientist and author Rachel Carson affirms the nurturing power of the natural world and urges us to appreciate the deep relationship between nature and the human spirit.

What is the value of preserving and strengthening this sense of awe and wonder, this recognition of something beyond the boundaries of human existence? Is the exploration of the natural world just a pleasant way to pass the golden hours of childhood or is there something deeper?

I am sure there is something much deeper, something lasting and significant. Those who dwell, as scientists or laymen, among the beauties and mysteries of the earth are never alone or weary of life. Whatever the vexations or concerns of their personal lives, their thoughts can find paths that lead to inner contentment and to renewed excitement in living. Those who contemplate the beauty of the earth find reserves of strength that will endure as long as life lasts. There is symbolic as well as actual beauty in the migration of the birds, the ebb and flow of the tides, the folded bud ready for spring. There is something infinitely healing in the repeated refrains of nature—the assurance that dawn comes after night, and spring after the winter.

SOURCE: Carson, R. 1956. *The Sense of Wonder.* New York: Harper & Row. Copyright © 1956 by Rachel Carson. Copyright © renewed 1984 by Roger Christie.

Clean Water

Few parts of the world have adequate quantities of safe, clean drinking water, and yet few things are as important to human health.

Water Contamination and Treatment Many cities rely at least in part on wells that tap local groundwater, but often it is necessary to tap lakes and rivers to supplement wells. Because such surface water is more likely to be contaminated with both organic matter and pathogenic microorganisms, it is purified in water-treatment plants before being piped into the community. At treatment facilities, the water is subjected to various physical and chemical processes, including screening, filtration, and disinfection (often with chlorine), before it is introduced into the water supply system. **Fluoridation,** a water-treatment process that reduces tooth decay by 15–40%, has been used successfully in the United States for more than 60 years.

In most areas of the United States, water systems have adequate, dependable supplies, are able to control waterborne disease, and provide water without unacceptable color, odor, or taste. However, problems do occur. In 1993, more than 400,000 people became ill and 100 died when Milwaukee's drinking water was contaminated with the bacterium *Cryptosporidium.* The Centers for Disease Control and Prevention (CDC) estimate that 1 million Americans become ill and 900–1000 die each year from microbial illnesses from drinking water. Pollution by hazardous chemicals from manufacturing, agriculture, and household wastes is another concern. (Chemical pollution is discussed later in the chapter.) The *Healthy People 2010* report sets the goal of increasing from 85% to 95% the proportion of Americans with drinking water that meets standards set by the U.S. Environmental Protection Agency (EPA). Worldwide, more than 2 million people, mostly children, die from water-related diseases each year.

Water Shortages Water shortages are also a growing concern. Some parts of the United States are experiencing rapid population growth that outstrips the ability of local systems to provide adequate water to all. Many proposals are being discussed to relieve these shortages, including long-distance transfers; conservation; the recycling of some water, such as the water in office-building air conditioners; and the sale of water by regions with large supplies to areas with less available water.

According to the World Health Organization (WHO), 1 billion people do not have safe drinking water and 2.6 billion do not have access to basic sanitation. Less than 1% of the world's fresh water—about 0.007% of all the water on Earth—is readily accessible for direct human use. Groundwater pumping and the diversion of water from lakes and rivers for irrigation are further reducing the amount of water available to local communities. In some areas, groundwater is being removed at twice the rate at which it is replaced. The Aral Sea, located in Kazakhstan and Uzbekistan, was once one of the world's largest inland seas. Since the 1960s, it has lost two-thirds of its volume to irrigation, and the exposed seabed is now as big as the Netherlands. People living in the area have experienced severe water and food shortages and increased rates of respiratory disease and throat cancer linked to dust storms from the dry seabed. Due to agricultural diversions, the Yellow River ran dry for the first time in China's 3000-year history in 1972, failing to reach the sea for 15 days that

Terms

environmental health The collective interactions of humans with the environment and the short-term and long-term health consequences of those interactions.

fluoridation The addition of fluoride to the water supply to reduce tooth decay.

year; now, the dry period extends for more than half of each year. In the United States, the Colorado River is now diverted to the extent that it no longer flows into the ocean.

What You Can Do to Protect the Water Supply

- Take showers, not baths, to minimize your water consumption. Don't let water run when you're not actively using it while brushing your teeth, shaving, or hand-washing clothes. Don't run a dishwasher or washing machine until you have a full load.

- Install sink faucet aerators and water-efficient shower heads, which use two to five times less water with no noticeable decrease in performance.

- Purchase a water-saver toilet, or put a displacement device in your toilet tank to reduce the amount of water used with each flush.

- Fix any leaky faucets in your house. Leaks can waste thousands of gallons of water per year.

- Use organic rather than chemical fertilizers, and don't overfertilize your lawn or garden; the extra could end up in the groundwater.

- Don't pour toxic materials such as cleaning solvents, bleach, or motor oil down the drain. Store them until you can take them to a hazardous waste collection center.

- Replant your lawn and garden with plants requiring less water. Avoid watering your lawn during the hottest part of the day to minimize evaporation.

Waste Disposal

Humans generate large amounts of waste, which must be handled in an appropriate manner if the environment is to be safe and sanitary.

Sewage Prior to the mid-nineteenth century, many people contracted diseases such as typhoid, cholera, and hepatitis A by direct contact with human feces, which were disposed of at random. Once the links between sewage and disease were discovered, practices began to change. People learned how to build sanitary outhouses and how to locate them so they would not contaminate water sources. As plumbing moved indoors, sewage disposal became more complicated. In rural areas, the **septic system,** a self-contained sewage disposal system, worked quite well. Today, many rural homes still rely on septic systems; however, in many areas more than 50% of old tanks are leaking contaminants into the environment.

Different approaches became necessary as urban areas developed. Most cities have sewage-treatment systems that separate fecal matter from water in huge tanks and ponds and stabilize it so that it cannot transmit infectious diseases. Once treated and biologically safe, the water is

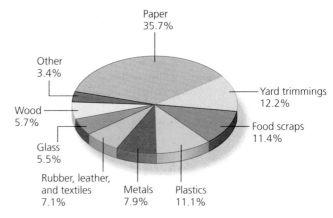

VITAL STATISTICS

Figure 23-1 Components of municipal solid waste, by weight. The total amount of trash produced by U.S. residences, businesses, and institutions is the equivalent of 4.4 pounds of waste per person, per day, up from 2.7 pounds in 1960. SOURCE: Environmental Protection Agency. 2004. *Municipal Solid Waste: Basic Facts* (http://www.epa.gov/epaoswer/non-hw/muncpl/facts.htm; retrieved March 6, 2005).

released back into the environment. The sludge that remains behind is often contaminated with **heavy metals** and is handled as hazardous waste; if not contaminated, sludge may be used as fertilizer. If incorporated into the food chain, heavy metals, such as lead, cadmium, copper, and tin, can cause illness or death; therefore, these chemicals must be prevented from being released into the environment when sludge is burned or buried.

In addition to regulating industrial discharge, many cities have now begun expanded sewage-treatment measures to remove heavy metals and other hazardous chemicals. This action has resulted from many studies linking exposure to chemicals such as mercury, lead, and **polychlorinated biphenyls (PCBs)** with long-term health consequences, including cancer and damage to the central nervous system. The technology to effectively remove heavy metals and chemicals from sewage is still developing, and the costs involved are immense.

Solid Waste The bulk of the organic food garbage produced in American kitchens is now dumped in the sewage system by way of the mechanical garbage disposal. The garbage that remains is not very hazardous from the standpoint of infectious disease because there is very little food waste in it, but it does represent an enormous disposal and contamination problem.

WHAT'S IN OUR GARBAGE? The biggest single component of household trash by weight is paper products, including junk mail, glossy mail-order catalogs, and computer printouts (Figure 23-1). Yard waste, plastic, metals, and glass are other significant components. About 1% of the solid waste is toxic; a new source of toxic waste is the disposal of computer components in both household and commercial waste. Burning, as opposed to burial, reduces the bulk of solid waste, but it may release hazardous material into the air.

Solid waste is not limited to household products. Manufacturing, mining, and other industries all produce large amounts of potentially dangerous materials that cannot simply be dumped. The experiences of communities like Love Canal (near Buffalo, New York) and Times Beach, Missouri, clearly demonstrated the dangers of the careless disposal of toxic wastes. At Love Canal, toxic industrial wastes had been dumped into a waterway for years until, in the 1970s, nearby residents began to suffer from associated birth defects and cancers. The government had to step in, people had to move from their homes, and huge costs were incurred.

DISPOSING OF SOLID WASTE Since the 1960s, much solid waste has been buried in **sanitary landfill** disposal sites. Careful site selection and daily management are an essential part of this approach to disposal. The site is thoroughly studied to ensure that it is not near groundwater, streams, or any other source of water that could be contaminated by leakage from the landfill. Sometimes protective liners are used around the site, and nearby monitoring wells are now required in most states. Layers of solid waste are regularly covered with thin layers of dirt until the site is filled. Some communities then plant grass and trees and convert the site into a park. Landfill is relatively stable; almost no decomposition occurs in the solidly packed waste.

Burying solid waste in sanitary landfills has several disadvantages. Much of this waste contains chemicals, ranging from leftover pesticides to nail polish remover to paints and oils, which should not be released indiscriminately into the environment. Despite precautions, buried contaminants do leak into the surrounding soil and groundwater. Burial is also expensive and requires huge amounts of space.

Industrial toxic waste poses an even greater disposal problem. In 1980, Congress enacted the Superfund program to clean up inactive hazardous waste sites that are a threat to human health and the environment. By 2004, cleanup was complete at 60% of priority sites, but further action was still needed at about 600 priority sites and nearly 10,000 other sites.

Because of the expense and potential chemical hazards of any form of solid waste disposal, many communities today encourage individuals and businesses to recycle their trash. Some cities offer curbside pickup of recyclables; others have recycling centers to which people can bring their waste. These materials are not limited to paper, glass, and cans but also include things such as discarded tires and used oils. Recycling programs have been successful in reducing the proportion of solid waste sent to landfills. In 1980, 81% went to landfills; in 2000, about 55%. (Currently, about 30% of solid waste is recycled and 17% is burned.) However, the total amount of garbage Americans generate will probably continue to rise as the population increases, and researchers estimate that 80% of the nation's landfills will be closed within 20 years.

What You Can Do to Reduce Garbage

- Buy products with the least amount of packaging you can, or buy products in bulk (see the box "How to Be a Green Consumer"). For example, buy large jars of juice, not individually packaged juice drinks. Buy products packaged in glass, paper, or metal containers; avoid plastic and aluminum (unless it's recycled). Reuse glass containers to store products bought in bulk or other nontoxic household items.

- Buy recycled or recyclable products. Avoid disposables; instead, use long-lasting or reusable products such as refillable pens and rechargeable batteries.

- Avoid using foam or paper cups and plastic stirrers by bringing your own china coffee mug and metal spoon to work or wherever you drink coffee or tea. Pack your lunch in reusable containers, and use a cloth or plastic lunch sack or a lunch box.

- To store food, use glass jars and reusable plastic containers rather than foil and plastic wrap.

- Recycle your newspapers, glass, cans, paper, and other recyclables. If your sanitation department doesn't pick up recyclables, take them to a local recycling center. If you receive something packaged with foam pellets, take them to a commercial mailing center that accepts them for recycling.

- Do not throw items such as computers, televisions, VCRs, cell phones, microwave ovens, digital cameras, household batteries, or fluorescent lights into the trash. Take all these to state-approved recycling centers; check with your local disposal service for more information.

- Start a compost pile for your organic garbage (non-animal food and yard waste) if you have a yard. If you live in an apartment, you can create a small composting system using earthworms, or take your organic wastes to a community composting center.

- Stop junk mail. To cancel your junk mail, send a request to Mail Preference Service, Direct Marketing Association, P.O. Box 643, Carmel, NY 10512 (http://www.dmaconsumers.org).

Terms

V w

septic system A self-contained sewage disposal system, often used in rural areas, in which waste material is decomposed by bacteria.

heavy metal A metal with a high specific gravity, such as lead, copper, or tin.

polychlorinated biphenyl (PCB) An industrial chemical used as an insulator in electrical transformers and linked to certain human cancers.

sanitary landfill A disposal site where solid wastes are buried.

Critical Consumer

It may seem like a hassle to consider the environmental impact of the things you buy, but a few simple choices can make a big difference without compromising your lifestyle. You can quickly and easily develop habits that direct your consumer dollar toward environmentally friendly products and companies.

- Remember the four Rs of green consumerism:
    Reduce the amount of trash and pollution you generate by consuming and throwing away less.
    Reuse as many products as possible—either yourself or by selling them or donating them to charity.
    Recycle all appropriate materials and buy recycled products whenever possible.
    Respond by educating others about reducing waste and recycling, by finding creative ways to reduce waste and toxicity, and by making your preferences known.

- Choose products packaged in refillable, recycled, reusable containers or in readily recyclable materials, such as paper, cardboard, aluminum, or glass. Don't buy products that are excessively packaged or wrapped; for specific guidelines, see the section "What You Can Do to Reduce Garbage."

- Look for products made with the highest possible content of recycled paper, metal, glass, plastic, and other materials.

- Choose simple products containing the lowest amounts of bleaches, dyes, and fragrances. Look for organically grown foods and clothes made from organically grown cotton or Fox Fibre or another naturally colored type of cotton.

- Buy high-quality appliances that have an Energy Star seal from the EPA or some other type of certification indicating that they are energy- and water-efficient.

- Get a reusable cloth shopping bag. Don't bag items that don't need to be bagged. If you forget to bring your bag to the store, it doesn't matter much if you use a paper or plastic bag to carry your purchases home. What's important is that you reuse whatever bag you get.

- Don't buy what you don't need—borrow, rent, or share. Take good care of the things you own, repair items when they break, and replace them with used rather than new items whenever possible. Sell or donate used items rather than throwing them out.

- Walk or bike to the store. If you must drive, do several errands at once to save energy and cut down on pollution.

- Look beyond the products to the companies that make them. Support those with good environmental records. If some of your favorite products are overpackaged or contain harmful ingredients, write to the manufacturer.

- Keep in mind that doing something is better than doing nothing. Even if you can't be a perfectly green consumer, doing your best on any purchase *will* make a difference.

SOURCES: U.S. Environmental Protection Agency. 2002. *Reduce, Reuse, and Recycle* (http://www.epa.gov/epaoswer/non-hw/reduce/catbook/the4.htm; retrieved March 6, 2005); Makower, J., J. Elkington, and J. Hailes. 1993. *The Green Consumer.* New York: Penguin Books; Madigan, C. O., and A. Elwood. 1995. *Life's Big Instruction Book.* New York: Warner Books.

Food Inspection

Diseases and death associated with foodborne illnesses and toxic food additives have decreased substantially ever since the passage of the Pure Food and Drug Act of 1906. Many agencies inspect food at various points in production. On the federal level, the U.S. Department of Agriculture (USDA) inspects grains and meats, and the U.S. Food and Drug Administration (FDA) is responsible for ensuring the wholesomeness of foods and regulating the chemicals that can be used in foods, drugs, and cosmetics. On the state level, public health departments inspect dairy herds, milking barns, storage tanks, tankers that transport milk, and processing plants. Local health departments inspect and license restaurants.

Overall, the food distribution system in the United States is safe and efficient, but cases of foodborne illness do occur. It is estimated that every American suffers an average of two or three episodes of foodborne illness every year. Recent outbreaks of serious illness have been traced to contaminated and undercooked fast-food hamburgers, unpasteurized juice, and imported produce. Many cases of foodborne illness can be prevented through

the proper storage and preparation of food. (For guidelines on avoiding foodborne illness and information on other food safety issues, see Chapter 12.)

Insect and Rodent Control

A great number of illnesses can be transmitted to humans by animal and insect vectors. In recent years, we have seen outbreaks of encephalitis transmitted by mosquitoes; Lyme disease from ticks in the Northeast, Midwest, and West; Rocky Mountain spotted fever from another type of tick in the Southeast; bubonic plague from fleas on wild mammals in the West; and West Nile virus transmitted by mosquitoes. Rodents carry forms of hantavirus, tapeworms, and *Salmonella.*

Disability and death from these diseases can be prevented by spraying insecticides when necessary, wearing protective clothing, and exercising reasonable caution in infested areas. Individuals should be concerned about possible exposure to rodentborne illnesses if they see rodents or rodent droppings in the home. In public facilities, such sightings should be reported to the local or state health department. Children should be warned to never play with

VITAL STATISTICS

Figure 23-2 World population growth.
The United Nations estimates that the world's population will continue to increase dramatically until it stabilizes above 10 billion people in 2200.   SOURCES: United Nations Population Division. 2005. *World Population Prospects: The 2004 Revision.* New York: United Nations; U.S. Bureau of the Census.

9 billion: 2048
8 billion: 2027
7 billion: 2013
6 billion: 1999
5 billion: 1987
4 billion: 1974
3 billion 1960
1 billion: 1804
2 billion 1927
0.3 billion: A.D.1
0.5 billion: 1500

sick animals. Travelers should be careful about mosquito bites, especially in developing countries and where disease warnings have been posted. For tips on avoiding tickborne and mosquitoborne illnesses, see Chapter 17.

POPULATION GROWTH

Throughout most of history, humans have been a minor pressure on the planet. About 300 million people were alive in the year A.D. 1; by the time Europeans were settling in the United States 1600 years later, the world population had increased gradually to a little over 500 million. But then it began rising exponentially—zooming to 1 billion by about 1800, more than doubling by 1950, and then doubling again in just 40 years (Figure 23-2).

The world's population, currently about 6.5 billion, is increasing at a rate of about 78 million per year—150 people every minute. The United Nations projects that world population will reach 9.1 billion by 2050 and will continue to increase until it levels off above 10 billion in 2200. Virtually all of this increase is taking place in less-developed regions. In 1950, the more-developed regions accounted for 32% of the world's population; their share dropped to 20% in 2000 and is expected to further decline to 13% in 2050. Changes are also projected for the world's age distribution: The proportion of people age 60 and over will increase from 10% in 2000 to about 21% in 2050, and by 2050 there will be more older persons than children.

This rapid expansion of population, particularly in the past 50 years, is generally believed to be responsible for most of the stress humans put on the environment. A large and rapidly growing population makes it more difficult to provide the basic components of environmental health discussed earlier, including clean and disease-free food and water. It is also a driving force behind many of the relatively more recent environmental health concerns, including chemical pollution, global warming, and the thinning of the atmosphere's ozone layer.

How Many People Can the World Hold?

No one knows how many people the world can support, but most scientists agree that there is a limit. The primary factors that may eventually put a cap on human population are the following:

• *Food.* Enough food is currently produced to feed the world's entire population, but economic and socio-political factors have led to food shortages and famine. Food production can be expanded in the future, but better distribution of food will be needed to prevent even more widespread famine as the world's population continues to grow. For all people to receive adequate nutrition, the makeup of the world's diet may also need to change. Because animal products require more resources to produce, the world could support nearly twice as many vegetarians as people eating a typical American diet, which is based heavily on animal products.

• *Available land and water.* Rural populations rely on trees, soil, and water for their direct sustenance, and a growing population puts a strain on these resources—forests are cut for wood, soil is depleted, and water is withdrawn at ever-rising rates. These trends contribute to local hardships and to many global environmental problems, including habitat destruction and species extinction (see the box "Natural Ecosystems and Biodiversity").

• *Energy.* Currently, most of the world's energy comes from nonrenewable sources: oil, coal, natural gas, and nuclear power. As nonrenewable sources are depleted, the world will have to shift to renewable energy sources, such as hydropower and solar, geothermal,

Our world supports an abundant variety of life. Scientists have identified some 1.75 million species, but they suspect that there are probably 10–80 million more. Different environments generate diverse life strategies, so that each **ecosystem**—from desert to tropical rainforest—contains a unique, close-knit community of organisms, linked together in a **food chain** or web. Plants use sunlight and soil for their needs. In turn, they sustain herbivores (plant eaters), which may themselves succumb to predators. When predators and surviving herbivores die, they become food for scavengers, then insect larvae, and finally bacteria, which break them down into organic substances. These substances, drawn from the soil by plants, help maintain the cycle. A similar system, based on plankton, exists in the oceans. Disruption at any point in this intricate, balanced cycle can alter or destroy an entire ecosystem.

Natural ecosystems provide humans with a wide variety of essential services. They maintain the climate and the composition of the atmosphere, cycle water and nutrients, produce food, dispose of organic wastes, generate and maintain soils, control pests, and pollinate crops; in addition, ecosystems support biological diversity, or **biodiversity**, represented by both the millions of different species on the earth and the genetic diversity within these species.

Biodiversity is critical as the basis for the future evolution of new species and as a genetic bank from which humans can draw useful genetic material and compounds. Although thus far we have examined few of these resources, the ones we have used provide many benefits, including medicines and pest and disease resistance for crops. For example, many children with leukemia can now be saved by drugs developed from the rosy periwinkle plant, and species of wild rice in India and wild tomato in Peru have provided domestic species with the disease resistance they need to be productive.

Human activity—driven by poverty and population growth in the developing world and excessive consumerism in the industrial nations—threatens biodiversity. Some species and populations are being lost through direct action, such as the overharvesting of whales, elephants, and certain fish; the overexploitation of musk deer, turtles, black bears, and certain plants has been linked to a growing worldwide demand for traditional Chinese medicines. But the major danger comes indirectly, from habitat destruction: We are paving over, chopping down, digging up, draining, and poisoning many areas. The destruction of tropical rainforests, which are disappearing at the rate of an acre every second, is of particular concern. Rainforests cover only about 7% of the planet but are thought to harbor more than half the world's species.

Extinction is irreversible, and species are disappearing far faster (50–100 a day) than they can be identified and assessed for useful properties. The current extinction rate is nearly 1000 times higher than the rate over the past 65 million years. Some scientists fear that humans are precipitating a wave of mass extinction so great that the diminished stock of species will not be an adequate base on which natural selection can work to rebuild biodiversity. Even if adequate, it could take more than 10 million years for biodiversity to be restored. And because of the many ties between organisms and the physical environment, mass extinction could also threaten the functioning of the entire biological world.

What can be done to maintain biodiversity? The United States has laws that protect specific endangered species, which by indirectly preserving natural communities help maintain biodiversity. International laws and conventions also protect certain rare species, although enforcement continues to be a problem. The Convention on Biological Diversity, signed by more than 185 countries (but *not* the United States) since the 1992 Earth Summit in Rio de Janeiro, deals specifically with the issue of biodiversity. It commits countries to preserving and managing biological resources and to integrating plant and animal preservation into economic planning. It also allows countries that are rich in species but poor in cash to share in the profits from the sale of medicines or other products derived from their biological resources. Although much still needs to be done to protect the biodiversity of our world, these actions are a step in the right direction.

---

wind, biomass, and ocean power. Supporting a growing population, maintaining economic productivity, and preventing further environmental degradation will require both greater energy efficiency and an increased use of renewable energy sources.

- *Minimum acceptable standard of living.* The mass media have exposed the entire world to the American lifestyle and raised people's expectations of living at a comparable level. But such a lifestyle is supported by levels of energy consumption that the earth cannot support worldwide. The United States has about 5% of the world's population but uses 25% of the world's energy. In contrast, India has 16% of the population but uses only 3% of the energy. If *all* people are to enjoy a minimally acceptable standard of living, the population must be limited to a number that the available resources can support.

Factors That Contribute to Population Growth

Although it is apparent that population growth must be controlled, population trends are difficult to influence and manage. A variety of interconnecting factors fuel the current population explosion:

- *High fertility rates.* The combination of poverty, very high child mortality rates, and a lack of social provisions of every type is associated with high fertility rates in the developing world. Families may have to have more children to ensure that enough survive childhood to work for the household and to care for parents in old age.

- *Lack of family planning resources.* Half the world's couples don't use any form of family planning, and 300 million couples worldwide say they want family planning services but cannot get them.
- *Lower death rates.* Although death rates remain relatively high in the developing world, they have decreased in recent years because of public health measures and improved medical care.

Changes in any of these factors can affect population growth, but the issues are complex. Increasing death rates through disease, famine, or war might slow population growth, but few people would argue in favor of these as methods of population control. (The latest United Nations population estimates already project that there will be 344 million fewer people alive in 2050 than there would have been without deaths from HIV/AIDS.) Although the increased availability of family planning services is a crucial part of population management, cultural, political, and religious factors also need to be considered.

To be successful, population management must change the condition of people's lives, especially poverty, to remove the pressures for having large families. Research indicates that the combination of improved health, better education, and increased literacy and employment opportunities for women works together with family planning to decrease fertility rates. Unfortunately, in the fastest-growing countries, the needs of a rapidly increasing population use up financial resources that might otherwise be used to improve lives and ultimately slow population growth.

POLLUTION

As mentioned earlier, the classic environmental health concerns are not merely historical. They still have the potential to cause serious problems today under certain circumstances, and they take on added significance as our population grows. At the same time, new problems are arising, and some long-standing problems are gaining increased public attention. Many of these modern problems are problems of pollution. The term *pollution* refers to any unwanted contaminant in the environment that may pose a health risk.

Air Pollution

Air pollution is not a human invention or even a new problem. The air is polluted naturally with every forest fire, pollen bloom, and dust storm, as well as with countless other natural pollutants. To these natural sources, humans have always contributed the by-products of their activities. During the Industrial Revolution, English cities had far more daily air pollution than we can observe or even imagine today. However, we now live long enough to experience both the short-term and the long-term conse-

quences of air pollution. Also, increased population growth, combined with more industrialization using old technologies, concentrates the problems and makes them more visible to the public—and possibly more dangerous. Recent studies have linked exposure to air pollution to reduced birth weight in infants, reduced lung capacity in teens, and atherosclerosis (thickening of the arteries) in adults.

Air Quality and Smog Air pollution can cause illness and death if pollutant levels are high; young children, older adults, and people with chronic health conditions are particularly at risk. The EPA uses a measure called the **Air Quality Index (AQI)** to indicate whether air pollution levels pose a health concern. The AQI is used for five major air pollutants:

- Carbon monoxide (CO): An odorless, colorless gas, CO forms when the carbon in **fossil fuels** does not completely burn. The primary sources of CO are vehicle exhaust and fuel combustion in industrial processes. CO deprives body cells of oxygen, causing headaches, fatigue, and impaired vision and judgment; it also aggravates cardiovascular diseases.

- Sulfur dioxide (SO_2): SO_2 is produced by the burning of sulfur-containing fuels such as coal and oil, during metal smelting, and by other industrial processes; power plants are a major source. SO_2 narrows the airways, which may cause wheezing, chest tightness, and shortness of breath, particularly in people with asthma; it may also aggravate symptoms of CVD.

- Nitrogen dioxide (NO_2): NO_2 is a reddish-brown, highly reactive gas formed when nitric oxide combines with oxygen in the atmosphere; major sources include motor vehicles and power plants. In people with respiratory diseases such as asthma, NO_2 affects lung function and causes symptoms such as wheezing and shortness of breath; NO_2 exposure may also increase the risk of respiratory infections.

Terms

ecosystem The community of organisms (plants and animals) in an area and the nonliving physical factors with which they interact.

food chain The transfers of food energy and other substances in which one type of organism consumes another.

biodiversity The variety of living things on the earth, including all the different species of flora and fauna and the genetic diversity among individuals of the same species.

Air Quality Index (AQI) A measure of local air quality and what it means for health. Concentrations of five major pollutants are measured and assigned index values between 0 and 500, with values above 100 considered unhealthy; the highest of the five values becomes the overall AQI for the day. Health warnings and recommendations may be issued when AQI values exceed 100.

fossil fuels Buried deposits of decayed animals and plants that are converted into carbon-rich fuels by exposure to heat and pressure over millions of years; oil, coal, and natural gas are fossil fuels.

• Particulate matter (PM): Particles of different sizes are released into the atmosphere from a variety of sources, including combustion of fossil fuels, crushing or grinding operations, industrial processes, and dust from roadways. PM can accumulate in the respiratory system and aggravate cardiovascular and lung diseases and increase the risk of respiratory infections. PM exposure is associated with increased rates of hospital admissions, physician visits, and premature death.

• Ground-level ozone: At ground level, ozone is a harmful pollutant; where it occurs naturally in the upper atmosphere, it shields the earth from the sun's harmful ultraviolet rays. (The health hazards from the thinning of this protective ozone layer are discussed later in the chapter.) Ground-level ozone is formed when pollutants emitted by cars, power plants, industrial boilers, refineries, chemical plants, and other sources react chemically in the presence of sunlight (photochemical reactions). Ozone can irritate the respiratory system, reduce lung function, aggravate asthma, increase susceptibility to respiratory infections, and damage the lining of the lungs. Short-term elevations of ozone levels have also been linked to increased death rates.

AQI values run from 0 to 500; the higher the AQI, the greater the level of pollution and associated health danger. When the AQI exceeds 100, air quality is considered unhealthy, at first for certain sensitive groups of people and then for everyone as AQI values get higher. For local areas, AQI values are calculated for each of the five pollutants listed above; the highest value becomes the AQI rating for that day. Depending on the AQI value, precautionary health advice may be provided; for example, see the AQI chart for ozone shown in Figure 23-3. Information on the AQI in your area is often available in newspapers, on television and radio, on the Internet, and from state and local telephone hotlines.

The term **smog** was first used in the early 1900s in London to describe the combination of smoke and fog. What we typically call smog today is a mixture of pollu-

Index Values	Levels of Health Concern	Cautionary Statements
0–50	Good	None
51–100*	Moderate	Unusually sensitive people should consider limiting prolonged outdoor exertion.
101–150	Unhealthy for sensitive groups	Active children and adults, and people with respiratory disease, such as asthma, should limit prolonged outdoor exertion.
151–200	Unhealthy	Active children and adults, and people with respiratory disease, such as asthma, should avoid prolonged outdoor exertion; everyone else, especially children, should limit prolonged outdoor exertion.
201–300	Very unhealthy	Active children and adults, and people with respiratory disease, such as asthma, should avoid all outdoor exertion; everyone else, especially children, should limit outdoor exertion.
301–500	Hazardous	Everyone should avoid all outdoor exertion.

*Generally, an AQI of 100 for ozone corresponds to an ozone level of 0.08 parts per million (averaged over 8 hours).

Figure 23-3 Air Quality Index (AQI) for ozone. SOURCE: U.S. Environmental Protection Agency. 2000. *Air Quality Index: A Guide to Air Quality and Your Health.* Pub. no. EPA-454/R-00-005.

tants, with ground-level ozone being the key ingredient. Major smog occurrences are linked to the combination of several factors: Heavy motor vehicle traffic, high temperatures, and sunny weather can increase the production of ozone. Pollutants are also more likely to build up in areas with little wind and/or where a topographic feature such as a mountain range or valley prevents the wind from pushing out stagnant air.

A weather event called a **temperature inversion** also contributes to smog buildup. A temperature inversion occurs when there is little or no wind and a layer of warm air traps a layer of cold air next to the ground. Normally, the sun heats the earth, making the air closest to the ground warmer than that just above it. Warm air rises and is replaced by cooler air, which in turn is warmed and rises, thereby producing a natural circulation. This circulation, combined with horizontal wind circulation, prevents pollutants from reaching dangerous levels.

When there is a temperature inversion, this replacement and cleansing action cannot occur. The effect is like covering an area with a dome that traps all the pollutants

Terms

V**i**w

smog Hazy atmospheric conditions resulting from increased concentrations of ground-level ozone and other pollutants. Smog most commonly occurs when oxides of nitrogen and hydrocarbons, primarily from motor vehicle exhaust, react in the presence of sunlight; also known as *photochemical smog*. (The term was first used to describe the combination of smoke and fog in early-twentieth-century London.)

temperature inversion A weather condition in which a cold layer of air is trapped by a warm layer so that pollutants cannot be dispersed.

greenhouse effect A warming of the earth due to a buildup of carbon dioxide and certain other gases.

global warming An increase in the earth's atmospheric temperature when averaged across seasons and geographical regions.

Smog tends to form over Los Angeles because of the natural geographical features of the area and because of the tremendous amount of motor vehicle exhaust in the air. The health effects of smog are most noticeable in people who already have some respiratory impairment.

and prevents vertical dispersion. If this condition persists for several days, the buildup of pollutants may reach dangerous levels and threaten people's health. Many cities have plans for shutting down certain industries and even curtailing transportation if unsafe levels are approached. State and federal governments have passed clean-air legislation that has helped improve U.S. air quality in the past 20 years. However, it is estimated that 60–130 million Americans still live in areas with unhealthy air. Many areas have elevated levels of ozone and/or particulate matter.

The Greenhouse Effect and Global Warming

The temperature of the earth's atmosphere depends on the balance between the amount of energy the planet absorbs from the sun (mainly as high-energy ultraviolet radiation) and the amount of energy radiated back into space as lower-energy infrared radiation. Key components of temperature regulation are carbon dioxide, water vapor, methane, and other greenhouse gases—so named because, like a pane of glass in a greenhouse, they let through visible light from the sun but trap some of the resulting infrared radiation and reradiate it back to the earth's surface. This reradiation causes a buildup of heat that raises the temperature of the lower atmosphere, a natural process known as the **greenhouse effect.** Without it, the atmosphere would be far cooler and much more hostile to life.

Human activity may be tipping this balance toward **global warming** (Figure 23-4). The concentration of

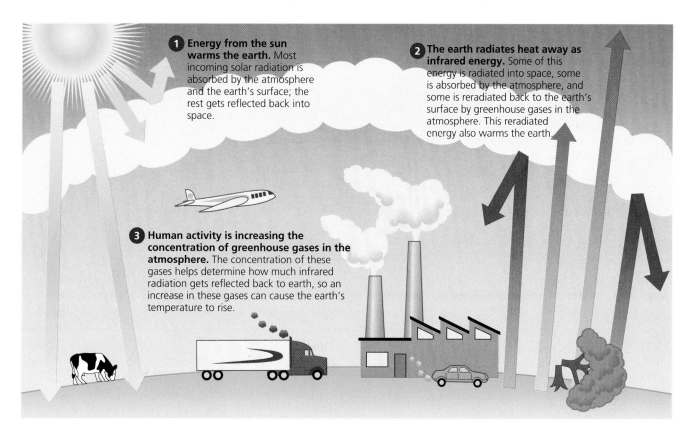

1 **Energy from the sun warms the earth.** Most incoming solar radiation is absorbed by the atmosphere and the earth's surface; the rest gets reflected back into space.

2 **The earth radiates heat away as infrared energy.** Some of this energy is radiated into space, some is absorbed by the atmosphere, and some is reradiated back to the earth's surface by greenhouse gases in the atmosphere. This reradiated energy also warms the earth.

3 **Human activity is increasing the concentration of greenhouse gases in the atmosphere.** The concentration of these gases helps determine how much infrared radiation gets reflected back to earth, so an increase in these gases can cause the earth's temperature to rise.

Figure 23-4   The greenhouse effect.

Table 23-1 Sources of Greenhouse Gases

Greenhouse Gas	Sources
Carbon dioxide	Fossil fuel and wood burning, factory emissions, car exhaust, deforestation
Chlorofluorocarbons (CFCs)	Refrigeration and air condition-ing, aerosols, foam products, solvents
Methane	Cattle, wetlands, rice paddies, landfills, gas leaks, coal and gas industries
Nitrous oxide	Fertilizers, soil cultivation, deforestation, animal feedlots and wastes
Ozone and other trace gases	Photochemical reactions, car exhaust, power plant emissions, solvents

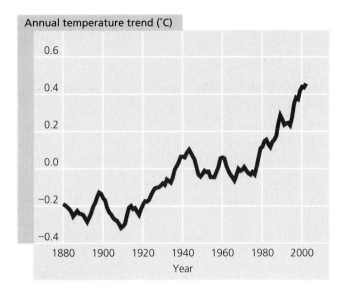

VITAL STATISTICS

Figure 23-5 Trend in annual mean temperature. This graph traces the trend in the annual mean temperature relative to the 1951–1980 mean value. There has been a strong warming trend over the past 30 years; variability within the overall trend is caused by such influences as large volcanic eruptions and periodic changes in ocean patterns (El Niño/La Niña). SOURCE: NASA Goddard Institute for Space Studies. 2005. *Global Temperature Trends: 2004 Summation* (http://www.giss.nasa.gov/data/update/gistemp/2004; retrieved March 5, 2005).

greenhouse gases is increasing because of human activity, especially the combustion of fossil fuels. Carbon diox-ide levels in the atmosphere have increased rapidly since the onset of the Industrial Revolution, and current levels are higher than at any time in the past 160,000 years. Deforestation, often by burning, also sends carbon dioxide into the atmosphere and reduces the number of trees available to convert carbon dioxide into oxygen. But energy use in the developed world is the primary cause of increases in the concentrations of greenhouse gases (Table 23-1). The United States alone is responsible for one-third of the world's total emissions of carbon dioxide.

According to a 2001 report from the United Nations–sponsored Intergovernmental Panel on Climate Change, the average global temperature will likely increase by about 2.5–10.4°F (1.4–5.8°C) by 2100, with a corresponding significant rise in sea level. Although the full implications of climate change are unknown, possible consequences include the following:

- Increased rainfall and flooding in some regions, in-creased drought in others. Coastal zones, where half the world's people live, would be severely affected.

- Increased mortality from heat stress, urban air pol-lution, and tropical diseases (due to the spread of

disease-carrying organisms like mosquitoes). Se-vere weather events such as hurricanes, tornadoes, droughts, and floods may also increase, along with associated deaths.

- A poleward shift of about 50–350 miles (150–550 km) in the location of vegetation zones, affecting crop yields, irrigation demands, and forest productivity.

Since record-keeping began in the mid-1800s, 9 of the 10 hottest years have occurred since 1990, the 3 hottest since 1997 (Figure 23-5). Data from tree rings, ice cores, and other sources suggest that recent temperatures are the warmest in 1000 years. For more on global warming, see the box "Climate Change: Politics and Science."

Thinning of the Ozone Layer Another air pol-lution problem is the thinning of the **ozone layer** of the atmosphere, a fragile, invisible layer about 10–30 miles above the earth's surface that shields the planet from the sun's hazardous ultraviolet (UV) rays. Since the mid-1980s, scientists have observed the seasonal appear-ance and growth of a hole in the ozone layer over Antarc-tica. More recently, thinning over other areas—including Canada, Scandinavia, the northern United States, Russia, Australia, and New Zealand—has been noted.

The ozone layer is being destroyed primarily by **chlo-rofluorocarbons (CFCs)**, industrial chemicals used as coolants in refrigerators and in home and automobile air conditioners; as foaming agents in some rigid foam

Terms

ozone layer A layer of ozone molecules (O_3) in the upper atmo-sphere that screens out UV rays from the sun.

chlorofluorocarbons (CFCs) Chemicals used as spray-can pro-pellants, refrigerants, and industrial solvents, implicated in the destruction of the ozone layer.

On February 16, 2005, the Kyoto Protocol to the United Nations Convention on Climate Change took effect. The protocol requires participating nations to reduce emissions of greenhouse gases by an average of 5.2% below 1990 levels by 2008–2012. Countries that miss their targets will be penalized with bigger cuts when the next set of emissions targets is set in 2012.

The pact was signed in 1997, but it could not take effect until countries accounting for at least 55% of global greenhouse emissions signed on; this hurdle was met when Russia ratified the protocol in 2004. The major industrialized countries that are *not* participating are the United States and Australia. If the United States had ratified the accord, it would have been required to reduce emissions by 6% below 1990 levels; U.S. emissions have actually increased significantly since 1990, including a more than 15% increase in carbon dioxide emissions.

Kyoto: Controversial but Critical?

Key areas of controversy relating to the Kyoto protocol include the following:

• *The science of climate change:* Critics of Kyoto, including the U.S. government, have argued that scientific knowledge regarding global warming is incomplete and it is therefore premature to set mandatory emissions cuts. However, as described in the chapter, scientific consensus on the human contribution toward climate change has been growing.

• *Kyoto's actual impact:* Even proponents acknowledge that the Kyoto protocol will have a relatively small impact. Current estimates have the Kyoto accord cutting just 0.1°C off the 1.4–5.8°C increase forecasted by 2100. However, supporters believe that the pact is a crucial first step and that it sets up a framework for more significant efforts in the future; its greatest immediate value may be symbolic.

• *The role of developing countries:* Developing countries were exempt from the Kyoto accord to give them an opportunity to pursue economic development and alleviate widespread poverty. These nations currently have far lower percapita energy use and greenhouse gas production than the United States. However, the combination of large population size and rapid industrial development means that any increase in greenhouse gas production in countries like India and China will have a substantial impact on worldwide emissions.

• *Economic costs:* The U.S. government argues that stiff limits on emissions would hurt economic growth; it favors voluntary cuts in emissions and investment in cleaner technologies. The Kyoto protocol does have mechanisms by which wealthy countries can, essentially, pay to pollute. It allows countries to meet their emission reduction goals through emissions trading, meaning they can buy credits from other countries that are surpassing their targets. Countries that invest in clean technologies would thus be able to sell emissions credits to other countries.

A Growing Scientific Consensus

The idea that human production of greenhouse gasses could lead to global warming was originally proposed in the 1890s, but the first major review of the evidence was not undertaken until the 1988 formation of the United Nations Intergovernmental Panel on Climate Change (IPCC). Based on complex climate models, the IPCC concluded that global temperatures are, indeed, increasing, and that human activity is responsible for a significant proportion of this increase. These conclusions have been supported by individual research and other agencies and organizations, including the National Academy of Sciences. Current scientific study and debate now appears to be focused not on whether human activity is causing global warming but rather on just how much human-caused warming will occur.

Where does the evidence for global warming come from? Firm world temperature data exists for the period since 1880, and that data shows a clear increase. For earlier periods, scientists use a variety of data sources, including tree rings and ice cores, to estimate past temperatures. Based on these data, temperatures are currently higher than at any point in the past 1000 years. Greenhouse gases are also at record-high concentrations in the atmosphere.

Researchers have also been able to measure declining amounts of infrared radiation escaping into space—and more trapped radiation leads to heating of the atmosphere. Another key piece of evidence was announced in early 2005, when researchers reported that computer climate models based on human-produced warming predicted with 95% accuracy actual changes seen in ocean temperatures throughout the world over the past 40 years.

We may already be seeing some of the early effects of global warming, ranging from earlier flowering of plants to increases in severe weather events. The Arctic is heating up nearly twice as fast as the rest of the planet, and problems related to thawing permafrost have already been reported—including the collapse of buildings and the destabilization of oil pipelines, roads, and airports. Glaciers and ice sheets are melting, with corresponding increases in sea level.

What Next?

Scientists continue to develop new and better climate models and to map the impacts of climate change. One key goal is to produce better models of how overall trends may affect specific regions. For example, 2003 was the third hottest year on record overall, but Europe experienced its hottest summer in 500 years, with about 30,000 deaths due to heat.

On the policy front, some European leaders have vowed to step up the campaign to involve the countries that have the greatest impact on greenhouse gas emissions. The United States, the European Union, Canada, Russia, Japan, China, and India together emit 75% of the world's greenhouse gasses. Proposals for involving developing countries include financial incentives and technology transfers to help them limit emissions without impacting their efforts to reduce poverty.

Despite the official U.S. position, some states are taking steps to limit greenhouse emissions on their own. For example, California is requiring stiff reductions in vehicle emissions, and several states in the Northeast are setting up an emissions trading system similar to that in the Kyoto accord. Individuals can also take steps to limit their contributions to global warming; try some of the lifestyle changes suggested in the sections on reducing air pollution and energy use.

SOURCES: United Nations. 2005. *United Nations Convention on Climate Change: Essential Background* (http://unfccc.int/essential_background/items/2877.php; retrieved March 6, 2005); Scripps Institution. 2005. *Scripps Researchers Find Clear Evidence of Human-Produced Warming in World's Oceans* (http://scrippsnews.ucsd.edu/article_detail.cfm?article_num=666; retrieved March 6, 2005); National Research Council. 2001. *Climate Change Science: An Analysis of Some Key Questions.* Washington, D.C.: National Academy Press; Intergovernmental Panel on Climate Change. 2001. *Climate Change 2001: Impacts, Adaptation, and Vulnerability.* Geneva: Intergovernmental Panel on Climate Change.

products, including insulation; as propellants in some kinds of aerosol sprays (most such sprays were banned in 1978); and as solvents. When CFCs rise into the atmosphere, winds carry them toward the polar regions. During winter, circular winds form a vortex that keeps the air over Antarctica from mixing with air from elsewhere. Ice crystals form in the Antarctic clouds during the cold, sunless months; chemical reactions taking place on these crystals, which wouldn't take place in air, free chlorine atoms from CFCs. When stimulated by the reappearance of the sun, the chlorine atoms begin destroying ozone. When the polar vortex weakens in the summer, winds richer in ozone from the north replenish the lost Antarctic ozone, but the ozone hole's growth each year may be contributing to the general thinning of the global ozone layer.

Since 1979, about 15% of Antarctic ozone has been destroyed, although locally and seasonally up to 95% of the ozone disappears (forming the hole). The size and shape of the hole are affected by meteorological factors as well as by the presence of ozone-destroying chemicals. The largest and deepest hole to date occurred in late 2000 over Antarctica. Spreading over 11 million square miles, an area three times larger than the landmass of the United States, the 2000 ozone hole extended over populated areas of South America, where residents were advised to stay indoors and take other measures to avoid UV exposure. (UV radiation levels under the hole were high enough to cause sunburn within 7 minutes.) In the Northern Hemisphere, ozone levels have declined by about 10% since 1980, and certain areas may be temporarily depleted in late winter and early spring by as much as 40%.

The loss of ozone is of concern because without the ozone layer to absorb the sun's UV radiation, life on Earth would be impossible. The potential effects of increased long-term exposure to UV light for humans include skin cancer, wrinkling and aging of the skin, cataracts and blindness, and reduced immune response. The United Nations Environment Programme predicts that a drop of 10% in overall ozone levels would cause a 26% rise in the incidence of nonmelanoma skin cancers. Some scientists blame ozone loss over Australia for a recent rise in melanoma cases there.

UV light may interfere with photosynthesis and cause lower crop yields; it may also kill phytoplankton and krill, the basis of the ocean food chain. And because heat generated by the absorption of UV rays in the ozone layer helps create stratospheric winds, the driving force behind weather patterns, a drop in the concentration of ozone could potentially alter the earth's climate systems.

Term

V w

acid precipitation Rain, snow, sleet, or hail with a low pH (acid), caused by atmospheric moisture combining with products of industrial combustion to form acids such as sulfur dioxide; harmful to forests and lakes, which cannot tolerate changes in acidity/alkalinity.

Worldwide production and use of CFCs have declined rapidly since the danger to the ozone layer was recognized. Industrialized nations agreed to eliminate CFC production and use by 2000, and limits have also been placed on other agents that destroy ozone. Metered-dose inhalers for conditions like asthma are the only significant commercial product to contain CFCs, and CFC-free inhalers are already available for some medications. However, use of some ozone-depleting agents, including bromine and halon-1211, is still increasing. In addition, CFCs persist in the atmosphere for long periods, and scientists estimate that the ozone layer will not significantly recover until about 2050.

Acid Precipitation   A by-product of many industrial processes, **acid precipitation** occurs when atmospheric pollutants combine with moisture in the air and fall to earth as highly acidic rain, snow, sleet, or hail. It occurs especially when coal containing large amounts of sulfur is burned and sulfur dioxide, sulfur trioxide, nitrogen dioxide, nitric acid, and other chemicals are released into the atmosphere. These concentrations can be carried great distances by the prevailing winds and form a highly acidic mixture containing sulfuric acid and nitric acid. Most of the pollutants in acid precipitation are produced by coal-burning electric power plants. Other sources are motor vehicles and certain industrial activities, such as smelting.

Acidification of lakes and streams due to acid precipitation has completely eradicated fish and other aquatic species in some areas. Trees are also affected because acid precipitation damages leaves, strips the soil of key nutrients, and releases toxic substances such as heavy metals from the soil; in some areas of central Europe, entire forests are dying. The air pollutants that cause acid precipitation reduce visibility and cause respiratory problems in some people. Acid precipitation also corrodes metals and damages stone and paint on buildings, monuments, and cars; repairs can cost billions of dollars. Acid precipitation appears to be causing the most damage in Canada, the northeastern United States, Scandinavia, and parts of central Europe. In the United States, the areas most affected are the Adirondacks, the mid-Appalachian highlands, the upper Midwest, and high elevations in the West.

Energy Use and Air Pollution   Americans are the biggest energy consumers in the world (Table 23-2). We use energy to create electricity, transport us, power our industries, and run our homes. About 85% of the energy we use comes from fossil fuels—oil, coal, and natural gas. The remainder comes from nuclear power and renewable energy sources (such as hydroelectric, wind, and solar power).

Energy consumption is at the root of many environmental problems, especially those relating to air pollution. Automobile exhaust and the burning of oil and coal by industry and by electric power plants are primary causes of smog, acid precipitation, and the greenhouse effect. The mining of coal and the extraction and transportation of oil

Table 23-2 | Energy Use in Selected Countries, 2002

	Per Capita Energy Use (million Btu)
United States	339
Australia	286
Russia	191
France	184
Japan	172
United Kingdom	162
South Africa	101
Mexico	65
China	33
India	13

SOURCE: Energy Information Administration. 2004. *International Total Primary Energy and Related Information* (http://www.eia.doe.gov/emeu/international/total.html; retrieved March 7, 2005).

cause pollution on land and in the water; coal miners often suffer from serious health problems related to their jobs. Nuclear power generation creates hazardous wastes and carries the risk of dangerous releases of radiation.

Two key strategies for controlling energy use are conservation and the development of nonpolluting, renewable sources of energy. Although the use of renewable energy sources has increased in recent years, renewables still supply only a small proportion of our energy, in part because of their cost. Some countries have chosen to promote energy efficiency by removing subsidies or adding taxes on the use of fossil fuels. This strategy is reflected in the varying prices drivers pay for gasoline. According to the U.S. Energy Information Agency, the average U.S. per gallon price of unleaded gasoline was $2.28 in April 2005. Although U.S. gas prices are higher than in the past, they are still several dollars a gallon lower than in many European and Asian countries. It is not surprising that per-capita energy use in the United States is twice that of many European countries. The International Center for Technology Assessment estimates that the actual price of gasoline—including tax breaks, government subsidies, and environmental, health, and social costs of gas usage—is as high as $15.14 per gallon.

Despite recent increases in U.S. consumer gas prices, more than 70% of commuters drive alone to work, and low-fuel-economy sport utility vehicles (SUVs) remain popular. Every gallon of gas burned puts about 20 pounds of carbon dioxide into the atmosphere; some SUVs average fewer than 10 miles per gallon, and the largest SUVs increase greenhouse gas emissions by 6 or more tons per year more than an average car. A more positive U.S. trend has been the introduction of hybrid electric vehicles (HEVs), which combine a conventional internal combustion engine with an electric motor, resulting in about twice the fuel economy of conventional vehicles. Researchers hope that hybrid technology can be extended to all classes of vehicles and that Americans can be convinced to use more fuel-efficient vehicles and to travel more frequently on public transportation, in carpools, or on foot.

Actions that individuals can take to promote energy efficiency and cut their use of energy are listed in the section "What You Can Do to Prevent Air Pollution."

Indoor Air Pollution Although most people associate air pollution with the outdoors, your home may also harbor potentially dangerous pollutants. Some of these compounds trigger allergic responses, and others have been linked to cancer. Common indoor pollutants include the following:

* *Environmental tobacco smoke (ETS),* a human carcinogen that also increases the risk of asthma, bronchitis, and cardiovascular disease (see Chapter 11). Several states and cities have passed legislation known as Clean Indoor Air Acts, which state that any enclosed, indoor areas used by the public shall be smoke-free except for certain designated areas.

* *Carbon monoxide and other combustion by-products,* which can cause chronic bronchitis, headaches, dizziness, nausea, fatigue, and even death. Common sources in the home are woodstoves, fireplaces, kerosene heaters and lamps, and gas ranges.

* *Formaldehyde gas,* which can cause eye, nose, and throat irritation; shortness of breath; headaches; nausea; lethargy; and, over the long term, cancer. This gas can seep from resins used in particle board, plywood paneling, and some carpeting and upholstery; it is also emitted by certain paints and floor finishes, permanent press clothing, and nail polish.

* *Biological pollutants,* including bacteria, dust mites, mold, and animal dander, which can cause allergic reactions and other health problems. These allergens need nutrients and moisture to survive and are typically found in bathrooms, damp or flooded basements, humidifiers, air conditioners, and even some carpets and furniture.

Asbestos and radon, two other dangerous indoor pollutants, are discussed later in the chapter.

What You Can Do to Prevent Air Pollution

* Cut back on driving. Ride your bike, walk, use public transportation, or carpool in a fuel-efficient vehicle.

* Keep your car tuned up and well maintained. Use only unleaded gas, and keep your tires inflated at recommended pressures. To save energy when driving, avoid quick starts, stay within the speed limit, limit the use of air conditioning, and don't let your car idle unless absolutely necessary. Have your car's air conditioner checked and serviced by a station

A key strategy for reducing air pollution and greenhouse gas emissions is to reduce energy consumption. Most people drive alone to commute to work or school; try to cut back on your solo driving time by riding your bike, walking, carpooling, or using public transportation.

that uses environmentally friendly refrigerants (car air conditioners made before 1994 are a major source of CFCs).

- Buy energy-efficient appliances, and use them only when necessary. Run the washing machine, dryer, and dishwasher only when you have full loads, and do laundry in warm or cold water instead of hot; don't overdry your clothes. Clean refrigerator coils and clothes dryer lint screens frequently. Towel or air-dry your hair rather than using an electric dryer.

- Replace incandescent bulbs with compact fluorescent bulbs (not fluorescent tubes). Although they cost more initially, they'll save you money over the life of the bulb. They produce a comparable light, last longer, and use only 25–35% of the energy of a regular bulb, thereby lowering carbon dioxide emissions from electric power plants.

- Make sure your home is well-insulated with ozone-safe agents; use insulating shades and curtains to keep heat in during winter and out during summer. Seal any openings that produce drafts. In cold weather, put on a sweater and turn down the thermostat. In hot weather, wear lightweight clothing and, whenever possible, use a fan instead of an air conditioner to cool yourself.

- Plant and care for trees in your own yard and neighborhood. Because they recycle carbon dioxide, trees work against global warming. They also provide shade and cool the air, so less air conditioning is needed.

- Before discarding a refrigerator, air conditioner, or humidifier, check with the waste hauler or your local government to ensure that ozone-depleting refrigerants will be removed prior to disposal. If you use a metered-dose inhaler, ask your physician if an ozone-safe inhaler is available for your medication.

- To prevent indoor air pollution, keep your house adequately ventilated, and buy some houseplants; they have a natural ability to rid the air of harmful pollutants.

- Keep paints, cleaning agents, and other chemical products tightly sealed in their original containers.

- Don't smoke, and don't allow others to smoke in your room, apartment, or home. If these rules are too strict for your situation, limit smoking to a single, well-ventilated room.

- Clean and inspect chimneys, furnaces, and other appliances regularly. Install carbon monoxide detectors.

Chemical Pollution

Chemical pollution is by no means a new problem. The ancient Romans were plagued by lead poisoning, and over 200 years ago in Europe, the phrase "mad as a hatter" came from the hatters' practice of preparing felt hats with mercury, which destroyed the central nervous system.

The difference today is that new chemical substances are constantly being created and introduced into the environment—as pesticides, herbicides, solvents, cleaning fluids, flame retardants, and hundreds of other products. We have many more chemicals, in more concentrated forms and in wider use, and larger numbers of people are exposed and potentially exposed to them than ever before.

Chemical pollutants have been responsible for several environmental disasters, including thousands of deaths and injuries among people in Bhopal, India, that occurred when a powerful chemical used in manufacturing the insecticide Sevin was released from a plant. Catastrophes illustrate the short-term potential for disaster, but the long-term health consequences may be just as deadly. The following are brief descriptions of just a few current problems.

Asbestos A mineral-based compound, asbestos was widely used for fire protection and insulation in buildings until the late 1960s. Microscopic asbestos fibers can be released into the air when this material is applied or when it later deteriorates or is damaged. These fibers can lodge in the lungs, causing **asbestosis,** lung cancer, and other serious lung diseases. Similar conditions expose workers to risk in the coal mining industry, from coal and silica dust (black lung disease), and in the textile industry, from cotton fibers (brown lung disease).

Asbestos can pose a danger in homes and apartment buildings, about 25% of which are thought to contain some asbestos. Areas where it is most likely to be found are insulation around water and steam pipes, ducts, and furnaces; boiler wraps; vinyl flooring; floor, wall, and ceiling insulation; roofing and siding; and fireproof board. An experienced contractor can pinpoint asbestos-

Dimensions of Diversity

Poverty and Environmental Health

Residents of poor and minority communities are often exposed to more environmental toxins than residents of wealthier communities, and they are more likely to suffer from health problems caused or aggravated by pollutants. Poor neighborhoods are often located near highways and industrial areas that have high levels of air and noise pollution; they are also common sites for hazardous waste production and disposal. Residents of substandard housing are more likely to come into contact with lead, asbestos, carbon monoxide, pesticides, and other hazardous pollutants associated with peeling paint, old plumbing, poorly maintained insulation and heating equipment, and attempts to control high levels of pests such as cockroaches and rodents. Poor people are more likely to have jobs that expose them to asbestos, silica dust, and pesticides, and they are more likely to catch and consume fish contaminated with PCBs, mercury, and other toxins.

The most thoroughly researched and documented link among poverty, the environment, and health is lead poisoning in children. Many studies have shown that children of low-income black families are much more likely to have elevated levels of lead in their blood than white children. One survey found that two-thirds of urban African American children from families earning less than $6000 a year had elevated lead levels. The CDC and the American Academy of Pediatrics recommend annual testing of blood lead levels for all children under age 6, with more frequent testing for children at special risk.

Asthma is another health threat that appears to be linked with both environmental and socioeconomic factors. The number of Americans with asthma has grown dramatically in the past 20 years; most of the increase has occurred in children, with African Americans and the poor hardest hit. Researchers are not sure what accounts for this increase, but suspects include household pollutants, pesticides, air pollution, cigarette smoke, and allergens like cockroaches. These risk factors are likely to cluster in poor urban areas where inadequate health care may worsen asthma's effects.

A new push for research on the health effects of exposure to toxins on low-income communities is being called for by the environmental justice movement. New studies are investigating the links between environmental factors and respiratory problems, skin diseases, and cancer. While health researchers seek to quantify the health effects, neighborhood activists continue to fight against the dumping of pollution in poor communities.

---

containing materials in a home; they can then be analyzed by a laboratory. If any of these materials begin to release asbestos fibers, the asbestos must be sealed off, encapsulated, or removed by a professional.

Lead   Lead poisoning continues to be a serious problem, particularly among children living in older buildings and adults who are exposed to lead in the workplace. When lead is ingested or inhaled, it can damage the central nervous system, cause mental impairment, hinder oxygen transport in the blood, and create digestive problems. Severe lead poisoning may cause coma or even death. Some symptoms of lead poisoning, including anemia, headaches, and abdominal pain, may cease if exposure stops, but neurological damage can be permanent. Lead damage to the brain can start even before birth if a pregnant woman has elevated levels of lead in her body.

The CDC estimates that as many as 500,000 children under age 6 may have unsafe lead levels in their blood. Many of these children live in poor, inner-city areas (see the box "Poverty and Environmental Health"). Long-term exposure to low levels of lead may cause kidney disease; it can also cause lead to buildup in bones, where it may be released into the bloodstream during pregnancy or when bone mass is lost from osteoporosis. The increased lead levels that occur as women age and lose bone mass can cause hypertension.

Young children can easily ingest lead from their environment by picking up dust and dirt on their hands and then putting their fingers in their mouth. Lead-based paints are believed to be the chief culprit in lead poisoning of children and were banned from residential use in 1978, but as many as 57 million American homes still contain lead paint. The use of lead in plumbing is now also banned, but some old pipes and faucets contain lead that can leach into drinking water.

Lead gets into the air from industrial and vehicle emissions, from tobacco smoke and paint dust, and from the burning of solid wastes that contain lead. Levels of lead in the air have dropped sharply as leaded gas use has declined, but many vehicles still use leaded fuel. Lead occurs naturally in soil, which also collects lead from the air and other sources. Other sources of lead are foods stored or served in lead-glazed pottery or lead crystal and processed foods sold in lead-soldered cans.

Pesticides   Pesticides are used primarily for two purposes: to prevent the spread of insectborne diseases and to maximize food production by killing insects that eat

---

Terms

asbestosis A lung condition caused by inhalation of microscopic asbestos fibers, which inflame the lung and can lead to lung cancer.

pesticides Chemicals used to prevent the spread of diseases transmitted by insects and to maximize food production by killing insects that eat crops.

crops. Both uses have risks as well as benefits. Take, for example, the pesticide DDT. Recognized as a powerful pesticide in 1939, DDT was extremely important in efforts to control widespread insectborne diseases in tropical countries and increase crop yields throughout the world. In 1962, biologist Rachel Carson questioned the safety of DDT in her book *Silent Spring*, pointing out that the pesticide disrupts the life cycles of birds, fish, and reptiles. DDT also builds up in the food chain, increasing in concentration as larger animals eat smaller ones, a process known as **biomagnification.** Despite its effectiveness as a pesticide, DDT was banned in the United States in 1972 because the costs associated with its use—to wildlife and potentially to humans—were too high. Most pesticide hazards to date have been a result of overuse, but there are concerns about the health effects of long-term exposure to small amounts of pesticide residues in foods, especially for children.

Mercury A naturally occurring metal, mercury is a toxin that affects the nervous system and may damage the brain, kidneys, and gastrointestinal tract; increase blood pressure, heart rate, and heart attack risk; and cause cancer. Mercury slows fetal and child development and causes irreversible deficits in brain function. As many as 600,000 babies are born each year after being exposed to levels of mercury that some studies have shown to have adverse health effects. A 2005 study estimated that the economic cost of the effects of mercury on children's brain development is $8.7 billion annually. Coal-fired power plants are the largest producers of mercury; other sources include mining and smelting operations and the disposal of consumer products containing mercury.

Mercury persists in the environment, and, like pesticides, it is bioaccumulative. In particular, large, long-lived fish may carry high levels of mercury. The FDA recommends that pregnant women, women of childbearing age who may become pregnant, women who are breastfeeding, and young children not consume shark, swordfish, king mackerel, and tilefish and limit total fish consumption to 12 ounces per week. Chapter 12 includes more information on safe fish consumption; see the box "Gender and Environmental Health" for more on issues affecting pregnant women.

Because of health concerns, some cities and stores have banned the sale of mercury fever thermometers, a small but significant source of mercury. If a thermometer breaks or is disposed of improperly, mercury can enter the environment; if it vaporizes into the atmosphere, it can be hazardous to health. To safely clean up mercury from a broken thermometer, increase ventilation in the room and pick up the mercury with an eyedropper or scoop up the beads with a piece of heavy paper. Dispose of it and any contaminated instruments by placing them in a plastic bag and taking them to an appropriate hazardous waste disposal site. Replace mercury thermometers with one of the many mercury-free alternatives.

The list of real and potential chemical pollution problems may well be as long as the list of known chemicals. To the preceding examples we can add recent concern about arsenic in drinking water, formaldehyde in synthetic building materials, prescription medications and hormones in streams, and other by-products of our industrial age. As mentioned earlier, hazardous wastes are also found in the home and should be handled and disposed of properly. They include automotive supplies (motor oil, antifreeze, transmission fluid), paint supplies (turpentine, paint thinner, mineral spirits), art and hobby supplies (oil-based paint, solvents, acids and alkalis, aerosol sprays), insecticides, batteries, computer and electronic components, and household cleaners containing sodium hydroxide (lye) or ammonia. These chemicals are dangerous when inhaled or ingested, when they contact the skin or the eyes, or when they are burned or dumped. Many cities provide guidelines about approved disposal methods and have hazardous waste collection days. Look in the government pages of your phone book under Environmental Health or Hazardous Waste.

What You Can Do to Prevent Chemical Pollution

- When buying products, read the labels, and try to buy the least toxic ones available. Choose nontoxic nonpetrochemical cleansers, disinfectants, polishes, and other personal and household products.

- Dispose of your household hazardous wastes properly. If you are not sure whether something is hazardous or don't know how to dispose of it, contact your local environmental health office or health department. Don't burn trash.

- Buy organic produce or produce that has been grown locally. Wash, scrub, and, if appropriate, peel fruits and vegetables. Consider eating less meat; animal products require more pesticides, fertilizer, water, and energy to produce.

- If you must use pesticides or toxic household products, store them in a locked place where children and pets can't get to them. Don't measure chemicals with food-preparation utensils, and wear gloves whenever handling them.

Terms

V w

biomagnification The accumulation of a substance in a food chain.

radiation Energy transmitted in the form of rays, waves, or particles.

radiation sickness An illness caused by excess radiation exposure, marked by low white blood cell counts and nausea; possibly fatal.

nuclear power The use of controlled nuclear reactions to produce steam, which in turn drives turbines to produce electricity.

Although many environmental health risks are shared by all, some risks disproportionately affect women or men. Women and men often have different roles and responsibilities with respect to family, community, and the workforce. These differences can determine the types of environmental hazards that individuals are exposed to and what the potential risks of those exposures are.

In many societies, women are more often involved in day-to-day activities associated with the environment, including food preparation, agricultural work, and tasks around the home. These activities can expose women to greater levels of indoor air pollution, water pollution, foodborne pathogens, agricultural chemicals, and waste contamination. Indoor pollutants, especially soot from burning wood, charcoal, and other solid fuels used for home heating and cooking, are a particular risk for women. Exposure to this particulate pollution increases the risk of respiratory diseases, lung cancer, and reproductive problems.

All humans are exposed to chemicals in air, food, and drinking water, and we all carry a body load of chemicals. Some of these chemicals bioaccumulate in our bones, blood, or fatty tissues. Women are smaller than men, on average, and have a higher percentage of body fat; so chemicals that accumulate in fatty tissue may pose a relatively greater risk for women. On the other hand, men may be more likely to work in industries that involve significant occupational exposures to disease-related toxins; for example, coal miners have an increased risk of lung cancer (black lung disease).

Although any chemical exposure can be a concern for health, women face the added risk of passing pollutants to a developing fetus during pregnancy or to an infant through breastfeeding. Even relatively low exposure to pollutants can result in a significant chemical body load in an infant or young child because of their small body size. And because infants and children are still developing, the effects of chemical exposure can be significant and devastating. It is not unusual for dangerous environmental toxin exposures to be first recognized through noticeable effects on infants or children.

Reproductive risks are not limited to women and infants in developing parts of the world. Even in industrialized countries with strong environmental laws, infants and children are affected by such chemicals as lead and mercury. In 2005, scientists announced that they had found elevated levels of the rocket fuel chemical perchlorate in human breast milk in amounts above the safe dose set by the National Academy of Sciences. Many other chemicals, including PCBs and pesticides, have already been found in breast milk.

Studies are ongoing to identify and reduce environmental hazards in the United States and throughout the world. However, many of the people most directly affected by environmental health problems—women, children, and people living in poor communities—have limited economic, social, and political power. It is important that everyone affected by environmental problems be given a voice in determining environmental policies.

SOURCES: Kirk, A. B., et al. 2005. Perchlorate and iodide in dairy and breast milk. *Environmental Science and Technology*, Web release, February 22; McCally, M., ed. 2002. *Life Support: The Environment and Human Health.* Cambridge, Mass.: MIT Press; Population Reference Bureau. 2002. *Women, Men, and Environmental Change: The Gender Dimensions of Environmental Policies and Programs.* Washington, D.C.: Population Reference Bureau.

- If you have your house fumigated for pest control, be sure to hire a licensed exterminator. Keep everyone, including pets, out of the house while the crew works and, if possible, for a few days after.

Radiation

Many people are afraid of **radiation,** in part because they don't understand what it is. Basically, radiation is energy. It can come in different forms, such as ultraviolet rays, microwaves, or X rays, and from different sources, such as the sun, uranium, and nuclear weapons (Figure 23-6, p. 712). These forms of electromagnetic radiation differ in wavelength and energy, with shorter waves having the highest energy levels. Of most concern to health are gamma rays produced by radioactive sources such as nuclear weapons, nuclear energy plants, and radon gas; these high-energy waves are powerful enough to penetrate objects and break molecular bonds. Although gamma radiation cannot be seen or felt, its effects at high doses can include **radiation sickness** and death; at lower doses, chromosome damage, sterility, tissue damage, cataracts, and cancer can occur. Other types of radiation can also affect health; for example, exposure to UV radiation from the sun or from tanning salons can increase the risk of skin cancer. The effects of some sources of radiation, such as cell phones, remain controversial.

Nuclear Weapons and Nuclear Energy Nuclear weapons pose a health risk of the most serious kind to all species. Public health associations have stated that in the event of an intentional or unintentional discharge of these weapons, the casualties would run into the hundreds of thousands or millions. Reducing these stockpiles is a challenge and a goal for the twenty-first century.

Power-generating plants that use nuclear fuel also pose health problems. When **nuclear power** was first developed as an alternative to oil and coal, it was promoted as clean, efficient, inexpensive, and safe. In general, this has proven to be the case. Power systems in several parts of the world rely on nuclear power plants. However, despite all the built-in safeguards and regulating agencies, accidents in nuclear power plants do happen, many due to human error (as at Three Mile Island in the United States and Tokaimura in Japan), and the consequences of such accidents are far more

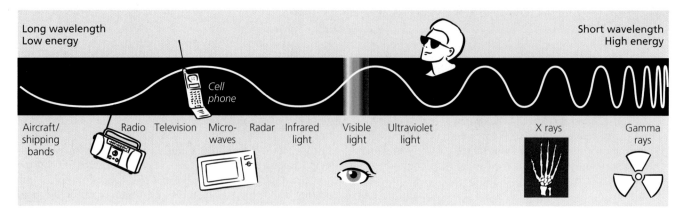

Long wavelength
Low energy

Short wavelength
High energy

Cell phone

Aircraft/
shipping
bands

Radio   Television   Micro-
                        waves

Radar   Infrared
         light

Visible
light

Ultraviolet
light

X rays

Gamma
rays

Figure 23-6   Electromagnetic radiation.   Electromagnetic radiation takes the form of waves that travel through space. The length of the wave determines the type of radiation: The shortest waves are high-energy gamma rays; the longest are radio waves and extremely low frequency waves used for communication between aircraft, ships, and submarines. Different types of electromagnetic radiation have different effects on health.

serious than those of similar accidents in other types of power-generating plants. The 1986 fire and explosion at the Chernobyl nuclear power station in Ukraine caused hundreds of deaths and increased rates of genetic mutation and cancer; the long-term effects are not yet clear. The zone around Chernobyl has been sealed off to human habitation and could be unsafe for the next 24,000 years.

An additional, enormous problem is disposing of the radioactive wastes these plants generate. They cannot be dumped in a sanitary landfill because the amount and type of soil used to cap a sanitary landfill are not sufficient to prevent radiation exposure. Deposit sites have to be developed that will be secure not just for a few years but for tens of thousands of years—longer than the total recorded history of human beings on this planet. To date, no storage method has been devised that can provide infallible, infinitely durable shielding for nuclear waste.

Medical Uses of Radiation   Another area of concern is the use of radiation in medicine, primarily the X ray. The development of machines that could produce images of internal bone structures was a major advance in medicine, and applications abounded. Chest X rays were routinely given to screen for tuberculosis, and children's feet were even X rayed in shoe stores to make sure their

new shoes fit properly. But, as is often the case, this new technology had disadvantages. As time passed, studies revealed that X ray exposure is cumulative and that no exposure is absolutely safe.

Early X ray machines are no longer used because of the high amounts of radiation they give off. Each new generation of X ray machines has used less radiation more effectively. From a personal health point of view, individuals should never have a routine X ray examination; each such exam should have a definite purpose, and its benefits and risks should be carefully weighed.

Radiation in the Home and Workplace   Recently, there has been concern about electromagnetic radiation associated with common modern devices such as microwave ovens, computer monitors, cell phones, and even high-voltage power lines. These forms of radiation do have effects on health, but research results are inconclusive.

Another area of concern is **radon,** a naturally occurring radioactive gas found in certain soils, rocks, and building materials. When the breakdown products of radon are inhaled, they cling to lungs and bombard sensitive tissue with radioactivity. Among miners, exposure to high levels of radon has been shown to cause lung cancer; overall, it is the second leading cause of lung cancer in the United States, after smoking tobacco. Radon can enter a home by rising through the soil into the basement through dirt floors, cracks, and other openings.

In 2005, the Surgeon General issued a national health advisory on radon, recommending that Americans test their homes for radon every 2 years, and retest any time they move, make structural changes to a home, or occupy a previously unused level of a residence. If elevated levels of radon are found (4 pCi/L or more), the problem should be dealt with as soon as possible through such measures as sealing cracks or installing basement ventilation systems.

Terms

V̇i̇w

radon A naturally occurring radioactive gas emitted from rocks and natural building materials that can become concentrated in insulated homes, causing lung cancer.

decibel A unit for expressing the relative intensity of sounds on a scale from 0 for the average least perceptible sound to about 120 for the average pain threshold.

tinnitus Ringing in the ears, a condition that can be caused by excessive noise exposure.

More information is available at the EPA Web site or by calling 1-800-SOS-RADON.

What You Can Do to Avoid Radiation

- If your physician orders an X ray, ask why it is necessary. Only get X rays that you need, and keep a record of the date and location of every X ray exam. Don't have a full-body CT scan for routine screening; the radiation dose of one full-body CT scan is nearly 100 times that of a typical mammogram.
- Follow the Surgeon General's recommendations for radon testing.
- Find out if there are radioactive sites in your area. If you live or work near such a site, form or join a community action group to get the site cleaned up.

Noise Pollution

We are increasingly aware of the health effects of loud or persistent noise in the environment. Concerns focus on two areas: hearing loss and stress. Prolonged exposure to sounds above 80–85 **decibels** (a measure of the intensity of a sound wave) can cause permanent hearing loss (Figure 23-7). The scream of an infant, the noise in a machine shop, and freeway traffic sounds can all exceed the safe range. Two common potential sources of excessive noise are the workplace and large gatherings of people at sporting events and rock concerts. The Occupational Safety and Health Administration (OSHA) sets legal standards for noise in the workplace, but no laws exist regulating noise levels at rock concerts, which often exceed OSHA standards for the workplace.

Most hearing loss occurs in the first 2 hours of exposure, and hearing usually recovers within 2 hours after the noise stops. But if exposure continues or is repeated frequently, hearing loss may be permanent. The employees of a club where rock music is played loudly are at greater risk than the patrons of the club, who might be exposed for only 2 hours at a time. Another possible effect of exposure to excessive noise is **tinnitus,** a condition of more or less continuous ringing or buzzing in the ears.

Excessive noise is also an environmental stressor, producing the typical stress response described in Chapter 2: faster heart rate, increased respiration, higher blood pressure, and so on. A chronic and prolonged stress response can have serious effects on health.

What You Can Do to Avoid Noise Pollution

- Wear ear protectors when working around noisy machinery.
- When listening to music on a headset with a volume range of 1–10, keep the volume no louder than 4; your headset is too loud if you are unable to hear people around you speaking in a normal tone of voice.

Figure 23-7   The intensity of selected sounds.   Hearing damage can occur after 8 hours of exposure to sounds louder than 80 decibels; regular exposure for longer than 1 minute to more than 100 decibels can cause permanent hearing loss. Children may suffer damage to their hearing at lower levels of sound than adults.

- Avoid loud music. Don't sit or stand near speakers or amplifiers at a rock concert, and don't play a car radio or stereo so high that you can't hear the traffic.

The following list of statements relates to your effect on the environment. Put a checkmark next to the statements that are true for you.

_____ I ride my bike, walk, carpool, or use public transportation whenever possible.

_____ I keep my car tuned up and well maintained.

_____ My residence is well insulated.

_____ Where possible, I use compact fluorescent bulbs instead of incandescent bulbs.

_____ I turn off lights and appliances when they are not in use.

_____ I avoid turning on heat or air conditioning whenever possible.

_____ I run the washing machine, dryer, and dishwasher only when they have full loads.

_____ I run the clothes dryer only as long as it takes my clothes to dry.

_____ I dry my hair with a towel rather than a hair dryer.

_____ I keep my car's air conditioner in good working order and have it serviced by a service station that recycles CFCs.

_____ When shopping, I choose products with the least amount of packaging.

_____ I choose recycled and recyclable products.

_____ I avoid products packaged in plastic and unrecycled aluminum.

_____ I store food in glass jars and waxed paper rather than plastic wrap.

_____ I take my own bag along when I go shopping.

_____ I recycle newspapers, glass, cans, and other recyclables.

_____ When shopping, I read labels and try to buy the least toxic products available.

_____ I dispose of household hazardous wastes properly.

_____ I take showers instead of baths.

_____ I take short showers and switch off the water when I'm not actively using it.

_____ I do not run the water while brushing my teeth, shaving, or hand-washing clothes.

_____ My sinks have aerators installed in them.

_____ My shower has a low-flow showerhead.

_____ I have a water-saver toilet or a water displacement device in my toilet.

_____ I snip or rip plastic six-pack rings before I throw them out.

_____ When hiking or camping, I never leave anything behind.

Statements you have not checked can help you identify behaviors you can change to improve environmental health.

For an overall estimate of how much land and water your lifestyle requires, take the Ecological Footprint quiz (www.myfootprint.org).

• Avoid exposure to painfully loud sounds, and avoid repeated exposure to any sounds above 80 decibels.

HEALING THE ENVIRONMENT

Faced with a vast array of confusing and complex environmental issues, you may feel overwhelmed and conclude that there isn't anything you can do about global problems. But this is not true. If everyone made individual changes in his or her life, the impact would be tremendous. (To assess your current lifestyle, refer to the box "Environmental Health Checklist.")

At the same time, it is important to recognize that large corporations and manufacturers are the ones primarily responsible for environmental degradation. Many of them have jumped on the environmental bandwagon with public relations and advertising campaigns designed to make them look good, but they haven't changed their practices nearly enough to make a difference. To influence them, people have to become educated, demand changes in production methods, and elect people to office who consider environmental concerns along with sound business incentives.

Large-scale changes and individual actions complement each other. What you do every day *does* count. Following the suggestions in the What You Can Do sections throughout this chapter will help you make a difference in the environment. In addition, you can become a part of larger community actions to work for a healthier world:

• Share what you learn about environmental issues with your friends and family.

• Join, support, or volunteer your time to organizations working on environmental causes that are important to you.

• Contact your elected representatives and communicate your concerns. For guidelines on how to be heard, see the box "Making Your Letters Count."

It takes only a few minutes to write to an elected official, but it can make a difference on an environmental issue you care about. When elected officials receive enough letters or e-mails on an issue, it does influence their vote—they want to be re-elected, and your vote counts! To give your letter the greatest possible influence, use these guidelines:

- Use your own words and your own stationery.

- Be clear and concise. Keep your letter to one or two paragraphs, never more than one page.

- Focus on only one subject in each letter, and identify it clearly. Refer to legislation by its name or number.

- Request a specific action—vote a particular way on a piece of legislation, request hearings, cosponsor a bill—and state your reasons for your position.

- If you live or work in the legislator's district, say so.

- Courteous letters work best. Don't be insulting or unnecessarily critical.

You can send letters via regular mail; however, increased security screenings often delay delivery. You can e-mail the president or vice president at the following addresses:

president@whitehouse.gov

vice-president@whitehouse.gov

To locate the contact information for your United States senators and representatives, visit the following Web sites:

Senate: www.senate.gov

House of Representatives: www.house.gov/writerep

Environmental health involves protecting ourselves from environmental dangers and protecting the environment from the dangers we ourselves create. The two are intimately connected, and both require that we take responsibility for our actions every day.

Right now you can

- Turn off the lights in any unoccupied rooms.

- Plan to buy compact fluorescent lightbulbs to replace incandescent bulbs.

- Turn down the heat a few degrees and put on a sweater, or turn off the air conditioner and change into shorts.

- Make an appointment to have your car checked if it's not running well or needs a tune-up.

- Check your trash can for recyclable items—soda cans, plastic water bottles, white paper, magazines—and put aside any you find for recycling or put them in your recycling bins.

SUMMARY

- Environmental health encompasses all the interactions of humans with their environment and the health consequences of those interactions.

- Concerns with water quality focus on pathogenic organisms and hazardous chemicals from industry and households, as well as on water shortages.

- Sewage treatment prevents pathogens from contaminating drinking water; it often must also deal with heavy metals and hazardous chemicals.

- The amount of garbage is growing all the time; paper is the biggest component. Recycling can help solid waste disposal problems.

- The world's population is increasing rapidly, especially in the developing world. Factors that may eventually limit human population are food, availability of land and water, energy, and minimum acceptable standard of living.

- Increased amounts of air pollutants are especially dangerous for children, older adults, and people with chronic health problems.

- Factors contributing to the development of smog include heavy motor vehicle traffic, hot weather, stagnant air, and temperature inversion.

- Carbon dioxide and other natural gases act as a greenhouse around the earth, increasing the temperature of the atmosphere. Levels of these gases are rising through human activity; as a result, the world's climate could change.

- The ozone layer that shields the earth's surface from the sun's UV rays has thinned and developed holes in certain regions.

- Acid precipitation occurs when certain atmospheric pollutants combine with moisture in the air.

- Environmental damage from energy use can be limited through energy conservation and the development of nonpolluting, renewable sources of energy.

- Indoor pollutants can trigger allergies and illness in the short term and cancer in the long term.

- Potentially hazardous chemical pollutants include asbestos, lead, pesticides, mercury, and many household products. Proper handling and disposal are critical.

- Radiation can cause radiation sickness, chromosome damage, and cancer, among other health problems.
- Loud or persistent noise can lead to hearing loss and/or stress; two common sources of excessive noise are the workplace and rock concerts.
- Most health advances today must come from lifestyle changes and improvements in the global environment. The effects of personal changes made by every concerned individual could be tremendous.

Take Action

1. **Inventory household hazardous chemicals:** Find out what hazardous chemicals you have in your household. Read the labels for disposal instructions. If there aren't any instructions, call your local health department and ask how to dispose of specific chemicals. Also ask if there are hazardous waste disposal sites in your community or special pickup days. If possible, get rid of some or all of the hazardous chemicals in your home.

2. **Identify recycling resources:** Investigate the recycling facilities in your community. Find out how materials are recycled and what they are used for in their recycled state. If recycling isn't available in your community, contact your local city hall to find out how a recycling program can be started.

3. **Track your trash output:** Keep track of exactly how many bags (or gallons) of trash your household produces per week. Is it more or less than the national weekly average of 6.73 bags (87.5 gallons) per three-person household? In either case, try to reduce it by recycling, composting, and buying and using fewer disposable products.

4. **Organize a cleanup day:** With a group of fellow students or coworkers, participate in an environmental cleanup event in your community. Depending on where you live, you might clean up trash along a beach, a river, a public park, or a roadside. You can tie your event to Earth Day or International Cleanup Day, or simply choose a day that works for your group.

For More Information

Books

Cunningham, W. P., et al. 2004. *Environmental Science: A Global Concern.* 8th ed. New York: McGraw-Hill. *A nontechnical survey of basic environmental science and key concerns.*

Getis, J. 1999. *You Can Make a Difference: Be Environmentally Responsible,* 2nd ed. New York: McGraw-Hill. *Describes environmental problems and suggestions for individual action.*

Maslin, M., 2005. *Global Warming: A Very Short Introduction.* New York: Oxford University Press. *A survey of the science and politics of global warming.*

McCally, M., ed. 2002. *Life Support: The Environment and Human Health.* Cambridge, Mass.: MIT Press. *Describes how humans affect the environment and how environmental problems affect health.*

Nadakavukaren, A. 2000. *Our Global Environment: A Health Perspective,* 5th ed. Prospect Heights, Ill.: Waveland Press. *A broad survey of major environmental issues and their effects on personal and community health.*

Useful annual or biennial publications include the following:

National Wildlife Federation. 2005. *2005 Conservation Directory.* Washington, D.C.: National Wildlife Federation.

World Resources Institute. 2003. *World Resources 2002–2004.* Washington, D.C.: World Resources Institute.

Worldwatch Institute. 2005. *Vital Signs 2005.* New York: Norton.

ViW Organizations, Hotlines, and Web Sites

CDC National Center for Environmental Health. Provides brochures and fact sheets on a variety of environmental issues.
http://www.cdc.gov/nceh/default.htm

Earth Times. An international online newspaper devoted to global environmental issues.
http://www.earthtimes.org

Ecological Footprint. Calculates your personal ecological footprint based on your diet, transportation patterns, and living arrangements.
http://www.myfootprint.org

Energy Efficiency and Renewable Energy Network (EREN). U.S. Department of Energy. Provides information about alternative fuels and tips for saving energy at home and in your car.
http://www.eere.doe.gov

Fuel Economy. Provides information on the fuel economy of cars made since 1985 and tips on improving gas mileage.
http://www.fueleconomy.gov

Indoor Air Quality Information Hotline. Answers questions, provides publications, and makes referrals.
800-438-4318

National Lead Information Center. Provides information packets and specialist advice.
800-LEAD-FYI

National Oceanic and Atmospheric Administration (NOAA): Climate. Provides information on a variety of issues related to climate, including global warming, drought, and El Niño and La Niña.
http://www.noaa.gov/climate.html

National Safety Council Environmental Health Center. Provides information on lead, radon, indoor air quality, hazardous chemicals, and other environmental issues.
http://www.nsc.org/ehc.htm

Student Environmental Action Coalition (SEAC). A coalition of student and youth environmental groups; the Web site has contact information for local groups.
215-222-4711
http://www.seac.org

United Nations. Several U.N. programs are devoted to environmental problems on a global scale; the Web sites provide information on current and projected trends and on international treaties developed to deal with environmental issues.

http://www.un.org/popin (Population Division)

http://www.unep.org (Environment Programme)

U.S. Environmental Protection Agency (EPA). Provides information about EPA activities and many consumer-oriented materials. The Web site includes special sites devoted to global warming, ozone loss, pesticides, and other areas of concern.

http://www.epa.gov

Worldwatch Institute. A public policy research organization focusing on emerging global environmental problems and the links between the world economy and the environment.

http://www.worldwatch.org

There are many national and international organizations working on environmental health problems. A few of the largest and best known are listed below:

Greenpeace: 800-326-0959; http://www.greenpeace.org

National Audubon Society: 212-979-3000; http://www.audubon.org

National Wildlife Federation: 800-822-9919; http://www.nwf.org

Nature Conservancy: 800-628-6860; http://www.tnc.org

Sierra Club: 415-977-5500; http://www.sierraclub.org

Selected Bibliography

American Council for an Energy-Efficient Economy. 2005. *Green Book: Market Trends* (http://www.greenercars.org/gctext.html; retrieved March 1, 2005).

Bell, M. L., et al. 2004. Ozone and short-term mortality in 95 U.S. urban communities, 1987–2000. *Journal of the American Medical Association* 292(19): 2372–2378.

CDC National Center for Environmental Health. 2004. *Children's Blood Lead Levels in the United States* (http://www.cdc.gov/nceh/lead/research/kidsBLL.htm; retrieved March 6, 2005).

Centers for Disease Control and Prevention. 2004. Adult blood lead epidemiology and surveillance. *Morbidity and Mortality Weekly Report* 53(26): 578.

Centers for Disease Control and Prevention. 2004. Surveillance for waterborne-disease outbreaks. *MMWR Surveillance Summaries* 53(SS-8).

Donohoe, M. 2003. Causes and health consequences of environmental degradation and social injustice. *Social Science and Medicine* 56(3): 573–587.

Energy Information Administration. 2005. *Impacts of Modeled Recommendations of the National Commission on Energy Policy.* Washington, D.C.: U.S. Department of Energy.

Energy Information Agency. 2005. *Gasoline and Diesel Fuel Update* (http://tonto.eia.doe.gov/oog/info/gdu/gasdiesel.asp; retrieved April 17, 2005).

Environmental Protection Agency. 2004. *Superfund National Accomplishments Summary Fiscal Year 2004* (http://www.epa.gov/superfund/action/process/numbers04.htm; retrieved March 6, 2005).

Environmental Protection Agency. 2005. *Municipal Solid Waste: Basic Facts* (http://www.epa.gov.epaoswer/non-hw/muncpl/facts.htm; retrieved March 1, 2005).

Environmental Protection Agency. 2005. *The Particle Pollution Report: Current Understanding of Air Quality and Emissions through 2003* (http://www.epa.gov/airtrends/pm.html; retrieved March 1, 2005).

Gauderman, W. J., et al. 2004. The effect of air pollution on lung development from 10 to 18 years of age. *New England Journal of Medicine* 351(11): 1057–1067.

Intergovernmental Panel on Climate Change. 2001. *Climate Change 2001: Impacts, Adaptation and Vulnerability.* Geneva: Intergovernmental Panel on Climate Change.

Ivanov, V. K., et al. 2003. Thyroid cancer incidence among adolescents and adults in the Bryansk region of Russia following the Chernobyl accident. *Health Physics* 84(1): 46–60.

Kunzli, N., et al. 2005. Ambient air pollution and atherosclerosis in Los Angeles. *Environmental Health Perspectives* 113(2): 201–206.

NASA Goddard Institute for Space Studies. 2005. *Global Temperature Trends: 2004 Summation* (http://www.giss.nasa.gov/data/update/gistemp/2004; retrieved March 5, 2005).

Nash, D., et al. 2003. Blood lead, blood pressure, and hypertension in perimenopausal and postmenopausal women. *Journal of the American Medical Association* 289(12): 1523–1532.

National Oceanic and Atmospheric Administration. 2005. *Billion Dollar U.S. Weather Disasters, 1980–2004* (http://www.ncdc.noaa.gov/oa/reports/billionz.html; retrieved March 1, 2005).

National Oceanic and Atmospheric Administration. 2005. *Northern Hemisphere Winter Summary* (http://www.cpc.ncep.noaa.gov/products/stratosphere/winter_bulletins/nh_03-04/index.html; retrieved March 1, 2005).

Parmesan, C., G. Yohe. 2003. A globally coherent fingerprint of climate change impacts across natural systems. *Nature* 421(6918): 37–42

Parker, J. D., et al. 2005. Air pollution and birth weight among term infants in California. *Pediatrics* 115(1): 121–128.

Pope, C. A., et al. 2002. Lung cancer, cardiopulmonary mortality, and long-term exposure to fine particulate air pollution. *Journal of the American Medical Association* 287(9): 1132–1141.

Trasande, L., P. J. Landrigan, and C. Schechter. 2005. Public health and economic consequences of methylmercury toxicity to the developing brain. *Environmental Health Perspectives* online, February 28.

United Nations Population Division. 2005. *World Population Prospects: The 2004 Revision.* New York: United Nations.

U.S. Department of Health and Human Services. 2005. *Surgeon General Releases National Health Advisory on Radon* (http://www.surgeongeneral.gov/pressreleases/sg01132005.html; retrieved January 24, 2005).

Uysal, N., and R. M. Shapira. 2003. Effects of ozone on lung function and lung diseases. *Current Opinion in Pulmonary Medicine* 9(2): 144–150.

Virtanen, J. K., et al. 2005. Mercury, fish oils, and risk of acute coronary events and cardiovascular disease, coronary heart disease, and all-cause mortality in men in eastern Finland. *Arteriosclerosis, Thrombosis, and Vascular Biology* 25(1): 228–233.

World Health Organization. 2005. *International Decade for Action: Water for Life 2005–2015* (http://www.who.int/water_sanitation_health/2005advocguide/en/index1.html; retrieved March 6, 2005).

Worldwatch Institute. 2004. *Vital Signs 2004.* New York: Norton.

Nutritional Content of Popular Items from Fast-Food Restaurants

Arby's

	Serving size (g)	Calories	Protein (g)	Total fat (g)	Saturated fat (g)	Total carbohydrate (g)	Sugars (g)	Fiber (g)	Cholesterol (mg)	Sodium (mg)	Vitamin A	Vitamin C	Calcium	Iron	% calories from fat
											(% RDI)				
Regular roast beef	154	320	21	13	6	34	5	2	45	950	0	0	6	20	34
Super roast beef	241	440	22	19	7	48	11	3	45	1130	2	2	8	25	39
Junior roast beef	125	270	16	9	4	34	5	2	30	740	0	0	6	15	33
Chicken fingers (4 pack)	192	640	31	38	8	42	0	3	70	1590	0	0	2	15	55
Market Fresh® Ultimate BLT	293	780	23	46	9	75	18	6	50	1570	15	30	15	25	53
Market Fresh® Roast Turkey & Swiss	357	720	45	27	6	74	16	5	90	1790	8	4	35	30	35
Market Fresh® Low Carbys™ Southwest chicken wrap	259	550	35	30	9	45	1	30	75	1690	10	10	40	10	49
Martha's Vineyard™ salad (w/o dressing)	291	250	26	8	4.5	23	23	4	60	490	60	40	20	10	28
Raspberry vinaigrette	57	172	0	12	1.5	16	14	0	0	344	0	4	0	0	63
Santa Fe™ salad (w/o dressing)	328	520	27	29	9	40	6	5	60	1120	130	45	25	20	50
Curly fries – medium	128	410	5	22	3	47	N/A	5	0	950	8	10	6	10	49
Jalapeno Bites® – regular (5)	110	310	5	19	7	29	3	2	30	530	15	0	4	6	55

SOURCE: Arby's © 2005, Arby's, Inc. (http://www.arbysrestaurant.com). Used with permission of Arby's, Inc.

Burger King

	Serving size (g)	Calories	Protein (g)	Total fat (g)	Saturated fat (g)	Trans fat (g)	Total carbohydrate (g)	Sugars (g)	Fiber (g)	Cholesterol (mg)	Sodium (mg)	Vitamin A	Vitamin C	Calcium	Iron	% calories from fat
												% Daily Value				
Original WHOPPER®	291	700	31	42	13	1	52	8	4	85	1020	20	15	10	30	54
Original WHOPPER® w/o mayo	270	540	30	24	10	1	52	8	4	75	900	10	15	10	30	40
Original DOUBLE WHOPPER® w/cheese	399	1060	56	69	27	2.5	53	9	4	185	1540	25	15	30	45	59
Original WHOPPER JR.®	158	390	17	22	7	0.5	31	5	2	45	550	10	6	8	15	51
BK VEGGIE® Burger*	215	420	23	16	3	0	46	7	7	10	1090	20	10	10	20	34
Original chicken sandwich	204	560	25	28	6	2	52	5	3	60	1270	8	0	6	15	45
CHICKEN TENDERS® (8 pieces)	123	340	22	19	5	3.5	20	0	<1	50	840	2	0	2	4	50
French fries (medium, salted)	117	360	4	18	5	4.5	46	<1	4	0	640	0	15	2	4	45
Onion rings (medium)	91	320	4	16	4	3.5	40	5	3	0	460	0	0	10	0	45
Chili (w/o cheese or crackers)	217	190	13	8	3	0	17	5	5	25	1040	25	60	8	8	38
Fire-grilled chicken caesar salad (w/o dressing or toast)	286	190	25	7	3	0	9	1	1	50	900	85	40	15	8	33
CROISSAN'WICH® w/bacon, egg, and cheese	126	340	14	20	7	1.5	26	7	<1	200	920	8	0	15	10	53
HERSHEY®'S sundae pie	79	300	3	18	10	1.5	31	23	1	10	190	2	0	4	6	54
Chocolate Shake (medium)	397	600	10	18	11	0	97	94	2	70	470	15	6	45	8	27

* Burger King Corporation makes no claim that the BK VEGGIE® Burger or any of its products meets the requirements of a vegan or vegetarian diet.

SOURCE: BURGER KING® nutritional information used with permission from Burger King Brands, Inc.

Domino's Pizza

(1 serving = 2 of 8 slices or ¼ of 14-inch pizza; 2 of 8 slices or ¼ of 12-inch pizza; 1 6-inch pizza)

	Serving size	Calories	Protein	Total fat	Saturated fat	Total carbohydrate	Sugars	Fiber	Cholesterol	Sodium	Vitamin A	Vitamin C	Calcium	Iron	% calories from fat
	g		g	g	g	g	g	g	mg	mg	\% Daily Value				
14-inch lg. hand-tossed cheese	219	516	21	15	7	75	6	4	32	1080	18	0	26	23	26
14-inch lg. thin crust cheese	148	382	17	17	7	43	6	2	32	1172	18	0	32	8	40
14-inch lg. deep dish cheese	256	677	26	30	11	80	9	5	41	1575	21	<1	33	31	40
12-inch med. hand-tossed cheese	159	375	15	11	5	55	5	3	23	776	13	0	19	17	26
12-inch med. thin crust cheese	106	273	12	12	5	31	4	2	23	835	13	0	23	5	40
12-inch med. deep dish cheese	181	482	19	22	8	56	6	3	30	1123	15	<1	24	22	41
Toppings: pepperoni	*	98	5	9	3	<1	<1	<1	20	364	<1	<1	<1	2	83
ham	*	31	5	2	<1	<1	<1	<1	12	292	<1	<1	<1	1	58
Italian sausage	*	110	5	9	3	3	<1	<1	22	342	<1	<1	2	3	74
bacon	*	153	8	13	4	<1	<1	<1	22	424	0	15	<1	2	77
beef	*	111	6	10	4	<1	<1	<1	21	309	<1	0	<1	3	81
anchovies	*	45	9	2	<1	<1	<1	<1	18	791	<1	0	5	6	40
extra cheese	*	68	6	6	3	<1	<1	<1	15	228	6	0	12	<1	79
cheddar cheese	*	71	5	6	3	<1	<1	<1	18	110	4	0	13	<1	76
Barbeque buffalo wings (1 piece)	25	50	6	2	<1	2	1	<1	26	175	<1	<1	<1	2	36
Buffalo chicken kickers™ (1 piece)	24	47	4	2	<1	3	<1	<1	9	163	0	0	<1	0	38
Blue cheese sauce	42	223	1	23	4	2	2	<1	20	417	1	0	2	<1	93
Breadsticks (1 stick)	37	116	3	4	<1	18	1	1	0	152	<1	<1	5	5	31
Double cheesy bread	43	142	4	6	2	18	<1	1	6	183	2	<1	5	5	38

* Topping information is based on minimal portioning requirements for one serving of a 14-inch large pizza; add the values for toppings to the values for a cheese pizza. The following toppings supply fewer than 15 calories per serving: green and yellow peppers, onion, olives, mushrooms, pineapple.

SOURCE: Domino's Pizza, 2005 (http://www.dominos.com). © Domino's Pizza, 2004. Reproduced with permission from Domino's Pizza LLC.

Jack in the Box

	Serving size	Calories	Protein	Total fat	Saturated fat	Trans fat	Total carbohydrate	Sugars	Fiber	Cholesterol	Sodium	Vitamin A	Vitamin C	Calcium	Iron	% calories from fat
	g		g	g	g	g	g	g	g	mg	mg	\% Daily Value				
Breakfast Jack®	129	305	13	14	4	0.5	34	3	0	205	715	N/A	N/A	N/A	N/A	41
Supreme croissant	155	475	16	27	8.5	3.5	41	4	1	220	815	N/A	N/A	N/A	N/A	51
Hamburger	119	310	17	14	5	0	30	6	0	45	590	N/A	N/A	N/A	N/A	41
Jumbo Jack® w/cheese	306	695	24	41.5	16	1	55	11	2	70	1305	N/A	N/A	N/A	N/A	54
Sourdough Jack®	246	715	26	51	18	2.5	36	7	2	75	1165	N/A	N/A	N/A	N/A	64
Chicken fajita pita	247	315	22	9	4	0	33	4	0	65	1080	N/A	N/A	N/A	N/A	26
Sourdough grilled chicken club	249	505	29	27	6.5	1.5	35	4	2	75	1220	N/A	N/A	N/A	N/A	48
Deli Trio Pannido™	271	645	30	34	8.5	0	53	4	2	95	2530	N/A	N/A	N/A	N/A	47
Jack's Spicy Chicken®	270	615	24	30.5	5.5	2.5	62	7	3	50	1090	N/A	N/A	N/A	N/A	45
Monster taco	110	240	8	14	5	2	20	4	3	20	390	N/A	N/A	N/A	N/A	53
Egg rolls (3)	198	445	14	19	6	3	55	10	6	15	1080	N/A	N/A	N/A	N/A	0
Chicken breast strips (5)	226	630	35	38	8	6	39	1	3	90	1470	N/A	N/A	N/A	N/A	54
Stuffed jalapeños (7)	168	530	15	30	13	4.5	51	5	4	45	1600	N/A	N/A	N/A	N/A	51
Barbeque dipping sauce	28	45	0	0	0	0	11	4	0	0	330	N/A	N/A	N/A	N/A	0
Seasoned curly fries (medium)	125	400	6	23	5	7	45	1	5	0	890	N/A	N/A	N/A	N/A	52
Onion rings	119	500	6	30	6	10	51	3	3	0	420	N/A	N/A	N/A	N/A	54
Side salad	164	155	5	7.5	2.5	0.5	16	3	0	10	290	N/A	N/A	N/A	N/A	44
Ranch dressing	71	390	1	41	6	0	4	2	0	30	590	N/A	N/A	N/A	N/A	95
Oreo® cookie ice-cream shake (small)	301	670	11	33	19	3	81	62	1	110	350	N/A	N/A	N/A	N/A	45

SOURCE: Jack in the Box, Inc. 2005 (http://www.jackinthebox.com). The following trademarks are owned by Jack in the Box, Inc.: Breakfast Jack,® Jumbo Jack,® Sourdough Jack,® Jack in the Box.® Reproduced with permission from Jack in the Box, Inc.

KFC

	Serving size (g)	Calories	Protein (g)	Total fat (g)	Saturated fat (g)	Trans fat (g)	Total carbohydrate (g)	Sugars (g)	Fiber (g)	Cholesterol (mg)	Sodium (mg)	Vitamin A	Vitamin C	Calcium	Iron	% calories from fat
													% Daily Value			
Original Recipe® breast	161	380	40	19	6	2.5	11	0	0	145	1150	0	0	0	6	45
Original Recipe® thigh	126	360	22	25	7	1.5	12	0	0	165	1060	0	0	0	6	63
Extra Crispy™ breast	162	460	34	28	8	4.5	19	0	0	135	1230	0	0	0	8	55
Extra Crispy™ thigh	114	370	21	26	7	3	12	0	0	120	710	0	0	0	6	63
Hot & Spicy breast	179	460	33	27	8	N/A	20	0	0	130	1450	0	0	0	6	53
Hot & Spicy thigh	128	400	22	28	8	N/A	14	0	0	125	1240	0	0	0	8	63
Tender Roast® sandwich w/sauce	196	390	31	19	4	0.5	24	0	1	70	810	0	0	4	10	44
Tender Roast® sandwich w/o sauce	177	260	31	5	1.5	0.5	23	0	1	65	690	0	0	4	10	17
Hot Wings™ (6)	134	450	24	29	6	4	23	1	1	145	1120	6	6	8	10	58
Colonel's Crispy Strips® (3)	151	400	29	24	5	4.5	17	0	0	75	1250	0	6	0	10	54
Popcorn chicken (large)	170	650	29	43	10	7	38	0	0	70	1530	0	4	4	35	60
Chicken pot pie	423	770	33	40	15	14	70	2	5	115	1680	200	0	0	20	47
Corn on the cob (5.5")	162	150	5	3	1	0	26	10	7	0	10	0	10	6	6	18
Mashed potatoes w/gravy	136	130	2	4.5	1	0.5	18	1	1	0	380	2	4	0	2	34
Baked beans	136	230	8	1	1	0.25	46	22	7	0	720	8	6	15	30	4
Cole slaw	130	190	1	11	2	0.25	22	13	3	5	300	25	40	4	0	52
Biscuit (1)	57	190	2	10	2	3.5	23	1	0	1.5	580	0	0	0	4	47
Potato salad	128	180	2	9	1.5	0.25	22	5	1	5	470	0	10	0	2	45

SOURCE: KFC Corporation, 2005. Nutritional information provided by KFC Corporation from its website www.kfc.com as of April 2005 and subject to the conditions listed therein. KFC and related marks are registered trademarks of KFC Corporation. Reproduced with permission from Kentucky Fried Chicken Corporation.

McDonald's

	Serving size (g)	Calories	Protein (g)	Total fat (g)	Saturated fat (g)	Trans fat (g)	Total carbohydrate (g)	Sugars (g)	Fiber (g)	Cholesterol (mg)	Sodium (mg)	Vitamin A	Vitamin C	Calcium	Iron	% calories from fat
													% Daily Value			
Hamburger	105	260	13	9	3.5	0.5	33	7	1	30	530	2	2	15	15	31
Quarter Pounder®	171	420	24	18	7	1	40	8	3	70	730	2	2	15	25	46
Quarter Pounder® w/cheese	199	510	29	25	12	1.5	43	9	3	95	1150	10	2	30	25	43
Big Mac®	219	560	25	30	10	1.5	46	8	3	80	1010	8	2	25	25	48
Big N' Tasty®	232	520	24	29	9	1.5	41	8	3	80	730	8	10	15	25	50
Filet-O-Fish®	141	400	14	18	4	1	42	8	1	40	640	2	0	15	10	40
McChicken®	147	420	15	22	4.5	1	41	5	1	45	760	0	2	15	15	48
Medium French Fries	114	350	4	16	3	4	47	0	5	0	220	0	10	2	6	43
Chicken McNuggets® (6 pieces)	96	250	15	15	3	1.5	15	0	0	35	670	2	2	2	4	52
Chicken Select® Premium Breast Strips (5 pieces)	221	630	39	33	6	4.5	46	0	0	90	1550	0	6	4	8	48
Tangy Honey Mustard Sauce	43	70	1	2	0	0	13	9	1	0	160	0	0	0	1	29
Bacon Ranch Salad w/Grilled Chicken (w/o dressing)	288	240	31	9	4	0	11	4	3	85	940	90	50	15	10	33
Caesar Salad w/Crispy Chicken (w/o dressing)	284	300	24	14	4.5	1.5	22	3	3	50	910	90	50	20	10	40
California Cobb Salad (w/o chicken and dressing)	214	150	11	9	4	0	7	4	3	85	400	100	45	15	8	53
Newman's Own® Ranch Dressing (2 oz)	56	170	1	15	2.5	0	9	4	0	20	530	0	0	4	0	76
Egg McMuffin®	138	290	17	11	4.5	0	30	2	2	235	850	10	2	30	15	34
Sausage Biscuit w/Egg	162	500	18	32	10	5	36	2	1	250	1080	6	0	8	20	58
Hotcakes (2 pats margarine & syrup)	228	600	9	17	4	4	102	45	2	20	620	8	0	15	15	27
Fruit 'n Yogurt Parfait	149	160	4	2	1	0	31	21	<1	5	85	0	15	15	4	13
Chocolate Triple Thick® Shake (16 oz)	448	580	13	14	8	1	102	84	<1	50	250	20	0	45	10	21

SOURCE: McDonald's Corporation, 2005 (http://www.mcdonalds.com). Used with permission from McDonald's Corporation.

Subway
Based on standard formulas with 6-inch subs on Italian or wheat bread

	Serving size	Calories	Protein	Total fat	Saturated fat	Trans fat	Total carbohydrate	Sugars	Fiber	Cholesterol	Sodium	Vitamin A	Vitamin C	Calcium	Iron	% calories from fat
	g		g	g	g	g	g	g	g	mg	mg		% Daily Value			
Italian BMT®	243	450	23	21	8	0	47	8	4	55	1790	8	30	15	25	42
Meatball Marinara	377	560	24	24	11	1	63	13	7	45	1610	15	50	20	40	39
Subway® Seafood Sensation	250	450	16	22	6	0.5	51	8	5	25	1150	8	30	15	25	44
Cheese steak	250	360	24	10	4.5	0	47	9	5	35	1090	8	30	15	45	25
Subway® melt	320	450	36	14	6	0	51	9	4	70	2330	8	30	15	30	28
Classic tuna	250	530	22	31	7	0	45	7	4	45	1030	8	30	10	30	53
Sweet onion chicken teriyaki	281	370	26	5	1.5	0	59	19	4	50	1220	6	40	8	25	12
Roast beef	224	290	19	5	2	0	45	8	4	20	920	4	30	6	30	16
Turkey breast	224	280	18	4.5	1.5	0	46	7	4	20	1020	4	30	4	25	14
Veggie Delite®	167	230	9	3	1	0	44	7	4	0	520	4	30	6	25	12
Turkey breast deli	152	210	13	3.5	1.5	0	36	4	3	15	730	4	15	10	25	15
Chicken Bacon Ranch Wrap (w/cheese)	256	440	41	27	10	0	18	1	9	90	1670	10	15	30	15	55
Turkey breast wrap	184	190	24	6	1	0	18	2	9	20	1290	4	10	10	15	28
Bacon and egg breakfast sandwich on Deli round	123	320	15	15	4.5	n/a	34	3	3	190	520	6	6	8	25	42
Grilled chicken & baby spinach salad (w/o dressing)	300	140	20	3	1	0	11	4	4	50	450	200	80	10	20	19
Tuna (w/cheese) salad (w/o dressing)	404	360	16	29	6	0.5	12	5	4	45	600	70	50	15	15	73
New England clam chowder	240	110	5	3.5	0.5	n/a	16	1	1	10	990	2	2	10	4	29
Chili con carne	240	240	15	10	5	0	23	14	8	15	860	15	0	6	10	38
Sunrise refresher (small)	341	120	1	0	0	0	29	28	1	0	20	4	210	2	0	0
Choclate chip cookie	45	210	2	10	4	1	30	18	1	15	160	4	0	0	6	43

SOURCE: Subway U.S. Nutrition Info as found on http://www.subway.com, 4/5/2005. Reprinted by permission of Subway.

Taco Bell

	Serving size	Calories	Protein	Total fat	Saturated fat	Trans fat	Total carbohydrate	Sugars	Fiber	Cholesterol	Sodium	Vitamin A	Vitamin C	Calcium	Iron	% calories from fat
	g		g	g	g	g	g	g	g	mg	mg		% Daily Value			
Taco	78	170	8	10	4	0.5	13	1	1	25	350	4	2	6	6	53
Taco Supreme®	113	220	9	14	7	1	14	2	1	35	360	8	6	8	6	57
Soft taco, beef	99	210	10	10	4	1	21	2	1	25	620	4	2	10	8	43
Gordita Supreme,® steak	153	290	16	13	5	0.5	28	7	2	35	520	6	6	10	15	37
Gordita Baja,® chicken	153	320	17	15	3.5	0	29	7	2	40	690	6	6	10	10	42
Gordita Baja,® chicken "Fresco Style"	153	230	15	6	1	0	29	7	2	25	570	6	10	6	10	23
Chalupa Supreme, beef	153	390	14	24	10	3	31	4	1	35	600	8	6	15	8	55
Chalupa Supreme, chicken	153	370	17	20	8	3	30	4	1	45	530	6	8	10	6	49
Bean burrito	198	370	14	10	3.5	2	55	4	8	10	1200	10	8	20	15	24
Burrito Supreme,® chicken	248	410	21	14	6	2	50	5	5	45	1270	15	15	20	15	31
Grilled stuffed burrito, beef	325	720	27	33	11	3.5	79	6	7	55	2090	15	6	35	25	41
Tostada	170	250	11	10	4	5	29	2	7	15	710	10	8	15	8	36
Zesty Chicken Border Bowl™ w/dressing	418	730	23	42	9	4	65	5	12	45	1640	20	15	15	20	52
Fiesta taco salad	548	870	31	47	16	9	80	10	12	65	1780	20	20	40	35	49
Steak quesadilla	184	540	26	31	14	2	40	4	3	70	1370	15	2	50	15	52
Nachos Supreme	195	450	13	26	9	5	42	3	5	35	810	8	8	10	10	58
Nachos BellGrande®	308	780	20	43	13	10	80	5	11	35	1300	8	8	20	15	50
Pintos 'n cheese	128	180	10	7	3.5	1	20	1	6	15	700	10	6	15	6	35
Mexican rice	131	210	6	10	4	1.5	23	1	3	15	740	20	8	10	10	43

SOURCE: Taco Bell Corporation, 2005 (http://www.tacobell.com). Reproduced courtesy of Taco Bell Corporation.

A
Wendy's

	Serving size g	Calories	Protein g	Total fat g	Saturated fat g	Trans fat g	Total carbohydrate g	Sugars g	Fiber g	Cholesterol mg	Sodium mg	Vitamin A	Vitamin C	Calcium	Iron	% calories from fat
												% Daily Value				
Classic Single® w/everything	218	410	25	19	7	1	37	8	2	70	910	N/A	N/A	N/A	N/A	42
Big Bacon Classic®	282	580	33	29	12	1.5	45	11	3	95	1430	N/A	N/A	N/A	N/A	45
Jr. hamburger	117	270	15	9	3.5	0.5	34	7	2	30	610	N/A	N/A	N/A	N/A	30
Jr. bacon cheeseburger	165	380	20	19	7	1	34	6	2	55	830	N/A	N/A	N/A	N/A	45
Ultimate Chicken Grill Sandwich	225	360	31	7	1.5	0	44	11	2	75	1100	N/A	N/A	N/A	N/A	18
Spicy Chicken Fillet Sandwich	225	510	29	19	3.5	1.5	57	8	2	55	1480	N/A	N/A	N/A	N/A	34
Homestyle Chicken Fillet Sandwich	230	540	29	22	4	1.5	57	2	2	55	1320	N/A	N/A	N/A	N/A	37
Caesar side salad (no toppings or dressing)	99	70	6	4.5	2	0	2	1	1	10	190	N/A	N/A	N/A	N/A	58
Chicken BLT salad (no toppings or dressing)	376	360	34	19	9	0.5	10	4	4	95	1140	N/A	N/A	N/A	N/A	48
Taco Supremo salad (no toppings or dressing)	495	360	27	16	8	1	29	8	8	65	1090	N/A	N/A	N/A	N/A	40
Creamy ranch dressing	64	230	1	23	4	0.5	5	3	0	15	580	N/A	N/A	N/A	N/A	90
Reduced fat creamy ranch dressing	64	100	1	8	1.5	0	6	3	1	15	550	N/A	N/A	N/A	N/A	72
Biggie® fries	159	440	5	19	3.5	5	63	0	7	0	380	N/A	N/A	N/A	N/A	39
Baked potato w/broccoli & cheese	411	440	10	15	3	0	70	6	9	10	540	N/A	N/A	N/A	N/A	31
Baked potato w/bacon & cheese	380	560	16	25	7	0	67	6	7	35	910	N/A	N/A	N/A	N/A	40
Chili, small, plain	227	200	17	5	2	0	21	5	5	35	870	N/A	N/A	N/A	N/A	23
Chili, large w/cheese	357	370	29	13	6.5	0	32	7	7	65	1420	N/A	N/A	N/A	N/A	32
Crispy Chicken Nuggets™ (5)	75	220	10	14	3	1.5	13	0	0	35	490	N/A	N/A	N/A	N/A	57
Barbecue sauce (1 packet)	28	40	1	0	0	0	10	5	0	0	160	N/A	N/A	N/A	N/A	0
Frosty,™ medium	298	430	10	11	7	0	74	55	0	45	200	N/A	N/A	N/A	N/A	23

SOURCE: Wendy's International, Inc., 2004 (http://www.wendys.com). Reproduced with permission from Wendy's International, Inc. The information contained in Wendy's Nutritional Information is effective as of March, 2005. Wendy's International, Inc., its subsidiaries, affiliates, franchisees and employees do not assume responsibility for a particular sensitivity or allergy (including peanuts, nuts or other allergies) to any food product provided in our restaurants. We encourage anyone with food sensitivities, allergies, or special dietary needs to check on a regular basis with Wendy's Consumer Relations Department to obtain the most up-to-date information.

Information on additional foods and restaurants is available online; see the Web sites listed with the tables in this appendix and the following additional sites: **Hardees:** http://www.hardees.com   **White Castle:** http://www.whitecastle.com

B A Self-Care Guide for Common Medical Problems

This self-care guide will help you manage some of the most common symptoms and medical problems:

- Fever
- Sore throat
- Cough
- Nasal congestion
- Ear problems
- Nausea, vomiting, or diarrhea
- Heartburn and indigestion
- Headache
- Low-back pain
- Strains and sprains
- Cuts and scrapes

Each symptom is described here in terms of what is going on in your body. Most symptoms are part of the body's natural healing response and reflect your body's wisdom in attempting to correct disease. Self-care advice is also given, along with some guidelines about when to seek professional advice. In most cases, the symptoms are self-limiting; that is, they will resolve on their own with time and simple self-care strategies.

No medical advice is perfect. You will always have to make the decision about whether to self-treat or get professional help. This guide is intended to provide you with more information so you can make better, more informed decisions. If the advice here differs from that of your physician, discuss the differences with him or her. In most cases, your physician will be able to customize the advice to your individual medical situation.

The guidelines given here apply to *generally healthy adults*. If you are pregnant or nursing or if you have a chronic disease, particularly one that requires medication, check with your physician for appropriate self-care advice. Additionally, if you have an allergy or suspected allergy to any recommended medication, check with your physician before using it.

If you have several symptoms, read about your primary symptom first and then proceed to secondary symptoms. Use your common sense when determining self-care. If you are particularly concerned about a symptom or confused about how to manage it, call your physician to get more information.

FEVER

A fever is an abnormally high body temperature, usually over 100°F (37.7°C). It is most commonly a sign that your body is fighting an infection. Fever may also be due to an inflammation, an injury, or a drug reaction. Chemicals released into your bloodstream during an infection reset the thermostat in the hypothalamus of your brain. The message goes out to your body to turn up the heat. The blood vessels in your skin constrict, and you curl up and throw on extra blankets to reduce heat loss. Meanwhile, your muscles begin to shiver to

generate additional body heat. The resulting rise in body temperature is a fever. Later, when your brain senses that the temperature is too high, the signal goes out to increase sweating. As the sweat evaporates, it carries heat away from the body surface.

A fever may not be all bad; it may even help you fight infections by making the body less hospitable to bacteria and viruses. A high body temperature appears to bolster the immune system and may inhibit the growth of infectious microorganisms.

Most generally healthy people can tolerate a fever as high as 103–104°F (39.5–40°C) without problems. Therefore, if you are essentially healthy, there is little need to reduce a fever unless you are very uncomfortable. Older adults and those with chronic health problems such as heart disease may not tolerate the increased metabolic demand of a high fever, and fever reduction may be advised.

Most problems with fevers are due to the excessive loss of fluids from evaporation and sweating, which may cause dehydration.

Self-Assessment

1. If you are sick, take your temperature several times throughout the day. Oral temperatures should not be measured for at least 10 minutes after smoking, eating, or drinking a hot or cold liquid. Mercury-containing glass thermometers are no longer recommended because of safety concerns; digital thermometers are accurate, easy to read, and relatively inexpensive. Follow the directions that came with your thermometer.

"Normal" temperature varies from person to person, so it is important to know what is normal for you. Your normal temperature will also vary throughout the day, being lowest in the early evening. If you exercise or if it is a hot day, your temperature may normally rise. Women's body temperature typically varies by a degree or more through the menstrual cycle, peaking around the time of ovulation. Rectal temperatures normally run about 0.5–1.0°F higher than oral temperatures. If your recorded temperature is more than 1.0–1.5°F above your normal baseline temperature, you have a fever.

2. Watch for signs of dehydration: excessive thirst; very dry mouth; infrequent urination with dark, concentrated urine; and light-headedness.

Self-Care

1. Drink plenty of fluids to prevent dehydration—at least 8 ounces of water, juice, or broth every 2 hours.

2. Take a sponge bath using lukewarm water; this will increase evaporation and help reduce body temperature naturally. Don't use alcohol rubs to reduce temperature.

3. Don't bundle up. This decreases the body's ability to lose excess heat.

4. Take aspirin substitute (acetaminophen, ibuprofen, or naproxen sodium). For adults, two standard-size tablets every 4–6 hours can be used to reduce the fever and the associated headache and achiness. Do not use aspirin in anyone younger than age 20 because some younger people with chicken pox, influenza, or other viral infections have developed a life-threatening complication, Reye's syndrome, after taking aspirin.

When to Call the Physician

1. Fever over 104°F (40°C), or 102°F (38.8°C) if over 60 years old

2. Persistent fever: 102° (38.8°C) or higher for 2 full days; 101° (38.3°C) or higher for 3 full days; or 100° or higher for 4 full days

3. Recurrent unexplained fevers

4. Fever accompanied by a rash, stiff neck, severe headache, difficulty breathing, cough with brown sputum, severe pain in the side or abdomen, painful urination, convulsions, or mental confusion

5. Fever with signs of dehydration

6. Fever after starting a new medication

SORE THROAT

A sore throat is caused by inflammation of the throat lining resulting from an infection, allergy, or irritation (especially from cigarette smoke). If you have an infection, you may also notice some hoarseness from swelling of the vocal cords and "swollen glands," which are enlarged lymph nodes that produce white blood cells to help fight the infection. The lymph nodes, part of your body's defense system, may become tender and remain swollen for weeks after the infection subsides.

Most throat infections are caused by viruses, so antibiotics are not effective against them. However, about 20–30% of throat infections are due to streptococcal bacteria. This type of microbe can cause complications such as rheumatic fever and rheumatic heart disease and therefore should be diagnosed by a physician and treated with antibiotics. Strep throat is usually characterized by very sore throat, high fever, swollen lymph nodes, a whitish discharge at the back of the throat, and the absence of other cold symptoms such as a cough and runny nose (which suggest a viral infection). Allergy-related sore throats are usually accompanied by running nose, sneezing, and watery, itchy eyes.

Self-Assessment

1. Take your temperature.

2. Look at the back of your throat in a mirror. Is there a whitish, puslike discharge on the tonsils or in the back of the throat?

3. Feel the front and back of your neck. Do you feel enlarged, tender lymph nodes?

Self-Care

1. If you smoke, stop smoking to avoid further irritation of your throat.

2. Drink plenty of liquids to soothe your inflamed throat.

3. Gargle with warm salt water (¼ tsp salt in 4 oz water) every 1–2 hours to help reduce swelling and discomfort.

4. Suck on throat lozenges, cough drops, or hard candies to keep your throat moist.

5. Use throat lozenges, sprays, or gargles that contain an anesthetic to temporarily numb your throat and make swallowing less painful.

6. Try aspirin substitute to ease throat pain.

7. For an allergy-related sore throat, try an antihistamine such as chlorpheniramine or lorantodine.

When to Call the Physician

1. Great difficulty swallowing saliva or breathing

2. Sore throat with fever over 101°F (38.3°C), especially if you do not have other cold symptoms such as nasal congestion or a cough

3. Sore throat with a skin rash

4. Sore throat with whitish pus on the tonsils

5. Sore throat and recent contact with a person who has had a positive throat culture for strep

6. Enlarged lymph nodes lasting longer than 3 weeks

7. Hoarseness lasting longer than 3 weeks

COUGH

A cough is a protective mechanism of the body to help keep the airways clear. There are two types of cough: a dry cough (without mucus) and a productive cough (with mucus). Common causes of cough include infection (viral or bacterial), allergies, and irritation from smoking and pollutants. If you have a cold, the cough may be the last symptom to improve, because the airways may remain irritated for several weeks after the infection has resolved.

Your airways are lined with hairlike projections called cilia, which move back and forth to help clear the airways of mucus, germs, and dust. Infections and cigarette smoking paralyze and damage this vital defensive mechanism.

Self-Assessment

1. Take your temperature.

2. Observe your mucus. Thick brown or bloody mucus suggests a bacterial infection.

Self-Care

1. If you are a smoker, stop smoking. Smoking irritates the airways and undermines your body's immune defenses, leading to more serious infections and longer-lasting symptoms. Most people do not feel like smoking when they have a cold with a cough. If you want to quit, a cold may provide an excellent opportunity to do so.

2. Drink plenty of liquids (at least six 8-ounce glasses a day) to help thin mucus and loosen chest congestion.

3. Use moist heat from a hot shower or vaporizer to help loosen chest congestion.

4. Suck on cough drops, throat lozenges, or hard candy to keep your throat moist and help relieve a dry, tickling cough.

5. If you have a dry, nonproductive cough or the cough keeps you from sleeping, you can use a cough syrup or lozenge that contains the nonprescription cough suppressant dextromethorphan. Because a cough that produces mucus is protective, it is generally not advisable to suppress a productive cough.

When to Call the Physician

1. Cough with thick brown or bloody sputum

2. Cough with high fever—above 102°F (38.8°C)—and shaking chills

3. Severe chest pains, wheezing, or shortness of breath

4. Cough that lasts longer than 3 weeks

NASAL CONGESTION

Nasal congestion is most commonly caused by infection or allergies. With infection, the nasal passages become congested because of increased blood flow and mucus production. This congestion is actually part of the body's defense to fight infection. The increased blood flow raises the temperature of the nasal passages, making them less hospitable to germs. The nasal secretions are rich in white blood cells and antibodies to help fight and neutralize the invading organisms and flush them away. Nasal congestion associated with sore throat, cough, and fever usually indicates a viral infection. Green nasal discharge is common with viral infections; it does not mean you need an antibiotic.

Nasal congestion caused by allergies is often accompanied by a thin watery discharge, sneezing, and itchy eyes; it is sometimes associated with a seasonal pattern. In an allergic reaction, the offending allergen (such as pollen, dust, mold, or dander) triggers the release of histamine and other chemicals from the cells lining the nose, throat, and eyes. These chemicals cause swelling, discharge, and itching. Antihistamine drugs block the release of these irritating chemicals.

Self-Assessment

1. Take your temperature.

2. Observe the color and consistency of your nasal secretions. A thick brown or bloody discharge suggests a bacterial sinus infection.

3. Tap with your fingers over the sinus cavities above and below the eyes. If the tapping causes increased pain, you may have a bacterial sinus infection.

Self-Care

1. If you smoke, stop smoking to prevent continuing irritation of the nasal passages.

2. Use moist heat from a hot shower or vaporizer to help liquefy congested mucus.

3. Use a decongestant nasal spray or drops to temporarily relieve congestion. However, if these decongestants are used for more than 3 days, they can cause "rebound congestion" that actually creates more nasal congestion. As an alternative, use saltwater nose drops (1/4 tsp salt in 1/2 cup boiled water, cooled before using) several times a day.

4. Try an oral decongestant such as pseudoephedrine (60 mg every 6 hours) to help shrink swollen mucous membranes and open nasal passages. In some people, these medications can cause nervousness, sleeplessness, or heart palpitations. If you have uncontrolled high blood pressure, heart disease, or diabetes, check with your physician before using decongestants.

When to Call the Physician

1. Nasal congestion with severe pain and tenderness in the forehead, cheeks, or upper teeth and a high fever (above 102°F or 38.8°C)

2. Thick brown or bloody nasal discharge

3. Nasal congestion and discharge unresponsive to self-care treatment and lasting longer than 3 weeks

EAR PROBLEMS

Ear symptoms include earache, discharge, itching, stuffiness, and hearing loss. They may be caused by problems in the external ear canal, eardrum, middle ear, or eustachian tube (the passageway that connects the middle ear space to the back of the throat). The ear canal can become blocked by excess wax, producing hearing loss and a sense that the ear is plugged. An infection of the external ear canal due to excessive moisture and trauma is often referred to as "swimmer's ear." It can cause pain, a sense of fullness, discharge, and itching. Congestion and blockage of the eustachian tube by a cold or allergy can result in pain, a sense of fullness, and hearing loss. A middle ear infection often produces severe pain, hearing loss, and fever.

Self-Assessment

1. Take your temperature. A fever may be a sign of infection.

2. Have someone look into the ear canal with a flashlight or otoscope. Look for wax blockage or a red, swollen canal indicating an external ear infection.

3. Wiggle the outer part of the ear. If this increases the pain, an infection or inflammation of the external canal is the likely cause.

Self-Care

1. If blockage of the ear canal with wax is the problem, first try a hot shower to liquefy the wax, and use a wash cloth to wipe out the ear canal. You can also use a few drops of an over-the-counter wax softener and then flush the canal gently with warm water in a bulb syringe. Do not use sharp objects or cotton swabs; they can scratch the canal or push the wax in deeper.

2. To treat mild infections of the external ear canal, you must thoroughly dry the ear canal. A few drops of a drying solution (1 part rubbing alcohol, 1 part white vinegar) on a piece of cotton gently inserted into the canal can act as a wick to dry the canal.

3. To relieve congestion and blockage of the eustachian tube, try a decongestant like pseudoephedrine or a nasal spray (but for no longer than 3 days). Hot showers or a vaporizer may help loosen secretions, and yawning or swallowing may help open the eustachian tube. For a mild plugging sensation without fever or pain, pinch your nostrils and blow gently to force air up the eustachian tube and "pop" your ears.

When to Call the Physician

1. Severe earache with fever

2. Puslike or bloody discharge from the ear

3. Sudden hearing loss, especially if accompanied by ear pain or recent trauma to the ear

4. Ringing in the ears or dizziness

5. Any ear symptom lasting longer than 2 weeks

NAUSEA, VOMITING, OR DIARRHEA

Nausea, vomiting, and diarrhea usually are defensive reactions of your body to rapidly clear your digestive tract of irritants. These symptoms may be caused by a viral infection, foodborne illness, medications, or other types of infection. Vomiting dramatically ejects irritants from your stomach, and nausea discourages eating to allow the stomach to rest. With diarrhea, overstimulated intestines flush out the offending irritants.

The major complications of vomiting and diarrhea are dehydration from fluid losses and decreased fluid intake and a risk of bleeding from irritation of the digestive tract.

Self-Assessment

1. Take your temperature. A fever is often a clue that an infection is causing the symptoms.

2. Note the color and frequency of vomiting and diarrhea. This will help you estimate the severity of fluid losses and check for bleeding (red, black, or "coffee grounds" material in the stool or vomit; iron tablets and Pepto-Bismol can also cause black stools).

3. Watch for signs of dehydration: very dry mouth; excessive thirst; infrequent urination with dark, concentrated urine; and light-headedness.

4. Look for signs of hepatitis, an infection of the liver: a yellow color in the skin and the white parts of the eyes.

Self-Care

1. To replace fluids, take frequent, small sips of clear liquids such as water, noncitrus juice, broths, flat ginger ale, or ice chips.

2. When the vomiting and diarrhea have subsided, try nonirritating, constipating foods like the BRAT diet: bananas, rice, applesauce, and toast.

3. For several days, avoid alcohol, milk products, fatty foods, aspirin, and other medications that might irritate the stomach. Do not stop taking regularly prescribed medications without discussing this change with your physician.

4. Medications are not usually advised for vomiting. Loperamide, available without a prescription, can be used to ease diarrhea.

When to Call the Physician

1. Inability to retain any fluids for 12 hours or signs of dehydration

2. Severe abdominal pains not relieved by the vomiting or diarrhea

3. Blood in the vomit (red or "coffee grounds" material) or in the stool (red or black tarlike material)

4. Vomiting or diarrhea with a high fever (above 102°F or 38.8°C)

5. Yellow color in skin or white parts of the eyes

6. Vomiting with severe headache and a history of a recent head injury

7. Vomiting or diarrhea that lasts 3 days without improvement

8. If you are pregnant or have diabetes

9. Recurrent vomiting and/or diarrhea

HEARTBURN AND INDIGESTION

Indigestion and heartburn are usually a result of irritation of the stomach or the esophagus, the tube that connects the mouth to the stomach. The stomach lining is usually protected from stomach acids, but the esophagus is not. Therefore, if stomach acids "reflux," or back up into the esophagus, the result is usually a burning discomfort beneath the breastbone. The esophagus is normally protected by a muscular valve that allows food to enter the stomach but prevents stomach contents from flowing upward into the esophagus. Certain foods (such as chocolate), medications, and smoking can loosen and open this protective sphincter valve. Overeating, lying down, or bending over can also cause the stomach acids to gain access to the sensitive lining of the esophagus.

Self-Assessment

1. Look for a pattern in the symptoms. Do they occur after eating certain foods, taking certain medications, or when you bend over or lie down? Do certain foods or an antacid relieve the symptoms?

2. Observe your bowel movements. Black tarlike stools may indicate bleeding in the stomach (iron tablets and Pepto-Bismol can also cause black stools).

Self-Care

1. Avoid irritants such as smoking, aspirin, ibuprofen, naproxen sodium, alcohol, caffeine (coffee, tea, cola), chocolate, onions, carbonated beverages, spicy or fatty foods, acidic

foods (vinegar, citrus fruits, tomatoes), or any other foods that seem to make your symptoms worse.

2. Take nonabsorbable antacids such as Maalox, Mylanta, or Gelusil every 1–2 hours and especially before bedtime, or try an acid reducer, now available without a prescription (Pepcid, Tagamet, Zantac, or Prilosec).

3. Avoid tight clothing.

4. Avoid overeating; eat smaller, more frequent meals.

5. Don't lie down for 1–2 hours after a meal. Elevate the head of your bed with 4- to 6-inch blocks of wood or bricks. Adding extra pillows usually makes things worse by creating a posture that increases pressure on the stomach. Using a waterbed also usually makes reflux worse. Try sleeping on your left side, which may reduce reflux compared to sleeping on your back or right side.

6. If you are overweight in the abdominal area, weight loss may help. Abdominal obesity can increase pressure on the stomach when you are lying down.

When to Call the Physician

1. Stools that are black and tarlike or vomit that is bloody or contains material that looks like coffee grounds

2. Severe abdominal or chest pain

3. Pain that goes through to the back

4. No relief from antacids

5. Difficulty swallowing solid foods

6. Symptoms lasting longer than 3 days

Recurrent or persistent abdominal pain may be a symptom of an ulcer, a raw area in the lining of the stomach or duodenum (the first part of the small intestine). About one in five men and one in ten women develop an ulcer at some time in their lives. Most ulcers are linked to infection with the bacterium *Helicobacter pylori;* people who regularly take nonsteroidal anti-inflammatory drugs like aspirin or ibuprofen are also at risk for ulcers because these drugs irritate the lining of the stomach. *H. pylori* infection is relatively easy to diagnose and treat, and other medications are available to treat ulcers linked to other causes. Many of the self-care measures described above are also frequently recommended for people with ulcers.

HEADACHE

Headache is one of the most common symptoms. There are four major types of headache: tension, migraine, cluster, and sinus. Tension headaches, migraines, and cluster headaches are described in Chapter 2 (p. 43). Sinus headaches are caused by blockage of the sinus cavities with resulting pressure and pain in the cheeks, forehead, and upper teeth. Headache caused by elevated blood pressure is very uncommon and occurs only with very high pressures.

Self-Assessment

1. Take your temperature. The presence of fever may indicate a sinus infection. Fever, severe headache, and a very stiff neck suggest meningitis, a rare but serious infection around the brain and spinal cord.

2. Tap with your fingers over the sinus cavities in your cheeks and forehead. If this causes increased pain, it may indicate a sinus infection.

3. For recurrent headaches, keep a headache journal. Record how often and when your headaches occur, associated symptoms, activities that precede the headache, and your food and beverage intake. Look for patterns that may provide clues to the cause(s) of your headaches.

Self-Care

1. Try applying ice packs or heat on your neck and head.

2. Gently massage the muscles of your neck and scalp.

3. Try deep relaxation or breathing exercises.

4. Take aspirin or aspirin substitute for pain relief. Over-the-counter products containing a combination of aspirin, acetaminophen, and caffeine are approved by the FDA for treating migraines.

5. If pain is associated with nasal congestion, try a decongestant medication like pseudoephedrine.

6. Try to avoid emotional and physical stressors (such as poor posture and eyestrain).

7. Try avoiding foods that may trigger headaches, such as aged cheeses, chocolate, nuts, red wine, alcohol, avocados, figs, raisins, and any fermented or pickled foods.

When to Call the Physician

1. Unusually severe headache

2. Headache accompanied by fever and a very stiff neck

3. Headache with sinus pain, tenderness, and fever

4. Severe headache following a recent head injury

5. Headache associated with slurred speech, visual disturbance, or numbness or weakness in the face, arms, or legs

6. Headache persisting longer than 3 days

7. Recurrent unexplained headaches

8. Increasing severity or frequency of headaches

9. Severe migraine headaches (In recent years, many new prescription medications have been approved for the prevention and treatment of migraines.)

LOW-BACK PAIN

Pain in the lower back is a very common condition; it is most often due to a strain of the muscles and ligaments along the spine, often triggered by bending, lifting, or other activity. Low-back pain can also result from bone growths (spurs) irritating the nerves along the spine or pressure from ruptured or protruding discs, the "shock absorbers" between the vertebrae. Sometimes back pain is caused by an infection or stone in the kidney. Fortunately, however, simple muscular strain is the most common cause of low-back pain and can usually be effectively self-treated.

Self-Assessment

1. Take your temperature. Back pain with high fever may indicate a kidney or other infection.

2. Check for blood in your urine or frequent, painful urination, which may also indicate a kidney problem.

3. Observe for tingling or pain traveling down one or both legs *below* the knee with bending, coughing, or sneezing. These symptoms suggest a disc problem.

Self-Care

1. Lie on your back or in any comfortable position on the floor or a firm mattress, with knees slightly bent and supported by a pillow. Rest for 1–3 days if the pain persists.

2. Use ice packs on the painful area for the first 3 days, and then continue with cold or change to heat, whichever gives more relief.

3. Take aspirin or aspirin substitute for pain relief as needed.

4. After the acute pain has subsided, begin gentle back and stomach exercises. Practice good posture and lifting techniques to protect your back. Try to resume gentle, everyday activities like walking as soon as possible. Bed rest beyond 3 days is no longer advised. To learn more about proper back exercises and use of your back, consult a physical therapist or your physician.

When to Call the Physician

1. Back pain following a severe injury such as a car crash or fall

2. Back pain radiating down the leg *below* the knee on one or both sides

3. Persistent numbness, tingling, or weakness in the legs or feet

4. Loss of bladder or bowel control

5. Back pain associated with high fever (above 101°F or 38.3°C), frequent or painful urination, blood in the urine, or severe abdominal pain

6. Back pain that does not improve after 2 weeks of self-care

STRAINS AND SPRAINS

Missteps, slips, falls, and athletic misadventures can result in a variety of strains, sprains, and fractures. A strain occurs when you overstretch a muscle or tendon (the connective tissue that attaches muscle to bone). Sprains are caused by overstretching or tearing ligaments (the tough fibrous bands that connect bone to bone). Depending on the severity and location, a sprain may actually be more serious than a fracture, because bones generally heal very strongly whereas ligaments may remain stretched and lax after healing. After a sprain, it may take 6 weeks for the ligament to heal.

After most injuries, you can expect pain and swelling. This is the body's way of immobilizing and protecting the injured part

so that healing can take place. The goal of self-assessment is to determine whether you have a minor injury that you can safely self-treat or a more serious injury to an artery, nerve, or bone that should be treated by your physician.

Self-Assessment

1. Watch for coldness, blue color, or numbness in the limb beyond the injury. These may be signs of damage to an artery or a nerve.

2. Look for signs of a possible fracture, which would include a misshapen limb, reduced length of the limb on the injured side compared to the uninjured side, an inability to move or bear weight, a grating sound with movement of the injured area, extreme tenderness at one point along the injured bone as you press with your fingers, or a sensation of snapping at the time of the injury.

3. Gently move the injured area through its full range of motion. Immobility or instability suggests a more serious injury.

Self-Care

1. Immediately immobilize, protect, and rest the injured area until you can bear weight on it or move it without pain. Remember: If it hurts, don't do it.

2. To decrease pain and swelling, immediately apply ice (a cold pack or ice wrapped in a cloth) for 15 minutes every hour for the first 24–48 hours. Then apply ice or heat as needed for comfort.

3. Immediately elevate the injured limb above the level of your heart for the first 24 hours to decrease swelling.

4. Immobilize and support the injured area with an elastic wrap or splint. Be careful not to wrap so tightly as to cause blueness, coldness, or numbness.

5. Take aspirin or aspirin substitute for pain as needed.

When to Call the Physician

1. An injury that occurred with great force, such as a high fall or motor vehicle crash

2. Hearing or feeling a snap at the time of the injury

3. A limb that is blue, cold, or numb

4. A limb that is bent, twisted, or crooked

5. Tenderness at specific points along a bone

6. Inability to move the injured area

7. A wobbly, unstable joint

8. Marked swelling of the injured area

9. Inability to bear weight after 24 hours

10. Pain that increases or lasts longer than 4 days

CUTS AND SCRAPES

Cuts and scrapes are common disruptions of the body's skin. Fortunately, the vast majority of these wounds are minor and don't require stitches, antibiotics, or a physician's care. An abrasion involves a scraping away of the superficial layers of skin. Abrasions, though less serious than cuts, are often more painful because they disrupt more skin nerves. There are two types of cuts: lacerations (narrow slices of the skin) and puncture wounds (stabs into deeper tissues).

Normal healing of a cut or abrasion is a remarkable process. After the bleeding stops, small amounts of serum, a clear yellowish fluid, may leak from the wound. This fluid is rich in antibodies to help prevent an infection. Redness and swelling may normally occur as more blood is shunted to the area, bringing white blood cells and nutrients to speed healing. There may also be some swelling of nearby lymph nodes, which are another part of your body's defense against infection. Finally, a scab forms. This is "nature's bandage," which protects the area while it heals.

The main concerns about cuts are the possibility of damage to deeper tissues and the risk of infection. Damage to underlying blood vessels may lead to severe bleeding as well as blueness and coldness in areas beyond the wound. Injured nerves may produce numbness and a loss of the ability to move parts of the body beyond the injured area. Damaged muscles, tendons, and ligaments can also result in inability to move areas beyond the cut.

Wound infection usually does not take place until 24–48 hours after an injury. Signs of infection include increasing redness, swelling, pain, pus, and fever. One of the most serious, though fortunately uncommon, complications of puncture wounds is tetanus ("lockjaw"). This bacterial infection thrives in areas not exposed to oxygen, so it is more likely to develop in deep puncture wounds or dirty wounds. Tetanus is not likely to develop in minor cuts or wounds caused by clean objects like knives. You need a tetanus immunization shot following a cut under the following conditions:

- If you have never had the basic series of three tetanus immunization injections
- If you have a dirty or contaminated wound and it has been longer than 5 years since your last injection
- If you have a clean, minor wound and it has been longer than 10 years since your last injection

Self-Assessment

1.   Look for warning signs of complications: persistent bleeding, numbness, an inability to move the injured area, or the later development of pus, increasing redness, and fever.

2.   Measure the size of the cut. If your cut is shallow, less than 1/4 inch deep, less than an inch long, and not in a high-stress area (such as a joint, which bends) and you can easily hold the edges of the wound closed, it probably won't need stitches.

Self-Care

1.   Apply direct pressure over the wound until the bleeding stops. The only exception is puncture wounds, which should be encouraged to bleed freely (unless spurting a large amount of blood) for a few minutes to flush out bacteria and debris.

2.   Try to remove any dirt, gravel, glass, or foreign material from the wound with tweezers or by gentle scrubbing.

3.   Wash the wound vigorously with soap and water, followed by an application of hydrogen peroxide solution as an antiseptic.

4.   If it is an abrasion, cover the area with a sterile adhesive bandage until a scab forms. For minor lacerations, close the cut with a butterfly bandage or a sterile adhesive tape, drawing the edges close together but not overlapping. If there is an extra flap of clean skin, leave it in place for extra protection. Do not attempt to close a puncture wound. Instead, soak the wound in warm water for 15 minutes several times a day for several days. Soaking helps keep the wound open and thus prevents infection.

When to Call the Physician

1.   Bleeding that can't be controlled with direct pressure

2.   Numbness, weakness, or an inability to move the injured area

3.   Any large, deep wound

4.   A cut in an area that bends and with edges that cannot easily be held together

5.   Cuts on the hands or face unless clean and shallow

6.   A contaminated wound from which you cannot remove the foreign material

7.   Any human or animal bite

8.   If you need a tetanus immunization (see indications noted earlier)

9.   Development of increasing redness, swelling, pain, pus, or fever 24 hours or more after the injury

10.   If the wound is not healing well after 3 weeks

Photo Credits

C-1

Index

Boldface numbers indicate pages on which glossary definitions appear.

AA (Alcoholics Anonymous), 261, 285–286, 287
abortifacients, **159**
abortion, 183–199
  complications of, 196–197
  current legal status of, 184–186
  current trends in, 191–192
  decision making and, 197–198
  defined, **184**
  history of, in the U. S., 184–185
  methods of, 194–195
  moral considerations in, 186–188
  personal considerations in, 189–191, 199
  public opinion on, 186–190
  spontaneous (*See* miscarriage)
abstinence, 143, **168**, 170, 561, 563, 577
Acceptable Macronutrient Distribution Ranges
    (AMDRs), 333, 334
acceptance, 65
accidents, 662. *See also* unintentional injuries
acculturation stress, 46
Accutane, 222, 223
acesulfame-K, 426
acid precipitation, **706**
acquaintance rape (date rape), 683–684
acquired immunity, **521**
acquired immunodeficiency syndrome (AIDS),
    548–562
  in children, 223, 553, 559–560
  defined, **549**
  diagnosis of, 556
  ethnicity and, 554, 555
  injection drug use and, 245
  reporting requirements for, 556–557
  statistics on, 549, 555, 573–574
  transmission of, 550, 551–553
  See also human immunodeficiency virus
acrylamide, 499
ACTH (adrenocorticotropic hormone), **34**
active euthanasia, **611**
active immunity, 522
acupuncture, 589, **645**, 646
added sugars, 337, 354, 355
addiction. *See* addictive behaviors, alcohol use,
    nicotine, psychoactive drugs
addictive behaviors, **236**, 236–239. *See also*
    addiction
additives in food, 365–366
Adequate Intake (AI), 343, 373–375
ADHD (attention-deficit/hyperactivity disorder),
    85, 241, 253
adipose tissue, 412
adolescence
  contraceptive education in, 176–177
  sexuality in, 138–139
adoption, 191
adrenal androgens, 396
adrenal glands, **34**, 127
adrenocorticotropic hormone (ACTH), **34**
adult day-care centers, 595
advance directives, **611**, 611–612
advertising
  for alcohol, 291
  false claims in, 644
  for foods, 367
  for medications, 632, 641
  for smoking, 302–303

AEDs (automated external defibrillators), 462
aerobic (cardiorespiratory) endurance exercise,
    379, 380
AFP (alpha-fetoprotein), 218
African Americans
  alcohol abuse among, 286–287
  asthma in, 525, 709
  body image in, 436
  breast cancer in, 496
  cardiovascular disease in, 458
  cervical cancer in, 489
  chlamydia in, 562
  cigarette advertisements and, 303
  contraceptive use among, 173
  depression in, 75
  diabetes in, 418, 458
  distribution in U.S. population, 9
  drug use in, 259
  glaucoma in, 588
  health concerns of, 9–10
  HIV/AIDS in, 554, 555
  homicide among, 676
  hypertension in, 449, 458
  lead poisoning in, 709
  lupus in, 542
  marriage law and, 111
  metabolic syndrome in, 458
  multiple myeloma in, 495
  obesity in, 422
  pancreatic cancer in, 493
  prostate cancer in, 488, 496, 504
  resting metabolic rate in, 422
  sexual decision making by, 142
  sickle-cell disease and, 207
  in single-parent families, 117
  sodium intake by, 349, 471
  tobacco use by, 304, 305, 307
  vitamin deficiencies in, 338
  See also ethnicity
African sleeping sickness, 539
age
  contraceptive use and, 173
  fertility and, 210
  health care visits and, 638
  health insurance coverage and, 655
  suicide rates and, 79
  See also aging
age-related macular degeneration (AMD), 588, **589**
aggressive driving, injuries from, 664–665
aging, 581–601
  caregiving for older adults, 595, 596
  elder abuse, 682
  Erikson's stages of development, 67–68
  government aid and policies, 597–598
  life-enhancing measures, 582–586
  life expectancy factors, 592
  medication issues, 596
  multicultural widsom on, 599
  nutritional needs, 357
  physical changes with, 584
  planning for social changes, 586–587
  sexuality and, 132
  statistics on, 594
  suicide and, 592
  theories of, 592–593
  See also age
agoraphobia, **76**
AI (Adequate Intake), 343, 373–375
AIDS. *See* acquired immunodeficiency syndrome
air bags, 667
air pollution, 701–708
  acid precipitation, 706
  asthma and, 525
  cancer and, 501–503
  energy use and, 706–707

greenhouse effect and global warming, 702,
    703–705
  indoor, 707
  preventing, 707–708
  smog, 701–703
Air Quality Index (AQI), **701**, 702
Al-Anon, 285
alarm stage of stress response, 39–40
Alaska Natives
  alcohol abuse among, 286, 287
  asthma in, 525
  distribution in U.S. population, 9
  drug use among, 259
  health concerns of, 9
  obesity in, 422
  See also ethnicity
alcohol abuse, 280, **281**. *See also* alcohol use
alcohol dependence, 280, **281**
Alcoholics Anonymous (AA), 261, 285–286, 287
alcoholism, 280, **281**, 282–288
alcohol-related neurodevelopmental disorder
    (ARND), 278, **279**
alcohol use, 269–295
  advertising and, 291
  aging and, 581, 585
  alcohol, defined, 270, **271**
  alcohol abuse, defined, 280, **281**
  alcoholism, 280, 282–286
  behavioral effects, 272
  binge drinking, 275, 278, 280–283
  blood alcohol concentration, 271–272, 665–666
  calories in, 328, 349
  cancer and, 483, 485, 499, 509
  cardiovascular disease and, 455, 471
  chemistry of, 270
  children of alcoholics, 284
  chronic effects of, 277–278
  combined with other drugs, 274
  driving and, 275–277, 283, 665–666
  effects on the body, 270–272
  gender differences in use of, 8, 286–287
  health benefits of, 279–280
  HIV infection and, 552, 561, 563
  immediate effects of, 273–275, 277
  poisoning by, 274
  during pregnancy, 221–223, 278–279
  responsible behavior for, 288–292, 293
  self-assessment on, 289
  sexual decision making and, 147, 275, 568, 576
  spirituality and, 244
  statistics on, 236, 270, 281
  stress and, 57
  violence and, 676, 687
  warning signs of dependence, 280
allergens, **523**, 523–524
allergic response, 524
allergies
  dealing with, 524–526
  defined, **523**
  to food, 366
  to latex, 561
  stress and, 41
  symptoms of, 533
  from tattoos and piercings, 537
  to vaccines, 523
allied health care providers, **637**
allostatic load, 40
allyl sulfides, 342
alpha-fetoprotein (AFP), 218
alpha-linolenic acid, 330–331, 332, 375
altered states of consciousness, 256–257, **257**
alternative medical systems, 644–647. *See also*
    complementary and alternative medicine
Alzheimer's disease (AD), **590**, 590–591
AMD (age-related macular degeneration), 588, **589**

AMDRs (Acceptable Macronutrient Distribution Ranges), 333, 334
amenorrhea, **419**
American Cancer Society dietary recommendations, 350
American College of Sports Medicine, 386, 388, 399
American Indians
  aging among, 599
  alcohol abuse among, 286, 287
  asthma in, 525
  body image in, 436
  diabetes in, 418
  distribution in U.S. population, 9
  drug use in, 259
  health concerns of, 9
  lupus in, 542
  obesity in, 422
  See also ethnicity
American Psychiatric Association (APA), 238, 240
amino acids, **329**, 396
amnesia, anterograde, 251, 683–684
amniocentesis, **218**
amniotic sac, **217**
amoebic dysentery, 539
amphetamines, 57, 81, 252–253
anabolic steroids, **396**, 468
analgesics, 533
anal intercourse, 143, 561, 563
anaphylaxis, 366, 524, **525**
androgens, **127**, 128
androgyny, 138
anemia, iron-deficiency, **340**, 356
anesthetics, **250**
aneurysms, **464**, 465
anger, 73–74
  assessment of, 455
  cardiovascular disease and, 454–455
  expressing, 73–74
  in intimate relationships, 104
  in other people, 74
  suppression of, 454
angina pectoris, **307**, **461**, 461–462
angiograms, **464**
anorexia nervosa, 435, **437**, 438
anterograde amnesia, 251, 683–684
anthrax, 541
anti-angiogenesis drugs, 507
antibiotics
  actions of, 530–531
  in agriculture, 531
  breast cancer and, 486
  defined, **639**
  resistance to, 528, 531, 541
  viruses and, 533
antibodies, 518–520, **519**, 556
anticarcinogens, **499**, 499–500
antidepressants, 81, 84–86, 641
antigens, defined, **519**
antihistamines, 525, 533, 666
antioxidants
  Alzheimer's disease and, 591
  cancer and, 499–500
  defined, **338**, **501**
  exercise and, 381
  functions of, 340–342
antipsychotics, 84
antiretroviral drugs, 223, 558–559
antiviral drugs, 223, 538, 558–559, 570
anxiety, defined, **74**
anxiety disorders, 74–78
  cardiovascular disease and, 454–455
  gender differences in, 80
  generalized anxiety disorder, 76
  obsessive-compulsive disorder, 76–77, 80, 435
  panic disorder, 75–76

prevalence of, 76
simple phobias, 74–75
social phobias, 75–77, 91
treatment for, 78, 86–87, 91
anxiolytics, 84–85
aorta, **446**, 447–448, 467
aortic aneurysms, 308
Apgar score, 228, **229**
apoptosis, **497**
appetite suppressants, 434
AQI (Air Quality Index), **701**, 702
Arby's, A–1
aristolochic acid, 650
ARND (alcohol-related neurodevelopmental disorder), 278, **279**
arrhythmias, 454, **462**, 468
ART (assisted reproductive technology), 211
arteries, **446**, 446–448, 460, 466–467. *See also* atherosclerosis
arthritis, 385, 529, 542, 588–589, **589**
artificial insemination, **210**
artificial sweeteners, 426
asanas, 55–56
asbestosis, 708–709, **709**
Asian Americans
  alcohol and, 272, 287
  cancer in, 496
  contraceptive use among, 173
  distribution in U.S. population, 9
  drug use among, 259
  health concerns of, 9
  metabolism of psychotropic drugs in, 75
  tobacco use in, 304, 305
  waist circumference in, 422
  See also ethnicity
Asian flu, 534. *See also* influenza
aspartame, 367, 426
aspirin, 474, 485, 486
assault, 676, 678
assertiveness, **72**
assessments
  aggressive driving, 665
  alcohol problems, 289
  anger, 455
  behavior change, 21
  cardiovascular disease risk, 470
  contraceptive method selection, 178
  drug problems, 245
  eating triggers, 424
  environmental health, 714
  family health trees, 209
  fitness, 402
  lifestyle evaluation, 16–17
  love maps questionnaire, 100
  mood disorders, 78
  nicotine dependence, 299
  personal health profile, 640
  sexual attitudes, 140
  sexually transmitted disease risk, 573
  stage of behavior change, 21
  stress level, 33
  of symptoms, 630–631
  ultraviolet radiation risk, 491
  your diet *vs.* MyPyramid, 356
assisted living facilities, 597
assisted reproductive technology (ART), 211
assisted suicide, 610–611
asthma
  allergies and, 524
  description of attacks, 525
  environmental tobacco smoke and, 314–315
  exercise and, 385
  poverty, ethnicity and, 525, 709
  stress and, 41
  treatment and prevention of, 525

asymptomatic phase, **551**
atherosclerosis
  chronic hostility and, 454
  defined, **41**, **307**, 449, 461
  environmental tobacco smoke and, 314
  high-density lipoproteins and, 450
  peripheral arterial disease, 460, 466–467
  stress and, 41
  tobacco use and, 307
athletes
  nutritional needs of, 337, 357
  sudden death in, 467–468
Atkins diet, 431
atria (*singular,* atrium), **446**, 447–448
attachment, after childbirth, 230–231
attachment styles, **96**, 101
attention-deficit/hyperactivity disorder (ADHD), 85, 241, 253
atypical sexual behaviors, **144**
authenticity, 66
autism, immunization and, 523
autoeroticism, **143**
autoimmune diseases, 8, 518, **519**, 542, 631
automated external defibrillators (AEDs), 462
automobile safety. *See* driving
autonomic nervous system, 33
autonomy, 65, 65–66
avian influenza, 534. *See also* influenza
ayurvedic medicine, 645, 650
AZT (zidovudine), 558

BAC. *See* blood alcohol concentration
back injuries, 672–673
bacteria (*singular,* bacterium)
  antibiotics and, 530–531
  defined, **526**
  diseases from, 223, 467–468, 489, 526–530
  as indoor air pollution, 707
  See also sexually transmitted diseases
bacterial vaginosis (BV), 572, **573**
balloon angioplasty, **464**
barbiturates, 249, 250
barrier methods of contraception
  cervical caps, 166, 170, 175
  defined, **153**
  diaphragms with spermicide, 164–166, 170
  female condoms, 162–164, 170
  male condoms, 161–162
  sponges, 163, 166–167, 170
  See also contraceptives
basal cell carcinoma, **490**, 491
battering, 678–680
Baumrind, Diana, 115–116
B cells, 518–520, **519**, 556
BDD (body dysmorphic disorder), 435
beans. *See* legumes (beans)
behavior change
  assessment of, 21
  continuing, 25–26
  motivation for, 15–20, 25–26
  personal contracts for, 23–24
  personalized plans for, 21–24
  readiness for, 20
  rewards for, 22–23
  sample plan for, 23–24
  self-efficacy and, 19
  target behaviors, 15
  weight-management programs, 441
  See also behavior change strategies
behavior change strategies
  adopting safer habits, 689
  changing your drug habits, 265
  choosing healthy beverages, 370
  complying with physicians' instructions, 658

dealing with social anxiety, 91
dealing with test anxiety, 60
developing responsible drinking habits, 293
incorporating more fruits and vegetables into the diet, 511
kicking the tobacco habit, 322–323
planning a personal exercise program, 406–407
reducing saturated and trans fats in the diet, 476–477
benign tumors, 480, **481**
Benson, Herbert, 53–54
benzodiazepines, 84–85, 250
benzo(a)pyrene, 308, 314, 497
bereavement, 620–621, **621**
beta-carotene, 342, 500
beverages, 349, 368, 370
Bextra (valdecoxib), 641
BHA, 366
BHT, 366
bicycle safety, 668–669
bidis, 313
bile acids, 498
Billings method, 169
binge drinking, 275, 278, 280–283, **281**
binge eating, 58, 437, 438, 439
binge-eating disorder, **437**, 439
biodiversity, 700, **701**
bioelectromagnetic-based therapies, **651**
bioengineering, 13
biofeedback, **56**, 56–57
biological-based therapies, **648**
biomagnification, **710**
biomedicine. *See* conventional medicine
biopsies, 480, **481**, 486
bioterrorism, 541
bipolar disorder, 81–82, **83**
birth control methods. *See* contraceptives
birth defects, 219, 220–221, 222, 223, 278–279, 338, 344
bisexuality, 110–111, 141
black lung disease, 708–709, 711
bladder cancer, 494
blastocysts, 208, **215**
blended families, 117
blood
    cardiovascular system, 446–448
    glucose levels in, 418
    HIV transmission through, 552–553
    platelets, 381, 448, 449, 454
    Rh factor, 196, 220
    viscosity of, 460
    white blood cells, 40, 518–520, 583
    See also blood clotting; blood pressure
blood alcohol concentration (BAC), 271–276. *See also* alcohol use
blood pressure
    cardiovascular disease and, 448–450, 472
    exercise and, 382, 385
    normal range, 449
    salt intake and, 348–349, 359
    See also high blood pressure
BMI. *See* body mass index
boating injuries, 671
body composition, **380**, 381–382, 398, 412, 415. *See also* body fat
body dysmorphic disorder (BDD), 435
body fat
    blood alcohol concentration and, 271
    calorie equivalent of, 412
    cancer and, 500
    dietary fat and, 425
    distribution of, 417
    fat cells, 421
    genetic factors in, 419–420
    health risks of excess, 416–417, 418, 420

hormones and, 421
liposuction and, 435
measurement of, 415
metabolism and, 420–421
percent, 271, 412–413, 415–416, 419
recommended amounts of, 416
types of, 412
very low levels of, 419
body image, **419**, 428, 435–437, 438
body mass index (BMI), 345, 414–415, **415**, 420, 422, 436
body piercing, 537
body weight
    blood alcohol concentration and, 271, 276
    body fat distribution, 417
    eating disorders and, 437–440
    evaluating, 414–415
    genetic factors in, 419–420
    psychoactive drug effects and, 247
    risk of death and, 382
    risks of excess body fat, 416, 420
    statistics on, 412
    See also body fat, weight management
bone marrow, **482**, 495, 506, 583, 613
bone marrow transplants, 506, 583, 613
bones
    bone mineral density testing, 590
    nutrition and, 340, 342
    osteoporosis, 340, 357, 383, 589–590
Bordetella pertussis, 529
Borna virus, 536
Borrelia burgdorferi, 529
botanicals, 648–650. *See also* herbal remedies
botulism (*Clostridium botulinum*), 361, 363, 365
bovine spongiform encephalopathy (BSE), 363, 539–540
brain
    in Alzheimer's disease, 591
    chronic alcohol use and, 278
    exercise and, 384
    hormones and, 128
    psychoactive drug effects on, 246
    stress and, 42
    tobacco use and, 307
brain cancer, 494, 503
brain damage, 365
brain death, **605**
Braxton Hicks contractions, **213**
BRCA1 (breast cancer gene 1), 497–498
breast cancer
    abortions and, 196
    breast self-exams, 486–487, 504
    detection of, 486, 504
    diet and, 499
    genes vs. lifestyle in, 12, 209
    genetic testing for, 498
    high birth weight and, 219–220
    risk factors for, 485–486
    treatment and prevention, 486–487
breastfeeding, 153, 229–230, 486, 559–560, 711
breast self-exams (BSE), 486–487, 504
breathing, 55, 395
"broken heart syndrome," 457
BSE (bovine spongiform encephalopathy), 363, 539–540
BSE (breast self-exams), 486–487, 504
Buddhism, 69, 300
bulimia nervosa, **437**, 438–439
bullying behavior, 677
buprenorphine, 260
bupropion (Wellbutin), 311, 321, 434
Burger King, A–1
burials, 614
Burkitt's lymphoma, 536

burnout, **45**. *See also* stress
BV (bacterial vaginosis), 572, 573

CAD (coronary artery disease), 307, 460. *See also* cardiovascular disease
caffeine
    bone health and, 342
    decreasing use of, 265
    dependence on, 235, 265
    during pregnancy, 222
    sources of, 254
    stimulant effects of, 253–254
    stress and, 49, 57
    in weight-loss products, 432
calcium, 131, 340, 341, 342, 357, 471, 485, 500, 590
calendar method, 168–169
calories
    defined, 328
    density in foods, 425
    energy balance, 413–414
    in fat and sugar substitutes, 426
    on food labels, 360
    intake goals, 334, 335, 353
    in nutrient classes, 328, 334
    sources of, 368
    weight management and, 412, 423
CAM. *See* complementary and alternative medicine
Campylobacter jejuni, 361, 363
Canadian drugs, 642
Canadian Society for Exercise Physiology, 389
cancer, 479–513
    benign *vs.* malignant tumors, 480, 481
    bladder, 494
    brain, 494, 503
    breast, 12, 196, 219–220, 485–487, 498
    cervical, 155, 311, 488–489, 496
    chronic alcohol use and, 278
    colon and rectal, 350, 382, 485, 497–499, 504
    coping with, 507–508
    defined, **481**
    detecting and diagnosing, 503–505
    diet and, 485, 486, 488, 498–500
    endometrial, 489, 504
    exercise and, 382–383, 500–501
    heredity and, 12, 485, 497, 504
    immune system and, 541
    incidence of, 482–484
    infectious agents in, 488–489, 536, 566
    kidney, 494
    larynx, 313
    leukemia, 480, 482, 494
    liver, 496, 501, 536–537
    lung, 308–309, 311, 314, 482–484, 501–503
    lymphomas, 482, 494–495, 501, 536
    metastasis of, 481
    multiple myeloma, 495
    obesity and, 500–501
    oral, 312, 313, 493, 499, 509
    ovarian, 489–490
    pancreatic, 313, 482, 493, 499
    prevention of, 507–510
    prostate, 487–488, 496, 499, 504–505
    role of DNA in, 495–498, 502
    skin, 482, 484, 490–493, 503
    stomach, 493–494, 496, 501
    stress and, 41
    testicular, 135, 493
    treatment of, 484, 485, 505–507, 646
    types of, 481–482
    uterine, 489, 504
    warning signs of, 503–504

Candida albicans, 538
Cannabis sativa. See marijuana
Cannon, Walter, 34
capillaries, **446**
capitation, **656**
carbohydrates
    cravings for, 421
    defined, 334, **335**
    as fat substitutes, 426
    glycemic index, 335–337, 472
    low-carbohydrate diets, 431
    menstrual disorders and, 131
    recommended intake, 334, 337,
        348–349, 375
    refined *vs.* whole, 335–336, 425
    stress and, 58
    weight management and, 425, 427, 431
carbon dioxide, as greenhouse gas, 704, 707
carbon monoxide, 314, 316, 670, 701, 707
carbon monoxide poisoning, 670
carboxyhemoglobin, 314
carcinogens
    in air pollution, 501–503, 509
    defined, **304**, **485**, 496
    environmental tobacco smoke as, 313
    ingested, 501
    radiation, 483, 484, 494, 503, 505
    in tobacco smoke, 304, 484, 497
carcinomas, **481**
cardiac arrest, signs of, 463
cardiac myopathy, 278, **279**
cardiopulmonary resuscitation (CPR), **462**, **686**,
    687–688
cardiorespiratory endurance, 378–380, **379**,
    388–389, 391–393, 397, 398, 453
cardiorespiratory endurance exercise, 380,
    388–389, **389**, 391–393, 397
cardiovascular disease (CVD)
    angina pectoris, 307, 461–462
    arrhythmias, 454, 462
    assessment of risk for, 470
    atherosclerosis (*See* atherosclerosis)
    cholesterol and, 450–451, 459,
        472–473
    chronic alcohol use and, 278
    congestive heart failure, 466, 467
    defined, **383**, **446**
    diabetes and, 453, 457
    diet and, 469–472
    emotions and, 454–455
    ethnicity and, 456, 457, 458, 461
    exercise and, 382, 451–452, 472
    gender differences in, 456–457
    heart attacks (*See* heart attacks)
    heart disease (*See* heart disease)
    heredity and, 456
    high blood pressure and, 448–450
    hormone replacement therapy and, 589
    hypertrophic cardiomyopathy, 466, 467–468
    infectious agents and, 459
    inflammation and C-reactive protein and,
        456–457
    metabolic syndrome and, 457–459
    obesity and, 452–453
    peripheral arterial disease, 460, 466–467
    protection against, 469–474
    statistics on, 446, 461
    stress and, 41, 454, 457
    strokes (*See* strokes)
    sudden cardiac death, 462
    time of day and year, 460
    tobacco use and, 307–310, 312, 448, 472
    triglyceride levels and, 453
    Vioxx and, 641

cardiovascular health, 445–477. *See also*
    cardiovascular disease
cardiovascular system, components of,
    446–448
caregiving, 595, 619
carotenoids, **499**, 499–500
carpal tunnel syndrome, 673, 673–674
car seats for children, 667
Carson, Rachel, 695, 710
case reports, 643
cataracts, 588, **589**
catecholamines, 434, **454**
Caucasians
    body image in, 436
    breast cancer in, 496
    cystic fibrosis in, 207
    distribution in U.S. population, 9
    drug use and, 259
    HIV/AIDS in, 555
    melanoma in, 490
    sexual decision making by, 142
    suicide in older men, 592
    testicular cancer in, 493
    tobacco use and, 304, 305
CCR-5 receptors, 558
CD4 T cells, **549**, 551, 556, 558
Celebrex (celecoxib), 641
celibacy, 142–143, **143**
cell phones, 503, 665
cellular death, 605
central nervous system (CNS), 249, **250**,
    250–254, 273
cerebral cortex, 307
cervical cancer, 155, 311, 488–489, 496, 504,
    566, 569
cervical caps, 166, **167**, 170, 175
cervical dysplasia, 489, 566
cervical mucus, 169
cervix, **124**, 125, 227
cesarean section, **229**
CFCs (chlorofluorocarbons), 704, 706, 708
CFS (chronic fatigue syndrome), 535
chancres, **571**
chancroid, 572, **573**
CHD (coronary heart disease). *See* coronary
    heart disease
chemical pollution, 708–711
chemotherapy, 484, **485**, 505, 646
Chernobyl nuclear accident, 503, 712
chewing (spit) tobacco, 298–299, 305,
    311–312, 316
chicken pox, 522, 535
child abuse, 682
childbirth, 224, 226–231
children
    advertising aimed towards, 368
    air bags and, 667
    of alcoholics, 284
    car seats, 667
    child abuse, 682, 685
    death of, 623
    depression in, 86
    developmental stages in, 67
    divorce and, 114
    environmental tobacco smoke and, 314–315
    grief in, 623
    health insurance coverage of, 654
    HIV infection in, 550
    nutrition in, 357, 373–375
    sexual abuse of, 685
    sexual behavior in, 138
    in single-parent families, 117
    temperaments of, 116
    violence against, 677, 682, 685

Chinese medicine, 644–646, 650
chiropractic, **651**
chlamydia, 223, 489, 562–565, **563**, 579
Chlamydia pneumoniae, 459, 527, 536
Chlamydia trachomatis, 562
chlorofluorocarbons (CFCs), **704**, 706, 708
choking, 671
cholera, 694
cholesterol
    cardiovascular disease and, 450–451,
        472–473
    defined, **331**
    dietary intake of, 348, 469, 471
    exercise and, 382
    on food labels, 360
    functions of, 451
    low-fat diets and, 431
    overview, 331–332
    recommended blood levels, 450, 452
    recommended intake, 348, 471
    reducing levels of, 450–451
    smoking and, 448
    stress and, 454
    types of lipoproteins, 331–332, 459
chondroitin sulfate, 589
chorionic villus sampling (CVS), **218**
Christianity, 69, 300
chromium picolinate, 396, 433
chromosomes, 127–128, **495**
chronic bronchitis, **309**
chronic diseases, coping with, 3, 41, 631. *See
    also* diseases
chronic fatigue syndrome (CFS), 535
chronic obstructive lung disease (COLD), 309
Cialis (tadalafil), 136
cigarettes. *See* tobacco use
cigarette tar, **304**, 312
cigars, 312–313
cilia, smoking and, 309–310
circumcision, 126–127, **127**, 138, 489, 552
cirrhosis, 277, 277–278, 536
civil unions, 111
CJD (Creutzfeldt-Jakob disease), 363, 539–540
climate change (global warming), 702, 703–705
clinical death, **605**
clitoris, **124**, 125
cloning, **210**, 211, 583
Clostridium botulinum (botulism), 361, 363
Clostridium perfringens, 363
Clostridium tetani, 529
clove cigarettes, 313
club drugs, 250, 251
cluster headaches, 8, 43
coarctation of the aorta, 467
cocaine, 223, 246–247, 251–252, 455
cocarcinogens, **304**
coccidioidomycosis, 539
cockroach allergies, 524, 525
coconut oil, 331
codependency, **261**, 261–262
cognitive-behavioral psychotherapy, 86–87
cognitive distortions, **70**, 70–71
cognitive functioning, exercise and, 384
cohabitation, 107–110, **108**
coitus, 144
coitus interruptus, 169
COLD (chronic obstructive lung disease), 309
colds, 41, 516, 532–533
cold sores, 535, 569
collagen, 593
collective violence, 678, 679
college students
    binge drinking by, 280–283
    body image in, 436

HIV transmission in, 562
human papillomavirus infections in, 566
nontraditional, 44
nutrition in, 357–358
staying safe on campus, 687
STDs in, 562, 566–567, 568
stress in, 39, 43–44
violence and, 675, 687
colon cancer, 350, 382, 485, 497–499, 504, 589
colostrum, **230**
commercial sex, 144–146
commitment, 98–100, 114
common colds, 41, 516, 532–533
communication
gender and, 103, 105
nonverbal, 102–103
relationship styles and, 106
sexual behavior and, 146
skills, 103–104
stress management and, 47–48
companionate love, 99
Compassionate Friends, 623
competitiveness, intimate relationships and, 100
complementary and alternative medicine (CAM),
634, 643–653
botanical remedies, 648–650
for cancer, 506
chiropractic, 651
defined, **633**
energy therapies, 651
evaluating, 644, 651–653
homeopathy, 644, 646–647
hypnosis, 647–648
mind-body interventions, 647–648
traditional Chinese medicine, 644–646, 650
complex carbohydrates, 335, 336. *See also*
carbohydrates
compulsions, 76, 238–239, 439
compulsive gambling, 238
compulsive overeating, 439
compulsive spending, 239
computed tomography (CT) scans, 415, **466**,
484, **505**
conception, 152, **153**, 206, 208
condoms, female, 162–164, 170
condoms, male
cervical cancer and, 479, 489
as contraceptives, 161–162
defined, **161**
in HIV infection prevention, 550, 561, 563
in other STD prevention, 170, 567, 568, 575–577
use of, 162–163, 563
conflict resolution, 103–106
congenital heart disease, 466, 467–468
congenital malformations, **221**
congestive heart failure, **466**, 467
conservation
air pollution and, 707–708
of energy, 707
green consumers, 698
reducing garbage amount, 697–698
of water, 696
consumer guidelines
alcohol advertising, 291
alternative remedies for depression, 83
bicycle helmets, 669
birth plans, 227
cold remedies, 533
contraceptives, 156, 163
dietary supplements and PMS, 131
drug-treatment programs, 262
exercise footwear, 401
fat and sugar substitutes, 426
food and supplement labels, 360, 362

funerals, 615
green consumers, 698
health care plans, 657
health fraud and quackery, 506, 644
health information evaluation, 18, 636
HIV tests, 557
mental health professionals, 89
smoking cessation products, 321
sunscreens and sun-protective clothing, 492
tattoos and body piercing, 537
weight-loss diets, 431
consummate love, 99
contagious diseases, defined, **531**. *See also*
infectious diseases
contemplation stage of behavior change, 20
continuation rate, **153**
contraceptive failure rate, **153**
contraceptive immunization, 175
contraceptive implants, 158, 175
contraceptives, 151–180
abstinence, 168, 170
cervical caps, 166, 170, 175
defined, **153**
diaphragms with spermicide, 164–166, 170
education on, 176–177
effectiveness of, 171
emergency, 159–160, 163
failure rate of, 153
female condoms, 162–164
fertility awareness method, 168–169
gender differences and, 175–176
hormonal contraceptives for men, 175
immunocontraceptives, 175
implants, 158, 175
injectable, 158–159, 175
intrauterine devices, 160–161
Lea's Shield, 166
male condoms, 161–162
method selection, 177–179
oral contraceptives, 154–156
principles of, 152–153
risks of, 157
skin patches, 156–157
spermicides, 163, 167–168, 170
sponges, 163, 166–167
sterilization, 170–174
vaginal contraceptive rings, 157
withdrawal method, 169
contraceptive skin patches, 156–157
contraceptive sponges, 163, 166–167, 170
contractions, **226**, 226–227
conventional medicine, **633**, 634–639, 643
Convention on Biological Diversity, 700
cooling down, 393
coping mechanisms
in challenges to self-esteem, 70–72
in death and dying, 616–619
in loss, 619–623
in weight management, 428
See also stress management
Copper T-380A IUD (ParaGard), 160–161
coronary arteries, **446**, 447–448, 452–454, 468
coronary artery disease (CAD), 307, 460. *See also*
coronary heart disease
coronary bypass surgery, **464**
coronary heart disease (CHD)
body composition and, 416
defined, **307**, **461**
depression and, 454
exercise and, 382
genetics and, 456
smoking and, 448
sudden cardiac death, 462
See also cardiovascular disease; heart disease

coronary thrombosis, **461**
corpus luteum, 129
cortisol, **34**, 40, 42, 219, 454, 543
coughs, self-care for, B–7 to B–8
Cowper's glands, 126
COX-2 inhibitors, 641
CPR (cardiopulmonary resuscitation), **462**, **686**,
687–688
crabs (pubic lice), 572, 573
crack cocaine, 252
C-reactive protein (CRP), 41, 456–457
creatine monohydrate, 396
creativity, 66–67
cremation, 614
Creutzfeldt-Jakob disease (CJD), 363, 539–540
cross-dressers, 137
cross-training, **404**
CRP (C-reactive protein), 41, 456–457
cruciferous vegetables, **342**
Cruzan, Nancy Beth, 609–610
crystal methamphetamine, 252–253, 561–562
CT (computed tomography) scans, 415, **466**,
484, **505**
culture
gender roles and, 137–138
obesity and, 422, 423
stress and, 38
See also ethnicity
cunnilingus, **143**
cuts, B–11 to B–12
CVD. *See* cardiovascular disease
CVS (chorionic villus sampling), **218**
cybersex, 144–145
cyberstalking, **680**, 680–682
cystic fibrosis, 9, 207
cytokines, **507**, **519**, 521, 543
cytomegalovirus (CMV), 223, 459, 535, 536

Daily Values, **344**
dairy products, recommended intake of,
348, 354
DASH eating plan, 345, 375, 449, 472
date rape, **683**, 683–684
date rape drugs, 251, 683–684
dating, 107, 109
DDT, 710
death, causes of
AIDS, 540, 550, 555
binge drinking, 281, 283
cancer, 480, 482–483
cardiovascular disease, 446, 461
chronic alcohol use, 278
current, 4–5
diabetes, 416
exercise and, 380, 382
gender differences in, 8
homicide, 664, 675
infant mortality, 225–226
infectious diseases, 526, 527, 528
injuries, 664, 666–671
smoking, 298, 448
vaccine-preventable diseases, 523
death and dying, 603–627
advance directives, 611–612
assisted suicide, 610–611
of children, 623
coping with dying, 616–619
coping with loss, 619–623
end-of-life care, 608, 618
funerals and memorial services, 614–616, 623
organ donors, 612–614
prolonging or hastening, 608–610
standards for defining, 604–605

death and dying *(continued)*
  tasks for survivors, 616
  trajectory of dying, 617–619
  wills, 606–607, 618
  withholding or withdrawing treatment, 610
  See also grief
Death with Dignity Act of 1994, 610
decibels, **712**, 713
decongestants, 533
deep breathing, 55
DEET, 492, 530
defense mechanisms, **70**, 70–72
Defense of Marriage Act (DOMA), 111
delirium tremens (DTs), **282**
delusions, 82
dementia, **590**, 596
demoralization, 70
dendritic cells, 518–519, **519**
denial, 72
dental diseases, tobacco and, 310, 312
dentists, **637**
deoxyribonucleic acid (DNA), **495**, 495–498, 506–507, 549
depersonalization, **255**
Depo-Provera, 158–159, 590
depressants, **250**
depression
  aging and, 591–592
  alternative remedies for, 83, 649
  antidepressants in young people, 86
  cardiovascular disease and, 454
  defined, 78, **79**
  exercise and, 383
  gender differences in, 80
  getting help for, 80–81
  pharmacological therapy for, 84–85, 434
  postpartum, 230
  seasonal affective disorder, 81
  suicide rates, 79–81
  symptoms of, 78–79
DES (diethylstilbestrol), 490, 493
designated drivers, 276
dexfenfluramine (Redux), 434
DHEA (dehydroepiandrosterone), 396
diabetes
  aging and, 593
  blood glucose levels in, 335
  cardiovascular disease and, 453, 457
  c-reactive protein levels and, 41
  ethnicity and, 458
  excess body fat and, 416–417, 500
  exercise and, 383, 385
  fiber and, 337
  gestational, 418
  nutritional needs in, 359
  pre-diabetes, 418
  during pregnancy, 223
  testicular cancer and, 493
  treatment of, 418
  type 1, 417, 418, 536
  type 2, 416–418
  warning signs and testing for, 418
Dia de los Muertos, 606, 607
diaphragm contraceptives, 164–166, **165**, 170
diarrhea, B–9
diastole, **446**, 448–449
diazepam (Valium), 286
diet
  aging and, 584–585
  average American, 355, 368
  cancer and, 485–486, 488, 498–500
  DASH eating plan, 345, 350, 375, 449, 472
  ethnic foods, 346
  in exercise programs, 400
  health journals, 21–22, 24, 356

Healthy Eating Pyramid, 375
heart-healthy, 469–472
improving one's, 23–24, 367–369, 370
incorporating fruits and vegetables into, 511
incorporating whole grains into, 336
low-carbohydrate, 431
low-fat diets, 431
MyPyramid, 343, 350–354
reducing saturated and trans fats, 349, 469, 471, 476–477
vegetarian, 354–356
weight management and, 421–422, 423–427, 429–430
  See also nutrition
dietary fats. *See* fats, dietary
dietary fiber. *See* fiber
Dietary Guidelines for Americans, **343**, 344–350
Dietary Reference Intakes (DRIs), **343**, 343–344, 373–375
dietary supplements
  for athletic performance, 395, 396
  herbal, 359, 361–362, 645–646, 648–650
  during pregnancy, 221, 222
  premenstrual syndrome and, 131
  reading labels on, 357–361
  reporting adverse reactions to, 644
  standardization of, 650
  for weight management, 430, 432–433
diet books, 430
diet formula drinks, 432
diethylstilbestrol (DES), 206, 210
digestion, 42, 277–278, 328–329, **329**
dilation and evacuation (D&E), **194**, 195
diphtheria, 522, 523
direct-to-consumer (DTC) advertising, 641
disabilities, people with, 11, 140, 385
discretionary calorie allowance, 354
discrimination, 10, 46, 458, 677
diseases. *See* genetic diseases and disorders; infectious diseases; sexually transmitted diseases
distress, **39**. *See also* stress
disulfiram (Antabuse), 272, 285–286
diversity issues
  abortion, 193
  alcohol metabolism, 272
  asthma and poverty, 525
  cancer and poverty, 496
  cardiovascular disease, 458
  contraceptive use, 173
  Dia de los Muertos, 607
  discrimination and stress, 46
  drug use, 259
  environmental health and poverty, 709
  ethnic foods, 346
  exercise for persons with disabilities, 385
  genetic diseases, 207
  health disparities among minorities, 10
  HIV/AIDS among African Americans and Latinos, 555
  HIV infection around the world, 550
  interfaith and intrafaith partnerships, 108
  multicultural wisdom about aging, 599
  overweight and obesity, 422
  psychological disorders, 75
  sexual decision making, 142
  smoking, 305
  socioeconomic status, 5
  uninsured Americans, 655
  violence and health, 679
  wellness and, 6–11
  See also ethnicity; gender differences
diverticulitis, 337
divorce, 114
DNA (deoxyribonucleic acid), **495**, 495–498, 506–507, 549

doctors, medical (M.D.), 635
doctors of chiropractic, 651
doctors of osteopathic medicine (D.O.), **635**, 637
domestic violence, 678–682
Domino's Pizza, A–1
dopamine, 246, 251, 330
dose-response function, **246**, 247, 275
double-blind studies, 636
double effect, doctrine of, 610, **611**
douching, 153, **167**, 572
Down syndrome, 205, 218
driving
  aggressive, 664–665
  alcohol use and, 275–277, 283, 665
  blood alcohol concentration and, 271–275
  cell phone use during, 665
  fatigue and, 665
  motor vehicle injuries, 664–668
drug abuse, defined, 240. *See also* psychoactive drugs
drug dependence, defined, 240–241. *See also* psychoactive drugs
Drug-Induced Rape Prevention and Punishment Act of 1996, 684
drugs, defined, **236**. *See also* psychoactive drugs
drug testing, 260
drug treatment, 260–262
drug use
  gender differences in, 243
  injectible, 245–246, 552, 562
  in older Americans, 581
  during pregnancy, 222
  prevention, 262
  self-assessment of, 245
  spirituality and, 244
  stress and, 57
  violence and, 676
  See also medications; psychoactive drugs
DTs (delirium tremens), **282**
dual (co-occurring) disorders, **243**
durable power of attorney for health care, 611–612
dust mite allergies, 524
dying
  end-of-life care, 608, 618
  prolonging or hastening, 608–610
  support for a dying person, 619
  tasks of coping with, 617
  See also death and dying
dysmenorrhea, 129
dysplasia, 481
dysthymic disorder, 79

E. coli, 361, 529, 531, 540
ear problems, B–8 to B–9
eating disorders
  anorexia nervosa, 435, 437, 438
  binge-eating disorder, 437, 439
  borderline disordered eating, 439
  bulimia nervosa, 437, 438–439
  defined, **437**
  distorted body image and, 435
  factors in developing, 437–438
  helping a friend with, 440
  statistics on, 437
  stress and, 58
  treatment for, 439–440
  triggers for, 424
Ebola hemorrhagic fever (EHF), 541
echinacea, 648–649
eclampsia, **225**
economic status. *See* poverty; socioeconomic status
ecosystems, biodiversity and, 700, **701**
ecstasy (MDMA), 251, 257

ECT (electroconvulsive therapy), **81**
ectopic pregnancy, 196, 224–225, **225**
educational attainment,
  drug use and, 259
  health disparities and, 9–11
  school violence, 677
  smoking and, 304
EEG (electronencephalogram), **605**, 651
EFM (electronic fetal monitoring), 226, 227
ejaculation, 134–135, **161**
ejaculatory duct, 126
EKG (electrocardiograms), 389, 462, 651
elder abuse, 682
elective surgeries, **643**
electrical impedance analysis, 415
electrocardiograms (ECG or EKG), 389,
  462, 651
electroconvulsive therapy (ECT), **81**
electromagnetic radiation, 711–712
electron-beam computed tomography
  (EBCT), 463
electronencephalogram (EEG), **605**, 651
electronic fetal monitoring (EFM), 226, 227
ELISA (enzyme-linked immunosorbent
  assay), **556**
embalming, 614, 615
embolic strokes, 464–465
embolus, **464**
embryo development, 208
embryonic stem cells, 583
embryos, 127–128, 208, **215**
emergencies, 463, 630–631, 680, 688. *See also*
  first aid
emergency contraceptives, 159–160, 163
emergency medical services (EMS) system,
  463, **688**
emergency preparedness, 680
emerging diseases, 540–541
emotional wellness, 2, 383, 384
emotions
  after childbirth, 230
  cardiovascular disease and, 454–455
  hormones and, 214
  pregnancy and, 214
  stress and, 35–38
  weight management and, 427–428
emphysema, **309**
employment, stress from, 44–45
"empty nest syndrome," 586
enabling behaviors, 261
encephalitis, **535**, 535–536
endemic diseases, 528, **529**
endocrine disrupters, 210
endocrine glands, **127**
endocrine system, 34, **34**, 42
end-of-life care, 608, 618
endometrial cancer, 489, 504
endometriosis, 135, 210
endometrium, 129, **206**, 488, 489
endorphins, **34**, 384
endoscopies, **639**
endothelial cells, **452**, 452–453
endurance athletes, 337, 359
endurance training, 379–383. *See also* cardiorespiratory endurance
energy (calories), 328, 329, 332, 420–421, 425.
  See also calories
energy balance, 413–414
energy consumption
  air pollution and, 706–707
  population growth and, 699–700
  statistics on, 707
energy therapies, **651**
Entamoeba histolytica, 539
environmental health, 693–717

acid precipitation, 706
air pollution, 701–708
  chemical pollution, 708–711
  defined, 694, **695**
  drinking water supply, 695–696
  food inspection, 698
  gender and, 711
  global warming, 702, 703–705
  healing the environment, 714–175
  insect and rodent control, 698–699
  noise pollution, 713–714
  ozone layer thinning, 704, 706
  population growth, 699–701
  poverty and, 709
  radiation, 711–713
  waste disposal, 696–697
environmental tobacco smoke (ETS)
  cervical cancer and, 489
  deaths from, 298
  defined, **313**
  effects of, 313–315
  heart disease and, 448
  indoor air pollution from, 707
  lung cancer and, 484
environmental wellness, 3
ephedra, 396, 432, 468
ephedrine, 253, 432
epidemics, 534, **535**
epididymis, 126
epididymitis, **563**
epidural, **226**, 227
epinephrine, 34, **34**, 40
episiotomy, **226**, 227
epithelial layer, **481**
Epstein-Barr virus, 501, 535, 536
erectile dysfunction, **135**, 135–136
erections, 138
Erikson, Erik, 67–68, 96
erogenous zones, **133**
erotic fantasy, **143**
erythropoietin (EPO), 396
Escherichia coli, 361, 529, 531, 540
essential amino acids, 329
essential fat, 412–413, 416, **423**
essential nutrients, defined, 328, **329**. *See also*
  nutrition
estate, **606**, 607
estradiol, 129
estrogens
  aging and, 132, 593
  breast cancer and, 485–486
  as cancer promoters, 497
  cardiovascular disease and, 457
  defined, **127**
  female sexual maturation and, 128
  lupus and, 542
  in menstrual cycle, 129
  stress and, 38
  See also hormone replacement therapy
ethnicity
  aging and, 599
  alcoholism and, 286–287
  asthma and, 525
  body image and, 436
  cancer and, 496
  cardiovascular disease and, 456, 457,
    458, 461
  contraceptive use among women, 173
  diabetes and, 418
  distribution in U.S. population, 9
  drug use and, 259
  ethnic foods, 346
  genetic diseases and, 9, 75, 207
  hate crimes and, 677
  health disparities and, 8–11
  health insurance coverage and, 655

HIV/AIDs and, 554, 555
  metabolic syndrome and, 458–459
  overweight and obesity and, 422
  psychological disorders and, 75
  sexual decision making and, 142
  smoking and, 304, 305
  stress and, 46
  suicide rates and, 79
  See also under specific ethnic groups
ethyl alcohol. *See* alcohol use
ETS. *See* environmental tobacco smoke
eugenol, 313
euphoria, **248**
European Americans. *See* Caucasians
eustress, **39**. *See also* stress
euthanasia, 610–611
exercise, 377–409
  aging and, 584, 588–590
  benefits of, 377, 380–384, 388, 390
  bone mass and, 342
  calories used in, 398–399
  cancer and, 486
  carbohydrates and, 335
  disabilities and special health concerns
    and, 385
  disease prevention and management, 382–383,
    451–452, 472
  eating and drinking for, 400
  immune system and, 544
  lifestyle approach to, 386–387
  menstrual disorders and, 131
  metabolism and, 421
  during pregnancy, 223–224
  recommended daily amount of, 347, 386–389
  self-esteem and, 384, 428
  stress management and, 48–49
  stretching, 392–393, 395–398
  weight management and, 347, 386, 422, 427
  See also exercise programs
exercise equipment, 399–400
exercise programs, 384–398
  basic principles of training, 389–391
  cardiorespiratory endurance exercise, 380,
    388–389, 391–393, 397
  disabilities and special health concerns and, 385
  duration (time), 392, 394–395, 397
  eating and drinking for, 400
  equipment for, 399–400
  fitness assessments, 402
  fitness centers, 400
  flexibility exercises, 395–397
  footwear for, 401
  frequency of, 391, 394, 396–397
  injuries and, 403–404
  instructors for, 398–399
  intensity in, 391–392, 394–395, 397
  lifestyle physical activity, 386–387
  medical clearance for, 388–389
  personal exercise plan, 406–407
  principles of physical training, 389–391
  recommended amount of activity, 387–389
  strength training, 393–395, 397
  warm-ups and cool-downs, 392–393
exhaustion stage of stress response, 40
expectations, unrealistic, 100
exposure, in behavioral model, 85
expressive writing, health and, 631
extinction, 700

fallopian tubes, 125, 172, **206**, 210
falls, 668–669
false negatives, **639**
false positives, **639**
FAM (fertility awareness method), 168–169, 170

families, 114–119
  becoming a parent, 114–115
  blended, 117
  caregiving for elderly in, 595
  child abuse in, 682, 685
  children's temperaments, 116
  parenting styles, 115–116
  recognizing the potential for abusiveness in a
    partner, 681
  single parents, 117
  statistics on, 95
  stepfamilies, 117
  stress management and, 48
  successful, 117–119
  violence in, 678–682, 682
  See also parents
family health tree, 11–12, 28, 209
FAS (fetal alcohol syndrome), 222, 278–279, 279
fast-food restaurants, 357, 358, A–1 to A–4
fat cells, 421
fathers, pregnancy tasks for, 215
fats, dietary
  calories in, 328, 425
  cancer and, 498–499
  cardiovascular disease and, 469, 471
  fat substitutes, 426
  on food labels, 360
  health and, 331–332
  low-fat diets, 431
  omega-3 (See omega-3 fatty acids)
  recommended intake of, 332–334, 348, 354,
    375, 469
  reducing saturated and trans, 349
  saturated, 327, 331–333, 347–348, 476–477
  trans, 327, 331–333
  unsaturated, 331–332, 333
  weight management and, 425, 431
  See also cholesterol
fat-soluble vitamins, 338, 339
fat substitutes, 426
fatty acids, 330–331
FDA. See Food and Drug Administration
fecal occult blood test (FOBT), 504
Federal Trade Commission (FTC), 615, 644
feedback, in intimate relationships, 103
fellatio, 143
female athlete triad, 419
female condoms, 162–164, 170
female genital mutilation, 138
female sex organs, 124–125
FemCap, 175
fenfluramine (Pondimin), 434
fertility, 155, 206–208, 310, 311
fertility awareness method (FAM), 168–169, 170
fertilization, 206, 208, 210–211
fertilized egg, 206
fetal alcohol syndrome (FAS), 222, 278–279, 279
fetal development, 214–220. See also pregnancy
fetal programming, 219–220
fetus, defined, 205
fevers, 519, 521, 630, B–6 to B–7. See also
    infectious diseases
fiber, 337–338
  cancer and, 499
  cardiovascular disease and, 471
  cholesterol control and, 450
  defined, 337
  on food labels, 360
  intake of, 337–338, 375
  for older adults, 585
  in weight management, 432
fibrinogen, 459–460
fight-or-flight reaction, 34, 34–35
firearms, 671, 676, 686–687

fires, injuries from, 669–670
first aid
  for alcohol poisoning, 274
  check-call-care system, 688
  for cuts and scrapes, B–11 to B–12
  defined, 686
  for exercise injuries, 403
  for heart attacks, 462–463
  Heimlich maneuver, 671
  home medical care kit, 633
  poison control hotline number, 670
  for strains and sprains, B–11
  when to consult a physician, 630–631, B–6 to
    B–12
fish, 221, 331–332, 333, 348, 364, 471, 710
fitness. See physical fitness
fitness centers, 399–400
fitness programs. See exercise programs
FITT (frequency, intensity, time, and type),
    380, 397
flashbacks, 257
flexibility
  defined, 380
  exercises for, 395–397
  proper stretching technique, 395–396
  recommendations for, 388–389, 397
flu. See influenza
fluid intelligence, 584
flukes, 539
flunitrazepam (Rohypnol), 250, 251, 683–684
fluoridation, 341, 348, 695
flushing syndrome, 272
FOBT (fecal occult blood test), 504
folic acid (folate)
  cancer and, 485, 500
  cardiovascular disease and, 338, 471
  functions of, 339
  during pregnancy, 206, 220
  for women, 206, 344, 357
follicles, ovarian, 129, 206
follicle-stimulating hormone (FSH), 129
food
  additives, 365–366
  allergies and intolerances, 366
  food inspection, 698
  food safety, 350, 361–365, 585, 698
  genetically modified, 366
  irradiated, 366
  organic, 365
  See also diet; nutrition
food allergies, 366, 523
Food and Drug Administration (FDA)
  food inspection by, 698
  herbal products and, 650
  supplement labels and, 359–362
  tobacco regulations, 303, 316–317
Food and Nutrition Board, 333–334
foodborne illnesses, 360–363
food chains, 700, 701
food intolerances, 366–367, 367
food irradiation, 366, 365
food labels, 336, 357–358
food safety, 350, 361–364, 585, 698
footwear, exercise, 401
foreplay, 143
formaldehyde, 304, 707
fossil fuels, 701, 704
Framework Convention on Tobacco Control
    (FCTC), 316, 317
fraternal twins, 208
free radicals, 340, 340–341, 381, 500, 501,
    591, 593
free weights, 395
fried foods, cancer and, 499

Friedman, Meyer, 37
friendships, 97, 98
fruits, 347, 351–352, 425, 499–500, 511
FSH (follicle-stimulating hormone), 129
FTC (Federal Trade Commission), 615, 644
functional fiber, 337
funerals, 614–616, 623
fungi (singular, fungus), 527, 538–539, 539
fusion inhibitors, 558, 559

GAD (generalized anxiety disorder), 76
gambling, compulsive, 238
gamete intrafallopian transfer (GIFT), 210, 211
gamma globulin, 523
gamma hydroxy butyrate (GHB), 249, 250, 251,
    396, 683
gang-related violence, 676–677
garbage, 696–698
Gardnerella vaginalis, 572
garlic supplements, 359, 649
GAS (general adaptation syndrome), 39, 39–40
gastric bypass surgery, 434–435
gays, 141. See also sexual orientation
gender, defined, 7, 137
gender differences
  in alcoholism, 286–287
  in autoimmune diseases, 8, 542
  in blood alcohol concentration, 271
  in blood pressure, 449
  in body composition, 412, 416
  in body image, 436
  in cancer deaths, 482–483
  in cardiovascular disease, 456–457, 461
  in communication, 103, 105
  contraception and, 175–176
  in depression and anxiety, 80, 82
  in drug use and abuse, 243
  in environmental health, 711
  in gender identity, 137–138
  in gender role flexibility, 138
  in grief, 620
  in health, 8
  in health care visits, 638
  in injuries, 663
  in leading causes of death, 5
  in life expectancy, 592–593
  in metabolism, 420
  in muscular strength, 393
  in nutritional needs, 357
  in obesity, 422, 423
  in patterns of health-related behaviors, 8
  in sexual decision making, 141–142
  in sexual differentiation, hormones, and the
    brain, 128
  in sexually transmitted diseases, 564
  in stress, 38–39
  in sudden death in athletes, 468
  in suicide rates, 79, 592
  in tobacco use, 311
  in violence, 675–676
  in wellness, 7
gender identity, 136, 137–138
gender roles
  cultural influences on, 137–138
  defined, 39, 96
  flexibility in, 138
  intimate relationships and, 96
  mass media and, 138
  risk-taking behavior and, 663
  stress and, 38
  transgendered individuals, 137
gene chips, 506, 507
general adaptation syndrome (GAS), 39, 39–40

generalized anxiety disorder (GAD), 76
generic drugs, 632, **633**, 643
genes, 11, 11–12, 128, 207, **208**, **495**, 593
gene therapy, 13, 505–506
genetically modified (GM) foods, 365–366
genetically modified (GM) organisms, 365–366
genetic counseling, 218–219, 498
genetic diseases and disorders
  Alzheimer's disease, 591
  androgen insensitivity syndrome, 128
  Down syndrome, 205, 218
  ethnicity and, 9, 75, 207
  family health tree, 209
  hemophilia, 209, 552
  hereditary nonpolyposis, 504
  hypertrophic cardiomyopathy, 467
  lifestyle and, 12
  psychological disorders and, 74–75
genetics
  alcoholism and, 284–285
  cancer and, 485
  cardiovascular disease and, 456
  colon cancer and, 485, 497
  eating disorders and, 437–438
  excess body fat and, 419–420
  family health tree, 209
  nicotine addiction and, 301
  wellness and, 11–12
  See also genetic diseases
genetic testing, for breast cancer, 498
genital herpes, 164, 222–223, 489, 535, **569**, 570
genital self-examination, 574
genital warts, 164, 538, **566**, 566–568. *See also*
  human papillomavirus (HPV)
genome, **11**
geriatricians, **598**
German measles virus, 221, 222–223, 522
germ cells, **124**
gerontologists, **598**
gestational diabetes, 418
GHB (gamma hydroxy butyrate), 249, 250, 251,
  396, 683
Giardia lamblia, 363, 539
giardiasis, **539**
GIFT (gamete intrafallopian transfer), 211
gingivitis, 312
Ginkgo biloba, 648–649
ginseng, 649
glans, 126, **127**
glaucoma, 584, 585
global warming (climate change), **702**, 703–705
glucosamine, 589
glucose, **335**, 418
gluten intolerance, 367
glycemic index, **335**, 335–337, 421
glycogen, **335**
gonads, **124**
gonococcal conjunctivitis, **565**
gonorrhea, 222–223, 531, 562, **565**, 575
"good death," 618
Gottman, John, 102, 106
grains, 335–337, 347, 351, 375, 425. *See also*
  carbohydrates
Graves' disease, 542
green consumers, 698
greenhouse effect, **702**, 703–704
grief
  aging and, 591
  in children, 623
  coping with, 623
  course of, 620–621
  from death of children, 226
  defined, **619**
  experiencing, 619–621

  gender and, 620
  support for a grieving person, 621, 623
Group B streptococcus (GBS), 222
Guillain-Barré syndrome, 361
guns, 671, 676, 686–687

H. pylori, 459, 493–494, 501
HAART (highly active antiretroviral therapy),
  558, 560
Haemophilus ducreyi, 572
Haemophilus influenzae type b (Hib), 522,
  527–528
Hahnemann, Samuel, 646
halfway houses, 261
hallucinations, from alcohol withdrawal, **282**
hallucinogens, **255**, 255–257
hand washing, 76, 538, 544
hangovers, 273–274
hantavirus pulmonary syndrome (HPS), 540–541
harassment, sexual, 686
hardiness, 37
harm reduction strategies, 261
Harvard Healthy Eating Pyramid, 350, 375
hashish, 254. *See also* marijuana
hate crimes, 677
hatha yoga, 55–56
HAV (hepatitis A), 363, 536, 570
Hawaiians, Native, 9, 259. *See also* ethnicity
hazardous wastes, 696–697, 710
HBV. *See* hepatitis B
HCG (human chorionic gonadotropin), 129, 212,
  213, 218
HCV. *See* hepatitis C
HDLs. *See* high-density lipoproteins
headaches, 42–43, B–10
health. *See* wellness
health care
  access to, 10–12, 496, 653–655
  appointments with physicians, 638–639
  choosing primary care physicians, 637–638
  for the elderly, 594, 597–598
  gender differences and, 638
  paying for, 653–657
  physician-patient relationship, 638
  self-care, 630–633
  when to consult a physician, 630, B–6 to B–12
  See also health insurance
health care providers, 635, 637–638
health care proxies, **611**
health information sources, 15, 18
health insurance, 496, 597–598, 609, 653–656
health journals, 21–22, 24, 356, 658
health maintenance organizations (HMOs), **656**
health news, evaluating, 636
health savings accounts (HSAs), **656**
Healthy Eating Pyramid, 375
Healthy People 2010
  on binge drinking, 281–282
  on calcium intake by women, 357
  on drinking water standards, 695
  on national wellness goals, 5–7
  on smoking by pregnant women, 315
hearing loss, 588, 596, 713–714
heart, 379, 380–381, 447–448, 467
heart attacks
  coronary thrombosis, 461
  defined, **461**
  exercise and, 382
  fiber and, 471
  gender differences in, 8
  helping victims of, 462–463
  iron and, 460
  oral contraceptives and smoking and, 457

  seasonal pattern of, 460
  stress and, 41
  sudden cardiac death, 462
  symptoms of, 461
  warning signs, 463
  See also cardiovascular disease; heart disease
heartburn, B–9 to B–10
heart disease
  anger and hostility and, 454–455
  angina pectoris, 461–462
  arrhythmias, 454, 462
  cholesterol and, 382
  congenital, 466, 467
  congestive heart failure, 466, 467
  detecting and treating, 463–464, 467
  dietary fats and, 332, 357
  exercise and, 382, 385, 451–452
  heart valve disorders, 468–469
  moderate alcohol use and, 280
  obesity and, 452–453
  personality types and, 37
  rheumatic, 467–468
  stress cardiomyopathy, 457
  sudden cardiac death, 462
  tobacco use and, 307–308
  vitamin deficiencies and, 338
  See also cardiovascular disease; heart attacks
heart transplants, 467
heart valve disorders, 468–469
heavy metals, 696, **697**
Hegar's sign, 213
height-weight charts, 414
Heimlich maneuver, **671**
Helicobacter pylori, 459, 493–494, 501, 529
helmet use, 667–668, 669, 672
helper T cells, 518–520, **519**, 542
helping others
  with alcohol use, 288
  with depression, 80–81
  with drug problems, 263
  with eating disorders, 440
  with heart attacks, 462–463
  helping yourself by, 587
  with psychological disorders, 88–89
  with suicidal thoughts, 80–81
  with tobacco use, 318
hematopoietic stem cells, 583
hemochromatosis, 207
hemophilia, 209, **552**
hemorrhagic fevers, 541
hemorrhagic strokes, **464**, 464–465, 466
hepatitis, **536**, 536–537, **571**. See also under
  specific types of hepatitis
hepatitis A (HAV), 363, 536, 570
hepatitis B (HBV), 222, 501, 536, **563**, 570–571
hepatitis C (HCV), 245, 278, 501, 536–537,
  570–571
herbal remedies, 361–362, 648–650
  government regulation of, 432, 650
  labels on, 359, 361–362
  reporting adverse reactions to, 644
  safety of, 644, 650
  in traditional Chinese medicine, 645–646, 650
  for weight loss, 432–433
heredity. *See* genetics
heroin, 248–250
herpes simplex virus (HSV), 222–223, 489, 535,
  569–570, 649. *See also* genital herpes
herpesviruses
  cancer and, 489, 501, 569
  cold sores from, 535, 569
  defined, **535**
  herpes simplex viruses, 222–223, 489, 535,
  569–570, 649

herpesviruses (*continued*)
  human herpesvirus 8, 501, 535
  in newborns, 222–223
  prevention of, 164
  transmission of, 535, 570
  treatment of, 535, 570
  Varicella-zoster virus, 522, 535
heterosexuality, **110**, 141. *See also* sexual orientation
HEVs (hybrid electric vehicles), 707
HHV-8 (human herpesvirus 8), 501, 535, 536
hierarchy of needs, 64–67
high, drug-induced, **248**
high blood pressure
  in African Americans, 349, 422, 458
  cardiovascular disease and, 448–450, 472
  diet and, 349, 375, 449–450, 471
  exercise and, 382, 385
  during pregnancy, 225
high-density lipoproteins (HDLs), **332**, 382, 432, 448, **450**, 450–452, 473
highly active antiretroviral therapy (HAART), 558, 560
Hinduism, 300
Hispanic Americans. *See* Latinos/Latinas
histamine, **519**, 524
histoplasmosis, 539
HIV antibody test, 556
HIV infection. *See* human immunodeficiency virus (HIV) infection
HIV-positive, defined, **556**
HIV Replication Capacity, 556
HIV RNA assay, **554**, 556, 575
HIV tests, 554, 556–557, 575
HMOs (health maintenance organizations), **656**
H5N1 influenza strain, 534
Hodgkin's disease, 495, 501
home injuries, **668**, 668–671
Homeland Security, Department of, 678
homeopathy, 644, 646–647, **647**
homeostasis, **34**, 34–35, 40
homicide, 664, 672, 675, 677–678
homocysteine, 41, 459
homophobia, 110–111, **141**
homosexuality, **110**, 141. *See also* sexual orientation
honesty, in relationships, 99
hormonal methods of contraception
  emergency, 159–160, 163
  implant, 158, 175
  injectable, 158–159
  oral, 154–156
  principles of, 152, 170
  skin patch, 156–157
  vaginal ring, 157
  See also contraceptives
hormone replacement therapy (HRT), 132, 136, 457, 485, 589, 590. *See also* estrogens
hormones
  asthma and, 525
  body fat and, 421
  breast cancer and, 219–220
  in contraceptives, 154–155, 158
  defined, **34**
  emotions and, 214
  endocrine disrupters, 210
  in the reproductive life cycle, 127–132
  sexual differentiation and, 128
  stress and, **34**, 38, 543
  See also hormone replacement therapy; *specific hormones*
hospice programs, **608**, 608–609
hostility, 454–455. *See also* anger
HPV. *See* human papillomavirus
HRT. *See* hormone replacement therapy

HSAs (health savings accounts), 656
HSV. *See* herpes simplex virus
HSV 1, 535, 569
HSV 2, 569. *See also* genital herpes
human chorionic gonadotropin (HCG), 129, 212, **213**, 218
human herpesvirus 8 (HHV-8), 501, 535, 536
human immunodeficiency virus (HIV) infection, 548–562
  anal sex and, 143
  circumcision and, 127
  costs of treatment, 560
  defined, **549**
  diagnosis of, 556–557
  education programs, 562, 573–574
  HIV infection process, 549–551
  injection drug use and, 245
  opportunistic infections with, 556
  populations of special concern for, 553–554
  pregnancy and, 222–223, 559–560
  prevention of, 147, 560–563, 575–577
  statistics on, 522, 548, 550, 553, 573
  symptoms of infection, 554, 556
  from tattoos and piercings, 537
  transmission of, 550, 551–553, 564, 569
  treatment of, 557–560
  tuberculosis and, 528
  vaccines for, 560
  See also acquired immunodeficiency syndrome
human papillomavirus (HPV)
  cervical cancer and, 488–489, 501, 536
  defined, **566**
  oral contraceptives and, 155
  p53 gene and, 497
  symptoms of, 567–568
  warts from, 538
humor, 52–53, 72
hybrid electric vehicles (HEVs), 707
hydrocodone, 248–250
hydrogenation, **331**
hydrostatic weighing, 415
Hypericum perforatum (St. John's wort), 81, 83, 359, 648–649
hypertension, defined, **449**. *See also* high blood pressure
hypertrophic cardiomyopathy (HCM), **466**, 467–468
hypertrophy, **452**
hypnosis, **647**, 647–648
hypnotics, 84–85
hypothalamus, **34**, **127**
hysterectomy, **174**

ibuprofen, 485, 589, 591
"ice," 252–253
identical twins, **208**
identity, adult, 67–68
identity crisis, 68
IDUs (injection drug users), 245–246, 552, 562
IgE (immunoglobulin E), 524
illnesses. *See* diseases; infectious diseases
immigrants
  access to health care by, 10
  cardiovascular disease in, 458
  tuberculosis in, 528
immune systems, 516–526
  allergies and, 523–526
  autoimmune diseases and, 8, 518, 519, 542
  chain of infection, 516–517
  components of, 518–519
  exercise and, 383
  gender differences in, 8, 542
  HIV infection and, 549–551, 554
  immune response, 519–520

immunity and, 520–521
  immunization and, 521–523
  inflammatory response, 519
  physical and chemical barriers, 517–518
  relationships and, 113
  stress and, 40–41, 543
  support for, 542–543
  T cells, 518–519, 543, 549
  See also infectious diseases
immunity, 520–523, **521**
immunization. *See* vaccines
immunocontraceptives, 175
immunoglobulin E (IgE), 524
immunotherapy, 525–526
impetigo, 528
Implanon, 158
impotence (erectile dysfunction), 135–136, 310, **488**
incest, **685**
incomplete proteins, 329
incontinence, **488**
incubation, **521**
indigestion, B–9 to B–10
indoor air pollution, 707
induction chemotherapy, **505**
infants
  environmental tobacco smoke and, 314–315
  genital herpes in, 222–223
  infant mortality, 10, 225–226
  intoxication in, 252
  nutritional needs of, 373–375
  vitamin K for, 344
infatuation, **98**
infection, chain of, **516**, 516–517. *See also* infectious diseases
infectious diseases, 526–542, 694–699
  antibiotic resistance and, 531
  chicken pox, 522, 535
  colds, 41, 516, 532–533
  defined, **3**
  emerging, 540–541
  encephalitis, 535–536
  fungal, 527, 538–539
  hepatitis, 222, 501, 536–537
  from herpesvirus, 222–223, 535
  in history, 3, 698
  infectious agents in chronic diseases, 536
  influenza, 532–535
  Lyme disease, 528–529, 698
  malaria, 13, 207, 526, 539
  measles, 522, 526, 535
  meningitis, 515, 526, 527–528
  mumps, 522, 526, 535
  pertussis, 529
  pneumonia, 526–527, 556, 559
  poliomyelitis, 531–532, 536, 537–538
  during pregnancy, 222
  prions and, 539–540
  protozoal, 527, 539
  rabies, 538
  Rocky Mountain spotted fever, 529, 698
  rubella, 221, 222–223, 522
  staphylococcal infections, 528
  statistics on, 526
  streptococcal infections, 467–468, 528
  tetanus, 529
  tuberculosis, 528, 529
  typhus, 529
  ulcers, 529
  urinary tract infections, 529–530
  warts, 538
  See also diseases; sexually transmitted diseases
infertility, 203, **208**, 210–212, 563
inflammation
  in allergic response, 524

Alzheimer's disease and, 591
in arthritis, 589
aspirin and, 474
cardiovascular disease and, 456–457, 460
colon cancer and, 485
COX-2 inhibitors for, 641
exercise and, 381
homocysteine and, 41, 459
in the immune response, 519
in lupus, 542
stress and, 41
influenza, 522–523, **532**, 532–535
inhalants, 257–258
injectable contraceptives, 158–159, 175
injection drug users (IDUs), 245–246, 552, 562
injuries
alcohol use and, 275
at-home, 668–671
bicycle, 668–669
causes of, 662–664
exercise, 403–404
falls, 668–669
fires, 669–670
gender differences in, 663
intentional vs. unintentional, 662
leisure time, 671–672
motor vehicle, 664–668
pedestrian, 668
poisoning, 670–671
prevention of, 383–384, 404, 667
smoking and, 310
statistics on, 662, 663, 664
suffocation and choking, 671
work-related, 672, 673
in-line skating injuries, 672
inner-directed, **66**
insect control, 698–699
insect repellent, 530
insect sting allergies, 523
insomnia, 42, 49, 50, 649
insulin
calming effect of foods and, 330
diabetes and, 416–417, 418
exercise and, 383
metabolic syndrome and, 457–459
stress and, 42
insulin resistance (pre-diabetes), 418, 453, 458–459
insulin resistance syndrome. *See* metabolic syndrome
integration, in self-concept, 69
intellectual wellness, 2
intensity, of exercise, 390, 391–392, 394–395, 397
intentional injuries, **662**. *See also* violence
intercourse, sexual, 144, 206
interferons, 519, 521
Intergovernmental Panel on Climate Change (IPCC), 705
interleukins, 519
Internet
addiction to, 239
counterfeit drugs on, 136
cybersex on, 145
cyberstalking, 680–682
evaluating health resources on, 18
online pharmacies, 641–642, 644
online relationships, 95, 109
pornography on, 144
shyness and, 77
social networks on, 45
weight management resources, 429, 433
interpersonal violence, 679
interpersonal wellness, 3
intersexed individuals, 137
interventions, 263
intestate, **606**, 607

intimate relationships, 95–119
capacity for, 66, 68
challenges in, 99–101
characteristics of friendships, 97
choosing a partner, 107
communication in, 102–106
conflict resolution, 103–106
dating and, 107
ending, 102
enhancing support in, 101
interfaith and intrafaith, 108
jealousy and, 101
living together, 107–110
love, sex, and intimacy in, 97–99
love maps questionnaire, 100
online relationships, 109
same-sex partnerships, 110–112
self-concept and self-esteem in, 96–97
sexual decision making in, 139, 174
sexual privacy in, 146
singlehood, 112
for single people, 106–107
successful, 101
unhealthy, 102
wellness and, 113
intoxication, **236**, 244, 248, 250, 252. *See also* alcohol use; psychoactive drugs
intracerebral hemorrhage, 465
intracytoplasmic sperm injection (ICSI), 211
intrauterine devices (IUDs), 160–161, **161**, 170
intrauterine insemination, 210
introverts, 77
in vitro fertilization (IVF), **210**, 210–211
Iraq war, trauma and loss in, 622
iron, 207, 340–341, 357, 460, 499
irradiated foods, 366
ischemic strokes, **464**, 464–465
Islam, 69, 300
isometric exercises, **393**
isotonic exercises, **394**
IUDs (intrauterine devices), 160–161, **161**, 170
IVF (in vitro fertilization), **210**, 210–211

Jack in the Box, A–1
Japan, social phobias in, 75
jaundice, **536**
jealousy, 101
Jewish people
breast cancer in, 498
metabolism of alcohol by, 272
paths to spiritual wellness in, 69
Tay-Sachs disease and, 207
tobacco use and, 300
jobs, stress from, 44–45
Judaism, 69, 300
junk mail, canceling, 697

Kaposi's sarcoma, 501, 536, **556**
Kegel exercises, 224
ketamine, 251, 257, 683
Kevorkian, Dr. Jack, 611
KFC, A–2
kidney cancer, 494
killer T cells, 518–519, **519**
kilocalories, 328–329, **329**. *See also* calories
Kobasa, Suzanne, 37
kreteks, 313
Kübler-Ross, Elizabeth, 617
Kyoto Protocol, 705

labels
false, 644
on foods and supplements, 336, 359–362

on OTC drugs, 632
on prescription medications, 640, 642–643
labor, **226**, 226–229
lactation, **230**
Lactobacillus, 526, 572
lacto-ovo-vegetarians, **355**
lactose intolerance, 207, 367
lacto-vegetarians, **355**
landfills, 697
laparoscopy, **172**
larynx cancer, 313
last rites, 614–616
Latinos/Latinas
aging, 599
alcohol abuse among, 286, 287
asthma in, 525
body image in, 436
cardiovascular disease in, 458
cervical cancer in, 496
contraceptive use among, 173
on death and dying, 607
diabetes in, 418, 422, 458
distribution in U.S. population, 9
drug use in, 259
health concerns of, 9–10
HIV/AIDS in, 554, 555
metabolic syndrome in, 458
obesity in, 422
sexual decision making by, 142
sickle-cell disease in, 207
in single-parent families, 117
tobacco use by, 304, 305
See also ethnicity
LBW (low-birth-weight), 225, 315
LDLs. *See* low-density lipoproteins
lead poisoning, 222–223, 708, 709
Lea's Shield, 166
legumes (beans), **329**, 333, 348, 351, 353, 354, 375
leisure injuries, **671**, 671–672
leptin, 421
lesbian, gay, or bisexual (LGB) orientation, 110, 141. *See also* sexual orientation
leukemia, 480, **482**, 494
leukoplakia, 312
Levitra (vardenafil), 136
Levonorgestral IUD (Mirena), 160–161
LGB (lesbian, gay, or bisexual) orientation, 110, 141. *See also* sexual orientation
LH (luteinizing hormone), 129
lice, 572, **573**
life expectancy
aging theories and, 592–593
AIDS and, 550
chronic alcohol use and, 278
defined, 592
exercise and, 380–381
factors influencing, 592
gender differences in, 8, 593
Healthy People initiative and, 5
obesity and, 416
quality of life and, 6
religion and, 473
smoking and, 297, 311
life span, **592**
lifestyle
culture and, 10
evaluation of, 16–17
exercise and, 386–387
leading causes of death and, 5–6
motivation for change, 15–20, 25–26
obesity and, 12, 421–423
personalized plans for change, 21–24
self-efficacy and, 19
wellness profile, 12–14

lifestyle physical activity, 386–387
life-support systems, 604–605, **605**, 609–610
lifting technique, 672–673
lightbulbs, 693, 708
"light" cigarettes, 306
lightening, 214, **215**
linoleic acid, 330–331, 332, 375
lipoprotein(a), 459
lipoproteins, 382, **383**, 450–451, 459
liposuction, 435
listening, intimate relationships and, 103–104
Listeria, 221, 361, 364
Listeria monocytogenes, 361
lithium carbonate, 82, 84
liver, 277–278, 536–537, 570–571, 649, 650
liver cancer, 496, 501, 536–537
living together, 107–110
living wills, **611**, 611–612
local anesthetic, **194**
lockjaw, 522, 526, 529
locus of control, **19**
loneliness, 73
loss, coping with, 619–623. *See also* grief
love
    addiction to, 238
    in intimate relationships, 97–99
    love maps questionnaire, 100
Love Canal, New York, 697
low-back pain, 383, B–10 to B–11
low-birth-weight (LBW), **225**, 315
low-carbohydrate diets, 431
low-density lipoproteins (LDLs), **332**, 382, 448,
    450, 450–452, 459, 472–473
low-fat diets, 431
low-tar cigarettes, 306
LSD (lysergic acid diethylamide), 246, 247, 251,
    256–257
lumpectomies, 486
Lunelle, 158–159, 175
lung cancer
    detection and treatment, 484
    environmental tobacco smoke and, 314
    pollution and, 501–503
    radon gas and, 503, 712
    risk factors for, 484, 500
    smoking and, 308–309, 311, 319
    trends in, 482–483
lupus, 542
luteinizing hormone (LH), 129
Lyme disease, 528–529
lymphatic system, 480–481, **481**, 516, 516–517, 519
lymph nodes, 519
lymphocytes, 40, 518, **519**
lymphomas, **482**, 494–495, 501, 536

macrophages, 309, 518–521, **519**
"mad cow disease," 363, 539–540
magnesium, 131, 341, 342, 485
magnetic resonance imaging (MRI), 415, **464**,
    505, 537
ma huang (ephedra), 396, 432
mainstream smoke, **314**
malaria, 13, 207, 526, **539**
male condoms. *See* condoms, male
male sex organs, 125–127
malignant tumors, 480, **481**
mammograms, 486, 504
managed-care plans, 654–656, **655**
mania, **81**, 81–82
manipulative therapies, 648, 651
manual vacuum aspiration (MVA), **194**, 194–195
marijuana
    dependence on, 255

effects and uses of, 254–256
    fertility and, 210
    placebo effect and, 248
    during pregnancy, 223
    properties of, 249
    statistics on, 235, 236
    stress and, 57
marriage
    abusive partners in, 678–680, 681
    benefits of, 112–113
    civil unions and, 111
    family life cycle and, 116–117
    interfaith, 108
    issues in, 113–114
    same-sex, 111
    separation and divorce, 114
    statistics on, 112
    See also intimate relationships
Maslow, Abraham, 64–65
mass media. *See* media
mast cells, 524
mastectomy, 486
Master Settlement Agreement (MSA), 315–316
masturbation, **136**, 137, 138, 143
mature understanding of death, **605**
maximal oxygen consumption (VO_{2max}), **391**
McDonald's, A–2
MDMA (ecstasy), 251, 257
measles, 522, 526, 535
meat, 353–354, 364, 498–499, 539–540
media
    body image and, 436
    gender, sexuality, and, 138
    portrayal of smoking in, 303
    violence in, 675
    See also advertising
Medicaid, **656**
medical abortion, 195. *See also* abortion
medical doctors (M.D.), **635**
medical ID bracelets, 643
Medicare, 597–598, 609, **656**
medications
    complying with physicians' instructions, 658
    costs of, 642
    errors in, 639–640
    generic, 632, 633, 643
    interactions with botanicals, 650
    labels on, 642–643
    off-label drug use, 640, 642
    over-the-counter, 631–633
    prescription, 639–643
    for psychological disorders, 84–85
    side effects of, 632, 641, 643
    Vioxx story, 641
    for weight management, 434
meditation, **54**, 54–55
MedWatch, 644
melanoma, **490**, 490–491, 493, 503, 507
memorial services, 614–616
memorial societies, 616–617, **617**
memory, 383, 590–591, 649
memory B cells, 518–519, **519**
memory T cells, 518–519, **519**
men
    abusive, 678–680, 681
    alcoholism in, 286–287
    body image in, 436
    cancer in, 483
    chlamydia in, 563
    circumcision of, 126–127, **127**, 489, 552
    communication advice for, 105
    date rape, 683–684
    fat distribution in, 417
    health-related behaviors in, 8

heart disease in, 456
    homocysteine levels in, 459
    injuries in, 663
    life expectancy in, 593
    male sex organs, 125–127
    male sexual maturation, 128–132
    nutritional needs of, 373–375
    obesity in, 422, 423
    sexual health problems in, 135
    sexual response cycle in, 133–135
    smoking by, 311
    statistics on marital status of, 105
    stress and, 39
    suicide among older, 592
    violence in, 675–676
    See also gender differences
menarche, 128
meningitis, 515, **526**, 526–528
menopause, 132, **133**, 589
menstruation
    in female athlete triad, 419
    iron supplements and, 344
    menopause and, 589
    menstrual cycle, 128–132
    menstrual disorders, 129–132, 419
    pregnancy and, 212
mental disorders. *See* psychological disorders
mental health. *See* psychological health
menthol in cigarettes, 306, 307
mercury
    from fish consumption, 221, 222, 365
    poisoning by, 223, 708, 710
    pollution by, 710
    during pregnancy, 221, 222, 223
    in vaccines, 523
mescaline, 257
metabolic rate, 381
metabolic syndrome
    characteristics of, 458–459
    cortisol levels in, 40
    diet types for, 431
    fat intake and, 469
    overview of, 458–459
    risk factors for, 417, 458–459
metabolism
    of alcohol, 271
    defined, **271**
    effects on, 420–421
    exercise and, 380–381
    resting metabolic rate, 420
metastasis, **481**
methadone treatment, 260, 261
methamphetamine, 252–253
methaqualone, 249, 250
methotrexate, 195, 224
Mexican Americans. *See* Latinos/Latinas
MI (myocardial infarction), 307, 461. *See also*
    heart attacks
microbicides, 560
middle knowledge, **617**
mifepristone, 186, 192, 195
migraines, 43
milk products, recommended intake of, 347,
    352–353
mind/body/spirit connections
    anger, hostility, and heart disease, 455
    coping with cancer, 508
    eating habits and total wellness, 330
    exercise, body image, and self-esteem, 428
    exercise and the mind, 384
    expressive writing and chronic
        conditions, 631
    healthy connections with others, 48
    helping yourself by helping others, 587

immunity and stress, 542
intimate relationships and health, 113
nature and the human spirit, 695
paths to spiritual wellness, 69
placebo effect, 647
religion and wellness, 473
in search of a good death, 618
sexual decision making, 139
spirituality and drug abuse, 244
stress and genital herpes, 570
stress and pregnancy, 219
stress and the brain, 42
tobacco use and religion, 300
warning signs of wellness, 4
mindfulness meditation, 54–55
minerals, **340**, 340–341
Mirena, 160–161
miscarriage, 184, 219, 224–225, 490
misoprostol, 195
mitochondrial DNA, 211
mitral valve prolapse (MVP), **468**, 469
MM (multiple myeloma), 495
moles, 491, 493
monkeypox, 540
monoclonal antibodies, 487
mononucleosis, 535
monosodium glutamate (MSG), 366, 367
monounsaturated fats, **331**, 331–332, 333
mood, 330, 384
mood disorders, 76, 78–82, 83
mood stabilizers, 84
mopeds, 667–668
moral development, 68–69
morphine, 249
mosquitoborne infections, 530, 540, 698–699
motivation for change, 15–20, 25–26
motorcycles, 667–668
motor vehicle injuries, **664**, 664–668
mourning, 620–621, **621**
mouth, pathogens and, 517–518
MRI (magnetic resonance imaging), 415, 464, 505
MS (multiple sclerosis), 536, 542
MSA (Master Settlement Agreement), 315–316
MSG (monosodium glutamate), 366, 367
mucus method, 169
multi-infarct dementia, 590
multiple births, 206, 208
multiple myeloma (MM), 495
mumps, 522, 526, 535
muscle dysmorphia, 435
muscular endurance, **380**
muscular strength
    defined, **379**
    developing, 393–395
    gender differences in, 393
    importance of, 379
    sports activities and, 398
    See also strength training
music, 56, 713
mutagens, 496, **497**
mutations, cancer and, 495–497
MVA (manual vacuum aspiration), **194**, 194–195
MVP (mitral valve prolapse), **468**, 469
Mycobacterium tuberculosis, 528
mycoplasmas, **526**, 527
myocardial infarction (MI), **307**, 461. *See also* heart attacks
myotonia, **133**
MyPyramid, **343**, 350–354
    discretionary calories, **354**
    energy intake, 353
    food groups, 351–354
    key messages, 350–351

Naltrexone, 286
narcotics, 248–250
Narcotics Anonymous (NA), 261
nasal congestion, B–8
National Center for Complementary and
    Alternative Medicine (NCCAM), 643
National Cholesterol Education Program (NCEP),
    469, 473
National Institutes of Health (NIH), 414
National Strength and Conditioning Association
    (NSCA), 399
National Weight Control Registry, 431
Native Americans. *See* American Indians
Native Hawaiians, 9, 259. *See also* ethnicity
natural killer cells, 518–519, **519**
nausea, 213, B–9
NCCAM (National Center for Complementary
    and Alternative Medicine), 643
NCEP (National Cholesterol Education Program),
    469, 473
necrotizing fasciitis, 528
Neisseria gonorrhoeae, 565
Neisseria meningitidis, 528
neoplasms, 480
neotame, 426
nervous system, 33–36, 250
neural tube defects, 206, 220, 344
neuropeptides, 40
neurotransmitters, 34, 37, 82, 330, **384**
neutrophils, 518–519, **519**
news, evaluating, 636
NHL (non-Hodgkin's lymphoma), 495
niacin, 339, 460
nicotine
    addiction to, 298–301
    addictive potential of, 235, 242
    defined, **299**
    immediate effects of, 307, 308, 448
    in reconstituted tobacco, 306
    in spit tobacco, 312
    stress and, 57
    treatment for addiction to, 311, 321
nicotine replacement therapy, 311, 321
NIH (National Institutes of Health), 414
nitrates, 365
nitrites, 350, 365, 493
nitrogen dioxide, 701
nitrosamines, **501**
NMR (nuclear magnetic resonance imaging), 415,
    464, 505, 651
nocturnal emissions, 139
noise pollution, 713–714
noncorporeal continuity, 605
nonessential (storage) fat, 412–413, **413**
non-Hodgkin's lymphoma (NHL), 495
nonnutritive sweeteners, 426
nonoxynol-9 (N-9), 151, 552, 561, 563
nonsteroidal anti-inflammatory drugs (NSAIDS),
    591, 641
nontraditional students, 44
nonverbal communication, 102–103
norepinephrine, **34**, 40, 251, 330
normality, compared with psychological health,
    64, **65**
Noroviruses, 363
Norplant contraceptive implant, 158, 175
NSAIDS (nonsteroidal anti-inflammatory drugs),
    591, 641
NSCA (National Strength and Conditioning
    Association), 399
nuclear magnetic resonance imaging (NMR), 415,
    464, 505, 651
nuclear power, **710**, 711–712
nuclear transfer, 211

nuclear weapons, 711–712
nurse-midwives, 226
nursing homes, 581, 597
nutrient density, 345, 349
nutrition, 327–375
    antioxidants, 338, 340–342, 499–500
    carbohydrates, 334–337 (*See also*
        carbohydrates)
    defined, 328, **329**
    Dietary Guidelines for Americans, 344–350
    dietary standards, 343–344
    ethnic foods and, 346
    at fast-food restaurants, A–1 to A–5
    fats, 330–334 (*See also* fats, dietary)
    fiber, 337–338, 360, 375
    fish consumption guidelines, 365
    food and supplement labels, 359–362
    gender differences in, 357
    Healthy Eating Pyramid, 375
    improving, 367–369, 370
    kilocalories, 328–329
    minerals, 340, 341
    MyPyramid, 350–354
    for older adults, 358–359
    phytochemicals, 342
    prenatal, 220–221
    proteins, 329–330, 334
    serving sizes, 353, 360
    stress management and, 49, 57–58
    total wellness and, 330
    vegetarian diets, 354–357
    vitamins, 338–340
    water and, 340
nutritional supplements. *See* dietary supplements
NuvaRing, 157

obesity
    aging and, 585
    BMI determination of, 414–415
    cancer and, 500–501
    cardiovascular disease and, 452–453
    contributing factors to, 413
    defined, 414, **415**
    Dietary Guidelines for Americans
        recommendations, 345–347
    exercise and, 385, 422
    fat cells and, 421
    genetic factors in, 419–420
    health risks of, 416, 420
    hormones and, 421
    lifestyle and, 12, 421–423
    metabolism and, 420
    psychosocial factors in, 423
    statistics on, 412
    surgery for, 434–435
    type 2 diabetes and, 383
    waist circumference and, 417, 420,
        422, 459
    See also body weight; weight management
obsessions, 76
obsessive-compulsive disorder (OCD), **76**, 76–77,
    80, 435, 536
Occupational Safety and Health Administration
    (OSHA), 672, 678
OCs. *See* oral contraceptives
off-label drug use, 640, 642
oils, dietary, 353–354. *See also* fats, dietary
olestra, 426
omega-3 fatty acids, **332**, 333, 459, 471, 499, 591
omega-6 fatty acids, 332, 333, 499
oncogenes, **497**
oncologists, **482**
online pharmacies, 641–642, 644

opioids, 57, **248**, 248–250
opportunistic infections, **551**, 559
optimism, 71–72
optometrists, **637**
oral cancer, 312, 313, 493, 499, 509
oral contraceptives (OCs), 154–156, **155**, 448, 457, 485, 489
oral-genital stimulation, 143
oral sex, STD transmission during, 552, 561, 562, 569, 571
Orasure tests, 557
Oregon Death with Dignity Act of 1994, 610
organ donors, 612–614
organic foods, **364**
organ transplants, 536–537, 612–614
orgasm, **133**, 133–135
orgasmic dysfunction, **136**, 137
orlistat (Xenical), 434
Ornish diet, 431
OrthoEvra, 156–157
OSHA (Occupational Safety and Health Administration), 672, 678
osteoarthritis (OA), 588
osteopenia, 590
osteoporosis
    calcium intake in women and, 357
    defined, **340**, **589**
    dietary guidelines for, 342
    exercise and, 383, 385
    overview, 589–590
OTC (over-the-counter) medications, 247, **631**, 631–633
other-directed, **66**
outpatient surgery, **643**
ovarian cancer, 489–490
ovaries, **124**, 125, **206**
overdosing, 248, 250
Overeaters Anonymous (OA), 432
overload, **389**, 389–390
over-the-counter (OTC) medications, 247, **631**, 631–633
overweight, 412, 414–416, **415**. *See also* obesity; weight management
oviduct, **206**
ovulation, 129, 152, **153**
oxycodone, 248–250
oxytocin, 38–39
ozone, 693, 702, 704, 706
ozone layer, **704**, 706

Pacific Islander Americans
    cancer in, 496
    distribution in U.S. population, 9
    drug use in, 259
    tobacco use by, 304, 305
    See also ethnicity
paclitaxel (Taxol), 487
PAD (peripheral arterial disease), 460, 466–467
pain management, 610–611, 618, 646, 648
palliative care, **608**, 618
palm oil, 331
pancreatic cancer, 313, 482, 493, 499
pandemics, influenza, 534, **535**
panic disorder, **74**, 75–76, 80
Pap tests, **155**, **488**, 489
ParaGard, 160–161
paraphilia, **144**
parasites, 363, 527, **531**, 539, 549, 572–573
parasitic worms, 527, **539**
parasympathetic division, 33
parenting styles, 115–116
parents
    becoming, 114–115
    children of alcoholic, 284

consent for abortion by, 198
family life cycle, 116–117
parenting styles, 115–116
pregnancy tasks for fathers, 215
preparation for parenthood, 204–206, 231
single, 117
stepfamilies, 117
violence against children by, 682, 685
See also families
Parkinson's disease, 647
parovirus B19, 205
partial birth abortion, 185, 195
partial vegetarians, **355**
particulate matter (PM), 702
Partnership for Healthy Weight Management, 432
PAS (physician-assisted suicide), 610, **611**
passion, 98–99. *See also* intimate relationships
passive-aggressive behavior, 72
passive euthanasia, 610, **611**
passive immunity, 522–523
pathogens, **361**, **516**. *See also* infectious diseases
pathological gambling, 238
Patriot Act, 678
PCBs (polychlorinated biphenyls), 364, **365**, 696, **697**
PCP, 257
pedestrian safety, 668
pedophiles, 685
peer counseling, 59, 88, 261, 286
pelvic exams, 156
pelvic inflammatory disease (PID), 135, 158, 160, 210, 563, **565**, 566
penicillins, 530
penis, **124**, 125–126, 134
Pennebaker, James, 52
PEP (post-exposure prophylaxis), 538, 559, 575
percent body fat, 271, 412–413, **413**, 415–416, 419. *See also* body fat
perchlorate, 711
perfectionism, 50
performance-enhancing drugs, 396
perinatal transmission, 552
peripheral arterial disease (PAD), 460, **466**, 466–467
persistent vegetative state, **608**, **609**
personal flotation device, **671**
personal health profile, 640
personality, 36, 36–38, 454
    Type A, 36–37, 454
    Type B, 36–37
    Type C, 37
    Type D, 454
    hardy, 37
personal safety, 661–691
    adopting safer habits, 689
    assault, 676, 678
    for children, 677
    emergency preparedness, 680
    factors contributing to violence, 674–676
    family violence, 678–682
    gang-related violence, 676–677
    hate crimes, 677
    home injuries, 668–671
    homicide, 672, 675, 677–678
    leisure time injuries, 671–672
    motor vehicle injuries, 664–668
    providing emergency care, 687
    public policies and, 686–687
    sexual violence, 682–686
    stalking and cyberstalking, 680–682
    statistics on, 662–664
    terrorism and, 47, 77, 678
    in the workplace, 677–678
    See also injuries
pertussis, 522, 526, 529
pescovegetarians, **355**

pessimism, 71–72
pesticides, **709**, 709–710
pet ownership, 587
p53 gene, 497
pharmaceuticals, in Western medicine, 634, **635**. *See also* medications
pharmacies, online, 642
pharmacological properties, **246**, 246–247
pharmacological therapy, for psychological disorders, 84–85
pharmacology, defined, 239
pharmacopoeia, **648**
pharmacy, defined, 239
phenylpropanolamine, 396, 432
phobias, 74–77, 91
phosphorus, 341, 342
physical activity
    cancer and, 500
    cardiovascular disease and, 451–452
    defined, 386
    lifestyle, 386–387, 427
    obesity and, 422
    physical activity pyramid, 388
    recommended amount of, 387–389
    See also exercise
Physical Activity and Health, 378
physical activity pyramid, 388
physical dependence, 240, **241**. *See also* addiction; psychoactive drugs
physical fitness
    aging and, 584
    amount of activity and, 387–388
    assessments of, 402
    body composition and, 380
    cardiorespiratory endurance and, 378–379
    defined, **379**
    flexibility and, 380
    muscular endurance and, 380
    muscular strength and, 379
    See also exercise; exercise programs
physical wellness, 2
physician-assisted suicide (PAS), 610, **611**
physicians, 630–631, 635, 637–639, 651–652
phytochemicals, 342, **343**, 500, **501**
phytoestrogens, 500, 589
PID. *See* pelvic inflammatory disease
"the pill," 154–156. *See also* oral contraceptives
pinworms, 539
pipe smoking, 312–313
pituitary gland, **34**, **127**
placebo, **83**
placebo effect, 83, **248**, 646–647
placenta, **217**, 228
Plan B, 159–160, 162
planetary wellness, 3
plant stanols and sterols, 471
plaques, 307, 460–462, **461**
Plasmodium, 539
platelets, 381, 448, **449**, 454
PMDD (premenstrual dysphoric disorder), **130**, 130–132
PMS (premenstrual syndrome), **130**, 130–132
Pneumocystis carinii pneumonia, **556**, 559
pneumonia, **526**, 526–527, 556, 559
PNI (psychoneuroimmunology), 40–41, **41**
podiatrists, **637**
point-of-service (POS) plans, **656**
poisoning, 670–671
poliomyelitis, 522–523, 531–532, **536**, 537–538
political violence, 679
pollen allergies, 523
pollution
    air, 701–708
    cancers from, 501–503
    chemical, 708–711

noise, 713–714
radiation, 711–713
water, 695
See also environmental health
polychlorinated biphenyls (PCBs), 364, **365**, 696, **697**
polyps, **485**
polyunsaturated fats, **331**, 331–332, 333
population growth, 699–701
pornography, **144**, 144–145
portion sizes. *See* serving sizes
post-exposure prophylaxis (PEP), 538, 559, 575
postpartum depression, **230**
postpartum period, **229**, 229–231
post-traumatic stress disorder (PTSD), 41–42, 47, 76, 77–78, 80, 622, 685
potassium, 342, 348, 349, 350, 450, 471, 585
poverty
age and, 594
AIDS/HIV and, 555
asthma and, 525, 709
cancer and, 496
drug use and, 259
emerging diseases and, 541
environmental health and, 709
gangs and, 676–677
health and, 10
health insurance coverage and, 496, 655
violence and, 675, 676–677, 679
See also socioeconomic status
preapproval drug studies, 641
preconception care, **205**, 205–206
precontemplation stage of behavior change, 20
pre-diabetes, 418, 453, 458
preeclampsia, **225**
preferred provider organizations (PPOs), **656**
pregnancy, 203–226
alcohol use during, 221–223, 278–279
bacterial vaginosis in, 52, 57
changes in the woman's body, 212–214
childbirth, 226–231
chlamydia transmission in, 563–564
complications of, 224–226
conception, 206–208
due date calculation, 213
emotional responses to, 214
exercise during, 223–224
fetal abnormality diagnosis, 217–219
fetal development, 214–220
fetal programming, 219–220
folic acid and, 206, 220, 357
healthy eating in, 220–221, 365, 373–375
hepatitis B in, 570
HIV transmission in, 553, 559–560
preconception care, 205–206
prenatal care, 220–224
psychoactive drugs during, 247–248, 251–253, 255
rates of, 152, 177
smoking and, 298, 315
stress and, 42, 219–220
tasks for fathers during, 215
teen, 177
tests, 212
unintended, 197–198
weight gain during, 213
pregnancy tests, 212
prehypertension, 449
premature ejaculation, **136**
premature infants, 225
premenstrual dysphoric disorder (PMDD), **130**, 130–132
premenstrual syndrome (PMS), **130**, 130–132
premenstrual tension, **130**, 130–132
prenatal care, 220–224

prenatal nutrition, 220–221
prepuce, **124**, 125–126
presbyopia, 588, **589**
prescription medications, 639–643. *See also* medications
Preven, 159
primary care physicians, 637–638
prions, 527, **539**, 539–540
problem-solving, 52
pro-choice position, 186–187, 189. *See also* abortion
procrastination, 25, 50–51
prodromal period, **521**
progesterone, 127–129, 158
progestins, **127**, 128, 158
progressive overload, 389–390
progressive relaxation, 53
pro-life position, 186, 188–189. *See also* abortion
proof value, 270, **271**
proprioception, 257
prostaglandins, 129–130, 136, 195
prostate cancer, 487–488, 496, 499, 504–505
prostate gland, 126, 647, 649
prostate-specific antigen (PSA) blood test, **488**, 504
prostatitis, 135
prostitution, **144**, 145–146
protease inhibitors, **507**, 558, **559**
proteins, dietary
amino acids, 329, 396
calcium loss and, 342
complete and incomplete, 329
defined, **329**
as fat substitutes, 426
mental boost from, 330
recommended intake, 329–330, 334, 375
supplements, 396
weight management and, 427
protozoa (*singular,* protozoan), 527, **539**
Prozac (fluoxetine), 82, 84, 86, 439
PSA (prostate-specific antigen) blood test, **488**, 504
psychiatrists, 89
psychoactive drugs, 235–267
abuse of, 240
addictive behaviors of, 236–239, 242–244
alcohol combined with other, 274
cardiovascular disease and, 455
club drugs, 251
CNS depressants, 249, 250
CNS stimulants, 250–254
date-rape drugs, 683–684
decision on use of, 262–264, 265
defined, **236**
dependence on, 240–241
drug testing, 260
economic cost of, 258
effects on body, 246–249
gender differences in use of, 243
hallucinogens, 255–257
HIV infection and, 550, 561–562
inhalants, 257–258
legalization of, 258–260
marijuana, 210, 223, 248–249, 254–256
method of use, 247
opioids, 57, 248–250
preventing drug abuse, 262
risks of, 244–246
self-assessment of problem with, 245
sexually transmitted diseases and, 550, 561–562, 568
sources of, 240
statistics on use of, 236, 259
stress and, 57
treatment for dependence on, 260–262
user and nonuser profiles, 241–242
psychodynamic model, 87

psychological disorders, 74–83
anxiety disorders, 74–78, 86–87, 91
ethnicity and, 10, 75
getting help for, 88–89
mood disorders, 78–82
neurotransmitters and, 82
prevalence in Americans, 76
statistics on, 63
stress and, 41–42
syphilis and, 572
treatment for, 78, 80–81, 83, 84–87
psychological health, 63–91
abortions and, 196–197
anger, 73–74
defense mechanisms, 70–72
defined, 64
Erikson's stages of development, 67–68
exercise and, 383, 384
healthy self-esteem, 69–71
honest communication, 72–73, 104
loneliness and, 73
Maslow's hierarchy of needs, 64–67
normality *vs.*, 64
optimism, 71–72
weight management and, 416, 427–428
psychologists, 89
psychoneuroimmunology (PNI), 40–41, **41**
psychosis, 253, 254
psyllium, 337
PTSD. *See* post-traumatic stress disorder
puberty, 128, 421
pubic lice, 572, **573**
public health systems, 4, 541, 634, 694
pulmonary circulation, **446**
pulmonary edema, **466**, 467
pulmonary heart disease, 308
purging, **438**

qi, 645–646
qigong, **651**
"quackery," 643
Quinlan, Karen Ann, 609
quitlines, 320–321

rabies, 522, 538
racism, health and, 10
radiation
avoiding, 713
cancer and, 483, 484, 494, 503, 505
defined, **710**
medical uses of, 712
nuclear power, 710, 711–712
nuclear weapons, 711
pregnancy and, 223
from radon gas, 503, 712–173
ultraviolet, 490–492, 497, 503, 704
radiation sickness, **710**, 711
radon gas, 503, **712**, 712–713
raloxifene (Evista), 487, 589, 590
randomized studies, 636
rape. *See* sexual assault
rape trauma syndrome, 685
rapid eye movement (REM) sleep, 49
rationalization, 72
realism, 65
recessive genes, 207
Recommended Dietary Allowances (RDAs), **343**, 343–344, 373–375
rectal cancer, 485, 504
recycling, 697–698
refractory period, 135
Reiki, **651**
reinforcement, in addiction, 237, 246, 301

reinforcement, in behavior model, **85**
relationships
  abusive, 678–680, 681
  adult identity and, 68
  being a good friend, 97–98
  characteristics of friendships, 97
  commitment in, 98
  infatuation, 98
  loneliness and, 73
  online, 109
  sexual decision making and, 139, 174
  strategies for enhancing support in, 101
  stress and, 44–45, 48
  unhealthy, 102
  wellness and, 113
  See also intimate relationships
relaxation response, **53**, 53–54
relaxation techniques, 53–57
  biofeedback, 56–57
  counterproductive coping strategies, 57–58
  deep breathing, 55
  hatha yoga, 55–56
  listening to music, 56
  meditation, 54–55
  progressive relaxation, 53
  systematic desensitization and, 60
  taijiquan, 56
  visualization, 54
religion
  circumcision and, 126–127
  interfaith and intrafaith partnerships, 108
  psychoactive drugs in, 244
  same-sex marriage and, 111
  spiritual wellness and, 69
  tobacco use and, 300
  See also spirituality
remission, 484, **485**
REM (rapid eye movement) sleep, 49
repetitive strain injuries (RSIs), **673**, 673–674
reproduction
  embryo differentiation, 127–128
  female sexual maturation, 128–132
  fetal development, 214–220
  male sexual maturation, 132
  menstrual cycle and, 128–132
  See also pregnancy
reproductive cloning, 583
reproductive systems. *See* sexual anatomy
residential care homes, 597
resistance exercise, **393**, 393–395
resistance stage of stress response, 40
resistance training, 386, 388–389, 395. *See also* strength training
respiratory system, 55, 308–310, 315, 395, 446, 517–518, 526–527, 687–688
response, in behavior model, **85**
resting metabolic rate (RMR), **420**, 422
retarded ejaculation, **136**
retirement, economics of, 586–587, 594
retirement communities, 595, 597
retroviruses. *See* human immunodeficiency virus (HIV) infection
reverse transcriptase inhibitors, 558, **559**
reversibility, in exercise, 390–391
reversible sterilization, 175
rewards for behavior change, 22–23
RHD (rheumatic heart disease), 467–468
rheumatic fever, **466**, 467–468
rheumatic heart disease (RHD), 467–468
rheumatoid arthritis, 542
Rh factor, 196, 220
R-I-C-E (rest-ice-compression-elevation), 403
rickettsias, **529**
right to die, 608–611

risk-taking behavior, 663
Ritalin, 253
RMR (resting metabolic rate), **420**, 422
road rage, 664–665
Rocky Mountain spotted fever, 529
rodent control, 698–699
Roe v. Wade (1973), 184–185, 188
Rohypnol (flunitrazepam), 250, 251, 683–684
role models, 19
romantic love, 98–99
rooming-in, **226**, 227
Rosenman, Ray, 37
Roux-en-Y gastric bypass, 434–435
RSIs (repetitive strain injuries), **673**, 673–674
RU-486 (mifepristone), 186, 192, 195
rubella (German measles) virus, 221, 222–223, 522, 535
"runner's high," 384
run-walk test, 1.5-mile, 402

saccharin, 426
SAD (seasonal affective disorder), 81
SADD (Students Against Destructive Decisions), 292
safer sex, 146–147, 561–562, 575–577
safety. *See* personal safety
safety belts, 666–667
safety seats, 667
Salmonella, 361, 363
salt intake. *See* sodium
same-sex partnerships, 110–112
sanitary landfills, **697**
sarcomas, **482**
sarcopenia, 379
SARS (severe acute respiratory syndrome), 540
saturated fats, 327, **331**, 331–333, 348, 349, 469, 471, 476–477
saw palmetto, 649
scabies, 572–573, **573**
scarlet fever, 528
schizophrenia, 75–76, 82–83, **83**, 536
school, violence, 677
scientific method, 634–635
scleroderma, 542
scooter injuries, 672
scrapes, B–11 to B–12
scrotum, **124**, 125, 126
scurvy, **338**
seasonal affective disorder (SAD), **81**
Seasonale, 154
seat belts, 666–667
secondary reinforcers, **301**
secondhand smoke. *See* environmental tobacco smoke
sedation, **250**
sedative-hypnotics, 250
selective estrogen-receptor modulators (SERMs), 486–487, 498, 589
selective serotonin reuptake inhibitors (SSRIs), 131
selenium, 341, 499–500
self-actualization, 64–66, **65**
self-assessments. *See* assessments
self-care, 88, 630–633, B–6 to B–12
self-concept
  defined, **65**
  developing, 69–70
  intimate relationships and, 96–97
  self-acceptance and, 65–66
self-disclosure, 103
self-efficacy, **19**
self-esteem
  challenges to, 70–71
  defined, **65**

  developing, 69–71
  exercise and, 384, 428
  intimate relationships and, 96–97
  jealousy and, 101
  weight management and, 423
self-help, for psychological disorders, 88
self-image, exercise and, 383
self-talk, 19, 52, 70–71, 428
self-treatment, 631–633
Seligman, Martin, 37, 72
Selye, Hans, 39–40
semen, 125, **135**
seminal vesicles, 126
semivegetarians, **355**
SEPs (syringe exchange programs), 245, 261
September 11, 2001 terrorist attacks, 454, 622, 678
septic systems, 696, **697**
SERMs (selective estrogen-receptor modulators), 486–487, 498, 589
seroconversion, **556**, 557
serotonin, 81, 82, 131, 251, 330, 384, 421, 434
serotonin reuptake inhibitors (SSRIs), 84, 86, 131
sertraline, 83
serving sizes
  estimating, 353
  on food labels, 360
  weight management and, 423, 425, 429
severe acute respiratory syndrome (SARS), 540
sewage treatment, 696
sex, 123–148
  defined, **7**, 137
  determination of, 128
  gender identity and, 137–138
  in intimate relationships, 97–98
  See also sexual behavior; sexual functioning; sexuality
sex addiction, 238
sex chromosomes, **127**, 127–128
sex therapy, 136
sexual anatomy
  circumcision, 126–127, **127**, 138, 489, 552
  female sex organs, 124–125
  intersexed individuals, 137
  male sex organs, 125–127
  sexual differentiation, 128
  sexual health problems, 135
sexual arousal, 133
sexual assault
  alcohol use and, 275, 568, 683–684
  child sexual abuse, 685
  date rape, 251, 683–684
  dealing with, 684–685
  defined, **683**
  effects of, 685
  HIV infection and, 550, 559
  men who commit, 683
  preventing, 684
  sexual harassment, 686
  statutory rape, 683
sexual behavior, 137–147
  abstinence, 143, 168, 170, 577
  age of first intercourse, 139
  anal intercourse, 143, 561, 563
  assessment of attitudes on, 140
  atypical and problematic, 144
  autoeroticism, 143
  celibacy, 142–143
  in childhood, 138
  contraceptive education, 176–177
  cybersex, 145
  decision making in, 139, 142, 174
  ethnicity and, 142
  gender roles and, 137–138
  HIV transmission and, 552, 561–562

masturbation, 137, 138, 143
  motivations for, 141
  oral-genital stimulation, 143
  oral sex, 552, 561, 562, 569, 571
  prostitution, 145–146
  responsible, 146–147
  sexual intercourse, 144, 206
  statistics on, 152
  talking with partners about contraception, 174
  touching and foreplay, 143
  unintended pregnancy and, 197–198
  See also sexual functioning
sexual coercion, 144. See also sexual assault
sexual differentiation, 128
sexual dysfunction, 132, 135, 136–137
sexual functioning, 132–137, 273
sexual harassment, 686
sexual intercourse, 144, 206
sexuality
  adolescent, 138–139
  adult, 139–140
  aging and, 132
  contraception education and, 176–177
  defined, 124
  in illness and disability, 140
  mass media and, 138
  sexual decision making, 139, 174
sexually transmitted diseases (STDs), 547–579
  antibiotic resistance in, 531
  bacterial vaginosis, 572, 573
  chancroid, 572, 573
  chlamydia, 223, 489, 562–565
  circumcision and, 127, 552
  defined, 153, 549
  diagnosis and treatment of, 574–575
  education about, 562, 573–574
  gender differences in, 8
  genital herpes, 222–223, 489, 535, 569–570
  genital warts, 164, 538, 566–568
  gonorrhea, 222–223, 531, 562, 565, 575
  infertility and, 210
  informing partners about, 574–575
  male-to-female transmission of, 547, 564
  pathogen entry in, 517
  pelvic inflammatory disease in, 135
  during pregnancy, 222–223
  prevention of, 146–147, 560–563, 567–568, 575–577
  pubic lice, 572, 573
  role of contraceptives in preventing, 170
  scabies, 572–573
  self-assessment of, 573
  statistics on, 548, 567
  syphilis, 222–223, 571–572
  testing for, 574
  treatment for, 575
  trichomoniasis, 572, 573
  See also human immunodeficiency virus (HIV) infection
sexual maturation, 128–132
sexual orientation
  defined, 110
  health concerns and, 11
  HIV transmission and, 554, 574
  origins of, 141–142
  same-sex partnerships, 110–112
  syphilis and, 571
  transgendered individuals, 137
  types of, 141
sexual privacy, 146
sexual response cycle, 133–135
sexual violence, 682–686
Shigella, 361
shingles, 535

shoes, athletic, 401
"Shoot for 9 for Better Health," 357
shopping, compulsive, 239
shyness, 75, 77, 85, 91
sibutramine (Meridia), 434
sickle-cell disease, 9, 13, 207
sidestream smoke, 306, 314
SIDS (sudden infant death syndrome), 203, 225, 225–226, 314
sigmoidoscopies, 485, 504
simple carbohydrates, 335, 336
simple (specific) phobia, 74, 74–76
singlehood, 112
single parents, 117
Sin Nombre virus (SNV), 540–541
sinsemilla, 254. See also marijuana
sinusitis, 311, 533
sinus node, 446, 447
skating injuries, 672
skin cancer, 482, 484, 490–493, 706
skinfold measurements, 415
skin patches, contraceptive, 156–157
sleep
  fatigue and driving, 665
  immune system and, 544
  stages of, 49
  stress management and, 49
small-cell lung cancer, 484
smog, 701–703, 702
smoke detectors, 670
smoking. See tobacco use
smoking cessation products, 320–322
snuff (spit tobacco), 298–299, 305, 311–312, 316
SNV (Sin Nombre virus), 540–541
social isolation, heart disease and, 455
social phobias, 74, 75–77, 91
social security, 594–595, 595, 597
social support. See support groups; supportive influences
social wellness, 3
socioeconomic status
  AIDS/HIV and, 555
  asthma and, 525
  cancer and, 496
  cardiovascular disease and, 455
  contraceptive use among women, 173
  drug use and, 259
  health disparities and, 5, 9–11
  health insurance coverage and, 655
  obesity and, 422, 423
  See also poverty
sodas, 349, 368, 370, 413
sodium
  African Americans and, 349, 458
  calcium loss and, 342
  cardiovascular disease and, 471
  functions of, 341
  hypertension and, 449–450
  monosodium glutamate, 366, 367
  for older adults, 585
  PMS and salt intake, 131
  recommended intake of, 348, 471
  reducing intake of, 348–350
soft drinks, 349, 368, 370, 413
solid waste, 696–698
somatic cell nuclear transfer, 583
somatic nervous system, 36
somatization, 75
sonograms (ultrasonography), 218, 486, 505
sore throat, 467–468, 521, 528, 533, 535, B–7
Southern Poverty Law Center, 677
soybean oil, 332–333
soy foods, 342, 355, 471, 589
Spanish flu, 534. See also influenza

special K (ketamine), 251
specificity, in exercise, 389
speeding, injuries from, 664
spending, compulsive, 239
sperm cells, 206, 210
sperm counts, 210
spermicides, 161, 163, 164–168, 170, 552, 561, 563
SPF (sun protection factor), 492
sphygmomanometers, 449
spina bifida, 206
spinal manipulation, 651
spirituality
  drug abuse and, 244
  interfaith and intrafaith partnerships, 108
  spiritual wellness, 2, 51–52, 69, 473
  stress management and, 51–52, 108
  wellness and, 2, 51–52, 69, 473
  See also mind/body/spirit connections; religion
spiritual wellness, 2, 51–52, 69, 473
spirochetes, 529, 571
spit tobacco, 298–299, 305, 311–312, 316. See also tobacco use
Splenda, 426
sponges, contraceptive, 163, 166–167, 167, 170
spontaneous abortion, 225. See also miscarriage
sports injuries, 671
sport utility vehicles (SUVs), 693, 707
sprains, B–11
squamous cell carcinoma, 490, 491
SSRIs (selective serotonin reuptake inhibitors), 84, 86, 131
St. John's wort, 81, 83, 359, 648–650
stages of development (Erikson), 67–68
stalking, 680, 680–682
standardization of herbal products, 650
standard Western medicine. See conventional medicine
Staphylococcus aureus, 361, 528
staphylococcus bacterium, 361, 528, 529
state dependence, 253
static exercises, 393
statistics
  on abortion, 190, 192, 197
  on aging, 594
  on alcohol abuse and dependence, 286
  on American diet, 355, 368
  on annual mean temperature, 704
  on binge drinking, 281, 283
  on cancer deaths, 480, 482
  on cardiovascular disease, 446, 461
  on causes of death among Americans, 5–6
  on contraceptive risks, 157
  on contraceptive use among American women, 173
  on drug use, 236
  on energy use, 707
  on health care costs, 654
  on infectious diseases, 526
  on injuries, 662, 663, 664
  on marital status, 112
  on organ donors, 612
  on overweight and obesity, 412
  on physical activity among American adults, 378
  on population growth, 699
  on prevalence of psychological disorders, 76
  on sexually transmitted diseases, 548
  on single-parent families, 117
  on smoking, 298, 304
  on solid waste components, 696
  on suicide rates, 79
  on tobacco use, 236, 298, 303–304, 313
  understanding, 636
  on use of complementary and alternative therapies, 634

statistics (*continued*)
  on violence, 673, 675, 679
  on worldwide sexual behavior, 152
  See also death, causes of
statutory rape, **683**
STDs. *See* sexually transmitted diseases
stem cells, 13, 207, 506, **507**, 583, 613
stepfamilies, 117
stereotyping, 7
sterilization, **170**, 170–175
Sternberg, Robert, 98–99
stevia, 426
stimulants, 250–254
  for ADHD in children, 85, 253
  amphetamines, 57, 81, 252–253
  athletic performance and, 396
  caffeine, 49, 222, 253–254, 265, 342
  cocaine, 223, 246–247, 251–252, 455
  defined, **85, 250**
  ephedra, 396, 432, 468
  stress and, 57
stimulus, in behavior model, 85
stomach cancer, 493–494, 496, 501
strains, B–11
strength. *See* muscular strength
strength training
  benefits of, 379, 381–382
  exercises for, 393–395
  gender differences and, 393
  recommendations for, 388–389, 397
  safety in, 395
streptococcal throat infections, 467–468, 528
streptococcus bacterium, 527, 528, **529**
Streptococcus pneumoniae, 527, 528
stress, 31–60
  aging and, 585–586
  alcohol use and, 282
  assessment of, 33
  behavior change and, 25
  cardiovascular disease and, 41, 454, 457
  common sources of, 42–46
  defined, **33**
  discrimination and, 46
  disease and, 39–43, 454
  divorce and, 114
  emotional and behavioral responses to, 35–38
  exercise and, 383, 384
  gender differences in, 38–39
  genital herpes and, 570
  immune system and, 543
  physical responses to, 32–35
  pregnancy and, 42, 219–220
  symptoms of, 33
  test anxiety, 60
  writing about, 631
  See also stress management
stress cardiomyopathy, 457
stress management, 46–58
  cognitive techniques, 52–53
  communication and, 47–48
  coping after mass violence, 47
  counterproductive coping strategies, 57–58
  exercise and, 48–49
  getting help, 58–59
  nutrition and, 49
  personal plan for, 58–59
  relaxation techniques, 53–57
  sleep and, 49
  social support, 46–47
  spirituality and, 51–52, 108
  systematic desensitization, 60
  test anxiety, 60
  time management and, 49–51
  weight management and, 429
  writing and, 52

stressors, 32, **33**, 42–46, 58
stress response, 32, **33**
stretching exercises, 392–393, 395–398
stretching technique, 395–396
strokes, 8, 308, 382, 458, 463, **464**, 464–466
students. *See* college students
Students Against Destructive Decisions
    (SADD), 292
subarachnoid strokes, 465
substance abuse, defined, 240–241, **241**.
    See also psychoactive drugs
substance dependence, defined, 240–241, **241**.
    See also addiction; psychoactive drugs
Subway, A–3
suction curettage, **194**
sudden cardiac death, **462**
sudden death in athletes, 467–468
sudden infant death syndrome (SIDS), 203, **225**,
    225–226, 314
suffocation, 671
sugar alcohols, 426
sugars
  added, 337, 354, 355
  as carbohydrates, 335
  dietary sources of, 327
  mood and, 330
  reducing intake of, 337, 354
sugar substitutes, 426
suicide
  antidepressants and, 86
  assisted, 610–611
  in compulsive gamblers, 238
  eating disorders and, 438
  in elderly people, 591–592
  gender differences in, 8, 80
  help for a friend, 80–81
  myths about, 81
  rates of, 79–80, 664
  schizophrenia and, 83
  at schools, 677
sulfites in food, 366, 367
sulforaphane, 342, 500, **501**
sulfur dioxide, 701, 706
suncreen, **490**, 491–492
sunlight, 491–492, 503
sun protection factor (SPF), 492
sun-protective clothing, 492
supplements. *See* dietary supplements
support groups
  for cancer, 508
  for genital herpes, 570
  for psychological disorders, 88
  for substance abuse, 261, 263
supportive influences
  for behavior change, 23, 25, 27
  for coping with stress, 46–48
  for a dying person, 619
  for a grieving person, 621, 623
  in relationships, 101
  wellness and, 113
suppressor T cells, 518, **519**, 542
Supreme Court. *See* U.S. Supreme Court
Surgeon General's report on physical activity, 386
surgery, 643
surgical methods of contraception, 152
surrogate motherhood, 211–212
surrogates, **611**, 611–612
SUVs (sport utility vehicles), 693, 707
sympathetic division, 33
symptoms, assessment of, 630–631
syndrome X. *See* metabolic syndrome
synesthesia, 256, **257**
synovial fluid, 392–393, **393**
syphilis, 222–223, 526, **571**, 571–572
syringe exchange programs (SEPs), 245, 261

systematic desensitization, 60
systemic circulation, **446**
systemic infection, **516**
systemic lupus erythematosus, 542
systole, **446**, 448–449

Taco Bell, A–3
taijiquan, 56
Take Charge
  in alcohol emergencies, 274
  becoming more active, 387
  being a good friend, 98
  breast self-examination, 487
  breathing for relaxation, 55
  choosing more whole-grain foods, 336
  communicating about sexuality, 146
  communication and care for older adults, 596
  communication guidelines, 104
  coping with grief, 623
  determining your target heart rate range, 392
  early treatment of STDs, 575
  eating for healthy bones, 342
  eating strategies for college students, 358
  enhancing support in relationships, 101
  healthy eating during pregnancy, 221
  heart attacks, cardiac arrests, or strokes, 463
  helping a friend stop using tobacco, 318
  helping a friend with an eating disorder, 440
  helping someone with a drug problem, 263
  intake goals for protein, fat, and
      carbohydrate, 334
  judging portion sizes, 353
  keeping well, 544
  maintaining your exercise program, 405
  making your letters count, 715
  meditation and relaxation response, in 54
  motivation boosters, 26
  motivation to quit smoking, 302
  online relationships, 109
  overcoming insomnia, 50
  preventing date rape, 684
  preventing HIV infection and other STDs, 563
  realistic self-talk, 71
  recognizing potential for abusiveness in a
      partner, 681
  reducing saturated and trans fats in diets, 348
  safe food handling, 363
  safe weight training, 395
  setting dietary intake goals, 334
  staying safe on campus, 687
  strategies of strong families, 118
  successful weight management, 429
  talking about condoms and safer sex, 576
  talking with a partner about contraception, 174
  tasks for survivors, 616
  testicle self-examination, 494
  tickborne and mosquitoborne infections, 530
tamoxifen, 486–487, 498, 502
tanning salons, 490, 492
tapeworms, 363, 539
tar, in cigarettes, **304**, 312
target behaviors, **15**
target heart rate range, **391**, 391–392
tattoos, 537
Tay-Sachs disease, 9, 207
TB (tuberculosis), 526, 528–529, **529**, 531, 556
T cells, 518–519, **519**, 543, 549
TCM (traditional Chinese medicine), 644–646,
    645, 650
teeth, 348, 439, 637
temperature inversions, **702**
temperature method, 169
tension headaches, 43
teratogens, 220–221, **221**, 223

terminal illnesses, 616–619. *See also* death and dying
terrorism, defined, 678
terrorist attacks, 47, 77, 622, 678, 680
test anxiety, 60
testators, **606**, 607
testes (*singular,* testis), **124,** 125, 126, **206**
testicle self-examination, 494
testicular atrophy, 273
testicular cancer, 135, 493
testosterone, 39, 128, **129,** 132, 136, 593, 663
testosterone replacement therapy, 132, 136
tetanus, 522, 526, 529
thalassemia, 207
THC (tetrahydrocannabinol), 254, 256. *See also* marijuana
therapeutic cloning, 583
Therapeutic Lifestyle Changes (TLC), 473
therapeutic touch, 651
thermometers, mercury, 710
thimerosol, 523
Three Mile Island nuclear accident, 711
thrombotic strokes, 464–465
thrombus, **464**
thyroid cancer, 503
thyroid gland, 212, 481
TIAs (transient ischemic attacks), 464, 465–466
tickborne infections, 528–530, 698–699
time-action function, **246,** 247
time management, stress and, 39, 44, 49–51
tinnitus, **712,** 713
Tips for Today
  abortion, 199
  aging, 599
  alcohol, 292
  cancer, 510
  cardiovascular disease, 474
  contraception, 179
  conventional and complementary medicine, 657
  death and dying, 624
  drug use and abuse, 264
  environmental health, 715
  exercise, 405
  immune system, 543
  intimate relationships, 119
  nutrition, 327
  personal safety, 688
  physical activity, 405
  positive choices in lifestyle, 27
  pregnancy, 231
  psychoactive drugs, 264
  psychological health, 90
  self-care, 657
  sexuality, 147
  sexually transmitted diseases, 577
  stress management, 59
  tobacco, 322
  weight management, 440
  wellness, 27
tissue plasminogen activator (TPA), 463
TLC (Therapeutic Lifestyle Changes), 473
TMS (triple marker screen), 218
tobacco companies, 315–316
tobacco use
  action and restrictions on, 317–319
  addiction to nicotine, 235, 242, 298–301
  additives in, 305–306
  advertisements for, 302–303
  aging and, 585
  cervical cancer and, 489
  cigars and pipes, 312–313
  costs of, 297, 310, 315–317
  cumulative effects of, 311
  demographics of use, 303–305
  diseases from, 5, 6, 307–311, 319, 448, 472

environmental tobacco smoke, 298, 313–317, 448, 484, 707
  gender differences in use of, 311
  heart disease and, 483–484
  immediate effects of smoking, 307–308
  lawsuits concerning, 315–316
  "light" and low-tar cigarettes, 306–307
  lung cancer and, 308–309, 311, 319, 483–484, 507–509
  menthol in, 306, 307
  new products, 316
  oral cancer from, 493, 499
  pelvic inflammatory disease and, 566
  pregnancy and, 203, 222–223, 315
  quitting use of, 302, 318, 319–323, 648
  reasons for use of, 298–304
  religion and, 300
  sexual dysfunction and, 136
  smoke toxicity, 304–307, 314, 497
  spit tobacco, 298–299, 305, 311–312, 316
  statistics on use of, 236, 298, 303–304, 313, 448
  stress and, 57
  tobacco, defined, **299**
  in unfiltered cigarettes, 306
  Vitamin C and, 344
Tokaimura, Japan nuclear accident, 711
Tolerable Upper Intake Level (UL), 343, 373–375
tolerance
  to alcohol, 282
  to drugs, 240–241, **241**
  to tobacco, 300–301
total fiber, 337
toxic shock syndrome (TSS), **165,** 528, **529**
toxic waste, 696–697
toxins, **516,** 529
toxoplasmosis, 205, 215, 221
traditional Chinese medicine (TCM), 644–646, **645,** 650
training intensity, 390, 391–392
trajectory of dying, **617,** 617–619
tranquilizers, 82, **250**
trans fats
  defined, **331**
  health risks of, 327, 331–333
  from hydrogenation, 331, 354
  recommended intake, 333, 348
  reducing intake of, 348, 469, 471, 476–477
transgendered individuals, 137
transient ischemic attacks (TIAs), **464,** 465–466
transition, **226,** 227
transmissible spongiform encephalopathies (TSEs), 539
transmission, of pathogens, 516
transportation for the elderly, 596–597
transsexual men and women, 137
transvestites, 137
trastuzumab (Herceptin), 487
trauma, 77–78, 80, 622, 631
Treponema pallidum, 571
Trichinella spiralis, 363
Trichomonas vaginalis, 572
trichomoniasis, 539, 572, **573**
triglycerides, 330–331, 382, 431, 452–453
trimesters, 212, **213**
triple marker screen (TMS), **218**
trypanosomiasis, 539
tryptophan, 131, 330
TSEs (transmissible spongiform encephalopathies), 539
TSS (toxic shock syndrome), **165,** 529
tsunamis, trauma and loss in, 622
tubal blockages, 210
tubal sterilization, **172,** 172–174
tuberculosis (TB), 526, 528–529, **529,** 531, 556
tumors, 480, 481

tumor suppressor genes, **497**
12-step programs, 261, 285
twins, 128, 208, 284–285
Type A, B, and C personalities, 36–37
Type D personalities, 454
type 1 diabetes, 417, 418, 536. *See also* diabetes
type 2 diabetes, 416–418. *See also* diabetes
typhus, 529

UL (Tolerable Upper Intake Level), 343, 373–375
ulcerative colitis, 485
ulcers, 310, 311, 529, 536
ultrasonography, **218,** 486, **486,** 505
Ultraviolet Protection Factor (UPF), 492
ultraviolet (UV) radiation, **490,** 491, 492, 497, 704, 706
umbilical cord, **217,** 228, 583
underwater weighing, 415
Uniform Donor Card, 614, **615**
unintentional injuries, 662–673
  defined, **662**
  at home, 668–671
  leisure time, 671–672
  motor vehicle, 664–668
  work-related, 672–673
  See also injuries
university students. *See* college students
unsaturated fatty acids, 331–332, 333
UPF (Ultraviolet Protection Factor), 492
urethritis, **563**
uric acid, 460
urinary tract infections (UTIs), 127, 529–530
U.S. Supreme Court
  Roe v. Wade, 184–185, 188
  Vacco v. Quill, 610
  Washington v. Glucksberg, 610
USDA MyPyramid, **343,** 350–354
USDA Organic seal, 365
USP-DSVP mark, 362
uterine cancer, 489, 504
uterus, **124,** 125, **206**
UV radiation. *See* ultraviolet (UV) radiation

vaccines
  contraceptive, 175
  defined, **521**
  issues in, 523
  preconception, 205
  table of recommended, 522
  types of, 522–523
Vacco v. Quill, 610
vacuum aspiration, 194
vagina, **124,** 125, 134
Vaginal Contraceptive Film (VCF™), 167
vaginal contraceptive ring, 157
vaginal infections, 143, 538–539
vaginal spermicides, 167–168
vaginismus, **136**
vaginitis, 135
Valium (diazepam), 85, 286
valley fever, 539
variant CJD (vCJD), 540
Varicella-zoster virus, 522, 535
vasa deferentia (*singular,* vas deferens), 126, **170,** 171
vasectomy, **170,** 171–172
vasocongestion, **133**
VBG (vertical banded gastroplasty), 434–435
VCF™ (Vaginal Contraceptive Film), 167
vectors, **516,** 698–699
vegans, **355**
vegetables, 340, 342, 347, 351, 352, 375, 425, 499–500, 511
vegetarian diets, 354–356